First published in the United Kingdom in 2010 by Informa Healthcare, Telephone House, 69-77 Paul Street, London EC2A 4LQ. Informa Healthcare is a trading division of Informa UK Ltd. Registered Office: 37/41 Mortimer Street, London W1T 3JH. Registered in England and Wales number 1072954.

Tel: +44 (0)20 7017 5000
Fax: +44 (0)20 7017 6699
Website: www.informahealthcare.com

A CIP record for this book is available from the British Library.
Library of Congress Cataloging-in-Publication Data

Data available on application

ISBN-10: 0 415 45167 1
ISBN-13: 978 0 415 45167 3

Book orders
Informa Healthcare
Sheepen Place
Colchester
Essex CO3 3LP
UK
Tel: +44 (0)20 7017 5540
Email: CSDhealthcarebooks@informa.com

Composition by Exeter Premedia Servies Private Ltd., Chennai, India
Printed and bound in Spain by Grafos SA

HUSBAND & REZNEK'S
IMAGING *in* ONCOLOGY
Third Edition

Edited by

Dame Janet E Husband DBE, FMedSci, FRCP, FRCR

*Emeritus Professor of Radiology, Institute of Cancer Research and
The Royal Marsden NHS Foundation Trust, London and Surrey, U.K.*

and

Rodney H Reznek MB ChB, FRANZCR (Hon), FRCP, FRCR

*Professor of Diagnostic Imaging, Cancer Imaging,
Institute of Cancer, Barts and The London School
of Medicine and Dentistry, London, U.K.*

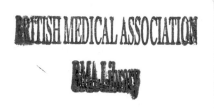
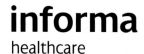
informa
healthcare

Contents

List of Contributors

Andreas Adam, MBBS(Hon), FRCP, FRCS, FRCR, FFRRCSI(Hon)
Professor of Interventional Radiology, Department of Radiology, St Thomas, Hospital, London, UK

Matthew Adams, MB, BChir, FRCR
Consultant Neuroradiologist, National Hospital for Neurology and Neurosurgery, Queen Square, London, UK

Gina Allen, BM, BCh, MRCGP, MRCP, FRCR, MFSEM
Consultant Musculoskeletal Radiologist, St Lukes Hospital, Oxford, UK Teaching Associate Green Templeton College, University of Oxford, Oxford, UK

Zahir Amin, MBBS, MRCP, MD, FRCR
Consultant Radiologist, Department of Imaging, University College Hospital, London, UK

Norbert Avril, MD
Reader in Nuclear Medicine, Department of Nuclear Medicine, Barts and The London School of Medicine and Dentistry, London, UK

Zelena Aziz, BSc(Hons), MB, BS, MRCP, FRCR
Consultant Radiologist, Department of Diagnostic Imaging, The London Chest Hospital, Barts and The London NHS Trust, London, UK

Richard L Baron, MD
Professor and Chair, Department of Radiology, University of Chicago, Chicago, Illinois, USA

Tristan Barrett, MBBS
Senior Radiology Registrar, Department of Radiology, Addenbrooke's Hospital, Cambridge University Teaching Hospitals NHS Foundation Trust, Cambridge, UK

Ahmed Ba-Ssalamah, MD
Associate Professor of Radiology, Department of Radiology, Medical University of Vienna, Vienna, Austria

Jonathan W Berlin, MD, MBA
Associate Professor of Clinical Radiology, University of Chicago, Evanston, Illinois, USA

Bobby Bhartia, MB BS, MRCP, FRCR
Consultant Radiologist, Department of Clinical Radiology, St James' University Hospital, Leeds, UK

Juliet Britton, MB, BS, FRCR, FRCP
Consultant Neuroradiologist, Department of Neuroradiology, Atkinson Morley Wing, St. George's Hospital, London, UK

Gina Brown, MB, MD, MRCP, FRCR,
Consultant Radiologist, Department of Diagnostic Radiology, The Royal Marsden NHS Foundation Trust, London and Surrey, UK

Guy J Burkill, BSc, MRCP, FRCR, MA
Consultant Radiologist, Department of Radiology, The Royal Sussex County Hospital, Eastern Hospital, Brighton, Sussex, UK

Bernadette M Carrington, MB ChB, MRCP, FRCR
Consultant Radiologist, The Christie NHS Foundation Trust, Manchester, UK

Roger Chinn, MB BS, MRCP, FRCR
Consultant Radiologist, Department of Radiology, Chelsea and Westminster Hospital, London, UK

Peter L Choyke, MD, FACR
Molecular Imaging Program, NCI, Bethesda, Maryland, USA

Richard H Cohan, MD
Professor of Radiology, Department of Radiology, University of Michigan Hospitals, Ann Arbor, Michigan, USA

Michel P Coleman, BA, BM, BCh, MSc, FPHM
Professor of Epidemiology and Vital Statistics, Non-Communicable Disease Epidemiology Unit, London School of Hygiene and Tropical Medicine, London, UK

Conor Collins, BSc, FRCPI, FRCR, FFRRCSI
Consultant Radiologist, St Vincent's University Hospital, Dubin, Ireland Hon. Senior Clinical Lecturer in Medicine, University College, Dublin, Ireland

Gary Cook, MBBS, MSc, MD, FRCP, FRCR
Consultant Radiologist, Department of Nuclear Medicine, The Royal Marsden NHS Foundation Trust, Sutton, Surrey, UK

A Mark Davies, MB ChB, FRCR
Department of Radiology, The Royal Orthopaedic Hospital, Northfield, Birmingham, UK

Johann S de Bono, MB ChB, FRCP, MSc, PhD
Senior Lecturer and Consultant Medical Oncologist, Section of Medicine, The Institute of Cancer Research, Sutton, Surrey, UK The Royal Marsden NHS Foundation Trust, Sutton, Surrey, UK

Sujal R Desai, MD, FRCP, FRCR
Consultant Radiologist and Honorary Senior Lecturer, Department of Radiology, King's College Hospital NHS Foundation Trust and Division of Gene and Cell Based Therapy, King's College, London, UK

Stephen M Ellis, BA MB BCh MRCP FRCR
Consultant Radiologist Department of Diagnostic Imaging, The London Chest Hospital, Barts and The London NHS Trust, London, UK

Jacques Estève, PhD
Professor of Biostatistics, Service de Biostatistique, Hospices Civils de Lyon, Lyon, France

Jane Evanson, MRCP, FRCR
Consultant Radiologist, Department of Neuroradiology, The Royal London Hospital, London, UK

James V Ferris, MD
Associate Professor of Radiology, University of Pittsburgh Medical Center, Pittsburgh, Pennsylvania, USA

Nicos Fotiadis, MD, FRCR
Consultant Interventional Radiologist, Department of Diagnostic Imaging, The Royal London Hospital, London, UK

Isaac R Francis, MD
Professor of Radiology, Department of Radiology, University of Michigan Hospitals, Ann Arbor, Michigan, USA

Christopher J Gallagher, MBBSc, PhD, FRCP
Consultant Medical Oncologist, Department of Medical Oncology, St Bartholomew's Hospital, London, UK

Alice R Gillams, MB ChB, MRCP, FRCR
Consultant Radiologist Senior Lecturer, UCL Medical School and Honorary Consultant, University College of London Hospital, London, UK

Matthew Gilman, MD
Assistant Radiologist, Massachusetts General Hospital and Instructor in Radiology, Harvard Medical School, Boston, Massachusetts, USA

Vicky Goh, MA, MBBChir, MD (Cantab), MRCP, FRCR
Consultant Radiologist, The Paul Strickland Scanner Centre, Mount Vernon Hospital, Northwood, Middlesex, UK

Jonathan Goldin, MD, PhD
Thoracic Imaging Research Group, Department of Radiological Sciences, UCLA, Los Angeles, California, USA

Richard M Gore, MD
Professor of Clinical Radiology, University of Chicago, Evanston, Illinois, USA
Chief, Gastrointestinal Radiology, Northshore University Health System, Evanston, Illinois, USA

Ashley B Grossman, BA, BSc, MD, FRCP, FMedSci
Professor of Neuroendocrinology, Centre for Endocrinology, Barts and The London School of Medicine, London, UK

David M Hansell, MD, FRCP, FRCR
Professor of Thoracic Imaging, National Heart and Lung Institute and Division of Investigative Science, Imperial College School of Medicine, London, UK
Department of Radiology, Royal Brompton Hospital, London, UK

Thomas F Hany, MD
Department of Medical Radiology, Division of Nuclear Medicine, University Hospital, Zurich, Switzerland

Robert Hermans, MD, PhD
Professor, Department of Radiology, University Hospitals Leuven, Leuven, Belgium

Alan Horwich, PhD, MBBS, FRCP, FRCR
Academic Unit of Radiotherapy and Oncology, The Royal Marsden NHS Trust and The Institute of Cancer Research, Sutton, Surrey, UK

Hedvig Hricak, MD, PhD
Chairman, Department of Radiology, Memorial Sloan-Kettering Cancer Center, New York, New York, USA

Robert Huddart, PhD, MBBS, MRCP, FRCR
Academic Unit of Radiotherapy and Oncology, The Royal Marsden NHS Foundation Trust and Institute of Cancer Research, Sutton, Surrey, UK

Tvrtko Hudolin, MD, PhD
Department of Radiology, Memorial Sloan-Kettering Cancer Center, New York, New York, USA

Paul A Hulse, BMed Sci, BM BS, MRCP, FRCR
Consultant Radiologist, The Christie NHS Foundation Trust, Manchester, UK

Janet E Husband, DBE, FMedSci, FRCP, FRCR, FFRRCSI (Hon), FRCPSG (Hon), FHKCR (Hon), FAMS (Hon)
Emeritus Professor of Radiology, Institute of Cancer Research and The Royal Marsden NHS Foundation Trust, London and Surrey, UK

Revathy B Iyer, MD
Associate Professor and Associate Division Head for Education, University of Texas, M.D. Anderson Cancer Center, Houston, Texas, USA

Steven LJ James, FRCR
Consultant Radiologist, Department of Radiology, The Royal Orthopaedic Hospital, Northfield, Birmingham, UK

R Brooke Jeffrey, MD
Professor of Radiology, Chief of Abdominal Imaging Section, Department of Radiology, Stanford University School of Medicine, Stanford, California, USA

Peter Johnson, MA, MD, FRCP
Professor of Medical Oncology, Somers Cancer Research Building, Southampton General Hospital, Southampton, UK

Harmeet Kaur, MD
Associate Professor, Department of Diagnostic Radiology, University of Texas, M.D. Anderson Cancer Center, Houston, Texas, USA

Stan B Kaye, MD, FRCP, FRCR, FRSE, FMedSci
Drug Development Unit, The Royal Marsden NHS Foundation Trust, Sutton, Surrey, UK
The Institute of Cancer Research, Sutton, Surrey, UK

Vincent Khoo, MBBS, FRACR, FRCR, MD
Consultant and Honorary Senior Lecturer in Clinical Oncology, Royal Marsden NHS Foundation Trust and Institute of Cancer Research, Chelsea, London, UK

D Michael King, MD, MS
Consultant Radiologist, Department of Radiology, The Royal Marsden NHS Foundation Trust, Chelsea London, UK

Claus Koelblinger, MD
Department of Radiology, Medical University of Vienna, Vienna, Austria

Dow-Mu Koh, MD, MRCP, FRCR
Consultant in Functional Imaging, Department of Diagnostic Radiology, The Royal Marsden NHS Foundation Trust, London and Surrey, UK

Gerald Lesnik, MD
Zentralröntgeninstitut, LKH Klagenfurt, Klagenfurt, Austria

Rebecca Leung, MBBS, FRCR
Department of Radiology, Great Ormond Street Hospital for Children, London, UK

Bruce F Levy, MBChB (Hons), MRCS, MSc.
Research Registrar, MATTU, Postgraduate Medical School, University of Surrey, Guildford, UK

Herman I Libshitz, MD, FACR
Chestertown, Maryland, USA

Sarah Lowndes, BM BCh, MA, MRCP
Specialist Registrar Medical Oncology, Somers Cancer Research Building, Southampton General Hospital, Southampton, UK

David MacVicar, MA, MRCP, FRCR
Consultant Radiologist, Department of Diagnostic Radiology, The Royal Marsden NHS Foundation Trust, London and Surrey, UK

Kieran McHugh, FACR, MRCPI
Consultant Paediatric Radiologist, Great Ormond Street Hospital for Children, London, UK

Alison M McLean, FRCP, FRCR
Consultant Radiologist, Department of Diagnostic Imaging, St Bartholomew's Hospital, London, UK

Uday K Mehta, MD
Assistant Professor of Clinical Radiology, University of Chicago, Evanston, Illinois, USA

Frank H Miller, MD
Professor of Radiology, Northwestern University Medical School, Chicago, Illinois, USA

Stephen Morris, MBBS, MRCP, FRCR
Department of Radiotheraphy, St. Thomas Hospital, London, UK

Eleanor Moskovic, FRCP, FRCR
Consultant Radiologist, Department of Radiology, The Royal Marsden NHS Foundation Trust, London, UK

Lia A Moulopoulos, MD
Associate Professor, Department of Radiology, Medical School, University of Athens, Athens, Greece

Reginald F Munden, MD, DMD
Professor and Chairman, Department of Radiology, University of Alabama at Birmingham, Birmingham, Alabama, USA

Priya Narayanan, BSc(Hons), MB BS(Hons), MRCP FRCR
Consultant Radiologist, Department of Radiology, Chelsea and Westminster Hospital, London, UK

Geraldine M Newmark, MD
Assistant Professor of Clinical Radiology, University of Chicago, Evanston, Illinois, USA
Section Head, Body Imaging, Northshore University Health System, Evanston, Illinois, USA

Matilde Nino-Murcia, MD
Professor of Radiology, Department of Radiology, Stanford University School of Medicine, Stanford, California, USA
Department of Radiology, Veterans Affairs Palo Alto Health Care System, Palo Alto, California, USA

Anwar Padhani, MBBS, MRCP, FRCR
Consultant Radiologist and Head of Imaging Research, The Paul Strickland Scanner Centre, Mount Vernon Hospital, Middlesex, UK

Simon Padley, MB BS, FRCP, FRCR
Consultant Radiologist, Department of Radiology, Chelsea and Westminster Hospital, London, UK

Jacqueline M Parkin, MBBS, PhD, FRCP
Vice President, Immuno-Inflammation Drug Discovery, Glaxo Smith Kline, UK

ADJ Pearson, MD
Professor of Paediatric Oncology, Institute of Cancer Research, Royal Marsden Hospital, Sutton, Surrey, UK

Sheila Rankin, DCH, FRCR
Consultant Radiologist, Guy's and St. Thomas Foundation Trust, Guy's Hospital, London, UK

Rodney H Reznek, MB ChB, FRANZCR(Hon), FRCP, FRCR, FFRRCSI(Hon)
Professor of Diagnostic Imaging, Cancer Imaging, Institute of Cancer, Barts and The London School of Medicine and Dentistry, London, UK

Polly S Richards, BA, MBBS, MRCP, FRCR
Consultant Radiologist, Department of Diagnostic Imaging, St. Bartholomew's Hospital, West Smithfield, London, UK

Andrea G Rockall, BSc, MBBS, MCRP, FRCR
Professor of Cancer Imaging, Department of Diagnostic Imaging, St Bartholomew's Hospital, London, UK

Timothy A Rockall, MB, BS, MD, FRCS
Professor of Surgery, Royal Surrey County Hospital, Guildford, UK

Tarun Sabharwal, FCRSI, FRCR
Consultant Interventional Radiologist, Department of Radiology, St Thomas' Hospital, London, UK

Anju Sahdev, MBBS, MRCP, FRCR
Consultant Radiologist, Department of Diagnostic Imaging, St Bartholomew's Hospital, London, UK

Debashis Sarker, MD
Clinical Research Fellow, Institute of Cancer Research and Royal Marsden Hospital, Sutton, Surrey, UK

Niklaus G Schaefer, MD
Nuclear Medicine, Department of Medical Radiology and Medical Oncology, Department of Internal Medicine, University Hospital, Zurich, Switzerland

Wolfgang Schima, MD, MSc
Associate Professor of Radiology, Abteilung für Radiologie und bildgebende Diagnostik, KH Göttlicher Heiland, Vienna, Austria

Lawrence H Schwartz, MD
Director, Magnetic Resonance Imaging (MRI), Memorial Sloan-Kettering Cancer Center, New York, New York, USA

Amita Sharma, MBBS, MRCP, FRCR
Assistant Radiologist, Massachusetts General Hospital and Instructor in Radiology, Harvard Medical School, Boston, Massachusetts, USA

Marilyn J Siegel, MD
Washington University School of Medicine, Mallinckrodt Institute of Radiology, St. Louis, Missouri, USA

Rod Skinner, MB ChB, PhD, FRCPCH, MRCP (UK), DCH
Consultant / Honorary Clinical Senior Lecturer in Paediatric and Adolescent Oncology / BMT, Department of Paediatric and Adolescent Oncology, Royal Victoria Infirmary, Newcastle upon Tyne, UK
Children's BMT Unit, Newcastle General Hospital, Newcastle upon Tyne, UK

S Aslam Sohaib, BSc, MRCP, FRCP
Consultant Radiologist, Department of Diagnostic Radiology, The Royal Marsden NHS Foundation Trust, London and Surrey, UK

John A Spencer, MD, FRCR
Consultant Radiologist, Department of Clinical Radiology, St James' University Hospital, Leeds, UK

David Stringer, BSc, MBBS, FRCR, FRCPC
Clinical Professor, (National University Singapore), Adjunct Clinical Professor, (Duke NUS Graduate Medical School), Head of Department, Department of Diagnostic Imaging, KK Women's and Children's Hospital, Singapore

Murali Sundaram, MBBS, FRCR
The Cleveland Clinic Foundation, Cleveland, Ohio, USA

M Ben Taylor, MRCP, FRCR
Consultant Radiologist, The Christie NHS Foundation Trust, Manchester, UK

Harvey Teo, MBBS, FRCR
Adjunct Associate Professor, (National University Singapore), Clinical Associate Professor, (Duke NUS Graduate Medical School), Deputy Head of Department, Department of diagnostic Imaging KK Women's and Children's Hospital, Singapore

Kiran H Thakrar, MD
Assistant Professor of Clinical Radiology, University of Chicago, Evanston, Illinois, USA

Datla GK Varma, MBBS
Professor of Radiology, Department of Radiology, M.D. Anderson Cancer Center, Houston, Texas, USA

Sarah J Vinnicombe, BSc(Hons), MRCP, FRCR
Consultant Radiologist, Department of Diagnostic Imaging, St Bartholomew's Hospital, London, UK

Ioannis Vlahos, B.Sc, MBBS, MRCP, FRCR
Consultant Radiologist, St George's Hospital, London, UK Assistant Professor, New York University, New York, USA

Gustav K von Schulthess, MD, PhD
Nuclear Medicine, Department of Medical Radiology, University Hospital, Zurich, Switzerland

Matthew Wheater, BM, MRCP
CRUK Clinical Research Fellow, Somers Cancer Research Building, Southampton General Hospital, Southampton, UK

Michael Williams, MD, FRCP, FRCR
Consultant Clinical Oncologist, Oncology Centre, Addenbrooke's NHS Trust, Cambridge, UK

David Wilson, MBBS, BSc, MFSEM, FRCP, FRCR
Consultant Musculoskeletal Radiologist, Nuffield Orthopaedic Centre NHS Trust, Oxford, UK Senior Clinical Lecturer, University of Oxford, Oxford, UK

Sandra Wong, MD, MS
Assistant Professor of Surgery, Division of Surgical Oncology, Department of Surgery, University of Michigan, Ann Arbor, Michigan, USA

Timothy A Yap, BSc(Hons), MBBS, MRCP
Drug Development Unit, The Royal Marsden NHS Foundation Trust, Sutton, Surrey, UK The Institute of Cancer Research, Sutton, Surrey, UK

Jingbo Zhang, MD
Department of Radiology, Memorial Sloan-Kettering Cancer Center, New York, New York, USA

Binsheng Zhao, DSc
Associate Attending Physicist, Departments of Medical Physics and Radiology, Memorial Sloan-Kettering Cancer Center, New York, New York, USA

Foreword

Imaging is fundamental to the management of almost all patients with cancer. It has important roles in screening of asymptomatic patients, diagnosis or exclusion of cancer in patients with symptoms, determining the extent of disease, selection of appropriate treatments, targeting of treatments to the right location, monitoring of response to treatment and detection of recurrence and metastasis. In addition, interventional radiology is increasingly playing a part in the direct treatment of cancer.

Imaging of cancer has developed remarkably during the 30 years of my career. CT was first introduced in the 1970s, MRI scanning in the 1980s, PET scanning in the 1990s and more recently the fusion of functional and anatomic imaging as with PET-CT. In addition to these major landmarks, incremental improvements in each technology have been introduced at more frequent intervals. The knowledge base related to imaging has also grown hugely, helping to define the optimal use of each modality for different cancers.

Given the diverse roles of imaging in the management of cancer and the rapid developments, it is unsurprising that radiologists are key members of specialist multidisciplinary cancer teams, working alongside pathologists, surgeons, oncologists, nurse specialists, palliative care specialists and others. During my training as a medical oncologist and subsequently as a consultant I was fortunate to work in several specialist cancer teams. Several of the authors of this textbook were members of those teams. Through them I have come to know how vital the expertise of the radiologist is to high-quality patient care. Equally I know that to undertake their role fully, radiologists need to keep up-to-date with progress on cancer generally and particularly with developments in their own discipline. Other cancer clinicians also need to keep abreast of developments in cancer imaging.

This third edition of *Imaging in Oncology* will be of enormous value both to radiologists and to other members of specialist cancer teams. The two editors, Janet Husband and Rodney Reznek, are internationally recognized as leading experts and teachers in their field. Alongside their own contributions to this textbook they have brought together a truly impressive array of other experts from across the world. The text is both authoritative and highly readable. Each chapter has a valuable introductory section as well as detailed information on imaging techniques. The illustrations are excellent, as are the lists of key points throughout the text.

In short this is a remarkable textbook. I strongly commend it both to radiologists working in the field of cancer and to their colleagues in specialist cancer teams.

Professor Mike Richards
National Cancer Director, England

Preface

Over the past several years, it has become clear that the optimal management of patients with cancer is best achieved by healthcare professionals working in a multidisciplinary team. During this evolution in cancer management, imaging technology has advanced markedly, largely but not wholly driven by expansion of computing power. Thus, multidetector computed tomography (CT) has become standard practice, allowing elegant, accurate 3D displays of anatomy and pathology, and new software for the accurate monitoring of treatment response has been introduced. In magnetic resonance (MR) imaging, new sequences and faster gradients have been developed, and in positron emission tomography-CT (PET-CT) refinements in technology have made a major impact on cancer assessment. These two latter developments have combined to make the specialist radiologist central to the multidisciplinary team; an individual who understands the clinical questions posed by the clinician, is skilled in cancer imaging interpretation, and is familiar with all the relevant recent technological advances.

As with previous editions, the aim of *Imaging in Oncology* is to provide an up-to-date text that addresses all these aspects of cancer imaging. All chapters included in the third edition of *Imaging in Oncology* have been revised, often extensively, to include the application of state-of-the-art imaging and to review its application to modern approaches in the management of patients with cancer. References have been updated to provide the reader with a current bibliography.

As with previous editions, *Imaging in Oncology* is divided into nine sections. The first section covers the general principles of the management of patients with cancer. As allied disciplines have become more aware of the importance of imaging in patient management, this section now includes separate chapters on cancer surgery, chemotherapy, and radiotherapy. Current thinking on trends in cancer incidence and the development of second malignancies has been addressed and particular focus has been placed on new developments in the assessment of treatment response.

Section 2, Staging Disease, is the largest section of *Imaging in Oncology*.

Each tumor site is dealt with separately in a set format that includes a diagrammatic illustration of the staging system together with an explanation followed by an evaluation of the role of imaging in demonstrating the extent of the disease. As a thorough understanding of the diagnostic performance of different imaging techniques is a crucial component of the radiologist's role in the multidisciplinary team, this aspect is stressed throughout the text.

The introduction of new and more successful therapies for many different types of cancer has encouraged earlier recognition of recurrent disease and therefore each chapter includes a section on the patterns of recurrence and their characteristic findings. Equally, with more aggressive management of metastatic disease,

great reliance is now placed on imaging for the accurate detection and delineation of metastases. Hence, this section has been updated to reflect modern imaging strategies and performance.

Since the second edition of *Imaging in Oncology*, great strides have been made in the localized treatment of tumors including targeted radiotherapy and percutaneous tumor ablation. These topics are considered in a separate section on "Imaging and Treatment."

Functional imaging is now becoming established as a valuable tool in the non-invasive assessment of metabolic and molecular processes, not only in the measurement of changes in response to therapy but also in the assessment of tumor aggressiveness and for targeting local therapies. MR imaging, CT, PET, and contrast-enhanced ultrasound have all been developed to assess functional processes, and several protocols are now moving from the research setting into routine clinical practice where they can be of real practical benefit. In this edition of *Imaging in Oncology* the final section is devoted to the principles of functional imaging because we believe that it is critically important for all cancer radiologists to become familiar with functional imaging techniques, and to have a broad understanding of their current benefits and limitations in the evaluation of various tumor types.

As in previous editions, salient points within the text have been highlighted as "Key Points" and a short summary is included at the end of each chapter in the same format as the Key Points. Several chapters include, where appropriate, color diagrams produced by Dee McLean to whom we owe a great debt of gratitude for her outstanding work. No one has worked harder to bring this third edition to fruition than Mrs. Maureen Watts, Mrs. Julie Jessop, and Mrs. Janet Macdonald. All found time in their busy working lives to contribute outstandingly to this project. Mrs. Watts co-ordinated the project from start to finish for Janet Husband, Mrs. Jessop did the same for Rodney Reznek. Mrs. Macdonald scrutinized all the images, working tirelessly to ensure that the highest possible quality has been achieved throughout the book.

Finally, we would like to acknowledge the enormous contribution of all the authors, and would like to thank them for sharing with us their valuable expertise and extensive experience. The high quality of their work has made the editing of this text informative, interesting, and a great pleasure.

We hope that this book will build on the previous editions of *Imaging in Oncology* to provide a useful reference text for all radiologists interested in cancer imaging. We hope too that it will make a contribution to the wider understanding of the ever increasing and constantly changing role that imaging plays in the management of patients with cancer.

Janet E Husband
Rodney H Reznek

32 Neuroendocrine Tumors
Andrea G Rockall, Norbert Avril, Ashley B Grossman, and Rodney H Reznek

INTRODUCTION

Neuroendocrine tumors (NETs), which include those that arise in the pancreas (also known as pancreatic neuroendocrine tumors or pancreatic NETs), the gastrointestinal tract and from neuroendocrine cells scattered in other tissues (carcinoids) are rare. These tumors were initially believed to arise from a putative common precursor, the amine precursor uptake and decarboxylation (APUD) cell, although this is now known not to be the case. These NETs are histologically closely related to melanoma, pheochromocytoma, and medullary carcinoma of the thyroid, which are described elsewhere (see chaps. 16, 30, and 48). All NETs have the potential to synthesize and secrete hormones. Functioning tumors are those in which hormone secretion by the tumor results in a clinical syndrome. Non-functioning tumors are those in which either there is no hormone secretion or hormone secretion does not result in a recognizable clinical syndrome. Functioning tumors usually present relatively early, due to the clinical syndrome, and may be a challenge for the radiologist to localize as they are often small. In contrast, non-functioning tumors generally go unrecognized for many years and present much later with mass effects.

The malignant potential of NETs varies. Malignancy is more common in some types, such as gastrinoma, whereas in others, such as insulinoma, malignancy is rare, but clinical behavior is often difficult to predict. In some cases, the tumors are associated with genetic disorders such as the multiple endocrine neoplasia type 1 (MEN 1) syndrome.

Imaging of functioning tumors, in particular, is primarily directed at localization and staging of the tumor. Preoperative localization reduces the likelihood of surgical complications and increases the chances of surgical resection, the only form of curative treatment for these tumors. Cross-sectional imaging is also valuable in the follow-up of recurrent or metastatic disease, and nuclear imaging techniques may be used to direct treatment with radiopharmaceuticals.

In this chapter, the clinical and imaging features of gastroenteropancreatic NETs will be described. The roles of the different imaging and radionuclide techniques used will be discussed.

CLINICAL FEATURES: PANCREATIC NEUROENDOCRINE TUMORS

Pancreatic neuroendocrine tumors (NETs) arise from the islet cells of Langerhans and include:

- Insulinoma
- Gastrinoma
- VIPoma
- Glucagonoma
- Somatostatinoma
- Pancreatic polypeptidoma (PPoma)

Epidemiology

Pancreatic NETs are rare, with a reported incidence of 1.2 to 1.6 per million and a prevalence of 10 per million of population (1,2). The incidence of clinically significant pancreatic NETs is four per million people per year. In early publications, the majority of pancreatic NETs were reported as functioning, with only 15% to 30% being non-functioning (3,4). However, in more recent data obtained from the Surveillance, Epidemiology and End Results (SEER) Program, a minority of cases were reported as functioning (2,5). The SEER database on islet cell tumors is the largest population-based study of islet cell tumors, with 1310 cases, but as this database only captures cases that were deemed to be malignant, it is unlikely to reflect the incidence of the small benign lesions, such as most insulinomas (2). The SEER data reports that 1.3% of all new pancreatic tumors are NETs. The peak incidence occurred in patients between 65 and 69 years of age with a median age at presentation of 59 and no sex prevalence. In other series, insulinomas, which are usually benign, are by far the most common pancreatic NETs, accounting for up to 50% of all cases (6). Benign insulinomas occur slightly more frequently in women (F3:M2), with an equal sex incidence in the rare malignant insulinomas. Other pancreatic NETs are more likely to be malignant, with gastrinoma being the next most common type. Gastrinomas account for 20% of pancreatic NETs (3), are seen in 0.5 to 3 patients per million people per year and slightly more commonly in males. In 10% to 20% of patients with a gastrinoma, there is a family history of disease and findings are consistent with MEN 1 (7). There is an equal sex incidence in the remainder of pancreatic NETs, PPomas being the next most common (although these do not produce a clinical syndrome). The other pancreatic NETs are rarer and may also be found in the context of MEN 1. Patients with MEN 1 generally present younger, usually have multiple tumors and may have prolonged survival compared to sporadic cases. Pancreatic NETs may also be associated with von Hippel–Lindau disease.

Etiology

The etiology of pancreatic NETs remains obscure. Abnormalities on chromosome 11q13 have been found in patients with MEN 1 and in patients with a sporadic gastrinoma (8,9). MEN 1 is inherited as an autosomal dominant trait: the syndrome comprises hyperplasia and/or tumors of several endocrine organs, the parathyroid gland being most commonly involved, followed by the pancreas, in which islet cell tumors are seen in over 50% of patients. Pituitary tumors, particularly prolactinomas, are the third major arm of the syndrome, but a variety of other tumors such as lipomas and adrenocortical tumors are also seen. One third of sporadic cases of gastrinoma have been shown to have similar chromosomal mutations to patients with MEN 1.

Histology, Classification, and Clinical Presentation (Table 32.1)

The histological appearance of pancreatic NETs is similar to that of other NETs, characterized by uniform sheets of small round cells.

Table 32.1 Classification of Pancreatic Neuroendocrine Tumors (3,4,6,7,21)

Tumor name	% frequency	Syndrome	Pancreatic islet cell	Hormone produced	% malignant	Anatomical location	Typical size
Insulinoma	50%	Insulinoma	B cell	Insulin	10–15%	Pancreas >99%	<2 cm 90%; <1 cm 40% (Head = body = tail)
Gastrinoma	20–30%	Zollinger–Ellison syndrome	G cell	Gastrin	60–75%	Pancreas 30–60%[a] Duodenum 30–40%[a] Lymph nodes 10–15%[a] Other <5	0.3–3.0 cm
Non-functioning and PPoma	15–30%	No syndrome	D1 cell	None or pancreatic polypeptide	60–90%	Pancreas (most frequently in the head)	Large
VIPoma	3%	Verner–Morrison syndrome; WDHA	D2 cell	Vasoactive intestinal peptide	50–80%	Pancreas 90% (usually tail) Adrenal 10%	Large
Glucagonoma	Rare	Glucagonoma	A cell	Glucagon	60%	Pancreas	2–10 cm
Somatostatinoma	Rare	Somatostatinoma[b]	D cell	Somatostatin	50–70%	Pancreas 56% Jejunum 44%	2–10 cm

[a]90% are within the gastrinoma triangle (see p. 764).
[b]Somatostatinoma may be associated with NF 1.

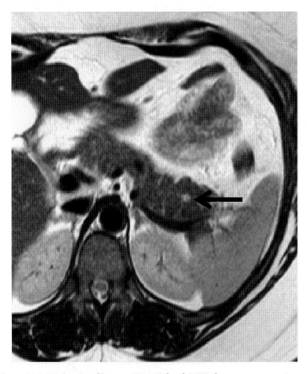

Figure 32.1 Benign insulinoma. T2-weighted MRI demonstrates an 8 mm high signal intensity lesion in the tail of pancreas (arrow). Most insulinomas are benign and measure less than 2 cm in diameter.

Several different patterns of growth have been described: a glandular pattern, a solid pattern, a gyriform pattern, and an unclassified pattern. However, the pattern of growth does not correlate with hormone production or malignant potential (7). In general, immunostaining with chromogranin and synaptophysin will confirm the neuroendocrine nature of the tumor, while special immunostains (insulin, gastrin, etc.) will identify specific secretory characteristics.

It is now recognized that most pancreatic NETs secrete a variety of hormonally active peptides. However, the classification of pancreatic

NETs is based on the presenting clinical syndrome, which is caused by the predominant hormone secreted by the tumor (Table 32.1). If no clinical syndrome is evident, the tumor is either classified by the hormone secreted (usually PPoma) or, if no hormone is secreted, it is called a non-functioning pancreatic NET.

The WHO clinicopathological classification of pancreatic NETs has three main divisions, well-differentiated endocrine tumor, well differentiated endocrine carcinoma, and poorly differentiated endocrine carcinoma-small cell carcinoma (10,11). Within each of these divisions, the tumors may be classified as functioning or non-functioning. A recently developed TNM classification, which is yet to be validated, has been found to be highly predictive of patient outcome and this may be combined with histopathological parmameters to classify pancreatic NETs (12).Well-differentiated endocrine tumors include those with benign behavior and those with uncertain behavior. Tumors with benign behavior are small (<2 cm), confined to the pancreas, have a low mitotic and proliferative index, and no angioinvasion. Those with uncertain behavior are confined to the pancreas but are >2 cm, have a slightly higher proliferative rate, or have angioinvasion.

Well-differentiated endocrine carcinomas of the pancreas are those which exhibit low-grade malignant signs with visible local invasion or metastases.

Poorly differentiated endocrine carcinoma-small cell carcinomas demonstrate high-grade malignant features and resemble small cell carcinoma of the lung. These tumors behave very aggressively and often present with widespread metastases.

Insulinomas (Figs. 32.1–32.4)
Insulinomas are solitary and intrapancreatic in over 90% of cases, with an equal distribution in the head, body, and tail of the gland (6,13). Of these tumors, 90% measure <2 cm and 40% <1 cm in diameter (4,14,15). Insulinomas almost invariably present with the clinical syndrome caused by hypoglycemia. The symptoms are variable and may be intermittent. There may be changes in personality or work performance, and in the elderly there may be confusion or dementia. The association of symptoms with fasting may

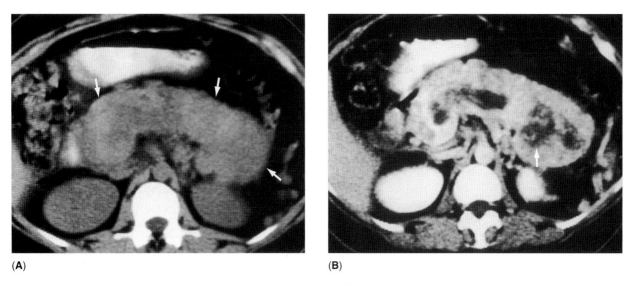

Figure 32.2 Malignant insulinoma. This 37-year-old male patient presented with vague abdominal pain. (A) Non-contrast CT at the level of the pancreas demonstrates diffuse enlargement of the entire pancreas (arrows). (B) Arterial phase contrast-enhanced image demonstrates diffuse heterogeneous enhancement of the gland with large areas of necrosis (arrow). The gland was infiltrated by a large malignant insulinoma, which was non-functioning.

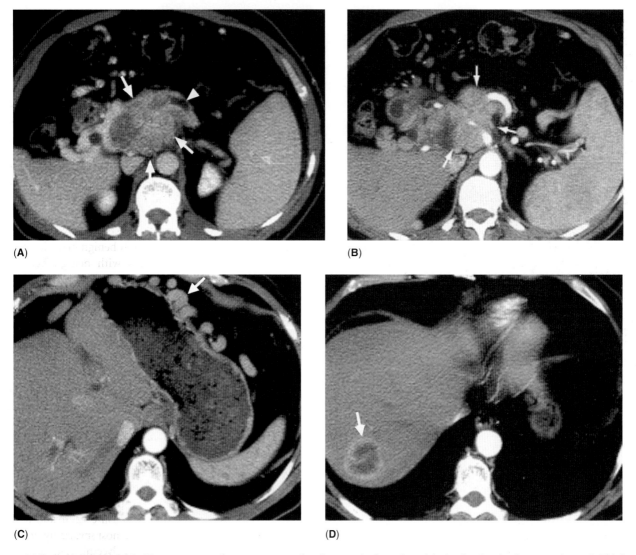

Figure 32.3 Malignant insulinoma. (A) CT, post-contrast, demonstrates an enhancing mass in the region of the head and neck of pancreas (arrows). This is causing obstruction of the main pancreatic duct, with atrophy of the tail (arrowhead). (B) At a slightly more cranial level, there is encasement of the celiac axis and the hepatic and splenic arteries (arrows). (C) Arterial phase (AP) CT through the stomach demonstrates large varices along the anterior wall of the stomach (arrow). This was secondary to portal vein thrombosis, due to tumor infiltration. (D) AP rim enhancement of a liver deposit indicates metastatic disease (arrow).

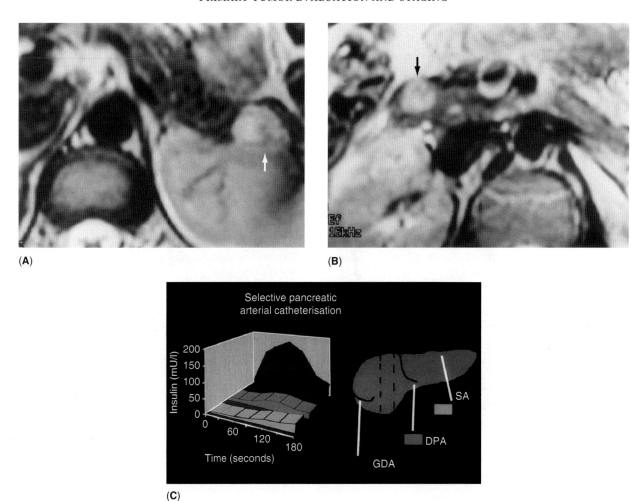

(A)

(B)

(C)

Figure 32.4 Multifocal insulinoma. (**A**) T2-weighted axial image through the tail of the pancreas. A well-defined high-signal lesion is demonstrated in the tail of pancreas (arrow). No other lesion was seen on T2-weighted images. (**B**) On T1 weighting, a second lesion is demonstrated in the head of pancreas, which has a high signal intensity on T1 weighting (arrow). This was initially missed. (**C**) Selective pancreatic arterial catheterization and venous sampling were performed. A secretagogue was injected into the splenic artery (SA), the duodenopancreatic artery (DPA) and the gastroduodenal artery (GDA). Venous sampling revealed no insulin surge from the region of the body or tail of pancreas, thus indicating that the lesion in the tail was non-functioning. However, there was marked insulin secretion following secretagogue injection in the region of the head of pancreas (via the GDA), indicating the presence of a functioning insulinoma in the head of the pancreas.

not be evident to the patient. The diagnosis is established clinically and biochemically prior to localization, on the basis of Whipple's triad, i.e., hypoglycemic attacks in the fasting state, blood glucose levels <2.2 mmol/l during an attack, with relief of symptoms following glucose administration. Other characteristic features include unusually high levels of insulin and C-peptide, and a negative screen for sulphonylureas or related drugs (16,17).

Key Points: Insulinomas

- The most common pancreatic NET is the insulinoma
- Diagnosis is made clinically and biochemically
- Ninety percent are benign, 90% measure <2 cm, 40% measure <1 cm
- The primary tumor is almost invariably located in the pancreas, whether single or multiple

Gastrinomas (Figs. 32.5–32.7)

Gastrinomas are the second most common pancreatic NETs, comprising some 20% to 30% of the total. About 60% of

gastrinomas are malignant with hepatic metastases at presentation, although there is a higher incidence of malignancy in those associated with MEN 1 (3,6). Metastases are usually to peripancreatic lymph nodes and liver, but bone metastases have been reported in approximately 30% of cases (18). About 90% of gastrinomas are located in the "gastrinoma triangle"; formed by the junction between the neck and body of the pancreas medially, the second and third parts of the duodenum inferiorly, and the junction of the cystic and common bile ducts superiorly (7).

Compared to insulinomas, these tumors tend to be even smaller, ranging in size from 0.3 to 3 cm, less vascular, and more often extrapancreatic (19). Patients generally present with recurrent, multiple or "ectopic" peptic ulceration, the Zollinger–Ellison syndrome (ZES), although in some cases ulceration may be mild. Diarrhoea and malabsorption due to acid inactivation of pancreatic enzymes may be predominant. The finding of an elevated gastrin level together with a high basal acid output is diagnostic of a gastrinoma (20). If possible, investigation should be undertaken in the absence of histamine

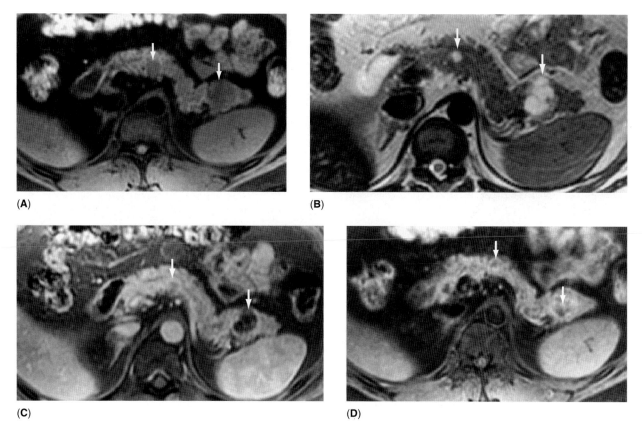

Figure 32.5 Multiple gastrinomas in a patient with MEN 1. (A) Axial T1-weighted scan with fat saturation demonstrates two lesions of low signal intensity within the body and tail of the pancreas (arrows). (B) On T2-weighted imaging, the lesions are of high signal intensity (arrows). (C) Dynamic T1-weighted image with fat saturation, 30 seconds following IV gadolinium administration. Both lesions demonstrate rim enhancement (arrows). (D) Dynamic T1-weighted image with fat saturation, 90 seconds following IV gadolinium administration. The lesions demonstrate further central enhancement (arrows).

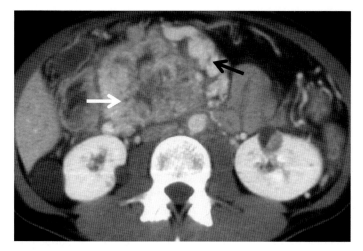

Figure 32.6 Malignant gastrinoma in a patient with von Hippel-Lindau disease. Portal venous-phase CT demonstrates a large mass in the region of the head of pancreas, which has heterogeneous enhancement and central necrosis (white arrow). Varices are seen around the periphery of the tumor (black arrow) due to obstruction of the SMV and portal vein. Note the cystic renal cell carcinoma in the left kidney, related to the VHL.

antagonists (>48 hours) or proton pump inhibitors (>2 weeks). Once the diagnosis of a gastrinoma has been confirmed, localization with imaging should be undertaken to identify the primary site and to stage the disease.

Key Points: Gastrinomas

- Sixty percent are malignant with hepatic metastases at presentation
- Ninety percent are located in the gastrinoma triangle
- Association with MEN 1 occurs frequently and features should be sought

Other Functioning Pancreatic NETs (Figs. 32.8 and 32.9)
The other functioning pancreatic NETs are very rare, frequently associated with MEN 1 and frequently malignant: 60% to 70% of glucagonomas, 50% to 80% of VIPomas and 50% to 70% of somatostatinomas are malignant (Table 32.1).

VIPomas (Fig. 32.8)
These comprise three percent of the total number of pancreatic NETs. Eighty percent are located within the pancreas (usually in the tail) but may also arise in the extrapancreatic tissue, particularly the retroperitoneal sympathetic chain and the adrenal medulla (6,7). The VIPoma syndrome, also known as WDHA (watery diarrhoea, hypokalemia, and achlorhydria), or the Verner–Morrison syndrome, is caused by the secretion of vasoactive intestinal peptide. The symptoms are of marked watery diarrhoea, causing hypokalemia which can be life-threatening. Death may occur due to cardiac arrest. The diagnosis is made on clinical and biochemical features, with the demonstration of an elevated plasma VIP. Other peptides such as neurotensin and PHM (peptidylglycine α-hydroxylating monooxygenase) may also

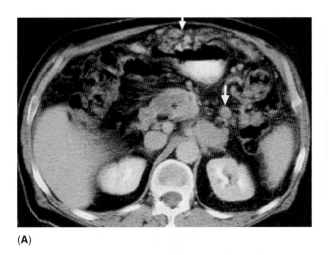

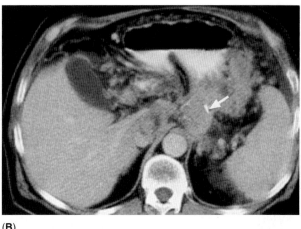

(A) **(B)**

Figure 32.7 Malignant gastrinoma. (**A**) Postcontrast CT demonstrates a central tumor mass (*) with extensive nodular deposits of tumor in the omental and peritoneal fat (arrows). (**B**) Following open biopsy, a diagnosis of malignant gastrinoma was confirmed (arrow indicates surgical clip).

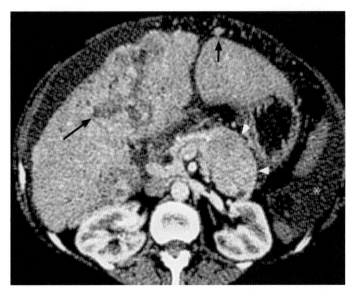

Figure 32.8 Malignant VIPoma. CT following IV contrast medium demonstrates an enhancing pancreatic mass (arrowheads), liver metastases (long arrow), a peritoneal deposit (short arrow), and ascites (*).

be elevated, but while they may be used as tumor markers their role in the presentation of the clinical syndrome is unclear.

Glucagonomas (Fig. 32.9)
These tumors often arise within the body or tail of the pancreas and they are usually large (2–10 cm) at the time of diagnosis (6,7,21). The glucagonoma syndrome presents with a characteristic necrolytic migratory erythematous rash, seen typically in the groin region in 75% of patients. This may be associated with glossitis and angular stomatitis. The diagnosis is confirmed by demonstrating elevated plasma glucagon levels. Glucagonomas tend to present late, usually with metastases, which are most frequently hepatic but may also be within lymph nodes or the mesentery. The prognosis is usually poor.

Somatostatinomas (Fig. 32.10)
Found in the pancreas in over half of affected individuals (most often in the pancreatic head), up to 50% of these tumors are located in the

duodenum and jejunum, where they may be associated with neurofibromatosis (7,22). Somatostatinomas are very slow-growing tumors with relatively mild non-specific symptoms (including diabetes mellitus, diarrhoea, steatorrhoea, and weight loss), and the tumors thus tend to be very large at presentation. Metastases are present in up to 90% of malignant somatostatinomas, most commonly to the liver, but also to lymph nodes, and bone (23). Duodenal somatostatinomas are sometimes associated with neurofibromatosis type 1.

Non-Functioning Pancreatic NETs (Fig. 32.11)
PPomas and pancreatic NETs that do not secrete any hormones do not result in a clinical syndrome and therefore sporadic cases present late as tumors causing mass effects (4). They are slow-growing tumors and tend to be large at diagnosis; approximately 60% to 90% are malignant (6,21). They usually lie in the pancreatic head and thus presentation may be similar to that of pancreatic adenocarcinoma, with biliary obstruction. In family groups with MEN 1, screening of the pancreas may identify non-functioning tumors at an early stage. They may also be seen in the von Hippel-Lindau syndrome.

Key Point

- Sixty to ninety percent of non-functioning pancreatic NETs are malignant and tend to be large at diagnosis

CLINICAL FEATURES: "CARCINOID" NEUROENDOCRINE TUMORS

The term "carcinoid" was first used in 1907 to describe a tumor of the gastro-intestinal (GI) tract that was slow-growing and not as aggressive as an adenocarcinoma. In the 1950s the tumors were found to contain serotonin, and the carcinoid syndrome was described, where patients with a small intestinal carcinoid tumor and liver metastases presented with the characteristic symptoms of diarrhoea, flushing, asthma, and right heart failure. However, overall only about 10% of such tumors are associated with the classical syndrome, although for small bowel carcinoids some elements of the syndrome may be present in around 30% of cases. The cells arise from the diffuse

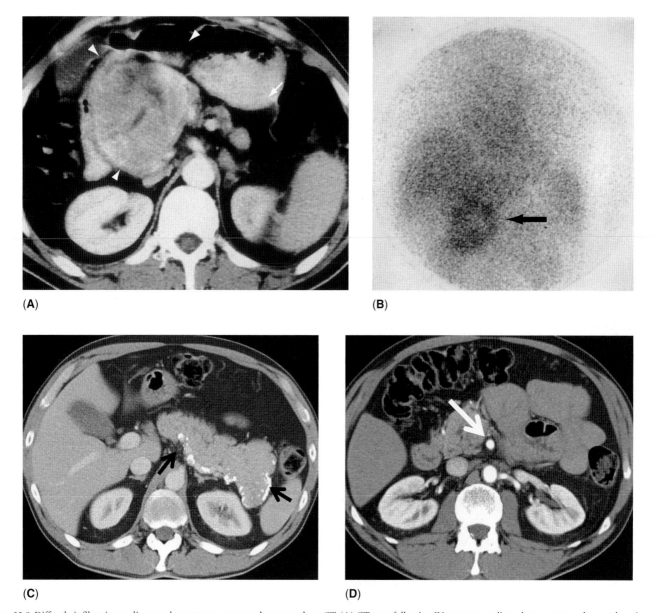

Figure 32.9 Diffusely infiltrating malignant glucagonoma on portal-venous phase CT. (A) CT scan following IV contrast medium demonstrates a large enhancing mass in the region of the head of pancreas (arrowheads). Areas of necrosis are seen in the central part of the mass. There is marked atrophy of the pancreatic tail, indicating the longstanding nature of the tumor (arrow). (B) In a different patient, the tumor was octreotide-avid (arrow). (C) In a different patient, the body and tail of pancreas are expanded by an ill-defined tumor. There is extensive calcification along the posterior margin of the tumor (arrows). (D) In a different patient, the tumor has infiltrated the head of pancreas, which is enlarged and heterogeneous (white arrow).

neuroendocrine system and have the potential to secrete a wide variety of amines and peptides, and therefore are now often referred to as NETs to reflect the wide range of clinical presentations (24,25).

Epidemiology (Table 32.2)

Carcinoid NETs occur much more frequently than pancreatic NETs and account for 2% of malignant tumors of the GI tract. The reported incidence of GI carcinoids is 7.1 per million people for men and 8.7 per million for women (26). However, the annual incidence is higher in autopsy studies, at 21 per million (27). NETs are most frequently diagnosed in the GI tract, where 66% are found. The second most common site is the bronchopulmonary system, accounting for 31% of NETs (28). Carcinoids present between the second and ninth decades of life, with certain sites being more

typical in certain age groups: carcinoids of the cervix present in the fourth decade, small intestine and respiratory tract in the early seventh, and rectal carcinoids in the late seventh decade (24,27,29).

Etiology

The etiology of carcinoids is not well understood. Certain disease states that result in hypergastrinemia, such as pernicious anemia and atrophic gastritis, appear to be predisposed to gastric carcinoids (see p. 770). In the Zollinger-Ellison syndrome, the development of a gastric carcinoid occurs most frequently in patients with MEN 1. Various tumor growth factors may influence the development of carcinoids and, as in patients with MEN 1, changes in chromosome 11q13 have been reported in patients with sporadic NETs, particularly foregut NETs, which are most commonly associated with

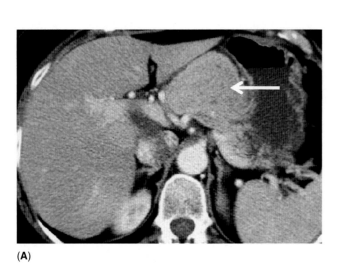

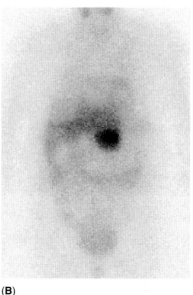

Figure 32.10 Somatostatinoma demonstrated on (**A**) portal-venous phase CT and (**B**) Octreotide scan. A large, relatively homogeneous mass in the body of pancreas is demonstrated (arrow). Over 50% of somatostatinomas arise in the pancreas, usually presenting as a mass. 80% are malignant and 95% are receptor-positive.

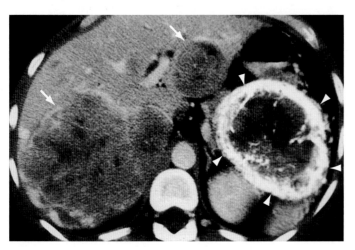

Figure 32.11 Non-functioning malignant PET. CT following IV contrast administration demonstrates a large mass in the tail of pancreas with extensive peripheral calcification (arrowheads), indicating the longstanding nature of the mass. Large necrotic liver metastases are present, with rim-enhancement (arrows). There was no clinical syndrome associated with this non-functioning endocrine tumor.

MEN 1 (25). NETs may also be seen in association with von Hippel-Lindau syndrome and neurofibromatosis (30).

Histology

Histologically, the tumor is comprised of sheets of uniform round cells arising from the enterochromaffin cells, which are APUD cells of the diffuse endocrine system. It is not possible to differentiate benign from malignant carcinoids based on histological features alone. It is the presence of local invasion or metastases that indicate malignancy. In addition, carcinoids cannot be differentiated histologically from pancreatic NETs. The tumors may be characterized by the histological staining patterns, which reflect the type of neurosecretory granules and cytoplasmic proteins. The tumor cells contain neurosecretory granules that contain a wide variety of

amines and peptides, such as 5-hydroxytryptamine (5-HT), neuron-specific enolase, hydroxytryptophan, synaptophysin, chromogranins A and C, and several hormones such as insulin, growth hormone, adrenocorticotrophic hormone (ACTH), and gastrin as well as many others. More recently, certain immunohistochemical markers have been used to categorize the tumors, including serotonin, chromogranin A and B, and neuron-specific enolase (NSE) (25,31,32). In general, most are diagnosed with the combination of chromogranin and synaptophysin immunostains, although others may be added to confirm suspicious or uncertain cases.

Classification and Clinical Presentation (Table 32.3)

Neuroendocrine carcinoid tumors are traditionally classified according to their site of origin: the secretory products and hence the clinical manifestations and immunohistochemical staining patterns are similar for tumors arising from particular anatomical sites (Table 32.3). Foregut carcinoids include NETs arising from the thymus, bronchus, gastric, or duodenal mucosa, and pancreas. Midgut carcinoids arise in the jejunum, ileum, and proximal colon; while hindgut tumors arise in the distal colon and rectum (33). A more recent classification has been proposed, replacing the term "carcinoid" with NETs (31). This WHO classification is based on the size, proliferative rate, location, differentiation, and hormone production. All GI and most other NETs can be categorized as:

- Well-differentiated endocrine tumors
- Well-differentiated endocrine carcinomas
- Poorly-differentiated endocrine carcinomas
- Mixed endocrine/exocrine tumors (WHO, 2005) (10)

Carcinoids can arise in a very wide variety of sites, but are most commonly reported at four sites (Table 32.2): bronchus (25%), jejuno-ileum (15%), appendix (2%), and rectum (19%), although in autopsy studies 76% are jejuno-ileal.

Table 32.2 Distribution of Carcinoids by Site at Presentation from the National Cancer Institute Database (28,47,152)

Location	Location (% of total)			Incidence of metastases (%)		
	1950–1971 (n = 4349)	1973–1991 (n = 5468)	1992–1999 (n = 4989)	1950–1971	1973–1991	1992–1999
Foregut						
Stomach	2	3.8	5.9	22	31	10–33
Duodenum	2.6	2.1	3.8	20	–	–
Bronchus, lung	11.5	32.5	25.3	20	27	27–35
Midgut						
Jejunum	1.3	2.3	1.5	35	70	58–64
Ileum	23	17.6	13.4	35		
Appendix	38	7.6	2.4	2	35	39–45
Colon	4.3	6.3	7.6	60	71	51–61
Hindgut						
Rectum	13	10	18.5	3	14	4–18

Table 32.3 Classification of Carcinoid Neuroendocrine Tumours (24,25)

Origin	Carcinoid syndrome	Metastases to bone	Organ	Clinical symptoms	Hormone production
Foregut	May occur; usually in cases with liver metastases	Occur	Thymus Lung	Cushing's syndrome Acromegaly Cushing's syndrome Acromegaly	CRH, ACTH, GHRH, (low 5-HT) CRH, ACTH, GHRH, PP, hCG alpha, neurotensin 5-HTP, (low 5-HT), histamine
			Stomach	Cushing's syndrome Pernicious anaemia Acromegaly, ZES	CRH, ACTH, GHRH, gastrin
			Duodenum	Somatostatinoma syndrome, ZES	Gastrin, somatostatin, neurotensin tachykinins, (low 5-HT)
Midgut "classical carcinoid"	Occurs frequently, in cases with metastases	Rare	Ileum Jejunum Proximal colon	Carcinoid syndrome	Tachykinins, bradykinins CGRP High 5-HT
			Appendix	Not hormone related	(Tachykinins, 5-HT)
Hindgut	Rare	Occur	Distal colon Rectum	Not hormone related	PP, HCG-alpha, PYY, somatostatin, (rarely 5-HT)

Abbreviations: ACTH, adrenocorticotrophic hormone; CGRP, calcitonin gene-related peptide; CRH, corticotrophin-releasing hormone; GHRH, growth hormone-releasing hormone; 5-HT, 5-hydroxytryptamine, serotonin; 5-HTP, 5-hydroxytryptophan; hCG, human chorionic gonadotrophin; PP, pancreatic polypeptide; PYY, peptide YY.

Foregut Carcinoids

Bronchial Carcinoids (Fig. 32.12)

Bronchial carcinoids, or bronchopulmonary NETs, are NETs of the bronchial epithelium arising from Kulschitsky cells, neuroepithelial bodies, or pluripotential bronchial epithelial stem cells (34,35). They have been classified into four groups by the WHO, (36) according to their malignant potential:

- Low grade typical carcinoid tumor (classical or benign bronchial carcinoid)
- Intermediate grade atypical carcinoid tumor
- Two high-grade malignancies: large cell neuroendocrine carcinoma (LCNEC) and small-cell carcinoma (SCLC)

The prognosis for bronchopulomary NETs has decreased considerably over the last 30 years, with the five-year survival rate (ysr) decreasing from 84.7% to 47.3%. This phenomenon may be due to changes in histopathology reporting (37). The prognosis is excellent for typical bronchial carcinoids (approximately 88% 5 ysr) and poor for small cell carcinomas (<5% 5 ysr) (38). Bronchial carcinoids now account for 25% of all carcinoid tumors (up from

11.5%, Table 32.2). This increase may also be due to changes in classification or increased recognition of broncopulmonary carcinoids by pathologists (38). Typical low-grade carcinoid tends to occur in younger patients between the fifth and sixth decade, and the relationship to smoking is uncertain (38,39). The high-grade LCNEC and SCLCs are more frequent in men and typically occur in the seventh decade, and are strongly correlated with a smoking history (40,41). Although 25% of patients are asymptomatic, clinical presentation is usually related to bronchial obstruction, with cough and wheezing, and hemoptysis occurs in 50% of patients, due to the highly vascular nature of the lesion. Cushing's syndrome (due to ACTH secretion) and carcinoid syndrome (in patients with liver metastases) occur in approximately 2% of cases (42). Metastases may be seen in the liver, bones, adrenal glands, and brain.

Thymic Carcinoids (Fig. 32.13)

NETs of the thymus are rare and may be part of MEN 1. The tumor is usually non-functioning and presents with an anterior mediastinal mass. If functioning, then the tumor usually secretes ACTH,

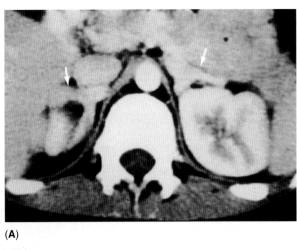

(A)

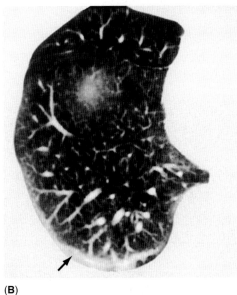

(B)

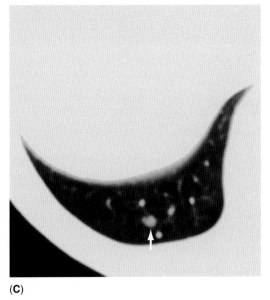

(C)

Figure 32.12 Bronchial carcinoid in a patient presenting with ACTH-dependent Cushing's syndrome. (A) There is marked bilateral adrenal hyperplasia secondary to ACTH production (arrows). No pituitary adenoma was identified and thus an ectopic source of ACTH was sought. (B) Supine CT of the thorax was unremarkable, apart from dependent changes at the bases (arrow). (C) Prone CT revealed a 5 mm solitary pulmonary nodule (arrow). This was resected and was confirmed to be a peripheral bronchial carcinoid.

causing ectopic ACTH-dependent Cushing's syndrome, which occurs in one third of patients with a thymic NET (42). In these cases, bilateral adrenal hyperplasia may be seen (43). Other hormones may also be produced, including corticotrophin-releasing hormone, growth hormone-releasing hormone, and 5-HT (44). The carcinoid syndrome has never been described in association with a thymic NET. The prognosis is generally poor (42).

Gastric Carcinoids (See Chap. 12) (Fig. 32.14)
NETs arising in the stomach are rare, accounting for 0.3% of gastric neoplasms but 11% to 41% of GI NETs (45). They have been divided into three subtypes based on predisposing factors, endoscopic appearances, and clinical course:

- *Type I gastric carcinoid* is the most common subtype and is associated with hypergastrinemia and chronic atrophic gastritis, with or without pernicious anemia. Hypergastrinemia results in hyperplasia of enterochromaffin-like cells, which may lead to the development of the carcinoid tumor. Tumors are multicentric lesions <1 cm predominantly found in the fundus and body of stomach, and are surrounded by enterochromaffin cell hyperplasia. The diagnosis is often made incidentally at endoscopy for dyspepsia. The disease is almost always benign, with metastases present in only 2% of cases.
- *Type II gastric carcinoids* are rare (5–10% of cases). They are associated with ZES and MEN 1: 30% of patients with MEN 1 have gastric carcinoids. Tumors arise from the enterochromaffin-like cells, are multicentric, but have an increased tendency to metastasize to regional lymph nodes, although the prognosis is generally good.
- *Type III gastric carcinoids* are sporadic, are not associated with hypergastrinemia and account for 13% of cases of gastric carcinoid. There is a strong male predominance (80%). The tumor is usually solitary, large and may ulcerate. Local invasion and metastases are common, and there is only a 20% five-year survival rate (45).

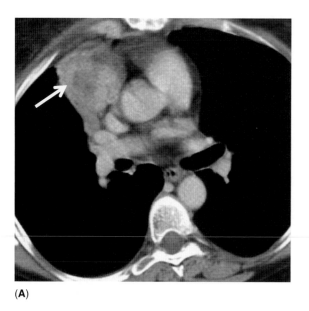
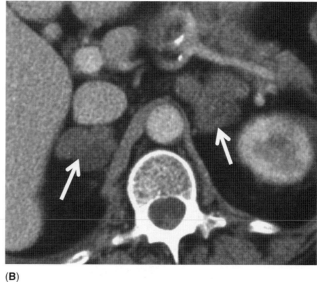

(A)   **(B)**

Figure 32.13 Thymic carcinoid on CT. (**A**) A large heterogeneous mass is demonstrated in the anterior mediastinum (arrow). There is no fat plane visible between the mass and the pericardium and pericardial invasion cannot be ruled out. (**B**) There is bilateral adrenal hyperplasia (arrows) secondary to ACTH production by the tumor (arrows).

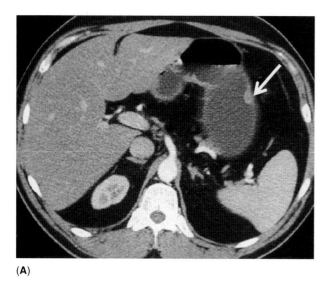
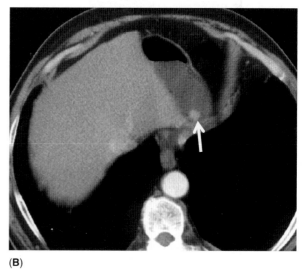

(A)   **(B)**

Figure 32.14 Gastric carcinoid type II in a patient with MEN 1. CT at the level of (A) the greater curve of the stomach (arrow) and (B) the gastro-esophageal junction. Multiple small enhancing lesions are demonstrated (arrows), arising from the gastric mucosa.

Key Points: Foregut Carcinoids

■ Bronchial carcinoids range from benign tumors (typical bronchial carcinoid) to highly malignant (poorly differentiated large or small cell carcinoma)

■ Thymic carcinoids are usually non-functioning and usually have a poor prognosis

■ Gastric carcinoids account for only 0.3% of all gastric neoplasms

Midgut Carcinoids (Figs. 32.15–32.19)

Midgut carcinoids are defined as NETs arising beyond the ligament of Treitz to the level of the mid-transverse colon and are the commonest primary malignant tumor of the small intestine. They tend to have a high serotonin content, with relatively high urinary 5-HIAA levels. Of all GI carcinoids, 42% arise in the small

bowel (28). Over the last 50 years, small bowel carcinoids account for approximately 20% to 30% of all carcinoid tumors and are the commonest cause of metastatic carcinoid (Table 32.2) (46,47). However, the percentage of all carcinoids that arise in the small bowel has decreased gradually during this period. This may be due to changes in classification. Abdominal pain is a relatively common presenting feature of carcinoid tumors of the GI tract and 40% present with symptoms of obstruction. Patients may have colicky abdominal pain and diarrhoea due to increased intestinal motility. Obstruction may be due to the primary tumor, either with or without intussusception, although frequently the tumor is very small. Tumor-associated desmoplastic fibrosis, which causes tethering and kinking of the small bowel mesentery, may also cause obstruction. It is probably due to local production of fibrogenic agents such as 5HT and TGF, and may compromise the arterial or venous vasculature. Dissemination of these agents beyond

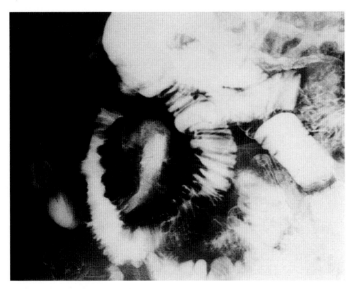

Figure 32.15 Midgut carcinoid. A barium follow-through study showing focal mesenteric thickening in the right iliac fossa with distortion of the surrounding loops of small bowel, which demonstrates spiculation, tethering, and slight fold thickening. The appearances are consistent with a desmoplastic response secondary to the presence of a mesenteric carcinoid tumor.

the liver into the venous circulation gives rise to right-sided cardiac valvular abnormalities. Metastases occur to liver (resulting in the carcinoid syndrome), bone, and lung (25). The incidence of metastases from midgut carcinoids is dependent on tumor size (25,46). In tumors <1 cm, 15% to 25% have metastases; in tumors between 1 and 2 cm, metastases are present in 58% to 80%; and in tumors >2 cm over 70% have metastases.

Key Points: Midgut Carcinoids

- This is the most common primary malignancy of the small intestine, and the commonest cause of metastatic carcinoid. It is frequently associated with the carcinoid syndrome
- It includes all the tumors from the ligament of Treitz to the mid-transverse colon

Hindgut Carcinoids

Hindgut carcinoids include those arising in the colon (distal to the mid-transverse colon) and rectum. Rectal carcinoids are the most common hindgut carcinoid and, in a large series between 1992 and 1999, these accounted for 27% of all GI carcinoid tumors (28). The proportion of GI carcinoids that are rectal has increased, as they

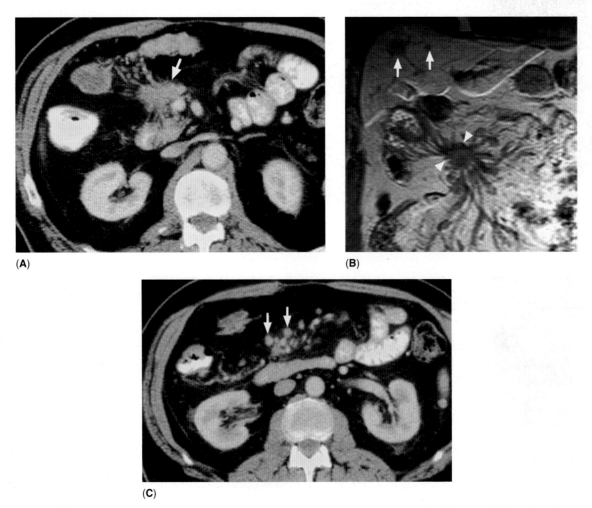

(A)   (B)

(C)

Figure 32.16 Midgut carcinoid. (**A**) CT following IV contrast medium demonstrates a mesenteric mass (arrow) which has a markedly spiculated appearance due to a fibrotic desmoplastic response in the surrounding tissues. (**B**) Coronal T1-weighted MR image demonstrates the marked spoke-wheel spiculation around the mesenteric mass (arrowheads). Liver metastases are also present (arrows). (**C**) Multiple enlarged mesenteric lymph nodes are seen within the mesenteric fat (arrows).

represented 17% of all GI carcinoids in the period between 1950 and 1969 (28). Rectal carcinoids account for 1% of all anorectal neoplasms (48). The tumors are usually slow-growing. However, in one large series, 30% of patients had metastatic disease at presentation (49). Metastases, which occur to the liver, lungs and bones, are more common in patients with atypical histology and the incidence increases with the size of the tumor (49,50).

Key Point: Hindgut Carcinoids

■ Rectal carcinoids are the commonest hindgut carcinoid and account for close to 30% of all GI carcinoids

IMAGING THE PRIMARY TUMOR: PANCREATIC NEUROENDOCRINE TUMORS

Localization

A wide variety of imaging methods are advocated in the literature for the localization of the primary site of disease and detection of

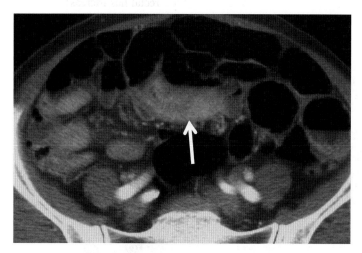

Figure 32.17 Ileal carcinoid on CT. There is a focal segment of thickened ileum (arrow). Several distended loops of small bowel are seen proximal to the lesion.

metastases. This reflects the difficulties encountered in satisfactorily demonstrating these tumors. The use of different modalities in the literature also reflects differences in local expertise and experience. In addition, the diagnostic performances that are quoted in the literature reflect techniques at different stages of development, making comparison of techniques challenging. The various techniques and imaging features of pancreatic NETs are now described, together with a discussion concerning the advantages and disadvantages of each technique.

Ultrasound

Transabdominal Ultrasound

Transabdominal ultrasound (US) is non-invasive and widely available, and does not use radiation, but has a relatively low sensitivity for localizing small pancreatic NETs, in the range of 20% to 86% (13,17,51). However, it has been shown to have a high specificity. The scanning technique should be tailored to optimize pancreatic visualization. The patient should drink water prior to scanning to allow the stomach to be used as an acoustic window; positioning the patient in both the standing position and lying in the left posterior oblique position may allow a more complete assessment. As with most of the imaging techniques available, sensitivity increases with the size of the lesion (51,52).

The tumor appearance is of a well-defined round mass, which is homogeneously hypoechoic in relation to the pancreas, and vascular on Doppler imaging. There may be a hyperechoic halo or distortion of the gland, an appearance that may help in detecting the lesion, particularly in younger patients, in whom the tumors tend to be less conspicuous due to the generally lower echogenicity of the pancreas. Tumors that lie along the surface of the pancreas or in the duodenum are less conspicuous. US contrast agents have been shown to have a high specificity of 90% to 100% in differentiating pancreatic ductal adenocarcinoma from other solid neoplastic masses, including NETs, on transabdominal US (53). Ductal adenocarcinomas are characterized by lesion hypovascuity in relation to the surrounding enhancing pancreatic parenchyma post-contrast medium administration. Conversely, iso- or hypervascularity is characteristic of other pancreatic neoplasms, including NETs.

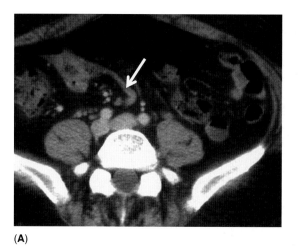

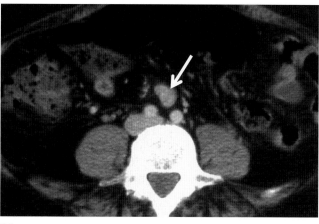

(A)   **(B)**

Figure 32.18 CT of appendiceal carcinoid in a patient with Cushing's syndrome. (A) The appendix is clearly demonstrated (arrow). (B) On the next slice superiorly, a mass is seen arising from the tip of the appendix, which contains speckled calcifications (arrow). A carcinoid tumor was confirmed at histology.

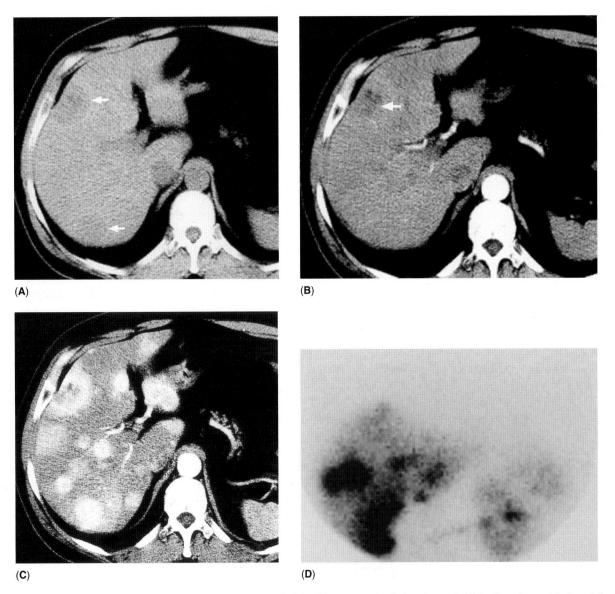

Figure 32.19 Carcinoid liver metastases. (**A**) Non-contrast CT demonstrates ill-defined low attenuation lesions (arrows). (**B**) In the early arterial-phase following contrast enhancement, the metastases are relatively poorly demonstrated. (**C**) In the late arterial phase (AP), extensive liver metastases are demonstrated, which enhance intensely. Many lesions could not be appreciated on the non-contrast or early AP CT. (**D**) Octreotide scanning demonstrates the multiple liver metastases, indicating that radiopharmaceutical therapy may be considered.

The patterns of enhancement of pancreatic lesions on contrast-enhanced ultrasound have been found to correlate with the enhancement on Computed Tomography (CT) (54).

Endoscopic Ultrasound
Endoscopic ultrasound (EUS) enables close proximity of the transducer to the pancreas, allowing a high frequency US probe to be used (7.5–10 mHz), resulting in greatly improved image resolution. The pancreatic head and duodenum are scanned with the probe positioned in the duodenum, and the body and tail are scanned through the stomach. Although EUS is invasive and operator-dependent, it greatly improves the sensitivity for the detection of small tumors (55,56). The advantages of the technique are:

- Localization of small tumors
- Localization of multiple tumors, particularly in MEN 1

- Detection of small tumors in the pancreatic head, which may be difficult to palpate at surgery
- Detection of tumors arising in the duodenal wall
- Detection of lymph node enlargement to improve staging accuracy
- Accurate depiction of the relations between vascular and biliary structures, and the tumor
- Fine needle aspiration biopsy can be undertaken

The disadvantages of the technique are:

- Technically challenging, requiring specialist training, and therefore not widely available; may not be suitable for all patients, for example, where there is duodenal scarring in ZES
- Reduced sensitivity in extrapancreatic lesions or in the tail of the pancreas
- The liver cannot be fully assessed

Although the diagnostic performance of EUS is difficult to evaluate, reports indicate that overall the technique is highly sensitive, with sensitivities as high as 79% to 100% reported (56,57). As on transabdominal US, pancreatic NETs are iso- or hypervascular following administration of US contrast medium. This feature is helpful in differentiating these lesions from ductal adenocarcinoma (53). Fine needle aspiration of suspected pancreatic NETs may be undertaken during EUS. There is a close correlation between the aspiration cytology and the final histology post-resection (58–60).

Intraoperative Ultrasound

This technique has similar advantages to EUS and may improve the intraoperative sensitivity for identifying small lesions in the head and multiple lesions to up to 92% to 97% and is a useful adjunct to palpation of the gland (17,61). It has been shown to change operative management in 10% of ZES cases, by identifying multiple gastrinomas or by demonstrating the malignant nature of a lesion (62). Intraoperative ultrasound (IOUS) has the advantage, over EUS, of being able to assess the liver. However, it is not as sensitive as surgical palpation in detecting extra-pancreatic lesions. The disadvantages of the technique are:

- Increased time and complexity of operation, as complete mobilization of the pancreas is required
- Specialist experience is required for performing and interpreting the scan
- Preoperative tumor localization is still needed
- Poor sensitivity in extrapancreatic/duodenal lesions

Overall, the technique is a useful addition to surgical palpation, particularly in small tumors such as insulinomas

---

Key Points: Pancreatic NETs on US

- Transabdominal US has high specificity but low sensitivity
- Lesion appears homogeneously hypoechoic in relation to the pancreas
- Lesion may have hyperechoic rim or cause distortion of the pancreas
- Lesion is iso- or hypervascular to the surrounding pancreas following enhancement
- EUS improves sensitivity for detection of small/multiple tumors in the head and neck of pancreas, but the tail of the pancreas is difficult to visualize
- IOUS improves sensitivity for the detection of small/multiple tumors in the head and neck of pancreas and the liver, and is a useful adjunct to palpation

---

Computed Tomography

CT is the most widely used diagnostic tool for the localization and staging of pancreatic NETs. It has the advantage of being widely available and is not subject to some of the difficulties encountered with US, such as potentially poor visibility and operator-dependence. Multidetector CT (MDCT) has enhanced the diagnostic strength of CT, allowing very rapid acquisition of the images, ensuring accurate arterial-phase images, and reduced movement artifact.

CT Technique

Optimal technique is essential for the accurate detection of these lesions. The patient should be fasted to ensure that the stomach and duodenum are emptied of their contents. The stomach is distended with water and IV hyoscine butylbromide or another anti-peristaltic agent is administered. An initial precontrast scan is performed to identify the level of the pancreas. Following IV administration of 150 ml of contrast medium at a rate of 3–5 ml/sec, biphasic scanning is recommended. Arterial-phase scanning is started either by bolus tracking or after a delay of approximately 30 seconds and portal venous scanning after a delay of 60 to 70 seconds. The section thickness should not exceed 5 mm and the entire liver should be included in all phases. The images are then reconstructed to 1 to 2 mm in slice thickness, and coronal or sagittal reformats may be made. Images should also be viewed on narrow window settings in order to augment the difference between the enhancing tumor and the pancreas (63–65).

CT Appearance

Functioning tumors are usually small (see p. 762–66 and Table 32.1) and subtle, with low inherent contrast between the tumor and surrounding pancreas. They are usually isodense with the pancreas on precontrast images and do not usually distort the contour of the pancreas. As in the angiography literature, a majority of islet cell tumors are hypervascular and will be best seen after intravenous injection of contrast medium. However, the best phase for the demonstration of those hyperattenuating small lesions is unclear. The authors' experience concurs with others who report that tumor-to-pancreas contrast is greatest on arterial-phase (AP) images compared to portal venous phase (PVP) imaging (66–68). However, others have found the PVP significantly more helpful in identifying these tumors (69). At present, therefore, we recommend biphasic imaging following IV injection of contrast medium to optimize the sensitivity of the technique. Narrow window settings may help to improve detection (Fig. 32.20). Rarely, insulinomas may be hypovascular or cystic and appear hypodense to the surrounding pancreas. Cystic pancreatic NETs represented four of 38 pancreatic NETs in one series, and these represented 14% of all pancreatic cystic lesions identified over a 10-year period (70). Cystic pancreatic NETs are usually benign and non-functioning, and cannot be reliably differentiated from other cystic pancreatic lesion neoplasms on imaging alone (70,71). In patients with a suspected gastrinoma, particular attention should be given to the "gastrinoma triangle" (see section "Gastrinomas" p. 770).

Large tumors are more likely to be non-functioning and necrotic centrally, and are more likely to be malignant (Fig. 32.2). The features that are associated with malignancy include large size, necrosis, overt infiltration of the surrounding retroperitoneal structures such as vessels, and calcification (Figs. 32.2, 32.3, and 32.11) (4,63). In one study, calcification was associated with well-differentiated tumors (72).

Diagnostic Performance of CT

Early studies using non-spiral CT techniques reported a relatively high sensitivity of 78% for the detection of lesions (4). Detection of the primary tumor is directly related to tumor size, with no tumors identified <1 cm, 30% of tumors detected between 1 and 3 cm, and 95% of tumors >3 cm in diameter demonstrated (4,7,73). The location of the tumor also influences the ability of CT to

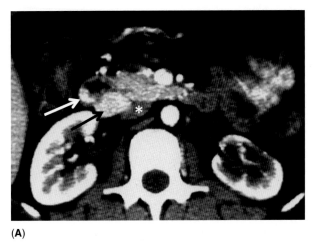
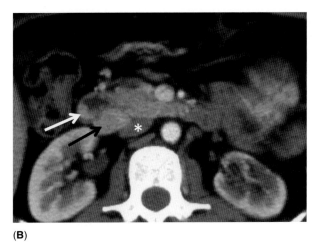

(A)   **(B)**

Figure 32.20 Multiple gastrinomas on CT: Importance of window settings. Arterial-phase CT on (**A**) narrow window settings and (**B**) wide window settings. Two brightly enhancing gastrinomas are seen; one shown here in the wall of the duodenum (white arrow) and another extrapancreatic gastrinoma adjacent to the uncinate process (black arrow). Note the unopacified IVC (asterisk). It is important to use oral water rather than Gastrografin in order to appreciate duodenal gastrinomas.

detect the lesion. One prospective study detected 68% of primary tumors and 86% of hepatic metastases (confirmed at surgery, autopsy or percutaneous biopsy), 90% of pancreatic head tumors, 80% of pancreatic body tumors, and 45% of pancreatic tail tumors (73,74). Small tumors of <1 cm in the duodenum are often missed on CT, and CT sensitivity for the detection of extrahepatic and extrapancreatic gastrinomas, which are often small at presentation, is only 30% to 50% (19,73). With the development of multidetector CT and the use of thin reformats, there has been a reported increase in sensitivity for the detection of insulinomas to 94% (75). In the same publication, a 100% sensitivity was achieved if the MDCT results were combined with EUS.

Key Points: Pancreatic NETs on CT

- Small functioning tumors are usually isodense to the pancreas and enhance strongly postcontrast
- Best visualization is on arterial phase but portal venous phase is complementary
- Cystic lesions occur but are rare
- Large tumors are more likely to be non-functioning
- Signs of malignancy include large size, necrosis, calcification, and invasion/infiltration of surrounding structures

Magnetic Resonance Imaging

Early studies with magnetic resonance (MR) imaging reported a lower sensitivity than CT for the detection of both the primary tumor and metastatic disease. However, with the marked improvements in MR technology that have occurred in the past decade, the diagnostic performance of MR has improved and in several studies has been shown to exceed or equal that of CT (69,76,77). MR has a higher sensitivity than angiography or CT for metastatic disease (78). However, angiography remains more sensitive than MR for identifying the primary tumor. A sensitivity of 94% for pancreatic lesions, but less for extra-pancreatic lesions, has been reported (76,79). As with the other cross-sectional modalities, tumor detection increases with tumor size. Multiple tumors, as in patients with MEN 1, are particularly difficult to detect.

The sensitivity of MR does depend on good quality images. Where there is image degradation due to movement artifact and a poor signal-to-noise ratio, for example, in obese patients, sensitivity may be reduced. Optimal technique requires a quadrature phased-array coil. The imaging sequences should include:

- Axial fat-suppressed T1-weighted spin-echo and gradient-echo
- Axial fast spin-echo, T2 weighted with and without fat suppression
- Axial dynamic contrast-enhanced gradient echo sequence

The tumors usually appear to be of low signal intensity on T1-weighted sequences and high on T2-weighted sequences in relation to the pancreas (Fig. 32.5). The tumors are most conspicuous on the fat-suppressed T1-weighted image whether spin-echo or gradient-recalled (76,79). Tumors that contain a high collagen or fibrous tissue content may return a low signal intensity on T2-weighted images, but this is rare (69). Following IV gadolinium administration, there is characteristic marked homogeneous enhancement, reflecting the highly vascular nature of these tumors (Fig. 32.5). In cystic lesions, rim enhancement may be seen (76). Liver-specific contrast agents, such as mangofadopir DPDP, may have a role in improved lesion detection, but this is currently under investigation (80,81).

Key Points: Pancreatic NETs on MR Imaging

- Best seen on fat-saturated T1-weighted sequences
- Usually hypointense to the pancreas on fat-saturated T1-weighted image
- Usually hyperintense to the pancreas on FSE T2-weighted image
- Homogeneous enhancement post gadolinium (rim enhanceent in cystic lesions)

Angiographic Techniques

Angiography

Angiography is rarely used nowadays in most centres and when used is usually combined with venous sampling. In order not to miss a lesion, detailed assessment of the vasculature is required with selective catheterization of all the branches of the coeliac and superior mesenteric arteries. Sensitivities are

fairly high. Both the primary tumor and liver metastases are seen as a well-defined blush in the capillary to early venous phases. Difficulties in diagnosis arise:

- When a tumor lies adjacent to a loop of bowel or spleen and the blush is not separately visible
- When the tumor is very small
- When there are multiple lesions
- When the tumor is hypovascular

All these problems may lead to false negative results. False positives arise from the blush of a splenunculus or normal pancreas or bowel.

Transhepatic Portal Venous Sampling

The principle of this technique is that the vein draining the tumor will have an abnormally high concentration of hormone. Transhepatic portal venous sampling (THPVS) may involve percutaneous catheterization of a portal venous branch. Blood is then sampled from the splenic vein, superior, and inferior mesenteric veins, pancreatic veins and portal trunk. Thus a tumor may be broadly localized to the tail, body or head of the pancreas/duodenum (these cannot be reliably distinguished using this technique). This method is only useful for tumors that secrete a hormone and false-negative results may occur if hormone secretion is intermittent. It has a limited role in patients with multiple tumors.

Arterial Stimulation and Venous Sampling

Arterial stimulation venous sampling (ASVS) combines simultaneous hepatic venous sampling with selective arterial injection of a pancreatic secretagogue, a technique that is less invasive than THPVS. Many different specific secretagogues have been used in the past, but generally now calcium gluconate is used regardless of the specific secretory product. Following injection of the secretagogue, hepatic venous sampling is performed every 30 seconds for two minutes (Fig. 32.4C). A two- or threefold increase in the level of hormone indicates the presence of tumor, allowing the depiction of the tumor region, as with THPVS. This technique is most useful in cases where the tumor remains occult on other imaging modalities, predominantly with very small functional tumors. It can be performed as part of pancreatic angiography and is liable to some of the risks associated with THPVS, such as hepatic arteriovenous fistulae, hematoma, and superior mesenteric arterial occlusion. Reported sensitivities are high, up to 93%, and the stimulation technique improves the sensitivity of angiography alone (7). In one case series, 10 of 11 insulinomas were correctly localized, with histological confirmation (82).

Key Points: Imaging of Functioning Pancreatic NETs

- These tumors are usually small (1–2 cm) at presentation
- They are markedly vascular
- Many different imaging techniques are advocated, including cross-sectional, interventional, and nuclear medicine
- Local expertise should guide the imaging algorithm

CHOICE OF IMAGING TECHNIQUE IN LOCALIZING PANCREATIC NETs

Several factors have to be taken into account when considering the choice of the most appropriate investigation for localizing biochemically proven pancreatic NETs, including such considerations as availability, cost, local experience, and expertise. Most investigators would initiate investigation with cross-sectional imaging, either CT or MR. Advantages and limitations of both are given above. This will clearly identify the largest lesions, allow assessment of the entire abdomen and provide valuable information on the presence of hepatic metastases. We believe that the investigation of choice for the precise localization of pancreatic NETs is EUS, which should follow cross-sectional imaging, especially where the findings are equivocal. In the context of multiple endocrine neoplasia it will help to identify whether the lesions are multifocal. Radionuclide scintigraphy (which is described on p. 783-86) is helpful in

- Associating an anatomical abnormality with functional evidence
- Identifying unsuspected metastases
- Assessing possible therapeutic options

The technique of ASVS, being more invasive, is used more sparingly. Where the imaging is unequivocal, it is not usually necessary to perform it. However, ASVS becomes extremely valuable in the context of MEN1, when the patient shows multifocal lesions and it is unclear which are responsible for a given hormonal hypersecretion. In such patients, pancreatic surgery may be limited to removal of selected lesions.

It has been argued in the past that for small pancreatic NETs, especially insulinomas, all that is needed is a confirmed biochemical diagnosis, and to proceed directly to surgery using IOUS. However, we believe that the treatment of NETs, in general, has become more individualized and precise radiological demonstration of the size, the functionality, and metastases will determine optimum outcomes, especially where a partial pancreatectomy or laparoscopic removal is the most appropriate procedure.

IMAGING THE PRIMARY TUMOR: CARCINOID NEUROENDOCRINE TUMORS

Localization

In some cases, the diagnosis of a carcinoid tumor is made at endoscopy, particularly for gastric, duodenal, rectal, or colonic lesions. Endobronchial carcinoids may be diagnosed bronchoscopically. However, imaging is used extensively for the localization of many primary NETs, as well as in staging the tumor. Many carcinoids do not present with a specific clinical syndrome, such as the carcinoid syndrome, and imaging may be performed to investigate nonspecific symptoms of abdominal discomfort or diarrhoea. Image-guided biopsy of a mass, liver lesions, or lymph nodes may help to establish the diagnosis. CT is the main cross-sectional imaging modality for localizing and staging carcinoid tumors (83). US is used predominantly in the detection of liver metastases and for guiding biopsy. It is not a primary diagnostic tool in localizing the tumor. Imaging is also useful in the investigation of second primary tumors,

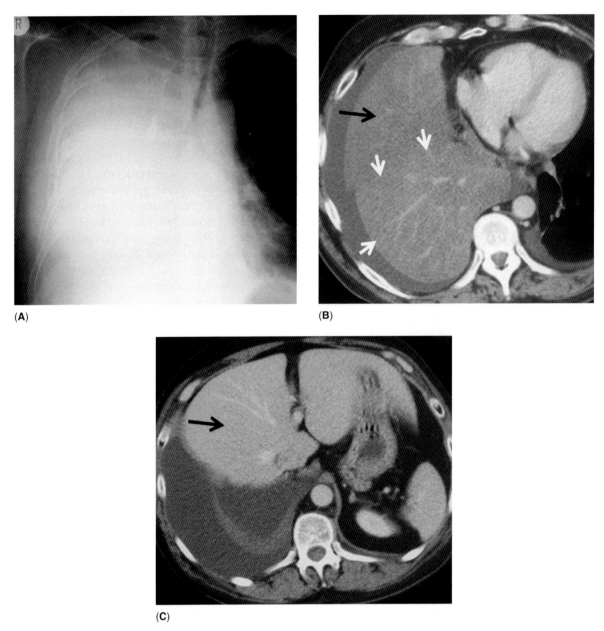

Figure 32.21 Large cell NET of the lung. (**A**) CXR demonstrates complete opacification of the right hemithorax. (**B**) CT at 25 minutes post-intravenous contrast medium administration demonstrates a very large tumor mass in the right lower thorax (white arrows). Multiple vessels are clearly seen running through the tumor, mimicking the configuration to the pulmonary vessels (the "pulmonary angiogram" sign). The liver is seen anteriorly on (**B**) arterial-phase and (**C**) portal-venous phase images (black arrow). There is an associated right pleural effusion.

such as GI and genitourinary tract adenocarcinoma, which are frequently described in association with carcinoid NETs (28,84).

Appearance of Primary Carcinoids

Foregut Carcinoids

Bronchial Carcinoid

Imaging features of the primary bronchial carcinoid are similar regardless of the grade of the tumor and the features depend on whether the tumor is located in the airways of the central/middle third of the lung (80% of cases) or the peripheral airways (Fig. 32.12) (39). The tumor may be detected with plain radiology with the appearance of a well-demarcated round or ovoid mass, often notched (85). Centrally located tumors may result in airways obstruction, with recurrent infection, lobar collapse, and a central mediastinal or hilar mass, which is usually smooth and lobulated, 2 to 5 cm in diameter (85). However, they are usually small and thus CT scanning is the most sensitive cross-sectional technique available. On CT, the mass may be visible within the bronchial lumen, usually with both an intra- and extraluminal component. A peripheral bronchial neuroendocrine lesion is seen in 20% of cases, with the appearance of a solitary pulmonary nodule (Fig. 32.12). The mass is typically round or ovoid with a smooth or lobulated border. Calcification is fairly common, either punctate or diffuse. Cavitation and hilar adenopathy are rare in typical carcinoids (85). Rarely, there may be two lesions, in which case it may be impossible to separate the appearance from pulmonary metastases (85). Aggressive lesions (large or small cell carcinomas) (Fig. 32.21) may demonstrate direct mediastinal invasion.

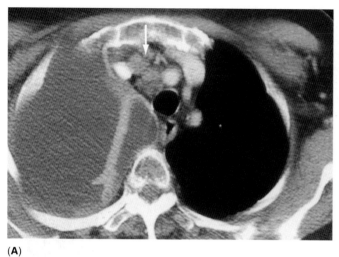

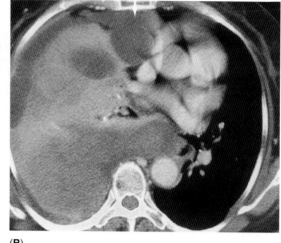

(A)   (B)

Figure 32.22 Foregut carcinoid. (A and B) CT of the thorax demonstrates a lobulated mass in the anterior mediastinum (arrow in B) that extends into the lower mediastinum and displaces the heart to the left. There is associated lymph node enlargement (arrow in A) and a large right pleural effusion.

Collapse or air trapping beyond the central lesion can be seen if there is a ball-valve obstruction of the bronchial lumen. Following IV contrast medium, there is usually intense homogeneous enhancement, although this is not seen in all cases. Marked enhancement can create diagnostic difficulty, as the appearance may mimic a pulmonary varix or pulmonary artery aneurysm, and a small vascular lesion may be overlooked or interpreted as a normal vessel (39). In patients with occult ectopic ACTH secretion, bronchial carcinoids are the most common source but can be elusive and difficult to identify (Fig. 32.12). When a pulmonary lesion is suspected but cannot be seen on CT, MR may play a role in localization. Bronchial carcinoids have high signal intensity on T2-weighted and short tau inversion recovery (STIR) images, allowing distinction between a small mass and the pulmonary vasculature of the central and middle third of the lung (86). In some cases, imaging with somatostatin receptor scintigraphy may help in the localization and characterization of a small peripheral lesion. Marked nodular adrenal hyperplasia may be incidentally noted, if the lesion secretes ACTH, causing Cushing's syndrome.

Key Points: Bronchial Carcinoids

- Eighty percent of bronchial carcinoids are located in the bronchi of the central or middle third of the lung
- Central lesions are small vascular masses, with intra- and extrabronchial components, which may cause signs of airways obstruction
- Thirty percent of these calcify
- MR imaging may help detect small, centrally located lesions in patients with an occult source of ectopic ACTH secretion
- Twenty percent are located peripherally and have the appearance of a solitary pulmonary nodule

Thymic Carcinoids

These tumors usually present as an anterior mediastinal mass (Fig. 32.13). The mass may be partly calcified and may cause SVC obstruction (43,87). There is usually evidence of invasive disease, with seven of eight patients in one series having extension into

the pleura, pericardium, great vessels, or regional lymph nodes (Fig. 32.22) (88). If the tumor is functioning and producing ACTH, then bilateral adrenal hyperplasia may also be seen (43). Bone metastases, which may be sclerotic, and lung and liver metastases may be present at the time of diagnosis (87–90).

Gastric Carcinoids (See Chap. 12)

Type I gastric carcinoids are small (<1 cm), multicentric, and predominantly found in the fundus and body of the stomach. The diagnosis is usually made endoscopically, not on imaging. The disease is almost always benign, with metastases present in only 2% of cases.

Type II gastric carcinoids, (Fig. 32.14) which are associated with the ZES and MEN-1, are multicentric. On CT, multiple masses are present within the gastric wall, which is diffusely thickened secondary to ZES. There is an increased tendency to metastasize to regional lymph nodes, although the prognosis is good (91).

Type III sporadic gastric carcinoids are usually solitary, large, and may ulcerate. Local invasion and metastases are common.

Midgut Carcinoids (Figs. 32.15–32.18)

The primary tumor may not be seen in midgut carcinoids as it is usually a small tumor that is not conspicuous against the small bowel or the ascending/transverse colon from which it arises. There may be multiple primary sites. The most frequent imaging findings are secondary features, which are described in detail later in the section on metastatic disease in NETs. Liver metastases are the most frequent finding, followed by tumor-associated desmoplastic fibrosis, which causes tethering and kinking of the small bowel mesentery and may also cause obstruction. Bone and lung metastases also occur. The incidence of metastases from midgut carcinoids is dependent on tumor size (25). In tumors <1 cm, 15% to 25% have metastases; in tumors between 1 and 2 cm, metastases are present in 58% to 80%; while in tumors >2 cm, over 70% have metastases.

CT

The primary bowel wall tumor is rarely demonstrated on CT and in one large series was only seen in one of 52 cases, where an ileal tumor was causing an intussusception into the cecum (92).

779

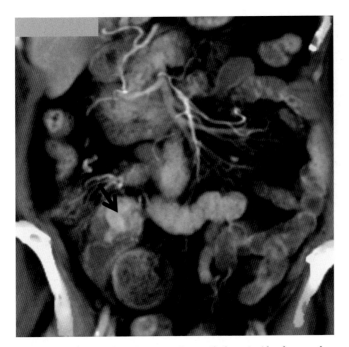

Figure 32.23 CT enteroclysis demonstrating an ileal carcinoid reformatted as a coronal MIP. The small bowel has been distended by an infusion through a naso-jejunal tube. An enhancing mass is seen in the region of the terminal ileum, which was confirmed to be a carcinoid neuroendocrine tumor at histology (arrow). *Source:* Courtesy of Dr. Martin Gore.

Detecting small primary tumors in the small bowel remains one of the most difficult challenges yet to be overcome on imaging (92,93).

Enteroclysis (Fig. 32.23)
There are a few reports of CT enteroclysis in the detection of small bowel carcinoid (94,95). On MDCT enteroclysis both transverse and multiplanar reformats were used to evaluate the small bowel: focal bowel wall thickening, small bowel masses, or stenosis, mesenteric stranding, lymph nodes or visceral metastases were recorded. In this series of 55 patients, carcinoid tumor was confirmed histologically in 19. Carcinoid tumors were seen as focal nodular lesions in the small bowel wall, demonstrating marked enhancement following IV contrast medium. In this series, there was an overall false-positive rate of 2.3% and false-negative rate of 4.1%, and there was an overall diagnostic accuracy of 84.7% (94).

MR
MR has been shown to demonstrate the primary tumor in 8 of 12 patients with a GI carcinoid (96). The best sequence for demonstrating the primary tumor was the post-gadolinium T1-weighted fat-suppressed image. In four cases, the tumor was a nodular mass arising from the bowel wall; in four cases there was regional uniform bowel wall thickening. The primary tumor enhanced moderately/intensely following gadolinium administration (96).

Other Imaging Techniques
Angiography of the superior and inferior mesenteric artery has a reasonable sensitivity for the localization of the primary tumor, lymph node and liver metastases. Rarely, THPVS may be helpful in localization of tumors in the upper abdomen, but this is no longer in common use. Barium follow-through may be abnormal if there is a fibrotic or desmoplastic reaction within the mesentery, resulting in distortion of the small bowel loops (Fig. 32.15). However, the technique is not sensitive in demonstrating the primary lesion. Echocardiography should be performed in all patients with carcinoid syndrome to identify signs of carcinoid heart disease. There is recent evidence that the presence of structural heart disease secondary to carcinoid syndrome is an independent poor prognostic factor (97).

Capsule Endoscopy
This novel technique requires ingestion of a capsule that transmits images by video-telemetry whilst travelling through the bowel. It has been shown to demonstrate the site of the primary small bowel NET in 45% of cases in one series of patients with metastatic small bowel NET in whom CT and enteroclysis were negative (98). In this series, nuclear imaging had a similar diagnostic yield, but could not differentiate a small bowel tumor from mesenteric disease.

Key Points: Imaging Midgut Carcinoids

- These are the commonest primary malignancy of the small bowel
- The primary bowel wall tumor mass is usually occult radiologically
- Liver metastases are common
- Mesenteric masses are common and usually have radiating strands of soft tissue and are often calcified
- Retroperitoneal or mesenteric lymphadenopathy is seen in 20% to 30% of cases

Hindgut Carcinoids
These lesions are usually diagnosed at endoscopy, although barium studies may demonstrate an extrinsic filling defect. At endoscopy, they appear as solitary yellowish submucosal lesions and are typically between 1 and 2 cm in diameter (48,99). As these lesions are small and disease is often confined to the rectum, minimally invasive techniques to allow local resection is the treatment of choice (99,100). However, these techniques are only suitable in Stage T1 (tumor confined to the mucosa and submucosa) and T2 (invasion of muscularis propria) disease, with no evidence of extension to the serosa. Imaging may be used to identify cases suitable for local resection. Endoscopic US demonstrates the lesion as a homogeneously hypoechoic submucosal mass (101). Endoscopic US may demonstrate invasion of the full rectal wall (Stage T3) and invasion into adjacent structures (T4) (100). In these cases, extended resection is required. MR may have a role in local staging of the primary mass. Both CT and MR can be used to stage lymph node disease and distant metastatic disease as part of the preoperative planning. In one large series, 30% of patients had metastatic disease at presentation (49,50).

METASTASES FROM PANCREATIC AND CARCINOID NETs

Metastases are a common finding in NETs. In a large autopsy series, 29% of patients with a carcinoid NET were found to have metastatic disease, the majority (61%) arising from small bowel carcinoids (27). In this series, 90% of metastases were in the lymph

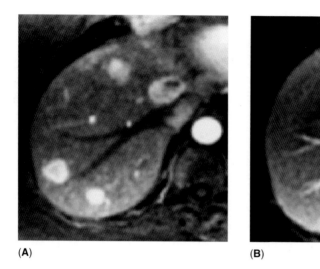

(A) **(B)**

Figure 32.24 Hypervascular liver metastases from a carcinoid tumor: importance of timing. (**A**) Arterial-phase T1-weighted MRI with fat saturation, acquired in the arterial phase following IV administration of gadolinium. Multiple brightly enhancing metastases are seen. (**B**) At the portal-venous phase several of the lesions are no longer visible and those that can be seen are isointense to the liver and are no longer conspicuous.

nodes, 44% in the liver, 14% in the lungs, 14% in the peritoneum, and 7% in the pancreas. The imaging appearances of metastatic disease from both pancreatic and carcinoid NETs are similar and will be considered together.

Liver Metastases

Liver metastases are seen in 40% to 80% of patients with a midgut carcinoid at presentation, depending on the site of the primary tumor. Liver metastases are present at the time of initial diagnosis in 40% of ileal lesions and up to 80% of caecal lesions (28). Liver metastases are the most common imaging finding (92). The extent of liver metastases is an important prognostic factor in pancreatic NETs (18). In patients with a malignant gastrinoma, the presence of liver metastases alone moderately decreases survival. However, the development of Cushing's syndrome or bone metastases in combination with liver metastases results in a markedly decreased survival rate (18). In patients with a metastatic carcinoid, the five-year survival rate of patients with no liver metastases is not significantly different to patients with a few liver metastases (fewer than five) (73% vs. 79%). However, there is a significant decrease in the five-year survival rate to 47% in patients with extensive liver metastases (more than five) (102).

Ultrasound

On transabdominal US, liver metastases tend to be hyperechoic, particularly in cases of metastatic gastrinoma, and are detected with a sensitivity of approximately 60%, although lesion conspicuity is reduced in patients with a fatty, hyperechoic liver (21,52). EUS is not reliable in detecting liver metastases, due to its limited depth of penetration. Intraoperative ultrasound can be helpful in the assessment of liver metastases, allowing accurate depiction of the relationship between a lesion and hepatic vessels, which may help in determining resectability (103).

CT

Neuroendocrine hepatic metastases may be difficult to identify and delineate on CT as they may be isointense to the liver on PVP imaging. A combination of precontrast, hepatic arterial-dominant phase (HAP), and PVP imaging will improve the sensitivity of detection, as in some cases a lesion may only be seen on one of the three phases (104). Evidence indicates that the HAP is particularly helpful in the detection of liver metastases (Fig. 32.19).

Liver metastases are most frequently of low attenuation in relation to the surrounding parenchyma on precontrast images and enhance strongly postcontrast, mimicking a hemangioma. Like the primary tumor, large lesions may become necrotic and may calcify. If the peak enhancement is missed due to the timing of the scan, the lesion may become isodense to the liver and thus lesion detection may be challenging.

In one study, CT was compared with selective angiography; the latter technique detected 20% more liver metastases than CT, with a very high rate of detection (74).

MR

On MR, 75% of neuroendocrine liver metastases appear as having low-signal intensity on T1- (Fig. 32.25) and high-signal intensity on T2-weighted images, with 94% of metastases being hypervascular on HAP post-gadolinium images (Fig. 32.24): 15% of hepatic metastases were only seen on the immediate post-gadolinium images in one series (96).

The use of mangofadopir-DPDP may increase the detection of small liver metastases and has been shown to be highly reproducible (Fig. 32.25) (80). In our institution, this technique is used prior to planning resection of liver metastases in order to ensure detection of all lesions.

Mesenteric Masses and Peritoneal Disease

Secondary mesenteric masses >1.5 cm are seen in approximately 50% to 75% of cases of midgut carcinoid, with a median size of 3 cm (92,96). Masses are of soft tissue density and commonly have a "spoke-wheel" appearance, with radiating strands of soft tissue (64–100%) (Fig. 32.16). The degree of radiating strands increases as the degree of fibrosis increases, as seen on histology, and is caused by hormonally active substances, particularly

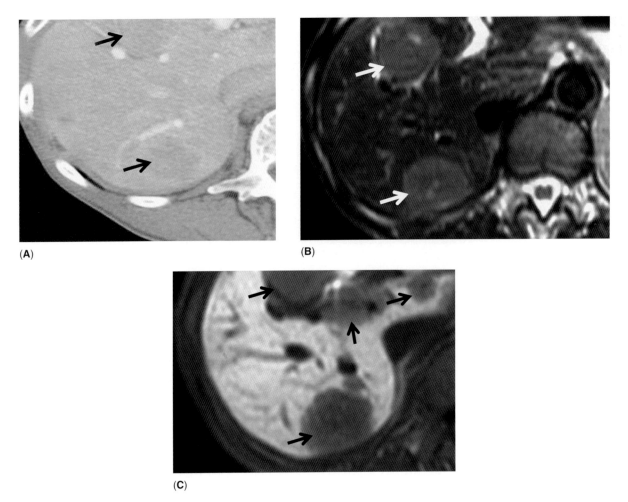

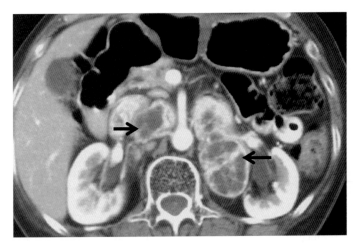

Figure 32.25 Liver metastases: use of liver-specific contrast medium. (A) Portal-venous phase CT demonstrates several poorly defined low attenuation liver metastases (arrows). (B) On T2-weighted MRI the metastases have a higher signal intensity than the surrounding liver. (C) T1-weighted image following administration of MnDPDP demonstrates enhancement of the liver parenchyma, increasing the liver-to-lesion signal intensity ratio. The liver metastases are highly conspicuous (arrows). Additional lesions could also be identified in this case.

Figure 32.26 Retroperitoneal nodes in a patient with metastatic carcinoid. There are bilateral para-aortic (arrows) and retro-caval nodes which demonstrate marked peripheral enhancement but have undergone central necrosis.

serotonin. Calcification is commonly seen within mesenteric masses (40–70%), and may be small stippled calcifications or bulky and conglomerate (32,92). On histology, calcification is localized within areas of mature fibrous scarring within the mass (32). Masses usually arise within the fat or nodal tissue of the small bowel mesentery, although the exact nidus of metastatic tumor growth in the mesentery is not certain (32).

Diffuse mesenteric/peritoneal disease, with peritoneal studding or ascites, is seen in 20% to 30% of patients with a GI carcinoid and may be associated with obstruction (Fig. 32.16C) (92,105). Peritoneal disease is less common in pancreatic NETs; it was seen in 11% of non-gastrinoma pancreatic NETs but did not occur in association with a gastrinoma in one series (Figs. 32.7 and 32.8) (105)

Lymph Node Metastases

Regional lymph node metastases are the most frequent metastatic site at autopsy (27). Retroperitoneal or mesenteric lymph node enlargement is seen in approximately 20% to 30% of patients with a midgut carcinoid (Figs. 32.16C and 32.26) (92). Retroperitoneal fibrosis may be seen in cases with retroperitoneal lymph node metastases and may cause ureteric obstruction. In thymic NETs, mediastinal lymph node metastases are present in 60% at the time of resection (Figs. 32.22 and 32.27) (106).

Lung Metastases

Lung metastases, which arise from a variety of NETs, may be hormone-secreting although in most patients they are

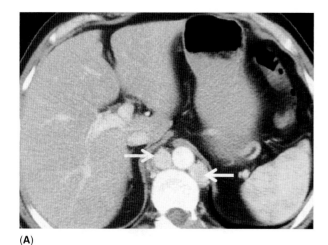

(A)

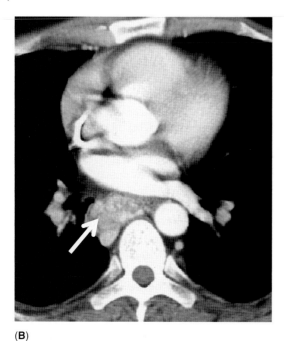

(B)

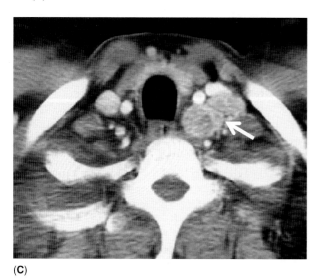

(C)

Figure 32.27 Nodal disease in a patient with a metastatic carcinoid of unknown primary site. Nodal metastases (arrows) are demonstrated (**A**) in the retrocrural nodes; (**B**) in the posterior mediastinum; and (**C**) in the left supraclavicular nodes.

asymptomatic. Diagnosis is accurately made on CT. Local metasta-sectomy, where clinically appropriate, has been shown to improve outcomes when compared with medical management (107).

Bone Metastases

Bone metastases are more commonly associated with foregut and hindgut carcinoids than midgut carcinoid tumors. The metastases are frequently sclerotic and may have the appearance of multiple small punctate sclerotic deposits (43). Bone metas-tases have been reported in up to 30% of patients with malignant gastrinoma and are indicative of a poor prognosis, particularly when associated with liver metastases (18). Whole-body MR and somatostatin receptor scintigraphy (SRS) have been used to detect bone metastases in patients with well-differentiated gas-tro-entero-pancreatic endocrine cancer and have been found to be equally sensitive (86% vs. 81%, p = 0.56) (108). The authors concluded that bone staging should be undertaken using SRS and spine MR in bronchial-thymic or unknown primary cases. In patients with a duodenal-pancreatic or ileal primary, bone staging may be restricted to those with liver metastases (108).

Key Points: Metastases from Pancreatic and Carcinoid NETs

- Liver metastases occur in 40% to 80% of midgut carcinoid tumors at presentation and are the most common imaging finding
- Liver metastases tend to be hypervascular on contrast-enhanced CT and MR, and are imaged optimally on the hepatic arterial phase following contrast medium injection
- Secondary mesenteric masses are common, usually of soft tissue density, often with a spoke-wheel appearance, and often with flecks of calcium
- Lymph node metastases are the most frequent metastatic site at autopsy

---

MOLECULAR IMAGING IN NETs

NETs often express high levels of peptide receptors, which can be targeted by radiolabeled receptor ligands. Successful approaches include the use of somatostatin (SST), vasoactive intestinal pep-tide (VIP), bombesin, and cholecystokinin-B/gastrin analogues. Both gamma camera imaging and positron emission tomography (PET) can be applied using appropriate radiolabeled receptor ligands. Gamma camera imaging generally includes planar scin-tigraphy often with additional Single Photon Emission Com-puted Tomography (SPECT). SPECT is being replaced by SPECT/CT, which provides co-registered functional and anatomical information. The most common radionuclides for gamma cam-era imaging are [111]Indium, [99m]Technetium and iodine radioiso-topes ([131]iodine and [123]iodine). PET radiopharmaceuticals include [18]fluorine-labelled fluorodeoxyglucose (FDG) and [68]gallium-la-belled peptides. Gamma camera imaging and PET provide an *in vivo* characterization of tissue and are often more sensitive and specific than conventional anatomical imaging modalities.

Regulatory peptides bind and act through transmembrane G protein coupled receptors. Peptides, in contrast to larger molecules such as antibodies and proteins, have the advantage of easily pen-

etrating into all tissues except the brain as they are hydrophilic (109). In order to fulfill their purpose for imaging, rapid degradation by peptidases, and thus fast inactivation, is very important. However, their short biological half-lives limit their use as radiopharmaceuticals. Hence a major focus of peptide research is the development of metabolically stable peptides for therapy and imaging.

Radiopeptide Scintigraphy

Although many regulatory peptide receptors are expressed on various tumors, to date somatostatin receptor analogues have gained the widest clinical application. Somatostatin receptors are present on many tumor types including carcinoma of the lung, breast, some sarcomas, and lymphoma. Five different subtypes of the human somatostatin receptor (SSTR1-5) are currently recognized, bound to varying degrees by the analogues ^{111}In-octreotide (also called pentetreotide), ^{111}In-lanreotide, and P829 (Neospect, Depreotide), a technetium-99m (^{99m}Tc) analogue (110).

[111]In-octreotide is the most widely available somatostatin analogue for imaging. The biologically active ring of octreotide is intact and a DTPA bridge is coupled to the phenylalanine group for labelling with [111]Indium. It has moderate affinity to SSTR2 and SSTR5 with virtually none to SSTR1, 3, and 4. ^{111}In-octreotide has an accepted role for tumor localization and staging, particularly in gastro-entero-pancreatic NETs. The role of ^{111}In-octreotide in NETs has been extensively reviewed (111–113) and shown to be of particular value in the localization of small lesions, in determining the local extent of disease, identification of metastases and detecting relapsed disease. Furthermore, it can be used to monitor results of surgery, radiotherapy, and chemotherapy. Occasionally it is shown to be of value in the detection of paragangliomas and pheochromocytomas if these tumors express somatostatin receptors (114–117).

Octreotide receptor imaging in NETs may therefore be used for:

- The detection of small primary or recurrent tumors, in the knowledge that a negative result is not exclusive, for example, gastrinoma, medullary thyroid carcinoma, insulinoma, and a proportion of other NETs (Fig. 32.9)
- The prediction of the success of therapeutic doses of unlabeled octreotide where the level of uptake of radiolabeled peptide ligands suggests therapy will be beneficial
- Guiding radiopeptide therapy with octreotide or lanreotide derivatives labeled with [90]Yttrium

The main limitation of radiolabeled octreotide as a diagnostic agent is its wide spectrum of activity with insufficient sensitivity for all tumors of a particular class, since some tumors will be receptor negative (Table 32.4).

Table 32.4 Percentage Frequency of Positive Imaging in NETs (85–88)

Type	^{123}I-MIBG (%)	^{111}In-octreotide (%)
Carcinoid tumors	50–75	67–96
Pancreatic neuroendocrine tumors	9–25	80–95
Medullary carcinoma of thyroid	35–50	71–100
Paraganglioma, pheochromocytoma	90–100	70–95
Neuroblastoma	88–95	80–90

Technique

Somatostatin receptor scintigraphy with ^{111}In-octreotide is generally performed as whole body planar scintigraphy approximately 24 hours after radiotracer injection. The addition of SPECT helps to localize potential abnormalities. The sensitivity can be further enhanced by fusion of SPECT imaging with CT. Since a new generation of combined SPECT/CT is now available, providing spatially co-registered SPECT and CT images, the addition of SPECT/CT is often very useful to differentiate normal from abnormal ^{111}In-octreotide uptake and to exactly localize disease.

PET Imaging

Recently, radiolabeled somatostatin receptor ligands for PET imaging have been developed of which ^{68}Ga-DOTATOC is the most commonly used (Fig. 32.28). Whole-body PET images are usually acquired 45–90 minutes following IV injection of ^{68}Ga-DOTATOC. Preliminary evidence indicates that ^{68}Ga-DOTATOC is more sensitive than ^{111}In-octreotide (118). For example, in a study of eight patients with metastatic carcinoids, a total of 207 lesions were located using ^{68}Ga-DOTATOC compared with only 124 detected by using ^{111}In-octreotide (119). The spatial resolution of ^{111}In-octreotide gamma camera imaging is limited, even with SPECT (approximately 1.5cm). In addition, PET offers a significantly higher sensitivity (counts per Bq) compared to gamma camera imaging. The latest PET and PET/CT scanner generation provides a spatial resolution of less than 0.5 cm.

Comparisons have been made between ^{111}In-octreotide and FDG-PET (120–123). In poorly differentiated tumors, when ^{111}In-octreotide imaging is negative, FDG-PET may localize disease. Well differentiated NETs, however, are often negative on FDG-PET. This is primarily due to the high differentiation grade and low anerobic glycolysis of these tumors (124). Nevertheless, FDG-PET appears to be the preferred functional imaging modality for staging and treatment monitoring of SDHB-related metastatic paraganglioma (see chap. 16).

Other PET somatostatin analogues such as ^{64}Cu-TETA-octreotide and [86]Y-DOTATOC have been found to be inferior to ^{68}Ga-DOTA-TOC (125–128). For these reasons, and the fact that several studies have already shown the benefit of this tracer, (118,119,129,130) ^{68}Ga-DOTATOC is currently the most attractive option for improving diagnosis and staging in patients with NETs.

Key Points: PET

- PET provides superior sensitivity and spatial resolution compared to conventional gamma camera imaging for detection of somatostatin receptor-positive tissue
- ^{68}Ga-DOTATOC is the preferred radiopharmaceutical for PET imaging of NETs
- Other PET somastostatin analogues have been found to be inferior to [68]GaDOTATOC

Other Radiolabeled Peptides

Cholecystokinin (CCK) and gastrin are gut-brain peptides with multiple functions in the gastrointestinal tract and in the brain. CCK2/Gastrin receptor expression has been demonstrated *in vitro* in medullary thyroid cancer, small cell lung cancer, astrocytomas, stromal ovarian carcinomas, NETs, and in very high densities in

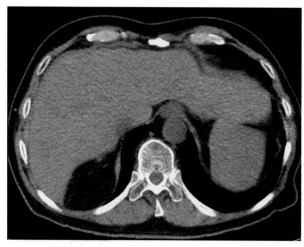

(A)

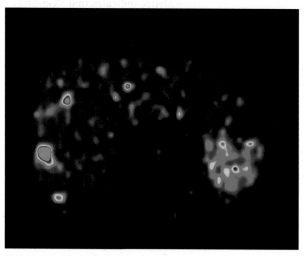

(B)

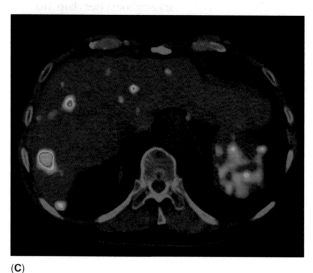

(C)

Figure 32.28 Patient with a midgut carcinoid. (A) The CT was difficult to interpret regarding the extent of liver metastases. (B) Unfused image and (C) fused image ^{68}Ga-DOTA-TOC PET/CT was performed. In these transaxial images at least four liver metastases are clearly depicted. *Source*: Courtesy of Dr. Anders Sundin.

gastrointestinal stromal tumors (131–133). Gastrin-releasing peptide (GRP) receptor is highly expressed in lung, breast, prostate, and pancreatic cancers. The neuropeptide bombesin has high affinity for GRP receptors and bombesin analogues are being developed for imaging labeled with Tc-99m, In-111, Ga-68, and F-18 (134,135). Many of the analogues have high hepatobiliary clearance limiting abdominal scintigraphy. VIP receptor expression is more widespread than somatostatin receptor expression particularly in common cancers such as breast and prostate (136). *In vivo* data with radio-iodinated VIP is encouraging with localization of most VIP expressing colorectal and pancreatic adenocarcinomas (137).

IMAGING WITH ^{123}I-MIBG

The first compounds which were evaluated for imaging the adrenal medulla were analogues of radiolabeled catecholamines. In 1980, Wieland and his colleagues found avid concentration of radioiodinated iodobenzylguanidines in the adrenal medulla with the metaisomer metaiodobenzylguanidine (MIBG) demonstrating faster uptake and less background activity *in vivo* (138). Radiolabeled MIBG is useful for imaging adrenal medullary tumors and shows increased uptake in medullary hyperplasia but far less uptake in the normal adrenal medulla. The uptake of radiolabeled MIBG is via the norepinephrine re-uptake mechanism with entry of MIBG into catecholamine storage vesicles. Therefore, drugs which interfere with norepinephrine re-uptake such as reserpine and tricyclic antidepressants, may cause false-negative results and need to be discontinued prior to imaging. In the past, ^{131}iodine was predominately used for labeling of MIBG, whereas ^{123}I-MIBG is now becoming more widely available. ^{123}I has several advantages over ^{131}I; ^{123}I is a pure gamma emitter and can therefore be administered in higher activities resulting in improved image quality. In addition, the photon energy of 159 keV is much better suited for gamma camera imaging.

There are two main indications for the use of ^{123}MIBG:

- Detection of amine-secreting NETs, for example, pheochromocytomas (Fig. 32.29) (see chap. 16)
- To test whether therapy with ^{131}I-MIBG would be appropriate in conditions where radiolabeled MIBG uptake is usual, as in malignant paragangliomas or, relatively less frequently, such tumors as carcinoids, medullary carcinomas of the thyroid or malignant pancreatic NETs

^{123}I-MIBG gamma camera imaging is generally performed as whole-body planar scintigraphy approximately 24 hours after radiotracer injection. The addition of SPECT/CT enhances the sensitivity and specificity, and has largely replaced more complex early and delayed gamma camera imaging to identify the position of the kidneys, renal pelvis, and other areas of normal radiolabeled MIBG uptake. Only tumors that show radiolabeled MIBG uptake at 24 hours are likely to benefit from ^{131}I-MIBG therapy.

MIBG Compared with Radiopeptide Scintigraphy

Many comparisons of ^{123}I-MIBG and ^{111}In-octreotide imaging in pancreatic and carcinoid NETs have been reported (114–117). A comparison of ^{99m}Tc-P829, Neospect, and ^{111}In-octreotide was made by Lebtahi et al. (139). ^{123}I-MIBG scintigraphy appeared to be more sensitive for sympatho-adrenomedullary tumors, but

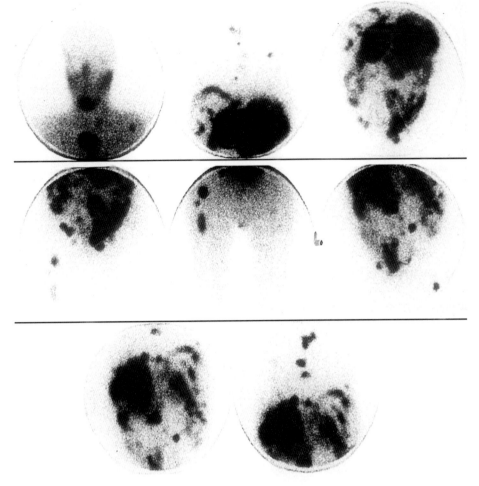

Figure 32.29 ^{123}I-MIBG scan. Extensive multiple metastases are demonstrated from an MIBG-avid neuroendocrine tumor.

[111]In-octreotide detects more tumors in all other neuroendocrine conditions (Table 32.4). The reason for imaging with ^{123}I-MIBG continues to be the availability of ^{131}I-MIBG therapy. This may change when ^{90}Y-octreotide therapy (or a related analog) becomes available on a regular basis. Potential future MIBG substitutes include ^{11}C-hydroxyephedrine (140), ^{11}C-DOPA (141), and ^{18}F-iodobenzylguanidine (142).

Key Points: Molecular Imaging in Neuroendocrine Tumors

- Radiolabeled somatostatin analogues for gamma camera imaging and PET bind to somatostatin receptors which are present in 80% to 90% of pancreatic NETs and 67% to 96% of carcinoids
- Imaging the level of uptake of radiolabeled somatostatin ligands is important as a guide to therapy with octreotide derivatives with pharmacologic agents or with therapeutic radiopharmaceuticals
- ^{123}I-MIBG is used in NETs as a guide to whether therapy with ^{131}I-MIBG is appropriate, even though it is substantially less sensitive than ^{111}In-octreotide in the detection of pancreatic and GI NETs
- FDG-PET is potentially useful in aggressive NETs

NET RADIONUCLIDE THERAPY (TABLE 32.5)

Molecular imaging identifies, by imaging with an appropriate radiopharmaceutical, whether NETs have particular antigens or receptors. The radionuclide used for imaging, which is either gamma- or positron-emitting, is then substituted with a therapy radionuclide. Generally, therapy radionuclides are beta-emitting, attached to the same molecular probe, so that only those patients who have been demonstrated by imaging to have tumors which show significant and specific uptake of the radiopharmaceutical are exposed to radionuclide therapy. Those with poor radiotracer uptake are considered unlikely to benefit and are saved from having unnecessary radiation. Beta-emitting radionuclides include [90]Ytrium (^{90}Y) and [177]Lutetium (^{177}Lu) which differ in their physical properties. The higher energy of [90]Ytrium results in longer ranges in tissue and may be preferable for treating larger tumors and tumors with heterogeneous receptor distribution (143). [90]Ytrium and [177]Lutetium form stable metal complexes with the chelator DOTA. DOTA coupled therapeutic radiopeptides include ^{90}Y-DOTA-octreotide ^{90}Y-DOTA-lantreotide and ^{177}Lu-DOTA-octreotate. These have different SSTR affinity profiles with the DOTATATE derivatives having highest affinity to SSTR 2 and the DOTA-lantreotide having considerable SSTR 5 affinity (136,144). In some series, 10% to 30% of patients achieved complete or

Table 32.5 Strategy for the Radionuclide Therapy
of Neuroendocrine Tumors

^{123}I-MIBG imaging	Avid	Æ	I-131 MIBG therapy
	Non-avid	Æ	^{111}In-octreotide Imaging
[111]In-octreotide	Avid	Æ	^{90}Y-octreother therapy
[99m]Tc-octreotide	Avid	Æ	^{90}Y-octreother therapy
	Non-avid	Æ	^{111}In-lanreotide imaging
[111]In-lanreotide	Avid	Æ	^{90}Y-lanreotide therapy
	Non-avid	Æ	Chemotherapy

partial responses following radiopeptide therapy (145–147). Gastro-ntero-pancreatic NETs seem to show better response rates, which are in the range of 36% to 38% (146,148,149).

FOLLOW-UP OF NEUROENDOCRINE TUMORS

Surgical resection is the only curative technique in pancreatic and carcinoid NETs. However, in non-resectable tumors, imaging may play a role in treatment planning. Palliation of symptoms may be achieved by embolization or chemo-embolization of hepatic metastases if the portal vein is patent (150).

Response to treatment of liver metastases following transcatheter arterial embolisation can be assessed on MR both following contrast enhancement MR and on diffusion-weighted imaging (151). In this study, 66 targeted neuroendocrine liver metastases were evaluated. The percentage enhancement in the arterial and portal-venous phase decreased significantly following treatment, as did the apparent diffusion coefficients. This finding was of particular importance as the use of RECIST criteria demonstrated partial response in only 23% of patients.

CT or MR is used to assess the response to therapy both in primary and metastatic disease. MR imaging is the preferred modality for following up patients with disorders such as MEN 1, where repeated imaging may be required for prolonged surveillance due to the often indolent nature of the disease.

Summary

- The majority of pancreatic NETs are functioning (only 15–30% are non-functioning) and the purpose of imaging is preoperative localization and staging.
- Insulinomas are the most common pancreatic NETs, usually small, solitary intrapancreatic and malignant in only 10% of cases; gastrinomas are often extrapancreatic and malignant in 60%.
- CT is the most widely used technique for detection of pancreatic NETs, and the majority are small and hypervascular. On MR a fat-suppressed T1-weighted sequence is the best for their detection.
- Carcinoid tumors arise from the diffuse neuroendocrine system, secrete a variety of amines and peptides, and most commonly arise from the bronchus (32.5%), jejuno-ileum (20%), appendix (8%), and rectum (10%).

- Metastases from NETs involve lymph nodes most frequently (90%) and liver (44%). Mesenteric masses > 1.5 cm are commonly seen in midgut carcinoids.
- Scintigraphy using radiolabeled somatostatin analogues and radio-iodinated met-iodobenzylguanidine are employed to localize functioning pathology, to detect metastases, and to predict suitability for octreotide or ^{131}I-MIBG therapy.

REFERENCES

1. Metz DC. Diagnosis and treatment of pancreatic neuroendocrine tumors. Semin Gastrointest Dis 1995; 6: 67–78.
2. Yao JC, Eisner MP, Leary C, et al. Population-based study of islet cell carcinoma. Ann Surg Oncol 2007; 14: 3492–500.
3. Kent RB, III, van Heerden JA, Weiland LH. Nonfunctioning islet cell tumors. Ann Surg 1981; 193: 185–90.
4. Stark DD, Moss AA, Goldberg HI, Deveney CW. CT of pancreatic islet cell tumors. Radiology 1984; 150: 491–4.
5. Halfdanarson TR, Rabe KG, Rubin J, Petersen GM. Pancreatic neuroendocrine tumors (PNETs): incidence, prognosis and recent trend toward improved survival. Ann Oncol 2008; 19: 1727–33.
6. Aldridge MC, Williamson RC. Surgery of endocrine tumours of the pancreas. In: Lynn J, Bloom SR, eds. Surgical Endocrinology. Oxford: Butterworth-Heinemann, 1996: 503–18.
7. Alexander HR, Jensen RT. Pancreatic endocrine tumors. In: Devita VT, Hellman S, Rosenberg SA, eds. Principles and Practice of Oncology. Philadelphia: Lippincott-Raven, 2001: 1788–813.
8. Chandrasekharappa SC, Guru SC, Manickam P, et al. Positional cloning of the gene for multiple endocrine neoplasia-type 1. Science 1997; 276: 404–7.
9. Zhuang Z, Vortmeyer AO, Pack S, et al. Somatic mutations of the MEN1 tumor suppressor gene in sporadic gastrinomas and insulinomas. Cancer Res 1997; 57: 4682–6.
10. Solcia E, Kloppel G, Sobin LH. Histological typing of endocrine tumours. World Health Organization. International Histological Classification of Tumours, 2nd edn. Berlin: Springer, 2000.
11. Rindi G, Capella C, Solcia E. Introduction to a revised clinicopathological classification of neuroendocrine tumors of the gastroenteropancreatic tract. Q J Nucl Med 2000; 44: 13–21.
12. La Rosa S, Klersy C, Uccella S, et al. Improved histologic and clinicopathologic criteria for prognostic evaluation of pancreatic endocrine tumors. Hum Pathol 2009; 40: 30–40.
13. van Heerden JA, Grant CS, Czako PF. Occult functioning insulinomas: which localizing studies are indicated? Surgery 1992; 112: 1010–15.
14. Service FJ, Dale AJ, Elveback LR, Jiang NS. Insulinoma: clinical and diagnostic features of 60 consecutive cases. Mayo Clin Proc 1976; 51: 417–29.
15. Berends FJ, Cuesta MA, Kazemier G, et al. Laparoscopic detection and resection of insulinomas. Surgery 2000; 128: 386–91.
16. Marks V. Insulinoma. In: Grossman AB, ed. Clinical Endocrinology. Oxford: Blackwell Science, 1998: 531–9.

17. Grant CS. Surgical aspects of hyperinsulinemic hypoglycemia. Endocrinol Metab Clin North Am 1999; 28: 533–54.

18. Yu F, Venzon DJ, Serrano J, et al. Prospective study of the clinical course, prognostic factors, causes of death, and survival in patients with long-standing Zollinger-Ellison syndrome. J Clin Oncol 1999; 17: 615–30.

19. Doppman JL, Shawker TH, Miller DL. Localization of islet cell tumors. Gastroenterol Clin North Am 1989; 18: 793–804.

20. O'Shea D, Wynick D, Bloom SR. Islet cell tumours (excluding insulinomas and carcinoids). In: Grossman AB, ed. Clinical Endocrinology. Oxford: Blackwell Science, 1998: 540–8.

21. King CM, Reznek RH, Dacie JE, Wass JA. Imaging islet cell tumours. Clin Radiol 1994; 49: 295–303.

22. Hammond PJ, Jackson JA, Bloom SR. Localization of pancreatic endocrine tumours. Clin Endocrinol (Oxf) 1994; 40: 3–14.

23. Vinik AI, Strodel WE, Eckhauser FE, Moattari AR, Lloyd R. Somatostatinomas, PPomas, neurotensinomas. Semin Oncol 1987; 14: 263–81.

24. Oberg K. Carcinoid syndrome. In: Grossman AB, ed. Clinical Endocrinology. Oxford: Blackwell Science, 1998: 607–20.

25. Jensen RT, Doherty GM. Carcinoid tumors and the carcinoid syndrome. In: Devita VT, Hellman S, Rosenberg SA, eds. Cancer: Principles and Practice of Oncology. Philadelphia: Lippincott-Raven, 2001: 1813–33.

26. Newton JN, Swerdlow AJ, dos SS, et al. The epidemiology of carcinoid tumours in England and Scotland. Br J Cancer 1994; 70: 939–42.

27. Berge T, Linell F. Carcinoid tumours. Frequency in a defined population during a 12-year period. Acta Pathol Microbiol Scand [A] 1976; 84: 322–30.

28. Modlin IM, Lye KD, Kidd M. A 5-decade analysis of 13,715 carcinoid tumors. Cancer 2003; 97: 934–59.

29. Norheim I, Oberg K, Theodorsson-Norheim E, et al. Malignant carcinoid tumors. An analysis of 103 patients with regard to tumor localization, hormone production, and survival. Ann Surg 1987; 206: 115–25.

30. Zikusoka MN, Kidd M, Eick G, Latich I, Modlin IM. The molecular genetics of gastroenteropancreatic neuroendocrine tumors. Cancer 2005; 104: 2292–309.

31. Capella C, Heitz PU, Hofler H, Solcia E, Kloppel G. Revised classification of neuroendocrine tumors of the lung, pancreas and gut. Virchows Arch 1995; 425: 547–60.

32. Pantongrag-Brown L, Buetow PC, Carr NJ, Lichtenstein JE, Buck JL. Calcification and fibrosis in mesenteric carcinoid tumor: CT findings and pathologic correlation. Am J Roentgenol 1995; 164: 387–91.

33. Williams ED, Sandler M. The classification of carcinoid tumours. Lancet 1963; 1: 238–9.

34. Paladugu RR, Benfield JR, Pak HY, Ross RK, Teplitz RL. Bronchopulmonary Kulchitzky cell carcinomas. A new classification scheme for typical and atypical carcinoids. Cancer 1985; 55: 1303–11.

35. Colby TV, Koss MN, Travis WD. Carcinoid and other neuroendocrine tumors. In: Colby TV, Koss MN, Travis WD, eds. Atlas to Tumor Pathology: Tumors of the Lower Respiratory Tract. Washington, DC: Armed Forces Institute of Pathology, 1995: 287–317.

36. Beasley MB, Brambilla E, Travis WD. The 2004 World Health Organization classification of lung tumors. Semin Roentgenol 2005; 40: 90–7.

37. Gustafsson BI, Kidd M, Modlin IM. Neuroendocrine tumors of the diffuse neuroendocrine system. Curr Opin Oncol 2008; 20: 1–12.

38. Gustafsson BI, Kidd M, Chan A, Malfertheiner MV, Modlin IM. Bronchopulmonary neuroendocrine tumors. Cancer 2008; 113: 5–21.

39. Jeung MY, Gasser B, Gangi A, et al. Bronchial carcinoid tumors of the thorax: spectrum of radiologic findings. Radiographics 2002; 22: 351–65.

40. Takei H, Asamura H, Maeshima A, et al. Large cell neuroendocrine carcinoma of the lung: a clinicopathologic study of eighty-seven cases. J Thorac Cardiovasc Surg 2002; 124: 285–92.

41. Govindan R, Page N, Morgensztern D, et al. Changing epidemiology of small-cell lung cancer in the United States over the last 30 years: analysis of the surveillance, epidemiologic, and end results database. J Clin Oncol 2006; 24: 4539–44.

42. Dusmet ME, McNeally MF. Pulmonary and thymic carcinoid tumors. World J Surg 1996; 20: 189–95.

43. Wollensak G, Herbst EW, Beck A, Schaefer HE. Primary thymic carcinoid with Cushing's syndrome. Virchows Arch A Pathol Anat Histopathol 1992; 420: 191–5.

44. Wilander E, Lundqvist M, Oberg K. Gastrointestinal carcinoid tumours. Histogenetic, histochemical, immunohistochemical, clinical, and therapeutic aspects. Prog Histochem Cytochem 1989; 19: 1–88.

45. Rindi G, Bordi C, Rappel S, et al. Gastric carcinoids and neuroendocrine carcinomas: pathogenesis, pathology, and behavior. World J Surg 1996; 20: 168–72.

46. Burke AP, Thomas RM, Elsayed AM, Sobin LH. Carcinoids of the jejunum and ileum: an immunohistochemical and clinicopathologic study of 167 cases. Cancer 1997; 79: 1086–93.

47. Modlin IM, Sandor A. An analysis of 8305 cases of carcinoid tumors. Cancer 1997; 79: 813–29.

48. Winburn GB. Multiple rectal carcinoids: a case report. Am Surg 1998; 64: 1200–3.

49. Koura AN, Giacco GG, Curley SA, et al. Carcinoid tumors of the rectum: effect of size, histopathology, and surgical treatment on metastasis free survival. Cancer 1997; 79: 1294–8.

50. Danikas D, Theodorou SJ, Matthews WE, Rienzo AA. Unusually aggressive rectal carcinoid metastasizing to larynx, pancreas, adrenal glands, and brain. Am Surg 2000; 66: 1179–80.

51. Bottger TC, Weber W, Beyer J, Junginger T. Value of tumor localization in patients with insulinoma. World J Surg 1990; 14: 107–12.

52. London JF, Shawker TH, Doppman JL, et al. Zollinger-Ellison syndrome: prospective assessment of abdominal US in the localization of gastrinomas. Radiology 1991; 178: 763–7.

53. Dietrich CF, Ignee A, Braden B, et al. Improved differentiation of pancreatic tumors using contrast-enhanced endoscopic ultrasound. Clin Gastroenterol Hepatol 2008; 6: 590–7.

54. Oshikawa O, Tanaka S, Ioka T, et al. Dynamic sonography of pancreatic tumors: comparison with dynamic CT. Am J Roentgenol 2002; 178: 1133–7.

55. Ueno N, Tomiyama T, Tano S, et al. Utility of endoscopic ultrasonography with color Doppler function for the diagnosis of islet cell tumor. Am J Gastroenterol 1996; 91: 772–6.

56. Rosch T, Lightdale CJ, Botet JF, et al. Localization of pancreatic endocrine tumors by endoscopic ultrasonography. N Engl J Med 1992; 326: 1721–6.

57. Fein J, Gerdes H. Localization of islet cell tumors by endoscopic ultrasonography. Gastroenterology 1992; 103: 711–12.

58. Baker MS, Knuth JL, DeWitt J, et al. Pancreatic cystic neuroendocrine tumors: preoperative diagnosis with endoscopic ultrasound and fine-needle immunocytology. J Gastrointest Surg 2008; 12: 450–6.

59. Jani N, Khalid A, Kaushik N, et al. EUS-guided FNA diagnosis of pancreatic endocrine tumors: new trends identified. Gastrointest Endosc 2008; 67: 44–50.

60. Chang F, van der WJ. Fine needle aspiration and core biopsy from a 43-year-old man with multiple abdominal masses. Cytopathology 2006; 17: 307–10.

61. Nikfarjam M, Warshaw AL, Axelrod L, et al. Improved contemporary surgical management of insulinomas: a 25-year experience at the Massachusetts General Hospital. Ann Surg 2008; 247: 165–72.

62. Norton JA, Cromack DT, Shawker TH, et al. Intraoperative ultrasonographic localization of islet cell tumors. A prospective comparison to palpation. Ann Surg 1988; 207: 160–8.

63. Buetow PC, Parrino TV, Buck JL, et al. Islet cell tumors of the pancreas: pathologic-imaging correlation among size, necrosis and cysts, calcification, malignant behavior, and functional status. Am J Roentgenol 1995; 165: 1175–9.

64. Kalra MK, Maher MM, Mueller PR, Saini S. State-of-the-art imaging of pancreatic neoplasms. Br J Radiol 2003; 76: 857–65.

65. Fidler JL, Fletcher JG, Reading CC, et al. Preoperative detection of pancreatic insulinomas on multiphasic helical CT. Am J Roentgenol 2003; 181: 775–80.

66. Stafford-Johnson DB, Francis IR, Eckhauser FE, Knol JA, Chang AE. Dual-phase helical CT of nonfunctioning islet cell tumors. J Comput Assist Tomogr 1998; 22: 335–9.

67. Van Hoe L, Gryspeerdt S, Marchal G, Baert AL, Mertens L. Helical CT for the preoperative localization of islet cell tumors of the pancreas: value of arterial and parenchymal phase images. Am J Roentgenol 1995; 165: 1437–9.

68. Chung MJ, Choi BI, Han JK, et al. Functioning islet cell tumor of the pancreas. Localization with dynamic spiral CT. Acta Radiol 1997; 38: 135–8.

69. Ichikawa T, Peterson MS, Federle MP, et al. Islet cell tumor of the pancreas: biphasic CT versus MR imaging in tumor detection. Radiology 2000; 216: 163–71.

70. Ahrendt SA, Komorowski RA, Demeure MJ, Wilson SD, Pitt HA. Cystic pancreatic neuroendocrine tumors: is preoperative diagnosis possible? J Gastrointest Surg 2002; 6: 66–74.

71. Imaoka H, Yamao K, Salem AA, et al. Pancreatic endocrine neoplasm can mimic serous cystadenoma. Int J Gastrointest Cancer 2005; 35: 217–20.

72. Rodallec M, Vilgrain V, Couvelard A, et al. Endocrine pancreatic tumours and helical CT: contrast enhancement is correlated with microvascular density, histoprognostic factors and survival. Pancreatology 2006; 6: 77–85.

73. Wank SA, Doppman JL, Miller DL, et al. Prospective study of the ability of computed axial tomography to localize gastrinomas in patients with Zollinger-Ellison syndrome. Gastroenterology 1987; 92: 905–12.

74. Maton PN, Miller DL, Doppman JL, et al. Role of selective angiography in the management of patients with Zollinger-Ellison syndrome. Gastroenterology 1987; 92: 913–18.

75. Gouya H, Vignaux O, Augui J, et al. CT, endoscopic sonography, and a combined protocol for preoperative evaluation of pancreatic insulinomas. Am J Roentgenol 2003; 181: 987–92.

76. Owen NJ, Sohaib SA, Peppercorn PD, et al. MRI of pancreatic neuroendocrine tumors. Br J Radiol 2001; 74: 968–73.

77. Semelka RC, Custodio CM, Cem BN, Woosley JT. Neuroendocrine tumors of the pancreas: spectrum of appearances on MRI. J Magn Reson Imaging 2000; 11: 141–8.

78. Pisegna JR, Doppman JL, Norton JA, Metz DC, Jensen RT. Prospective comparative study of ability of MR imaging and other imaging modalities to localize tumors in patients with Zollinger-Ellison syndrome. Dig Dis Sci 1993; 38: 1318–28.

79. Thoeni RF, Mueller-Lisse UG, Chan R, Do NK, Shyn PB. Detection of small, functional islet cell tumors in the pancreas: selection of MR imaging sequences for optimal sensitivity. Radiology 2000; 214: 483–90.

80. Rockall AG, Planche K, Power N, et al. Detection of neuroendocrine liver metastases with MnDPDP-enhanced MRI. Neuroendocrinology. In press.

81. Wang C. Mangafodipir trisodium (MnDPDP)-enhanced magnetic resonance imaging of the liver and pancreas. Acta Radiol Suppl 1998; 415: 1–31.

82. Chavan A, Kirchhoff TD, Brabant G, et al. Role of the intra-arterial calcium stimulation test in the preoperative localization of insulinomas. Eur Radiol 2000; 10: 1582–6.

83. Modlin IM, Latich I, Zikusoka M, et al. Gastrointestinal carcinoids: the evolution of diagnostic strategies. J Clin Gastroenterol 2006; 40: 572–82.

84. Habal N, Sims C, Bilchik AJ. Gastrointestinal carcinoid tumors and second primary malignancies. J Surg Oncol 2000; 75: 310–16.

85. Nessi R, Basso RP, Basso RS, et al. Bronchial carcinoid tumors: radiologic observations in 49 cases. J Thorac Imaging 1991; 6: 47–53.

86. Doppman JL, Pass HI, Nieman LK, et al. Detection of ACTH-producing bronchial carcinoid tumors: MR imaging vs CT. Am J Roentgenol 1991; 156: 39–43.

87. Brown LR, Aughenbaugh GL, Wick MR, Baker BA, Salassa RM. Roentgenologic diagnosis of primary corticotropin-producing carcinoid tumors of the mediastinum. Radiology 1982; 142: 143–8.

88. Wang DY, Chang DB, Kuo SH, et al. Carcinoid tumors of the thymus. Thorax 1994; 49: 357–60.

89. Brown LR, Aughenbaugh GL. Masses of the anterior mediastinum: CT and MR imaging. Am J Roentgenol 1991; 157: 1171–80.

90. Fujiwara K, Segawa Y, Takigawa N, et al. Two cases of atypical carcinoid of the thymus. Intern Med 2000; 39: 834–8.

91. Binstock AJ, Johnson CD, Stephens DH, Lloyd RV, Fletcher JG. Carcinoid tumors of the stomach: a clinical and radiographic study. Am J Roentgenol 2001; 176: 947–51.

92. Woodard PK, Feldman JM, Paine SS, Baker ME. Midgut carcinoid tumors: CT findings and biochemical profiles. J Comput Assist Tomogr 1995; 19: 400–5.

93. Sugimoto E, Lorelius LE, Eriksson B, Oberg K. Midgut carcinoid tumors. CT appearance. Acta Radiol 1995; 36: 367–71.

94. Pilleul F, Penigaud M, Milot L, et al. Possible small-bowel neoplasms: contrast-enhanced and water-enhanced multidetector CT enteroclysis. Radiology 2006; 241: 796–801.

95. Minordi LM, Vecchioli A, Guidi L, et al. Multidetector CT enteroclysis versus barium enteroclysis with methylcellulose in patients with suspected small bowel disease. Eur Radiol 2006; 16: 1527–36.

96. Bader TR, Semelka RC, Chiu VC, Armao DM, Woosley JT. MRI of carcinoid tumors: spectrum of appearances in the gastrointestinal tract and liver. J Magn Reson Imaging 2001; 14: 261–9.

97. Moller JE, Connolly HM, Rubin J, et al. Factors associated with progression of carcinoid heart disease. N Engl J Med 2003; 348: 1005–15.

98. van Tuyl SA, van Noorden JT, Timmer R, et al. Detection of small-bowel neuroendocrine tumors by video capsule endoscopy. Gastrointest Endosc 2006; 64: 66–72.

99. Maeda K, Maruta M, Utsumi T, et al. Minimally invasive surgery for carcinoid tumors in the rectum. Biomed Pharmacother 2002; 56(Suppl 1): 222s–226s.

100. Schindl M, Niederle B, Hafner M, et al. Stage-dependent therapy of rectal carcinoid tumors. World J Surg 1998; 22: 628–33.

101. Matsumoto T, Iida M, Suekane H, et al. Endoscopic ultrasonography in rectal carcinoid tumors: contribution to selection of therapy. Gastrointest Endosc 1991; 37: 539–42.

102. Janson ET, Holmberg L, Stridsberg M, et al. Carcinoid tumors: analysis of prognostic factors and survival in 301 patients from a referral center. Ann Oncol 1997; 8: 685–90.

103. Zeiger MA, Shawker TH, Norton JA. Use of intraoperative ultrasonography to localize islet cell tumors. World J Surg 1993; 17: 448–54.

104. Paulson EK, McDermott VG, Keogan MT, et al. Carcinoid metastases to the liver: role of triple-phase helical CT. Radiology 1998; 206: 143–50.

105. Vasseur B, Cadiot G, Zins M, et al. Peritoneal carcinomatosis in patients with digestive endocrine tumors. Cancer 1996; 78: 1686–92.

106. Fukai I, Masaoka A, Fujii Y, et al. Thymic neuroendocrine tumor (thymic carcinoid): a clinicopathologic study in 15 patients. Ann Thorac Surg 1999; 67: 208–11.

107. Khan JH, McElhinney DB, Rahman SB, et al. Pulmonary metastases of endocrine origin: the role of surgery. Chest 1998; 114: 526–34.

108. Leboulleux S, Dromain C, Vataire AL, et al. Prediction and diagnosis of bone metastases in well-differentiated gastro-entero-pancreatic endocrine cancer: a prospective comparison of whole body magnetic resonance imaging and somatostatin receptor scintigraphy. J Clin Endocrinol Metab 2008; 93: 3021–8.

109. Behr TM, Gotthardt M, Barth A, Behe M. Imaging tumors with peptide-based radioligands. Q J Nucl Med 2001; 45: 189–200.

110. Menda Y, Kahn D. Somatostatin receptor imaging of non-small cell lung cancer with 99mTc depreotide. Semin Nucl Med 2002; 32: 92–6.

111. Krenning EP, Kwekkeboom DJ, Bakker WH, et al. Somatostatin receptor scintigraphy with [111In-DTPA-D-Phe1]- and [123I-Tyr3]-octreotide: the Rotterdam experience with more than 1000 patients. Eur J Nucl Med 1993; 20: 716–31.

112. Kwekkeboom D, Krenning EP, de Jong M. Peptide receptor imaging and therapy. J Nucl Med 2000; 41: 1704–13.

113. Kwekkeboom DJ, Krenning EP. Somatostatin receptor imaging. Semin Nucl Med 2002; 32: 84–91.

114. Hoefnagel CA. MIBG and radiolabeled octreotide in neuroendocrine tumors. Q J Nucl Med 1995; 39(4 Suppl 1): 137–9.

115. Ramage JK, Williams R, Buxton-Thomas M. Imaging secondary neuroendocrine tumours of the liver: comparison of I123 metaiodobenzylguanidine (MIBG) and In111-labelled octreotide (Octreoscan). QJM 1996; 89: 539–42.

116. Kaltsas G, Korbonits M, Heintz E, et al. Comparison of somatostatin analog and meta-iodobenzylguanidine radionuclides in the diagnosis and localization of advanced neuroendocrine tumors. J Clin Endocrinol Metab 2001; 86: 895–902.

117. Bombardieri E, Maccauro M, De Deckere E, Savelli G, Chiti A. Nuclear medicine imaging of neuroendocrine tumours. Ann Oncol 2001; 12(Suppl 2): S51–61.

118. Gotthardt M, Boermann OC, Behr TM, Behe MP, Oyen WJ. Development and clinical application of peptide-based radiopharmaceuticals. Curr Pharm Des 2004; 10: 2951–63.

119. Mariani G, Erba PA, Signore A. Receptor-mediated tumor targeting with radiolabeled peptides: there is more to it than somatostatin analogs. J Nucl Med 2006; 47: 1904–7.

120. Adams S, Baum R, Rink T, et al. Limited value of fluorine-18 fluorodeoxyglucose positron emission tomography for the imaging of neuroendocrine tumours. Eur J Nucl Med 1998; 25: 79–83.

121. Pasquali C, Rubello D, Sperti C, et al. Neuroendocrine tumor imaging: can 18F-fluorodeoxyglucose positron emission tomography detect tumors with poor prognosis and aggressive behavior? World J Surg 1998; 22: 588–92.

122. Le Rest C, Bomanji JB, Costa DC, et al. Functional imaging of malignant paragangliomas and carcinoid tumours. Eur J Nucl Med 2001; 28: 478–82.

123. Virgolini I, Patri P, Novotny C, et al. Comparative somatostatin receptor scintigraphy using in-111-DOTA-lanreotide and in-111-DOTA-Tyr3-octreotide versus F-18-FDG-PET for evaluation of somatostatin receptor-mediated radionuclide therapy. Ann Oncol 2001; 12(Suppl 2): S41–S45.

124. Reubi JC. Regulatory peptide receptors as molecular targets for cancer diagnosis and therapy. Q J Nucl Med 1997; 41: 63–70.

125. Reubi JC, Schar JC, Waser B, et al. Affinity profiles for human somatostatin receptor subtypes SST1–SST5 of somatostatin radiotracers selected for scintigraphic and radiotherapeutic use. Eur J Nucl Med 2000; 27: 273–82.

126. de Herder WW, Hofland LJ, van der Lely AJ, Lamberts SW. Somatostatin receptors in gastroentero-pancreatic neuro-endocrine tumours. Endocr Relat Cancer 2003; 10: 451–8.

127. Blum J, Handmaker H, Lister-James J, Rinne N. A multicenter trial with a somatostatin analog (99m)Tc depreotide in the evaluation of solitary pulmonary nodules. Chest 2000; 117: 1232–8.

128. Ruszniewski P, Ducreux M, Chayvialle JA, et al. Treatment of the carcinoid syndrome with the longacting somatostatin analogue lanreotide: a prospective study in 39 patients. Gut 1996; 39: 279–83.

129. Valkema R, de Jong M, Bakker WH, et al. Phase I study of peptide receptor radionuclide therapy with [In-DTPA]oct-reotide: the Rotterdam experience. Semin Nucl Med 2002; 32: 110–22.

130. Anthony LB, Woltering EA, Espenan GD, et al. Indium-111-pentetreotide prolongs survival in gastroenteropancreatic malignancies. Semin Nucl Med 2002; 32: 123–32.

131. Reubi JC, Schaer JC, Waser B. Cholecystokinin(CCK)-A and CCK-B/gastrin receptors in human tumors. Cancer Res 1997; 57: 1377–86.

132. Reubi JC, Korner M, Waser B, Mazzucchelli L, Guillou L. High expression of peptide receptors as a novel target in gastro-intestinal stromal tumors. Eur J Nucl Med Mol Imaging 2004; 31: 803–10.

133. Behr TM, Behe MP. Cholecystokinin-B/Gastrin receptor-targeting peptides for staging and therapy of medullary thy-roid cancer and other cholecystokinin-B receptor-expressing malignancies. Semin Nucl Med 2002; 32: 97–109.

134. Lin KS, Luu A, Baidoo KE, et al. A new high affinity tech-netium-99m-bombesin analogue with low abdominal accu-mulation. Bioconjug Chem 2005; 16: 43–50.

135. Zhang H, Schuhmacher J, Waser B, et al. DOTA-PESIN, a DOTA-conjugated bombesin derivative designed for the imaging and targeted radionuclide treatment of bombesin receptor-positive tumours. Eur J Nucl Med Mol Imaging 2007; 34: 1198–208.

136. Heppeler A, Froidevaux S, Eberle AN, Maecke HR. Receptor targeting for tumor localisation and therapy with radio-peptides. Curr Med Chem 2000; 7: 971–94.

137. Virgolini I, Raderer M, Kurtaran A, et al. Vasoactive intestinal peptide-receptor imaging for the localization of intestinal adenocarcinomas and endocrine tumors. N Engl J Med 1994; 331: 1116–21.

138. Wieland DM, Brown LE, Tobes MC, et al. Imaging the pri-mate adrenal medulla with [123I] and [131I] meta-iodo-benzylguanidine: concise communication. J Nucl Med 1981; 22: 358–64.

139. Lebtahi R, Le Cloirec J, Houzard C, et al. Detection of neuro-endocrine tumors: 99mTc-P829 scintigraphy compared with 111In-pentetreotide scintigraphy. J Nucl Med 2002; 43: 889–95.

140. Shulkin BL, Wieland DM, Baro ME, et al. PET hydroxyephe-drine imaging of neuroblastoma. J Nucl Med 1996; 37: 16–21.

141. Ahlstrom H, Eriksson B, Bergstrom M, et al. Pancreatic neu-roendocrine tumors: diagnosis with PET. Radiology 1995; 195: 333–7.

142. Vaidyanathan G, Affleck DJ, Zalutsky MR. Validation of 4-[fluorine-18]fluoro-3-iodobenzylguanidine as a positron-emitting analog of MIBG. J Nucl Med 1995; 36: 644–50.

143. de Jong M, Breeman WA, Valkema R, Bernard BF, Krenning EP. Combination radionuclide therapy using 177Lu- and 90Y-la-beled somatostatin analogs. J Nucl Med 2005; 46(Suppl 1): 13S–17S.

144. Krenning EP, Teunissen JJ, Valkema R, et al. Molecular radio-therapy with somatostatin analogs for (neuro-)endocrine tumors. J Endocrinol Invest 2005; 28(11 Suppl Int): 146–50.

145. Paganelli G, Bodei L, Handkiewicz JD, et al. 90Y-DOTA-D-Phe1-Try3-octreotide in therapy of neuroendocrine malig-nancies. Biopolymers 2002; 66: 393–8.

146. Waldherr C, Pless M, Maecke HR, et al. Tumor response and clinical benefit in neuroendocrine tumors after 7.4 GBq (90) Y-DOTATOC. J Nucl Med 2002; 43: 610–16.

147. Bodei L, Cremonesi M, Zoboli S, et al. Receptor-mediated radionuclide therapy with 90Y-DOTATOC in association with amino acid infusion: a phase I study. Eur J Nucl Med Mol Imaging 2003; 30: 207–16.

148. Kwekkeboom DJ, Mueller-Brand J, Paganelli G, et al. Over-view of results of peptide receptor radionuclide therapy with 3 radiolabeled somatostatin analogs. J Nucl Med 2005; 46(Suppl 1): 62S–66S.

149. Bodei L, Cremonesi M, Grana C, et al. Receptor radionuclide therapy with 90Y-[DOTA]0-Tyr3-octreotide (90Y-DOTA-TOC) in neuroendocrine tumours. Eur J Nucl Med Mol Imaging 2004; 31: 1038–46.

150. Wallace S, Ajani JA, Charnsangavej C, et al. Carcinoid tumors: imaging procedures and interventional radiology. World J Surg 1996; 20: 147–56.

151. Liapi E, Geschwind JF, Vossen JA, et al. Functional MRI evaluation of tumor response in patients with neuro-endocrine hepatic metastasis treated with transcatheter arterial chemoembolization. Am J Roentgenol 2008; 190: 67–73.

152. Godwin J D. Carcinoid tumors. An analysis of 2,837 cases. Cancer. 1975; 36: 560–9.

Lymphoma
Sarah J Vinnicombe, Rodney H Reznek, and Norbert Avril

INTRODUCTION

The lymphomas, Hodgkin's lymphoma (HL) and non-Hodgkin's lymphoma (NHL), are a diverse group of neoplasms that vary widely in age of presentation, patterns of tumor growth, and survival rates. Hodgkin's disease, or HL was first described by Thomas Hodgkin in 1832, but it is only during the last two decades that the prognosis has improved so that currently HL is curable in the majority of patients. NHL has a variable course, ranging from slow and indolent to aggressive and rapidly fatal. As with HL, improvements in survival rates are largely attributed to advances in therapy. However, the impact of modern imaging methods on the accurate delineation of disease extent and identification of risk factors, both of which facilitate optimized individualized risk-adapted treatment with resultant survival benefits, cannot be understimated.

In the lymphomas, imaging plays a vital role in the correct deployment of combined modality treatment at the time of diagnosis and staging, in monitoring response to therapy and in the detection of disease relapse.

The objectives of initial staging are to define as accurately as possible the local extent of clinically overt disease and to search for occult disease elsewhere with a full knowledge of the likely pattern of tumor spread (1). It should also identify adverse prognostic features such as extranodal disease and factors which may influence delivery of therapy, such as venous obstruction or hydronephrosis. Choice of the appropriate imaging method requires an appreciation of:

- The likelihood of particular sites being affected given the patterns of tumor spread
- The sensitivity and specificity of particular tests chosen to investigate those sites
- The likely impact of a positive result on treatment choice

INCIDENCE

Lymphoma accounts for 5% to 6% of all malignancies in adults in the United Kingdom and about 10% of all childhood cancers (2,3). In the United States in 2008 it was estimated that there would be 66,120 new cases of NHL and 19,160 deaths (4). Each year in the United States NHL accounts for 5% of new cancers in men and 4% of new cancers in women. According to the National Cancer Institute, the United States age-adjusted incidence rate for NHL was 15.5 per 100,000 people in 1996 (5). HL is less common than NHL, accounting for about 15% of all lymphomas. It was estimated that in the United States there would be 8220 new cases of HL and 1350 deaths in 2008 (4). In the United Kingdom there were 10,003 new cases of NHL and 1519 new cases of HL in 2004; there were 4451 deaths from NHL and 291

deaths from HL in 2005. The lifetime risk of developing NHL is approximately 1 in 83, and males are affected slightly more often than females in both types of lymphoma with the following ratios (2):

- Hodgkin's lymphoma M:F 1.4:1
- Non-Hodgkin's lymphoma M:F 1.1:1

In the United States, while the incidence of HL has remained approximately stable, that of NHL has risen by approximately 60% since 1960. The increased incidence is evident for all age groups, but particularly for the elderly (6). It is also more marked in men than in women, and in White more than non-White ethnic groups. Internationally, the incidence of NHL varies 8 to 10 fold, being much more common in the West (7), but even so this markedly increased incidence has been noted in international cancer registries of seven European countries (8) as well as in all geographical areas of the Unites States (5). The overall mortality for NHL has also increased steadily over the last few decades, and in the United States this trend in mortality is most evident in the elderly. Despite this, the survival rate for each subtype of NHL has increased with time, reflecting steady advances in treatment.

Several hypotheses have been used to explain the striking increase in incidence. Some may be artifactual, where new NHL classification techniques and systems have led to a diagnosis of NHL in some patients who would previously have had other diagnoses (9). Improved imaging techniques have undoubtedly led to more NHL diagnoses, particularly lymphoma of the central nervous system (CNS) (9). It has also been estimated that in 10% to 15% of cases a reclassification of cases previously diagnosed as HL contributes to the apparent increase in NHL incidence (10). Part of the increase in the late 80s and early 90s was a consequence of the increased incidence of lymphomas associated with immune deficiency, particularly secondary to human immunodeficiency virus (HIV) infection. However, the incidence of those cases of NHL associated with HIV (primary CNS lymphoma or PCNSL, Burkitt lymphoma and immunoblastic lymphoma) has been falling since the introduction of highly active antiretroviral therapies in 1995 (11). Even when factors such as accuracy of diagnosis, the effect of HIV and occupational exposures are considered, the reason for most of the increase in NHL remains unexplained (12).

HL used to show an obvious bimodal peak distribution, the first in the third decade of life, and the second between 65 and 75 years of age; but in recent years this has become less obvious, with a decrease in the incidence in patients over 55 years. In part this is attributable to the reclassification of cases that would previously have been called HL as NHL, as described above. NHL is a disease mainly of the elderly with an increasing incidence over the age of 50 years (13) and a median age at diagnosis of 65 years (14).

Key Points: Incidence

- The incidence of NHL has increased by 60% over the last two decades in the United States and United Kingdom, while the incidence of HL is stable
- HL has a peak incidence between the ages of 30 and 40 years and also in those aged over 65 years. NHL is seen in children and in those over 50 years of age

ETIOLOGY

There is an association between the Ebstein-Barr virus (EBV) and HL but debate continues regarding the exact etiological role of EBV in this disease. It is interesting that the suggestion of EBV infection having a causal relationship with HL was originally made by Hodgkin himself in his first description of the morbid anatomy of the condition. Patients with HL have a higher antibody titer to the EBV viral capsular antigen than normal adults and the risk of HL amongst patients who have had infectious mononucleosis is trebled (15). EBV can be found in the malignant cells of HL (the Hodgkin's and Reed-Sternberg cells). There is some evidence for the role of other infective agents such as human herpes virus 6 (HHV) and also HIV1, which is associated with the mixed cellularity subtype of classical HL.

Infective agents are also implicated in the development of NHL. EBV may be an important etiological factor in Burkitt lymphoma (BL), particularly in the endemic African form where virtually 100% of cases have EBV. In the sporadic form the incidence is 15% to 30%. The rare primary effusion lymphomas are associated with HHV 8. *Helicobacter pylori* infection is necessary for the development of gastric lymphoma of mucosa-associated lymphoid tissue (MALT) type. The HTLV-1 retrovirus is known to have a causal relationship with adult T-cell leukemia/lymphoma, which is seen in South Japan and the Caribbean (16). It is thought that the disease represents a clonal expansion of HTLV1 infected T lymphocytes. *Borrelia burgdorferi* infection is associated with a low-grade cutaneous B cell lymphoma which can resolve once the infection is eradicated (17).

Genetic factors have limited importance in the etiology of HL, with approximately 5% of cases being familial. The incidence is increased in siblings, first-degree relatives of affected individuals and in monozygotic twins of sufferers. This may relate to changes in the HLA class 1 region of chromosome 6. Genetic studies have also revealed the importance of mutation, altered expression and loss of function of genes in the development and progression of NHL (18) and familial aggregation of NHL is well recognized. Immunosuppression is a very important etiological factor in NHL, with a high incidence in AIDS patients and those on long-term immunosuppressant therapy; for example, following renal transplantation (19,20). The latter is associated with diffuse large B cell lymphoma (DLBCL), extranodal and central nervous system disease. Up to 25% of patients with congenital immunodeficiency syndromes such as ataxia-telangiectasia, Wiskott-Aldrich syndrome and X-linked immunodeficiencies will develop malignancies. Lymphoproliferative disorders (including HL and EBV-driven NHL), account for over 50% of these (21). Non organ-specific autoimmune diseases such as rheumatoid arthritis are associated with DLBCL, whereas organ-specific autoimmune diseases predispose to the development of extranodal marginal zone lymphomas of MALT type within the affected organs (for example, the thyroid and salivary glands).

Key Points: Etiology

- There is a link between the Epstein–Barr virus (EBV), HL, and NHL
- Various other infective agents are associated with a number of specific types of NHL
- Congenital and acquired immunodeficiency states predispose to the development of lymphoproliferative disorders

PATHOLOGY

Classification

Non-Hodgkin Lymphoma

A robust classification has to be clinically relevant and must be translatable to allow communication of new knowledge and comparison of clinical results (22). In this context, the reproducibility and widespread use of the Rye modification of the Luke–Butler classification (introduced in 1966) has proved to be reliable for HL (Table 33.1) (23,24). This contrasts greatly with the profusion of classifications for NHL, although since its introduction in 1982 the working formulation, described below, has resulted in some degree of consensus (25). The functional anatomy of the lymph node and its relationship to lymphoma is shown in Figure 33.1. The recognition that most NHLs arise from the cells of the germinal follicle of the lymph node led to the development of a Working Formulation of NHL for clinical usage (25). This classification was widely employed, until the introduction of the REAL (Revised European American Classification of Lymphoid Neoplasms) classification, and completely superseded the plethora of previous classifications, which were largely unsatisfactory (26,27). The Working Formulation was based upon the idea that lymphoma is a result of clonal expansion of T or B lymphocytes at a particular point in their normal maturation (28). B lymphocytes (bone marrow-derived) are concerned with antibody production and develop into plasma cells that produce immunoglobulin. If normal maturation is prevented, the arrested cell multiplies. This results in lymphoma whose type and grade depends on the stage of maturation at the time of insult. T lymphocytes (thymic-derived) do not contain immunoglobulin but are also concerned with immune response. T-cell lymphomas are either central T-cell lymphomas that are immature (e.g., diffuse lymphoblastic lymphoma), or those derived from more mature T lymphocytes, which are termed peripheral T-cell lymphomas. Histiocytic lymphomas do not fall into either of these categories.

Table 33.1 Rye Classification of Hodgkin's Lymphoma with Approximate Distribution of Frequency (23,24)

Histology	Frequency (%)
Lymphocyte predominance	5
Nodular sclerosis	65
Mixed cellularity	25
Lymphocyte depletion	5

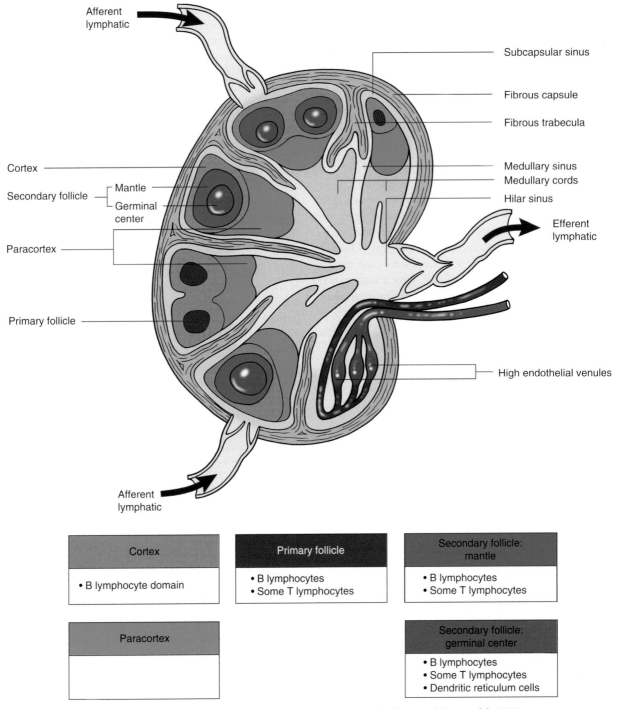

Figure 33.1 Relationship of functional lymph node anatomy to normal cell type and lineage of the NHLs.

The majority of NHL (over 90%) are B-cell lymphomas. NHLs which arise at stages of development occurring within the germinal center of the node have a follicular pattern, whereas those that arise outside the germinal center have a diffuse architectural pattern. The Working Formulation designated each lymphoma according to characteristics of the cell type at the time of arrested maturation and overall divided NHL into low-grade, intermediate, and high-grade tumors. The "miscellaneous" group did not fulfil all the requirements of the three main categories.

The Working Formulation had important practical implications:

- Therapy was based on the grade of lymphoma
- The grade of lymphoma carried important prognostic significance
- The classification of lymphoma predicted possible transformation into a higher grade
- The detailed subclassification of lymphomas allowed standardization of therapies and comparison of results from different centers

However, since the classification was based upon treatment outcomes rather than the recognition of the cell of origin or of discrete disease entities, it was difficult to gain an understanding of the pathogenesis of the various conditions. Many common entities were not recognized at all, which hindered research into tumor biology.

More recently, in 1994, improvement in the understanding of NHL and the recognition of new clinico-pathological entities resulted in the introduction of the REAL classification by the International Lymphoma Study Group, which was adopted internationally (29). The REAL classification is a consensus list of all lymphoid neoplasms that appear to be distinct clinical entities. Unlike the Working Formulation, it utilizes all available features (morphology, immunophenotype, genetics, and clinical features) to define each entity according to cell of origin (principally B or T cell) and stage of differentiation, if known. This practical consensus approach differentiated it from previous morphological classifications and enabled widespread usage by pathologists and clinicians.

In 1995, under the auspices of the WHO, the European Association for Haematopathology and the Society for Hematopathology collaborated on a project to classify all tumors of hematopoietic and lymphoid lineages. The proposals were reviewed by a Clinical Advisory Committee (CAC) and the result is the WHO Classification of Tumors of Hematopoietic and Lymphoid Tissues (30), which is an updated version of the REAL classification (Table 33.2).

The WHO classification stratifies neoplasms by lineage: myeloid, lymphoid, histiocytic/dendritic, and mast cell. The classification is a list of over 40 disease entities with distinct clinical features defined by a combination of morphology, immunophenotype, and genetic features. It recognizes three major groups of lymphoid neoplasms: B cell, T cell, and natural killer (NK) cell; and HL. It is now clear that the malignant cell in HL is lymphoid, hence its inclusion in the classification. Indeed, the distinction between HL and NHL is not always straightforward, with composite and sequential cases occurring. It includes the leukemias, as they represent circulating phases of particular neoplasms. Thus B-cell chronic lymphocytic leukemia and B-cell small lymphocytic lymphoma are the same entity, as are lymphoblastic lymphoma and lymphoblastic leukemia. Within the B and T/NK categories two major groups are recognized—precursor neoplasms (corresponding to the early stages of differentiation) and mature or peripheral neoplasms, corresponding to more differentiated stages. Furthermore, many entities such as follicular lymphoma have a range of grade and aggressiveness. Since variations in cytological grade can inform treatment decisions, grading schemes and other prognostic markers are included in the classification. The main lymphoid groups are shown in Table 33.2.

The approach is thought to represent a significant advance in the ability to identify and treat disease entities, with international consistency. A study to address this issue of consistency showed that expert hematopathologists, given adequate material, agreed on the classification of the entity in over 95% of cases (31,32). A key advantage of the classification is that it permits refinement or elaboration. A second edition is in the process of being drafted and within it there are a number of new entities. For example, it has recently been shown that gene expression profiling in DLBCL with cDNA microarrays enables the recognition of a number of discrete

subsets (germinal center B-cell type and activated B-cell type) which have independent prognostic significance (33), and this is likely to be included in the next iteration of the classification. Other additions include pediatric follicular lymphoma, primary DLBCL of the central nervous system (PCNSL), B-cell lymphoma with features intermediate between DLBCL and classical HL, and B-cell lymphoma with features intermediate between DLBCL and BL.

Hodgkin's Lymphoma

Since biological and clinical studies have shown that HL is a true lymphoma, the term HL is preferred to "Hodgkin's disease". Central to the diagnosis of HL is the demonstration of the neoplastic Reed–Sternberg (Fig. 33.2) and Hodgkin cells in a background of non-neoplastic inflammatory cells. The Rye modification of the Luke–Butler classification divides HL into four subgroups based on the proportion of lymphocytes in relation to the number of Hodgkin and Reed–Sternberg cells, and the type of connective tissue background. However, as recognized in the REAL and WHO classifications, HL comprises two distinct entities:

- Nodular lymphocyte predominant Hodgkin's lymphoma (NLPHL) (5%)
- Classical Hodgkin's lymphoma (CHL) (95%)

Table 33.2 Summary of the Who Classification of Tumors of Lymphoid Tissues

B-cell neoplasms	T-cell and NK-cell neoplasms
Precursor B-cell neoplasm	Precursor T-cell neoplasms
Precursor B lymphoblastic leukemia/lymphoma	Precursor T lymphoblastic leukemia/lymphoma
Mature B-cell	Blastic NK cell lymphoma
CLL/small lymphocytic lymphoma	**Mature T-cell and NK neoplasms**
B-cell prolymphocytic leukemia	T-cell prolymphocytic leukemia
Lymphoplasmacytic lymphoma	T-cell large granular lymphocytic leukemia
Splenic marginal zone lymphoma	Aggressive NK cell leukemia
Hairy cell leukemia	Adult T-cell leukemia/lymphoma
Plasma cell myeloma	Extranodal NK/T-cell lymphoma, nasal type
Solitary plasmacytoma of bone	Enteropathy-type T-cell lymphoma
Extraosseous plasmacytoma	Hepatosplenic T-cell lymphoma
Extranodal marginal zone B-cell lymphoma of	Subcutaneous panniculitis-like T-cell lymphoma
mucosa associated lymphoid tissue (MALT)	Mycosis fungoides
Nodal maginal zone B-cell lymphoma	Sezary syndrome
Follicular lymphoma	Primary cutaneous anaplastic large cell lymphoma
Mantle cell lymphoma	Peripheral T-cell lymphoma, unspecified
Diffuse large B-cell lymphoma	Angioimmunoblastic T-cell lymphoma
Mediastinal (thymic) large B-cell lymphoma	Anaplastic large cell lymphoma
Intravascular large B-cell lymphoma	**T-cell proliferation of uncertain malignant potential**
Primary effusion lymphoma	Lymphoid papulosis
Burkitt's lymphoma/leukemia	**Hodgkin's lymphoma**
B-cell proliferations of uncertain malignant potential	Nodular lymphocyte predominant HL
Lymphomatoid granulomatosis	Classical HL
Post-transplant lymphoproliferative disorder, polymorphic	Nodular sclerosis classical HL
	Lymphocyte rich classical HL
	Mixed cellularity classical HL
	Lymphocyte depleted classical HL

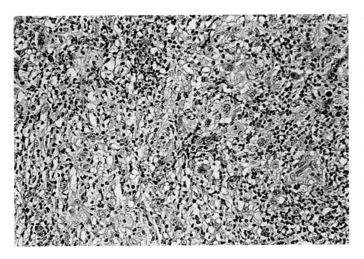

Figure 33.2 Histological section of mixed cellularity HL showing Reed–Sternberg cells, lymphocytes, and neutrophils.

These two differ in clinical features, behavior, morphology, and immunophenotype, whereas the four CHL subtypes all share the same immunophenotype.

Most cases of NLPHL were probably misclassified as lymphocyte predominance Hodgkin's disease in the past. It represents 5% of all HL. Patients are mostly male in the 30 to 50-year age group. Most patients present with Stage I or II peripheral adenopathy affecting one or two nodal groups only (axillary, cervical, or inguinal); mediastinal, splenic, and marrow involvement are rare. Latent EBV infection is not seen in the malignant cells. The disease has an indolent course with a high relapse rate but, paradoxically, excellent survival even with relapsed disease.

CHL accounts for 95% of all cases. Patients with infectious mononucleosis have a higher incidence, and familial and geographic clustering is seen. The cervical lymph nodes are involved in over 75% of cases. Overall, the incidence of splenic and bone marrow involvement at presentation is low (25% and 5%, respectively).

In *nodular sclerosing* HL, nodules of lymphoid tissue are separated by dense bands of collagen. It is the most frequent subgroup, accounting for approximately 70% of CHL. The median age is around 25 years and it is the only form of HL without a male preponderance. Anterior mediastinal disease occurs in 80% of cases, bulky disease in around 50%, splenic and/or lung involvement in 10%. Most patients are Stage II at presentation with disease confined to two nodal groups on the same side of the diaphragm, and B symptoms are seen in 40%. Males are affected as often as females in this subtype.

Mixed cellularity HL comprises 20% to 25% of CHL. It is more common in HIV patients and in developing countries. Of those affected, 70% are male. Stage III or IV disease is common, as are B symptoms. Peripheral nodal disease is frequent, splenic involvement occurs in up to 30%, and marrow involvement in 10% of affected individuals. Mediastinal disease is uncommon. This subtype is most commonly associated with EBV positivity.

Lymphocyte-rich CHL comprises 5% of all HL; 70% of these are male with a higher median age. Stage I or II peripheral nodal disease is typical, without mediastinal involvement or B symptoms. Survival appears slightly better in this subtype.

Lymphocyte-depleted CHL is the rarest subtype, accounting for less than 5% of cases; 75% of the affected individuals are male,

with a median age of 35 to 40 years. It is often associated with HIV infection and is seen more often in developing countries. Peripheral lymph nodes are relatively spared, with involvement instead of abdominal organs, retroperitoneal nodes and bone marrow. Stage III or IV disease is common (70%) as are B symptoms (80%). Most HIV-positive cases are EBV infected and have relatively aggressive courses. This is now an infrequent diagnosis, as in the past this condition was often misdiagnosed; many cases were in fact NHL.

Key Points: Classification of Lymphomas

■ HL comprises two distinct entities: NLPHL and CHL
■ CHL is made up of four subtypes: nodular sclerosing (70%), mixed cellularity (20–25%), lymphocyte rich (5%), and lymphocyte-depleted (<5%)
■ The WHO update of the REAL classification stratifies lymphoma by myeloid, lymphoid, histiocytic/dendritic and mast cell lineage, and provides a list of distinct disease entities

STAGING CLASSIFICATIONS

The Ann Arbor staging system was introduced for HL in 1970. It takes into account the extent of nodal disease and the presence of extranodal extension. However, an increasing recognition of the influence of tumor bulk as an independent prognostic indicator within each stage, and the routine application of new diagnostic techniques, such as computed tomography (CT) or magnetic resonance (MR) imaging led to a modification of the Ann Arbor classification in 1989 called the Cotswolds classification (Table 33.3) (34). This system is similar to the Ann Arbor classification, but Stage III is subdivided and an additional qualifier "X" denotes bulky disease. Both the Ann Arbor and Cotswolds systems are applied to NHL, but are of less value, as the prognosis in NHL is

Table 33.3 Staging of Lymphoma (Cotswolds Classification) (34)

Stage	Area of involvement
I	One lymph node region or extralymphatic site
II	Two or more lymph node regions on the same side of the diaphragm
III	Involvement of lymph node regions or structures on both sides of diaphragm, subdivided thus:
III(1ᵃ)	With involvement of spleen and/or splenic hilar, coeliac, and portal nodes
III(2ᵃ)	With para-aortic, iliac, or mesenteric nodes
IV	Extranodal sites beyond those designated E
Additional qualifiers	
A	No symptoms
B	Fever, sweats, weight loss (to 10% of body weight)
E	Involvement of single extranodal site, contiguous in proximity to a known nodal site
Xᵃ	Bulky disease
	Mass >1/3 thoracic diameter at T5
	Mass >10 cm maximum dimension
CEᵃ	Clinical stage
PSᵃ	Pathological stage: PS at a given site denoted by a subscript (i.e., M, marrow; H, liver; L, lung; O, bone; P, pleural; D, skin)

ᵃModifications from Ann Arbor system.

more dependent on histological grade and other parameters such as tumor bulk and specific organ involvement, than on stage (35,36). In NHL, the critical question is whether or not disease is limited and, therefore, potentially treatable with radiotherapy, or whether it is disseminated.

Childhood NHL exhibits a clinical spectrum somewhat different to adult lymphoma with more frequent extranodal involvement, there being a very high incidence of lymphoma in the gastro-intestinal tract, solid abdominal viscera including the kidneys and pancreas, and extranodal sites in the head and neck (37,38). The staging system of Murphy is most widely used (Table 33.4).

CLINICAL FEATURES

HL and NHL are diseases of the lymph nodes, both of which may present as truly localized processes involving a single nodal group or organ, or as widely disseminated disease. However, recognizable differences distinguish the clinical presentation in the two diseases (Table 33.5). Broadly, NHL is disseminated at presentation more frequently than HL and, although the majority of adult patients with NHL present with superficial lymphadenopathy, involvement of the viscera is more common in all types of NHL than it is in HL.

Hodgkin's Lymphoma

Most patients with HL present with painless asymmetrical lymph node enlargement, which may be accompanied with sweats, fever, weight loss, and pruritus in about 40% of patients. Alcohol-induced pain is a rare complaint.

On clinical examination the commonest site of nodal involvement is the cervical region, present in 60% to 80% of patients. Axillary nodal involvement is also common, occurring in 6% to 20% of patients, and inguinal/femoral nodal disease is seen in 6% to 15%. Exclusive infradiaphragmatic lymphadenopathy occurs in less than 10% of patients at diagnosis. Splenomegaly is found on clinical examination in about one third of patients.

HL tends to spread in a contiguous fashion from one lymph node group to the next adjacent group. Primary extranodal HL is very rare and can only be diagnosed after a thorough search for disease in other sites.

Non-Hodgkin's Lymphoma

As in HL, the majority of patients with NHL present with nodal enlargement, but extranodal disease is far commoner and the overwhelming majority has advanced stage disease at presentation.

In low-grade lymphoma, lymphadenopathy may be intermittent and the median age at diagnosis is between 55 and 60 years. They are rarely diagnosed under the age of 30 years and account for 30% to 45% of all lymphomas.

Intermediate-grade lymphoma usually includes both follicular and diffuse forms. The diffuse large B-cell lymphoma (DLBCL) accounts for 35–40% of all NHL and is the commonest B-cell NHL, usually presenting with rapidly enlarging lymph nodes. Together with follicular lymphoma (FL), these tumors comprise 70% to 80% of all lymphomas. FL accounts for around 30% of all newly diagnosed NHL and the WHO classicification includes three grades depending on the number of centroblasts per high power field. Grade 3 is further subdivided into a and b depending on the presence or absence of centrocytes in addition to centroblasts. FL grade 3b may be more closely related to DLBCL (39). They usually present between the ages of 50 and 55 years and may be associated with extranodal disease at presentation. DLBCL is aggressive but responds well to therapy. Recent work on gene expression profiling has resulted in the recognition of two main variants of DLBCL: germinal center-like signature, which has a relatively good outcome, and activated B cell signature, with a poorer prognosis (33).

High-grade lymphomas are the most aggressive tumor subtype but many patients have apparently localized disease at the time of presentation. Overall, approximately 20% of patients with NHL have systemic symptoms such as fever, sweat, and weight loss, compared to 40% of patients with HL. NHL is a disseminated disease involving lymph node groups haphazardly, multiple organs and bone marrow (40).

Table 33.4 Murphy's Staging System for Childhood NHL

Stage	Criteria for extent of disease
I	A single tumor (extranodal) or single anatomical area (nodal) with the exclusion of the mediastinum or abdomen
II	A single tumor (extranodal) with regional nodal involvement
	Two or more nodal areas on the same side of the diaphragm
	Two single (extranodal) tumors with or without regional node involvement of the same side of the diaphragm
	A primary GI tract tumor, usually in the ileocaecal area, with or without involvement of associated mesenteric nodes only, grossly completely resected
III	Two single tumors (extranodal) on opposite sides of the diaphragm
	Two or more nodal areas above and below the diaphragm
	ALL primary intrathoracic tumors (mediastinal, pleural, thymic)
	ALL extensive primary intra-abdominal disease, unresected
	ALL paraspinal or epidural tumors, regardless of other tumor site(s)
IV	Any of the above with initial CNS and/or bone marrow involvement

Table 33.5 Key Differences Between the Clinical Features of HL and NHL

	HL	NHL
Clinical features		
Fever, night sweats, loss of weight	40%	20%
Spread	Tends to be contiguous	Multiple remote nodal groups are often involved
Age	Uncommon in childhood	More frequent 40–70 yr
Nodal groups		
Thoracic	65–85%	25–40%
Para-aortic	25–35%	45–55%
Mesenteric	5%	50–60%
Extranodal disease		
CNS	<1%	2%
GI tract	<1%	5–15%
Genitourinary tract	<1%	1–5%
Bone marrow	3%	20–40%
Lung parenchyma	8–12%	3–6%
Bone	<1%	1–2%
Stage at diagnosis	>80% Stages I–II	>85% Stages III–IV

Key Points: Clinical Aspects

■ The majority of patients with HL and NHL present with painless enlargement of a group of lymph nodes

■ In HL, most patients present with Stage I or II disease, and in NHL the majority of patients have Stage III or IV disease at diagnosis

■ Systemic symptoms are seen more frequently in HL than NHL

PROGNOSIS AND TREATMENT OPTIONS

Hodgkin's Lymphoma

There has been a dramatic improvement in survival from HL in the past 30 years, mortality rates falling by more than 60% from the late 1960s to the 1990s. Current mortality rates are around 0.5/100,000 for men and 0.3/100,000 for women. For early stage disease, there is a five year survival rate of over 90% (41). The prognosis of HL depends upon a number of factors (15), including:

- Age—Older patients have a worse prognosis (for early stage disease, five year survival is 45% over the age of 65, cf > 90% for younger patients)
- Tumor subtype—Those with mixed cellularity and lymphocyte depletion have a worse prognosis than with nodular sclerosis and lymphocyte-predominant HL
- Raised erythrocyte sedimentation rate (ESR)
- Multiple sites of involvement
- Bulky mediastinal disease
- Systemic symptoms

Patients with HL have traditionally been divided into two or three prognostic groups, chiefly according to stage and B symptoms, but also taking various other factors into consideration. Each group is associated with a typical standard treatment strategy, but this strategy has changed quite markedly since the advent of effective combination chemotherapy. HL is highly radiosensitive and can be cured by radiotherapy alone (34). Hence, the standard treatment for early-stage HL used to be radiotherapy to the involved nodes as well as the adjacent lymph node chains (extended field radiotherapy). Administration of mantle radiotherapy for cervical lymphadenopathy included irradiation to the bilateral cervical nodes, the supraclavicular and axillary nodes, together with mediastinal nodes, extending down to the lower border of the vertebral body of T10. The overall 10-year survival rate in patients with Stages I and II HL treated with radiotherapy is greater than 90% (42,43). However, increasing recognition of the long-term toxicity from radiotherapy — including a vast excess of breast cancer in women and thyroid cancer in both men and women who have received mantle radiotherapy — has prompted development of efficacious chemotherapeutic regimens which reduce the need for radiotherapy (44). Thus, major developments in treatment have been aimed at reducing toxicity while at the same time maintaining efficacy. The different regimes have different side effects ranging from nausea, vomiting, and hair loss to bone marrow suppression, sterility and leukemogenesis (45–47). Only in nodular lymphocyte predominant HL, which commonly presents with stage I disease involving the groin or axilla, would

radiotherapy alone be considered now. Treatment according to prognostic grouping is summarized below:

- Early stages, favorable: combination chemotherapy plus involved field radiotherapy
- Early stages, unfavorable: more intense chemotherapy plus radiotherapy
- Advanced stages: extensive chemotherapy with or without consolidatory (usually local) radiation to sites of bulk disease or a residual mass

In the past, staging laparotomy was routinely undertaken in patients with HL to identify splenic involvement and intra-abdominal lymph node spread. Although it is known that the spleen is involved in about 30% of patients with Stage I and Stage II HL, the technique has been abandoned for the following reasons:

- Combination chemotherapy is more frequently used in the treatment of HL, thereby obviating the need for splenectomy
- In the rare instance of patients treated with radiotherapy alone, subsequent infradiaphragmatic relapse can be successfully salvaged with subsequent chemotherapy
- Staging laparotomy is a major procedure, and splenectomy increases the risk of overwhelming infection and may have a causal relationship with the subsequent development of leukemia (48)

HL is chemosensitive and chemotherapy combined with radiotherapy is widely used in patients with unfavorable prognostic indicators in early-stage disease, for example, those presenting with bulky mediastinal masses or multiple sites of involvement. Omission of radiotherapy altogether in this situation has been shown to give poorer results. Chemotherapy with or without irradiation is also the standard approach for the treatment of Stages III and IV disease. In patients with bulky disease the aim is to use chemotherapy to reduce bulk, followed by radiotherapy to that site, in order to avoid excessive irradiation of lung parenchyma and subsequent radiation fibrosis. Thus, the role of radiotherapy has become more consolidatory reducing the relapse rate by 25% and increasing overall survival. The commonest treatment is six courses of ABVD chemotherapy (doxorubicin or Adriamycin®, bleomycin, vinblastine, and dacarbazine) whereas the Stanford V protocol utilizes a shorter course of chemotherapy with irradiation of all sites originally larger than 5 cm, or to the spleen if clinically involved.

Overall, in patients with more advanced disease (bulky Stage II, Stage III, and IV), 50% to 80% will achieve complete remission following multi-agent chemotherapy, but of these 30% to 50% will subsequently relapse within five years. Combination chemotherapy for recurrence after primary treatment with radiotherapy alone has been successful in achieving a prolonged second remission (49). Patients failing initial chemotherapy for advanced HL have a poor prognosis, but high-dose chemotherapy with hemopoietic stem cell rescue is being increasingly employed, although its long-term benefits are yet to be established (50).

Second Malignancies After HL

HL is curable in the vast majority of patients and with such prolonged survival, long-term consequences of the disease and the

treatment have become more apparent. Indeed, in those patients with early stage disease treated when they were younger than 50, the absolute excess risk of mortality actually increases with time because of the increased incidence of cardiac disease and second tumors as a result of treatment (51). The most important long-term complication of treatment is the development of a second malignancy. The commonest malignancies are acute myeloid leukemia (AML) and NHL (DLBCL or Burkitt-like) (52). AML usually develops two to five years after successful treatment. The risk of NHL is relatively low (2% for classical HL), but increased after combined chemoradiation. This may in part be secondary to the immunodeficiency associated with HL. Large B cell lymphomas can occur after NLPHL and this may represent clonal expansion of the original malignancy, since composite forms can occur (53).

Non-Hodgkin's Lymphoma

The prognosis of NHL varies hugely. Unlike HL, histological subtype is the major determinant of treatment, and prognosis and treatment are dependent on a combination of histological subtype and stage. Low-grade lymphomas, although incurable, often have a prolonged indolent course. For example the median survival for patients with follicular lymphoma is 10 years, but some live more than 15 years. It is slowly progressive and has a tendency to become histologically more diffuse, with a greater number of large blast cells with time. Such transformation to large B cell NHL has grave implications for prognosis and therefore an impact on treatment strategy. It may be a terminal event in up to 70% of cases (54). Intermediate and high-grade lymphomas carry a worse prognosis, especially those with larger cells and blast forms. In these patients, however, cure is possible with advanced chemotherapeutic regimens. Untreated, the median survival for patients with DLBCL is under one year. Over 40% of patients with DLBCL are cured with anthracycline-based combination chemotherapy and can expect long-term disease-free survival; the rest eventually succumb to the disease. The International Prognostic Index (IPI) was developed by an international collaborative group in recognition of the fact that appropriate choice of therapy for a patient and comparison of therapies can only be achieved with a uniform prognostic system in place (55). In aggressive lymphomas such as DLBCL, five factors were found to have prognostic significance:

- Age >60 years
- Elevated serum lactate dehydrogenase (LDH)
- Eastern Cooperative Oncology Group (ECOG) performance status >1 (i.e., non-ambulatory) (56)
- Advanced Stage (III or IV)
- Presence of >1 extranodal site of disease

Four risk groups are recognized depending on the number of prognostic features that are present. Prognostic stratification in this way enables choice of more aggressive therapies for those at higher risk. Patients in the low risk group (0 or 1 prognostic factor present) have an 87% complete response rate with five year survival greater than 70%. In contrast, patients in the high-risk group (4 or 5 factors present) have only a 25% five year survival. The IPI is, strictly speaking, only applicable to DLBCL and does not have sufficient discriminatory ability for low-grade lymphomas. More recently, a similar prognostic index has been developed for FL (57), where the important factors are considered to be:

- Age >60 years
- Elevated serum LDH
- Hemoglobin <12g/dl
- Advanced Stage 3 or 4
- More than 4 nodal sites of disease

For the purposes of this index, nine nodal sites are recognized: right and left cervical, right and left axillary, mediastinal, para-aortic (including iliac), mesenteric, right and left inguinal.

Although the REAL and WHO classifications have changed our understanding of the clinical pattern and prognosis of the disease, the treatment in the individual NHL subtypes is still largely dictated by the previous broad categorization into low- and high-grade lymphomas, as well as the sites of involvement. At one end of the scale, asymptomatic patients presenting with low-grade lymphomas may simply be followed without treatment until symptoms develop or transformation occurs. At the other end of the scale, patients presenting with high-grade disease may be successfully treated with multi-agent anthracycline-containing chemotherapy with most attaining a remission and up to 50% of patients achieving long-term disease-free survival (58).

The development of antibody therapies has added a new dimension to NHL and the immunological subtype is now a critical consideration in defining treatment, particularly for B-cell lymphomas, which express a variety of surface antigens against which monoclonal antibodies may be raised. There are a number which have NICE and FDA approval. The best known is rituximab, a chimeric monoclonal antibody against CD20, which is found in more than 95% of B-cell tumors. It can be used as a single agent, for example in indolent NHL, but is also additive with chemotherapy. Thus CHOP-rituximab (CHOP-R) is now standard treatment for advanced stage DLBCL and for early stage bulky DLBCL. It is also possible to combine monoclonal antibodies with toxins, to form immunotoxins, and with radioactive isotopes, to form radioimmunoconjugates. The anti-CD20 antibody, tositumomab, combined with iodine[131] (Bexxar®), is used to treat follicular lymphoma. As it is a gamma emitter it can be used for imaging as well as treatment. The combination of an anti-CD20 antibody, ibritumomab, with yttrium[90] (ibritumomab tiuxetan or Zevalin®) is also used for FL. This is a beta emitter, which has higher energies and is better for larger tumors. It has the advantage of being safe to administer on an outpatient basis. Both drugs show response rates of 65% to 80% in relapsed lymphoma.

Most relapses occur within the first two years after treatment. Once relapse occurs, particularly if remission is short, it is difficult to sustain further response to salvage chemotherapy, with or without immunotherapy. Current investigation is directed towards high-dose therapy with autologous bone marrow transplant after pre-conditioning with second-line chemotherapy (59).

Radiotherapy has a role in localized low and intermediate-grade NHL, for example in some MALT lymphomas and in rare instances of Stage 1 or 2 FL, where regional or involved field radiotherapy may be the treatment of choice if surgical excision is not an option. As 80% of NHL are widespread at presentation, it is usually inappropriate for first line therapy, but it is

frequently used as consolidatory therapy in many forms of NHL; for example, in primary mediastinal large B-cell lymphoma (PMBCL). It also has a role in high-dose salvage therapies and is extremely useful in local palliation, most NHL being very radiosensitive.

Key Points: Prognosis and Treatment

- In HL, disease stage is the most important prognostic factor and determines the intensity and nature of treatment
- HL is curable in the vast majority of cases
- In NHL, the histological subtype is the major determinant of treatment
- Paradoxically, cure is is most often achieved in the more aggressive large cell lymphomas

NODAL DISEASE

In HL, lymph node involvement is usually the only manifestation of disease, whereas in NHL nodal disease is frequently associated with extranodal sites of tumor. Lymph node enlargement tends to be greater in NHL than HL, but both types may produce either huge conglomerate tumor masses or no significant nodal enlargement. In nodular sclerosing and lymphocyte-depleted HL, involved lymph nodes tend to be normal in size or only moderately enlarged. A characteristic feature of lymphoma is that involved nodes tend to displace structures rather than invade them and in this respect they differ from carcinomas, an exception being the large cell high-grade lymphomas that are often locally invasive.

Imaging Techniques

Cross-Sectional Imaging

The introduction of *computed tomography* (CT) had a major impact on the way lymphoma was staged, rendering staging laparotomy largely redundant. Furthermore, the therapeutic impact of CT increased with time, as newer generation scanners were introduced (60). The ability of CT to demonstrate enlarged lymph nodes throughout the body and detect associated pathology in soft tissue structures, together with its reproducibility, has contributed to CT becoming the modality of choice for the staging and follow-up of lymphoma. Not only does it accurately demonstrate the full extent of disease, it also enables localization of the most appropriate lesion for consideration of percutaneous image-guided biopsy.

Ultrasound (US) will readily show lymph node enlargement in the celiac region, splenic hilum and porta hepatis (61–65). Frequently, however, the entire retroperitoneum cannot be shown, limiting its value in staging. Typically, lymphomatous nodal involvement produces uniformly hypoechoic, lobulated masses, appearances that are non-specific. The pattern of nodal vascular perfusion as assessed by power Doppler sonography may suggest a diagnosis of lymphoma, lymphomatous nodes being highly perfused in both the nodal center and periphery (66). The main value of US in lymphoma lies not in routine staging (67), for which it is not sufficiently reliable, but in confirming that a palpable mass is in fact nodal. It helps in solving specific problems in the liver,

spleen, or kidneys (68), and in providing image guidance for biopsy at many sites.

Although the accuracy of MR in detecting lymph node involvement is equal to that of CT (69–71), it has no particular advantage over CT. Its role is essentially adjunctive, used to solve problems in the identification of lymph node pathology (for example in the pelvis or supraclavicular fossa) or in monitoring response to treatment (72). As with CT and US, involved lymph nodes can be diagnosed only by size criteria (73). They are easily identified as relatively low/intermediate signal intensity masses on T1-weighted images and are of intermediate/high signal intensity in T2-weighted images (Fig. 33.3). As a result of advances in scanner technology, whole-body MR imaging has now become feasible for staging lymphoma. A combination of T1 weighted and fluid-sensitive short-tau inversion recovery (STIR) sequences enables identification of nodal enlargement as well as marrow infiltration. On STIR sequences, enlarged nodes may have very high signal intensity. Though whole body scanning at 3 T is faster, there is insufficient evidence for its superiority over conventional 1.5 T scanning (74). Similarly, there is no robust data on whole-body diffusion weighted imaging of lymphoma, though it may have a role in the differentiation of lymphoma from other causes of malignant nodal enlargement (75). At present, MR-specific lymphographic agents in the form of ultra-small superparamagnetic iron oxide particles do not have a role in the detection of lymphomatous involvement of normal-sized nodes (76,77). Though magnetic resonance spectroscopy (MRS) is not used for staging of lymphoma, preliminary evidence indicates a potential role in evaluation of response to treatment (78). Treated nodes, particularly in nodular sclerosing HL, may become necrotic and the nodes then have a signal intensity similar to that of fluid (Fig. 33.4). Calcification may occasionally develop following treatment for HL, which is clearly seen on CT. On MR the signal intensity of calcified nodes is markedly reduced.

Nuclear Medicine

For all three of the anatomical cross-sectional imaging modalities, recognition of nodal disease depends almost entirely on size criteria, and detection of disease in normal-sized nodes is not possible (though clustering of multiple small prominent nodes, for example in the anterior mediastinum or mesentery, is suggestive). Conversely, it is not possible to differentiate between nodes that are enlarged by lymphoma or reactive hyperplasia. Both distinctions are possible with functional radioisotope studies. Gallium-67 (Ga-67) and the positron emitter 2-[F-18]fluoro-2-deoxy-d-glucose (^{18}FDG) can demonstrate viable tumor cells within nodes with high sensitivity (79,80). Ga-67 is a cyclotron-produced radionuclide with a half-life of 3.2 days, which can be used in the citrate form as a tumor- and inflammation-localizing radiotracer. The accuracy of Ga-67 is dependent on several factors including cell type, and the location and size of the lesions. Its accuracy is greater for HL and high-grade lymphoma than for other forms. Its sensitivity diminishes for lesions under 2 cm in size, especially below the diaphragm, because of the limited resolution of gamma camera imaging and confounding bowel and splenic uptake. Furthermore some lymphomas, especially low-grade NHL, are non-gallium avid, resulting in too many false negative studies to render it effective as an isolated staging tool in NHL or HL (81–83). Thus, Ga-67 imaging has largely been

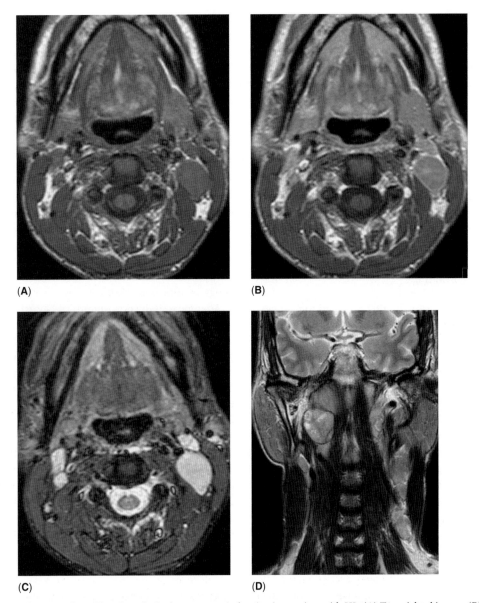

(A)　　　　　　　　　　　(B)

(C)　　　　　　　　　　　(D)

Figure 33.3 Axial MR images showing enlarged lymph nodes in the upper cervical region in a patient with HL. (**A**) T1-weighted image. (**B**)T1-weighted image post-intravenous gadolinium-DTPA. Note moderate uniform enhancement. (**C**) STIR image. Note marked T2 hyperintensity of right and left level 2 lymph nodes. (**D**) Coronal T2-weighted MR showing bilateral enlarged lymph nodes from level 2 to 4. Notice heterogeneous T2 hyperintensity of the large left level 2 node.

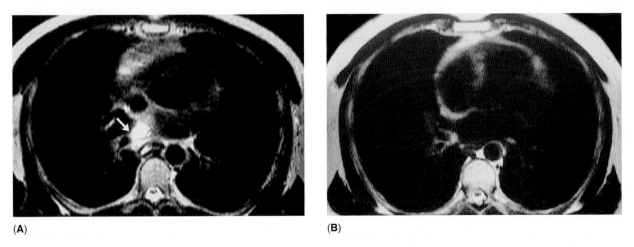

(A)　　　　　　　　　　　(B)

Figure 33.4 MR images of a patient with HL. (**A**) Pretreatment turbo spin-echo T2-weighted image shows a high signal intensity residual lymph node in the subcarinal space (arrowed). No further treatment was given. (**B**) A follow-up examination four months later shows complete resolution of the node, presumed to be necrotic.

replaced by positron emission tomography using 2-[F-18]fluoro-2-deoxy-D-glucose (FDG).

Positron Emission Tomography

In the last decade there have been numerous studies of the efficacy of 2-[F-18]fluoro-2-deoxy-D-glucose positron emission tomography (FDG PET) in the staging and re-staging of HL and NHL. Glucose metabolism is often increased in malignant tumors including HL and NHL, resulting in increased cellular uptake of FDG. Recent studies give results at least comparable to or better than CT for the detection of nodal and extranodal disease (84,85), with a trend to greater positivity for FDG PET on a lesion-by-lesion or site-based analysis. FDG PET tends to demonstrate a higher site positivity rate than Ga-67 (86,87), resulting in clinically significant upstaging in 10% to 20% of patients. It is more sensitive than Ga-67 for small masses (1–2 cm), below the diaphragm, and in the assessment of low-grade lymphomas (88–90).

In HL, upstaging as a result of FDG PET can lead to changes in therapy, for example, from radiotherapy to chemotherapy, or alteration of radiotherapy portals (91,92), but it is not recommended as an isolated staging tool (91), because of rare instances of false negative studies in specific anatomical sites such as the lung parenchyma.

In NHL, staging FDG PET gives important information for all grades of tumors by indicating tumor burden as well as the presence of extranodal disease. Most low-grade tumors do show increased uptake, the exceptions being some mucosa-associated lymphoid tissue (MALT) types, cutaneous lymphomas and small lymphocytic types (93,94). As with HL, it is not recommended for use as an isolated staging tool for this reason.

An important limitation of using FDG PET alone is its lack of precision in localization of abnormalities due to the lack of reliable anatomical landmarks, and the limited spatial resolution of current PET scanner technology. FDG PET imaging is particularly challenging in the neck, abdomen, and pelvis due to variable physiologic FDG uptake in lymphatic, bowel, and muscle tissue as well as by the renal excretion of the radiotracer, which can confound image interpretation. The introduction of PET/CT into clinical practice undoubtedly heralds a new era in staging HL and NHL, allowing accurate localization of morphological abnormalities together with their associated functional changes. Combined PET/CT devices acquire PET and CT images that are concurrent and co-registered, merging the functional information from PET with the anatomical information from CT. PET/CT is unique because it provides tissue characterization as well as assessment of the exact localization and the extent of tumor tissue. Debate is now centerd on whether it is necessary to carry out a full diagnostic CT scan as part of the PET/CT study, or whether a low dose CT for the purposes of attenuation correction and anatomical correlation, possibly in combination with a high resolution CT of the lungs, is sufficient (95,96).

After the introduction of third and fourth generation CT scanners and highly effective combination chemotherapy, lymphangiography as a method of evaluating non-enlarged infradiaphragmatic retroperitoneal lymph nodes was essentially abandoned. Though it remains the only imaging technique that demonstrates nodal architecture, the complementary yield over CT for lymph nodes of 1 cm or less is negligible (Fig. 33.5) (97). A recent study comparing FDG PET with lymphangiography in 28 patients with HL and a normal abdominal CT did not show any advantage for lymphangiography over FDG PET, but it was responsible for one false positive FDG PET finding as a result of inflammation produced by the lymphangiogram (98).

Nodal disease in HL and NHL may involve any site where lymph nodes are found anatomically, but for convenience this description is divided into the following sections: neck, thorax, abdomen, and pelvis.

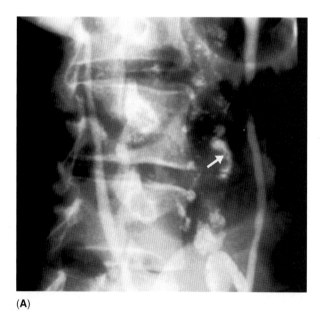

(A)

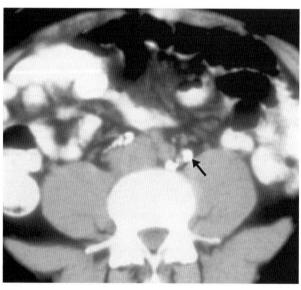

(B)

Figure 33.5 Lymphangiogram in Hodgkin's lymphoma. (A) Oblique view of the lumbar spine showing filling defects in involved left para-aortic lymph nodes (arrow). (B) Computed tomographic scan in the same patient as (A) performed on the same day, showing opacified unenlarged lymph nodes shown to be involved on LAG (arrow).

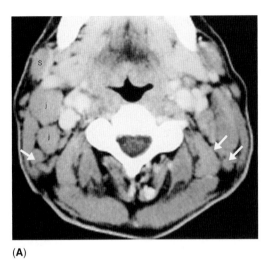
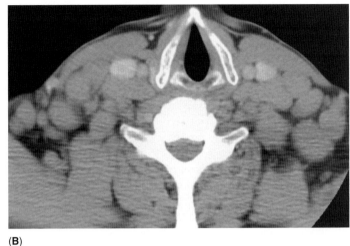

(A)   (B)

Figure 33.6 NHL involving lymph nodes in the neck. (**A**) Contrast-enhanced CT shows discrete enlargement of lymph nodes bilaterally at presentation. The involved nodes are larger on the right. Submandibular nodes (s), jugular node (j), spinal accessory node (arrows); (**B**) Contrast-enhanced CT in a patient with low-grade NHL showing bilateral midjugular and posterior triangle nodes.

Key Points: Nodal Imaging: General

- Recognition of nodal disease with CT and MR depends on size criteria alone
- CT and MR are equally efficacious in the depiction of lymph node enlargement above and below the diaphragm
- US is too insensitive to be used as a staging tool, but has a role in problem-solving and guidance for biopsy
- Functional techniques particularly FDG PET, enable identification of disease in normal-sized lymph nodes
- PET-CT provides unique information on disease extent and localization

Neck

Patients with HL most commonly present with a group of enlarged cervical lymph nodes, seen in 60% to 80% of cases. It may also be the presenting feature in NHL. HL typically involves the internal jugular chain of nodes initially, with further spread to the spinal accessory chain and the transverse cervical chain, these nodes forming the deep lymphatic chains of the neck (99). The internal jugular chain follows the course of the internal jugular vein, the spinal accessory nodes are found between the sternocleidomastoid and trapezius muscles in the posterior triangle, and the transverse cervical nodes join the internal jugular and spinal accessory nodes in the lower neck (Fig. 33.6). Nodes in the submandibular, submental, parotid, and retropharyngeal regions are occasionally involved. Patients with bulky supraclavicular or bilateral neck adenopathy are at increased risk of infradiaphragmatic disease.

The pattern of NHL is more haphazard than HL because of hematogenous spread and is more likely to be associated with extranodal and bulky disease.

Lymph nodes greater than 1 cm in short axis diameter are generally considered enlarged on CT. Although level 2 jugulodigastric lymph nodes may normally have a short axis diameter greater than 1 cm, most authorities would still call these enlarged if they exceed 1 cm short axis diameter. Minimally enlarged discrete lymph nodes seen in the neck in patients with lymphoma usually have a well-defined contour, but once the tumor has broken beyond the confines of the node, the fat planes between the nodal mass and adjacent structures are lost. Fibrosis following radiotherapy may also eliminate the fat planes, making post-treatment assessment difficult on clinical examination and CT. This is one anatomical area where the routine use of IV contrast material undoubtedly facilitates nodal evaluation. Central necrosis within a lymph node is rarely seen in the lymphomas, a striking contrast to the typical features seen in squamous carcinoma nodal metastasis on contrast-enhanced CT. Enhancement following IV injection of contrast medium is usually mild to moderate though occasionally marked (100).

Imaging, particularly CT, has a useful role in evaluating the neck in patients with lymphoma as it may:

- Identify involved nodes that are clinically impalpable
- Provide a baseline for assessing treatment response, particularly in patients treated with radiotherapy
- Identify recurrence in patients with thickened tissues due to previous radiotherapy (Fig. 33.7)

MR imaging may be particularly useful for defining the extent of lymphomatous masses in the lower neck and supraclavicular fossa (Fig. 33.8) (101).

Thorax

The frequency and distribution of intrathoracic lymph node involvement in HL and NHL differ, although the appearances on imaging are similar. As in the neck, lymph nodes >1 cm in diameter are considered enlarged both on CT and MR. However, the number of nodes present should also be taken into account; multiple nodes under 1 cm in diameter within the anterior mediastinum should certainly be regarded as suspicious. Nodes within the thorax are involved at the time of presentation in 60% to 85% of patients with HL and 25% to 40% of patients with NHL (36,102–103). Any intrathoracic group of nodes may be involved

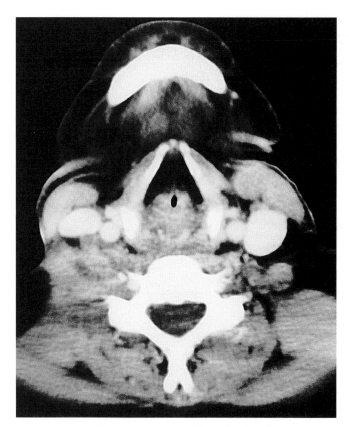

Figure 33.7 Recurrent low-grade NHL. A nodal mass on the right side of the neck is seen on contrast-enhanced CT, which has an ill-defined contour. The patient had previously been treated with radiotherapy.

in patients with lymphoma, but all the mediastinal sites are more frequently involved by HL than NHL, except the paracardiac and posterior mediastinal nodes, where the reverse is the case. The frequency of nodal involvement in HL is as follows:

- Prevascular and paratracheal (84%)
- Hilar (28%)
- Subcarinal (22%) (Fig. 33.9)
- Other sites (approx. 5%)
  o Aortopulmonary window
  o Anterior diaphragmatic
  o Internal mammary
  o Posterior mediastinal

The frequency of intrathoracic nodal involvement in NHL was analysed by Castellino et al. (104) as follows:

- Superior mediastinal (34%)
- Hilar (9%)
- Subcarinal (13%)
- Other sites (up to 10%) (Fig. 33.10)

In most cases lymphadenopathy is bilateral but asymmetric. Almost all patients with nodular sclerosing HL have disease in the anterior mediastinum. The great majority of cases of HL show enlargement of two or more nodal groups, whereas only one nodal group is involved in up to half of the cases of NHL. Hilar nodal enlargement is rare without associated mediastinal involvement, particularly in HL. The posterior mediastinum is infrequently involved but if disease is present in the lower part of the mediastinum, contiguous retrocrural disease is likely (105). Although nodes in the internal mammary chains and paracardiac regions

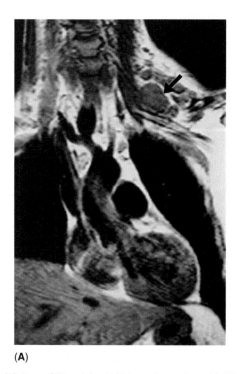

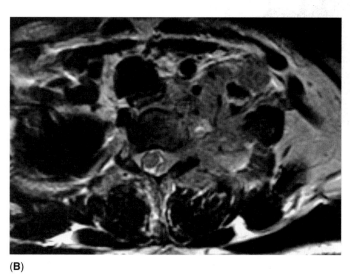

(A)   **(B)**

Figure 33.8 (**A**) Coronal T1-weighted MR image in a patient with HL. The nodes are seen as intermediate signal intensity masses (arrowed). (**B**) Axial T2-weighted image in a different patient with NHL. There is excellent soft tissue contrast between the infiltrative mass in the left supraclavicular fossa, the adjacent musculature and fat. Note extension of tumour into the intervertebral foramen and vertebral body.

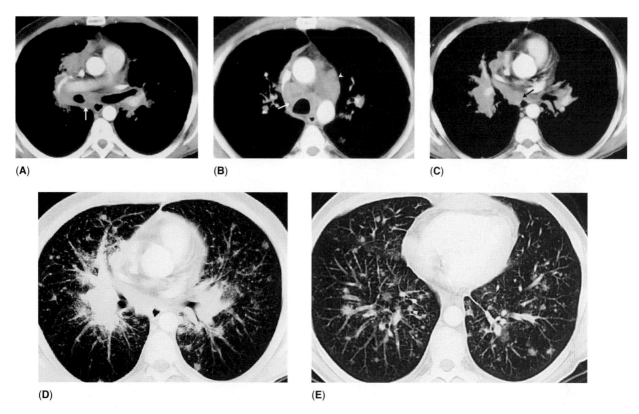

(A) (B) (C)

(D) (E)

Figure 33.9 Extensive mediastinal lymph node and lung parenchymal involvement in NHL. (A) Subcarinal lymph node enlarged (arrowed). (B) Scan above the level at (A) showing lymph node enlargement in the paratracheal region (arrow) and in the aortopulmonary region (arrowhead). (C) Lymph node enlargement in the azygo-esophageal region in the same patient as (A). (D) In the same patient as shown in (A–C) when viewed on lung settings, there is peribronchial and juxtamediastinal lung parencymal involvement with linear shadowing and more discrete peripheral nodularity also shown in Figure 33.9 (E).

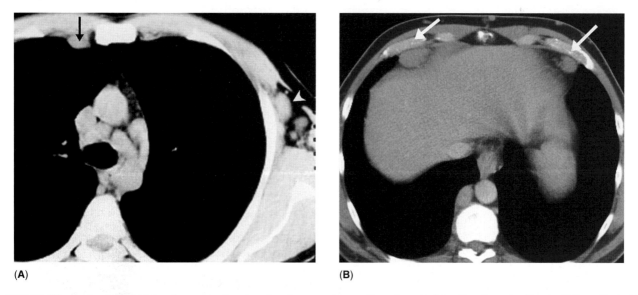

(A) (B)

Figure 33.10 (A) CT scan showing right internal mammary lymph node enlargement (arrowed) together with left axillary (arrowhead) and middle mediastinal lymph node enlargement. (B) CT scan of a patient with NHL. There are bilateral peridiaphragmatic nodes (arrows) in addition to a large right retrocrural node.

are rarely involved at presentation, they become important as sites of recurrence as they may not be included in conventional radiation fields (Fig. 33.10) (106).

On CT, enlarged nodes may be discrete or matted together, and usually show only minor enhancement after injection of IV contrast medium (Fig. 33.11). Calcification prior to therapy is extremely rare, and does not appear to have any prognostic implications, though it is common in more aggressive subtypes (107,108). It is seen occasionally following therapy. Cystic degeneration seen rarely in both HL and NHL may persist following therapy when the rest of the nodal masses shrink away (Fig. 33.4) (109). Cystic change is more likely with large anterior mediastinal

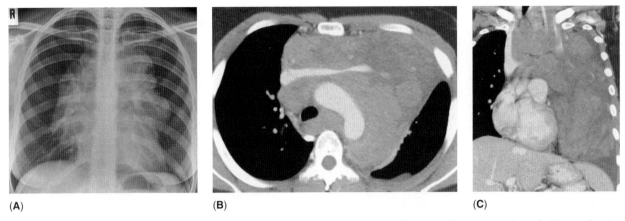

(A)   **(B)**   **(C)**

Figure 33.11 Massive mediastinal lymph node enlargement in a patient with HL. (A) Plain chest radiograph. (B) Contrast-enhanced CT scan showing anterior mediastinal lymph node mass. (C) Coronal reformatted image in another patient with HL beautifully demonstrates the effect of the mass on the mediastinal structures.

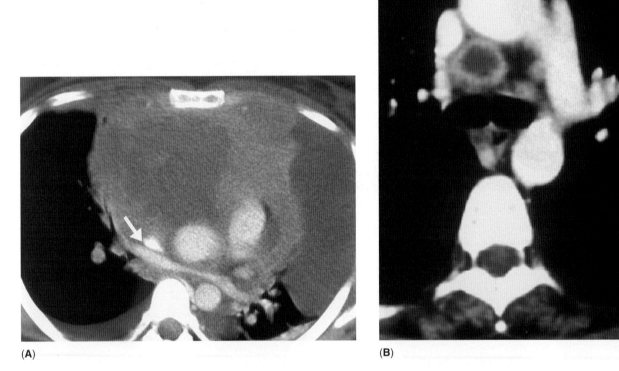

(A)   **(B)**

Figure 33.12 Cystic change within lymph nodes. (A) Cystic change within a mediastinal mass of nodes. Notice also severe extrinsic compression of the superior vena cava (arrowed). (B) Ring enhancement following IV injection of contrast medium due to cystic change within a paratracheal lymph node.

masses, but again this does not have any prognostic significance, nor does it indicate a particular pathological subtype, occurring in both nodular sclerosing HL and primary mediastinal large B-cell lymphoma (Fig. 33.12) (109).

In about 10% of patients with HL, CT demonstrates enlarged mediastinal nodes despite a normal chest radiograph (Fig. 33.13) (103). Patients with HL who have even a moderate volume of unsuspected intrathoracic disease at CT have a poorer prognosis (110). CT will change clinical stage in up to 16% of patients with lymphoma and management may be altered in up to 25%, particularly where radiotherapy is planned. Thus, the effect of

CT is more pronounced in patients with HL than NHL (103,104,111–113).

Even in patients with bulky disease, CT frequently provides additional information such as:

- The inferior extent of the mass and its relationship to the heart
- The presence of pericardial thickening and effusion, which can be distinguished from lymphadenopathy
- The presence of significant airway narrowing and central venous occlusion

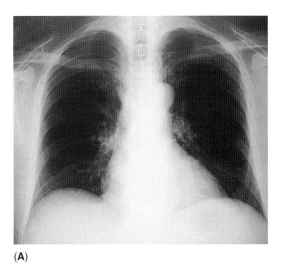
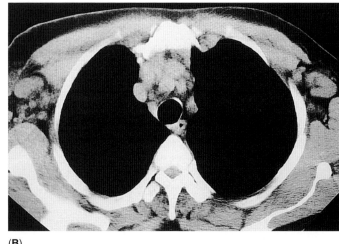

(A) **(B)**

Figure 33.13 (A) Plain chest radiograph and (B) CT scan in a patient with NHL. The plain chest radiograph appears normal but CT shows multiple enlarged lymph nodes in the mediastinum, indicating intrathoracic disease. Note left internal mammary and bilateral axillary lymph node enlargement.

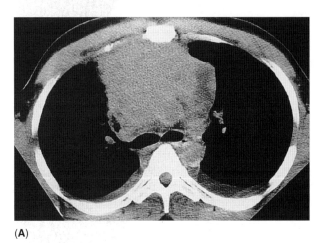
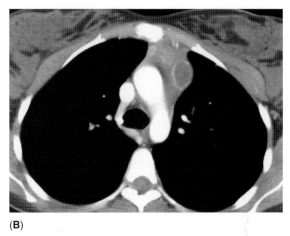

(A) **(B)**

Figure 33.14 CT scans in two patients with HL. (A) Before treatment there is a large anterior mediastinal mass, probably involving the thymus. Note an area of low density within the mass on the left which either represents necrosis or cystic change. (B) Following treatment in a different patient there is a small residual mass containing a central low attenuation area surrounded by a rim of calcification.

Large anterior mediastinal masses usually represent thymic infiltration as well as a nodal mass (114) (Fig. 33.14). Enlarged nodes can usually be distinguished from a thymic mass but in up to 30% of cases, thymic involvement can only be diagnosed on evaluation of follow-up studies after treatment, when the thymus has resumed its normal shape (115). Thymic infiltration may be seen in both HL and NHL. Although the thymus is usually seen on CT as a homogeneous soft tissue mass, cystic areas within the mass may be identified both on CT and MR, especially with primary mediastinal large B-cell lymphoma (Fig. 33.12) (116). These cysts are more frequently detected on MR (117). It has been shown that in NHL high-grade tumors tend to be more heterogeneous on pre- and post-contrast CT scans than low-grade tumors of comparable size, but the clinical relevance of this is uncertain (118). Similarly, there is some evidence that heterogeneous high T2 signal intensity within mediastinal masses is associated with high-grade tumors and poorer survival (119,120). A large anterior mediastinal mass, especially when it exceeds one third of the transthoracic diameter at the level of T6, is an adverse prognostic factor in HL, as recognized in the Ann Arbor classification. CT also depicts local complications of the more aggressive lymphomas, such as airway compromise and central venous obstruction, both of which are particular features of primary mediastinal large B cell lymphoma (121).

Impalpable axillary nodal enlargement is also frequently detected on CT in HL and NHL, and may be unilateral or bilateral (Figs. 33.10 and 33.13b). Occasionally uninvolved nodes contain fat centrally, helping distinguish nodes involved by lymphoma from those with benign reactive hyperplasia.

MR imaging of the chest may provide additional information to CT in a problem-solving role, for example in the demonstration of nodal enlargement in areas where CT evaluation is difficult, such as the subcarinal space and aortopulmonary window (Fig. 33.15). MR imaging is also helpful for defining the full extent of disease, for example infiltration of the chest wall.

When reporting thoracic CT for staging HL or NHL, it is always important to check all possible sites of involvement because minimally enlarged nodes in such sites as the internal

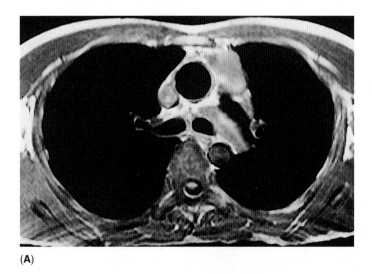

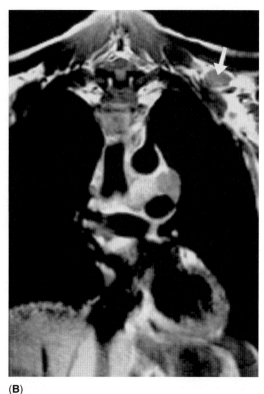

(A)   **(B)**

Figure 33.15 MR images in a patient with HL showing nodal enlargement in the anterior mediastinum and aortopulmonary window. Turbo spin-echo T1-weighted images: (**A**) axial; (**B**) coronal. The enlarged nodes have an intermediate signal intensity lower than that of fat but higher than that of muscle. Note an enlarged lymph node in the left supraclavicular fossa (arrowed).

mammary group or diaphragmatic nodes are easily overlooked (Fig. 33.10A and B).

Key Points: Supradiaphragmatic Nodal Disease

- Sixty to eighty percent of patients with HL present with enlarged neck nodes. It is also a common presentation in NHL
- Sixty to eighty percent of patients with HL and 25% to 40% of patients with NHL have prevascular and paratracheal lymphadenopathy at diagnosis
- Ten percent of patients with HL have enlarged nodes detected on CT but a normal chest radiograph
- Hilar lymphadenopathy is rarely seen in isolation
- A large anterior mediastinal mass may represent lymphomatous infiltration of the thymus
- Enlarged axillary nodes are found in 6% to 20% of HL at diagnosis

Abdomen and Pelvis

At presentation, the retroperitoneal nodes are involved in 25% to 35% of patients with HL, and 45% to 55% of patients with NHL (122–124). Mesenteric lymph nodes are involved in more than half of patients with NHL and <5% of patients with HL (122–125). Other sites, as in the porta hepatis and around the splenic hilum, are also less frequently involved in HL than NHL. In HL, nodal spread is predictably from one lymph node group to contiguous groups (126,127). In this context, the term "contiguous" does not mean physical contiguity but through directly connected lymphatic pathways. Thus, involvement of retrocrural nodes should prompt close scrutiny of the coeliac axis nodes. Nodes are frequently of normal size or only minimally enlarged (97). In NHL, nodal involvement is frequently non-contiguous, bulky, and is more frequently associated with extranodal disease.

In HL the coeliac axis, splenic hilar and porta hepatis nodes are involved in about one third of patients, and splenic hilar nodal involvement is almost always associated with diffuse splenic infiltration (Figs. 33.16 and 33.17). In the porta hepatis, the node of the foramen of Winslow (portocaval node) is important. It lies between the portal vein and inferior vena cava (Fig. 33.18) and has a triangular or lozenge shape; its normal transverse diameter is up to 3 cm and in the anterio-posterior plane is approximately 1 cm (128). Enlargement of this node is easily overlooked, which is particularly important if it is the only site of relapse. In the coeliac axis, multiple normal-sized nodes may be seen, which can be difficult to evaluate because involved normal-sized nodes are frequent in HL (127). In this context, the functional information provided by FDG PET can be extremely helpful.

In NHL, discrete mesenteric nodal enlargement or masses may be seen with or without retroperitoneal nodal enlargement (Fig. 33.19). Large-volume nodal disease in both the mesentery and retroperitoneum, may give rise to the so-called "hamburger" sign, in which a loop of bowel is compressed between the two large nodal masses (Fig. 33.19C). In NHL, regional nodal involvement is frequently seen in patients with primary extranodal lymphoma involving an abdominal viscus. Enhancement following IV injection of contrast medium is mild and calcification is rare before treatment. Analysis of enhancement characteristics of nodes may

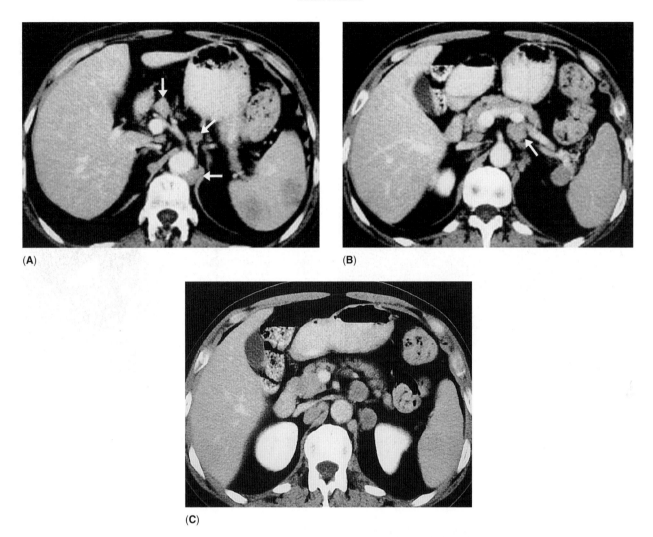

Figure 33.16 HL. CT scans showing involvement of (**A**) coeliac axis lymph nodes and a retrocrural lymph node on the left (arrowed). Note focal deposits in the spleen. (**B**) At a lower level there is an enlarged lymph node at the splenic hilum and a further enlarged node is seen in the superior mesenteric group (arrowed). The portal node is prominent but not enlarged on CT criteria. (**C**) At the level of the upper poles of the kidneys, enlarged retroperitoneal lymph nodes are seen.

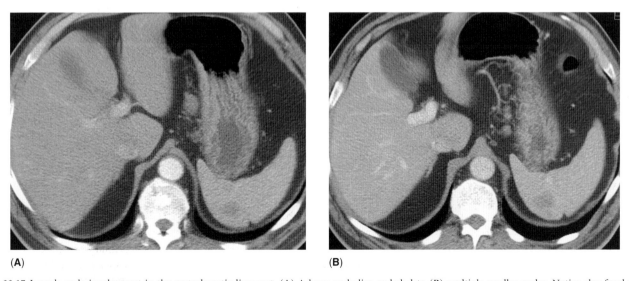

Figure 33.17 Lymph node involvement in the gastrohepatic ligament. (**A**) A large node lies cephalad to (**B**) multiple smaller nodes. Notice also focal splenic lesion.

help differentiate lymphoma from infectious causes such as TB or atypical infections. Central necrosis, peripheral or multilocular enhancement favor infection (129). Multiple normal-sized mesenteric nodes should be regarded with suspicion for the diagnosis of lymphoma, as should nodularity and streakiness within the mesentery. The latter presumably reflects dilatation and obstruction of lymphatic vessels.

In the pelvis all nodal groups may be involved in both HL and NHL (Fig. 33.20). Presentation with enlarged inguinal/femoral lymphadenopathy is seen in less than 20% of cases of HL. However when it does occur, careful attention must be paid to the evaluation of pelvic nodes on imaging as these will be the next contiguous sites of tumor spread. In patients with massive pelvic disease, MR is helpful for delineating the full extent of tumor in the coronal and axial planes. It can also help differentiate between engorged venous tributaries and lymph nodes, and in problem-solving (69,71).

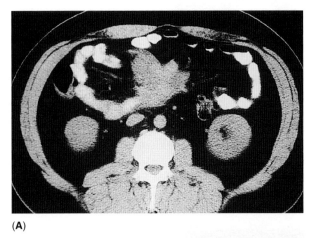

Figure 33.18 A patient with NHL showing an enlarged portocaval lymph node (arrowed). There is also nodal enlargement in the porta hepatis, around the coeliac axis and the aorta, as well as multiple small focal splenic lesions.

Key Points: Abdominal Nodal Disease

- Retroperitoneal lymphadenopathy is more commonly seen in NHL than HL
- Mesenteric lymphadenopathy is seen in over 50% of cases in NHL
- The coeliac, splenic hilar, and porta hepatis nodes are involved in about 30% of HL patients. Splenic hilar lymphadenopathy is almost invariably accompanied by splenic infiltration

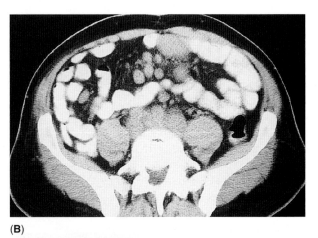

(A)

(B)

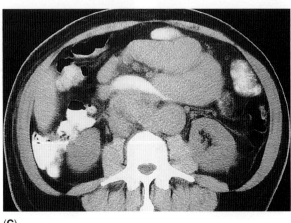

(C)

Figure 33.19 CT scans in three different patients with NHL. (A) A large mesenteric mass without evidence of retroperitoneal lymph node involvement. (B) Discrete nodal enlargement of mesenteric lymph nodes associated with retroperitoneal lymphadenopathy. (C) A large mass in the mesentery associated with a mass of retroperitoneal lymph nodes. These masses compress an opacified loop of bowel, giving rise to the "hamburger" sign.

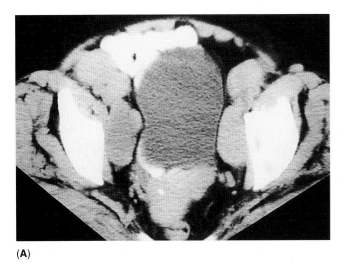

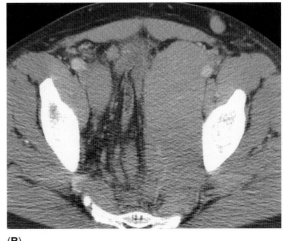

(A)   (B)

Figure 33.20 Pelvic lymph node enlargement in two different patients with NHL. (A) Moderate obturator and external iliac disease on the right. (B) Massive disease on the left more than the right, displacing and compressing the pelvic viscera.

EXTRANODAL DISEASE

In about 40% of cases, the vast majority of which are NHL, lymphoma arises primarily in extranodal sites. The pathological subtypes that most commonly arise extranodally are DLCBL, mucosa-associated lymphoid tissue (MALT) types and FL. The most common locations affected in decreasing order of frequency are Waldeyer's ring, the stomach and small intestine, the soft tissues and the orbit. There is a propensity for lymphomas associated with immunodeficiency and also those that develop in childhood to arise extranodally. Secondary extranodal lymphoma occurs due to spread of lymph node disease into adjacent structures and organs, and may be seen in both HL and NHL. The presence of extranodal disease is an adverse prognostic factor as recognized in the IPI (55), though localized DLBCL (stage I or IIE) does not have a worse prognosis than stage IV disease unless it arises in the testis. The increase in incidence of NHL has been much more marked for extranodal sites, especially in the gastrointestinal (GI) tract, central nervous system (CNS), and eyes (6). Furthermore, visceral lymphoma can mimic many other disease entities, making recognition of the radiological appearances of extranodal lymphoma increasingly important.

As with nodal disease, CT is generally excellent in the depiction of extranodal lymphoma. There are specific areas where MR and US perform better, as indicated in the relevant sections. In addition, FDG PET is generally more sensitive and accurate in the staging of extranodal disease, largely because of its ability to demonstrate bone marrow involvement (85). Data also indicates that FDG PET and PET-CT are more sensitive than CT in identifying organ involvement, reaching sensitivities of 86% and 73% for PET and PET-CT respectively, with only 37% sensitivity for CT (130,131). The use of PET or PET-CT can result in disease being upstaged in up to 40% of cases, most frequently secondary to demonstration of splenic or extranodal disease undetected by CT (130, 131). However, there are certain areas where CT is more sensitive than FDG PET, for example in the depiction of miliary pulmonary parenchymal involvement. The advantages of PET/CT over isolated FDG PET or CT are obvious in this respect, enabling accurate anatomical localization of extranodal, and nodal, disease.

A modified Ann Arbor staging classification is used, with isolated involvement of one extranodal site generally being regarded as stage IE disease. Concomitant involvement of locoregional lymph nodes is stage IIE. However, some authorities consider any bone marrow involvement, even if associated with primary bone lymphoma, as stage IV.

Thorax

Lung

Secondary involvement of the lung parenchyma at presentation in HL is most commonly by direct invasion from involved hilar and mediastinal nodes, hence the frequent perihilar or juxtamediastinal location. In this situation, there is no effect on staging: the "E" lesion. However, peripheral subpleural masses or consolidation without a visible connection to enlarged nodes in the mediastinum or hila also occur in both HL and NHL, indicating stage IV disease. On chest radiography, lung parenchymal involvement is seen three times more frequently in HL (12%) than in NHL (102) (Fig. 33.21). Parenchymal involvement in HL is almost invariably accompanied by intrathoracic adenopathy, whereas in NHL pulmonary or pleural lesions may be seen without mediastinal or hilar lymphadenopathy in as many as 50% of cases (132). However, if the mediastinal and hilar nodes have been previously irradiated, recurrence confined to the lungs may be seen in both HL and NHL (133). Thus, in a patient with HL who has not received radiotherapy, in whom there is no evidence of hilar or mediastinal disease, a pulmonary abnormality probably represents pathology other than HL (103,132). In the presence of widespread extrathoracic disease, parenchymal involvement is more common, especially in AIDS-related lymphoma (ARL) (134).

The radiographic changes in both HL and NHL are varied and difficult to characterize. Pulmonary involvement is frequently perihilar or juxtamediastinal (Fig. 33.9) (135). The most common pattern is one or more discrete nodules resembling primary or

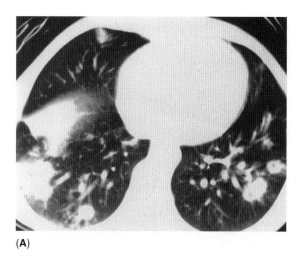
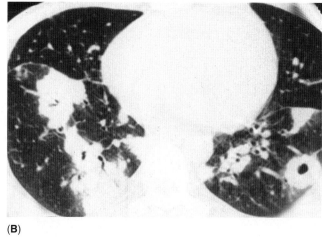

(A)   **(B)**

Figure 33.21 (**A**), (**B**) CT scan at two different levels showing pulmonary involvement in a patient with HL. There are multiple areas of consolidation and poorly defined nodules, some of which are cavitating.

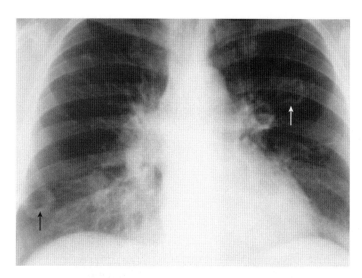

Figure 33.22 Chest radiograph on a patient with HL, bilateral hilar lymph node enlargement and cavitating lung nodules in both lungs (arrowed).

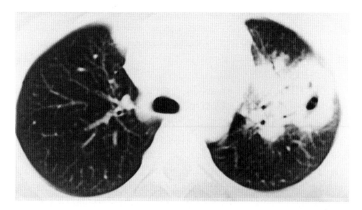

Figure 33.23 Pulmonary involvement in a patient with high-grade NHL. The CT scan shows consolidation with air bronchograms and cavitation.

metastatic carcinoma, but usually less well-defined, which may also cavitate (Figs. 33.9, 33.21, and 33.22) (136–138).Rounded or segmental consolidation with visible air bronchograms, often subpleural, is another common pattern (Figs. 33.23 and 33.24). Peribronchial pulmonary nodules (Fig. 33.25) extending from the

hila, or focal streaky shadowing, also peribronchial, may be seen in association with the consolidation, reflecting spread along the peribronchial lymphatics. The least common pattern is widespread reticulonodular (lymphangitic) shadowing. This is sufficiently rare in HL to necessitate excluding other conditions causing interstitial lung disease. Endobronchial disease causing atelectasis is extremely rare, but is still more likely than extrinsic occlusion by neighboring lymph node enlargement (139).

Primary (or isolated) pulmonary lymphoma is uncommon (1% of all extranodal presentations), and is usually due to NHL. Low-grade B-cell lymphomas comprise the majority of primary NHL of the lung. Most are lymphomas of mucosa- (or bronchus-) associated lymphoid tissue (MALT or BALT), the so-called extranodal marginal zone lymphomas (140,141). These low-grade lymphomas occur most frequently in patients in their fifth to sixth decades of life, the clinical course is indolent, and there is an 80% to 90% survival rate at five years. Many patients are asymptomatic. As with other subtypes, the radiographic findings are non-specific. Solitary nodules are identified on chest radiographs in >50% of cases, ranging from 2 to 20 cm. Multiple nodules may occur, or there may be localized or multiple areas of consolidation (142). Ill-defined alveolar multifocal opacities are also seen (143). Imaging appearances are variable, but focal consolidation is more common than nodulation, and both are more often multiple than solitary (144). Bronchiolitis and interstitial disease are infrequent. Fairly low level FDG uptake has also been described (144). Hilar or mediastinal lymph nodes are rarely involved.

MALT lymphoma constitutes the majority of primary pulmonary lymphomas, high-grade DLBCL accounting for the remaining 15% to 20% (142). These patients are usually symptomatic with dyspnea, cough, and B symptoms. Solitary or multiple nodules are the most common radiographic pattern, and rapid growth is a feature that can cause diagnostic confusion (145). These tumors are often locally aggressive with involvement of adjacent structures including the chest wall.

Primary pulmonary HL is extremely rare (142). The most common findings are single or multiple nodules with an upper zone predominance and a relatively high incidence of cavitation (146,147).

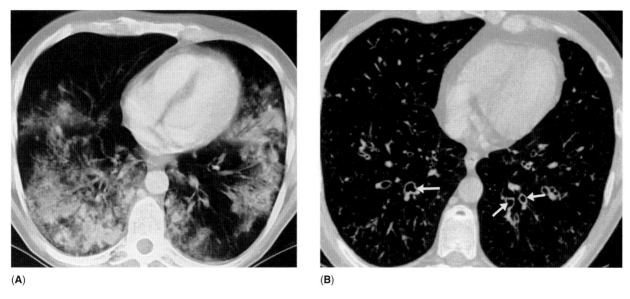

Figure 33.24 (A) Segmental consolidation bilaterally in a patient with NHL. (B) The same patient as in (A) following treatment showing almost complete resolution of the parenchymal disease, but with residual mild bilateral bronchiectasis (arrowed).

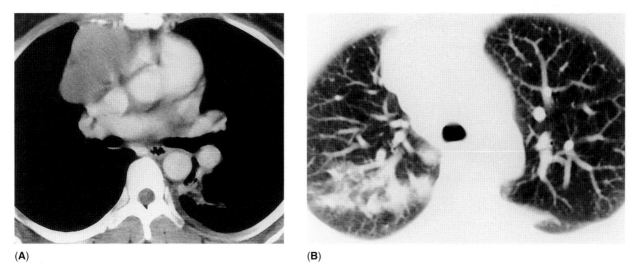

Figure 33.25 Pulmonary involvement in a patient with HL. (A) A predominantly right-sided anterior mediastinal mass. (B) A CT scan showing peribronchial pulmonary nodules extending from the hila.

The diverse appearances of pulmonary lymphoma provide a particular diagnostic challenge because many of these patients have other reasons for developing lung disease, such as:

- Opportunistic infection either following or during chemotherapy
- Pneumonitis following radiotherapy
- Drug-related pulmonary fibrosis

In one study of 60 patients with HIV, cavitation, size <1 cm and centrilobular distribution favored infection rather than lymphoma (148). However, a differential diagnosis is difficult and the diagnosis of pulmonary lymphoma, particularly in previously treated patients, must take into account full clinical information. Diagnosis requires an adequate biopsy specimen and though percutaneous or transbronchial biopsy will often establish the diagnosis, open biopsy may be necessary.

Pleural Disease

Pleural effusions due to lymphoma occur in up to 10% of patients at presentation and are nearly always accompanied by mediastinal lymph node enlargement, and sometimes by pulmonary involvement, visible on a chest radiograph (102). Most effusions are unilateral, are usually exudates and may disappear with irradiation of mediastinal nodes. Such effusions probably result from venous or lymphatic obstruction by enlarged mediastinal nodes, rather than direct neoplastic involvement, and may be detected on CT in over 50% of patients with mediastinal nodal involvement (Fig. 33.26) (137). Chylothorax is only occasionally encountered. Solid soft tissue pleural masses are rare at presentation and are seen more often in recurrent disease, usually accompanied by an effusion. In one review, 40% of patients with an effusion had adjacent extrapleural or pleural soft tissue disease, with nodules or thickening of the parietal pleura being a common finding (Fig. 33.26B) (149).

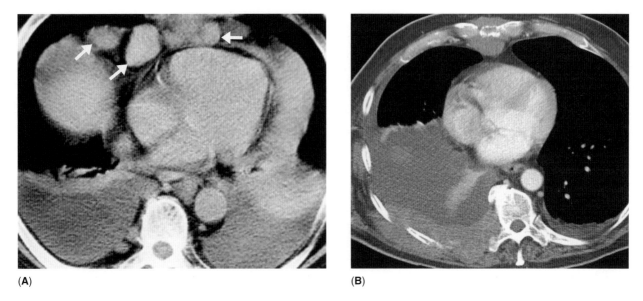

Figure 33.26 Pleural and pericardial involvement in two different patients with NHL. (**A**) Pericardial involvement in a high-grade NHL. The CT scan shows massive pericardial disease with a large soft tissue mass encasing the pericardium. There is also discrete paracardiac lymph node enlargement (arrows). Note too, the bilateral pleural effusions. (**B**) A large pleurally based mass posteriorly invades the chest wall. There is an associated pleural effusion. A second mass is involving the sternum.

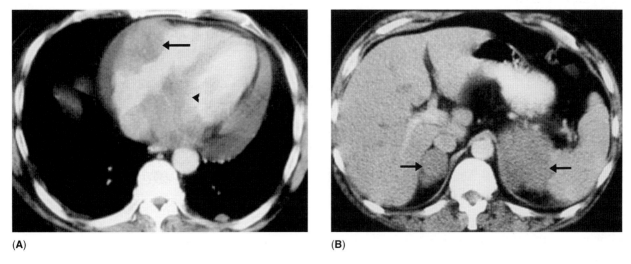

Figure 33.27 Pericardial, cardiac, and adrenal involvement in NHL. (**A**) CT scan through the heart following IV injection of contrast medium showing a moderate-sized pericardial effusion and mass lesions involving the right ventricle (arrow) and left ventricle (arrowhead). (**B**) CT scan of the abdomen in the same patient showing lymphomatous masses in both adrenal glands (arrowed).

Chest Wall

Involvement of the chest wall occurs most commonly in HL as a result of direct extension from an anterior mediastinal mass. Less commonly, large masses of NHL may arise primarily in the soft tissues of the thoracic wall. Both direct invasion and primary chest wall lymphoma are better demonstrated on MR than CT. T2-weighted images are preferable to T1-weighted images because of excellent contrast between the high signal intensity mass and the low signal intensity of the normal muscles of the chest wall. In this way MR may allow more accurate planning of radiotherapy portals (150,151). Bony destruction is uncommon and suggests infection or carcinoma.

Pericardium and Heart

Pericardial effusions are seen on CT in 6% of patients with HL at presentation (152). Effusions are presumptive evidence of pericardial involvement and in all such patients there is coexistent large mediastinal adenopathy extending over the cardiac margins. Pericardial effusions are frequently seen in patients undergoing therapy for HL and NHL. They are usually distinguishable from pericardial lymphomatous involvement (Figs. 33.26 and 33.27) because they develop when the patient is on chemotherapy and are usually small and resolve spontaneously.

Direct invasion of the heart may be seen in patients with aggressive, bulky mediastinal masses and in this rare situation MR is the best technique for defining the presence and extent of cardiac involvement (Fig. 33.27) (153). Intracardiac masses can occur with high-grade T-cell lymphomas and large B-cell lymphoma, especially in the setting of ARL or post-transplant lymphoproliferative disorder (PTLD).

Thymus

Thymic involvement occurs in 30% to 50% of patients with newly diagnosed HL (114). It may be impossible to distinguish the

enlarged thymus on CT or MR from adjacent lymph node enlargement, which is usually but not invariably present (Fig. 33.14). On CT, the gland may be of homogeneous soft tissue density, similar to adjacent lymph nodes. On MR too the signal intensity on both T1- and T2-weighted images is similar to that of enlarged nodes. Primary mediastinal B-cell lymphoma also involves the thymus, and in contradistinction to most other types of lymphoma can cause vascular occlusion and airway obstruction. SVCO is present in over 40% of affected individuals (Fig. 33.12A). Cysts and calcification may be seen within the enlarged gland, either at presentation or during follow-up on both CT and MR (115,117). Cysts are better appreciated on MR but calcification is more easily recognized on CT (117). As with other malignancies, benign thymic rebound hyperplasia can develop after completion of chemotherapy, which can be difficult to differentiate from recurrent disease. Unfortunately, functional imaging with Ga-67 or FDG PET may not always differentiate between the two and clinical correlation combined with follow-up studies may be necessary.

Key Points: Extranodal Thoracic Disease

- Secondary involvement of the lung parenchyma is seen three times more frequently in HL than NHL. Lung involvement in HL is almost invariably associated with mediastinal lymphadenopathy
- Most primary low-grade lymphomas of the lung are MALT or BALT tumors
- Pleural effusions are associated with mediastinal lymphadenopathy in over 50% of cases
- Chest wall invasion occurs most commonly in HL by direct extension of a mediastinal mass
- Thymic infiltration occurs in 30% to 50% of patients newly diagnosed with HL

Breast

Primary breast lymphoma is rare, accounting for less than 1% of all breast tumors and approximately 2% of all lymphomas. In the majority of cases of primary breast lymphoma, masses are solitary, but synchronous bilateral disease and metachronous contralateral disease are well recognized. Utrasound demonstrates fairly well-defined hypoechoic lesions, often with pronounced vascularity on power Doppler (154). An echogenic rim and posterior acoustic enhancement occur in approximately one third of cases (155). A more diffuse pattern is occasionally seen resembling inflammatory carcinoma (156). This is well recognized in pregnancy and lactation, especially in cases of Burkitt's and other high-grade lymphomas. In secondary lymphoma, multiple masses (not infrequently impalpable) with associated large volume axillary adenopathy are seen. Masses tend to be better defined than in primary disease (157). Calcification and distortion are rare in primary and secondary forms, and as anticipated, lesions usually enhance markedly at dynamic contrast-enhanced MR and are FDG-avid.

Abdomen

Spleen

The spleen is involved in 30% to 40% of patients with HL (124,158). In the majority of cases this occurs in the presence of nodal disease above and below the diaphragm (159). It is the sole abdominal focus of disease in 10% of adults presenting with HL clinically confined to sites above the diaphragm. For the purposes of staging, the spleen is regarded as a lymph node in the Ann Arbor classification and therefore, a patient with supradiaphragmatic nodal disease and splenic involvement would be stage III$_{(s)}$. To date, all imaging techniques have been unreliable in the detection of splenic involvement, partly because in the vast majority of cases of splenic HL, infiltration is usually microscopic, or there are nodules under 1 cm in size. An enlarged spleen is not a reliable indicator of disease as one third of patients with HL and splenomegaly do not have involvement of the spleen. However, one third of normal-sized spleens in patients with HL or NHL are found to contain tumor at laparotomy (123,124).

Occasionally, focal splenic nodules >1 cm are seen on cross-sectional imaging (Figs. 33.16 and 33.17). These lesions have a non-specific appearance, are usually hypoechoic on US, isodense on unenhanced CT, and enhance to a lesser extent than normal parenchyma following IV injection of contrast medium (Fig. 33.16). Splenic lymphoma can take the form of a solitary lesion, miliary nodules or multiple low-attenuation masses. Detection of such lesions has improved with the advent of multidetector CT, since the entire spleen can be imaged in the portal venous phase of enhancement, and lesions no larger than a few millimeters can be identified. The differential diagnosis of focal lesions includes opportunistic infection, and occasionally sarcoid or metastases, which can appear identical. Infectious nodules tend to be smaller and more uniform in size (160).

In early studies, the sensitivity of US in demonstrating splenic involvement was extremely low (not exceeding 35%) (61), although in a more recent study US was more sensitive than CT (63% vs. 37%), detecting nodules down to 3 mm in size and identifying diffuse infiltration more often than CT (63). Although this low sensitivity for the detection of splenic involvement on imaging is disappointing, failure to detect splenic infiltration in HL is now of less clinical importance than before, since most patients with early-stage disease who have occult splenic infiltration will be treated with multi-agent chemotherapy. This has also resulted in the cessation of staging laparotomy for Stages I and II HL in Europe.

Up to 40% of patients with NHL have splenic involvement at some stage. Primary splenic NHL is rare, accounting for 1% to 2% of all NHL. It is a particular feature of mantle cell and splenic marginal zone lymphoma, where massive splenomegaly can occur. In contradistinction to HL, the presence of splenomegaly generally indicates involvement by lymphoma, and infarction is a frequent complication (Fig. 33.28). Primary disease usually presents as a mass or masses rather than splenomegaly alone (161). Serial measurements of splenic volume during treatment may be helpful in the assessment of response to treatment where there is diffuse infiltration (162). However, despite excellent results in some series, splenic volumes and indices have not gained widespread acceptance, as measurement is somewhat cumbersome (163–165). Unfortunately, the intrinsic tissue contrast of MR is insufficient for consistent recognition of diffuse infiltration (73), though IV superparamagnetic iron oxide (SPIO) may improve detection of diffuse and focal infiltration (166–168). FDG PET detects splenic infiltration more accurately than CT or Ga-67 scintigraphy (85,169).

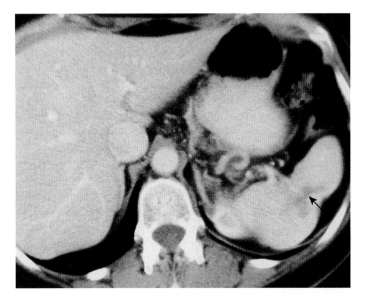

Figure 33.28 Post-contrast CT scan showing splenic infarction (arrow) in a patient with mantle-cell NHL.

Key Points: Splenic Involvement

■ In 10% of HL, the spleen is the only site of subdiaphragmatic disease
■ An enlarged spleen is not a reliable indicator of disease in HL
■ Staging laparotomy is no longer undertaken because early relapse due to undetected splenic involvement can be salvaged by treatment with chemotherapy

Liver

In HL, around 5% of patients have liver involvement at presentation, nearly always associated with splenic involvement (159,170). In NHL about 15% of patients have hepatic infiltration, though the incidence is higher in the pediatric population and in recurrent disease. True primary lymphoma of the liver is extremely rare, though the incidence is increasing, especially in immunocompromised patients. It is indistinguishable radiologically from other forms of hepatic malignancy such as hepatocellular carcinoma or metastatic disease. Up to 25% of patients are hepatitis B or C positive.

As with splenic disease, in untreated patients, hepatic lymphoma usually takes the form of microscopic infiltration with small foci of tumor confined to the portal triad (171).

Detection of liver involvement by cross-sectional imaging is usually difficult. Large focal areas of involvement, detectable on US, CT or MR, are seen in only 5% to 10% of patients with liver disease and resemble metastatic disease from other sources (Fig. 33.29). In both HL and NHL, the lesions are well-defined, frequently large, hypoechoic on US and hypodense relative to the normal parenchyma on both enhanced and unenhanced CT scans. As in metastatic disease, on MR images the lesions display T1 hypointensity and T2 hyperintensity relative to the liver parenchyma. It has been suggested that MR may be more sensitive than CT in the detection of focal hepatic pathology (172). Occasionally, especially in children, a form of liver infiltration is demonstrated as low density soft tissue infiltrating the porta hepatis and the margins of the portal veins (Fig. 33.30) (38,173).

Cross-sectional imaging is relatively insensitive to the detection of the more common diffuse microscopic liver infiltration. However, in contradistinction to the unreliability of splenomegaly, liver enlargement is strongly suggestive of infiltration, particularly in NHL. To date, despite initial enthusiasm (174), attempts to detect the diffuse form on MR have not been successful (73,175), though some work suggests that SPIO may increase the sensitivity of MR for small focal lesions (176).

Involvement of the bile ducts and gall bladder is rare, but has been described in AIDS-related lymphoma (see section on "AIDS-Related Lymphomas").

Key Points: Liver Involvement

■ Liver involvement is almost invariably associated with splenic infiltration
■ Only 5% to 10% of patients with liver disease have focal lesions detectable on cross-sectional imaging
■ Enlargement of the liver is a strong indicator of lymphomatous infiltration
■ Periportal low attenuation may be a feature of NHL

Gastro-Intestinal Tract

The GI tract (GIT) is the most common site of primary extra-nodal lymphoma, being the initial site of involvement in 5% to 10% of adult patients (177). HL of the GIT is extremely rare.

Primary GI lymphomas develop from the lymphoid elements in the lamina propria and constitute about 1% of GI tumors. They occur most frequently in two age-related peaks, the first below the age of 10 years, usually Burkitt lymphoma (BL), and a second between the ages of 50 and 60 years (most of which are the MALT type and also high-grade intestinal T-cell type associated with enteropathy). Primary lymphomas of the GIT usually involve only one site. The criteria for the diagnosis of primary GI lymphoma include:

- Absence of superficial or intrathoracic lymph nodes
- Normal white cell count
- No involvement of liver or spleen
- Lymph node involvement, if present, must be confined to the drainage area of the involved segment of gut (178)

A modified Ann Arbor staging system takes account of these criteria. Stage I is where disease is confined to the visceral wall, and Stage II where there is local extension to adjacent organs (IIE) or draining lymph nodes (179).

Secondary GI involvement is common because of the frequent origin of lymphoma in the mesenteric or retroperitoneal nodes. Typically, multiple sites are involved.

In both the primary and secondary forms, the stomach is the most commonly involved organ (50%), followed by the small bowel (35%), large bowel (15%), and esophagus (<1%). In 10% to 50% of cases the involvement is multicentric (177). In children, the disease appears almost exclusively in the ileum and ileocaecal region.

Stomach (See also Chap. 12, "Gastric Cancer")

Primary lymphoma of the stomach accounts for about 2% to 5% of gastric tumors (177,180) and the incidence appears to be rising. Pathologically, the commonest sybtypes are DLBCL and MALT type lymphomas. In DLCBL, the radiological appearances reflect

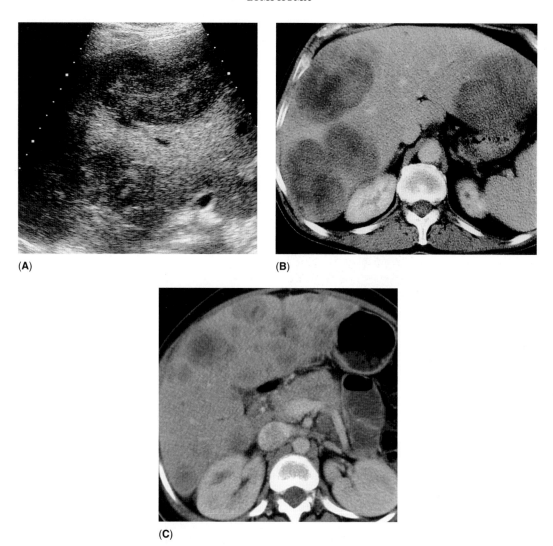

Figure 33.29 Liver involvement in a patient with NHL. (**A**) Transverse ultrasound scan showing multiple large inhomogeneous focal abnormalities of varying echogenicity. (**B**) Post-contrast CT scan in the same patient also showing multiple focal partially enhancing lesions of decreased attenuation within the liver. (**C**) Contrast-enhanced CT scan in a different patient showing multiple hepatic masses, some of which have a target-like appearance.

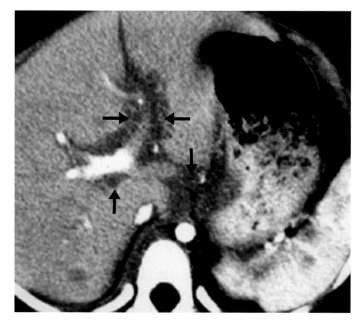

Figure 33.30 CT in a child with NHL, showing periportal infiltration by low-density lymphomatous tissue (arrowed).

the gross pathological findings. Common appearances are multiple nodules, some with central ulceration, seen readily at endoscopy or barium meal, or a large fungating lesion with or without ulceration. About one third of cases present with diffuse infiltration with marked thickening of the wall and narrowing of the lumen, sometimes with extension into the duodenum, indistinguishable from scirrhous carcinoma. Localized polypoid forms have also been described (181). Only about one-tenth are characterized by diffuse enlargement of the gastric folds (Fig. 33.31), similar to the pattern seen in hypertrophic gastritis and Ménétrièr's disease.

Because the disease originates in the submucosa, these features are best demonstrated endoscopically or on barium studies, but these studies do not demonstrate the extent of the disease (Fig. 33.31). CT has proved particularly valuable, often showing extensive gastric wall thickening with a smoothly lobulated border. Unlike gastric carcinoma, the walls of the stomach are usually clearly separable from the surrounding organs (Fig. 33.32) (182).

Gastric MALT lymphomas, especially low-grade ones, are localized at diagnosis in more than two-thirds of cases and usually result in minimal gastric mural thickening, which may not be recognizable even with dedicated CT studies utilizing an oral water load

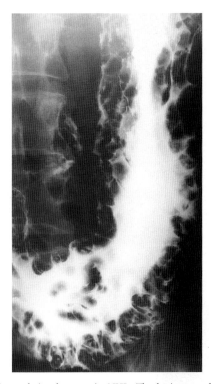

Figure 33.31 Stomach involvement in NHL. The barium meal shows diffuse enlargement of the gastric folds due to submucosal infiltration.

and IV smooth muscle relaxants (183). Endoscopic US is of more value in local staging and assessment of response to treatment, but since multi-organ involvement occurs in up to 25% of patients, extensive imaging for staging may be necessary (184,185).

Small Bowel

Lymphoma accounts for up to 50% of all primary tumors of the small bowel (178), occurring most frequently in the terminal ileum and becoming less frequent proximally. It accounts for up to 35% of all cases of GI lymphoma. Of the tumors in this region, over 60% are of B-cell lineage, usually DLBCL but also mantle cell lymphoma. Patients with AIDS are prone to GI lymphoma and the pattern resembles that found in immunocompetent patients (186). Multifocal disease is present in up to 50% of cases. As it usually originates in the lymphoid follicles, mural thickening is typical and results in constriction of segments of bowel with obstructive symptoms, which are common at presentation. Thickening of the bowel is well demonstrated on CT (Figs. 33.33 and 33.34) with displacement of adjacent loops. Alternating areas of dilatation and constriction are the most common manifestation (178). Occasionally, the lymphomatous infiltration is predominantly submucosal, resulting in multiple nodules or polyps of varying size, scattered throughout the small bowel but predominantly in the terminal ileum. This form is particularly prone to intussusception, which is a classical mode of presentation

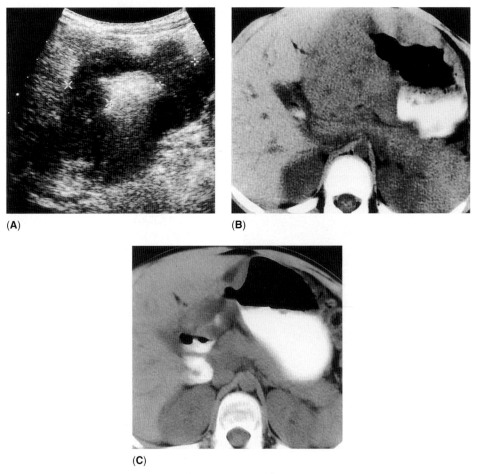

(A)   (B)

(C)

Figure 33.32 Burkitt's lymphoma of the stomach in a child. (**A**) Transverse ultrasound scan showing massive thickening of the wall of the body of the stomach. (**B**) CT scan correlating with the ultrasound appearances in (**A**), again showing massive thickening of the wall, which is clearly separable from the surrounding organs. (**C**) Follow-up CT scan following chemotherapy two months after (**B**) showing an excellent response to chemotherapy. Only a minor amount of thickening of the wall of the gastric antrum persists.

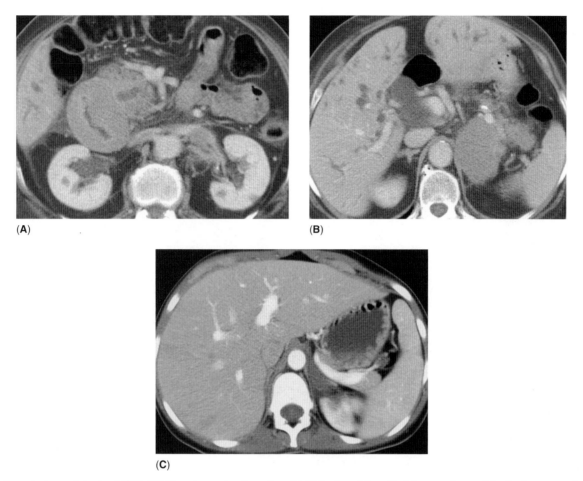

Figure 33.33 A rare instance of duodenal NHL. (**A**) There is massive circumferential thickening of the wall of the second part of the duodenum, causing biliary and pancreatic ductal obstruction. (**B**) At a higher level there is massive dilatation of the common bile duct and a large left adrenal mass. (**C**) After treatment the biliary obstruction has completely resolved and there is a small low density residual mass in the left adrenal gland, which has assumed a more adreniform shape.

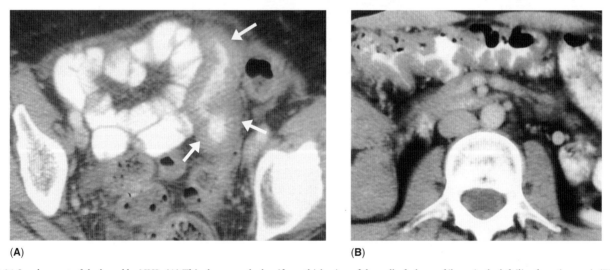

Figure 33.34 Involvement of the bowel by NHL. (**A**) This shows marked uniform thickening of the wall of a loop of ileum in the left iliac fossa (arrows). (**B**) CT scan of the same patient showing diffuse uniform thickening of the transverse colon due to infiltration by NHL.

(Fig. 33.35), usually ileocecal or ileoileal. This is the commonest cause of intussusception in children older than six. Barium studies may show multiple polypoid filling defects, with or without irregular thickening and ulceration of the valvulae. The nature and extent of intestinal lymphoma may also be demonstrated with MR enterography (187).

Enteropathy-associated T-cell lymphoma (associated with gluten-sensitive enteropathy) and immunoproliferative small intestinal disease (alpha-chain disease) affect the jejunum and ileum; malabsorption and acute abdominal presentations secondary to perforation are common. This form of lymphoma may result in aneurysmal dilatation of the small bowel, where the tumor spreads

through the submucosa and muscularis propria, creating a tube-like segment that ultimately becomes aneurysmal, presumably because of destruction of the muscularis and autonomic plexus in the affected segment. Long segments of affected bowel also suggest this diagnosis (187). Immunoproliferative small intestinal disease is thought to be a MALT type lymphoma, possibly related to *Campylobacter jejuni* infection (188).

Secondary invasion of the small bowel by large mesenteric lymph node masses causing displacement, encasement or compression may also be seen. Omental thickening, peritoneal enhancement and ascites cannot be differentiated from peritoneal carcinomatosis and usually occur in advanced abdominal disease, though they may be seen at presentation in BL (Fig. 33.36) (189).

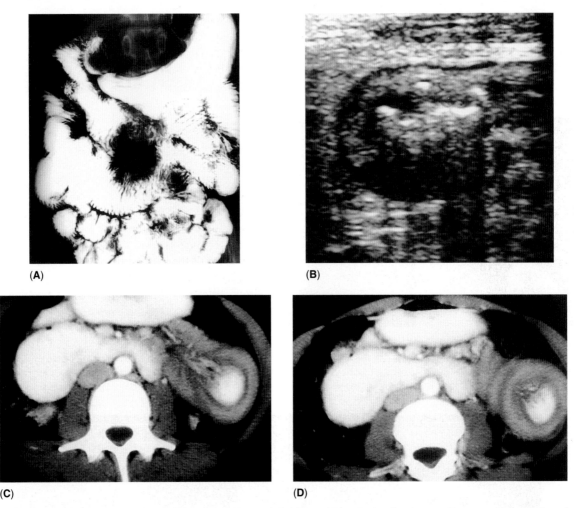

Figure 33.35 Duodeno-jejunal intussusception due to lymphoma. (A) A barium follow-through examination showing an apparent mass lesion in the region of the jejunum with dilatation of the jejunum proximal to this "mass." Note too the thickening of the valvulae conniventes. (B) Ultrasound examination in the mid-abdomen in the region of the "mass" showing marked thickening of the wall of the loop of small bowel. (C and D) CT scans showing thickening of the wall of the loop of jejunum with a classic "coiled spring" appearance due to intussusception.

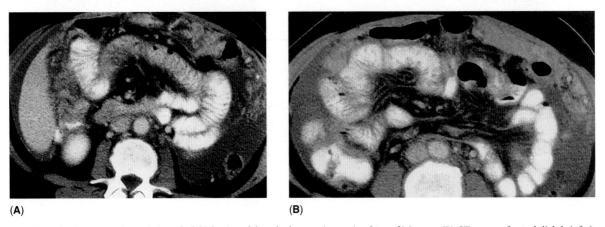

Figure 33.36 Small bowel infiltration in NHL. (A) Marked thickening of the valvulae conniventes in a loop of jejunum. (B) CT scan performed slightly inferior to (A) also shows thickening of the valvulae in the ileum. Note in (A) and (B) the extensive infiltration of the omentum, perivascular thickening and thickening of the peritoneum.

Colon and Rectum

Primary lymphoma accounts for only 0.05% of all colonic neoplasms and usually involves the caecum and rectum rather than other parts of the colon. Conversely, secondary involvement is usually widely distributed and multicentric. The most common form of the disease is a diffuse or segmental distribution of nodules 0.2 to 2 cm in diameter, typically with the mucosa intact (Fig. 33.34B). A focal form appears as a large polypoid mass, often in the caecum, where it is indistinguishable from colonic cancer unless there is concomitant involvement of the terminal ileum, which is more suggestive of lymphoma. Elsewhere, concentric structuring masses are seen (Fig. 33.37). The mass may

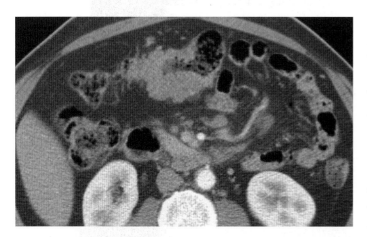

Figure 33.37 Primary colonic NHL. There is a constricting mass of the transverse colon with transmural spread into the adjacent pericolonic fat, radiologically indistinguishable from a colonic carcinoma.

have a large intraluminal component. In very advanced disease, there may be marked thickening of the colonic or rectal folds, resulting in focal strictures or ulcerative masses with fistula formation (Fig. 33.38). Colonic involvement is a particular feature of ARL and BL, but MALT types also occur, usually causing nodularity (see section on "MALT Lymphoma").

Esophagus

Intrinsic esophageal involvement is extremely uncommon, usually involves the distal third of the esophagus and can result in a smooth tapered narrowing. Occasionally, both the fundus and distal esophagus are involved by a bulky fungating tumor.

Pancreas

Primary pancreatic lymphoma is extremely rare and accounts for only 1.3% of all cases of pancreatic malignancy (190) and 2% of patients with NHL (191). Secondary pancreatic involvement usually occurs in association with disease elsewhere, most commonly due to direct infiltration from adjacent nodal masses, which may be focal or massive (192). Intrinsic involvement of the pancreas most commonly results in a solitary mass lesion, indistinguishable from a primary adenocarcinoma on US, CT, or MR (Fig. 33.39) (192). Biliary and pancreatic ductal obstruction as well as invasion or narrowing of the portal vein are commonly seen at CT (193). Calcification and necrosis are rare. The presence of a large mass in the head of the pancreas, with only mild biliary or pancreatic ductal dilatation, should raise the possibility of lymphoma, especially if there is retroperitoneal nodal enlargement below the level of the renal veins (194). Less commonly, diffuse palpable masses or diffuse uniform enlargement of the pancreas is seen. Involvement is far more common in NHL than HL, particularly in ARL.

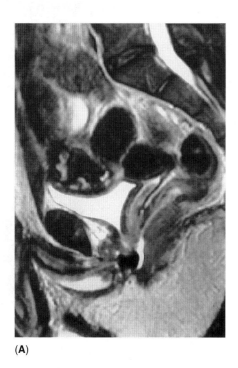
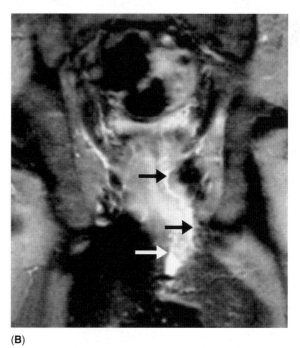

(A)   **(B)**

Figure 33.38 Rectal involvement in a patient with lymphoma and AIDS. (**A**) A sagittal fast spinecho T2-weighted MR image showing thickening of the rectal wall and a high-signal intensity fistula extending into the perineum. (**B**) A coronal STIR image in the same patient showing the marked thickening and a marked increase in signal intensity of the rectal wall. This scan also shows the high signal intensity of the complex fistula extending from the left side of the rectal wall into the perineum (arrowed).

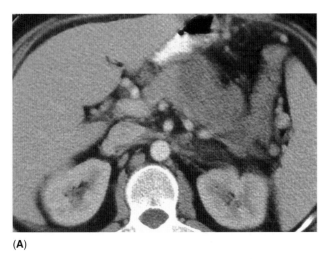
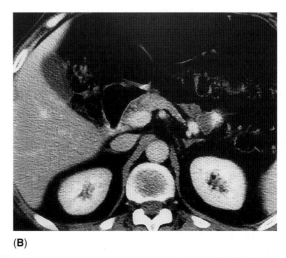

(A)   **(B)**

Figure 33.39 Primary pancreatic lymphoma. (A) Note a large mass of decreased attenuation following contrast medium replacing the normal body of the pancreas due to primary pancreatic NHL. (B) A CT scan performed three months following chemotherapy shows complete resolution of the lymphomatous mass with marked atrophy of the remaining pancreas.

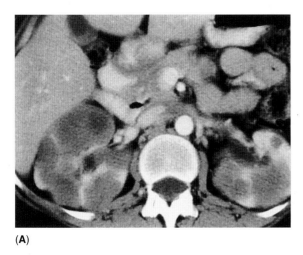
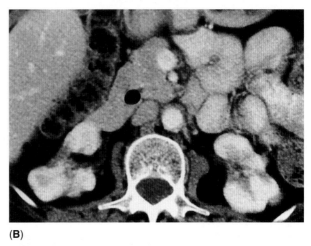

(A)   **(B)**

Figure 33.40 Renal lymphoma. (A) CT scan showing multiple masses enhancing less than the adjacent renal parenchyma following IV injection of contrast medium. Note the absence of retroperitoneal lymph node enlargement. (B) CT scan performed four months after (A) following chemotherapy shows complete resolution of the multiple renal masses with marked scarring of the kidneys following treatment.

Key Points: Gastro-Intestinal Tract

- The stomach is the most frequent site of either primary or secondary GI lymphoma
- Lymphoma accounts for up to 50% of all primary tumors of the small bowel and is multifocal in 50% of cases
- Intussusception is a characteristic feature at presentation with predominantly submucosal nodular/polypoid lymphoma
- Involvement of the colon and rectum accounts for only 0.5% of colonic neoplasms
- Pancreatic lymphoma is usually secondary due to invasion by adjacent lymph node masses

Genitourinary Tract

The genitourinary tract is infrequently involved at the time of presentation, although in end-stage disease more than 50% of cases will have involvement of some part of the genitourinary tract. The testicle is the most commonly involved organ, followed by the kidney and perirenal space. Involvement of the bladder, prostate, uterus, vagina, and ovaries is extremely rare (195).

Kidney

Renal involvement is detected in about 3% of all patients undergoing abdominal imaging for the staging of lymphoma (196–198). Primary or isolated renal lymphoma is rare. Although CT is more sensitive in identifying lymphomatous renal masses than US or urography, a large discrepancy exists between the radiological detection and incidence at autopsy (up to 50% having involvement in autopsy series), presumably because renal involvement is a late phenomenon. It is extremely unusual for the detection of renal involvement to alter the disease stage. Close to 90% of cases are due to high-grade NHL, renal function is usually normal and in more than 40% of patients the disease occurs at the time of recurrence only. DLBCL and BL are the histological subtypes that most commonly involve the kidneys.

Multiple masses is the most frequent pattern of disease, seen in up to 60% of cases. CT may show a typical "density reversal pattern" before and after contrast administration. The lesions are more dense than the surrounding parenchyma before contrast medium administration and less dense after contrast medium administration (Fig. 33.40) (196).

Solitary masses occur less frequently (10–20%) and may be indistinguishable from renal cell carcinoma (196). An important feature of renal masses occurring in NHL is that in over 50% of cases there is no evidence of retroperitoneal lymph node enlargement on CT, suggesting that the kidneys are involved by hematogenous spread.

Direct infiltration of the kidney is the secondmost common type of renal involvement, occurring in 25% of cases. Invasion occurs from the retroperitoneum into the renal hilum and sinus, encasing the renal vessels and simulating a transitional cell carcinoma, an important differential diagnosis (Fig. 33.41). Frequently, a soft tissue mass is seen in the perirenal space, occasionally encasing the kidney without evidence on CT of invasion of the parenchyma (Fig. 33.42).

Diffuse infiltration of the kidneys (Fig. 33.43) with global renal enlargement without focal nodules is a less common manifestation, usually without lymph node enlargement. The appearance after IV contrast medium injection is variable, but usually the normal parenchymal enhancement is replaced by homogeneous non-enhancing tissue. This pattern can be seen with BL. After successful treatment, the appearance can revert entirely to normal. A particularly rare form of disease is isolated periureteric lymphoma, which has been described in NHL and HL (199).

Bladder and Prostate

Although primary lymphoma of the bladder is extremely rare, secondary lymphoma of the bladder is more common and is found in 10% to 15% of patients with lymphoma at autopsy (195,200). Such secondary involvement can affect the wall of the bladder intrinsically or in contiguity from adjacent involved nodes. Microscopic involvement is far more common than gross involvement, but this too can be associated with hematuria. The appearances on CT and MR are non-specific (Fig. 33.44) with either diffuse widespread thickening of the bladder wall or a large nodular mass, both patterns indistinguishable from transitional cell carcinoma (201).

Primary bladder lymphoma accounts for less than 1% of all bladder tumors. There is a female preponderance in the sixth and seventh decades, and a history of cystitis is common, explaining the high incidence of MALT-type lymphomas. Solitary or occasionally multiple sessile masses are most often seen (202).

Unlike primary lymphoma of the bladder, where the response to chemotherapy/radiotherapy is good, lymphomatous involvement of the prostate carries a poor prognosis. It is usually intermediate or high grade and produces irritative obstructive symptoms. Solitary nodules are uncommon and in the majority of cases there is diffuse infiltration throughout the prostate and periprostatic tissue. Secondary involvement of the prostate is far more common than primary prostatic involvement and direct extension into the prostate from pelvic lymph nodes is often seen in very advanced disease.

Testis

Testicular lymphoma is the most common testicular tumor occurring in individuals over the age of 60, but accounts for only 5% of all testicular neoplasms (203). The vast majority are DLBCL. At presentation it is seen in about 1% to 2% of men with NHL (more commonly in BL) but is practically non-existent in HL. At presentation 80% are localized to the testis and abdominal or

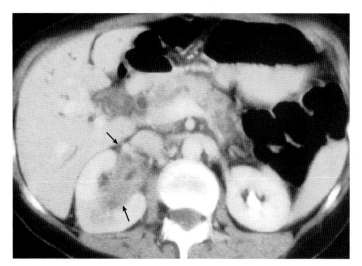

Figure 33.41 Renal lymphoma simulating transitional cell tumor. CT scan on a patient with NHL showing a mass within the right renal pelvis (arrowed), extending into the renal parenchyma.

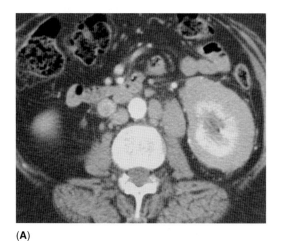

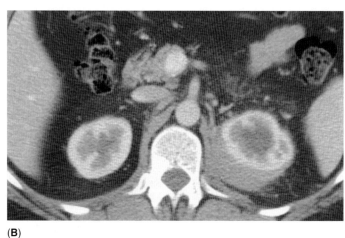

(A)   **(B)**

Figure 33.42 Perirenal lymphomatous infiltration. Two different instances, (A) with and (B) without accompanying retroperitoneal lymph node enlargement.

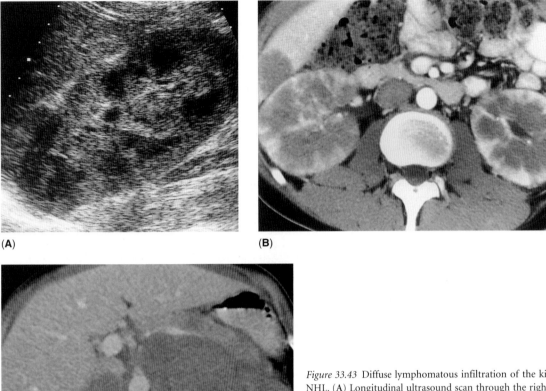

(A)

(B)

(C)

Figure 33.43 Diffuse lymphomatous infiltration of the kidney in a patient with high-grade NHL. (**A**) Longitudinal ultrasound scan through the right kidney showing marked enlargement of the kidney (the right kidney measures 16 cm, the left 16.5 cm). There is diffuse increased reflectivity of the renal parenchyma with resultant prominent lucency of the renal papillae. The normal outline of the kidney is preserved. (**B**) CT scan following IV injection of contrast medium in the same patient as (**A**), showing diffuse infiltration of both kidneys by lymphomatous tissue. There is preservation of a rim of normal renal parenchyma. Note the absence of retroperitoneal lymph node enlargement and the presence of a focal lesion in the inferior aspect of the right lobe of the liver. (**C**) Post-contrast CT scan demonstrating massive bilateral renal infiltration, more marked on the left than the right, with virtually no normally enhancing renal parenchyma.

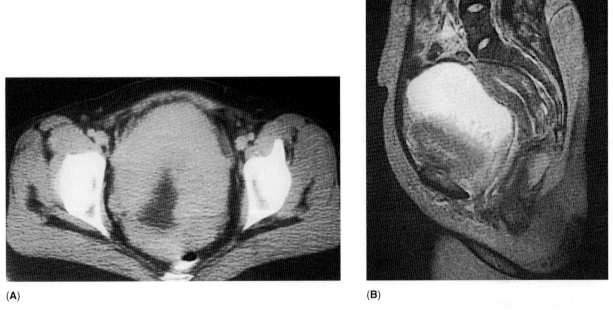

(A)

(B)

Figure 33.44 NHL of the bladder. (**A**) CT scan showing large soft tissue mass occupying a major part of the base of the bladder. (**B**) Sagittal spin-echo T2-weighted MR image showing extensive involvement of the anterior abdominal wall in the same patient.

pelvic lymph nodes (Stage IIE). As in other sites of lymphomatous involvement of the genitourinary tract, the frequency of involvement discovered at autopsy is much higher: 18% of men with NHL. There is an association with lymphoma of Waldeyer's ring, the CNS, and skin. The outcome is poorer than other DLBCL of equivalent stage, probably because of the tendency for CNS relapse.

On US, the lesions usually have a non-specific appearance, with focal areas of decreased echogenicity. However, a well-recognized pattern is a diffuse decrease in reflectivity of the testicle without any focal abnormality. As involvement is bilateral in 10% to 25% of cases, it is extremely important to examine the contralateral side. MR offers little advantage over US in evaluation of the testis (204).

Female Genitalia

In advanced, widespread lymphomatous disease, the female genital organs are frequently involved secondarily (26). However, isolated lymphomatous involvement is rare, accounting for approximately 1% of extranodal NHL. Most are diffuse large B cell in type. Around 70% of women affected are postmenopausal and present with vaginal bleeding. The tumors originate predominantly in the uterine cervix, where on CT and MR a large mass can be seen (Fig. 33.45). Involvement of the uterine body usually produces diffuse enlargement, often with a lobular contour similar to a fibroid, with relatively homogeneous signal intensity on all sequences in spite of the large tumor size (205). Similarly, primary lymphoma of the cervix and/or vagina is characterized by a large, exophytic, soft tissue mass.

Involvement of these gynecological structures is best demonstrated by MR, since masses are seen as intermediate to high signal intensity lesions on T2 weighting and are therefore clearly distinguished from the surrounding normal tissues, including the

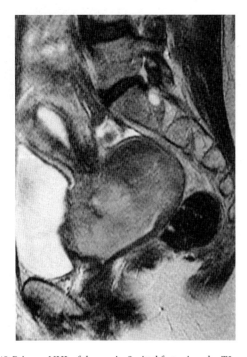

Figure 33.45 Primary NHL of the cervix. Sagittal fast spin-echo T2- weighted MR image showing a very large mass in the uterine cervix due to high-grade NHL. There was no evidence of disease elsewhere in this patient.

uterus, cervix, and vaginal wall. MR is excellent in follow-up and assessment of response to treatment (206). Ovarian lymphoma is less common and carries a worse prognosis than uterine lymphoma because the tumors are usually more advanced at the time of discovery. The appearance on cross-sectional imaging is indistinguishable from primary epithelial ovarian carcinoma (207). Involvement is often bilateral, and DLBCL or BL are the usual subtypes. The presence of large bilateral homogeneous masses with moderate enhancement on MR, without hemorrhage, necrosis or calcification, may suggest this diagnosis (208).

Key Points: Genitourinary Tract

- Renal involvement is seen in about 3% of cases undergoing abdominal CT
- Lymphomatous involvement of the kidneys is not usually associated with renal impairment
- Primary lymphoma of the prostate carries a poor prognosis whereas primary lymphoma of the bladder has a good prognosis
- The testis is the most frequent site of involvement of the genitourinary tract with lymphoma
- Lymphoma of the testis accounts for only 5% of all testicular tumors
- Primary lymphoma of the female genital tract is rare and is best demonstrated on MR

Adrenal Glands

Primary adrenal lymphoma is rare, usually occurring in men over the age of 60. Secondary involvement of the adrenal glands in lymphoma is usually demonstrated on routine abdominal CT for staging (where it is seen in up to 6% of cases of NHL) as presentation with adrenal insufficiency is extremely rare (195,207). Involvement is usually bilateral and the appearances are indistinguishable from bilateral metastases, but readily distinguishable from adenomas (Figs. 33.27B and 33.33). Non-lymphomatous bilateral hyperplasia of the adrenal glands has been described (209). The reason for this is unclear, but probably due to ectopic production of an ACTH-like substance (210).

Central Nervous System
Primary

Primary CNS lymphoma (PCNSL) is initially localized to the CNS at presentation. It occurs almost exclusively within the brain, as the spinal cord is only very rarely the site of origin (<1%) (211, 212). Although in the mid-1980s primary lymphoma accounted for only 1.5% of all brain tumors, its frequency increased markedly in the early 1990s, partly due to an association with immunosuppressive therapy following cardiac or renal transplants and acquired immunodeficiency. Up to 5% of AIDS patients can be expected to develop primary CNS lymphoma during the course of the disease (213), but the introduction of HAART has resulted in a decline in the incidence of AIDS-related PCNSL. Cases of PCNSL have been reported from the age of two months to 90 years, but presentation between the fourth and sixth decades appears to be the most frequent. There is a separate peak in the first decade of life. It now accounts for over 3% of brain tumors

and up to 30% of cases of NHL in some series. There are differences in the clinical features of AIDS-related PCNSL and PCNSL in immunocompetent patients. The former are younger, more likely to be male and to present with fits and altered mental status rather than focal neurology and signs of raised intracranial pressure.

On CT or MR, more than 50% of lesions occur within the cerebral white matter, close to or within the corpus callosum (212). Most abut the ependyma of the ventricles or the ependymal surface. A butterfly distribution with spread across the corpus callosum is seen (214). In about 15% of cases, the deep cortical grey matter of the basal ganglia, thalamus and hypothalamus are involved. In 10% of cases, lymphoma develops in the posterior fossa and is multifocal in a further 20% of cases. In AIDS-related PCNSL, multifocality is much more common, being seen in up to 50% of cases. On CT, the tumor mass is typically of increased density on unenhanced CT and the majority of lesions enhance homogeneously after IV injection of contrast medium. Only about 10% of lesions do not enhance (211). Calcification is very rare and surrounding vasogenic edema relatively mild (214). On MR, the typical appearance is of a tumor mass hypo- or isointense relative to the surrounding normal tissue on T1-weighted sequences. There is usually uniform enhancement after injection of gadolinium–DTPA (Fig. 33.46), but ring enhancement can be a feature of AIDS-related primary CNSL. The appearance of primary and secondary lymphoma within the brain is essentially similar on CT and MR.

Secondary

Cerebral involvement occurs in 10% to 15% of patients with NHL at some time during the course of their disease (71,215). Certain groups are at risk: those with stage IV disease, testicular or ovarian

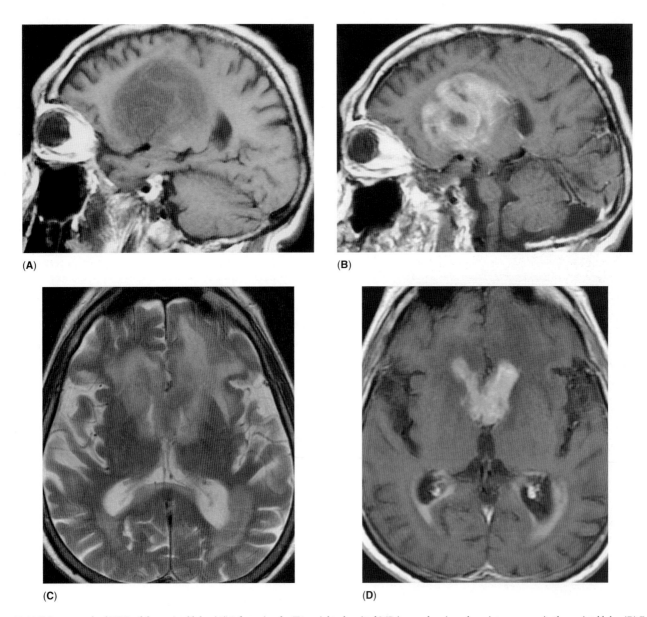

(A)

(B)

(C)

(D)

Figure 33.46 Primary cerebral NHL of the parietal lobe. (A) A fast spinecho T1-weighted sagittal MR image showing a hypointense mass in the parietal lobe. (B) Following IV administration of gadolinium-DTPA, the mass enhances intensely. (C) Axial T2-weighted MR showing a mass in the genu of the corpus callosum with marked surrounding vasogenic edema. (D) T1-weighted post-contrast MR showing enhancing mass in typical butterfly distribution in the corpus callosum.

presentations, high-grade T-cell lymphomas, immunoblastic, and BL (216). Secondary cerebral involvement is so rare in HL that a space-occupying lesion in the brain of a patient with known HL should prompt a second diagnosis (217). Secondary lymphoma is distinguishable from the primary form to some extent by its propensity to involve the extracerebral spaces (epidural, subdural, and subarachnoid) (Fig. 33.47) and the spinal epidural and subarachnoid spaces (211). MR imaging with direct multiplanar imaging is ideal for detecting extracerebral plaque-like tumor deposits in the subdural or epidural spaces. Typically, these plaques are hypo- to isodense on all pulse sequences, but they are made more obvious on gadolinium–DTPA-enhanced T1-weighted images (Fig. 33.47). CT is less sensitive, not only in the detection of these extracerebral lesions, but also in demonstrating leptomeningeal deposits of lymphoma coating the cranial nerves (218), particularly when resulting in cranial nerve palsies.

Gadolinium-enhanced MR is also a relatively sensitive, non-invasive method for demonstrating spinal leptomeningeal involvement by lymphoma and involvement of the spinal cord and nerve roots. Nonetheless, there is a significant false negative rate that is higher than that for leptomeningeal carcinomatosis (219). Epidural extension of tumor into the spinal canal from a paravertebral nodal mass may also be elegantly demonstrated on MR. Although extension through the intervertebral foramina may also be clearly depicted on CT, subtle disease is easily missed (Fig. 33.48) (220).

Compression of the spinal cord or cauda equina due to lymphomatous disease is a late manifestation of HL, but is often an earlier manifestation of NHL. In both types of lymphoma, extension of nodal spread through the intervertebral neural foramina is the most common cause. Tumor compresses the dura, but the dura itself usually acts as an effective barrier to the intrathecal spread of tumor. Vertebral collapse with cord compression may be seen in some of the aggressive forms of NHL, but it is less common than compression due to an epidural mass (Fig. 33.48). On occasion, patients can present with epidural disease causing back pain and paresis, for example in endemic BL.

The Orbit

NHL is the most common primary orbital malignancy in adults, accounting for 10% to 15% of orbital masses (211) and about 5% of all primary extranodal NHL. *Primary* orbital lymphomas occur most commonly in patients between 40 and 70 years of age, and most typically present as a slow-growing, diffusely infiltrative tumor for which the main differential diagnosis is from the non-malignant condition known as "orbital pseudotumor." They can arise from the conjunctiva, eyelids, lacrimal glands, or retrobulbar soft tissues. Retrobulbar lymphoma infiltrates around and through the extraocular muscles causing proptosis and ophthalmoplegia, but visual acuity is rarely disturbed. In patients with an orbital lymphomatous mass, up to 50% will be found to have an extra-central nervous system primary site of origin.

Secondary orbital involvement occurs in approximately 3.5% to 5% of both HL and NHL. In both the primary and secondary forms, the clinical manifestations will depend on the site of involvement. Involvement of the lacrimal glands is bilateral in over 20% of cases; the presenting features are those of bilateral masses with downward displacement of the globe (Fig. 33.49). The prognosis is generally good (even with bilateral disease). Relapse in the contralateral orbit is not uncommon. Involvement of the eyelids and subconjunctival spaces is readily assessed on clinical examination, whereas MR best depicts the presence and extent of any intracranial extension.

> ### Key Points: Central Nervous System
>
> - Primary CNS lymphoma almost exclusively involves the cerebral white matter
> - Primary cerebral lymphoma is increasing in incidence
> - Secondary lymphoma preferentially involves the extracerebral spaces and the spinal epidural and subarachnoid spaces
> - Spinal cord compression results from nodal spread through the intervertebral neural foramina in both HL and NHL
> - NHL is the most common primary orbital malignancy in adults

Head and Neck Lymphoma

Although HL typically involves the cervical lymph nodes as the presenting feature, true extranodal involvement of sites in the head and neck region is rare. Extension from nodal masses in the neck to Waldeyer's ring may occur, but this is seen in less than 1% of patients.

In NHL, extranodal head and neck tumor involvement is relatively common and indeed 10% of patients present with extranodal disease in the head and neck; on investigation about half will have disseminated lymphoma. Extranodal NHL accounts for approximately 5% of head and neck cancers (221).

Waldeyer's ring comprises lymphoid tissue in the nasopharynx, oropharynx, the faucial and palatine tonsil, and the lingual tonsil on the posterior third of the tongue. It is the most common site of head

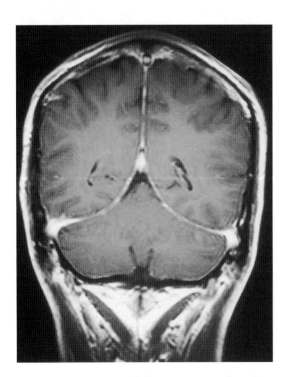

Figure 33.47 NHL showing meningeal disease on a coronal MR image using a T1-weighted sequence following injection of IV contrast medium (gadolinium–DTPA). Note intense enhancement of the thickened meninges over the cerebral hemispheres, cerebellum, and tentorium.

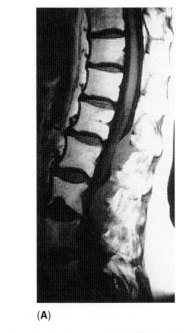

(A)

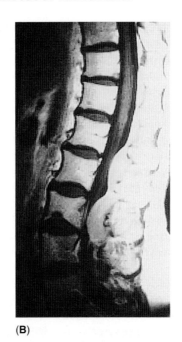

(B)

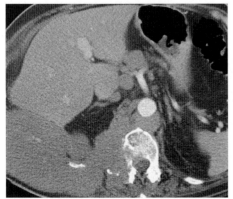

(C)

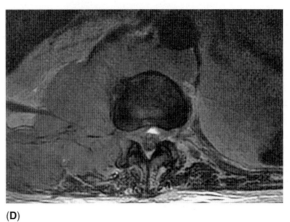

(D)

Figure 33.48 T1-weighted MR images of the lumbar spine (**A**) pre- and (**B**) post-contrast showing extensive enhancing epidural disease. (**C**) Axial contrast-enhanced CT scan (same patient as Fig. 33.26B) showing extension of tumour into the epidural space on the right. However, this is much more clearly depicted on (**D**) the axial T2-weighted MR scan on the same patient.

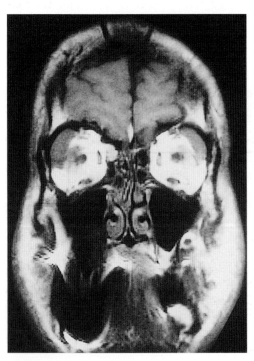

Figure 33.49 Orbital lymphoma. T1-weighted coronal MR image. There are bilateral orbital masses of homogeneous low signal intensity. The masses are symmetrical and occupy the superolateral orbital compartments. There is no evidence of bone erosion.

and neck lymphoma and there is a pronounced link with involvement of the GIT, which may be synchronous, or metachronous; this is partly a reflection of the fact that some are of the MALT type. Hence most centers include a full staging CT and/or endoscopy as part of staging, since up to 30% will have advanced disease at presentation. A diagnosis of NHL is suggested by circumferential involvement or multifocality. Middle-aged women are most often affected and a history of Sjögren's syndrome should be sought. The majority are DLCBL, 60% of which are localized. Secondary invasion from adjacent nodal masses is also a common occurrence.

NHL comprises 8% of tumors of the paranasal sinuses. In the West, the disease affects middle-aged men and the maxillary sinus is most commonly involved, nearly always with DLBCL, whereas the aggressive diffuse T-cell type (that formed part of the "lethal midline granuloma" syndrome) affects younger Asians and is linked to EBV. Whilst paranasal sinus involvement often presents with acute facial swelling and pain, and disease often spreads from one sinus to the other in a contiguous fashion, bony destruction is considerably less marked than in squamous cell carcinomas (222). Nevertheless, these tumors are aggressive and can transgress normal anatomical barriers, as a consequence of which intracranial spread through the base of the skull is seen in up to 40% of cases. Thus, CNS prophylaxis is an important component of treatment.

MR imaging is the preferred imaging technique for evaluating head and neck lymphoma due to high tissue contrast between tumor and normal structures; its multiplanar capability allows clear demonstration of the full extent of disease within the intricate anatomy of the facial region (Fig. 33.50). It also permits detection of tumor spread into the cranial cavity from the infratemporal fossa, orbit, and soft tissue of the face. Fat-suppressed T1 weighted sequences pre-and post intravenous gadolinium-based contrast medium is most helpful.

Salivary Glands

All the salivary glands may be involved in lymphoma but the parotid gland is the most frequent site (223). Most are MALT type. The patient presents with single or multiple well-defined masses that are of higher density than the surrounding gland on CT, hypoechoic on US, and of intermediate signal intensity on T1- and T2-weighted MR sequences.

Thyroid

NHL accounts for 2% to 5% of malignant tumors of the thyroid (224). There is an association with Hashimoto's disease, so the disease tends to occur in women in their 60s with MALT types. However, DLBCL also occurs, and these patients present with a rapidly growing mass and obstructive symptoms. Direct spread of tumor beyond the gland and involvement of adjacent lymph nodes is common. On CT these masses usually have a lower attenuation than the normal gland and they may show peripheral enhancement following injection of IV contrast medium (Fig. 33.51). MR can delineate the local effects on adjacent soft tissues more accurately than CT, though this is not generally necessary unless radiotherapy is being contemplated (225). Most present with stage I or II disease and as would be expected, MALT types have a better prognosis than DLBCL.

Key Points: Head and Neck

- Extranodal NHL accounts for approximately 5% of all head and neck cancers
- Waldeyer's ring is the most common site of head and neck lymphoma
- The parotid is the most frequent salivary gland involved by lymphoma
- NHL accounts for up to 5% of all malignant thyroid tumors

Musculoskeletal System

Skeletal involvement may occur in both HL and NHL. Since the bone marrow is an integral part of the reticuloendothelial system, lymphomas may arise within the marrow as a true primary disease. More often, however, the marrow is involved as part of a

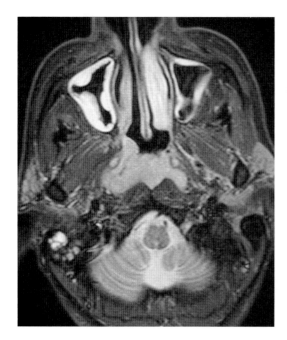

Figure 33.50 Axial T2-weighted MR image with fat suppression demonstrating massive soft tissue thickening of the nasopharynx with resultant obstruction of the mastoid air cells on the right.

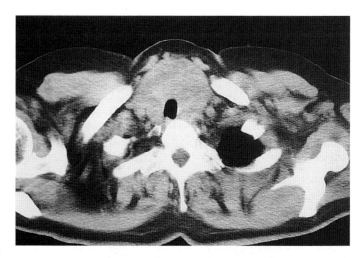

Figure 33.51 CT scan showing primary lymphoma of the thyroid. On staging, no other evidence of disease was found in this patient with biopsy-proven disease.

disseminated process and this is categorized as Stage IV disease. The majority of those with "apparent" primary lymphomas usually have widespread disease and, therefore, in reality have secondary involvement. This is particularly true in children. Hence this diagnosis is made very rarely, not least because better imaging enables detection of synchronous disease elsewhere.

Bone and bone marrow are important sites of disease relapse and any skeletal symptoms following previous treatment for lymphoma should raise the suspicion of bone disease. Involvement of osseous bone is less widespread and does not necessarily imply bone marrow involvement (226), nor does skeletal radiography have any predictive value in determining marrow involvement. Infiltration of bone may also occur by direct invasion of adjacent soft tissue masses. This is designated with the suffix "E" after the appropriate stage of disease elsewhere, e.g., Stage IIE. For the purposes of clarity, involvement of the bone is distinguished in this description from diffuse involvement of the bone marrow.

Bone
Primary lymphoma of bone is almost exclusively due to NHL as primary HL of bone is extremely rare. The criteria for the diagnosis of primary lymphoma require that:

- Only a single bone is involved
- There is unequivocal histological evidence of lymphoma
- Other disease is limited to regional areas at the time of presentation
- The primary tumor precedes metastasis by at least six months

The average age at presentation is 24 years; 50% of cases occur in patients between 10 and 30 years of age. Males are affected more often than females. Primary lymphoma affects the appendicular skeleton involving the femur, tibia, and humerus, in descending order of frequency. Primary lymphoma of bone accounts for about 1% of all NHL (227), and under 5% of cases of localized primary extranodal lymphoma. Nearly all are DLBCL and patients typically present with localized bone pain, with or without a palpable mass.

Secondary involvement of bones is present in 5% to 6% of patients with NHL (226,227), although less present with symptoms due to a skeletal lesion. Bone involvement is more frequent in children with NHL (38). Radiographic evidence of bone involvement is present in 20% of patients, in HL appearing as the initial presentation in 4% of cases (226). Systemic (secondary) NHL involves the axial skeleton more frequently than the appendicular skeleton.

Appearances
Primary NHL of bone is radiologically indistinguishable from systemic NHL, HL and other bone tumors. While the bone lesions in NHL (primary or secondary) are usually permeative osteolytic (77%) (Fig. 33.52), sclerotic in only 4% and mixed in 16%, bony involvement in HL typically gives a sclerotic or mixed sclerotic and lytic (86%) and infrequently lytic (14%) picture (228). Bone scintigraphy is more sensitive than plain radiography, but MR is the imaging modality of choice for staging and follow-up, depicting the extent of marrow involvement and muscle infiltration much more accurately (229,230). It has been suggested that FDG PET is more sensitive and specific than bone scintigraphy, with a high positive predictive value (PPV) for the detection of osseous

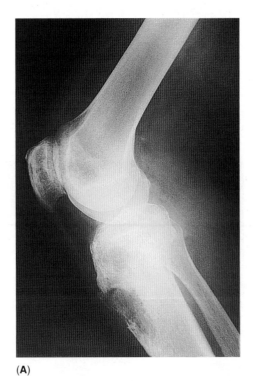

(A)

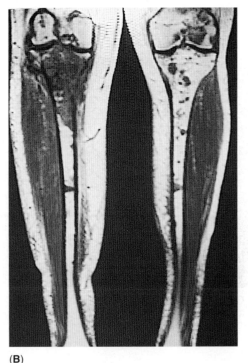

(B)

Figure 33.52 NHL of upper tibia. (**A**) Lateral plain radiograph showing a destructive lesion in the upper aspect of the tibia. (**B**) Coronal T1-weighted MR image showing a large area of abnormal low signal intensity in the upper tibia that corresponds to the abnormal bone on the plain radiograph. However, in addition, multiple lesions of low signal intensity are seen throughout both femoral condyles and tibiae, indicating much more extensive disease than had been appreciated clinically and on skeletal radiographs.

involvement (231). There is also some evidence that FDG PET can demonstrate response to treatment earlier and more accurately than conventional modalities including MR (232).

In HL, soft tissue disease typically may involve adjacent bones; anterior mediastinal and paravertebral masses frequently invade the sternum and vertebrae, respectively, resulting either in destruction or scalloping. A classic finding is the sclerotic "ivory vertebra." Direct invasion of bone by local lymph node disease is denoted by the suffix "E" added to the appropriate stage.

Because of the relatively low incidence of bone lesions at presentation, screening for bone involvement is not routine but is reserved for patients with specific complaints.

Bone Marrow
Involvement of the bone marrow indicates Stage IV disease. It is rare at presentation in HL but is found in 20% to 40% of patients with NHL at presentation (128,233–237) and is associated with a worse prognosis than involvement of the liver, lung, or osseous bone (236). During the course of HL, marrow involvement occurs in 5% to 15% of patients (237). Because of these figures, bone marrow biopsies are not indicated as part of the initial staging of early stage HL, but the high incidence in NHL justifies its use as a staging procedure (238), increasing the stage in up to 30% of cases, mainly from Stage III to Stage IV (238). Bone marrow involve-ment in low-grade NHL is typically diffuse but in intermediate- and high-grade lymphoma it is more likely to be focal. Therefore, not surprisingly, the performance of bilateral rather than single-site biopsies increases the pick-up rate by up to 20% (239).

MR imaging is undoubtedly an extremely sensitive technique in the demonstration of bone marrow involvement (Fig. 33.53). On T1-weighted images, tumor infiltration is of low signal (Figs. 33.52 and 33.53) (240) and of high signal intensity on STIR. In one recent study, T1-weighted spin-echo was the most sensitive sequence, whereas fast STIR and echo-planar imaging (EPI) sequences were most specific for infiltration (241,242). MR imaging can upstage as many as 33% of patients with negative iliac crest biopsies. Focal desposits as small as 5 mm can be identified though false negative studies do occur with microscopic infiltration (under 5%) and low-grade lymphoma. Compared to CT, whole-body MR can upstage nearly 20% of patients through demonstration of bone marrow disease (237,240,241,243). Patients with a positive MR study appear to have a poorer prognosis, regardless of bone marrow biopsy findings (244).

FDG PET to date has shown reasonable sensitivity and specificity for bone marrow disease. A small number of false negative PET findings occur with low-grade lymphoma, often PET negative elsewhere (245), or with microscopic infiltration. In one study, FDG PET alone resulted in change of stage twice as often as bone marrow

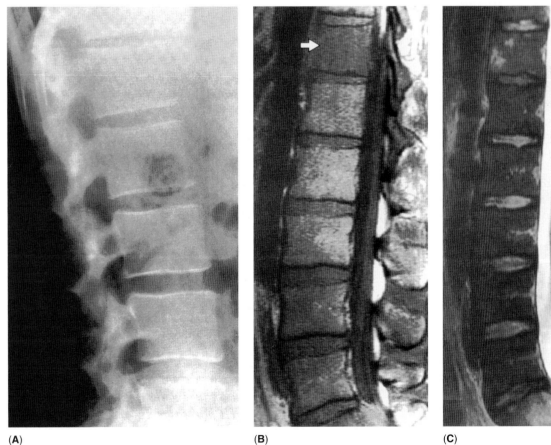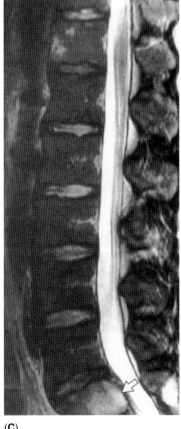

(A)   **(B)**   **(C)**

Figure 33.53 Bone involvement in a patient with NHL. (**A**) Normal skeletal radiograph in a patient with NHL and back pain. The radio-isotope scan was also normal. (**B**) T1-weighted sagittal MR image showing loss of the normal high-signal intensity of fat in the body of L1 (arrowed). (**C**) Fast spin-echo T2-weighted sagittal MR image showing areas of high-signal intensity within the body of L1 vertebra and also the body of S1 (arrowed). A bone biopsy of S1 showed involvement of the cortical bone as well as of the bone marrow.

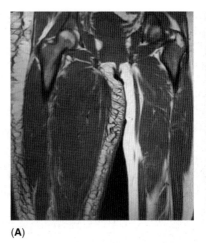 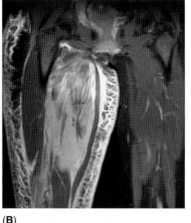 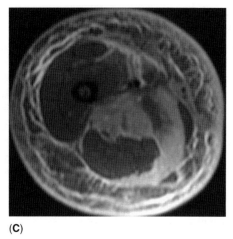

(A) (B) (C)

Figure 33.54 Soft tissue involvement by lymphoma. (**A**) Coronal T1-weighted image, (**B**) coronal (**B**) and (**C**) axial T2-weighted images with fat suppression of the thigh in a patient with massive lymphomatous infiltration of the medial and adductor compartment of the right thigh, with marked accompanying edema.

biopsy. In another, PET/CT changed stage in 21 of 50 patients compared with combined CT and bone marrow biopsy and in 7 of the 21, this was significant (from early stage I or II to stage IV) (246). In this study, a CT counterpart of the FDG-avid focus was rare, but the CT facilitated confirmatory image-guided biopsy of the FDG-positive foci. However, FDG PET has not been shown to be consistently reliable in detecting bone marrow involvement (247,248). A recent meta-analysis of 13 studies of FDG PET in the evaluation of bone marrow infiltration, including 587 patients and using bone marrow biopsy as the reference standard, showed that only half the patients with a positive bone marrow biopsy were detected by FDG PET, whilst more than 90% of cases with a negative bone marrow biopsy also had a negative PET scan (249).

Preliminary data suggest that superparamagnetic iron oxides may have a role in the differentiation of normo- and hypercellular marrow after treatment from persistent or residual infiltration, a distinction which is difficult with conventional MR imaging and FDG PET scanning (particularly if granulocyte colony-stimulating factor has been administered) (250).

Despite the sensitivity (and in some cases specificity) of these imaging techniques to detect bone marrow infiltration their precise role in the staging of patients with lymphoma has not yet been defined, given the obvious need to examine the cytology of bone marrow in these patients.

Soft Tissues

Soft tissue masses may develop in both HL and NHL, either as tumor extension from bone involvement, or as an isolated mass within the muscles. Primary muscle lymphoma is extremely rare and is based on the absence of clinical or imaging features of lymphoma elsewhere. Patients with soft tissue lymphoma usually present with pain or neurological deficit, but occasionally a palpable mass may be present (251). The commonest radiological manifestation is muscle enlargement secondary to diffuse infiltration, with or without regional adenopathy (252). Without question, MR is the technique of choice for investigating patients with persistent pain, and even though a mass may be detected in retrospect on CT, the lack of contrast between the mass and adjacent muscle groups may lead to difficulties in diagnosis (Fig. 33.54).

Key Points: Bone and Bone Marrow

- Primary lymphoma of bone accounts for only 1% of all cases of NHL, whereas secondary involvement is seen in 5% to 6% of cases
- Secondary bone involvement is seen in 20% of patients with HL. Primary HL of bone is extremely rare
- In HL, soft tissue disease may invade adjacent bone but this is rare in NHL
- Bone marrow involvement indicates Stage IV disease and is present in 20% to 40% of patients with NHL at presentation
- Bone marrow biopsy in NHL increases the stage of disease in up to 30% of cases (Stage III to IV)
- In HL, bone marrow involvement occurs in 5% to 15% of patients during the course of disease
- Though FDG PET is more sensitive than CT or bone scintigraphy, false negative examinations occur with microscpic infiltrations and low-grade lymphomas
- MR is the method of choice for detecting soft tissue lymphomatous masses, which are usually due to secondary NHL

MUCOSA-ASSOCIATED LYMPHOID TISSUE (MALT) LYMPHOMA

Whilst extranodal involvement can be seen in any subtype of NHL, some forms of B-cell NHL occur exclusively in extranodal locations—the extranodal marginal zone lymphomas. They represent around 8% of all types of lymphoma and, for convenience, are divided into MALT types and generic types (31,32).

Pathology and Clinical Features

The MALT lymphomas arise from mucosal sites that normally have no organized lymphoid tissue, but within which acquired lymphoid tissue has arisen as a result of chronic inflammation or autoimmunity. Examples include Hashimoto's thyroiditis, Sjögren's syndrome and *Helicobacter*-induced chronic follicular gastritis. The association between gastric MALT lymphoma and *H. pylori* infection was

established in 1991 by Wotherspoon et al. (253), who found the organism in over 90% of cases. The detectability of *H. pylori* has been shown to diminish as lymphoma evolves from chronic gastritis (254). Remission of gastric MALT lymphoma can be achieved in over 60% of patients treated with antibiotics against *H. pylori.*

Patients with Sjögren's syndrome or lymphoepithelial sialadenitis have 44 times the risk of developing lymphoma, of which over 80% is MALT type. Patients with Hashimoto's thyroiditis have a 70-fold increased risk of thyroid lymphoma.

The histological hallmark of MALT lymphoma is the presence of lymphomatous cells in a marginal zone around reactive follicles, which can spread into the epithelium of glandular tissues to produce the characteristic lymphoepithelial lesion. In up to 30%, transformation to large cell lymphoma occurs, for example in the stomach.

The commonest site of involvement is the GIT (50% of cases), within which the stomach is most often affected (around 85% of cases). The small bowel and colon are involved in immunoproliferative small intestinal disease (IPSID), previously known as alpha-chain disease. Other sites commonly affected include the lung, head, neck, ocular adnexae, skin, thyroid, and breast.

Most cases occur in adults with a median age of 60 and there is a slight female preponderance. Most patients present with stage IE or IIE disease, which tends to be indolent. Bone marrow involvement is seen in 20%, but the frequency varies depending on the primary site, being higher with MALT lymphoma of the lung and ocular adnexae. Multiple extranodal sites are involved in up to 10%, but this does not appear to have the same poor prognostic import as in other forms of NHL, as it may not reflect truly disseminated disease (255). Nonetheless, extensive staging investigations may be necessary (185).

Imaging Features

GI Tract

Often gastric MALT lymphoma, especially low grade, causes minimal mucosal thickening, and CT may be normal (183), even if dedicated gastric CT is carried out with an oral water load and IV smooth muscle relaxants (256). It has been suggested that low-grade MALT lymphoma is more likely to cause shallow ulceration and nodulation, whereas higher grade ones are more likely to produce more massive gastric infiltration and polypoid masses (257). Endoscopic US is more accurate than CT pre- and post-treatment, defining wall depth and lymph node involvement (Fig. 33.55) (184,258). In addition, staging with EUS can help predict response to treatment of *H. pylori* (259).

In the colon and small bowel, MALT lymphoma is manifest as mucosal nodularity, which can be appreciated in barium studies (260).

Respiratory Tract

Mucosa-associated lymphoid tissue or BALT lymphoma represents 60% of all primary pulmonary lymphomas. The radiological pattern is similar to that of other lymphomas, being quite variable. The commonest patterns are masses, areas of consolidation and nodules with or without air bronchograms, and the CT angiogram sign (144,261–263). Multiple lesions are present in up to 80% of cases and lesions are often bilateral. Peribronchovascular nodularity and thickening is much less common. Lesions tend to

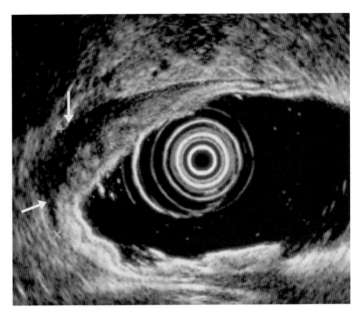

Figure 33.55 MALT lymphoma of the stomach. Endoscopic ultrasound examination showing a submucosal mass of low reflectivity (arrowed).

be indolent, whether nodular or consolidative. Associated pleural effusions occur in up to 20%.

Other Sites

In the thyroid, MALT lymphomas can present as diffuse enlargement or as large nodules that are hypoechoic at US and relatively hypodense at CT.

Mucosa-associated lymphoid tissue lymphomas of the lacrimal glands present as a mass or periorbital swelling. As with gastric MALT lymphoma, regional lymph node involvement is common in salivary gland MALT lymphomas. CT and MR depict uni- or bilateral enhancing masses with a non-specific appearance.

Up to 20% of lymphomas involving Waldeyer's ring are of MALT type. The tonsils are most commonly affected, the commonest pattern being asymmetric thickening of the pharyngeal mucosa. This is well shown by CT and MR.

Key Points: MALT Lymphoma

- These arise from mucosal sites that normally have no organized lymphoid tissue, but arise as a result of chronic inflammation or autoimmunity
- The commonest site of involvement is the GI tract; the stomach is involved in 85% of cases
- Other sites include the thyroid (Hashimoto's), respiratory tract, and lacrimal gland (Sjögren's)

BURKITT LYMPHOMA (BL)

Burkitt lymphoma is a highly aggressive B-cell variant of NHL, associated with EBV in a variable proportion of cases. Nearly all have genetic translocations involving the *c-myc* oncogene.

Three clinical variants are recognized:

- Endemic (African) type (264)–EBV positive in 50% to 70%
- Sporadic (non-endemic) (265)–EBV positive in 15% to 20%
- Immunodeficiency associated

These tumors are extremely aggressive and rapidly growing, but they are potentially curable. Though they account for only 2% to 3% of NHL in immunocompetent adults, 30% to 50% of all childhood lymphomas are BL. Immunodeficiency associated BL is seen chiefly in association with HIV infection and may be the initial manifestation of AIDS. EBV is identified in up to 40% of these cases. Extranodal disease is common and all three variants are at risk for CNS disease (266).

In the endemic form, the jaws, maxilla, and orbit are involved in 50% of cases, producing the "floating tooth sign" on plain radiography. The ovaries, kidneys, and breast may be involved. The sporadic forms have a predilection for the ileocecal region and patients can present with acute abdominal emergencies such as intussusception. Again, ovaries, kidneys, and breasts are commonly involved. Retroperitoneal and paraspinal disease can cause paraplegia, the presenting feature in up to 15% of affected individuals. Thoracic disease is relatively rare; in a recent series, 50% had disease confined to the abdomen (267). Leptomeningeal disease can be seen at presentation and is a site of relapse.

LYMPHOMA IN THE IMMUNOCOMPROMISED (SEE ALSO CHAPS. 57–60)

The WHO classification recognizes four broad groupings associated with an increased incidence of lymphoma and lymphoproliferative disorders (268):

- Primary immunodeficiency syndromes
- Infection with HIV
- Iatrogenic immunosuppression after solid organ or bone marrow allografts
- Iatrogenic immunosuppression from methotrexate (usually for autoimmune disorders)

The development of lymphoma in these settings is multifactorial, but mostly related to defective immune surveillance, with or without chronic antigenic stimulation.

AIDS-Related Lymphomas (ARL) (See also Chaps. 59 and 60)

The incidence of all subtypes of NHL is increased 60 to 200 fold in patients with HIV, and lymphoma is the first AIDS-defining illness in up to 5% of HIV patients. The incidence of HL is also increased up to eight-fold. Various types of NHL are seen, including those seen in immunocompetent patients, such as BL, DLBCL (especially in the CNS), but some occur much more frequently in the HIV population (e.g., primary effusion lymphoma and plasmablastic lymphoma of the oral cavity). Compared with non-HIV associated high-grade NHL, the prognosis is poorer with more frequent relapses and shorter overall survival. Since the advent of highly active antiretroviral therapy (HAART), the incidence of ARL have decreased from 6.2 to 3.6 per 1000 person-years (11),

but despite this, the proportion of patients for whom NHL is AIDS-defining has increased (269).

Most ARL have a marked propensity to involve extranodal sites, especially the GI tract, CNS (less frequent with the advent of highly active antiretroviral therapy), liver, and bone marrow. Multiple sites of extranodal involvement are seen in over 75% of cases (270). Peripheral lymph node enlargement is seen in only 30% of cases at presentation.

Most tumors are aggressive, with advanced stage bulky disease and a high serum LDH at presentation. DLBCL tends to occur later on, when CD4 counts are under 100×10^6/L, whereas BL occurs in less immunodeficient patients. EBV positivity occurs in up to 70% of cases depending on the precise morphological variant, whereas PCNSL is associated with EBV in over 90% of cases; interestingly, EBV positivity is seen in nearly all cases of HL associated with HIV.

In the chest, NHL is usually extranodal; pleural effusion and lung disease are common, often with nodules, acinar and interstitial opacities. Hilar and mediastinal nodal enlargement is generally mild. There is a wide differential diagnosis and in one study the presence of cavitation and nodal necrosis predicted for mycobacterial infection rather than lymphoma (271).

Within the abdomen, the GI tract, liver, kidneys, adrenal glands, and lower genitourinary tract are commonly involved. Mesenteric and retroperitoneal nodal enlargement is less common than in immunocompetent patients, but there are no apparent differences in the CT features of patients with or without AIDS, at least in relation to the small bowel (186).

Regarding PCNSL, certain features such as rim enhancement and multifocality are seen more often than in the immunocompetent population. This can cause confusion with cerebral toxoplasmosis, though the location of PCNSL in the deep white matter is suggestive (272). Quantitative FDG PET uptake can help in the differentiation of PCNSL, toxoplasmosis and progressive multifocal leucoencephalopathy (PML), being higher in the former (273).

Post-Transplant Lymphoproliferative Disorders (Fig. 33.56)

These occur in 2% to 4% of solid organ transplant recipients depending on the type of transplant, the lowest frequency being seen in renal transplant recipients (1%) and the highest in heart–lung or liver–bowel allografts (5%). Marrow allograft recipients in general have a low risk (1%). Most are associated with EBV infection and appear to represent EBV-induced monoclonal or, more rarely, polyclonal B-cell or T-cell proliferation in a setting of reduced immune surveillance as a consequence of immune suppression. The clinical features are variable, correlating with the type of allograft and type of immunosuppression. Post-transplant lymphoproliferative disorders develop earlier in patients receiving cyclosporin A (mean interval 15 months) rather than azathioprine (mean interval 48 months). Epstein–Barr-positive cases occur earlier than EBV-negative cases, the latter occurring four to five years after transplantation. In all cases, extranodal disease is common. In patients receiving azathioprine, the allograft itself and the CNS are often involved, whereas in patients who have received cyclosporin A, the GI tract is affected more often than the CNS. The bone marrow, liver, and lung are often affected, as are the tonsils.

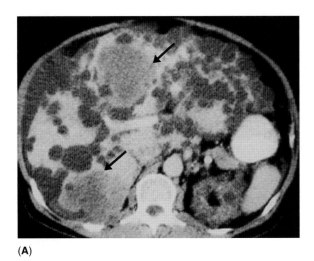
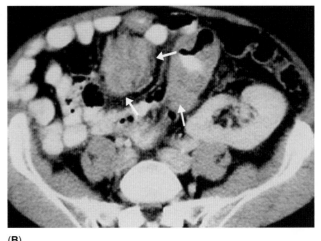

(A)   (B)

Figure 33.56 Post-transplant lymphoproliferative disorder of the liver. (**A**) CT scan in patient with known autosomal dominant cystic disease of the kidneys who underwent a renal transplant (see **B**). Multiple lymphomatous foci are demonstrated within the liver (arrowed) together with the associated benign liver cysts. Note the associated ascites and the cystic disease of the native left kidney. (**B**) Renal transplant in the left iliac fossa. A large mesenteric mass is also demonstrated (arrowed) together with infiltration of the small bowel.

In the lung, multiple or solitary pulmonary nodules occur, with or without mediastinal adenopathy. Pleural effusions are common and confluent; patchy airspace opacity is another pattern (274–276). Reticulonodular opacity is rare.

Abdominal PTLD is characterized by a relatively high frequency of extranodal disease, especially of the GI tract and liver (Fig. 33.56). Multiple segments of bowel may be affected and there is a propensity for PTLD to develop in the allograft itself (277,278).

Key Points: Lymphoma in the Immunocompromised

■ Lymphomas associated with HIV have a propensity to involve extranodal sites (especially the GI tract, CNS, liver, and bone marrow) and multiple sites. Most tumors are aggressive with advanced stage, bulky disease

■ Post-transplant lympoproliferative disorder occurs in 2% to 4% of solid organ and 1% of marrow allograft recipients and typically causes solitary or multiple lung nodules. In the abdomen this disorder is characterized by involvement of the GI tract and liver

POST-TREATMENT EVALUATION

With the advent of FDG PET and now FDG PET/CT, there has been a paradigm shift in response assessment in lymphoma. Before the introduction of FDG PET into clinical practice, CT was the main tool available for this purpose. Cross-sectional imaging still plays a vital role in monitoring response to therapy during and at the end of treatment. Once treatment is completed, periodic surveillance studies help in detection of potential relapse. Where there is clinical evidence of relapse, imaging studies are performed to evaluate the extent of the disease.

Monitoring Response to Therapy

Achievement of a complete remission following treatment is the most important factor for prolonged survival in both HL and

NHL. Thus, final evaluation of response at or within one month of completion of therapy is critical.

"Complete remission" is diagnosed only when no abnormality is seen at the site of previously demonstrated disease. The chest radiograph is useful in assessing response when there is intrathoracic disease and is repeated at each monthly visit. Although the chest radiograph will show response early in the treatment, changes due to radiotherapy often make the mediastinum difficult to assess. Other mediastinal changes associated with treatment such as rebound hyperplasia or thymic cyst formation cannot be reliably identified on the chest radiograph and therefore response cannot be monitored reliably. CT therefore remains essential in the monitoring of response to treatment for mediastinal disease, especially when the chest radiograph is indeterminate (279). In patients with intra-abdominal disease, serial CT is essential in monitoring response. For the purpose of assessment of response to treatment, it is often necessary to measure a number of marker lesions before and after therapy. Modern CT scanners permit accurate reproducible measurements of well defined nodal masses provided scan parameters (narrow collimation slices, with overlapping reconstructions) and techniques are optimized. However, there is significant interobserver variation, which is even more pronounced with irregular masses or when there is poor lesion–background contrast, which may occur even with adequate bowel and vascular opacification (280).

The optimal and exact timing of such scans for reassessment has not been widely investigated (281,282). In many centers, the practice is to assess patients fully one month after completion of therapy. Others favor an interim CT study during initial chemotherapy for lymphoma after two cycles of chemotherapy; the timing will often depend on local clinical practice, the availability of resources, and on whether the patient is participating in a clinical trial. The speed of modern CT scanners has largely removed the need for limited scans advocated in the past, and though it has been argued that routine administration of IV contrast medium is unnecessary for follow-up scans, in practice, multislice technology allows the acquisition of scans with optimal vascular and parenchymal enhancement throughout the neck, chest, abdomen, and pelvis, facilitating follow-up of nodal and particularly, extranodal disease.

Criteria of Response

International standardized response criteria are essential for clinical research, facilitating data interpretation and comparison of therapies. A report published in 1999 set out new criteria for assessment of response in NHL, bringing it into line with those already in use for HL (283). The International Workshop radiological criteria (IWC) are defined as follows:

- Complete remission (CR): complete disappearance of all radiographic evidence of disease. Nodes and nodal masses of disease regressed to <1.5 cm in greatest transverse diameter for nodes >1.5 cm before therapy. Previously involved nodes 1.1 to 1.5 cm in greatest transverse diameter regressed to <1 cm in greatest transverse diameter after therapy. The spleen, if enlarged by CT criteria, must have regressed
- Complete remission, unconfirmed (CR$_u$): where there is a residual nodal mass >1.5 cm maximum transverse diameter that has regressed by >75% of sum of products of greatest diameters (SPD)
- Partial remission (PR): >50% decrease in SPD of largest nodes/masses. No increase in size of spleen, lymph nodes, liver. Splenic and hepatic nodules decreased by 50%
- Stable disease (SD): decrease in SPD less than a PR and no evidence of progressive disease
- Progressive disease (PD): 50% or greater increase from nadir in the SPD of any previously identified abnormal node for PRs or non-responders—appearance of any new lesion during or at the end of therapy
- Relapse from CR or CR$_u$ requires: appearance of any new lesion or increase by 50% or more in the size of previously involved sites. Fifty percent increase in greatest diameter of any previously identified node >1 cm in its short axis or in the SPD of more than one node

Assessment of Residual Masses

Although successfully treated enlarged nodes often return to normal, in HL and NHL a residual mass of "sterilized" fibrous tissue can persist. On a chest radiograph such a residual mass may remain following treatment in 12% to 88% of patients (284). Such residual masses occur more frequently in patients with bulky rather than non-bulky disease, in HL and NHL. Residual masses are seen at CT in up to 20% to 50% of patients in clinical CR after treatment for NHL (285,286). It is uncertain whether relapse is more common in patients with residual masses; the literature on this subject is conflicting (282,287). There is no obvious correlation between the size of the residual mass and the relapse rate. Determining the nature of such residual masses and excluding the possibility of active disease by imaging remains a major challenge in monitoring patients with lymphoma.

Computed Tomography

Using the International Workshop criteria, residual masses at CT are those that have reduced by up to 75% but which are nonetheless more than 1.5 cm in maximum transverse diameter (Fig. 33.14). CT cannot distinguish between fibrotic tissue, necrosis, and residual active disease on the basis of density alone, hence the very low specificity and PPV of CT after treatment in every series published to date. Nevertheless, serial CT performed every two to three months has been the most widely used method of determining the true nature of a residual mass. Masses that remain static after one year are considered to be inactive, whereas any increase in size is highly suggestive of relapse. Relapse following satisfactory response to initial treatment occurs in 10% to 40% of patients with HL and in around 50% of patients with NHL (126). In HL, relapse usually occurs within the first two years following treatment and patients are followed up closely during this period, although CT examinations are not usually required unless clinical features suggest the possibility of recurrence.

Magnetic Resonance Imaging

There is now substantial data investigating the value of MR in identifying residual active neoplasm within residual masses (71,72,288,289). In general, a reduction in signal intensity on T2-weighted images is seen during or following successful treatment (Fig. 33.57).

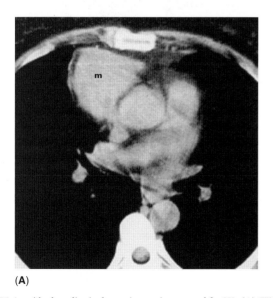

(A)

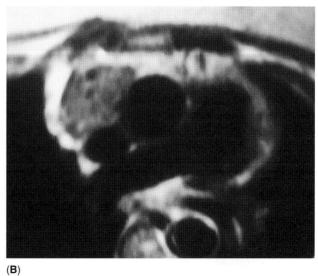

(B)

Figure 33.57 A residual mediastinal mass in a patient treated for HL. (**A**) CT scan. (**B**) Conventional spin-echo T2-weighted MR image. The residual mass (m) measures approximately 5 × 5 cm in diameter and has a homogeneous intensity, suggesting that the mass is inactive. A CT-guided core biopsy was obtained. On histological examination there was no evidence of active HL.

Persistent heterogeneous or recurrent high signal intensity on T2-weighted sequences following treatment appears to have a high specificity and PPV for residual active disease (289). False positives do arise due to inflammatory edema or cyst formation (117,288,290). However, not surprisingly, the sensitivity for the detection of active disease is low, as small foci of persistent tumor within a low signal intensity mass cannot be identified reliably on T2-weighted images (71,72,290). Furthermore, with increasing availability of PET/CT, it is likely that this modality will supercede MR in the assessment of the residual mass.

Functional Imaging
In the past decade, there has been an explosion of interest in the use of functional imaging (notably, FDG PET) for response assessment and evaluation of the residual mass. Gallium scintigraphy is no

longer the investigation of choice in this setting. Though persistent positive uptake usually indicates persistent active neoplasm (reflected in a PPV for relapse double that of CT) (291,292), the value of gallium scanning is limited by both its lower sensitivity and specificity, by the significant proportion of non-gallium-avid tumors, and by the imaging characteristics of the isotope (82,291). Furthermore, the radiation dose imparted is much higher than that from a PET scan. Indeed, in a recent study of patients with HL and residual mediastinal masses, there was a non-significant trend towards greater accuracy with MR compared to Ga-67, with greater predictive powers for two year progression-free survival (293). For all these reasons, Ga-67 today is not widely used to evaluate the residual mass.

On the other hand, FDG PET has been shown to have a high predictive value in the differentiation between active tumor and fibrosis in patients with a residual mass (Figs. 33.58 and 33.59) (80).

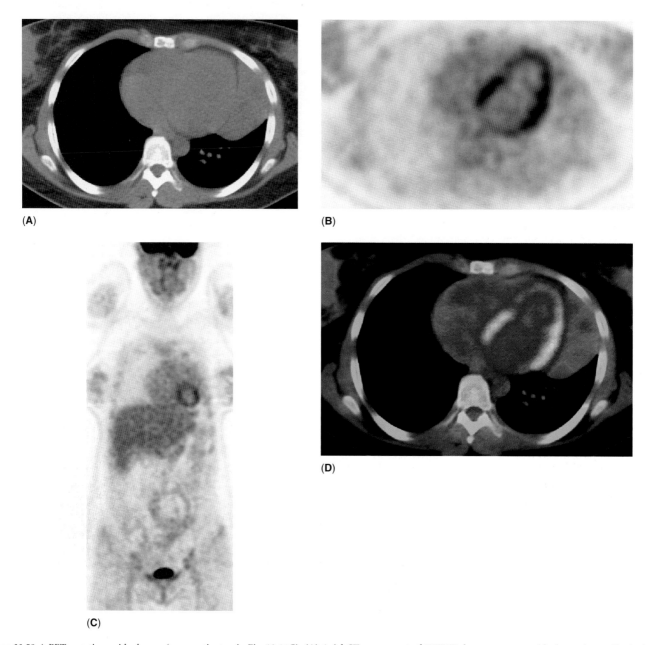

(A)

(B)

(C)

(D)

Figure 33.58 A PET negative residual mass (same patient as in Fig. 33.11C). (**A**) Axial CT component of PET/CT demonstrates a residual anterior mediastinal mass. (**B**) Axial FDG-PET scan. (**C**) Coronal FDG-PET scan. (**D**) Fused axial image. There is no significant metabolic activity within the residual mass.

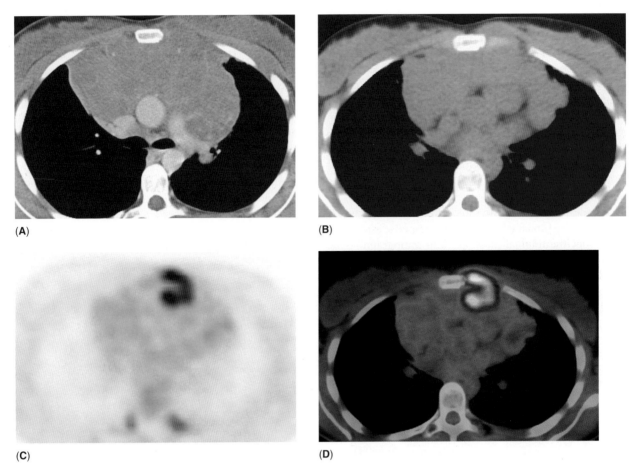

Figure 33.59 A PET-positive residual mass in a patient with primary mediastinal large B cell lymphoma. (A) Pre-treatment axial contrast-enhanced CT scan. (B) Post-treatment CT component of PET/CT scan demonstrates an irregular residual mass. (C) The axial FDG-PET scan demonstrates a focus of intense metabolic activity within part of the residual mass. (D) Fused image. The focus of residual disease involves the chest wall. Symmetrical moderate activity around the costo-transverse joints posteriorly is within brown fat.

Indeed, FDG PET has a high PPV for relapse, with or without a residual mass at CT, allowing directed biopsies, or consolidative therapy as appropriate (294–300). There are a few pitfalls in that small volumes of disease can produce false negative examinations (in around 5%), whereas reactive and inflammatory changes (for example in the lungs, thymus, and bone marrow) are causes of false positive examinations. Thus, it is essential that clinical correlation be made when interpreting FDG PET results (301). In one study directly comparing Ga-67 and FDG PET, the latter was more sensitive, and though there were more false positive findings with FDG PET, these were readily interpreted as such when reference was made to the clinical history and other findings (302).

FDG PET in Response Assessment
Generally, a positive FDG PET scan at the end of therapy strongly predicts for early relapse (298) for HL and NHL. In one follow-up study, all PET-positive/CT-negative patients relapsed, whereas only 5% of PET-negative/CT-positive patients relapsed (303). Jerusalem and colleagues showed the PPV of FDG PET to be 100%, compared with 42% for CT, in the post-treatment assessment of patients with HL or NHL (297). In a similar study including 93 patients with NHL, Spaepen et al. demonstrated the predictive value for progression-free survival (PFS) of FDG

PET at the end of first-line therapy, with a two year PFS of 4% for patients with a positive FDG PET, compared with 85% for patients with a negative FDG PET (304). Ultimately, all patients with a positive PET scan relapsed, but under 50% of relapses would have been predicted by conventional imaging. Similar results were reported by the same group in patients with HL, two year PFS being 0% for patients with a positive FDG PET in comparison with 91% for the group with a negative FDG PET (305).

Incorporation of the end-of-treatment FDG PET scan result into the standard response criteria has a significant impact on response categorization. In a retrospective study of 54 patients with DLBCL treated with CHOP, and followed up for 18 months, Juweid et al. found that the assessment based on IWC and PET provided a more accurate response classification that correlated better with clinical outcome than the standard response criteria (306). Patients with a PR by standard IWC, who were FDG PET negative, did as well as those who were in CR by IWC and IWC and PET, indicating superior discriminative ability. The category CR$_u$ was abolished by the inclusion of FDG PET.

As a result of the increasing evidence for the use of FDG PET in response assessment, an International Harmonization Project was convened to revise the standard response criteria (307). These guidelines support the use of FDG PET for end of therapy response assessment in DLBCL and HL. However, they state that the role

of FDG PET for response assessment of "aggressive" NHL subtypes other than DLBCL and "indolent" lymphomas is less clear-cut, and that FDG PET should be used only if overall response rate and CR rate are important end-points of clinical studies. The revised criteria specify that patients can be assigned to the CR category with a residual mass of any size, provided that it is PET negative at the end of treatment and was, or can reasonably expected to have been, FDG PET positive before treatment. The CR$_u$ category is eliminated. For patients with FDG-avid lymphomas, a partial response exists where there is residual FDG PET positivity in at least one previously involved site. The group has also issued guidance on performance and interpretation of FDG PET scans (308).

FDG PET in Prognostication

One of the most exciting applications of FDG PET scanning is in early prediction of response to treatment, which is quite different from assessment of treatment response after completion of therapy. Prediction of response refers to FDG PET imaging after one or two cycles of systemic therapy. Early prediction of response to treatment may be of value in the identification of patients who are unlikely to respond, allowing early discontinuation of ineffective therapy before toxicity has resulted (309). Several studies have shown early FDG PET (after 2 or 3 cycles of chemotherapy) in "aggressive" NHL to be a more accurate predictor of PFS and overall survival than other known prognostic indictors, such as the IPI, especially for diffuse histologies (294,310). Haioun et al. found that PFS at two years was 82% for patients with a negative interim FDG PET, whereas it was 43% for patients with a positive FDG PET (311). Similar studies of early interim FDG PET in patients with HL have also shown a strong association between FDG PET result after two to three cycles and PFS and overall survival (OS) (312,313). There is some evidence that FDG PET performed after just one cycle of chemotherapy has high prognostic value both in DLBCL and HL, but the optimum timing of early response assessment still needs to be evaluated in larger studies with longer follow-up (314).

Most of these studies have used qualitative interpretation of FDG uptake and there is limited data utilizing quantitative assessment. Calculation of standardized uptake values (SUV) by normalization of tumor FDG uptake to injected activity and body weight is the most common method for tumor quantification. Naumann and colleagues reported that a cut-off of 3.0 for the SUV was able to differentiate between active lymphoma and sterile residual masses with a sensitivity of 100% and a specificity of 93% (298). The percentage reduction in SUV from baseline may also be used to differentiate responders from non-responders. Thus, Torizuka et al. clearly separated responders from the non-responders using a 60% reduction in the SUV from baseline to post one to two cycles of chemotherapy (315). At present, there is no consensus on which method should be used for early prediction of response, and therefore, interim FDG PET should only be performed as part of a clinical trial.

FDG PET can also be used to predict outcome prior to high-dose treatments (316). Patients who commence high-dose therapies with a positive pre-treatment PET scan have a much poorer prognosis.

Key Points: Functional Imaging

- Residual masses are seen in up to 50% of patients successfully treated for HL and NHL
- Functional imaging with FDG PET distinguishes between residual disease and sterilized fibrous tissue much more accurately than anatomical cross-sectional imaging
- Incorporation of end-of-treatment PET result into the standardized response criteria for NHL improves correlation with clinical outcome
- Early interim PET scans after one to two cycles of treatment for aggressive NHL can confer important prognostic information
- A positive FDG PET scan at completion of therapy predicts for early relapse and reduced progression-free survival, regardless of the CT findings

Follow-up and Surveillance

Strategies for follow-up with imaging vary between institutions and, in addition, in patients with residual masses in HL and NHL, follow-up depends on the size of the mass, the sites of involvement, and the extent of disease. It is therefore impossible to define strict guidelines for each clinical situation.

For patients who attain CR or CR$_u$ (i.e., where there is a Ga-67 or a FDG PET-negative residual mass), it has been argued that routine imaging is desirable to detect asymptomatic early relapse, so that salvage therapy can be offered. In this situation, CT may be of limited value, since it may take some time before there is an appreciable increase in the size of the residual mass.

In one series of patients with NHL who attained CR, only two of 36 relapses were diagnosed before patients were symptomatic, and only one was identified by imaging alone. This study did not include functional imaging. Of the relapses, 25% were in new sites alone, whereas the previous site was involved in the remainder (317). Front et al. (79) found that Ga-67 scintigraphy indicated relapse on average seven months before the development of clinical signs or an abnormality on CT and in this setting, the sensitivity of Ga-67 was 95%. In another study, the quoted sensitivities and specificities for recurrence were 59% and 72% for CT, and 88% and 100% for Ga-67, respectively (318).

There are other studies suggesting that conventional imaging follow-up with CT is rarely rewarding. Radford et al. found that 86% of relapses in a cohort of patients with HL were detected as a result of investigation of new symptoms rather than by routine follow-up studies (319), and Guadagnolo et al. calculated that there was very little benefit from routine CT in the surveillance of asymptomatic patients in CR after treatment for HL (320). In another series of patients with treated intermediate and high-grade NHL, only 17% of relapses were detected by routine CT (13%) or laboratory tests (4%) alone (321).

Given the wealth of comparative data consistently showing a higher sensitivity for FDG PET in the detection of disease compared to CT, especially at extranodal sites, and the lower radiation dose (9 mSv vs. 30 mSv), there are theoretical reasons for choosing PET as a routine surveillance procedure—but there is as yet little evidence to support the role of PET in this situation. Jerusalem et al. evaluated FDG PET in the detection of preclinical relapse in

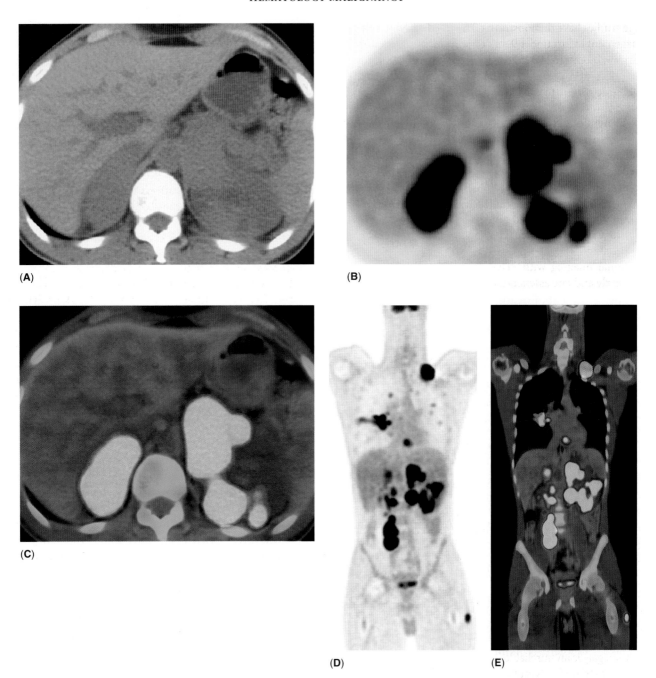

Figure 33.60 Relapsed high-grade NHL. (**A**) Axial CT component of PET/CT scan.(**B**) Corresponding FDG-PET scan. (**C**) Fused dataset. There are renal and adrenal FDG-avid masses as well as a small coeliac axis lymph node which also displays moderate activity. (**D**) Coronal FDG-PET scan and (**E**) corresponding fused dataset demonstrate nodal and extranodal relapse in multiple supra- and infradiaphragmatic nodal groups, the lungs, major viscera and also within the musculature of the thigh.

a cohort of patients treated for HL (322). In this series, all relapses were identified by PET before there was any other evidence of relapse. There was a significant number of false positive scans but in each of these, a confirmatory scan four to six weeks later was normal, and there were no false negative studies. In this setting, FDG PET will only be useful if there is a survival advantage to be gained from starting salvage therapy sooner rather than later, and if the rate of false positive studies is acceptably low. However, in cases of suspected relapse, the development of a positive PET scan is highly suggestive (Fig. 33.60). There is a need for multicenter prospective randomized trials to establish the role, if any, of routine imaging surveillance of asymptomatic patients.

Role of Percutaneous Biopsy

Percutaneous core biopsy using imaging guidance is now established as a valuable method of determining the nature of soft tissue masses in lymphoma. The indications for its use include:

- Defining the nature of a residual mass following treatment
- Detection of transformation of NHL to a higher grade (323,324)
- Primary diagnosis in patients who present with unusual manifestations of disease

Two large studies have demonstrated that core biopsy is sufficient for management in just under 90%, enabling around 80% to avoid open surgical biopsy (324,325)

Key Points: Post-Treatment Evaluation

- Achievement of CR following treatment is the most important prognostic indicator in both HL and NHL
- Relapse following initial treatment occurs in up to 40% of patients with HL and over 50% of patients with NHL
- Relapse usually occurs within the first two years following treatment of HL
- Residual masses in HL and NHL may contain active malignancy that cannot be detected on anatomical cross-sectional imaging alone
- Functional imaging with FDG-PET is more accurate than CT in early and late assessment of response to treatment

Summary

- NHL and HL are a heterogeneous diverse group of malignancies that predominantly involves the lymph nodes
- In HL, most patients present with early-stage malignancy, whereas in NHL most patients present with advanced disease
- The incidence of NHL is increasing but the incidence of HL is stable
- In NHL, the prognosis varies widely according to tumor grade and stage at diagnosis
- HL tends to spread from one lymph node to the next in a contiguous manner, whereas NHL spreads in a more haphazard manner
- Involvement of intrathoracic lymph nodes is more common in HL than NHL
- Involvement of retroperitoneal and mesenteric nodes is more common in NHL than HL
- Extranodal sites of involvement are more common in NHL than HL
- The spleen is involved in 10% of patients with HL as isolated infradiaphragmatic disease
- Splenomegaly is an unreliable indicator of splenic lymphoma
- Primary extranodal lymphoma is almost exclusively seen in NHL

REFERENCES

1. Reznek RH, Richards MA. The radiology of lymphoma. Baillière's Clin Haematol 1987; 1: 77–107.
2. CancerStats—Incidence UK. Cancer Research UK, February 2008.
3. Callender ST, Vaneghan RI. The lymphomas. In: Weatherall DJ, Ledingham JG, Warrell DA, eds. Oxford Textbook of Medicine. Oxford: Oxford University Press, 1983: 160–74.
4. Jemal A, Siegel R, Ward E, et al. Cancer Statistics, 2008. CA Cancer J Clin 2008; 58: 71–96.
5. Ries LA, Kosary CL, Hankey BF, et al. SEER Cancer Statistics Review, 1973–1996. Bethesda, MD: National Cancer Institute, 1999.
6. Devesa SS, Fears T. Non-Hodgkin's lymphoma time trends: United States and international data. Cancer Res 1992; 52: 5432s–5440s.
7. Muir C, Waterhouse J, Mack T, et al. Cancer incidence in five continents, Vol V. IARC Scientific Publication 42. Lyon: International Agency for Research on Cancer, 1987.
8. Cartwright R, Brincker H, Carli PM, et al. The rise in incidence of lymphomas in Europe 1985–1992. Eur J Cancer 1999; 35: 627–33.
9. Rabkin CS, Devesa SS, Zahm SH, Gail MH. Increasing incidence of non-Hodgkin's lymphoma. Semin Hematol 1993; 30: 286–96.
10. Banks PM. Changes in diagnosis of Non-Hodgkin's lymphomas over time. Cancer Res 1992; 52: 5453s–5455s.
11. International collaboration on HIV and cancer. Highly active antiretroviral therapy and the incidence of cancer in HIV-infected adults. J Natl Cancer Inst 2000; 92: 1823–30.
12. Hartge P, Devesa SS. Quantification of the impact of known risk factors on time trends in non-Hodgkin's lymphoma incidence. Cancer Res 1992; 52: 5566s–5569s.
13. Barnes N, Cartwright RA, O'Brien C, et al. Rising incidence of lymphoid malignancies—true or false? Br J Cancer 1986; 53: 393–8.
14. Glass AG, Karnell LH, Menck HR. The National Cancer Data Base report on non-Hodgkin's lymphoma. Cancer 1997; 80: 2311–20.
15. Horwich A. Hodgkin's disease. In: Horwich A, ed. Oncology: A Multidisciplinary Textbook. London: Chapman and Hall, 1995: 235–50.
16. Kuefler PR, Bunn PA Jr. Adult T cell leukaemia/lymphoma. Clin Haematol 1986; 15: 695–726.
17. De la Fouchardiere A, Vandenesch F, Berger F. Borrelia-associated primary cutaneous MALT lymphoma in a non-endemic region. Am J Surg Pathol 2003; 27: 702–3.
18. Skibola CF, Curry JD, Nieters A. Genetic susceptibility to lymphoma. Haematologica 2007; 92: 960–9.
19. Ballerini P, Gaidano G, Gong JZ, et al. Multiple genetic lesions in acquired immunodeficiency syndrome-related non-Hodgkin's lymphoma. Blood 1993; 81: 166–76.
20. Cleary ML, Sklar J. Lymphoproliferative disorders in cardiac transplant recipients are multiclonal lymphomas. Lancet 1984; 2: 489–93.
21. Filipovich AH, Mathur A, Kamat D, Shapiro RS. Primary immunodeficiencies: genetic risk factors for lymphoma. Cancer Res 1992; 52(19 Suppl): 5465s–5467s.
22. Osborne BM. Contextual diagnosis of Hodgkin's disease and non-Hodgkin's lymphoma. Radiol Clin North Am 1990; 28: 669–82.
23. Lukes RJ, Butler JJ. The pathology and nomenclature of Hodgkin's disease. Cancer Res 1966; 26: 1063–83.
24. Lukes RJ, Craver LF, Hall TC, et al. Report of the Nomenclature Committee. Cancer Res 1966; 26: 1311.
25. National Cancer Institute sponsored study of classifications of Non-Hodgkin's lymphomas: summary and description of a working formulation for clinical usage. The Non-Hodgkin Lymphoma Pathologic Classification Project. Cancer 1982; 49: 2112–35.
26. Rosenberg SA, Diamond HD, Jaslowitz B, Craver LF. Lymphosarcoma: a review of 1269 cases. Medicine 1961; 40: 31–84.

27. Rappaport H. Tumors of the hematopoietic system. In: Atlas of Tumor Pathology. Section 2, Fascicle 8. Washington, DC: Armed Forces Institute of Pathology, 1966.

28. Cossman J, Uppenkamp M, Sundeen J, Coupland R, Raffeld M. Molecular genetics and the diagnosis of lymphoma. Arch Pathol Lab Med 1988; 112: 117–27.

29. Harris NL, Jaffe ES, Stein H, et al. A revised European-American classification of lymphoid neoplasms: a proposal from the International Lymphoma Study Group. Blood 1994; 84: 1361–92.

30. Harris NL, Jaffe ES, Diebold J, et al. World Health Organization classification of neoplastic diseases of the hematopoietic and lymphoid tissues: report of the Clinical Advisory Committee meeting—Airlie House, Virginia, November 1997. J Clin Oncol 1999; 17: 3835–49.

31. A clinical evaluation of the International Lymphoma Study Group classification of non-Hodgkin's lymphoma. The Non-Hodgkin's Lymphoma Classification Project. Blood 1997; 89: 3909–18.

32. Armitage JO, Weisenburger DD. New approach to classifying non-Hodgkin's lymphomas: clinical features of the major histologic subtypes. Non-Hodgkin's Lymphoma Classification Project. J Clin Oncol 1998;16: 2780–95.

33. Alizadeh AA, Eisen MB, Davis RE, et al. Distinct types of diffuse large B-cell lymphoma identified by gene expression profiling. Nature 2000; 403: 503–11.

34. Lister TA, Crowther D, Sutcliffe SB, et al. Report of a committee convened to discuss the evaluation and staging of patients with Hodgkin's disease: Cotswolds meeting. J Clin Oncol 1989; 7: 1630–6.

35. Cabanillas F, Fuller LM. The radiologic assessment of the lymphoma patient from the standpoint of the clinician. Radiol Clin North Am 1990; 28: 683–95.

36. Marglin SI, Castellino RA. Selection of imaging studies for the initial staging of patients with Hodgkin's disease. Semin Ultrasound CT MR 1985; 6: 393.

37. Murphy SB. Childhood non-Hodgkin's lymphoma. N Engl J Med 1978; 299: 1446–8.

38. Ng YY, Healy JC, Vincent JM, et al. The radiology of non-Hodgkin lymphoma in childhood: a review of 80 cases. Clin Radiol 1994; 49: 594–600.

39. Ott G, Katzenberger T, Lohr A, et al. Cytomorphologic, immunohistochemical and cytogenetic profiles of follicular lymphoma: 2 types of follicular lymphoma grade 3. Blood 2002; 99: 3806–12.

40. Price CG. Non-Hodgkin's lymphoma. In: Price CG, Sikora K, eds. Treatment of Cancer. London: Chapman and Hall, 1995: 881–97.

41. Kennedy BJ, Loeb V Jr, Peterson VM, et al. National survey of patterns of care for Hodgkin's disease. Cancer 1985; 56: 2547–56.

42. Hellman S, Mauch P. Role of radiation therapy in the treatment of Hodgkin disease. Cancer Treat Rep 1982; 66: 915–23.

43. Tubiana M, Henry-Amar M, Carde P, et al. Toward comprehensive management tailored to prognostic factors of patients with clinical stages I and II in Hodgkin's disease. The EORTC Lymphoma Group controlled clinical trials: 1964–1987. Blood 1989; 73: 47–56.

44. Henry-Amar M. Second cancer after the treatment for Hodgkin's disease: a report from the International Database on Hodgkin's Disease. Ann Oncol 1992; 3(Suppl 4): 117–28.

45. Chabner BA, Fisher RI, Young RC, DeVita VT. Staging of non-Hodgkin's lymphoma. Semin Oncol 1980; 7: 285–91.

46. Bonadonna G, Santoro A, Bonfante V, Valagussa P. Cyclic delivery of MOPP and ABVD combinations in Stage IV Hodgkin disease: rationale, background studies, and recent results. Cancer Treat Rep 1982; 66: 881–7.

47. Canellos GP, Anderson JR, Propert KJ, et al. Chemotherapy of advanced Hodgkin's disease with MOPP, ABVD, or MOPP alternating with ABVD. N Engl J Med 1992; 327: 1478–84.

48. Gupta RK, Lister TA. Hodgkin's disease. In: Price CG, Sikora K, eds. Treatment of Cancer. London: Chapman & Hall, 1995: 851–80.

49. Healey EA, Tarbell NJ, Kalish LA, et al. Prognostic factors for patients with Hodgkin disease in first relapse. Cancer 1993; 71: 2613–20.

50. Desch CE, Lasala MR, Smith TJ, Hillner BE. The optimal timing of autologous bone marrow transplantation in Hodgkin's disease patients after a chemotherapy relapse. J Clin Oncol 1992; 10: 200–9.

51. Ng AK, Bernardo MP, Weller E, et al. Long-term survival and competing causes of death in patients with early-stage Hodgkin's disease treated at age 50 or younger. J Clin Oncol 2002; 20: 2101–8.

52. Kaufman D, Longo D. Hodgkin's disease. Crit Rev Oncol/Hematol 1992; 13: 135–87.

53. Sundeen JT, Cossman J, Jaffe ES. Lymphocyte predominant Hodgkin's disease, nodular subtype with coexistent "large cell lymphoma". Histological progression or composite malignancy? Am J Surg Pathol 1988; 12; 599–606.

54. Bastion Y, Sebban C, Berger F, et al. Incidence, predictive factors and outcome of lymphoma transformation in follicular lymphoma patients. J Clin Oncol 1997; 15: 1587–94.

55. The International Non-Hodgkin's Lymphoma Prognostic Factors Project. A predictive model for aggressive non-Hodgkin's lymphoma. N Engl J Med 1993; 329: 987–94.

56. Oken MM, Creech RH, Tormey DC, et al. Toxicity and response criteria of the Eastern Cooperative Oncology Group. Am J Clin Oncol 1982; 5: 649–55.

57. Solal-Celigny P. Follicular Lymphoma International Prognostic Index. Curr Treat Option Oncol 2006; 7: 270–5.

58. Dyer MJ. Non-Hodgkin's lymphoma. In: Horwich A, ed. Oncology: A Multidisciplinary Textbook. London: Chapman and Hall, 1995: 251–9.

59. McMillan AK, Goldstone AH. Autologous bone marrow transplant for non-Hodgkin's lymphoma. Eur J Haem 1991; 46: 129–35.

60. Fineberg HV, Wittenberg J, Ferrucci JT Jr, et al. The clinical value of body computed tomography over time and technologic change. Am J Roentgenol 1983; 141: 1067–72.

61. Carroll BA. Ultrasound of lymphoma. Semin Ultrasound 1982; III: 114–22.

62. Beyer D, Peters PE. Real-time ultrasonography—an efficient screening method for abdominal and pelvic lymphadenopathy. Lymphology 1980; 13: 142–9.

63. Munker R, Stengel A, Stäbler A, Hillere E, Brehm G. Diagnostic accuracy of ultrasound and computed tomography in the staging of Hodgkin's disease. Verification by laparotomy in 100 cases. Cancer 1995; 76: 1460–6.

64. Clouse ME, Harrison DA, Grassi CJ, et al. Lymphangiography, ultrasonography, and computed tomography in Hodgkin's disease and non-Hodgkin's lymphoma. J Comput Tomogr 1985; 9: 1–8.

65. Magnusson A, Erikson B, Hemmingsson A. Investigation of retroperitoneal lymph nodes in Hodgkin's disease. Ups J Med Sci 1984; 89: 205–12.

66. Steinkamp HJ, Wissgott C, Rademaker J, Felix R. Current status of power Doppler and color Doppler sonography in the differential diagnosis of lymph node lesions. Eur Radiol 2002; 12: 1785–93.

67. Neumann CH, Robert NJ, Rosenthal D, Canellos G. Clinical value of ultrasonography for the management of non-Hodgkin's lymphoma patients as compared with abdominal computed tomography. J Comput Assist Tomogr 1983; 7: 666–9.

68. Reznek RH, Husband JE. The radiology of lymphoma. Curr Imaging 1990; 2: 9–17.

69. Lee JK, Heiken JP, Ling D, et al. Magnetic resonance imaging of abdominal and pelvic lymphadenopathy. Radiology 1984; 153: 181–8.

70. Dooms GC, Hricak H, Crooks LE, Higgins CB. Magnetic resonance imaging of the lymph nodes: comparison with CT. Radiology 1984; 153: 719–28.

71. Greco A, Jelliffe AM, Maher EJ, Leung AW. MR imaging of lymphomas: impact on therapy. J Comput Assist Tomogr 1988; 12: 785–91.

72. Hill M, Cunningham D, MacVicar D, et al. Role of magnetic resonance imaging in predicting relapse in residual masses after treatment of lymphoma. J Clin Oncol 1993; 11: 2273–8.

73. Nyman R, Rhen S, Ericsson A, et al. An attempt to characterize malignant lymphoma in spleen, liver and lymph nodes with magnetic resonance imaging. Acta Radiol 1987; 28: 527–33.

74. Shmidt GP, Wintersperber B, Graser A, et al. High-resolution whole-body magnetic resonance imaging applications at 1.5 and 3 Tesla: a comparative study. Invest Radiol 2007; 42: 449–59.

75. King AD, Ahuja AT, Yeung DK, et al. Malignant cervica lymphadenopathy: diagnostic accuracy of diffusion-weighted MR Imaging. Radiology 2007; 245: 806–13.

76. Weissleder R, Elizondo G, Wittenberg J, et al. Ultrasmall superparamagnetic iron oxide: an intravenous contrast agent for assessing lymph nodes with MR imaging. Radiology 1990; 175: 494–8.

77. Bellin MF, Roy C, Kinkel K, et al. Lymph node metastases: safety and effectiveness of MR imaging with ultrasmall superparamagnetic iron oxide particles – initial clinical experience. Radiology 1998; 207: 799–808.

78. Griffiths JR, Tate AR, Howe FA, Stubbs M. Magnetic resonance spectroscopy of cancer: practicalities of multi-centre trials and early results in non-Hodgkin's lymphoma. Eur J Cancer 2002; 38: 2085–93.

79. Front D, Bar-Shalom R, Epelbaum R, et al. Early detection of lymphoma recurrence with gallium-67 scintigraphy. J Nucl Med 1993; 34: 2101–4.

80. Newman JS, Francis IR, Kaminski MS, Wahl RL. Imaging of lymphoma with PET with 2-[F-18]-fluoro-2-deoxy-D-glucose: correlation with CT. Radiology 1994; 190: 111–16.

81. Front D, Israel O, Epelbaum R, et al. Ga-67 SPECT before and after treatment of lymphoma. Radiology 1990; 175: 515–19.

82. Gallamini A, Biggi A, Fruttero A, et al. Revisiting the prognostic role of gallium scintigraphy in low-grade non-Hodgkin's lymphoma. Eur J Nucl Med 1997; 24: 1499–506.

83. Hussain R, Christie DR, Gebski V, Barton MB, Gruenewald SM. The role of the gallium scan in primary extranodal lymphoma. J Nucl Med 1998; 39: 95–8.

84. Moog F, Bangerter M, Diederichs CG, et al. Lymphoma: role of whole-body 2-deoxy-2-[F-18]fluoro-D-glucose (FDG) PET in nodal staging. Radiology 1997; 203: 795–800.

85. Moog F, Bangerter M, Diederichs CG, et al. Extranodal malignant lymphoma: detection with FDG PET versus CT. Radiology 1998; 206: 475–81.

86. Wirth A, Seymour JF, Hicks RJ, et al. Fluorine-18 fluorodeoxyglucose positron emission tomography, gallium-67 scintigraphy, and conventional staging for Hodgkin's disease and non-Hodgkin's lymphoma. Am J Med 2002; 112: 262–8.

87. Kostakoglu L, Leonard JP, Kuji I, et al. Comparison of fluorine-18 fluorodeoxyglucose positron emission tomography and Ga-67 scintigraphy in evaluation of lymphoma. Cancer 2002; 94: 879–88.

88. Bangerter M, Moog F, Buchmann I, et al. Whole-body 2-[18F]-fluoro-2-deoxy-D-glucose positron emission tomography (FDG-PET) for accurate staging of Hodgkin's disease. Ann Oncol 1998; 9: 1117–22.

89. Hoh CK, Glaspy J, Rosen P, et al. Whole-body FDG-PET imaging for staging of Hodgkin's disease and lymphoma. J Nucl Med 1997; 38: 343–8.

90. Jerusalem G, Warland V, Najjar F, et al. Whole-body 18F-FDG PET for the evaluation of patients with Hodgkin's disease and non-Hodgkin's lymphoma. Nucl Med Commun 1999; 20: 13–20.

91. Weihrauch MR, Re D, Bischoff S, et al. Whole-body positron emission tomography using 18F-fluorodeoxyglucose for initial staging of patients with Hodgkin's disease. Ann Hematol 2002; 81: 20–5.

92. Menzel C, Döbert N, Mitrou P, et al. Positron emission tomography for the staging of Hodgkin's lymphoma—increasing the body of evidence in favor of the method. Acta Oncol 2002; 41: 430–6.

93. Hoffmann M, Kletter K, Diemling M, et al. Positron emission tomography with fluorine-18-2-fluoro-2-deoxy-D-glucose (F18-FDG) does not visualize extranodal B-cell lymphoma of the mucosa-associated lymphoid tissue (MALT)-type. Ann Oncol 1999; 10: 1185–9.

94. Jerusalem G, Beguin Y, Najjar F, et al. Positron emission tomography (PET) with 18F-fluorodeoxyglucose (18F-FDG) for the staging of low-grade non-Hodgkin's lymphoma (NHL). Ann Oncol 2001; 12: 825–30.

95. Rodríguez-Vigil B, Gómez-León N, Pinílla I, et al. PET/CT in lymphoma: prospective study of enhanced full-dose PET/CT versus unenhanced low-dose PET/CT. J Nucl Med 2006; 47: 1643–8.

96. La Fougère C, Hundt W, Bröckel N, et al. Value of PET/CT versus PET and CT performed as separate investigations in patients with Hodgkin's disease and non-Hodgkin's lymphoma. Eur J Nucl Med Mol Imaging 2006; 33: 1417–25.

97. Stomper PC, Cholewinski SP, Park J, Bakshi SP, Barcos MP. Abdominal staging of thoracic Hodgkin disease: CT-lymphangiography-Ga-67 scanning correlation. Radiology 1993; 187: 381–6.

98. Valette F, Querellou S, Oudoux A, et al. Comparison of positron emission tomography and lymphangiography in the diagnosis of infradiaphragmatic Hodgkin's disease. Acta Radiol 2007; 48: 59–63.

99. DePena CA, Van Tassel P, Lee YY. Lymphoma of the head and neck. Radiol Clin North Am 1990; 28: 723–43.

100. Pombo F, Rodriguez E, Caruncho MV, Villalva C, Crespo C. CT attenuation values and enhancing characteristics of thoracoabdominal lymphomatous adenopathies. J Comput Assist Tomogr 1994; 18: 59–62.

101. Dooms GC, Hricak H, Crooks LE, Higgins CB. Magnetic resonance imaging of the lymph nodes: comparison with CT. Radiology 1984; 153: 719–28.

102. Filly R, Bland N, Castellino RA. Radiographic distribution of intrathoracic disease in previously untreated patients with Hodgkin's disease and non-Hodgkin's lymphoma. Radiology 1976; 120: 277–81.

103. Castellino RA, Blank N, Hoppe RT, Cho C. Hodgkin disease: contributions of chest CT in the initial staging evaluation. Radiology 1986; 160: 603–5.

104. Castellino RA, Hilton S, O'Brien JP, Portlock CS. Non-Hodgkin's lymphoma: contribution of chest CT in the initial staging evaluation. Radiology 1996; 199: 129–32.

105. Grossman H, Winchester PH, Bragg DG, Tan C, Murphy ML. Roentgenographic changes in childhood Hodgkin's disease. Am J Roentgenol Radium Ther Nucl Med 1970; 108: 354–64.

106. Jochelson MS, Balikian JP, Mauch P, Liebman H. Peri- and paracardial involvement in lymphoma: a radiographic study of 11 cases. Am J Roentgenol 1983; 140: 483–8.

107. Strijk SP. Lymph node calcification in malignant lymphoma. Presentation of nine cases and a review of the literature. Acta Radiol Diagn (Stockh) 1985; 26: 427–31.

108. Apter S, Avigdor A, Gayer G, et al. Calcification in lymphoma occurring before therapy: CT features and clinical correlation. Am J Roentgenol 2002; 178: 935–8.

109. Hopper KD, Diehl LF, Cole BA, et al. The significance of necrotic mediastinal lymph nodes on CT in patients with newly diagnosed Hodgkin disease. Am J Roentgenol 1990; 155: 267–70.

110. North LB, Fuller LM, Hagemeister FB, et al. Importance of initial mediastinal adenopathy in Hodgkin disease. Am J Roentgenol 1982; 138: 229–35.

111. Gallagher CJ, White FE, Tucker AK, Malpas JS, Lister TA. The role of computed tomography in the detection of intrathoracic lymphoma. Br J Cancer 1984; 49: 621–9.

112. Khoury MB, Godwin JD, Halvorsen R, Hanun Y, Putman CE. Role of chest CT in non-Hodgkin's lymphoma. Radiology 1986; 158: 659–62.

113. Hopper KD, Diehl LF, Lesar M, et al. Hodgkin disease: clinical utility of CT in initial staging and treatment. Radiology 1988; 169: 17–22.

114. Heron CW, Husband JE, Williams MP. Hodgkin disease: CT of the thymus. Radiology 1988; 167: 647–51.

115. Wernecke K, Vassallo P, Rutsch F, Peters PE, Potter R. Thymic involvement in Hodgkin disease: CT and sonographic findings. Radiology 1991; 181: 375–83.

116. Shaffer K, Smith D, Kirn D, et al. Primary mediastinal large-B-cell lymphoma: radiologic findings at presentation. Am J Roentgenol 1996; 167: 425–30.

117. Spiers AS, Husband JE, MacVicar AD. Treated thymic lymphoma: comparison of MR imaging with CT. Radiology 1997; 203: 369–76.

118. Rodriguez M, Rehn SM, Nyman RS, et al. CT in malignancy grading and prognostic prediction of non-Hodgkin's lymphoma. Acta Radiol 1999; 40: 191–7.

119. Rehn S, Sperber GO, Nyman R, et al. Quantification of inhomogeneities in malignancy grading of non-Hodgkin's lymphoma with MR imaging. Acta Radiol 1993; 34: 3–9.

120. Rehn SM, Nyman RS, Glimelius BL, Hagberg HE, Sunström JC. Non-Hodgkin's lymphoma: predicting prognostic grade with MR imaging. Radiology 1990; 176: 249–53.

121. Lazzarino M, Orlandi E, Paulli M, et al. Primary mediastinal B-cell lymphoma with sclerosis: an aggressive tumor with distinctive clinical and pathological features. J Clin Oncol 1993; 11: 2606–13.

122. Harell GS, Breiman RS, Glatstein EJ, Marshall WH Jr, Castellino RA. Computed tomography of the abdomen in the malignant lymphomas. Radiol Clin North Am 1977; 15: 391–400.

123. Castellino RA, Marglin S, Blank N. Hodgkin disease, the non-Hodgkin's lymphomas, and the leukemias in the retroperitoneum. Semin Roentgenol 1980; 15: 288–301.

124. Kadin MD, Glatstein EJ, Dorfman RF. Clinicopathologic studies in 117 untreated patients subject to laparotomy for the staging of Hodgkin's disease. Cancer 1980; 27: 1277–94.

125. Goffinet DR, Warnke R, Dunnick NR, et al. Clinical and surgical (laparotomy) evaluation of patients with non-Hodgkin's lymphomas. Cancer Treat Rep 1977; 61: 981–92.

126. Rosenberg SA, Kaplan HS. Evidence for an orderly progression in the spread of Hodgkin's disease. Cancer Res 1966; 26: 1225–31.

127. Urba WJ, Longo DL. Hodgkin's disease. N Engl J Med 1992; 326: 678–87.

128. Weinstein JB, Heiken JP, Lee JK, et al. High resolution CT of the porta hepatis and hepatoduodenal ligament. Radiographics 1986; 6: 55–74.

129. Yang ZG, Min PQ, Sone S, et al. Tuberculosis versus lymphomas in the abdominal lymph nodes: evaluation with contrast-enhanced CT. Am J Roentgenol 1999; 172: 619–23.

130. Hutchings M, Loft A, Hansen M, et al. Position emission tomography with or without computed tomography in the primary staging of Hodgkin's lymphoma. Haematologica 2006; 91: 482–9.

131. Partridge S, Timothy A, O'Doherty MJ, et al. 2-Fluorine-18-fluoro-2-deoxy-D glucose positron emission tomography in the pretreatment staging of Hodgkin's disease: influence on patient management in a single institution. Ann Oncol 2000; 11: 1273–9.

132. Kaplan HS. Contiguity and progression in Hodgkin's disease. Cancer Res 1971; 31: 1811–13.

133. Cobby M, Whipp E, Bullimore J, et al. CT appearances of relapse of lymphoma in the lung. Clin Radiol 1990; 41: 232–8.

134. Eisner MD, Kaplan LD, Herndier B, Stulbarg MS. The pulmonary manifestations of AIDS-related non-Hodgkin's lymphoma. Chest 1996; 110: 729–36.

135. MacDonald JB. Lung involvement in Hodgkin's disease. Thorax 1977; 32: 664–7.

136. Burgener FA, Hamlin DJ. Intrathoracic histiocytic lymphoma. Am J Roentgenol 1981; 136: 499–504.

137. Lewis ER, Caskey CI, Fishman EK. Lymphoma of the lung: CT findings in 31 patients. Am J Roentgenol 1991; 156: 711–14.

138. Jackson SA, Tung KT, Mead GM. Multiple cavitating pulmonary lesions in non-Hodgkin's lymphoma. Clin Radiol 1994; 49: 883–5.

139. Isaacson PG, Norton AJ. General features of extranodal lymphoma. In: Isaacson PG, ed., Extranodal Lymphomas. London: Churchill-Livingstone, 1994: 1–14.

140. Cordier JF, Chailleux E, Lauque D, et al. Primary pulmonary lymphomas. A clinical study of 70 cases in nonimmunocompromised patients. Chest 1993; 103: 201–8.

141. Peterson H, Snider HL, Yam LT, et al. Primary pulmonary lymphoma. A clinical and immunohistochemical study of six cases. Cancer 1985; 56: 805–13.

142. Murray KA, Chor PJ, Turner JF Jr. Intrathoracic lymphoproliferative disorders and lymphoma. Curr Probl Diagn Radiol 1996; 25: 78–106.

143. Ooi GC, Ho JC, Khong PL, et al. Computed tomography characteristics of advanced primary pulmonary lymphoepithelioma-like carcinoma. Eur Radiol 2003; 13: 522–6.

144. Bae YA, Lee KS, Han J, et al. Marginal zone B-cell lymphoma of bronchus-associated lymphoid tissue: imaging findings in 21 patients. Chest 2008; 133: 433–40.

145. Dunnick NR, Parker BR, Castellino RA. Rapid onset of pulmonary infiltration due to histiocytic lymphoma. Radiology 1976; 118: 281–5.

146. Radin AI. Primary pulmonary Hodgkin's disease. Cancer 1990; 65: 550–63.

147. Cartier Y, Johkoh T, Honda O, Muller NL. Primary pulmonary Hodgkin's disease: CT findings in three patients. Clin Radiol 1999; 54: 182–4.

148. Edinburgh KJ, Jasmer RM, Huang L, et al. Multiple pulmonary nodules in AIDS: usefulness of CT in distinguishing among potential causes. Radiology 2000; 214: 427–32.

149. Celikoglu F, Teirstein AS, Krellenstein DJ, Strauchen JA. Pleural effusion in non-Hodgkin's lymphoma. Chest 1992; 101: 1357–60.

150. Bergin CJ, Healy MV, Zincone GE, Castellino RA. MR evaluation of chest wall involvement in malignant lymphoma. J Comput Assist Tomogr 1990; 14: 928–32.

151. Carlsen SE, Bergin CJ, Hoppe RT. MR imaging to detect chest wall and pleural involvement in patients with lymphoma: effect on radiation therapy planning. Am J Roentgenol 1993; 160: 1191–5.

152. North LB, Libshitz HI, Lorigan JG. Thoracic lymphoma. Radiol Clin North Am 1990; 28: 745–62.

153. Tesoro-Tess JD, Biasi S, Balzarini L, et al. Heart involvement in lymphomas. The value of magnetic resonance imaging and two-dimensional echocardiography at disease presentation. Cancer 1993; 72: 2484–90.

154. Tohno E, Cosgrove DO, Sloan JP. Malignant disease—local recurrence and metastases. In: Tohno E, Cosgrove DO, Sloan JP, eds. Ultrasound Diagnosis of Breast Diseases. Edinburgh: Churchill Livingstone, 1994: 186.

155. Yang WT, Lane DL, Le-Petross HT, Abruzzo LV, Macapinlac HA. Breast lymphoma: imaging findings of 32 tumors in 27 patients. Radiology 2007; 245: 692–702.

156. Paulus DD. Lymphoma of the breast. Radiol Clin North Am 1990; 28: 833–40.

157. Sabaté JM, Gómez A, Torrubia S, et al. Lymphoma of the breast: clinical and radiologic features with pathologic correlation in 28 patients. Breast J 2002; 8: 294–304.

158. Thomas JL, Bernardino ME, Vermess M, et al. EOE-13 in the detection of hepatosplenic lymphoma. Radiology 1982; 145: 629–34.

159. Bonadonna G, Santoro A. Clinical evolution and treatment of Hodgkin's disease. In: Wiernik PH, Canellos G, Kyle RA, Schiffer CA, eds. Neoplastic Disease of the Blood. Edinburgh: Churchill Livingstone, 1985: 789.

160. Warshauer DM, Molina PL, Worawattanakul S. The spotted spleen: CT and clinical correlation in a tertiary care center. J Comput Assist Tomogr 1998; 22: 694–702.

161. Dachman AH, Buck JL, Krishnan J, Aguilera NS, Buetow PC. Primary non-Hodgkin's splenic lymphoma. Clin Radiol 1998; 53: 137–42.

162. Daskalogiannaki M, Prassopoulos P, Katrinakis G, et al. Splenic involvement in lymphomas. Evaluation on serial CT examinations. Acta Radiol 2001; 42: 326–32.

163. Strijk SP, Wagener DJ, Bogman MJ, de Pauw BE, Wobbes T. The spleen in Hodgkin disease: diagnostic value of CT. Radiology 1985; 154: 753–7.

164. Strijk SP, Boetes C, Bogman MJ, de Pauw BE, Wobbes T. The spleen in non-Hodgkin's lymphoma. Diagnostic value of computed tomography. Acta Radiol 1987; 28: 139–44.

165. Hess CF, Kurtz B, Hoffmann W, Bamberg M. Ultrasound diagnosis of splenic lymphoma: ROC analysis of multi-dimensional splenic indices. Br J Radiol 1993; 66: 859–64.

166. Harisinghani MG, Saini S, Weissleder R, et al. Splenic imaging with ultrasmall superparamagnetic iron oxide ferumoxtran-10 (AMI-7227): preliminary observations. J Comput Assist Tomogr 2001; 25: 770–6.

167. Weissleder R, Elizondo G, Stark DD, et al. The diagnosis of splenic lymphoma by MR imaging: value of superparamagnetic iron oxide. Am J Roentgenol 1989; 152: 175–80.

168. Weissleder R, Hahn PF, Stark DD, et al. Superparamagnetic iron oxide: enhanced detection of focal splenic tumors with MR imaging. Radiology 1988; 169: 399–403.

169. Rini JN, Manalili EY, Hoffman MA, et al. F-18 FDG versus Ga-67 for detecting splenic involvement in Hodgkin's disease. Clin Nucl Med 2002; 27: 572–7.

170. Kaplan HS, Dorfman RF, Nelsen TS, Rosenberg SA. Staging laparotomy and splenectomy in Hodgkin's disease: analysis of indications and patterns of involvement in 285 consecutive, unselected patients. Natl Cancer Inst Monogr 1973; 36: 291–301.

171. Maher MM, McDermott SR, Fenlon HM, et al. Imaging of primary non-Hodgkin's lymphoma of the liver. Clin Radiol 2001; 56: 295–301.

172. Weissleder R, Stark DD, Elizondo G, et al. MRI of hepatic lymphoma. Magn Reson Imaging 1988; 6: 675–8.

173. Coakley FV, O'Reilly EM, Schwartz LH, Panicek DM, Castellino RA. Non-Hodgkin's lymphoma as a cause of intrahepatic periportal low attenuation on CT. J Comput Assist Tomogr 1997; 21: 726–8.

174. Richards MA, Webb JA, Reznek RH, et al. Detection of spread of malignant lymphoma to the liver by low field strength magnetic resonance imaging. Br Med J (Clin Res Ed) 1986; 293: 1126–8.

175. Weinreb JC, Brateman L, Maravilla KR. Magnetic resonance imaging of hepatic lymphoma. Am J Roentgenol 1984; 143: 1211–14.

176. Stark DD, Weissleder R, Elizondo G, et al. Superparamagnetic iron oxide: clinical application as a contrast agent for MR imaging of the liver. Radiology 1988; 168: 297–301.

177. Brady LW, Asbell SO. Malignant lymphoma of the gastrointestinal tract. Erskine Memorial Lecture, 1979. Radiology 1980; 137: 291–8.

178. Dodd GD. Lymphoma of the hollow abdominal viscera. Radiol Clin North Am 1990; 28: 771–83.

179. Rohatiner A, d'Amore F, Coiffier B, et al. Report on a workshop convened to discuss the pathological and staging classifications of gastrointestinal tract lymphoma. Ann Oncol 1994; 5: 397–400.

180. Dragosics B, Bauer P, Radaszkiewicz T. Primary gastrointestinal Non-Hodgkin's lymphomas. A retrospective clinicopathologic study of 150 cases. Cancer 1985; 55: 1060–73.

181. Fishman EK, Urban BA, Hruban RH. CT of the stomach: spectrum of disease. Radiographics 1996; 16: 1035–54.

182. Megibow AJ, Balthazar EJ, Naidich DP, Bosniak MA. Computed tomography of gastrointestinal lymphoma. Am J Roentgenol 1983; 141: 541–7.

183. Kessar P, Norton A, Rohatiner AZ, Lister RA, Reznek RH. CT appearances of mucosa-associated lymphoid tissue (MALT) lymphoma. Eur Radiol 1999; 9: 693–6.

184. Fujishima H, Chijiiwa Y. Endoscopic ultrasonographic staging of primary gastric lymphoma. Abdom Imaging 1996; 21: 192–4.

185. Raderer M, Vorbeck F, Formanek M, et al. Importance of extensive staging in patients with mucosa-associated lymphoid tissue (MALT)-type lymphoma. Br J Cancer 2000; 83: 454–7.

186. Balthazar EJ, Noordhoorn M, Megibow AJ, Gordon RB. CT of small-bowel lymphoma in immunocompetent patients and patients with AIDS: comparison of findings. Am J Roentgenol 1997; 168: 675–80.

187. Lohan DG, Alhajeri AN, Cronin CG, Roche CJ, Murphy JM. MR enterography of small bowel lymphoma: potential for suggestion of histologic subtype and the presence of underlying celiac disease. Am J Roentgenol 2008; 190: 287–93.

188. Lecuit M, Abachin E, Martin A. Immunoproliferative small intestinal disease associated with Campylobacter jejuni. N Engl J Med 2004; 350: 239–48.

189. Kim Y, Cho O, Song S, et al. Peritoneal lymphomatosis: CT findings. Abdom Imaging 1998; 23: 87–90.

190. Reed K, Vose PC, Jarstfer BS. Pancreatic cancer: 30 year review (1947 to 1977). Am J Surg 1979; 138: 929–33.

191. Webb TH, Lillemoe KD, Pitt HA, Jones RA, Cameron JL. Pancreatic lymphoma. Is surgery mandatory for diagnosis or treatment? Ann Surg 1989; 209: 25–30.

192. Shirkhoda A, Ros PR, Farah J, Staab EV. Lymphoma of the solid abdominal viscera. Radiol Clin North Am 1990; 28: 785–99.

193. Van Beers B, Lalonde L, Soyer P, et al. Dynamic CT in pancreatic lymphoma. J Comput Assist Tomogr 1993; 17: 94–7.

194. Prayer L, Schurawitzki H, Mallek R, Mostbeck G. CT in pancreatic involvement of non-Hodgkin's lymphoma. Acta Radiol 1992; 33: 123–7.

195. Charnsangavej C. Lymphoma of the genitourinary tract. Radiol Clin North Am 1990; 28: 865–77.

196. Reznek RH, Mootoosamy I, Webb JA, Richards MA. CT in renal and perirenal lymphoma: a further look. Clin Radiol 1990; 42: 233–8.

197. Hartman DS, David CJ Jr, Goldman SM, Friedman AC, Fritzsche P. Renal lymphoma: radiologic-pathologic correlation of 21 cases. Radiology 1982; 144: 759–66.

198. Heiken JP, Gold RP, Schnur MJ, et al. Computed tomography of renal lymphoma with ultrasound correlation. J Comput Assist Tomogr 1983; 7: 245–50.

199. Connor SE, Umaria N, Guest PJ. Case report: extranodal peripelvic and periureteric lymphoma—demonstration with CT. Clin Radiol 2001; 56: 422–4.

200. Aigen AB, Phillips M. Primary malignant lymphoma of urinary bladder. Urology 1986; 28: 235–7.

201. Yeoman LJ, Mason MD, Olliff JF. Non-Hodgkin's lymphoma of the bladder—and MRI appearances. Clin Radiol 1991; 44: 389–92.

202. Tasu JP, Geffroy D, Rocher L, et al. Primary malignant lymphoma of the urinary bladder: report of three cases and review of the literature. Eur Radiol 2000; 10: 1261–4.

203. Mostofi FK. Proceedings: Testicular tumors. Epidemiologic, etiologic, and pathologic features. Cancer 1973; 32: 1186–201.

204. Thurnher S, Hricak H, Carroll PR, Pobiel RS, Filly RA. Imaging the testis: comparison between MR imaging and US. Radiology 1988; 167: 631–6.

205. Kim YS, Koh BH, Cho OK, Rhim HC. MR imaging of primary uterine lymphoma. Abdom Imaging 1997; 22: 441–4.

206. Jenkins N, Husband J, Sellars N, Gore M. MRI in primary non-Hodgkin's lymphoma of the vagina associated with a uterine congenital anomaly. Br J Radiol 1997; 70: 219–22.

207. Glazer HS, Lee JK, Balfe DM, et al. Non-Hodgkin's lymphoma: computed tomographic demonstration of unusual extranodal involvement. Radiology 1983; 149: 211–17.

208. Ferrozzi F, Tognini G, Bova D, Zuccoli G. Non-Hodgkin's lymphomas of the ovaries: MR findings. J Comput Assist Tomogr 2000; 24: 416–20.

209. Vincent JM, Morrison ID, Armstrong P, Reznek RH. Computed tomography of diffuse, non-metastatic enlargement of the adrenal glands in patients with malignant disease. Clin Radiol 1994; 49: 456–60.

210. Jenkins PJ, Sohaib SA, Trainer PJ, et al. Adrenal enlargement and failure of suppression of circulating cortisol by dexamethasone in patients with malignancy. Br J Cancer 1999; 80: 1815–9.
211. Zimmerman RA. Central nervous system lymphoma. Radiol Clin North Am 1990; 28: 697–721.
212. Hobson DE, Anderson BA, Carr I, West M. Primary lymphoma of the central nervous system: Manitoba experience and literature review. Can J Neurol Sci 1986; 13: 55–61.
213. Snider WD, Simpson DM, Nielsen S, et al. Neurological complications of acquired immune deficiency syndrome: analysis of 50 patients. Ann Neurol 1983; 14: 403–18.
214. Jenkins CN, Colquhoun IR. Characterization of primary intracranial lymphoma by computed tomography: an analysis of 36 cases and a review of the literature with particular reference to calcification haemorrhage and cyst formation. Clin Radiol 1998; 53: 428–34.
215. Herman TS, Hammond N, Jones SE, et al. Involvement of the central nervous system by non-Hodgkin lymphoma: the Southwest Oncology Group experience. Cancer 1979; 43: 390–7.
216. Kotasek D, Albertyn LE, Sage RE. A five-year experience with central nervous system lymphoma. Med J Aust 1986; 144: 299–303.
217. Bragg DG, Colby TV, Ward JH. New concepts in the non-Hodgkin's lymphomas: radiologic implications. Radiology 1986; 159: 291–304.
218. Chamberlain MC, Sandy AD, Press GA. Leptomeningeal metastasis: a comparison of gadolinium-enhanced MR and contrast-enhanced CT of the brain. Neurology 1990; 40: 435–8.
219. Yousem DM, Patrone PM, Grossman RI. Leptomeningeal metastases: MR evaluation. J Comput Assist Tomogr 1990; 14: 255–61.
220. MacVicar D, Williams MP. CT scanning in epidural lymphoma. Clin Radiol 1991; 43: 95–102.
221. Evans C. A review of non-Hodgkin's lymphomata of the head and neck. Clin Oncol 1981; 7: 23–31.
222. Robbins KT, Fuller LM, Vlasak M, et al. Primary lymphomas of the nasal cavity and paranasal sinuses. Cancer 1985; 56: 814–19.
223. Shikhani A, Samara M, Allam C, Salem P, Lenhard R. Primary lymphoma in the salivary glands: report of five cases and review of the literature. Laryngoscope 1987; 97: 1438–42.
224. Takashima S, Ikezoe J, Morimoto S, et al. Primary thyroid lymphoma: evaluation with CT. Radiology 1988; 168: 765–8.
225. Takashima S, Nomura N, Noguchi Y, Matsuzuka F, Inoue T. Primary thyroid lymphoma: evaluation with US, CT and MRI. J Comput Assist Tomogr 1995; 19: 282–8.
226. Braunstein EM. Hodgkin disease of bone: radiographic correlation with the histological classification. Radiology 1980; 137: 643–6.
227. Cooley BL, Higinbotham NL, Groesbeck HP. Primary reticulum cell sarcoma of bone: classification. Radiology 1950; 50: 641–58.
228. Ngan H, Preston BJ. Non-Hodgkin's lymphoma presenting with osseous lesions. Clin Radiol 1975; 26: 351–6.
229. Stroszczynski C, Oellinger J, Hosten N, et al. Staging and monitoring of malignant lymphoma of the bone: comparison of ^{67}Ga scintigraphy and MRI. J Nucl Med 1999; 40: 387–93.
230. Mengiardi B, Honegger H, Hodler J, et al. Primary lymphoma of bone: MRI and CT characteristics before and after successful treatment. Am J Roentgenol 2005; 184: 185–92.
231. Moog F, Kotzerke J, Reske SN. FDG PET can replace bone scintigraphy in primary staging of malignant lymphoma. J Nucl Med 1999; 40: 1407–13.
232. Park YH, Kim S, Choi SJ, et al. Clinical impact of whole-body FDG-PET for evaluation of response and therapeutic decision-making of primary lymphoma of bone. Ann Oncol 2005; 16: 1401–2.
233. Castellino RA, Goffinet DR, Blank N, Parker BR, Kaplan HS. The role of radiography in the staging of non-Hodgkin's lymphoma with laparotomy correlation. Radiology 1974; 110: 329–38.
234. Chabner BA, Johnson RE, Young RC, et al. Sequential non-surgical and surgical staging of non-Hodgkin's lymphoma. Ann Intern Med 1976; 85: 149–54.
235. Glatstein E, Guernsey JM, Rosenberg SA, Kaplan HS. The value of laparotomy and splenectomy in the staging of Hodgkin's disease. Cancer 1969; 24: 709–18.
236. Kaplan HS. Essentials of staging and management of the malignant lymphomas. Semin Roentgenol 1980; 15: 219–26.
237. Linden A, Zankovich R, Theissen P, Diehl V, Schicha H. Malignant lymphoma: bone marrow imaging versus biopsy. Radiology 1989; 173: 335–9.
238. Pond GD, Castellino RA, Horning S, Hoppe RT. Non-Hodgkin's lymphoma: influence of lymphography, CT, and bone marrow biopsy on staging and management. Radiology 1989; 170: 159–64.
239. Wang J, Weiss LM, Chang KL, et al. Diagnostic utility of bilateral bone marrow examination: significance of morphologic and ancillary technique study in malignancy. Cancer 2002; 94: 1522–31.
240. Döhner H, Gückel F, Knauf W, et al. Magnetic resonance imaging of bone marrow in lymphoproliferative disorders: correlation with bone marrow biopsy. Br J Haematol 1989; 73: 12–17.
241. Hoane BR, Shields AF, Porter BA, Shulman HM. Detection of lymphomatous bone marrow involvement with magnetic resonance imaging. Blood 1991; 78: 728–38.
242. Yasumoto M, Nonomura Y, Yoshimura R, et al. MR detection of iliac bone marrow involvement by malignant lymphoma with various MR sequences including diffusion-weighted echo-planar imaging. Skeletal Radiol 2002; 31: 263–9.
243. Shields AF, Porter BA, Churchley S, et al. The detection of bone marrow involvement by lymphoma using magnetic resonance imaging. J Clin Oncol 1987; 5: 225–30.
244. Tsunoda S, Takagi S, Tanaka O, Miura Y. Clinical and prognostic significance of femoral marrow magnetic resonance imaging in patients with malignant lymphoma. Blood 1997; 89: 286–90.
245. Moog F, Bangerter M, Kotzerke J, et al. 18-F-fluorodeoxy-glucose-positron emission tomography as a new approach to detect lymphomatous bone marrow. J Clin Oncol 1998; 16: 603–9.

246. Schaefer NG, Stroble K, Taverna C, Hany T. Bone involvement in patients with lymphoma: the role of FGD-PET/CT. Eur J Nucl Med Mol Imaging 2007; 34: 60–7.

247. Elstrom R, Guan L, Baker G, et al. Utility of FDG-PET scanning in lymphoma by WHO classification. Blood 2003; 101: 3875–6.

248. Carr R, Barrington SF, Madan B, et al. Detection of lymphoma in bone marrow by whole-body positron emission tomography. Blood 1998; 91: 3340–6.

249. Pakos EE, Fotopoulos AD, Ioannidis JP. 18F-FDG PET for evaluation of bone marrow infiltration in staging of lymphoma: a meta-analysis. J Nucl Med 2005; 46: 958–63.

250. Daldrup-Link HE, Rummeny EJ, Ihssen B, et al. Iron-oxide-enhanced MR imaging of bone marrow in patients with non-Hodgkin's lymphoma: differentiation between tumor infiltration and hypercellular bone marrow. Eur Radiol 2002; 12: 1557–66.

251. Williams MP, Olliff JF. Magnetic resonance imaging in extranodal pelvic lymphoma. Clin Radiol 1990; 42: 264–8.

252. Malloy PC, Fishman EK, Magid D. Lymphoma of bone, muscle, and skin: CT findings. Am J Roentgenol 1992; 159: 805–9.

253. Wotherspoon AC, Ortiz-Hidalgo C, Falzon MR, Isaacson PG. Helicobacter pylori-associated gastritis and primary B-cell gastric lymphoma. Lancet 1991; 338: 1175–6.

254. Nakamura S, Aoyagi K, Furuse M, et al. B-cell monoclonality precedes the development of gastric MALT lymphoma in Helicobacter pylori-associated chronic gastritis. Am J Pathol 1998; 152: 1271–9.

255. Thieblemont C, Bastion Y, Berger F, et al. Mucosa-associated lymphoid tissue gastrointestinal and nongastrointestinal lymphoma behavior: analysis of 108 patients. J Clin Oncol 1997; 15: 1624–30.

256. Vorbeck F, Osterreicher C, Püspök A, et al. Comparison of spiral-computed tomography with water-filling of the stomach and endosonography for gastric lymphoma of mucosa-associated lymphoid tissue-type. Digestion 2002; 65: 196–9.

257. Park MS, Kim KW, Yu JS, et al. Radiographic findings of primary B-cell lymphoma of the stomach: low-grade versus high-grade malignancy in relation to the mucosa-associated lymphoid tissue concept. Am J Roentgenol 2002; 179: 1297–304.

258. Palazzo L, Roseau G, Ruskone-Fourmestraux A, et al. Endoscopic ultrasonography in the local staging of primary gastric lymphoma. Endoscopy 1993; 25: 502–8.

259. Sackmann M, Morgner A, Rudolph B, et al. Regression of gastric MALT lymphoma after eradication of Helicobacter pylori is predicted by endosonographic staging. MALT Lymphoma Study Group. Gastroenterology 1997; 113: 1087–90.

260. Lee HJ, Han JK, Kim TK, et al. Primary colorectal lymphoma: spectrum of imaging findings with pathologic correlation. Eur Radiol 2002; 12: 2242–9.

261. King LJ, Padley SP, Wotherspoon AC, Nicholson AG. Pulmonary MALT lymphoma: imaging findings in 24 cases. Eur Radiol 2000; 10: 1932–8.

262. Lee DK, Im JG, Lee KS, et al. B-cell lymphoma of bronchus-associated lymphoid tissue (BALT): CT features in 10 patients. J Comput Assist Tomogr 2000; 24: 30–4.

263. Vincent JM, Ng YY, Norton AJ, Armstrong P. CT "angiogram sign" in primary pulmonary lymphoma. J Comput Assist Tomogr 1992; 16: 829–31.

264. Burkitt DP. Classics in oncology. A sarcoma involving the jaws in African children. CA Cancer J Clin 1972; 22: 345–55.

265. O'Connor GT, Rappaport H, Smith EB. Childhood lymphoma resembling "Burkitt tumour" in the United States. Cancer 1965; 18: 411–17.

266. Ziegler JL, Bluming AZ, Morrow RH, Fass L, Carbone PP. Central nervous system involvement in Burkitt's lymphoma. Blood 1970; 36: 718–28.

267. Johnson KA, Tung K, Mead G, Sweetenham J. The imaging of Burkitt's and Burkitt-like lymphoma. Clin Radiol 1998; 53: 835–41.

268. World Health Organization Classification of Tumours. Pathology & Genetics. Tumours of Haematopoietic and Lymphoid Tissues. Lyon: IARC Press, 2001.

269. Dal Maso L, Franceschi S. Epidemiology of non-Hodgkin's lymphoma and other haemolymphopoietic neoplasms in people with AIDS. Lancet Oncol 2003; 4: 110–19.

270. Radin DR, Esplin JA, Levine AM, Ralls PW. AIDS-related non-Hodgkin's lymphoma: abdominal CT findings in 112 patients. Am J Roentgenol 1993; 160: 1133–9.

271. Jasmer RM, Gotway MB, Creasman JM, et al. Clinical and radiographic predictors of the etiology of computed tomography-diagnosed intrathoracic lymphadenopathy in HIV-infected patients. J Acquir Immune Defic Syndr 2002; 31: 291–8.

272. Cordoliani Y-S, Derosier C, Pharaboz C, et al. Primary cerebral lymphoma in patients with AIDS: MR findings in 17 cases. Am J Roentgenol 1992; 159: 841–7.

273. O'Doherty MJ, Barrington SF, Campbell M, Lowe J, Bradbeer CS. PET scanning and the human immunodeficiency virus-positive patient. J Nucl Med 1997; 38: 1575–83.

274. Dodd GD III, Ledesma-Medina J, Baron RL, Fuhrman CR. Posttransplant lymphoproliferative disorder: intrathoracic manifestations. Radiology 1992; 184: 65–9.

275. Carignan S, Staples CA, Muller NL. Intrathoracic lymphoproliferative disorders in the immunocompromised patient: CT findings. Radiology 1995; 197: 53–8.

276. Lim GY, Newman B, Kurland G, Webber SA. Posttransplantation lymphoproliferative disorder: manifestations in pediatric thoracic organ recipients. Radiology 2002; 222: 699–708.

277. Lee DA, Hartman RP, Trenkner SW, Leone JP, Gruessner R. Lymphomas in solid organ transplantation. Abdom Imaging 1998; 23: 553–7.

278. Pickhardt PJ, Siegel MJ. Abdominal manifestations of posttransplantation lymphoproliferative disorder. Am J Roentgenol 1998; 171: 1007–13.

279. Heron CW, Husband JE, Williams MP, Cherryman GR. The value of thoracic computed tomography in the detection of recurrent Hodgkin's disease. Br J Radiol 1988; 61: 567–72.

280. Hopper KD, Kasales CJ, Van Slyke MA, et al. Analysis of interobserver and intraobserver variability in CT tumor measurements. Am J Roentgenol 1996; 167: 851–4.

281. DeVita VT Jr, Hellman S, Rosenberg SA, eds. Non-Hodgkin's lymphomas (Chapter 45.3) and Lymphoma (Chapter 45.6). In: Cancer—Principles and Practice of Oncology. Toronto: J B Lippincott Co, 2001: 2339, 2256.

282. North LB, Fuller LM, Sullivan-Halley JA, Hagemeister FB. Regression of mediastinal Hodgkin disease after therapy: evaluation of time interval. Radiology 1987; 164: 599–602.

283. Cheson BD, Horning SJ, Coiffier B, et al. Report of an international workshop to standardize response criteria for non-Hodgkin's lymphomas. NCI Sponsored International Working Group. J Clin Oncol 1999; 17: 1244.

284. Radford JA, Cowan RA, Flanagan M, et al. The significance of residual mediastinal abnormality on the chest radiograph following treatment for Hodgkin's disease. J Clin Oncol 1988; 6: 940–6.

285. Surbone A, Longo DL, Devita VT Jr, et al. Residual abdominal masses in aggressive non-Hodgkin's lymphoma after combination chemotherapy: significance and management. J Clin Oncol 1988; 6: 1832–7.

286. Lewis E, Bernardino ME, Salvador PG, et al. Post-therapy CT-detected mass in lymphoma patients: is it viable tissue? J Comput Assist Tomogr 1982; 6: 792–5.

287. Coiffier B, Gisselbrecht C, Herbrecht R, et al. LNH-84 regimen: a multicenter study of intensive chemotherapy in 737 patients with aggressive malignant lymphoma. J Clin Oncol 1989; 7: 1018–26.

288. Nyman RS, Rehn SM, Glimelius BL, et al. Residual mediastinal masses in Hodgkin's disease: prediction of size with MR imaging. Radiology 1989; 170: 435–40.

289. Rahmouni A, Tempany C, Jones R, et al. Lymphoma: monitoring tumor size and signal intensity with MR imaging. Radiology 1993; 188: 445–51.

290. Rodriguez M. Computed tomography, magnetic resonance imaging and positron emission tomography in non-Hodgkin's lymphoma. Acta Radiol Suppl 1998; 417: 1–36.

291. Kaplan WD, Jochelson MS, Herman TS, et al. Gallium-67 imaging: a predictor of residual tumor viability and clinical outcome in patients with diffuse large-cell lymphoma. J Clin Oncol 1990; 8: 1966–70.

292. Front D, Ben-Haim S, Israel O, et al. Lymphoma: predictive value of Ga-67 scintigraphy after treatment. Radiology 1992; 182: 359–63.

293. Herman M, Paucek B, Raida L, et al. Comparison of magnetic resonance imaging and (67)gallium scintigraphy in the evaluation of posttherapeutic residual mediastinal mass in the patients with Hodgkin's lymphoma. Eur J Radiol 2007; 64: 432–8.

294. Mikhaeel NG, Timothy AR, O'Doherty MJ, Hain S, Maisey MN. 18-FDG-PET as a prognostic indicator in the treatment of aggressive non-Hodgkin's lymphoma—comparison with CT. Leuk Lymphoma 2000; 39: 543–53.

295. Cremerius U, Fabry U, Neuerburg J, et al. Positron emission tomography with 18F-FDG to detect residual disease after therapy for malignant lymphoma. Nucl Med Commun 1998; 19: 1055–63.

296. de Wit M, Bumann D, Beyer W, et al. Whole-body positron emission tomography (PET) for diagnosis of residual mass in patients with lymphoma. Ann Oncol 1997; 8(Suppl 1): 57–60.

297. Jerusalem G, Beguin Y, Fassotte MF, et al. Whole-body positron emission tomography using 18F-fluorodeoxyglucose for posttreatment evaluation in Hodgkin's disease and non-Hodgkin's lymphoma has higher diagnostic and prognostic value than classical computed tomography scan imaging. Blood 1999; 94: 429–33.

298. Naumann R, Vaic A, Beuthien-Baumann B, et al. Prognostic value of positron emission tomography in the evaluation of post-treatment residual mass in patients with Hodgkin's disease and non-Hodgkin's lymphoma. Br J Haematol 2001; 115: 793–800.

299. Schöder H, Meta J, Yap C, et al. Effect of whole-body (18) F-FDG PET imaging on clinical staging and management of patients with malignant lymphoma. J Nucl Med 2001; 42: 1139–43.

300. Weihrauch MR, Re D, Scheidhauer K, et al. Thoracic positron emission tomography using 18F-fluorodeoxyglucose for the evaluation of residual mediastinal Hodgkin disease. Blood 2001; 98: 2930–4.

201. Bakheet SM, Powe J. Benign causes of 18-FDG uptake on whole body imaging. Semin Nucl Med 1998; 28: 352–8.

302. Van Den Bosche B, Lambert B, De Winter F, et al. 18FDG PET versus high-dose 67Ga scintigraphy for restaging and treatment follow-up of lymphoma patients. Nucl Med Commun 2002; 23: 1079–83.

303. Zinzani PL, Chierichetti F, Zompatori M, et al. Advantages of positron emission tomography (PET) with respect to computed tomography in the follow-up of lymphoma patients with abdominal presentation. Leuk Lymphoma 2002; 43: 1239–43.

304. Spaepen K, Stroobants S, Dupont P, et al. Prognostic value of positron emission tomography (PET) with fluorine-18 fluorodeoxyglucose ([18F]FDG) after first-line chemotherapy in non-Hodgkin lymphoma: is [18F]FDG-PET a valid alternative to conventional diagnostic methods? J Clin Oncol 2001; 19: 414–19.

305. Spaepen K, Stroobants S, Dupont P, et al. Can positron emission tomography with [(18)F]-fluorodeoxyglucose after first-line treatment distinguish Hodgkin's disease patients who need additional therapy from others in whom additional therapy would mean avoidable toxicity? Br J Haematol 2001; 115: 272–8.

306. Juweid M, Wiseman GA, Vose J, et al. Response assessment of aggressive non-Hodgkin's lymphoma by Integrated International Workshop criteria and fluorine-18-fluordeoxyglucose positron emission tomography. J Clin Oncol 2005; 23: 4652–61.

307. Cheson BD, Pfistner B, Juweid ME, et al. Revised response criteria for malignant lymphoma. J Clin Oncol 2007; 25: 579–86.

308. Juweid ME, Stroobants S, Hoekstra OS, et al. Use of positron emission tomography for response assessment of lymphoma: consensus of the Imaging Subcommittee of International Harmonization Project in Lymphoma. J Clin Oncol 2007; 25: 571–8.

309. Kostakoglu L, Coleman M, Leonard JP, et al. PET predicts prognosis after 1 cycle of chemotherapy in aggressive lymphoma and Hodgkin's disease. J Nucl Med 2002; 43: 1018–27.

310. Spaepen K, Stroobants S, Dupont P, et al. Early restaging positron emission tomography with (18)F-fluorodeoxy-glucose predicts outcome in patients with aggressive non-Hodgkin's lymphoma. Ann Oncol 2002; 13: 1356–63.

311. Haioun C, Itti E, Rahmouni A, et al. [18F]fluoro-2-deoxy-D-glucose positron emission tomography (FDG-PET) in aggressive lymphoma: an early prognostic tool for predicting patient outcome. Blood 2005; 106: 1376–81.

312. Hutchings M, Loft A, Hansen M, et al. FDG-PET after two cycles of chemotherapy predicts treatment failure and progression-free survival in Hodgkin lymphoma. Blood 2006; 107: 52–9.

313. Gallamini A, Hutchings M, Rigacci L, et al. Early interim 2-[18F]fluoro-2-deoxy-D-glucose positron emission tomography is prognostically superior to international prognostic score in advanced-stage Hodgkin's lymphoma: a report from a joint Italian-Danish study. J Clin Oncol 2007; 25: 3746–52.

314. Kostakoglu L, Goldsmith SJ, Leonard JP, et al. FDG-PET after 1 cycle of therapy predicts outcome in diffuse large cell lymphoma and classic Hodgkin disease. Cancer 2006; 107: 2678–87.

315. Torizuka T, Nakamura F, Kanno T, et al. Early therapy monitoring with FDG-PET in aggressive non-Hodgkin's lymphoma and Hodgkin's lymphoma. Eur J Nucl Med Mol Imaging 2004; 31: 22–8.

316. Becherer A, Mitterbauer M, Jaeger U, et al. Positron emission tomography with [18F]2-fluoro-D-2-deoxyglucose (FDG-PET) predicts relapse of malignant lymphoma after high-dose therapy with stem cell transplantation. Leukemia 2002; 16: 260–7.

317. Weeks JC, Yeap BY, Canellos GP, Shipp MA. Value of follow-up procedures in patients with large-cell lymphoma who achieve a complete remission. J Clin Oncol 1991; 9: 1196–203.

318. Setoain FJ, Pons F, Herranz R, et al. 67Ga scintigraphy for the evaluation of recurrences and residual masses in patients with lymphoma. Nucl Med Commun 1997; 18: 405–11.

319. Radford JA, Eardley A, Woodman C, Crowther D. Follow up policy after treatment for Hodgkin's disease: too many clinic visits and routine tests? A review of hospital records. Br Med J 1997; 314: 343–6.

320. Guadagnolo BA, Punglia RS, Kuntz KM, Mauch PM, Ng AK. Cost-effectiveness analysis of computerized tomography in the routine follow-up of patients after primary treatment for Hodgkin's disease. J Clin Oncol 2006; 24: 4116–22.

321. Elis A, Blickstein D, Klein O, et al. Detection of relapse in non-Hodgkin's lymphoma: role of routine follow-up studies. Am J Hematol 2002; 69: 41–4.

322. Jerusalem G, Beguin Y, Fassotte MF, et al. Early detection of relapse by whole-body positron emission tomography in the follow-up of patients with Hodgkin's disease. Ann Oncol 2003; 14: 123–30.

323. Whelan JS, Reznek RH, Daniell SJ, et al. Computed tomography (CT) and ultrasound (US) guided core biopsy in the management of non-Hodgkin's lymphoma. Br J Cancer 1991; 63: 460–2.

324. Pappa VI, Hussain HK, Reznek RH, et al. Role of image-guided core-needle biopsy in the management of patients with lymphoma. J Clin Oncol 1996; 14: 2427–30.

325. Ben Yehuda D, Polliack A, Okon E, et al. Image-guided core-needle biopsy in malignant lymphoma: experience with 100 patients that suggests the technique is reliable. J Clin Oncol 1996; 14: 2431–4.

34 Multiple Myeloma
Conor Collins

INTRODUCTION

Multiple myeloma is the second most common form of hematological malignancy in the western world after non-Hodgkin's lymphoma, accounting for approximately 10% of hematological malignancies and 1% of all malignancies (1). It is a disease of later life with 98% of patients aged 40 or older at presentation (median age 70 years) (2). The etiology is unknown though there is an increased risk in those who have a past history of radiation exposure.

Multiple myeloma is characterized by uncontrolled proliferation of plasma cells within the marrow (mature antibody producing B cells). This leads to disruption of the subtle balance between osteoblastosis and osteoclastosis within bone by overproduction of TRANCE (tumor necrosis factor-related induced cytokine) and inactivation of osteoprotegerin resulting in unrestricted osteoclastic activity manifest as lytic deposits. An unwanted secondary effect is the promotion of further clonal proliferation of myeloma cells thus augmenting the disease process (3). Multiple myeloma should not be confused with the condition known as monoclonal gammopathy of undetermined significance (MGUS). In this disease the serum paraprotein level is <3 g/dl with no evidence of myeloma or a related disorder. The risk of MGUS progressing to myeloma or a related condition is low: 16% at 10 years, 33% at 20 years, and 40% at 25 years (4).

Diagnosis is based on laboratory and radiographic findings and depends on three abnormal results:

- Bone marrow containing more than 10% plasma cells (normally no more than 4% of the cells in the bone marrow are plasma cells)
- Generalized osteopenia and/or lytic bone deposits on plain film radiography
- Blood serum and/or urine containing an abnormal protein

In about 75% of all cases of multiple myeloma the paraprotein present (M protein) will correspond with one type of immunoglobulin. In about 60% of cases an abnormal protein, known as Bence-Jones protein may also be found in the urine. Measuring the amount of paraprotein in the blood or urine is of value in the diagnosis of myeloma and in monitoring the response to treatment.

STAGING

The clinical staging system devised by Durie and Salmon distinguishes different patient subgroups in terms of tumor mass and disease aggression and even now frequently determines management (Table 34.1) (5). Patients with at least two lytic foci are classified in advanced disease subgroups and aggressive systemic treatment is usually indicated. Subsequently, the scientific advisers of the International Myeloma Foundation proposed a new staging system called "Durie and Salmon PLUS" based on the traditional Durie and Salmon system integrated by ^{18}F-fluoro-2-deoxyglucose

positron emission tomography (FDG PET) or magnetic resonance (MR) imaging of the spine (Table 34.2) (6). This system attributes an equal relevance to both FDG PET and MR imaging of the spine, which can be used, as suggested by the guidelines, in a flexible fashion. However, this staging system has recently been replaced by one based entirely on serum β2 microglobulin and serum albumin levels (Table 34.3) (7). Patient outcome in myeloma may be affected by abnormalities of chromosome 13 but this does not add to the prognostic power of the new international staging system (7,8). Despite the new system many physicians still find that information regarding imaging status influences their management, so the Durie-Salmon PLUS is a more relevant system for radiologists (Table 34.2).

THERAPY

The International Myeloma Foundation and U.K. Myeloma Forum (with the support of the British Committee for Standards in Haematology) should be regarded as the preferred source of detailed guidance on treatment (6,9,10). Treatment strategy is directed towards adequate analgesia, rehydration, management of hypercalcemia and renal impairment, and treatment of infection. The response categories (complete, near complete, partial, minimal, stable, and progressive) are determined primarily by the level of M protein present. M protein is the level of monoclonal protein measured by protein electrophoresis in serum or 24 hour urine. Changes in M protein should be supported with other evidence of treatment benefit to confirm response (6).

Chemotherapy is indicated for management of symptomatic myeloma. High dose therapy using melphalan and prednisolone can produce complete remission in up to 75% of patients (11,12). In recent years thalidomide (and its more potent immunomodulatory analogue lenalidomide) has been recognized as a valuable drug for the treatment of myeloma (13–15). A newer class of drug Bortezomib (a proteasome inhibitor) is effective for treatment of relapsed refractory myeloma and is superior to dexamethasone in progression-free and overall survival (16–19). Other new agents entering clinical trials include conventional drugs (Doxil), cytokines (Avastin), biological agents (Betathine), and agents such as arsenic trioxide (15,20,21). Animal studies using the novel recombinant vesicular stomatitis virus have proved encouraging and point to the likely direction of future therapies (22).

The most serious morbidity in these patients arises from destructive bone deposits which cause severe intractable pain and pathological fractures often resulting in deformity and disability. Vertebroplasty and kyphoplasty have been performed to alleviate bone pain from collapsed vertebrae and restore vertebral body height (23–25). A recently published retrospective review of outcome data from 67 myeloma patients treated with vertebroplasty demonstrated significant improvement in rest pain, activity pain, narcotic use, and mobility (26). The introduction of the bisphosphonate group of drugs has transformed this aspect of the disease.

Table 34.1 Durie and Salmon Staging System for Multiple Myeloma (5)

Stage[a]	Criteria	Cell Mass
I	All of the following	Low
	Hemoglobin >10 g/100 ml	$<0.6 \times 10^{12}$ cells per mm^2
	Normal serum calcium <12 mg/100 ml	
	Normal bone structure or solitary bone lesion only on radiography	
	Low M component production rates	
	IgG <5 g/100 ml	
	IgA <3 g/100 ml	
	Urine light chain M component on electrophoresis <4 g/24 hr	
II	Fitting neither stage I nor stage III	Intermediate
III	One or more of the following:	High
	Hemoglobin <8.5 g/100 ml	$>1.2 \times 10^{12}$ cells per mm^2
	Serum calcium >12 mg/100 ml	
	Advanced lytic bone lesion	
	High M component production rates	
	IgG >7 g/100 ml	
	IgA >5 g/100 ml	
	Urine light chain M component on electrophoresis >12 g/24 hr	

[a]Subclassifications: A, relatively normal renal function [serum creatinine value <20 mg/100 ml (175 mol/l)]; B, abnormal renal function [serum creatinine value >20 mg/100 ml (175 mmol/l)].

Table 34.2 Durie and Salmon PLUS Staging System for Symptomatic Multiple Myeloma (6)

Laboratory findings	Imaging findings (including MR and FDG PET)
Stage I clinical criteria	<5 focal spine lesions ± mild diffuse spine disease
Stage II clinical criteria	5–20 focal lesions ± moderate diffuse spine disease
Stage III clinical criteria	>20 focal lesions ± severe diffuse spine disease

Table 34.3 New International Staging System (7)

Stage I	Serum β2 microglobuli <3.5 mg/L (average survival 62 mo) Serum albumin >3.5 g/dL
Stage II	Not I or III[a] (average survival 44 mo)
Stage III	Serum β2 microglobulin >5.5 mg/L (average survival 29 mo)

[a]There are two categories for stage II
• Serum β2 microglobulin <3.5 mg/L but serum albumin <3.5 g/dL
Or
• Serum β2 microglobulin 3.5–5.5 irrespective of the serum albumin level.

They bind to the bone at sites of active bone remodeling and can therefore inhibit myelomatous bone damage, thereby arresting the destructive cycle described above (27,28). These agents (used in conjunction with cytotoxic chemotherapy) have been found to be superior to chemotherapy alone in decreasing the incidence of pathological fractures and bone pain and may lead to prolonged survival (29–32). Recently published guidelines recommend that bisphosphonate therapy be discontinued after two years in patients with stable or responsive disease (33).

Autologous transplantation has an established place in the treatment of myeloma. It is the treatment of choice for patients aged under 65 years and can be considered in older age groups (with good performance status) carrying a procedure related mortality

of less than 5% (15,34,35). At present the added benefit of double or tandem transplantation versus a single autologous transplant is not known.

Radiation therapy is reserved for patients with spinal cord compression secondary to vertebral body collapse associated with a soft tissue mass or to pathological fractures elsewhere associated with a soft tissue mass. It can be very effective but permanently destroys normal bone marrow stem cells in the treatment field.

Myeloma is generally considered incurable. It is a slowly progressing disease with long periods of relative inactivity. Relapse occurs in virtually all cases. On current treatment regimens patients younger than 70 years can expect a median survival of five years (depending on stage) (11,21). Death results from bacterial infection, renal insufficiency, and thromboembolism.

Key Points: General Features

■ Multiple myeloma is the second most common form of hematological malignancy in the Western world after non-Hodgkin's lymphoma
■ Multiple myeloma is an uncontrolled proliferation of a clone of plasma cells
■ Myeloma is characterized by (*i*) plasma cell proliferation of the bone marrow, (*ii*) lytic bone deposits, and (*iii*) myeloma protein in the serum or urine
■ Myeloma should not be confused with monoclonal gammopathy of uncertain significance (MGUS)
■ The Durie and Salmon PLUS staging system intergrates the traditional Durie–Salmon staging system with ^{18}F-FDG PET or MR imaging of the spine
■ Treatment comprises chemotherapy for symptomatic myeloma and supportive measures to reduce pain, renal impairment, and infection. Surgery also has a place in the management of complications such as pathological fractures

RADIOLOGY AND CROSS-SECTIONAL IMAGING

Radiology plays an important role in staging, monitoring treatment response, detection of relapse, and assessing complications. The various imaging techniques employed and their associated findings are described more fully below.

Conventional Radiography (Skeletal Survey)
Almost 80% of patients with multiple myeloma will have radiological evidence of skeletal involvement at diagnosis which is manifested in four different appearances—solitary deposit (plasmacytoma), diffuse skeletal involvement (myelomatosis), generalized osteopenia, and sclerosing myeloma (36). Views acquired should be posteroanterior chest, anteroposterior and lateral views of cervical spine (including an open mouth view), thoracic spine, lumbar spine, humeri, and femora, AP and lateral views of skull, and AP view of pelvis (Fig. 34.1) (37). Additional views of any symptomatic area should also be acquired. The most common sites include the vertebrae, ribs, skull, and pelvis whereas involvement of the distal bones is unusual. In early stage disease the role of the plain radiograph is limited because myeloma deposits are often not visualized (38,39).

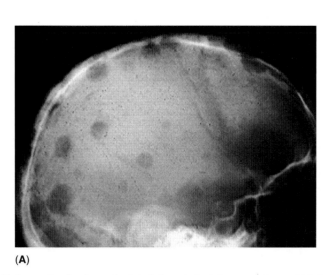

(A)

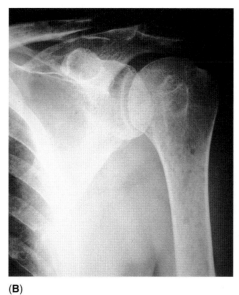

(B)

Figure 34.1 (A) Conventional radiograph of skull (lateral view) demonstrating multiple lytic deposits. (B) Conventional radiograph of left shoulder demonstrating multiple lytic deposits in left humerus, clavicle, and scapula.

Sites of involvement include

- Vertebrae in 66% of patients
- Ribs (45%)
- Skull (40%)
- Shoulder (40%)
- Pelvis (30%)
- Long bones (25%)

Myeloma lesions are sharply defined, small lytic areas (average size 20 mm) of bone destruction with no reactive bone formation. At post mortem these lesions are due to nodular replacement of marrow and bone by plasma cells. Although myeloma arises within the medulla, disease progression may produce infiltration of the cortex, invasion of the periosteum, and large extraosseous soft tissue masses. The pattern of destruction may be geographic, moth-eaten, or permeated. Pathological fractures are common and the probability of occurrence can be calculated using a scoring system (Fig. 34.2) (Table 34.4) (40,41).

When the skeletal survey has been obtained any further imaging should be discussed in the context of a multidisciplinary setting that includes an appropriately experienced radiologist, hemato-oncologist, and sometimes the contribution of an orthopedic surgeon may also be valuable (42). The expertise of the latter is useful in deciding if surgical stabilization of any bones is required. A major disadvantage of the skeletal survey is its relatively low sensitivity, with lytic deposits only becoming visible once 30% of the trabecular bone substance has been lost. Particular difficulty may arise in the sternum, sacrum, scapulae, and ribs. In addition, accurate assessment of osteopenia is not possible.

Generalized osteopenia may be the only bone manifestation of myeloma in up to 15% of patients. At post mortem these patients show diffuse replacement of marrow with plasma cells but have less severe bone resorption when compared with lytic deposits (40). Vertebral body collapse is the usual manifestation of this subtype which should not be confused with non-myelomatous osteoporosis which occurs in many older patients. Normal bone

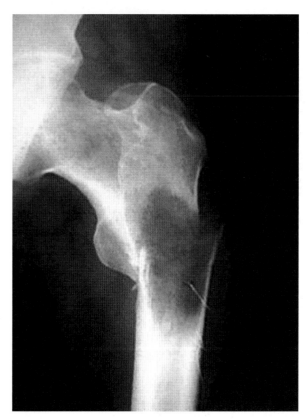

Figure 34.2 Conventional radiograph of proximal left femur (AP view) demonstrating a large deposit associated with a pathological fracture.

Table 34.4 Scoring System for Diagnosing Impending Pathological Fractures (41)

Variable	Score		
	1	2	3
Site	Upper limb	Lower limb	Peritrochanteric
Pain	Mild	Moderate	Functional
Lesion	Blastic	Mixed	Lytic
Size	<1/3 diameter	1/3–2/3 diameter	>2/3 diameter

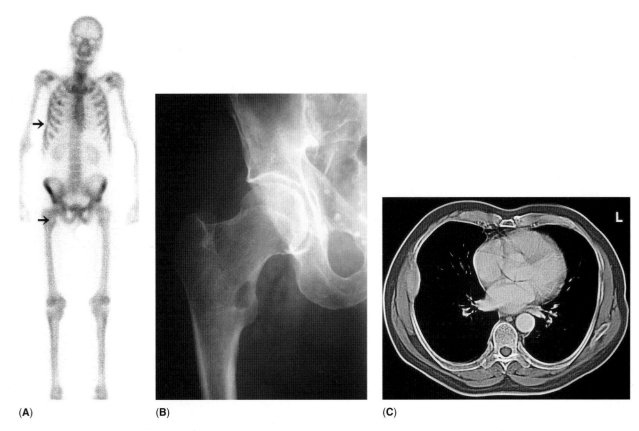

(A)   (B)   (C)

Figure 34.3 (A) Technetium-99m disphosphonate isotope bone scan showing photopenic regions affecting mid-right rib (arrow) and lesser trochanter of right femur (arrow). There is also a recent fracture affecting third right anterior rib. (B) Plain radiograph confirms presence of lytic deposit in lesser trochanter of right femur. (C) CT demonstrates an expansile myelomatous deposit arising from mid right rib.

surveys are noted in 10% of myeloma patients although this has not always been associated with improved survival (43).

Radionuclide Imaging

In multiple myeloma the osteoblastic response to bone destruction is negligible and the bone scan (using Technetium-99m labeled diphosphonate) is therefore frequently normal or may show areas of decreased uptake (photopenia) (Fig. 34.3) (Table 34.5). Most studies have shown that the sensitivity of skeletal scintigraphy for detecting individual deposits ranges from 40% to 60% (44,45). However, skeletal scintigraphy may be helpful in evaluating areas not well visualized on plain film radiographs such as the ribs, sacrum, scapulae, and sternum.

Technetium-99m-2-methoxyisobutlisonitrile (Tc99m-MIBI) has been shown to be superior to conventional radiography and skeletal scintigraphy in detecting bone and bone marrow involvement (46,47). Alterations in cell metabolism which occur in malignant cells (including plasma cells) can affect the membrane potential of the cell wall and mitochondrion leading to accumulation of Tc99m-MIBI within the cell (48). Different patterns of Tc99m-MIBI uptake have been described with multiple myeloma (negative, diffuse, focal, combined focal and diffuse) and semi-quantitative evaluation of these patterns showed a significant correlation with clinical status and stage of the disease (49). A negative scan in a patient with multiple myeloma indicates early stage disease or post treatment remission while the presence of focal uptake and/or intense diffuse bone marrow uptake suggests an advanced stage of active

Table 34.5 Multiple Myeloma Vs. Bone Metastases

Radiological features	Multiple myeloma	Bone metastases
Involvement of intervertebral discs	Yes	No
Involvement of mandible	Yes	No
Involvement of vertebral pedicles	No	Yes
Associated paraspinal soft tissue mass	Yes	No
Isotope bone scan	Frequently negative	Frequently positive

disease (91% of patients with a positive scan had active myeloma). The semi-quantitative score of diffuse Tc99m-MIBI bone marrow uptake (based on intensity and extension of uptake) correlates with the amount of monoclonal component and with the percentage of bone marrow plasma cells. These results suggested a potential role for Tc99m-MIBI in the prognosis and follow-up of patients with multiple myeloma (currently based on measurement of the monoclonal component, skeletal survey, and bone marrow biopsy).

Thallium-201 has also been described in multiple myeloma but due to limitations of the isotope its use has not been widespread nor has it been shown to be superior to Tc99m-MIBI (50,51). As a result the technique has largely fallen into disuse.

Positron emission tomography (PET) using the glucose analogue ^{18}F-fluorodeoxyglucose (FDG) has both the functional and morphological capacity to identify the extent and activity of multiple myeloma for staging and monitoring purposes. The ability of PET to perform whole body examinations is a major advantage

over conventional imaging techniques. In one series comprising 28 patients, PET was true positive in almost 93% of the radiographically documented osteolytic deposits and demonstrated a greater extent of disease than plain film radiography in 61% of patients (52). Another study confirmed its reliability in detecting active myeloma both within bone and at extramedullary sites and its ability to differentiate between new active disease and inactive (treated) sites (53,54). It is extremely useful in the evaluation of non-secretory myeloma and in identifying patients with a poor prognosis (residual myeloma post-stem cell transplantation and extramedullary myeloma). A negative ^{18}F-FDG PET strongly supports the diagnosis of MGUS (53,55). In a recent study of 49 patients with plasma cell malignancies only 5% relapsed after a negative FDG PET scan post therapy (55). The more recently available technology of PET combined with computed tomography (PET-CT) is now being used in the assessment of multiple myeloma (Fig. 34.4). In a small study of 16 patients comparing FDG PET-CT with the skeletal survey, CT and MR imaging was shown that FDG PET-CT led to management changes in nine patients but that MR imaging revealed diffuse bone involvement in five patients not evident on PET-CT (56). A larger study of 46 patients comparing FDG PET-CT with MR imaging of spine and pelvis and skeletal survey revealed that in 30% of patients PET-CT failed to show abnormalities visible on the MR imaging (57). However, PET-CT identified deposits outside the spine and pelvis in 35% of patients. Combining both techniques enabled identification of 92% of medullary and extramedullary sites of active disease. A further study comparing FDG PET-CT with Tc99m-MIBI and MR imaging in 33 patients demonstrated that PET-CT performed better than MIBI in the detection of focal deposits whereas MIBI was superior in the visualization of diffuse disease (58). MR imaging was comparable to both techniques in the spine and pelvis in the detection of focal and diffuse disease. Therefore, in the diagnostic work-up of multiple myeloma, the ability of MR imaging to accurately detect both focal and diffuse disease in the spine and pelvis means that it should be reserved for the evaluation of bone marrow involvement in these regions. Until whole-body MR imaging with reasonably short imaging times, good spatial resolution, and standardized sequences for multiple myeloma becomes widely available, the main drawback of MR imaging of spine and pelvis will be the limited field of

view which could lead to understaging of newly diagnosed multiple myeloma because deposits located outside these regions are inevitably missed. Therefore, in the whole-body evaluation of multiple myeloma patients at diagnosis, ^{18}F-FDG PET-CT can contribute to a more accurate assessment of disease, especially in a clinical context highly suggestive of focal involvement of the appendicular skeleton, such as the presence of bone pain or pathologic fractures in long bones or in the case of discrepancies between clinical status and hematological readings. On the other hand, despite the limited capacity in detecting focal lesions, Tc99m-MIBI still remains the most rapid and inexpensive technique for whole-body evaluation and may be an alternative option when a PET facility is not available. No formal study comparing whole body MR imaging with PET-CT is yet available although the usefulness of both techniques in this setting has been acknowledged (59,60).

It is worth remembering that false positive PET scans using FDG may arise from inflammatory changes due to active infection, chemotherapy within the previous three to four weeks or radiotherapy within the previous two to three months (61,62).

A study comparing ^{18}F FDG PET-CT with ^{11}C-Choline PET-CT in 10 patients demonstrated a higher sensitivity for ^{11}C-Choline in the detection of myelomatous deposits but the difference was not significant (63). Increased methionine uptake has also been demonstrated in plasma cells enabling imaging to be undertaken using ^{11}C-methionine PET-CT to identify disease at medullary and extra-medullary sites (64).

Cross-Sectional Imaging
Computed Tomography
A wide range of findings have been described in CT of myeloma. These include sharp, lytic foci of small and relatively homogenous size with no sclerotic rim, diffuse faint osteolysis fan angioma-like appearance due to the presence of thickened vertical trabeculae and expansile deposits (Fig. 34.4) (65). Myelomatous marrow often shows an abnormally high attenuation value compared with normal marrow. Discrete interruption of the cortical contour may be seen. CT can accurately depict the extent of associated soft tissue masses and can direct needle biopsy for histological diagnosis. For detection of small lytic bone deposits of less than 1 cm, narrow collimation protocols at a high tube current and tube voltage are

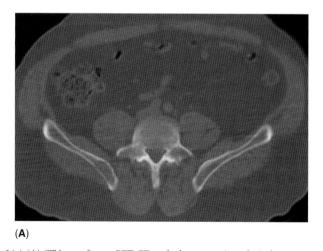

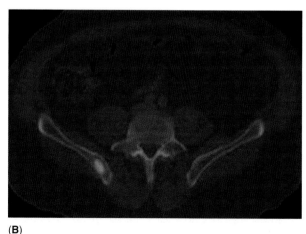

(A)   **(B)**

Figure 34.4 (A) CT image from a PET-CT study demonstrating a lytic deposit in posterior right ilium. (B) Fused PET-CT image demonstrates active disease at this site.

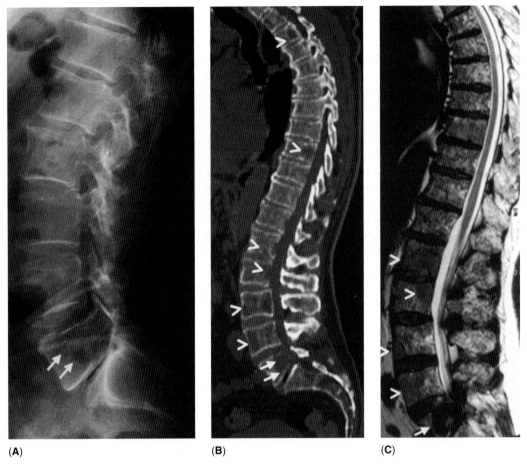

(A)   (B)   (C)

Figure 34.5 Sixty-eight-year-old man with newly diagnosed multiple myeloma, Stage III. (A) Lateral radiograph of lumbar spine [corresponding to multidetector CT (MDCT) and MR image] shows large osteolytic deposit affecting L5 (arrows). Further deposits larger than 1 cm in diameter in lumbar spine and in T3 and T9 are not recognizable on conventional radiographs. (B) MDCT image depicts deposits diameter larger than 10 mm in L5 (arrows) as well as in L1–L4, T3, and T9 (arrowheads). Diffuse osteopenia or deposits with diameters between 5 mm and 1 cm are visible in all vertebrae depicted. (C) Sagittal T2-weighted MR image (TR/TE 2957/120) shows tumor infiltration of all depicted vertebrae. Lesions larger than 1 cm in lumbar spine (arrowheads), especially in L5 (arrow), are clearly depicted. *Source*: From Ref. 66.

mandatory, because these parameters determine the resolution and image noise. Advances in X-ray tube technology with high heat storage capacities and simultaneous acquisition of multiple slices per rotation allows scanning time to be shortened significantly to less than a minute for a complete body scan. The advent of multidetector CT (MDCT) provides more detailed information on the risk of vertebral fractures compared with conventional radiography and MR imaging (66). In patients who are severely disabled or who are unable to undergo MR imaging examination this is a useful alternative imaging technique (67).

A study using MDCT in patients with Stage III myeloma provided more detailed information on the risk of vertebral fractures compared with plain film radiography and MR imaging (Fig. 34.5). Upward stage migration occurred in 17% of patients (66). More recently, a study comparing MDCT (64 × 0.6 mm collimation) with conventional radiography demonstrated a significant increase in detection of myelomatous deposits in spine, pelvis, and ribs (p < 0.001) necessitating a change in management in 18% of patients (68). MDCT also allows for improved imaging of patients with scoliosis due to its ability to adapt the dataset to the individual patient's features. As the degree of osseous infiltration in myeloma has a significant influ-

ence on therapy, it is likely there will be an increasing role for this technique in patients who are severely disabled or who are unable to undergo MR imaging examination. As most patients are elderly, dose considerations are not a major drawback and its ability to provide high quality images of the ribs, sternum, scapulae, and sacrum in addition to the fact that intravenous contrast medium is not necessary makes MR imaging a realistic alternative in the clinical scenarios outlined above. A large study comparing whole body low dose unenhanced MDCT in 131 patients with multiple myeloma with conventional hematological parameters demonstrated that the combination provided significantly greater diagnostic accuracy compared with laboratory testing alone particularly in monitoring patients post-therapy (69). A study comparing the efficacy of MDCT with MR imaging and FDG PET for detection of spinal bone marrow involvement in 10 patients demonstrated that MDCT was superior to FDG PET overall and to MR imaging in the detection of spinal deposits less than 5 mm (p = 0.031) (70). Although some groups use MDCT routinely in the assessment of multiple myeloma patients, this is not universal practice with others preferring to use the CT images from an FDG PET-CT examination in the context of follow-up evaluation (60,66,67,69,71).

MDCT has an important role in evaluating suspected spinal cord compression in cases when MR imaging is contraindicated (e.g., cardiac pacemaker, intraorbital metallic foreign body), or impossible due to patient intolerance or when facilities are unavailable.

Magnetic Resonance Imaging

MR imaging is used routinely in many centers as a diagnostic technique due to its high sensitivity and its ability to directly visualize bone marrow. The role of MR imaging (and PET imaging) is acknowledged by their inclusion in the Durie-Salmon Plus staging system (6). In this system the number of lytic lesions is counted leading to possible upstaging and altered therapy (71). In patients with suspected cord compression MR imaging is the examination of first choice. Bone deposits have been shown by MR imaging in about 50% of asymptomatic myeloma patients with normal plain radiographs. In a recent study of over 600 patients it was shown that focal deposits detected by MR imaging (but not on skeletal survey) independently affected survival (72). Complete resolution of focal lesions visualized on MR imaging also conferred superior survival. MR imaging can detect bone marrow infiltration in 29% to 50% of patients with Durie-Salmon Stage I disease and negative conventional radiographs (73). Nonetheless, the skeletal survey retains an important role in myeloma and remains on the list of recommended investigations (Fig. 34.6) (37).

Sagittal studies of the spine enable screening of a high proportion of hematopoietic marrow in a limited time and detection of any potential threat to the spinal cord. Additional coronal images of the pelvis and proximal femora enable evaluation of about an extra one-third of red marrow in an adult. These images may enable detection of deposits potentially at risk of fracture. Whole body MR imaging (WB-MRI) can be performed although its

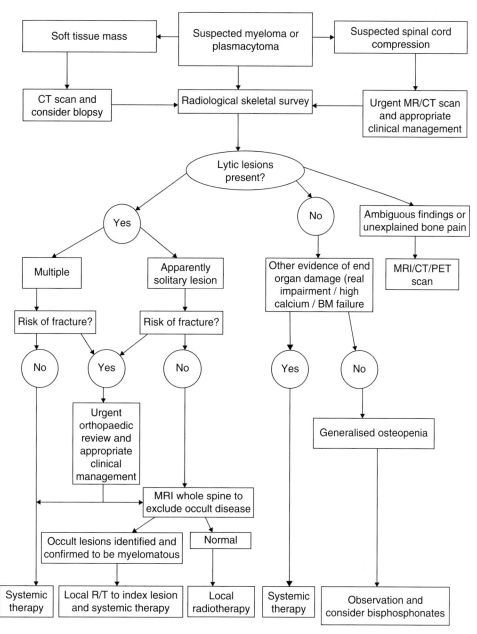

Figure 34.6 Suggested algorithm for imaging multiple myeloma (37).

clinical benefit has not yet been fully evaluated in myeloma (60,74–76). In one study comparing WB-MRI and the skeletal survey in 54 patients (47 myeloma, 7 MGUS), WB-MRI correctly demonstrated marrow deposits in 74% of patients versus 55% for the skeletal survey (Fig. 34.7) (77). WB-MRI also showed greater extent of infiltration in 90% of concordant deposits.

The imaging patterns in multiple myeloma can be classified as normal, focal, diffuse, and variegated (78,79). Others have added a further classification of combined diffuse and focal infiltration (80). Normal marrow is present on MR imaging at diagnosis in 50% to 75% of patients with early untreated (Stage I) myeloma and in about 20% of patients with advanced and treated (Stage III)

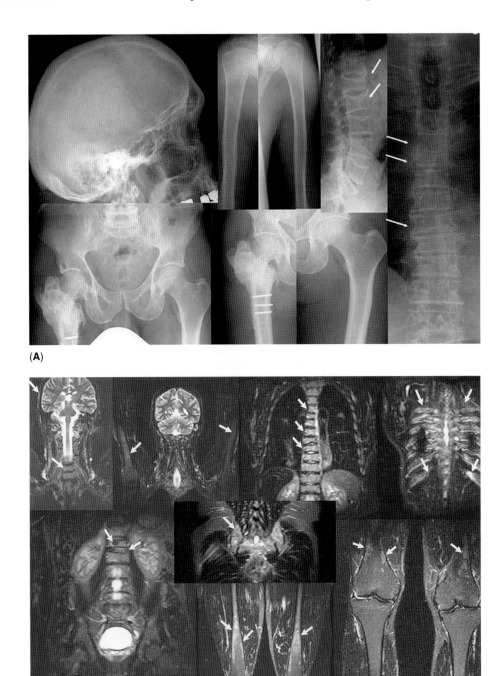

(A)

(B)

Figure 34.7 A 58-year-old male with Stage III disease of IgG myeloma. Bone marrow specimen revealed a bone marrow infiltration of 50%. Whole-body MRI and the radiographic skeletal survery (RSS) were performed within 12 days. (A) The RSS reveals no osteolytic bone lesion of the skull, upper, and lower extremities and pelvis. Note pinned healed fracture of the right femur. On plain films of the axial skeleton, no diffuse osteoporosis was detected. The thoraco-lumbar spine is characterized by degenerative change, although a height decrease of the different multiple vertebra at levels T12, L1, and L2 is seen, indicating bone involvement for multiple myeloma with pathological fractures (arrows). (B) Whole-body MRI shows a combined homogeneous and inhomogeneous pattern, indicating disseminated bone marrow infiltration (arrows). A homogeneous diffuse bone marrow infiltration of both humeri, the rib cage, and the cervical spine is depicted by whole body MRI. The vertebral bodies of the thoracic and lumbar spine, which are characterized by morphological changes of the adjacent endplates and a height decrease, exhibit a diffuse inhomogeneous appearance. Pathological fractures at levels L1 and L2 are depicted with whole body MRI in agreement with the RSS. Diffuse bone marrow infiltration of the sacrum, pelvis, and femora is also seen on MRI. In the clinical follow-up of 18 months, this patient had a progressive disease. *Source:* From Ref. 77.

disease. Monoclonal plasma cells arrange themselves so as not to displace the fat cells and the ratio of hematopoietic (and myeloma) to fat cells in bone marrow does not exceed that of healthy individuals (81). Hematopoietic marrow in adults between 40 and 70 years old is composed of approximately 20% to 25% bone substance, 40% to 45% fat, and 30% to 35% cellular marrow (82).

Fast and complete assessment can be achieved using a combination of a T1-weighted sequence and a fat suppression technique (Fig. 34.8) (73). The focal pattern consists of localized areas of decreased signal intensity on T1-weighted images and increased signal intensity on T2-weighted images. Myelomatous deposits are generally sharply demarcated on a background of an otherwise normal appearing bone marrow. Homogeneous enhancement occurs on T1-weighted images following intravenous contrast injection. Dynamic contrast-enhanced MR imaging has been shown to correlate with vessel density and paraprotein level (83). In a recent study using WB-MRI in 23 patients the highest sensitivity and reliability was achieved using a T2-weighted inversion recovery sequence (84).

The diffuse pattern is characterized by a diffuse and homogeneous decrease in marrow signal intensity which becomes identical to or lower than that of adjacent intervertebral discs on a T1-weighted image and on a T2-weighted image by a diffuse or patchy increase in signal intensity (Fig. 34.9). Marked enhancement is usually seen on T1-weighted images following intravenous contrast medium. The increased contrast between enhancing marrow and the lower signal intervertebral discs allows more subtle forms of infiltration to be identified (85).

The variegated pattern is characterized by the presence of multiple foci of low signal intensity on T1-weighted images, intermediate to high signal intensity on T2-weighted images, and enhancement following IV contrast T1-weighted images. This pattern is seen almost exclusively in an early stage of the disease (86).

These patterns of marrow involvement do not seem to correlate with the interstitial, nodular, and diffuse patterns of marrow infiltration seen at microscopy. However, they show a positive correlation with some laboratory parameters. Patients with the normal and variegated patterns tend to have a lower tumor burden than those with the focal and diffuse marrow involvement patterns. Higher cellularity, higher plasmacytosis, and more severe signs of bone failure are usually found in patients with the diffuse pattern (87).

The lack of specificity of the MR imaging patterns should be noted. The focal and diffuse patterns may be observed in both metastatic disease from primary solid tumors and in other hematological malignancies, especially lymphoma, and leukemia. Differentiation between red marrow hyperplasia secondary to anemia, infection, malignant or treated marrow infiltration can be extremely difficult. Normal marrow heterogeneities may mimic the variegated pattern although in most cases high signal intensity on T2-weighted images and contrast enhancement help distinguish relevant small marrow abnormalities from normal hematopoietic foci that generally show intermediate signal intensity on T2-weighted images and no contrast enhancement on T1-weighted images. The advent of diffusion-weighted imaging promised an effective method for differentiating benign from malignant compression fractures (88,89). However, only variable

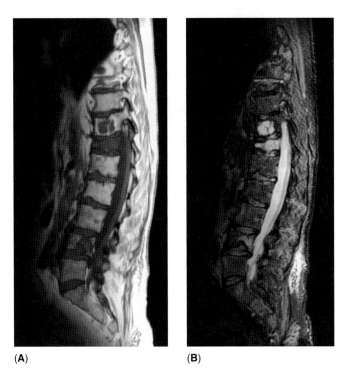

(A)   **(B)**

Figure 34.8 (A) Sagittal T1-weighted and (B) STIR MR images of lower thoracic and lumbar spine showing focal and diffuse myelomatous infiltration affecting multiple vertebrae with marked compression affecting T12.

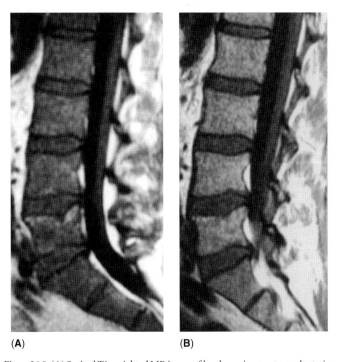

(A)   **(B)**

Figure 34.9 (A) Sagittal T1-weighted MR image of lumbar spine pre-transplantation demonstrating diffuse abnormal low signal intensity in vertebral bodies. (B) Sagittal T1-weighted MR image of lumbar spine post-transplantation shows conversion to normal high signal marrow. *Source:* From Ref. 131.

success has been reported since then and as a result it is not used routinely (90,91).

Key Points: Radiological Features

- Eighty percent of patients have radiological evidence of skeletal disease with four patterns of disease; solitary deposit, diffuse involvement, generalized osteopenia, and sclerosing myeloma. 66% of patients have vertebral deposits
- Myeloma lesions are sharply defined, small (20 mm), and lytic. They are only visible when 30% of the trabecular bone has been destroyed
- Osteopenia may be the only manifestation of disease in up to 15% of patients
- Conventional bone scintigraphy is frequently normal as the osteoblastic reaction around deposits is negligible. Skeletal scintigraphy may be helpful for evaluating areas difficult to display on conventional films such as the ribs, sternum, scapulae, and sacrum
- PET and PET-CT technology using ^{18}F-FDG has a growing role in the management of multiple myeloma. It may identify more extensive disease than on plain radiographs and may distinguish new active disease and inactive deposits
- A negative PET scan indicates the diagnosis of MGUS
- MDCT is a useful imaging tool for the assessment of patients at risk of vertebral fractures or those with obvious fractures. It can demonstrate the presence and extent of the soft tissue component and is able to assess suspected spinal cord compression. It is a realistic alternative in patients who are unable to undergo MR imaging
- MR imaging shows bone abnormalities in 50% of asymptomatic patients with normal conventional radiography
- Focal deposits show a low signal intensity on T1 and a high signal intensity on T2 weighting. Uniform enhancement occurs after injection of intravenous contrast medium
- The MR imaging patterns are non-specific and may be observed in both metastatic disease from primary solid tumors and other hematological malignancies
- WB-MRI shows promise but is not yet fully established in practice
- Combining MR imaging with FDG PET-CT enables identification of more than 90% of active medullary and extramedullary sites

Compression Fractures in Multiple Myeloma

Compression fractures arise from extensive osteoclastic bone resorption or replacement of bone by a growing plasma cell tumor mass. Several criteria exist for differentiating benign from malignant vertebral body compression fractures (Table 34.6) (92) (Fig. 34.10). However, these should be applied with caution to patients with multiple myeloma as normal signal intensity within a compressed vertebral body on spinal MR images does not preclude the diagnosis of multiple myeloma. In a study of 224 vertebral fractures in patients with known multiple myeloma, Lecouvet et al. found that 67% appeared benign on MR imaging and 38% of their 37 patients had benign fractures only at diagnosis (93).

Table 34.6 MRI Criteria for the Differential Diagnosis of Benign Vs. Malignant Vertebral Fractures (95)

Variable	Osteoporotic fractures	Malignant fractures
Marrow Signal	Normal on all sequences (old fracture)	Diffusely low on T1-weighted images
	Band-like low SI adjacent to fracture (acute)	High or heterogeneous on T2-weighted images
	Normal SI preserved opposite the fractured end plate	Round or irreglar foci of marrow replacement
		Posterior elements involved
		Soft tissues/epidural involvement
Contrast enhancement	Homogenous "return to normal" SI after injection	High or heterogeneous
Vertebral contours	Retropulsion of a posterior bone fragment (often postero-superior)	Convex posterior cortex

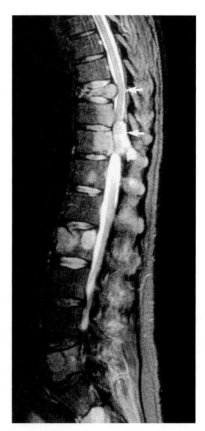

Figure 34.10 Sagittal MRI STIR image of the spine showing malignant vertebral body compression at T9 and T11 in addition to spinal cord compression at these sites (arrows).

In patients with osteoporotic or post-traumatic vertebral compression of recent onset, MR imaging will usually show signal alteration that parallels one of the endplates, involves less than half of the vertebral body, does not extend to the pedicles and enhances homogeneously following intravenous contrast. Diffusion-weighted MR imaging may also prove to be a useful method to apply to the differential diagnosis of compression fractures (88).

Patients being treated for multiple myeloma may suffer acute back pain secondary to vertebral body collapse even after effective

chemotherapy. This is due to resolution of the tumor mass that was supporting the bony cortex. Thirty-five new vertebral compression fractures were discovered on post-treatment MR images of 29 patients with multiple myeloma in remission (94). In another study, 131 vertebral compression fractures appeared in 37 patients with multiple myeloma after the onset of therapy (88). Conversely, progression of disease may also be responsible for a new compression fracture and MR imaging may be useful in differentiating between these two clinical settings. It has been shown that patients with either normal marrow appearance or less than ten focal lesions on pre-treatment MR images had significantly longer fracture-free survival than patients with more than 10 focal lesions or with diffuse patterns on pre-treatment MR images (87).

Key Points: Compression Fractures

- Criteria for differentiating benign and malignant vertebral compression fractures should be applied with caution in patients with multiple myeloma
- A normal signal intensity of a compressed vertebral body does not preclude the diagnosis of multiple myeloma.
- New compression fractures may arise following treatment as a result of resolving soft tissue masses which formerly supported bone. Progression of disease may also result in compression fractures and MR imaging is helpful in distinguishing these two different entities

SIDE EFFECTS OF THERAPY AND COMPLICATIONS: THE ROLE OF RADIOLOGY

Drug Therapy

Infection is the single most dangerous complication for myeloma patients with the patient most at risk in the first three months of front-line therapy and is a recognized cause of bone pain in its own right (6,95). Myeloma is associated with a higher incidence of infective discitis and cerebritis in part due to cytotoxic therapy induced immunosuppression associated with corticosteroid therapy (96–98). Central venous catheters represent a potential source of bacteremia (99). MR imaging enables early identification followed by percutaneous needle aspirate using CT to confirm the diagnosis and provide information regarding choice of antibiotic (100). Melphalan is associated with increased risk of pancytopenia, mucositis, and pulmonary complications (101–104). Conventional radiography and CT scanning are the appropriate imaging investigations. High doses of corticosteroids may cause spinal fractures and avascular necrosis of the femoral heads (amongst other bones). MR imaging is useful for assessing both these conditions. When thalidomide is used in combination with dexamethasone it carries a 16% incidence of deep vein thrombosis (DVT) (105,106). Abdominal discomfort resulting from constipation is also a well-recognized side effect of thalidomide and can be readily assessed radiologically using a supine plain radiograph of abdomen. A reported side-effect is interstitial pneumonitis which can be identified on high resolution CT (107). The drug Bortezomib is associated with cytopenia and a decrease in platelet count to $<50,000 \, mm^3$ occurs in almost 30% of patients increasing the risk of hemorrhage (108). This drug has not been associated with an increased incidence of DVT in trials reported to date (21). Other reported adverse effects are sensory neuropathy and pseudomembranous colitis (109). Chronic bisphosphonate use is associated with renal damage (monitored with regular serum creatinine levels) and osteonecrosis of the mandible (110–113). Regular dental check-ups in association with an orthopantomogram and a CT scan enable early diagnosis of the latter (114).

Marrow Transplantation

Allogeneic transplant is a high risk procedure with reported encephalopathic changes (reversible) which may develop as result of cyclosporin therapy (115). In patients undergoing non-myeloablative or "mini" allogeneic transplants there is a high risk of acute (32–39%) and chronic (32–46%) graft versus host disease in reported series (15). Autologous stem cell transplantation is also available but it is not curative with a median relapse time of three years (116). Imaging depends on symptomatology and consists of plain film radiography, CT, and MR imaging as required.

Spinal Cord Compression

Spinal cord compression resulting from vertebral body collapse may occur in up to 25% of patients and has been described as the presenting feature in 12% of patients (117–119). Early recognition of back pain and neurological symptoms is essential. MR is the imaging investigation of choice (Fig. 34.10). Pathological fractures are common occurring in 50% of patients (40). Fractures of the tubular bones heal readily with normal amounts of callus but extensive fractures may require insertion of intra-medullary nails. Myelofibrosis manifest by diffuse low signal on both T1-weighted and STIR sequences and amyloidosis manifest by focal areas of decreased signal on T1-weighted and STIR sequences are other recognized complications (36).

Osteopenia

In myeloma, osteopenia may be confined to bones where myeloma is active leaving the remaining bony skeleton unaffected. Insufficiency fractures may arise in the sacrum, pubic rami, or acetabular roof with the latter having a characteristic appearance (Fig. 34.11) (120). Although dual energy X-ray absorptiometry (DEXA) is the best technique for diagnosing osteoporosis and for fracture risk assessment no reliable data exists currently to differentiate between benign osteoporosis and myeloma induced osteoporosis. One study comprising 30 patients has demonstrated that lumbar DEXA scans at diagnosis can identify patients at risk from early vertebral body compression (121). Newer scanners allow estimation of vertebral bone mineral density from a lateral view (with the patient supine) but accuracy of the analysis is affected if spinal osteophytes, pre-existing vertebral body compression, or spondylosis are present precluding its use routinely. A further complicating factor is the widespread use of bisphosphonates in symptomatic myeloma patients.

Patients being treated for multiple myeloma may suffer acute back pain secondary to vertebral body collapse even after effective chemotherapy. This is due to resolution of the tumor mass that was supporting the bony cortex. Thirty-five new vertebral compression fractures were discovered on post-treatment MR images of 29 patients with multiple myeloma in remission (94). In another study, 131 vertebral compression fractures appeared in 37 patients

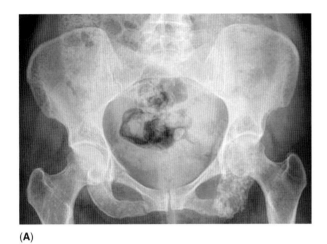

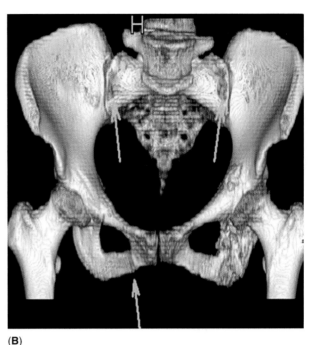

(A)   (B)

Figure 34.11 A 56-year-old woman with known multiple myeloma and new right groin pain. Pelvic radiograph (**A**) shows fractures of right superior and inferior pubic rami. 3D CT image (**B**) constructed from whole body PET-CT examination data shows fractures of pubic rami and both sacral alae (arrows). These fractures were considered to be insufficiency fractures through areas of myelomatous foci rather than pathological fractures. *Source:* From Ref. 60.

with multiple myeloma after the onset of therapy (88). Conversely, progression of disease may also be responsible for a new compression fracture and MR imaging may be useful in differentiating between these two clinical settings. It has been shown that patients with either normal marrow appearance or less than ten focal lesions on pre-treatment MR images had significantly longer fracture-free survival than patients with more than 10 focal lesions or with diffuse patterns on pre-treatment MR images (87).

The most sensitive and specific imaging technique for the diagnosis of avascular necrosis of the femoral head is MR imaging which is manifest by a characteristic double-line sign on T2-weighted images (122). This condition may result from high dose steroid therapy or radiotherapy and its early recognition before the development of subchondral fractures is important for the success of conservative management.

Renal Impairment

Renal impairment is common in myeloma and affects up to half of all patients at some stage in their illness. This is usually a consequence of amyloisosis rather than plasma cell infiltration (123). Other possible causes include hypercalcemia, dehydration, hyperuricemia, infection or the action of nephrotoxic drugs. Unfortunately several of the drugs that are used to treat myeloma have an adverse effect on kidney function. Secondary amyloid occurs in approximately 10% of cases and in the early stages ultrasound demonstrates enlarged kidneys with increased cortical reflectivity. Amyloid protein is deposited mainly in the cortex so that corticomedullary differentiation is preserved and the pyramids are normal in size (124). Radiolabeled serum amyloid P component scintigraphy is a non-invasive and quantitative method for imaging amyloid deposits though it is less effective in myeloma associated amyloid than other forms of amyloid (125). Cardiac involvement is

difficult to demonstrate due to motion artefact and blood pooling in addition to proximity of the spleen (126). Unfortunately, this examination is only available in a few specialist centers.

Key Points: Side Effects of Therapy: The Role of Radiology

■ Infective discitis is a serious complication, and MR imaging and CT have a key role in identifying the site of disease and in guiding needle aspiration
■ High dose steroid therapy may induce avascular necrosis and spinal fractures are best investigated with MR imaging

RADIOLOGY OF RESPONDING/RELAPSING DISEASE

The role of radiology in the assessment of treatment response is limited and sequential quantification of biological markers of disease (monoclonal protein levels and bone marrow plasmacytosis) are usually sufficient to assess response to chemotherapy. The choice of imaging technique for assessing disease response depends on the findings from the initial work-up and treatment received.

Conventional Radiography

A repeat skeletal survey is not routinely indicated as lytic bone deposits often show little evidence of healing radiographically (manifest by shrinkage or sclerosis) even in those patients achieving a complete remission (37,71). The addition of bisphosphonate compounds as antiosteoclast agents leads to bone strengthening which may further accentuate these features. New or enlarging deposits signify disease progression. New vertebral body compression fractures on conventional radiography do not necessarily

indicate disease progression as they may arise due to resolution of the tumor mass formerly supporting the bony cortex. Persistence of radiological abnormalities should not be considered evidence of active disease, since they may represent residual osteolysis in the absence of plasma cell proliferation. There is insufficient evidence to recommend routine skeletal surveys in untreated asymptomatic patients in the absence of any evidence of disease progression (37). If this situation changes the skeletal survey should be repeated with targeted views of any symptomatic region.

Computed Tomography

Current evidence does not support the use of CT for routine follow-up assessment. However, in selected cases particularly those with a substantial soft tissue component it is reasonable to use CT to monitor treatment response. In these cases there is disappearance of extra-osseous or extra-medullary masses and the reappearance of a continuous cortical outline with fatty marrow content (79). CT should also be considered if there are persistent unexplained symptoms, concern about a risk of fracture or lack of response to therapy.

Magnetic Resonance Imaging

There is insufficient evidence to recommend routine MR imaging for the follow-up of treated disease (37). Interpretation of post-treatment MR imaging changes can be difficult as there is a wide spectrum of possible treatment induced changes on MR imaging depending on the pattern of bone marrow infiltration. Although MR imaging is more sensitive than the skeletal survey it is often difficult to differentiate inactive from active disease. Focal marrow lesions may remain identical or decrease in size (94,127). Changes in contrast enhancement between the pre- and post-treatment MR examinations have been studied (128). The lack of lesion enhancement or only a peripheral rim enhancement seen after treatment can be indicative of responsive deposits. Other features suggestive of a good response include decreased signal intensity on T2-weighted images (73). Local radiation therapy of focal complex deposits induces a rapid decrease in the soft tissue extension and appearance of presumably necrotic, avascular central areas within the deposit on T1-weighted images with a later decrease in lesion size (129). In diffuse marrow abnormalities, increased marrow signal is usually observed on post-treatment T1-weighted images due to reappearance of fat cells within more hydrated cellular components (Fig. 34.9). Conversion of a diffuse to a focal or variegated pattern is also frequent (94). Post-treatment MR imaging of the bone marrow may provide important information for patients with equivocal clinical and laboratory results as well as for patients with non-secretory myeloma.

In contrast to patients with advanced disease stages treated with conventional chemotherapy, patients with normal MR findings at diagnosis have better response to treatment and a longer survival than those with focal or diffuse marrow abnormalities at MR imaging (85). This feature has not yet been assessed in patients treated with marrow transplantation. Patients undergoing therapy with thalidomide have more favorable outcomes (better overall survival rate and prolonged event-free survival) with normal post-treatment MR imaging than those with persistent focal deposits (13).

After bone marrow transplantation, the bone marrow generally has a high signal on T1-weighted images but focal residual deposits are frequent (130). The prognostic significance of these abnormalities is uncertain as patients with these residual abnormalities did not always have a poorer outcome than those with normal post-transplantation MR imaging examinations (36,131). Increased marrow cellularity due to marrow stimulating factors and decreased signal due to marrow hemosiderosis resulting from repeated transfusions may also be present on post-transplantation MR images. Despite the superiority of MR imaging over conventional radiography for spinal and pelvic lesion detection, an MR imaging survey limited to these areas may be less sensitive than the conventional skeletal survey which may detect deposits in the skull and rib (132).

In patients with clinical relapse new focal deposits or an increase in size of deposits previously present can be identified with MR imaging. Conversion of a normal or variegated pattern to a diffuse pattern indicates severe relapse on follow-up MR imaging. MR imaging is also useful in assessing status of leptomeninges as abnormal enhancement representing tumor spread has been reported in 18 out of 1856 treated patients in one series (133). In patients with a solitary bone plasmacytoma MR screening of the spine and pelvis will usually reveal radiographically unsuspected deposits in up to 80% of patients thus suggesting true myeloma from the outset. This finding is associated with a poor response to localized radiotherapy and an earlier development of systemic disease than in patients with a negative MR imaging survey (134).

MR imaging has been useful in the assessment of patients following transplantation. The bone marrow evolution index based on comparison of pre- and post-transplant MR imaging combines findings related to the number of deposits, deposit size, contrast enhancement, and marrow background (131). A score of 0, 1, or 2 is given depending on whether there is improvement, stability or deterioration. A score below 4 had superior treatment response and was more successful than evaluating each parameter individually. However, diffuse or focal marrow changes following granulocyte colony stimulating factor (GCSF) treatment may mimic active disease and limit its effectiveness (135).

High levels of serum $\beta2$ microglobulin correlate with a poor prognosis and remain the single most powerful determinant of outcome (136). No correlation between this finding and appearances on MR imaging has yet been demonstrated. Long term prospective studies are required to establish the significance and prognostic value of the different MR imaging patterns of marrow involvement and their correlation with various laboratory values particularly in patients undergoing transplantation.

Functional Imaging

Conventional Scintigraphy

Although abnormal tracer uptake has been shown to indicate residual activity on conventional skeletal scintigraphy, osteoblastic activity due to healing vertebral body fractures, fractures elsewhere in bony skeleton, and drug therapy (particularly bisphosphonates) will also give rise to increased isotope uptake (27,28,45). ^{99m}Tc-MIBI has been shown to be superior to plain film radiography and skeletal scintigraphy in detecting bone and bone marrow involvement (46–48,137). A negative scan in a patient with multiple myeloma indicates early stage disease or post-treatment remission while the presence of focal uptake and/or intense diffuse bone marrow uptake suggests an advanced stage of active disease (49). A subsequent follow-up study involving

22 patients showed a significant correlation between the scintigraphic findings and clinical status post-chemotherapy (138). More recent studies have demonstrated significant correlation between the extent of disease within bone marrow and serum β2 microglobulin levels (p = 0.012) in 25 patients (139). A further study involving 24 patients correlating Tc99m-MIBI with MR imaging scans and skeletal survey demonstrated no significant difference between the Tc99m-MIBI scan and MR imaging in predicting the extension of bone marrow infiltration and was significantly better than the skeletal survey (p = 0.021) (140). The post-treatment Tc99m-MIBI score also correlated significantly with post-treatment response (p = 0.016). In the largest study comprising 397 scans, 40% of asymptomatic patients were upstaged as a result of the Tc99m-MIBI scan (141). Of 168 scans performed during follow-up, the specificity of Tc99m-MIBI was 86% in patients demonstrating a complete response. These results indicate a role for this examination particularly in patients who are unable to undergo MR imaging or PET-CT. However, evaluation of the treated patient using this tracer may be compromised if drug resistance is present. If this is manifest as Pgp expression dual phase imaging (at 10 minutes and four hours following injection) helps to differentiate but if Bcl-2 is expressed correlation with other imaging methods is necessary (142). MIBI has also been found to be predictive of disease relapse (143). Despite the volume of published work supporting MIBI it is likely to be superseded by PET-CT in major oncology centers in the coming years.

FDG-PET and PET-CT
Studies have demonstrated its reliability in detecting active myeloma both within bone and at extramedullary sites and its ability to differentiate between new active disease and inactive treated sites (53,144,145). In a study involving 13 patients using FDG PET, nine of whom had undergone therapy, PET proved superior to anatomical imaging in identifying sites of active residual disease (54). Patients showing no abnormal or decreased FDG uptake demonstrated clinical improvement. In a recent study of 49 patients with plasma cell malignancies only 5% relapsed after a negative FDG PET post therapy (55). False negative results may occur due to limitations with spatial resolution, resulting in deposits less than 0.5 cm not being detected. If relapse is suspected PET may identify new sites of disease and unsuspected sites of extramedullary disease. If FDG uptake is present in medullary or extramedullary compartment following high dose therapy and stem cell transplantation then prognosis is adversely affected (53). GCSF can cause changes mimicking active disease on PET scans which can last for up to one month following discontinuation of treatment (146). In many centers PET-CT is becoming the imaging study of choice for post-transplant patients. Deposits in the range of 0.5 to 1 cm ($SUV_{max} > 2.5$) can be identified (83). FDG PET-CT has an advantage over MR imaging in the post transplantation patient by more accurately reflecting disease status (Fig. 34.12) (57,147). Given the range of newer therapies now available the identification of occult active disease may allow for targeted multimodal therapy. Non-secretory myeloma patients should get PET-CT during their initial staging since PET-CT will be the imaging study of choice after treatment (60). Despite much anecdotal evidence for its success, PET is not yet recommended for use in routine follow-up in treated myeloma patients (37).

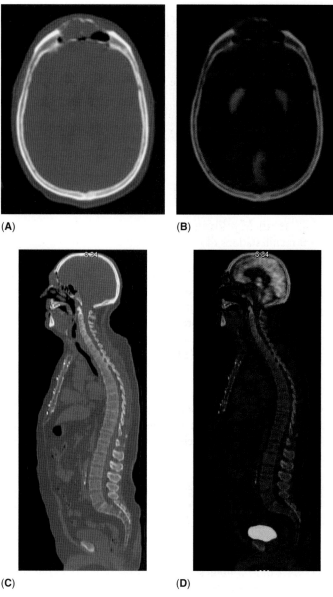

(A)   (B)

(C)   (D)

Figure 34.12 Axial CT scan (**A**) from a 57-year-old male post treatment demonstrating a residual soft tissue mass within right frontal bone. Fused PET-CT image (**B**) demonstrates no abnormal FDG uptake indicating the absence of active disease. Sagittal CT image from PET-CT study (**C**) shows no evidence of lytic deposits. Sagittal fused PET-CT image (**D**) demonstrates active focus of myeloma within body of sternum.

Key Points: Post-Treatment Evaluation

- Role of radiology in assessment of treatment response is limited; routine use of conventional radiography, MDCT, or MR imaging is not recommended
- Sequential analysis of biological markers is more frequently employed
- A wide spectrum of findings is present on post-treatment MR imaging
- Conversion of diffuse to a focal or variegated pattern on MR imaging is frequent
- Lack of contrast enhancement on MR imaging can be indicative of responsive deposits

- Focal residual deposits are frequent on MR imaging following bone marrow transplantation but are not necessarily associated with a poorer outcome
- ^{99m}Tc-MIBI is superior to plain film radiography and skeletal scintigraphy in detecting bone and bone marrow involvement post-treatment
- FDG PET-CT is now becoming the imaging technique of choice in treated patients as it can distinguish active disease from inactive disease

UNCOMMON VARIANTS OF MYELOMA

Extraosseous Myeloma

Clinical manifestations of extraosseous myeloma are rare, occurring in less than 5% of patients with multiple myeloma. Extraosseous myeloma deposits have been reported at multiple sites with the breast, lymph nodes, and spleen most frequently involved. It may also occur in the epidural region causing cord compression (148). Extraosseous myeloma is more aggressive, occurs in a younger age group (average age 50 years), and is associated with worse survival than conventional myeloma (149).

Sclerotic Myeloma

Primary sclerotic manifestations are rare and occur only in 3% of patients. It may take the form of diffuse osteosclerosis, patchy sclerotic areas throughout the skeleton or very small numbers of focal sclerotic lesions (150).

Summary

- Multiple myeloma is characterized by the classic triad of bone marrow infiltration by plasma cells, lytic bone deposits on conventional radiography (skeletal survey), and the presence of M protein serum or urine
- Durie-Salmon PLUS staging system remains the preferred choice of many oncologists as it combines imaging and laboratory findings
- MDCT is a realistic alternative for imaging in severely disabled patients or those unable to undergo MR imaging examination
- FDG PET-CT reliably detects active and inactive myeloma within bone and at extramedullary sites
- Improvements in PET-CT technology allow the CT component of the examination to be used for anatomical assessment of the bony skeleton
- No role for routine imaging in the assessment of treatment response—sequential analysis of biological markers is preferred
- Marrow deposits demonstrated on post-transplantation MR imaging are not necessarily associated with a poorer outcome
- Skeletal survey will be superseded by whole body-MRI and FDG PET-CT
- Serum beta microglobulin levels remain the single most powerful prognostic determinant

REFERENCES

1. Cancer Facts and Figures 2007. American Cancer Society, Inc. Atlanta, Georgia, U.S.A. [Available from: www.cancer.org].
2. Phekoo KJ, Schey SA, Richards MA, et al. A population study to define the incidence and survival of multiple myeloma in a National Health Service Region in UK. Br J Haematol 2004; 127: 299–304.
3. Tricot G. New insights into role of microenvironment in multiple myeloma. Lancet 2000; 355: 248–50.
4. Kyle RA, Rajkumar SV. Monoclonal gammopathies of undetermined significance. Hematol Oncol Clin North Am 1999; 13: 1181–202.
5. Durie BG, Salmon SE. A clinical staging system for multiple myeloma. Correlation of measured myeloma cell mass with presenting clinical features, response to treatment, and survival. Cancer 1975; 36: 842–54.
6. Durie BG, Kyle RA, Belch A, et al. Myeloma management guidelines: a consensus report from the Scientific Advisors of the International Myeloma Foundation. Haematol J 2003; 4: 379–98.
7. Greipp PR, San Miguel J, Durie BG, et al. International staging system for myeloma. J Clin Oncol 2005; 23: 3412–20.
8. Facon T, Avet-Loiseau H, Guillerm G, et al. Intergroupe Francophone du Myélome. Chromosome 13 abnormalities identified by FISH analysis and serum beta2-microglobulin produce a powerful myeloma staging system for patients receiving high dose therapy. Blood 2001; 97: 1566–71.
9. Samson D. Diagnosis and management of multiple myeloma. Br J Haematol 2001; 115: 522–40.
10. Smith A, Wisloff F, Samson D. Guidelines on the diagnosis and management of multiple myeloma 2005. Br J Haematol 2006; 132: 410–51.
11. Sirohi B, Powles R. Multiple myeloma. Lancet 2004; 363: 875–87.
12. Barlogie B, Shaughnessy J, Tricot G, et al. Treatment of multiple myeloma. Blood 2004; 103: 20–32.
13. Barlogie B, Zangari M, Spencer T, et al. Thalidomide in the management of multiple myeloma. Semin Hematol 2001; 38: 250–9.
14. Cavenagh JD, Oakervee H. Thalidomide in multiple myeloma: current status and future prospects. Br J Haematol 2003; 120: 18–26.
15. Harousseau JL, Shaughnessy J Jr, Richardson P. Multiple myeloma. Hematology (Am Soc Hematol Educ Program) 2004: 237–56.
16. Dicato M, Boccadoro M, Cavenagh J, et al. Management of multiple myeloma with bortezomib: experts review the data and debate the issues. Oncology 2006; 70: 474–82.
17. Popat R, Joel S, Oakervee H, Cavenagh J. Bortezomib for multiple myeloma. Expert Opin Pharmacother 2006; 7: 1337–46.
18. Oakervee H, Popat R, Cavenagh JD. Use of bortezomib as induction therapy prior to stem cell transplantation in frontline treatment of multiple myeloma: impact on stem cell harvesting and engraftment. Leuk Lymphoma 2007; 48: 1910–21.

19. Morgan GJ, Davies FE, Cavenagh JD, Jackson GH. Position statement on the use of bortezomib in multiple myeloma. Int J Lab Hematol 2008; 30: 1–10.

20. Bruno B, Rotta M, Giaccone L et al. New drugs for treatment of multiple myeloma. Lancet Oncology 2004; 5: 430–42.

21. Morgan GJ, Davies FE. Evolving treatment strategies for myeloma. Br J Cancer 2005; 92: 217–21.

22. Goel A, Carlson SK, Classic KL, et al. Radioiodide imaging and radiovirotherapy of multiple myeloma using VSV(Delta51)-NIS, an attenuated vesicular stomatitis virus encoding the sodium iodide symporter gene. Blood 2007; 110: 2342–50.

23. Cotten A, Dewatre F, Cortet B, et al. Percutaneous vertebroplasty for osteolytic metastases and myeloma: effects of the percentage of lesion filling and the leakage of methyl methacrylate at clinical follow-up. Radiology 1996; 200: 525–30.

24. Theodorou DJ, Theodorou SJ, Sartoris DJ. Treatment of osteoporosis: current status and recent advances. Compr Ther 2002; 28: 109–22.

25. Dudeney S, Lieberman IH, Reinhardt MK, Hussein M. Kyphoplasty in the treatment of osteolytic vertebral compression fractures as a result of multiple myeloma. J Clin Oncol 2002; 20: 2382–7.

26. McDonald RJ, Trout AT, Gray LA, et al. Vertebroplasty in multiple myeloma: outcomes in a large patient series. AJNR Am J Neuroradiol 2008; 29: 642–8.

27. Conte P, Coleman R. Bisphosphonates in the treatment of skeletal metastases. Semin Oncol 2004; 31: 59–63.

28. Lipton A. Pathophysiology of bone metastases: how this knowledge may lead to therapeutic intervention. J Support Oncol 2004; 2: 205–13; discussion 213–14, 216–17, 219–20.

29. Kanis JA, McCloskey EV. Bisphosphonates in multiple myeloma. Cancer 2000; 88: 3022–32.

30. Theriault RL, Hortobagyi GN. The evolving role of bisphosphonates. Semin Oncol 2001; 28: 284–90.

31. Berenson JR, Hillner BE, Kyle RA, et al. American Society of Clinical Oncology clinical practice guidelines: the role of bisphosphonates in multiple myeloma. J Clin Oncol 2002; 20: 3719–36.

32. Durie BG, Jacobson J, Barlogie B, Crowley J. Magnitude of response with myeloma frontline therapy does not predict outcome: importance of time to progression in Southwest Oncology Group Chemotherapy Trials. J Clin Oncol 2004; 22: 1857–63.

33. Kyle RA, Yee GC, Somerfield MR, et al. American Society of Clinical Oncology 2007 clinical practice guideline update on the role of bisphosphonates in multiple myeloma. J Clin Oncol 2007; 25: 2464–72.

34. Barlogie B, Jagannath S, Vesole DH, et al. Superiority of tandem autologous transplantation over standard therapy for previously untreated multiple myeloma. Blood 1997; 89: 789–93.

35. Zaidi AA, Vesole DH. Multiple myeloma: an old disease with new hope for the future. CA Cancer J Clin 2001; 51: 273–85.

36. Angtuaco EJ, Fassas AB, Walker R, Sethi R, Barlogie B. Multiple myeloma: clinical review and diagnostic imaging. Radiology 2004; 231: 11–23.

37. D'Sa S, Abildgaard N, Tighe J, Shaw P, Hall-Craggs M. Guidelines for the use of imaging in the management of myeloma. Br J Haematol 2007; 137: 49–63.

38. Moulopoulos LA, Dimopoulos MA, Smith TL, et al. Prognostic significance of magnetic resonance imaging in patients with asymptomatic multiple myeloma. J Clin Oncol 1995; 13: 251–6.

39. Mariette X, Zagdanski AM, Guermazi A, et al. Prognostic value of vertebral lesions detected by magnetic resonance imaging in patients with stage I multiple myeloma. Br J Haematol 1999; 104: 723–9.

40. Kapadia SB. Multiple myeloma: a clinicopathologic study of 62 consecutively autopsied cases. Medicine (Baltimore) 1980; 59: 380–92.

41. Mirels H. Metastatic disease in long bones. A proposed scoring system for diagnosing impending pathologic fractures. Clin Orthop Relat Res 1989; (249): 256–64.

42. Singh J, Fairbairn KJ, Williams C, et al. Expert radiological review of skeletal surveys identifies additional abnormalities in 23% of cases: further evidence for the value of myeloma multi-disciplinary teams in the accurate staging and treatment of myeloma patients. Br J Haematol 2007; 137: 172–3.

43. Smith DB, Scarffe JH, Eddleston B. The prognostic significance of X-ray changes at presentation and reassessment in patients with multiple myeloma. Haematol Oncol 1988; 6: 1–6.

44. Ludwig H, Kupman W, Sinzinger H. Radiography and bone scintigraphy in multiple myeloma: a comparative analysis. Br J Radiol 1982; 55: 173–81.

45. Bataille R, Chevalier J, Rossi M, Sany J. Bone scintigraphy in plasma-cell myeloma. A prospective study of 70 patients. Radiology 1982; 145: 801–4.

46. Catalano L, Pace L, Califano C, et al. Detection of focal myeloma lesions by technetium-99m-sestaMIBI scintigraphy. Haematologica 1999; 84: 119–24.

47. Alexandrakis MG, Kyriakou DS, Passam F, Koukouraki S, Karkavitsas N. Value of Tc-99m sestamibi scintigraphy in the detection of bone lesions in multiple myeloma: comparison with Tc-99m methylene diphosphonate. Ann Haematol 2001; 80: 349–53.

48. Fonti R, Del Vecchio S, Zannetti A, et al. Bone marrow uptake of 99mTc-MIBI in patients with multiple myeloma. Eur J Nucl Med 2001; 28: 214–20.

49. Pace L, Catalano L, Pinto A, et al. Different patterns of technetium-99m sestamibi uptake in multiple myeloma. Eur J Nucl Med 1998; 25: 714–20.

50. Ishibashi M, Nonoshita M, Uchida M. Bone marrow uptake of thallium-201 before and after therapy in multiple myeloma. J Nucl Med 1998; 39: 473–5.

51. Chun KA, Cho IH, Won KC, et al. Comparison of Tc-99m sestamibi and Tl-201 uptake in multple myeloma. Clin Nucl Med 2001; 26: 212–15.

52. Schirrmeister H, Bommer L, Buck AK, et al. Initial results in the assessment of multiple myeloma using 18F-FDG PET. Eur J Nucl Med Mol Imaging 2002; 29: 361–6.

53. Durie BG, Waxman AD, D'Agnolo A, Williams CM. Whole body (18)F-FDG PET identifies high-risk myeloma. J Nucl Med 2002; 43: 1457–63.

54. Bredella MA, Steinbach L, Caputo G, Segall G, Hawkins R. Value of FDG PET in the assessment of patients with multiple myeloma. AJR Am J Roentgenol 2005; 184: 1199–204.

55. Adam Z, Bolcak K, Stanicek J, et al. Fluorodeoxyglucose positron emission tomography in multiple myeloma, solitary plasmocytoma and monoclonal gammapathy of unknown significance. Neoplasma 2007; 54: 536–40.

56. Breyer RJ 3rd, Mulligan ME, Smith SE, Line BR, Badros AZ. Comparison of imaging with FDG PET/CT with other imaging modalities in myeloma. Skeletal Radiol 2006; 35: 632–40.

57. Zamagni E, Nanni C, Patriarca F, et al. A prospective comparison of 18F-fluorodeoxyglucose positron emission tomography-computed tomography, magnetic resonance imaging and whole-body planar radiographs in the assessment of bone disease in newly diagnosed multiple myeloma. Haematologica 2007; 92: 50–5.

58. Fonti R, Salvatore B, Quarantelli M, et al. 18F-FDG PET/CT, 99mTc-MIBI, and MRI in evaluation of patients with multiple myeloma. J Nucl Med 2008; 49: 195–200.

59. Lin C, Luciani A, Itti E, Haioun C, Rahmouni A. Whole body MRI and PET/CT in haematological malignancies. Cancer Imaging 2007; 7 Spec No A: S88–93.

60. Mulligan ME, Badros AZ. PET/CT and MR imaging in myeloma. Skeletal Radiol 2007; 36: 5–16.

61. Mahfouz T, Miceli MH, Saghafifar F, et al. 18F-fluorodeoxyglucose positron emission tomography contributes to the diagnosis and management of infections in patients with multiple myeloma: a study of 165 infectious episodes. J Clin Oncol 2005; 23: 7857–63.

62. Juweid ME, Cheson BD. Positron-emission tomography and assessment of cancer therapy. N Engl J Med 2006; 354: 496–507.

63. Nanni C, Zamagni E, Cavo M, et al. 11C-choline vs. 18F-FDG PET/CT in assessing bone involvement in patients with multiple myeloma. World J Surg Oncol 2007; 5: 68.

64. Dankerl A, Liebisch P, Glatting G, et al. Multiple Myeloma: Molecular Imaging with 11C-Methionine PET/CT—Initial Experience. Radiology 2007; 242: 498–508.

65. Helms CA, Genant HK. Computed tomography in the early detection of skeletal involvement with multiple myeloma. JAMA 1982; 248: 2886–7.

66. Mahnken AH, Wildberger JE, Gehbauer G, et al. Multidetector CT of the spine in multiple myeloma: comparison with MR imaging and radiography. AJR Am J Roentgenol 2002; 178: 1429–36.

67. Horger M, Claussen CD, Bross-Bach U, et al. Whole-body low-dose multidetector row-CT in the diagnosis of multiple myeloma: an alternative to conventional radiography. Eur J Radiol 2005; 54: 289–97.

68. Kröpil P, Fenk R, Fritz LB, et al. Comparison of whole-body 64-slice multidetector computed tomography and conventional radiography in staging of multiple myeloma. Eur J Radiol 2008; 18: 51–8.

69. Horger M, Kanz L, Denecke B, et al. The benefit of using whole-body, low-dose, nonenhanced, multidetector computed tomography for follow-up and therapy response monitoring in patients with multiple myeloma. Cancer 2007; 109: 1617–26.

70. Hur J, Yoon CS, Ryu YH, Yun MJ, Suh JS. Efficacy of multidetector row computed tomography of the spine in patients with multiple myeloma: comparison with magnetic resonance imaging and fluorodeoxyglucose-positron emission tomography. J Comput Assist Tomogr 2007; 31: 342–7.

71. Mulligan ME. Imaging techniques used in the diagnosis, staging, and follow-up of patients with myeloma. Acta Radiol 2005; 46: 716–24.

72. Walker R, Barlogie B, Haessler J, et al. Magnetic resonance imaging in multiple myeloma: diagnostic and clinical implications. J Clin Oncol 2007; 25: 1121–8.

73. Baur-Melnyk A, Buhmann S, Dürr HR, Reiser M. Role of MRI for the diagnosis and prognosis of multiple myeloma. Eur J Radiol 2005; 55: 56–63.

74. Schmidt GP, Schoenberg SO, Reiser MF, Baur-Melnyk A. Whole-body MR imaging of bone marrow. Eur J Radiol 2005; 55: 33–40.

75. Johnston C, Brennan S, Ford S, Eustace S. Whole body MR imaging: applications in oncology. Eur J Surg Oncol 2006; 32: 239–46.

76. Schmidt GP, Reiser MF, Baur-Melnyk A. Whole-body imaging of the musculoskeletal system: the value of MR imaging. Skeletal Radiol 2007; 36: 1109–19.

77. Ghanem N, Lohrmann C, Engelhardt M, et al. Whole-body MRI in the detection of bone marrow infiltration in patients with plasma cell neoplasms in comparison to the radiological skeletal survey. Eur Radiol 2006; 16: 1005–14.

78. Dimopoulos MA, Moulopoulos LA, Datseris I, et al. Imaging of myeloma bone disease—implications for staging, prognosis and follow-up. Acta Oncol 2000; 39: 823–7.

79. Lecouvet FE, Vandeberg BC, Malghem J, Maldague BM. Magnetic resonance and computed tomography imaging in multiple myeloma. Semin Musculoskelet Radiol 2001; 5: 43–55.

80. Baur-Melnyk A, Reiser M. [Staging of multiple myeloma with MRI: comparison to MSCT and conventional radiography]. Radiologe 2004; 44: 874–81.

81. Stäbler A, Baur A, Bartl R, et al. Contrast enhancement and quantitative signal analysis in MR imaging of multiple myeloma: assessment of focal and diffuse growth patterns in marrow correlated with biopsies and survival rates. AJR Am J Roentgenol 1996; 167: 1029–36.

82. Bartl R, Frisch B, Fateh-Moghadam A, et al. Histologic classification and staging of multiple myeloma. A retrospective and prospective study of 674 cases. Am J Clin Pathol 1987; 87: 342–55.

83. Nosàs-Garcia S, Moehler T, Wasser K, et al. Dynamic contrast-enhanced MRI for assessing the disease activity of multiple myeloma: a comparative study with histology and clinical markers. J Magn Reson Imaging 2005; 22: 154–62.

84. Weininger M, Lauterbach B, Knop S, et al. Whole-body MRI of multiple myeloma: Comparison of different MRI sequences in assessment of different growth patterns. Eur J Radiol 2008; 69: 339–45.

85. Lecouvet FE, Vande Berg BC, Michaux L, et al. Stage III multiple myeloma: clinical and prognostic value of spinal bone marrow MR imaging. Radiology 1998; 209: 653–60.

86. Van de Berg BC, Lecouvet FE, Michaux L, et al. Stage I multiple myeloma: value of MR imaging of the bone marrow

in the determination of prognosis. Radiology 1996; 201: 243–6.

87. Lecouvet FE, Malghem J, Michaux L, et al. Vertebral compression fractures in multiple myeloma. Part II. Assessment of fracture risk with MR imaging of spinal bone marrow. Radiology 1997; 204: 201–5.

88. Baur A, Stäbler A, Bruning R, et al. Diffusion-weighted MR imaging of bone marrow: differentiation of benign versus pathologic compression fractures. Radiology 1998; 207: 349–56.

89. Le Bihan DJ. Differentiation of benign versus pathologic compression fractures with diffusion-weighted MR imaging: a closer step toward the "holy grail" of tissue characterization? Radiology 1998; 207: 305–7.

90. Baur A, Huber A, Ertl-Wagner B, et al. Diagnostic value of increased diffusion weighting of a steady-state free precession sequence for differentiating acute benign osteoporotic fractures from pathologic vertebral compression fractures. AJNR Am J Neuroradiol 2001; 22: 366–72.

91. Castillo M. Diffusion-weighted imaging of the spine: is it reliable? AJNR Am J Neuroradiol 2003; 24: 1251–3.

92. Cuénod CA, Laredo JD, Chevret S, et al. Acute vertebral collapse due to osteoporosis or malignancy: appearance on unenhanced and gadolinium-enhanced MR images. Radiology 1996; 199: 541–9.

93. Lecouvet FE, Vande Berg BC, Maldague BE, et al. Vertebral compression fractures in multiple myeloma. Part I. Distribution and appearance at MR imaging. Radiology 1997; 204: 195–9.

94. Moulopoulos LA, Dimopoulos MA, Alexanian R, Leeds NE, Libshitz HI. Multiple myeloma: MR patterns of response to treatment. Radiology 1994; 193: 441–6.

95. Desikan R, Barlogie B, Sethi R, et al. Infection—an under-appreciated cause of bone pain in multiple myeloma. Br J Haematol 2003; 120: 1047–50.

96. Burton CH, Fairham SA, Millet B, DasGupta R, Sivakumaran M. Unusual aetiology of persistent back pain in a patient with multiple myeloma: infectious discitis. J Clin Pathol 1998; 51: 633–4.

97. Tung GA, Rogg JM. Diffusion-weighted imaging of cerebritis. AJNR Am J Neuroradiol 2003; 24: 1110–13.

98. Desikan R, Barlogie B, Sawyer J, et al. Results of high-dose therapy for 1000 patients with multiple myeloma: durable complete remissions and superior survival in the absence of chromosome 13 abnormalities. Blood 2000; 95: 4008–10.

99. Bucher E, Trampuz A, Donati L, Zimmerli W. Spondylodiscitis associated with bacteraemia due to coagulase-negative staphylococci. Eur J Clin Microbiol Infect Dis 2000; 19: 118–20.

100. Chew FS, Kline MJ. Diagnostic yield of CT-guided percutaneous aspiration procedures in suspected spontaneous infectious diskitis. Radiology 2001; 218: 211–14.

101. Williams L, Beveridge RA, Rifkin RM, et al. Increased pulmonary toxicity results from a 1-day versus 2-day schedule of administration of high-dose melphalan. Biol Blood Marrow Transplant 2002; 8: 334–5.

102. Srkalovic G, Elson P, Trebisky B, Karam MA, Hussein MA. Use of melphalan, thalidomide, and dexamethasone in treatment of refractory and relapsed multiple myeloma. Med Oncol 2002; 19: 219–26.

103. Palumbo A, Bringhen S, Bertola A, et al. Multiple myeloma: comparison of two dose-intensive melphalan regimens (100 vs 200 mg/m(2)). Leukemia 2004; 18: 133–8.

104. Carlson K, Hjorth M, Knudsen LM. Toxicity in standard melphalan-prednisone therapy among myeloma patients with renal failure—a retrospective analysis and recommendations for dose adjustment. Br J Haematol 2005; 128: 631–5.

105. Osman K, Comenzo R, Rajkumar SV. Deep venous thrombosis and thalidomide therapy for multiple myeloma. N Engl J Med 2001; 344: 1951–2.

106. Rajkumar SV. Thalidomide: tragic past and promising future. Mayo Clin Proc 2004; 79: 899–903.

107. Onozawa M, Hashino S, Sogabe S, et al. Side effects and good effects from new chemotherapeutic agents. Case 2. Thalidomide-induced interstitial pneumonitis. J Clin Oncol 2005; 23: 2425–6.

108. Kyle RA, Rajkumar SV. Multiple myeloma. N Engl J Med 2004; 351: 1860–73.

109. Moon SJ, Min CK, Lee DG, et al. Pseudomembranous colitis following bortezomib therapy in a myeloma patient. Acta Haematol 2007; 117: 211–14.

110. Lugassy G, Shaham R, Nemets A, Ben-Dor D, Nahlieli O. Severe osteomyelitis of the jaw in long-term survivors of multiple myeloma: a new clinical entity. Am J Med 2004; 117: 440–1.

111. Vannucchi AM, Ficarra G, Antonioli E, Bosi A. Osteonecrosis of the jaw associated with zoledronate therapy in a patient with multiple myeloma. Br J Haematol 2005; 128: 738.

112. Kelleher FC, McKenna M, Collins C, et al. Bisphosphonate induced osteonecrosis of the jaws: unravelling uncertainty in disease causality. Acta Oncol 2007; 46: 702–4.

113. Kelleher FC, McKenna M, Collins CD, Crown JP. A potential anatomic cause of mandibular osteonecrosis in patients receiving bisphosphonate treatment. Mayo Clin Proc 2007; 82: 134; author reply 134–5.

114. Phal PM, Myall RW, Assael LA, Weissman JL. Imaging findings of bisphosphonate-associated osteonecrosis of the jaws. AJNR Am J Neuroradiol 2007; 28: 1139–45.

115. Aydin K, Donmez F, Tuzun U, Minareci O, Atamer T. Diffusion MR findings in cyclosporin-A induced encephalopathy. Neuroradiology 2004; 46: 822–4.

116. Attal M, Harousseau JL. Role of autologous stem-cell transplantation in multiple myeloma. Best Pract Res Clin Haematol 2007; 20: 747–59.

117. Woo E, Yu YL, Ng M, Huang CY, Todd D. Spinal cord compression in multiple myeloma; who gets it? Aus N Z J Med 1986; 16: 671–5.

118. Speiss JL, Adelstein DJ, Hines JD. Multiple myeloma presenting with spinal cord compression. Oncology 1988; 45: 88–92.

119. Loughrey GJ, Collins CD, Todd SM, Brown NM, Johnson RJ. Magnetic resonance imaging in the management of suspected spinal canal disease in patients with known malignancy. Clin Radiol 2000; 55: 849–55.

120. Theodorou SJ, Theodorou DJ, Schweitzer ME, Kakitsubata Y, Resnick D. Magnetic resonance imaging of para-acetabular

insufficiency fractures in patients with malignancy. Clin Radiol 2006; 61: 181–90.

121. Abildgaard N, Brixen K, Eriksen EF, et al. Sequential analysis of biochemical markers of bone resorption and bone densitometry in multiple myeloma. Haematologica 2004; 89: 567–77.

122. Lafforgue P, Dahan E, Chagnaud C, et al. Early-stage avascular necrosis of the femoral head: MR imaging for prognosis in 31 cases with at least 2 years of follow-up. Radiology 1993; 187: 199–204.

123. Kyle RA. Multiple myeloma: review of 869 cases. Mayo Clin Proc 1975; 50: 29–40.

124. Subramanyam BR. Renal amyloidosis in juvenile rheumatoid arthritis: sonographic features. AJR Am J Roentgenol 1981; 136: 411–12.

125. Hawkins PN. Serum amyloid P component scintigraphy for diagnosis and monitoring amyloidosis. Curr Opin Nephrol Hypertens 2002; 11: 649–55.

126. Hachulla E, Maulin L, Deveaux M, et al. Prospective and serial study of primary amyloidosis with serum amyloid P component scintigraphy: from diagnosis to prognosis. Am J Med 1996; 101: 77–87.

127. Lecouvet FE, De Nayer P, Garbar C, et al. Treated plasma cell lesions of bone with MRI signs of response to treatment: unexpected pathological findings. Skeletal Radiol 1998; 27: 692–5.

128. Rahmouni A, Divine M, Mathieu D, et al. MR appearance of multiple myeloma of the spine before and after treatment. AJR Am J Roentgenol 1993; 160: 1053–7.

129. Lecouvet F, Richard F, Vande Berg B, et al. Long-term effects of localised spinal radiation therapy on vertebral fractures and focal lesions appearance in patients with multiple myeloma. Br J Haematol 1997; 96: 743–5.

130. Agren B, Rudberg U, Isberg B, Svensson L, Aspelin P. MR imaging of multiple myeloma patients with bone marrow transplants. Acta Radiol 1998; 39: 36–42.

131. Lecouvet FE, Dechambre S, Malghem J, et al. Bone marrow transplantation in patients with multiple myeloma: prognostic significance of MR imaging. AJR Am J Roentgenol 2001; 176: 91–96.

132. Lecouvet FE, Malghem J, Michaux L, et al. Skeletal survey in advanced multiple myeloma: radiographic versus MR imaging survey. Br J Haematol 1999; 106: 35–39.

133. Fassas AB, Muwalla F, Berryman T, et al. Myeloma of the central nervous system: association with high-risk chromosomal abnormalities, plasmablastic morphology and extramedullary manifestations. Br J Haematol 2002; 117: 103–8.

134. Moulopoulos LA, Dimopoulos MA, Weber D, et al. Magnetic resonance imaging in the staging of solitary plasmacytoma of bone. J Clin Oncol 1993; 11: 1311–15.

135. Hartman RP, Sundaram M, Okuno SH, Sim FH. Effect of granulocyte-stimulating factors on marrow of adult patients with musculoskeletal malignancies: incidence and MRI findings. AJR Am J Roentgenol 2004; 183: 645–53.

136. Sezer O, Niemöller K, Jakob C, et al. Relationship between bone marrow angiogenesis and plasma cell infiltration and serum beta2-microglobulin levels in patients with multiple myeloma. Ann Haematol 2001; 80: 598–601.

137. Alper E, Gurel M, Evrensel T, et al. 99mTc-MIBI scintigraphy in untreated stage III multiple myeloma: comparison with X-ray skeletal survey and bone scintigraphy. Nucl Med Commun 2003; 24: 537–42.

138. Pace L, Catalano L, Del Vecchio S, et al. Predictive value of technetium-99m sestamibi in patients with multiple myeloma and potential role in the follow-up. Eur J Nucl Med 2001; 28: 304–12.

139. Koutsikos J, Grigoraki V, Athanasoulis T, et al. Scintigraphy with technetium-99m methoxyisobutylisonitrile in multiple myeloma patients: correlation with the International Staging System. Hell J Nucl Med 2006; 9: 177–80.

140. Erten N, Saka B, Berberoglu K, et al. Technetium-99m 2-methoxy-isobutyl-isonitrile uptake scintigraphy in detection of the bone marrow infiltration in multiple myeloma: correlation with MRI and other prognostic factors. Ann Hematol 2007; 86: 805–13.

141. Mele A, Offidani M, Visani G, et al. Technetium-99m sestamibi scintigraphy is sensitive and specific for the staging and the follow-up of patients with multiple myeloma: a multicentre study on 397 scans. Br J Haematol 2007; 136: 729–35.

142. Pace L, Del Vecchio S, Salvatore M. Technetium 99m sestamibi in multiple myeloma. Radiology 2005; 234: 312–13; author reply 313.

143. Fallahi B, Saghari M, Fard Esfahani A, et al. The value of 99mTc-MIBI whole body scintigraphy in active and in remission multiple myeloma. Hell J Nucl Med 2005; 8: 165–8.

144. Jadvar H, Conti PS. Diagnostic utility of FDG PET in multiple myeloma. Skeletal Radiol 2002; 31: 690–4.

145. Orchard K, Barrington S, Buscombe J, et al. Fluorodeoxyglucose positron emission tomography imaging for the detection of occult disease in multiple myeloma. Br J Haematol 2002; 117: 133–5.

146. Kazama T, Swanston N, Podoloff DA, Macapinlac HA. Effect of colony-stimulating factor and conventional- or high-dose chemotherapy on FDG uptake in bone marrow. Eur J Nucl Med Mol Imaging 2005; 32: 1406–11.

147. Wiesenthal AA, Nguyen BD. F-18 FDG PET/CT staging of multiple myeloma with diffuse osseous and extramedullary lesions. Clin Nucl Med 2007; 32: 797–801.

148. Okacha N, Chrif E, Brahim E, et al. Extraosseous epidural multiple myeloma presenting with thoracic spine compression. Joint Bone Spine 2008; 75: 70–72.

149. Patlas M, Hadas-Halpern I, Libson E. Imaging findings of extraosseous multiple myeloma. Cancer Imaging 2002; 2: 120–2.

150. Grover SB, Dhar A. Imaging spectrum in sclerotic myelomas: an experience of three cases. Eur Radiol 2000; 10: 1828–31.

35 Leukemia
Dow-Mu Koh and Janet E Husband

INTRODUCTION

Leukemias are a group of diverse neoplasms which are derived from the arrested or aberrant development of a clone of normal hemopoietic cells. These immature cells proliferate progressively within the bone marrow replacing normal hemopoietic tissue and circulate within the peripheral blood becoming deposited in various organs and tissues, such as the spleen and lymph nodes. Leukemic cells are incapable of normal function and many of the clinical features and complications arising from this condition are a direct result of the failure of normal hemopoietic activity.

There are four major groups of leukemia, categorized according to the predominant type of proliferating cell:

- Acute myelogenous leukemia (AML)
- Acute lymphoblastic leukemia (ALL)
- Chronic myelocytic leukemia (CML)
- Chronic lymphocytic leukemia (CLL)

A complete classification of the leukemias has become increasingly complex as new methods of discriminating different subtypes, such as immunophenotyping and cytogenetic studies, have been developed. Thus the subclassification and characterization of the leukemias continues to evolve (1,2). Two major classification systems are in use: the French-American-British (FAB) classification system and the World Health Organization (WHO) classification system. The classification shown in Table 35.1 is illustrative of the wide-ranging heterogeneity of these diseases, but a detailed review of the two classification systems is beyond the scope of this chapter.

While the radiologist working in oncological practice does not need to have a full understanding of the different subtypes of leukemia, some knowledge of the subtypes is useful as they manifest different radiological appearances.

There is some overlap between leukemias and lymphomas. However, in general, ALL is distinguished from lymphomas on the basis of cellular maturity and by the fact that at least initially lymphomas mainly involve extramedullary sites. The lymphoblastic lymphomas and Burkitt's lymphoma have features of both leukemia and lymphoma. Adult T-cell leukemia/lymphoma (ATLL) is a distinct variety of leukemia/lymphoma that is characterized by lymphadenopathy and hepatosplenomegaly and is endemic in certain parts of the world including Japan and the Caribbean basin.

Myelodysplasia is a syndrome characterized by pancytopenia or chronic anemia which results from dysfunction of the bone marrow. Transformation into acute leukemia may develop during the course of disease.

Cross-sectional imaging, as well as conventional radiology, has an important place in the management of leukemia. However, it is impossible to define strict algorithms for the use of imaging because the disease is manifested in many different organs and organ systems and the complications of leukemia are common and diverse. As in other malignant tumors, close liaison between clinician and radiologist is essential to determine the most appropriate use of imaging for individual patient care.

INCIDENCE AND ETIOLOGY

Acute leukemias account for less than 3% of all cancers in the United States but are a leading cause of cancer death in patients under the age of 35 years. The estimated number of new cases of leukemia in the United States in 2008 was 44,270. Chronic leukemias accounted for 7% more cases than acute leukemias. The total number of deaths was estimated at approximately 21,700 (3). Interestingly, mortality from CML has decreased due to improved treatment outcome using the multi-kinase inhibitor Imatinib.

Subtype	New cases (3)	Deaths (3)
Acute myeloid leukemia	13,290	8,820
Chronic lymphatic leukemia	15,110	4,390
Chronic myeloid leukemia	4,830	450
Acute lymphocytic leukemia	5,430	1,460
Other leukemias	5,610	6,590

The most common type of leukemia in children under 19 years of age is ALL. Acute myelogenous leukemia is more common than ALL in adults. In adults, the most common subtypes of leukemia are AML and CLL.

In the United Kingdom, the incidence of leukemia in relation to other cancers and the distribution of subtypes is similar to that in the United States. There are about 7300 new cases diagnosed annually and in 2006 there were 4292 deaths in the United Kingdom (4). Leukemia incidence rates in Great Britain increased slowly until the end of the 1990s. However, the last few years have started to see a fall in the incidence rates. The current overall lifetime risk of developing leukemia is 1.0% in males and 0.8% in females.

More recently, enormous strides have been made in understanding the molecular biology and cytogenetics of leukemia. Various chromosomal abnormalities have been identified which have helped to define the subsets of AML and ALL listed in the classification (e.g., Philadelphia chromosome-positive). These subsets of leukemia have various clinical features and different patterns of response to therapy. This information is used to direct patients to particular therapeutic regimens and, in the longer-term, may allow appropriate targeting of new therapies.

While the importance of genetic changes in the development of the leukemias is well-established, the underlying causes initiating these changes are largely unknown. Down's syndrome and certain other genetic syndromes are linked to leukemia. Excessive exposure to ionizing radiation (5), chronic exposure to low-dose radiation in the environment, chemicals, and smoking (6) have now been established as important causes. It is worth pointing out that many people with risk factors do not develop the disease, and many patients diagnosed with leukemia do not have any apparent risk factors.

Table 35.1 Classification of Leukemia

Acute
Acute myelogenous leukemia (AML)
  Acute myeloblastic leukemia
  Acute promyelocytic leukemia
  Acute myelomonocytic leukemia
  Acute monoblastic leukemia
  Acute erythroleukemia
  Acute megakaryoblastic leukemia
Acute lymphoblastic leukemia (ALL)
  Pre-B-cell acute lymphoblastic leukemia
    Common acute lymphoblastic leukemia
    Cytoplasmic immunoglobulin (+) ALL
    Philadelphia chromosome (+) ALL
  T-cell
  B-cell
Acute unclassifiable leukemia (AUL)
Chronic
Chronic myelocytic leukemia (CML)
  Chronic phase of CML
  Metamorphosis of CML
    Accelerated ± myelofibrosis
    Lymphoblastic transformation
    Myeloblastic transformation
    Megakaryoblastic transformation
Juvenile chronic granulocytic leukemia
Chronic eosinophilic leukemia
Chronic lymphocytic leukemia (CLL)
  B-cell
  T-cell
Hairy cell leukemia
Polymorphocytic leukemia
Plasma cell leukemia
Sézary syndrome[a]
Adult T-cell leukemia/lymphoma

[a]Leukemic phase of mycosis fungoides.

Secondary AML may develop after treatment of childhood acute leukemia and following therapy for other cancers such as tumors of the breast and ovary, and Hodgkin's disease (7–10).

A human retrovirus (HTLV-1) has been identified as a cause of human T-cell leukemia/lymphoma (ATLL) (11,12). The cumulative risk of an infected individual developing ATLL is estimated to be between 0.5% and 5% (13,14).

Key Points: General Features

- Leukemias are derived from the arrested or aberrant development of a clone of normal hemopoietic cells
- Various subtypes are recognized which have different clinical features, and radiological features, prognosis, and therapeutic implications
- ALL is the most common subtype in childhood
- AML and CLL are the most common subtypes in adults
- Various chromosomal abnormalities have been identified in the leukemias
- Acute leukemias account for about 3% and chronic leukemias for about 7% of all cancers in the United States
- Down's syndrome is strongly linked with acute leukemia
- Ionizing radiation, chemicals, and smoking cause leukemia
- The human retrovirus (HTLV-1) infection causes human T-cell leukemia/lymphoma

CLINICAL FEATURES

The replacement of normal hemopoietic cells within the bone marrow by an excessive number of abnormal functionless cells is responsible for the major clinical features of leukemias:

- Anemia
- Infection
- Hemorrhage

In acute leukemia, patients usually present with a one month to three months history of weight loss, fatigue, bruising, or signs of infection such as fever. In chronic leukemias, the onset of disease is more insidious but fever may be observed without an obvious infective cause. Occasionally, the diagnosis of chronic leukemia is made on routine examination of the peripheral blood in an otherwise asymptomatic patient.

In all patients, the diagnosis is confirmed by examination of the peripheral blood and bone marrow biopsy. Immunophenotyping and cytogenetic studies are performed to discriminate between the different subsets of the disease. A majority of patients have anemia and thrombocytopenia. The peripheral white cell blood count may be normal, raised, or reduced but blast cells are seen in the peripheral blood of almost all the patients.

Certain clinical features of leukemia are more prevalent in one subtype than another, and the frequency of involvement of different organs and sites also varies (Table 35.2) (15).

In acute leukemias, central nervous system (CNS) involvement is more common in ALL than AML but is also seen in chronic leukemias. The CNS is resistant to chemotherapy and is therefore termed a "sanctuary site" of disease.

Hepatosplenomegaly due to leukemia infiltration is seen in almost all cases but the degree of enlargement is greater in chronic than in acute leukemias (Fig. 35.1).

Lymphadenopathy is most frequently seen in CLL and in juvenile CML (Figs. 35.2 and 35.3). It is rare in adult Philadelphia chromosome-positive CML. The incidence of enlarged lymph nodes at presentation in the acute leukemias is as follows:

- Acute lymphoblastic leukemias (50%) (usually T-cell or B-cell)
- Acute monoblastic leukemias (15–20%)
- Other subtypes of acute myelogenous leukemia (8%) (16)

Fever is a common feature of all the leukemias whether due to infection or not. In those without documented infection, fever may be caused by increased metabolism due to the leukemic process.

Anemia is present in the majority of patients and is caused by inadequate erythrocyte production, bleeding, hypersplenism, or hemolysis.

Bleeding is more common in the acute leukemias than in the chronic subtypes and usually takes the form of small petechial hemorrhages. Occasionally, a patient may present with a catastrophic intracranial hemorrhage.

In the acute leukemias hemorrhage is a major cause of death and morbidity. Hemorrhage results from coagulation defects associated with the disease, thrombocytopenia, and the effects of chemotherapy. The acute promyelocytic form of leukemia is particularly prone to hemorrhage and, in one study, intracranial hemorrhage was the cause of death in 60% of patients (17). Another group of patients at

particularly high risk of intracranial hemorrhage are those with acute leukemia in "blast" crisis. In such patients the excessive numbers of leucocytes form tiny foci which plug small arterioles and destroy the vascular walls, leading to hemorrhage (18).

Table 35.2 Organ Involvement by Leukemia Cell Type (1958–1982) (15)

Organ/sites	AML (%)	CML (%)	ALL (%)	CLL[a] (%)
CNS (sanctuary sites)				
Brain	9	11	14	7
Dura mater	14	14	26	21
Leptomeninges	12	10	34	8
Lymphoreticular sites				
Liver	41	55	63	83
Lymph nodes	45	59	55	76
Spleen	58	68	70	76
Cardiopulmonary				
Pericardium	8	6	11	14
Heart	15	11	21	22
Pleura	8	5	11	16
Lungs	28	29	41	41
Gastro-intestinal				
Esophagus	17	9	16	19
Stomach	11	11	17	11
Large bowel	15	9	20	15
Pancreas	8	6	18	12
Endocrine				
Pituitary	9	10	15	20
Thyroid	6	3	5	7
Adrenals	15	22	21	33
Genito-urinary				
Kidneys	33	38	53	63
Bladder	7	6	9	8
Prostate	9	5	12	22
Uterus	11	4	25	14
Gonads (sanctuary sites)				
Testes	20	16	40	15
Ovaries	11	9	21	22
Total number of cases	585	204	308	109

[a]Percentage of all cases examined.

Patients with intracranial hemorrhage present acutely with headaches, seizures, and deterioration of neurological functions. Rarely, intracranial hemorrhage may lead to the diagnosis of acute leukemia.

Bone pain is a common presenting feature in children with ALL, occurring in 25% to 30% of cases, whereas in adults it is only seen in approximately 5% of patients (19,20). Bone pain is characteristically migratory and periarticular (21). It is probably due to lifting of the periosteum by infiltration of leukemic cells or to the development of bone infarction (22). Monoarthralgia or polyarthralgia is not an uncommon presenting feature.

Abdominal and chest pain are also relatively common and are related to a variety of problems. For example, abdominal pain may result from stretching of the splenic capsule due to its rapid enlargement or from intestinal obstruction due to leukemic infiltration of the bowel wall. Chest pain may be caused by a large mediastinal mass compressing adjacent structures.

Granulocytic sarcoma (chloroma) is a mass composed of leukemic cells. These tumors are usually seen in patients with AML but may also occur in CML and other myeloprolific disorders such as polycythemia rubra vera (23). They consist of myeloblasts, promyelocytes, and myelocytes and are most frequently found in the orbits, subcutaneous tissues, paranasal sinuses, lymph nodes, and bones but many other sites have also been described (24). In a series of 728 patients with childhood myelogenous leukemia, Pui et al. found an incidence of 4.7% of granulocytic sarcoma developing at some point during the course of disease. Others have reported an incidence ranging from 2.5% to 8% (25,26). Rarely, these tumors may be the presenting feature of leukemia occurring before the onset of clinically overt disease (27). They were first described by Burns in 1811 (28) but it was not until 1853 that the term chloroma was coined by King to describe their typical greenish color (29). However, in 1966, the term chloroma was replaced by granulocytic sarcoma because fewer than half of them actually display the characteristic greenish color.

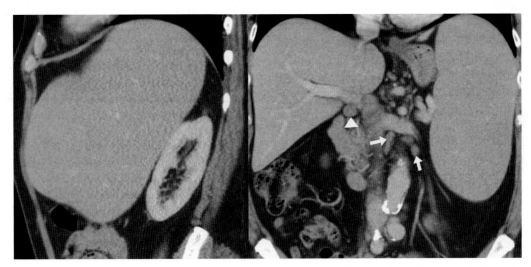

Figure 35.1 A 54-year-old man with acute lymphoblastic leukemia. Coronal and sagittal CT reformats allow the volume of the enlarged spleen to be calculated. Note also the enlarged portal lymph node (arrowhead) and retroperitoneal lymph nodes (arrows).

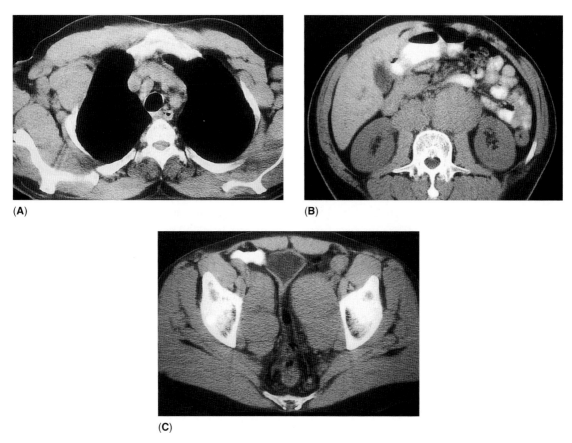

Figure 35.2 A male patient with CLL showing multiple enlarged lymph nodes on CT. (**A**) in the mediastinum and axillae, (**B**) in the retroperitoneum, and (**C**) in the pelvis.

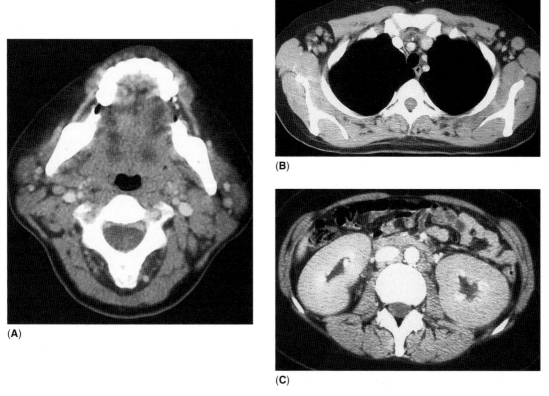

Figure 35.3 In this 24-year-old patient with ALL, there is nodal enlargement seen (**A**) along the deep cervical chain of lymph nodes in the neck, (**B**) both axillae, and (**C**) within the retroperitoneum. Note also the diffusely enlarged kidneys due to leukemic infiltration.

STAGING AND TREATMENT

At diagnosis, the leukemias are usually widely disseminated. Consequently, conventional staging using tumor size measurement, nodal dissemination, and metastatic involvement (TNM classification) is inappropriate. Laboratory tests rather than imaging are used to determine the type of leukemia, which in turn influences the choice of treatment. However, in clinical practice, the leukemias are still often classified or staged, because this provides important prognostic information as well as giving an indication of the likelihood of response to treatment.

Treatment of acute leukemia aims to induce a remission as quickly as possible and then to maintain remission. The success of therapy depends as much on the treatment of non-leukemic-related problems as on the eradication of leukemia itself.

In the acute leukemias, certain features are important prognostic factors and determine the detailed approach to management. These include patient age (older patients are less likely to achieve complete remission) or previous myelodysplasia. Certain cytogenetic subtypes have a poorer prognosis. For example, in adult patients with ALL, the Philadelphia chromosome (a translocation between chromosomes 9 and 22) can be detected in 20% to 25% of cases, which is a poor prognostic indicator.

Acute lymphoblastic leukemia (common ALL) is the most successfully treated of all the leukemias (30–33). Complete remission can be achieved in over 90% of children and in up to 80% of adults (30).

IMAGING IN LEUKEMIA

Leukemia is diagnosed and monitored by hematological studies of the peripheral blood and bone marrow and imaging therefore plays a lesser role in the diagnosis and staging of this disease than in the lymphomas. However, the importance of radiology in the management of leukemia has increased over the last two decades, mainly due to the advent of cross-sectional imaging and also to improvements in therapy. Imaging is used to evaluate the leukemic process itself or to investigate its complications. Thus the imaging findings in leukemia can be broadly categorized into two groups, those related to:

- Direct involvement of organs and tissues by leukemic cells
- Indirect involvement of organs and tissues due to complications

In this text, direct and indirect imaging findings will be discussed in relation to different anatomical sites and organ systems.

Central Nervous System
Direct Involvement by Leukemia

Central nervous system (CNS) involvement is usually seen in acute leukemia. It may be a manifestation of disease at diagnosis or may herald relapse in patients believed to be in remission. At diagnosis, less than 10% of adults with ALL have CNS involvement and it does not appear to be an independent prognostic indicator (34). The number of patients who relapse with CNS involvement has been dramatically reduced by the introduction of CNS prophylactic therapy (35).

Leukemic spread to the CNS is presumed to be by direct infiltration from involved bone marrow of the cranium (or vertebrae) or by the hematogenous route whereby circulating leukemia cells enter the CNS by migration through spaces in the venous endothelium (36,37).

The leukemic process may involve the leptomeninges, dura, or both, and may be diffuse or focal. Meningeal involvement occurs in up to 10% of patients with acute leukemia and begins in the superficial arachnoid membrane; leukemic cells then invade the cerebrospinal fluid (CSF) space and pia mater (38,39). Extradural (parameningeal) masses (granulocytic sarcoma) may also be observed in intracranial or intraspinal sites. Involvement of the brain parenchyma is rare but when it does occur, it probably results from perivascular extension of the disease across the Virchow–Robin spaces through the pia–glial membrane (40). Intracerebral and meningeal granulocytic sarcomas are a rare occurrence in myelogenous leukemias.

Meningeal and Dural Disease

Symptoms of meningeal involvement of the brain include headache, nausea, vomiting, and lethargy. Signs of intracranial pressure and cranial nerve palsies may be apparent on clinical examination (35). Meningeal involvement is diagnosed based on the finding of leukemic cells within CSF. However, analysis of the CSF is often negative and several repeat lumbar punctures may be required to establish the diagnosis of meningeal disease.

Imaging is complementary to lumbar puncture but the detection of diffuse meningeal involvement with computed tomography (CT) has been disappointing due to insufficient contrast enhancement of the abnormal meninges (41). CT is more accurate in carcinomatous meningitis and inflammatory conditions because the contrast enhancement is usually more intense (40).

Magnetic resonance (MR) imaging is the method of choice for the detection of intracranial and spinal leptomeningeal disease and occasionally may demonstrate leukemic infiltration in the presence of multiple negative cytological analyses (35). The technique is considerably more sensitive than CT, myelography or CT myelography, and so has replaced these techniques in the investigation of CNS leukemia (42,43). Although T2-weighted spin-echo sequences may reveal abnormal signal intensity within the CSF space, meningeal disease is best demonstrated on gadolinium-enhanced T1-weighted images. Axial and coronal images of the head and sagittal images of the spine provide the best imaging planes to survey all the meningeal surfaces. Leukemic infiltration is seen as abnormal nodular thickening of the meninges which enhances after injection

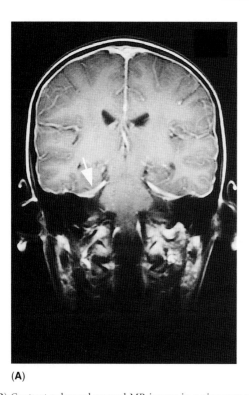

(A)

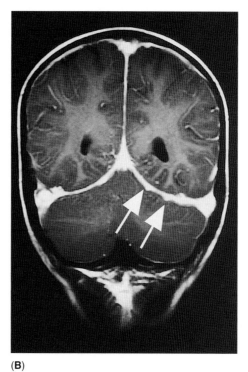

(B)

Figure 35.4 (A) and (B) Contrast-enhanced coronal MR images in a nine-year-old boy with AML. There is extensive contrast-enhanced nodual thickening of the leptomeninges (arrows), representing leukemic infiltration.

of intravenous (IV) contrast medium (Fig. 35.4). Thickening and enhancement of nerve roots, particularly in the region of the cauda equina, is shown on MR imaging but may also be demonstrated on CT myelography. Diffuse dural infiltration is less common than leptomeningeal disease, but is also seen as thickening and enhancement of the dural surfaces. In patients with leukemia, the observation of thickened enhancing meninges is not pathognomonic of leukemic infiltration as it may also be seen in other conditions associated with leukemia such as infectious meningitis, drug reactions, and meningeal fibrosis following hemorrhage (35).

Parameningeal Disease
Intracranial and spinal parameningeal disease usually takes the form of a mass of leukemic cells known as granulocytic sarcoma (chloroma).

The majority of intracranial granulocytic sarcomas are durally-based lesions and are believed to develop by direct spread from the bone marrow. The CT and MR imaging appearances of granulocytic sarcomas are variable and they may mimic meningiomas, other tumors, or abscesses (44,45). For example, Moudden et al. describe a case of granulocytic sarcoma in ALL mimicking a falx meningioma (46,47).

On unenhanced CT, intracranial granulocytic sarcomas are isodense or slightly hyperdense compared to a normal brain but frequently show intense enhancement following injection of IV contrast medium (Fig. 35.5) (47,48). On MR imaging, these lesions may be of high signal intensity on T1-weighted images and bright on T2-weighting. As with CT, they show intense contrast enhancement (44).

Spinal granulocytic sarcomas may be paraspinal or intraspinal (Fig. 35.6). Soft tissue masses in the paravertebral region extend into the spinal canal via the intervertebral foraminae (Fig. 35.7) (49). These masses invade the dura and may cause spinal cord compression, nerve root compression, and bone destruction.

Although CT may show paravertebral masses and extension into the spinal canal or discrete intraspinal masses (Fig. 35.7A), MR imaging is the preferred technique for demonstrating these lesions because the whole spine can be examined at a single investigation (Fig. 35.7B). The multiplanar capability of MR imaging is also an advantage as it allows clear delineation of tumor extent. Granulocytic sarcomas have a low signal intensity on T1-weighted images and a relatively high or intermediate signal intensity on T2-weighted images (49). They often show intense contrast enhancement.

Key Points: Central Nervous System

- CNS involvement is usually a manifestation of acute leukemia
- Approximately 3% of all children with ALL have CNS disease
- The leukemic process may involve the leptomeninges, dura, or extradural space
- Disease may be diffuse or focal
- Granulocytic sarcomas are usually durally-based lesions
- MR is the best imaging method for detecting intracranial meningeal and dural infiltration as well as granulocytic sarcoma

Indirect Effects of Leukemia
The indirect effects of leukemia on the CNS include vascular events, infection, and toxic effects related to therapy.

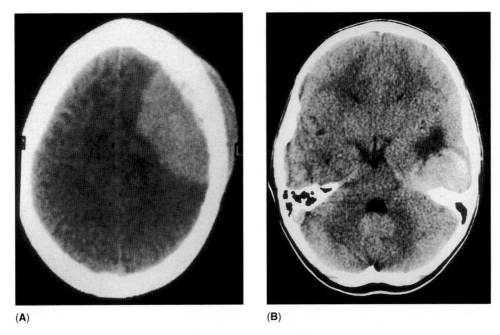

(A)   **(B)**

Figure 35.5 Intracranial granulocytic sarcoma. (**A**) CT of the brain in a 14-year-old boy with relapsed ALL. The mass which probably arises from the left parietal bone extends both intracranially and into the subcutaneous soft tissues. There is homogeneous intense contrast enhancement. (**B**) CT of an eight-year-old girl who relapsed following initial therapy for ALL with a large durally-based lesion in the temporal lobe. Note homogeneous enhancement and surrounding edema.

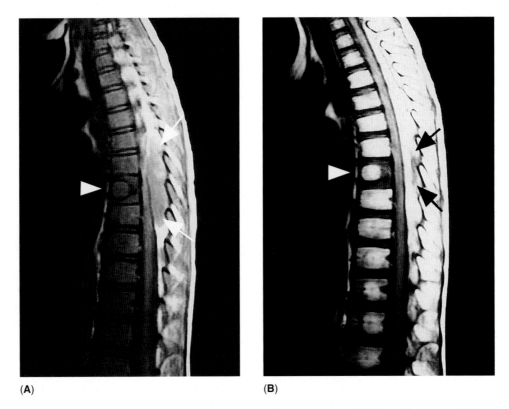

(A)   **(B)**

Figure 35.6 A nine-year-old boy who presented with acute back pain and signs of spinal cord compression. (**A**) T1-weighted sagittal MR image showing an intraspinal extradural soft tissue mass in the mid-thoracic region (arrows). Note partial collapse of the vertebral body of T5 (arrowhead). A diagnosis of AML with a granulocytic sarcoma was made on investigation. There is diffuse abnormally low signal intensity throughout the vertebral bodies indicating diffuse leukemic infiltration. (**B**) Repeat T1-weighted MR scan six weeks later shows an excellent response to treatment. The granulocytic sarcomatous mass has almost completely resolved (arrows) and the signal intensity of the bone marrow has increased markedly indicating reduction in bone marrow infiltration. The vertebral body of T5 still shows abnormal signal intensity posteriorly.

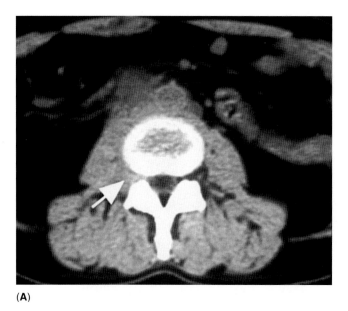

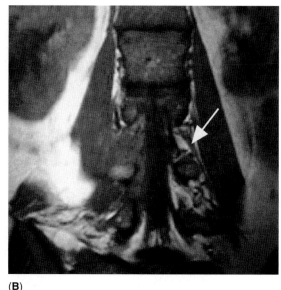

(A)   **(B)**

Figure 35.7 An adult male patient who presented with back pain due to a granulocytic sarcoma before clinical manifestation of AML. (A) CT, and (B) T1-weighted coronal MR image. In (A) a soft tissue mass is seen surrounding the inferior vena cava and obscuring the contour of the aorta. The mass extends posteriorly deep to the right psoas muscle and enters the spinal canal through the intervertebral foramen (arrow). In (B) the coronal MR image shows the cranio-caudal extent of the mass and clearly delineates the intraspinal component at the level of L3/L4 and L4/L5 intervertebral foraminae. Tumor surrounds the exit nerve roots. Note normal nerve roots on the left side (arrow).

Vascular Complications

Hemorrhage. CT or MR imaging is essential in patients suspected of intracranial hemorrhage. In most cases, CT will be undertaken, as this is more readily available and generally quicker than MR examinations. Unenhanced CT will show the classic features of subarachnoid and/or intracerebral hemorrhage, which includes the presence of high-density material in the subarachnoid space, in the brain parenchyma and ventricular system. There may be mass effect with some surrounding edema. On MR imaging, fresh blood has high signal intensity on T1 and T2 weighting. Breakdown products of hemoglobin (hemosiderin) may also be present giving low signal intensity on T2 weighting.

CT and MR imaging are not only valuable for demonstrating the presence of intracranial hemorrhage but also for excluding hemorrhage in patients in whom the diagnosis is questionable on clinical grounds. Furthermore, imaging may show other associated abnormalities such as sinovenous thrombosis.

Sinovenous Thrombosis. Sinovenous thrombosis, another vascular complication of acute leukemia, may be related to treatment with L-asparaginase as well as to leukemic infiltration (41,49). Both CT and MR imaging are useful non-invasive methods of detecting sinovenous thrombosis. On CT, postcontrast-enhanced images may show a low density filling defect within the sinus and, on precontrast images, the sinus may be abnormally hyperdense. On MR imaging, loss of the normal signal void is apparent on T2-weighted sequences and, on postcontrast images, a filling defect may be observed, as on CT. Gradient-echo or other flow sensitive techniques such as fast fluid-attenuated inversion recovery (FLAIR) may also demonstrate sinovenous thrombosis on MR imaging (41,50). Leukemic infiltration of meninges and sinus thrombosis may coexist.

Cerebral Infarction. Patients with leukemia are at an increased risk of cerebral infarction for several reasons, which include: (41)

- General risks—patient age, atherosclerosis
- Intravascular coagulation
- Sinovenous occlusion
- Tumor emboli
- Septic emboli
- Effects of therapy (17)

As in the diagnosis of intracranial hemorrhage, CT and MR imaging are valuable for demonstrating the presence of cerebral infarction and for distinguishing infarcts from other intracranial lesions such as hemorrhage, infection, and drug-related toxicity.

Infection

In leukemic patients, intracranial infection results from direct spread of infection from the paranasal sinuses or by the hematogenous route. Sinusitis is usually aggressive in immunocompromised patients and infection with organisms such as Aspergillus results in invasion of local structures and destruction of bone (Fig. 35.8), thereby giving access to the dura, meninges, and underlying brain parenchyma. Other organisms including bacteria (e.g., Klebsiella pneumonii) and viruses are also associated with intracranial infection in leukemia (51). Abscesses may develop and, whether solitary or multiple, may simulate parenchymal leukemic deposits (51). On CT, abscesses usually show rim enhancement with a relatively low-density center; on MR imaging these masses have a high signal intensity on T2 weighting and a relatively low signal intensity on T1 weighting. As on CT rim enhancement is noted following injection of IV contrast medium.

Treatment-Related Complications

There are many neurological complications associated with the treatment of leukemia but such complications are related particularly to the treatment or prophylaxis of the CNS. Different syndromes and

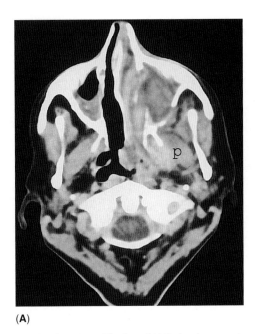
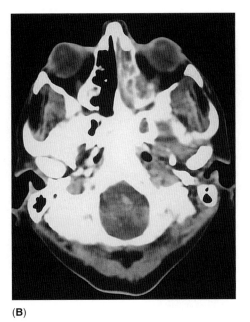

(A)   **(B)**

Figure 35.8 CT in a 53-year-old male patient with relapsed AML showing extensive paranasal sinus infection with Aspergillus. (A) The soft tissue mass occupies the left maxillary sinus. There is almost complete destruction of the medial wall of the maxillary sinus with extension of the soft tissue mass into the nasal cavity and nasopharynx. There is also destruction of the lateral wall of the maxillary sinus with extension of disease into the pterygoid region. Note enlargement and poor definition of the lsteral pterygoid muscle (p). (B) The soft tissue mass is also seen extending into the posterior aspect of the left orbit. The left ethmoid sinuses are replaced by soft tissue and there is destruction of the medial wall of the orbit.

clinical features are associated with particular drugs or radiotherapy. In general, CNS toxicity can be divided into acute, subacute, and chronic forms (52).

Acute or subacute neurological complications are more likely to be reversible than the complications which develop in the longer term. Patients present with symptoms and signs of raised intracranial pressure and on examination neurological deficit is common (53). After bone marrow transplantation for CML, MR imaging may show acute ventricular enlargement and cortical atrophy which progress over time (54). On clinical evaluation, it may be impossible to distinguish CNS leukemic relapse from the effects of therapy and, in this situation, imaging plays a key role. Delayed or chronic toxic effects are more likely to be irreversible and may develop several years after initial treatment.

Radiotherapy neurotoxicity is usually subacute, developing several weeks after treatment. It is characterized by drowsiness, nausea, and malaise, as well as somnolence (35). Imaging is not usually required to reach a definitive diagnosis.

The delayed effects of radiotherapy include cerebral atrophy and necrosis (52). This results in growth disturbance, intellectual impairment, neuroendocrine problems, and even second cancers (52). MR shows abnormally high signal intensity in the white matter following cranial irradiation and may demonstrate abnormalities even in patients without clinical evidence of toxicity. CT may reveal areas of low attenuation within the white matter and calcifications. Long-term survivors of childhood ALL treated with cranial irradiation and intrathecal methotrexate frequently show abnormalities on MR imaging. This is more common in patients treated with both modalities than with intrathecal methotrexate alone (55,56). A study reported by Laitt and colleagues (57) revealed an incidence of significant abnormalities in the brain on MR imaging in 26% of 35 long-term survivors. These abnormalities included three tumors (meningioma,

rhabdomyosarcoma, and anaplastic astrocytoma) as well as large vessel vasculopathy, small cystic infarcts and diffuse white matter change. Recently, long-term cerebral metabolic changes have been demonstrated with proton MR spectroscopy (MRS) in patients treated with intrathecal methotrexate and cranial irradiation prophylaxis for ALL. These abnormalities were found in brains with hemosiderin and were reflected by decreasing N-acetylaspartate (NAA)/creatine (Cr) and choline (Cho)/creatine (Cr) from diagnosis (58).

Intrathecal methotrexate may cause acute arachnoiditis and imaging is not required in the diagnostic work-up. Subacute neurotoxicity and delayed reactions are characterized by seizures and other manifestations of motor dysfunction such as paraplegia. Imaging may be required to exclude direct involvement of the CNS by leukemia, for example the presence of a granulocytic sarcoma. Delayed effects of methotrexate include white matter ischemia and imaging shows intracerebral calcifications and cerebral atrophy. Both CT and MR imaging are useful for demonstrating the extent of these abnormalities.

Disseminated necrotising leucoencephalopathy is more likely to develop when CNS irradiation is combined with intrathecal methotrexate and high-dose methotrexate but may occur without cranial irradiation (Fig. 35.9) (35,53,59–61). This condition may be fulminating and rapidly fatal, or less severe leading to chronic neurological deficit. Leucoencephalopathy affects the white matter of the brain and is seen on CT as multifocal areas of low attenuation and on MR imaging as areas of high signal intensity on spin-echo T2-weighted images. Enhancement of these lesions can sometimes be seen on CT and MR imaging (61–64). Calcification may also be observed in the basal ganglia and in the subcortical white matter (61). It may be difficult to distinguish leucoencephalopathy from underlying disease. However, on MR imaging, a new focus in the periventricular white matter, especially the corpus callosum may be considered suspicious

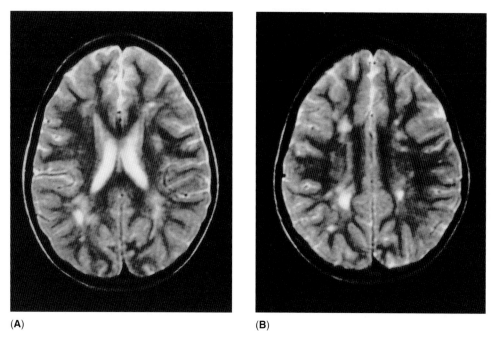

Figure 35.9 Necrotizing leucoencaphalopathy. (A) and (B) T2-weighted axial MR images of the brain showing abnormal high signal intensity in the white matter following cranial irradiation and methotrexate therapy.

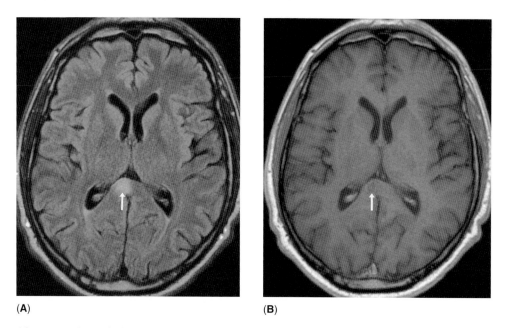

Figure 35.10 (A) FLAIR axial MR image shows a high signal intensity focus within the posterior corpus callosum (arrow). (B) T1-weighted MR image acquired at the same level shows no appreciable enhancement (arrow) following intravenous gadolinium contrast administration. The appearance is in keeping with leucoencephalopathy.

of leucoencephalopathy because the periventricular white matter is highly susceptible to radiation necrosis (Fig. 35.10). Radiation necrosis is also more likely to have a nodular or swiss-cheese appearance.

Other drugs such as cytarabine and cyclosporin A are also associated with severe neurotoxicity (34). Vera et al. (65) investigated SPECT in the diagnosis of CNS toxicity following therapy with a cytarabine-containing regimen and found that diffuse heterogeneous low perfusion levels may be the only abnormal feature on imaging.

Neuropsychological disorders developing as a result of treatment of childhood leukemia are well-recognized (66). Earlier imaging studies, such as that reported by Harila-Saari et al. (67) showed no significant correlation between neuropsychological outcome and morphological MR imaging findings of white matter change, atrophy, old hemorrhage, and calcifications. However, a subsequent investigation of the long-term cognitive effects of intrathecal methotrexate and cranial irradiation in a group of 21 children cured of ALL showed that poor performance was associated with white matter changes in 50% of cases (68). Furthermore, there was good correlation between the presence of calcifications and the number of methotrexate injections. There is now some evidence to suggest that diffusion-tensor imaging (DTI), an MR imaging technique used to study the diffusivity and orientation of the white matter tracts in the brain, can demonstrate potential relationships between changes observed at DTI and neurocognitive performance (69). Microscopic damage in

the normal-appearing white matter, in children treated with cranial irradiation for pediatric tumors, was reflected as lower diffusion fractional anisotrophy (FA), which were in turn correlated with poorer IQ scores compared to the age-matched controls (69,70). Thus, DTI appears to have the potential to quantify the degree of treatment related damage to the normal brain non-invasively.

Key Points: CNS Complications

- Hemorrhage is a major cause of death in acute leukemia, particularly in acute promyelocytic leukemia and patients in "blast" crisis
- Sinovenous thrombosis may be demonstrated by MR imaging and CT, but may co-exist with leukemic meningeal infiltration
- Cerebral infarction has an increased incidence in patients with leukemia
- Intracranial infection usually results from spread of infection from paranasal sinuses directly by organisms such as Aspergillus
- CNS toxicity is related to irradiation, intrathecal methotrexate, and high-dose methotrexate
- Disseminating necrotizing leucoencephalopathy affects the white matter of the brain and is demonstrated on MR imaging as areas of high signal intensity with foci on T2-weighted images, which have a predilection for periventricular white matter and may have a nodular or swiss-cheese appearance. Enhancement of the lesions may be seen
- Long-term cognitive impairment can result from intrathecal methotrexate and cranial irradiation. Changes may be demonstrated on CT and MR imaging

Head and Neck

Direct Involvement by Leukemia

The most important extracranial site of leukemia of the head and neck region is the orbit. Leukemic deposits may infiltrate around the optic nerve, often in association with meningeal disease and the choroid and retina may also be involved by diffuse infiltration. The orbit is a well-recognized site of granulocytic sarcoma (chloroma) (45,71,72). On both CT and MR imaging, intraorbital granulocytic sarcomas enhance with IV contrast medium and are usually seen as soft tissue masses related to the intraocular muscles (Fig. 35.11) (24). Granulocytic sarcoma in the paranasal sinuses may spread by direct extension into the orbit.

Key Point: Granulocytic Sarcoma

- The orbit is a common site of granulocytic sarcoma

Indirect Effects of Leukemia

Two major indirect effects of leukemia in the head and neck are hemorrhage and infection. Infection of the paranasal sinuses may be extremely aggressive, resulting in intracranial disease as described above. Imaging with CT or MR may be required to define the extent of infection extracranially as well as the presence of meningeal or brain involvement (73).

Intrathoracic Disease

The vast majority of pulmonary abnormalities detected in leukemic patients are due to indirect causes related to complications

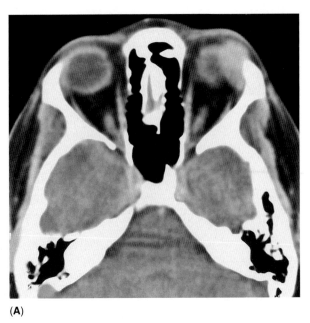

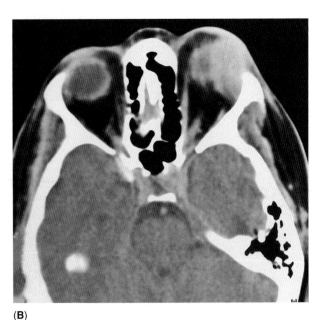

(A)   **(B)**

Figure 35.11 Orbital chloroma in a young man with ALL. (**A**) Contrast-enhanced CT showing an enhancing mass arising from the superolateral corner of the left orbit, with displacement of the underlying globe. The appearance is typical for orbital granulocytic sarcoma. (**B**) CT of the orbits obtained three months later showed progression of disease.

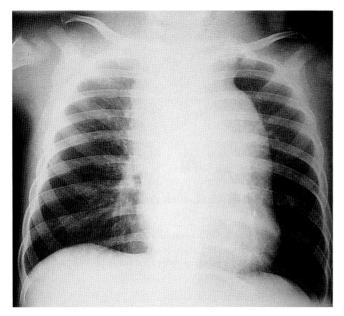

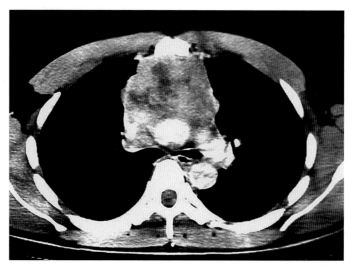

Figure 35.13 CT in a male patient with T-cell leukemia showing bulky heterogeneous anterior mediastinal lymphadenopathy, resulting in widening of the mediastinum.

Figure 35.12 Chest radiograph in a four-year-old boy with ALL showing a large mediastinal mass at presentation.

of therapy, whereas mediastinal abnormalities, although much less common, are usually the result of nodal involvement. Chest radiographs play an important role in the assessment of leukemic patients, especially during therapy at the time of immunosuppression. High resolution CT (HRCT) of the lungs can also provide additional useful information in selected cases but should be used as an adjunct to plain chest radiographs and not as a substitute investigation (74).

Direct Involvement by Leukemia

Mediastinal lymphadenopathy is a common feature of ALL as well as CLL (Fig. 35.12). A large anterior mediastinal mass on plain chest films is a characteristic feature of childhood T-cell leukemia, and over 50% of patients with adult T-cell leukemia also have mediastinal disease (Fig. 35.13) (16,75). These large masses may cause superior vena caval obstruction or tracheal compression. Hilar lymphadenopathy may also be seen.

Pulmonary leukemic infiltration is only rarely diagnosed on plain chest radiographs but is found more commonly at autopsy (76). On a plain chest film, leukemic infiltration appears as diffuse peribronchial infiltration accompanied by septal lines. The findings are usually indistinguishable from infection or pulmonary edema and therefore the diagnosis is rarely made radiologically. In those cases detected while the patient is alive, the diagnosis is readily made at transbronchial biopsy and bronchial lavage (77). In a series of 109 patients reported by Green and Nichols, 30 had autopsy evidence of pulmonary infiltration but only two of these patients showed evidence of infiltration on chest radiographs (78). HRCT may show diffuse nodular lesions along peribronchovascular bundles, but biopsy is required for a definitive diagnosis (79).

Indirect Effects of Leukemia

Mediastinal widening may be due to hemorrhage within the mediastinum, thrombus within the superior vena cava (usually as a result of central line insertion) or to mediastinitis (this may be associated with central line insertion due to an extraluminal placement of a catheter tip or infection). The cause can be detected on contrast-enhanced CT and is readily distinguished from lymphadenopathy (Fig. 35.14).

Pulmonary infection is a major cause of abnormal shadowing detected on plain chest radiographs in leukemic patients. These infections result from immunosuppression and may be bacterial, viral, or fungal (Fig. 35.15). The most common organisms with a predilection for immunosuppressed hosts include cytomegalovirus (CMV), *Pneumocystis carinii*, and fungal infection by organisms such as Aspergillus and Cryptococcus (80–82). On occasion, HRCT may be useful in the differential diagnosis of pulmonary infiltration, for example CT may demonstrate the rounded lesions of *Aspergillus fumigatus* not visualized on plain chest films. Invasive aspergillosis is an increasingly common and frequently fatal complication in children with hematological disorders (83). Oropharyngeal and esophageal infection with *Candida albicans* is common and results from antibiotic therapy as well as the impaired immune response (80).

Pulmonary hemorrhage should be considered in the differential diagnosis of abnormal air space pulmonary shadowing on plain chest films, particularly if accompanied by hemoptysis. Pulmonary edema may mimic infection and indeed may coexist with an inflammatory process.

Treatment-related pulmonary damage is important in the differential diagnosis of abnormal pulmonary shadowing and chest symptoms in the leukemic patient.

Drugs cause pulmonary edema and vasculitis. In the early stages of lung toxicity, plain chest radiographs are usually normal. Alveolar damage is usually a generalized process at the lung bases and, in moderate to severe cases, is seen as bilateral

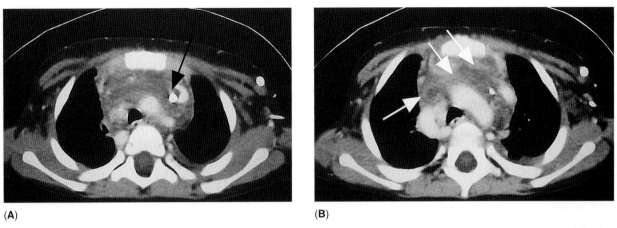

Figure 35.14 (A) and (B) Contrast-enhanced CT in a three-year-old child with massive mediastinal widening due to extrusion of the central line from the left innominate vein into the mediastinal soft tissues. Note thrombus in the left innominate vein shown as tubular low attenuation (arrows). Thrombus is also present in the superior vena cava (arrow). The mediastinum is widened and contains generalized increased soft tissue density due to mediastinitis. Central venous line (black arrow).

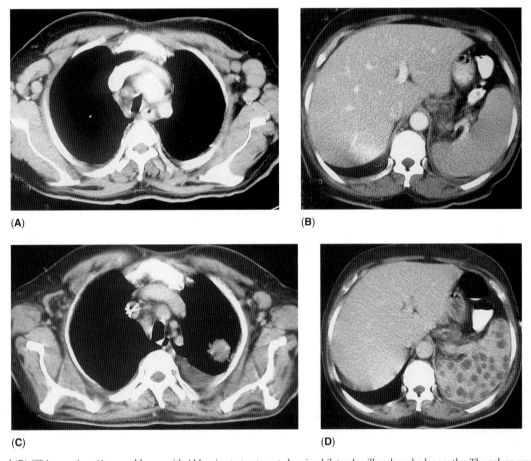

Figure 35.15 (A) and (B) CT images in a 41-year-old man with ALL prior to treatment showing bilateral axillary lymphadenopathy. The spleen was normal in appearance. (C) CT performed two months after commencing chemotherapy revealed reduction in the axillary lymphadenopathy, but a new mass was visible within the left upper lobe associated with a small pleural effusion. (D) In addition, multiple low attenuation lesions were also noted within the spleen. Biopsy of the lung mass confirmed infection with mycobacterium tuberculosis.

abnormal non-specific shadowing both on plain films and on CT. Such injury may be caused by busulphan, carmustine (BCNU), and methotrexate. Pulmonary vasculitis leads to infarction and, in some cases, cavitation may result. Pulmonary vascular damage may occur with busulphan therapy (84).

Chronic graft versus host disease (GVHD) is characterized by lymphocytic infiltration of the interstitial tissues and bronchial walls. Bronchiolitis obliterans is also seen (85). Plain chest radiographs may be normal but abnormal shadowing around peripheral bronchi may be observed on CT (86).

Key Points: Thoracic Manifestations

- Mediastinal lymphadenopathy is a common feature of ALL and CLL
- Mediastinal lymphadenopathy is also seen in T-cell childhood leukemia and in adult T-cell leukemia/lymphoma
- Leukemic infiltration of the lungs is rarely diagnosed during life. The appearances are often indistinguishable from infection or pulmonary edema
- Mediastinal widening may be due to mediastinitis, hemorrhage, or superior vena caval thrombosis as well as lymphadenopathy
- Pulmonary infection is a major cause of morbidity in leukemic patients. Organisms include CMV, *P. carinii*, and fungal infections such as invasive pulmonary aspergillosis

Abdomen and Pelvis

Direct Involvement by Leukemia

Hepatosplenomegaly due to diffuse involvement of the liver and spleen is a frequent manifestation of leukemia (Fig. 35.1). Imaging is not usually undertaken to evaluate these organs but both CT and ultrasound (US) will demonstrate hepatosplenomegaly. Focal lesions within the liver and spleen due to leukemia are rarely seen. Splenic infarction may be associated with gross splenomegaly. These lesions appear as an irregular, relatively low-density area within a massively enlarged spleen on CT and as hypoechoic lesions on US.

Renal involvement in leukemia is common, occurring in approximately 50% of cases at autopsy (16). As in patients with lymphoma, leukemia may involve the kidneys by:

- Diffuse parenchymal infiltration (bilateral or unilateral) (Fig. 35.16)
- Discrete renal mass or masses
- Obstruction due to lymphadenopathy at the hilum

In a review of 700 cases of the renal manifestations of non-Hodgkin's lymphoma and lymphocytic leukemia by Da'as et al. (87) no cases of primary renal involvement were found. Acute renal failure was seen in 83 patients but leukemic infiltration was shown to be the cause in only five (87).

US is a useful technique for detecting leukemic infiltration. The kidneys are diffusely enlarged and show patchy areas of low echogenicity. On contrast-enhanced CT, the parenchyma shows an inhomogeneous pattern with areas of diminished density interspersed with areas of enhancement, findings similar to those seen in lymphoma (88). Solid renal masses may also be observed on CT.

The gastrointestinal tract is involved in leukemia in about 25% of cases (89). Leukemia infiltrates spread through the lamina propria or submucosa of the bowel wall producing localized areas of bowel wall thickening. Imaging is seldom required as it is unusual for such lesions to become clinically manifest. Occasionally, a granulocytic sarcoma may develop within the bowel wall and may present as abdominal pain or intestinal obstruction.

As in other anatomical sites, abdominal lymph node involvement is more commonly seen in the acute lymphoblastic and chronic lymphocytic leukemias than in the myelogenous leukemias. Multiple enlarged nodes may be seen within the retroperitoneum, mesentery, splenic hilum, porta hepatis, and other intra-abdominal and pelvic sites (Figs. 35.2, 35.16, and 35.17). Nodes are usually discretely enlarged and, on imaging, the appearances are indistinguishable from those of non-Hodgkin's lymphoma.

Other sites of involvement in the abdomen and pelvis include the prostate gland, uterus, and adrenal glands. The testis and ovary are sanctuary sites and are therefore relatively resistant to chemotherapy (Table 35.2) (15).

Key Points: Abdominal/Pelvic Manifestations

- Hepatosplenomegaly is a common feature of all the leukemias
- Splenic infarcts may be demonstrated on imaging
- Renal involvement is seen in 50% of cases at autopsy
- Renal involvement may be diffuse or focal
- Enlarged lymph nodes in the abdomen and pelvis occur in multiple sites in ALL and CLL
- The gastro-intestinal tract is involved in approximately 25% of cases. In the majority of patients the disease is silent

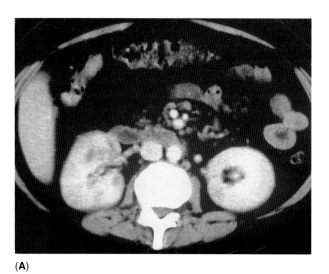

(A)

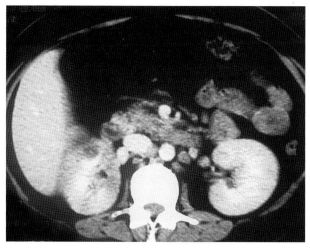

(B)

Figure 35.16 (A) and (B) CT in a 40-year-old female patient with AML showing bilateral renal infiltration. Both kidneys are enlarged and demonstrate multiple ill-defined low attenuation areas. Note the presence of small volume retroperitoneal lymph nodes.

Indirect Effects of Leukemia

The most important indirect effects of leukemia within the abdomen and pelvis are GVHD, neutropenic enterocolitis, hemorrhage, and infection.

Graft vs. Host Disease

Graft versus host disease most commonly affects the skin, gastrointestinal tract, and liver. This disease is a major complication of allogeneic BMT, occurring in about 50% of patients. The phenomenon is a manifestation of graft rejection in which the immunocompetent donor lymphoid cells react against host antigens. The

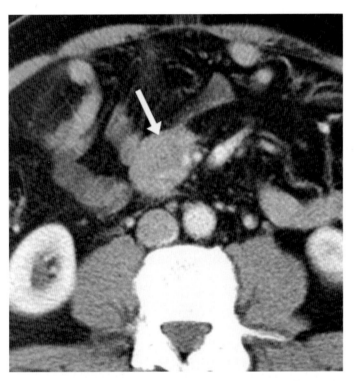

Figure 35.17 Contrast-enhanced CT in a 34-year-old man with ALL demonstrating a mesenteric mass (arrow).

principal bowel abnormalities are those of lymphocytic infiltration of the lamina propria, crypt dilatation and necrosis, and focal micro-abscess formation (90,91). Involvement of the bowel can be demonstrated on conventional plain abdominal radiographs, barium studies, and on CT (92).

On plain radiography, air-fluid levels, bowel wall and mucosal fold-thickening, and ascites may be seen (93). On barium studies, the small bowel shows thickening and flattening of the mucosal folds, a rapid transit time, and air-fluid levels (94). Pneumatosis intestinalis may be observed in severe cases (95). Graft versus host disease may resolve completely, in which case the abnormal plain film and barium findings return to normal. CT findings of GVHD include bowel wall thickening, stenosis of small bowel loops and edema of the bowel wall. Edema is typically seen as a "target sign" with decreased attenuation centrally bounded by high attenuation on both the serosal and mucosal surfaces of the bowel (Fig. 35.18). In addition, there is usually generalized increased density within the mesenteric fat (96). These findings are non-specific and may be seen in other benign and malignant conditions.

Neutropenic Enterocolitis

Neutropenic enterocolitis is a severe complication of intensive chemotherapy for acute leukemia and is difficult to confidently diagnose clinically. Patients present with abdominal pain, fever, and diarrhea, and imaging with US and CT can play a useful role in the diagnosis by demonstrating bowel wall thickening. Cartoni et al. (97) found that US was able to determine bowel wall thickening and that the degree of thickness correlated well with the clinical course and disease outcome. Patients with bowel wall thickening greater than 10 mm had a significantly poorer prognosis than those with lesser degrees of thickening.

Hemorrhage

Occasionally, imaging is required to investigate clinical features suggestive of intra-abdominal hemorrhage in leukemic patients. This is usually manifested by acute abdominal pain together with clinical features of blood loss. Retroperitoneal hemorrhage may present as acute back pain and, in such patients, CT is the ideal imaging modality to demonstrate the presence of fresh blood and the extent of hemorrhage (Fig. 35.19).

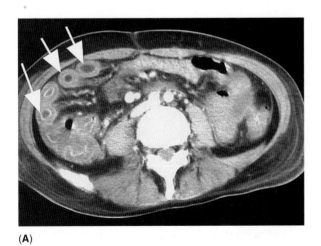

(A)

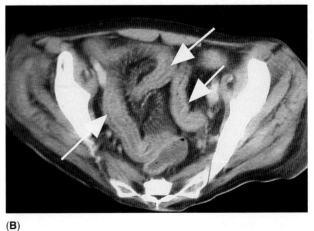

(B)

Figure 35.18 In this 38-year-old man with previous history of an allogenic bone marrow transplant for CML, CT (**A**) and (**B**) shows multiple thickened small bowel loops exhibiting "target sign" (arrows) due to low attenuation edema within the bowel wall adjacent to the enhancing mucosal and serosal surfaces. The CT appearance is suggestive of graft versus host disease.

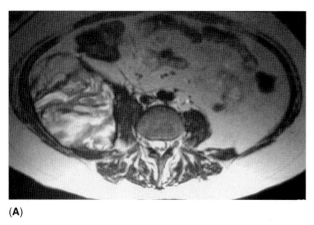
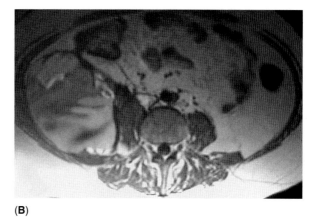

(A) **(B)**

Figure 35.19 (**A**) T1-weighted and (**B**) T2-weighted axial MR images in a 53-year-old man with ALL, presenting with acute right flank pain. The images show a large right retroperitoneal hematoma, which appears of high signal intensity on both T1- and T2-weighted imaging, indicating the presence of blood within the lesion.

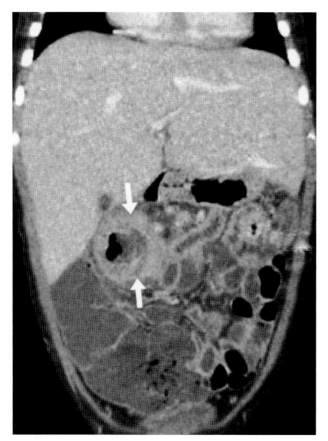

Figure 35.20 Coronal reformatted CT image of the abdomen in a three-year-old girl with acute lymphocytic leukemia. Note abnormal thickening of transverse colon (arrows) due to an infective colitis.

Infection

Intra-abdominal infection is an important cause of abdominal pain in leukemic patients. Infectious cecitis (typhlitis), perirectal abscesses, and appendicitis may all complicate the clinical picture of leukemia (Fig. 35.20). CT may be helpful in the management of these patients because hemorrhage may be distinguished from infection and the site of infection localized.

Liver infection is a serious complication of treatment. Candidiasis may involve the liver and spleen and is recognized on imaging as multiple small focal lesions throughout the organ parenchyma. Diagnosis must be made by biopsy or blood culture in the presence of abnormal imaging findings. MR imaging is a sensitive method of identifying these focal liver abnormalities and may also be used to monitor therapy.

Key Points: Abdominal/Pelvic Complications

- GVHD is a major complication of allogeneic BMT
- Acute GVHD most commonly affects the skin, liver, and gastrointestinal tract
- Plain radiographs, barium studies, and CT may all show dilatation, stenosis, and thickening of small bowel loops with air-fluid levels
- Ascites and pneumatosis intestinalis are seen in severe cases
- Neutropenic enterocolitis is a serious complication of intensive treatment as it is manifested by bowel wall thickening
- Intra-abdominal/retroperitoneal hemorrhage may account for the onset of abdominal pain in leukemic patients
- Intra-abdominal infection such as cecitis (typhlitis) may complicate acute leukemia
- Liver infection with candidiasis can be detected and monitored with imaging; MR is a sensitive technique to monitor response

Skeletal System

Direct Involvement of Leukemia

The incidence and radiographic manifestations of skeletal involvement in leukemia vary with patient age and subtype of the disease.

Radiographic Findings

In children, leukemic infiltration of the long bones produces characteristic appearances on plain radiographs (Fig. 35.21), which include:

- Diffuse osteoporosis
- Transverse metaphyseal bands of diminished density
- Dense transverse metaphyseal lines of arrested growth
- Subperiosteal new bone formation
- Osteolytic lesions
- Osteosclerotic lesions in less than 2% of patients (20)

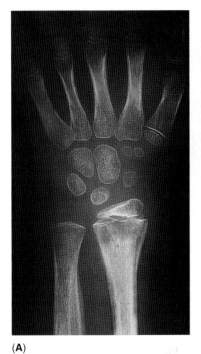
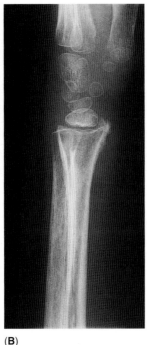

(A)   **(B)**

Figure 35.21 Plain radiographs of the wrist in a four-year-old boy with ALL. (A) Anterior/posterior view; (B) lateral view, showing diffuse osteoporosis throughout the radius and ulna as well as the bones of the wrist. Transverse metaphyseal bands of diminished density are noted. There is an extensive periosteal reaction on the distal surfaces of the radius and ulna.

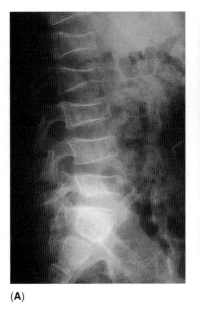
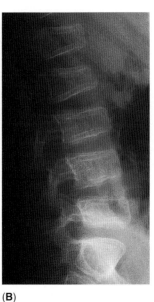

(A)   **(B)**

Figure 35.22 Lateral plain radiographs in a four-year-old boy who presented with back pain due to ALL. (A) At presentation, partial collapse of the lumbar vertebral bodies is noted. The most severely affected vertebra is L2. (B) Two years later following treatment, there has been remodeling of the bone. Note the thin dense lines adjacent to the vertebral end-plates giving the appearance of a bone within a bone. There is still extensive osteoporosis.

Diffuse osteoporosis is the most common skeletal abnormality in childhood ALL, occurring in up to 60% of cases, and is most obvious in the spine.

In adults, osteoporosis and cortical thinning of long bones due to expansion of the marrow space are common. Other characteristic features of childhood leukemia such as metaphyseal bands, are not seen in adults. In adult T-cell leukemia/lymphoma, lytic bone lesions are common (75). Subperiosteal bone resorption may be seen in this subtype of leukemia and probably results from hypercalcemia (75).

In children with acute leukemia presenting with backache, plain radiographs may show collapse of one or several vertebral bodies (Fig. 35.22A). This is either due to vertebral compression fractures as a result of osteoporosis or from destruction of bone trabeculae by leukemic infiltration. With treatment, remodeling of the vertebral body with reconstitution of the vertebral height may be observed (Fig. 35.22B). A characteristic but unusual feature is that of a "bone" within a bone (98).

Submetaphyseal bands are seen in approximately 40% of children and probably represent osteoporosis in the rapidly growing region of the long bone. They are seen most frequently in the distal femur, proximal tibia, proximal humerus, and vertebral bodies.

Focal lytic lesions are less common in AML than in ALL (Fig. 35.23) but may develop in CML during the accelerated growth phase and, in this group of patients, hypercalcemia may also be evident (99). Focal lesions are usually permeative and may show cortical destruction with pathological fracture. In the skull, lucent areas with a "moth-eaten" appearance may be identified due to leukemic infiltration. In children, widening of the sutures is associated with underlying meningeal disease. This has been less commonly observed since the introduction of CNS prophylaxis.

Bone is one of the most frequent sites for development of granulocytic sarcoma. An area of bone destruction is seen on plain radiographs which may be accompanied by a soft tissue mass. The lesions are most commonly found in the skull, spine, ribs, and sternum (100). Unusually, leukemic infiltration may affect the periosteum and para-osteal soft tissue (Fig. 35.24).

CT is indicated for the evaluation of leukemic masses (granulocytic sarcoma) in various sites, as the technique can define the soft tissue disease as well as the extent of bone destruction.

Neither radionuclide bone scanning with technetium-99m-diphosphonate, nor bone marrow imaging with colloid, is required in the routine management of leukemia (101,102). However, bone scans may be helpful in patients suspected of harboring occult bone infection.

When MR imaging was first introduced into clinical practice over a decade ago there was considerable enthusiasm regarding its potential to evaluate diffuse bone marrow disease. Certainly, diffuse infiltration of the bone marrow can be elegantly demonstrated on spin-echo imaging as diffuse abnormally low signal intensity on T1-weighted images accompanied by intermediate signal intensity on T2-weighted images. In leukemia, the axial skeleton is mainly involved (Fig. 35.25). However, MR imaging is non-specific, as both benign and malignant disorders give similar appearances (Fig. 35.26) (103,104). Clear advantages of MR imaging are the ability to survey large volumes of the bone marrow at a single investigation and the high sensitivity of the technique in detecting bone marrow pathology.

MR imaging may demonstrate changes within the bone marrow in leukemic patients in response to treatment (Fig. 35.27) and some authors have used quantitative measurements of T1 relaxation times to evaluate therapeutic response (105,106). Van de Berg et al. (107) showed that sequential quantitative MR imaging during therapy for ALL and AML revealed significant differences in the initial bulk values of T1 relaxation between these subtypes of leukemia and also in the changes observed in T1 between the two groups during therapy. As a

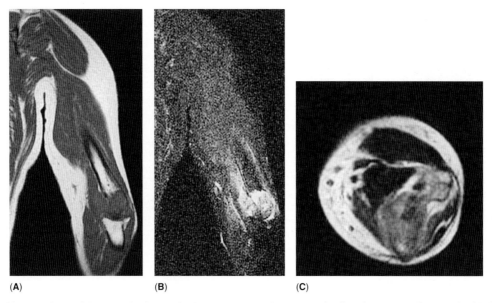

Figure 35.23 A 42-year-old man with ALL. (A) T1-weighted coronal, (B) STIR coronal, and (C) T1-weighted axial MR images showing a focal leukemic deposit replacing the normal marrow signal within the condyles of the distal left humerus. The mass infiltrates into the adjacent soft tissues.

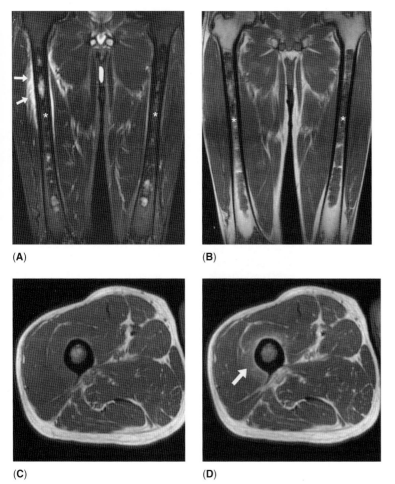

Figure 35.24 (A) STIR and (B) T1-weighted coronal MR images through both femur show irregular low T1-signal changes within the marrow cavity in keeping with bone infarcts (*). In addition there is abnormal high signal intensity in the periosteum and paraosteal soft tissue on STIR imaging around the shaft of the upper right femur (arrows). T1-weighted axial MR image obtained (C) before and (D) after gadolinium contrast shows abnormal enhancement (arrow) in the area. Biopsy confirmed leukemic infiltration.

result, these authors suggest that bone marrow imaging with MR may be a useful method of predicting response in ALL (107). However, Lecouvet et al. (108) have shown that quantitative MR imaging failed to identify bone marrow abnormalities in 41% of patients with CLL. Diffusion-weighted imaging may be applied to examination of the bone marrow in leukemic patients (109). Measured signal-to-noise ratios agreed with an estimate of percentage cellularity and, in addition, the signal-to-noise ratios were also dependent on time

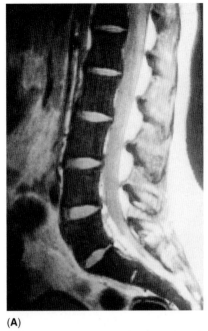

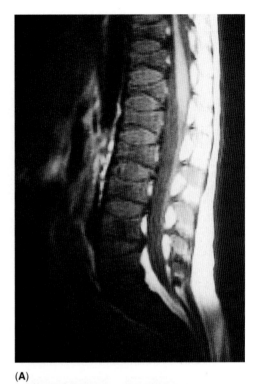

(A)

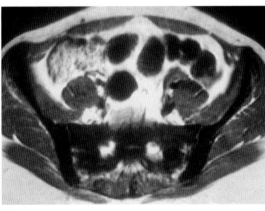

(B)

Figure 35.25 T1-weighted spin-echo MR images in a 21-year-old female with ALL. (A) Sagittal image of the spine; (B) axial image through the pelvis. The MR examination shows widespread diffuse abnormal low signal intensity throughout the vertebral bodies and pelvis, indicating extensive bone marrow infiltration.

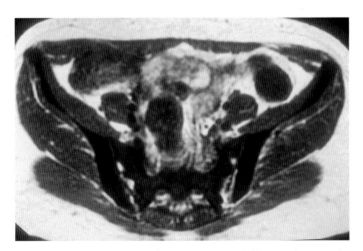

Figure 35.26 A 50-year-old female patient with myelofibrosis. The spin-echo T1-weighted axial MR image of the pelvis shows diffuse abnormal low signal intensity throughout the iliac bones and sacrum. The appearances are identical to those of leukemic infiltration.

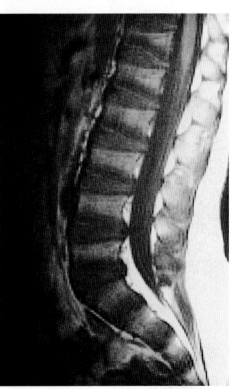

(B)

Figure 35.27 MR images in a four-year-old boy with ALL. This is the same patient as shown in Figure 35.22 T1-weighted sagittal images through the thoracic and lumbar spine, (A) before treatment, (B) two years after treatment. The MR image at presentation shows diffuse abnormal low signal intensity throughout the vertebral bodies indicating leukemic infiltration. Note that the signal intensity of the bone marrow is lower than that of the adjacent intervertebral discs. There is partial collapse of multiple vertebrae. Two years later the signal intensity of the vertebral bodies is higher than the adjacent intervertebral discs. This represents response to treatment.

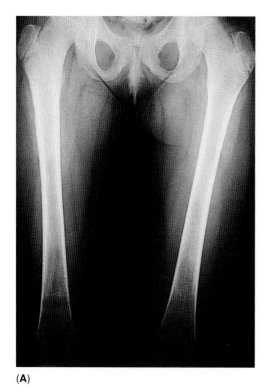
(A)

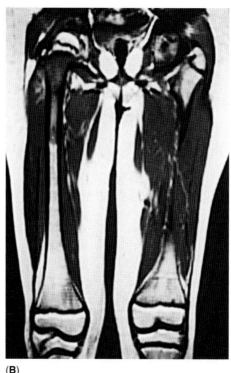
(B)

Figure 35.28 A 10-year-old boy treated three years previously for ALL with CNS relapse. He represented with right leg pain. (A) Plain radiograph of the femora did not reveal any abnormality. (B) Coronal T1-weighted MR image of the femora showing extensive abnormal low signal intensity throughout the metaphyseal region and upper diaphysis of the right femur. This represented leukemic relapse.

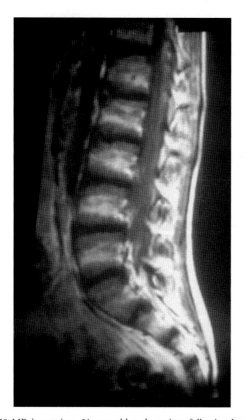

Figure 35.29 MR image in a 21-year-old male patient following bone marrow transplant. T1-weighted sagittal image showing typical "bandlike" pattern of repopulation of bone marrow with areas of low signal intensity adjacent to the vertebral end-plates. Higher signal intensity centrally represents fat.

after commencement of treatment (109). Dynamic contrast-enhanced MR imaging (DCE-MRI) has also been investigated as a method of measuring angiogenic activity of bone marrow as a predictor of adverse clinical outcome. Shih et al. (110) have shown that DCE-MRI proved to be an independent prognostic indicator in 78 patients with acute myeloid leukemia.

Despite these interesting results, the current role of MR imaging in the evaluation of leukemia is limited as clinical and hematological investigations usually direct patient management. Although MR imaging seems to have little role in the routine evaluation of the bone marrow in leukemia, it is useful in patients suspected of relapse. It is useful for patients believed to be in remission who present with bone pain (Fig. 35.28), or in patients at high risk of relapse in whom serial bone marrow biopsies are negative.

Key Points: Skeletal Involvement

- Osteoporosis occurs in up to 60% of childhood ALL cases
- Metaphyseal translucencies are seen in the long bones in approximately 40% of children with ALL
- Focal bone lesions are more common in ALL than AML
- Granulocytic sarcoma in AML occurs most frequently in the skull, ribs, and sternum
- MR imaging shows diffuse bone marrow abnormality in acute leukemia but the appearances are non-specific
- MR imaging has a valuable role in the detection of leukemic relapse in patients with bone pain

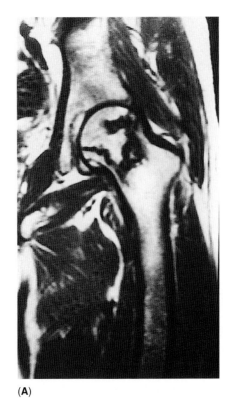
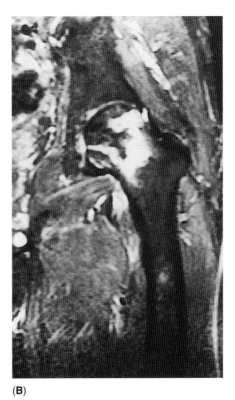

(A)　　　　　　　　　　　　　**(B)**

Figure 35.30 An adult male patient with ALL with avascular necrosis of the femoral head. (**A**) Coronal T1-weighted MR image, (**B**) turbo STIR image. The T1-weighted image shows classic signs of avascular necrosis with irregular areas of low signal intensity within the femoral heads bilaterally. The STIR image shows abnormal high signal intensity areas within the femoral heads and also in the femoral neck on the right, indicating associated edema.

Indirect Effects of Leukemia

Following therapy with BMT, repopulation of the bone marrow gives rise to striking appearances with bands of low signal intensity adjacent and bands of high signal intensity central to the vertebral end-plates on MR imaging (Fig. 35.29). These appearances are related to repopulation of the marrow in the region of the capillary network which lies adjacent to the vertebral end-plates (111,112). Treatment with steroids may lead to avascular necrosis of the femoral head (Fig. 35.30). Bony infarcts may also be detected on MR imaging. MR is well-established as the best imaging technique for detecting avascular necrosis and is indicated in all symptomatic patients with normal plain films. As in other areas of the body, infection is a major hazard in the acute leukemias and bone pain may represent osteomyelitis as well as leukemic relapse (Fig. 35.31).

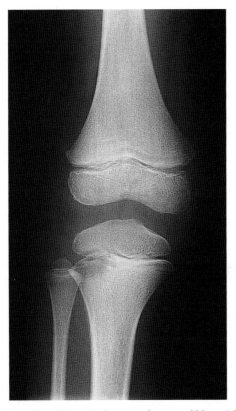

Figure 35.31 Plain film of the right knee in a five-year-old boy with ALL complaining of severe bone pain around the knee joint. There is a destructive lytic lesion in the lateral aspect of the tibial metaphysis. This was due to osteomyelitis and was surgically drained.

Summary

- Acute lymphoblastic leukemia (ALL) is the most common subtype in childhood
- Acute myelogenous leukemia (AML) and chronic lymphocytic leukemia (CLL) are the most common subtypes in adults
- Chromosomal abnormalities have been identified in many of the subtypes of leukemia, which is of prognostic importance
- The major clinical features of leukemia relate to anemia, infection, and hemorrhage

- Bone pain is a common presenting feature in children with ALL but is rare in adults
- Granulocytic sarcoma (chloroma) is a mass composed of precursors of myelocytes. It occurs in AML and in other myeloprolific disorders
- Granulocytic sarcoma most commonly involves the orbits
- In the CNS, leukemia involves the leptomeninges, dura and, rarely, the brain parenchyma. It may be diffuse or focal
- Hemorrhage, sinovenous thrombosis and cerebral infarction, as well as infection, are all indirect effects of leukemia on the CNS
- Intrathoracic leukemia usually involves mediastinal and hilar lymph nodes. Pulmonary complications include infection, hemorrhage, edema, and graft versus host disease (GVHD)
- Diffuse involvement of intra-abdominal organs is common (liver, spleen, kidneys, gastrointestinal tract, intra-abdominal lymph nodes)
- GVHD and neutropenic enterocolitis are important intra-abdominal complications which can be assessed with CT and US
- Skeletal manifestations of childhood leukemia are seen in up to 60% of patients and include osteoporosis, transmetaphyseal bands, and subperiosteal new bone formation

REFERENCES

1. Caligiuri MA, Ritz J. Immunology. In: Henderson ES, Lister TA, eds. Leukaemia, 5th edn. Philadelphia: W B Saunders, 1990; 103–30.
2. Garson CM. Cytogenetics of leukemic cells. In: Henderson ES, Lister TA, eds. Leukaemia, 5th edn. Philadelphia: W B Saunders, 1990; 131–52.
3. Cancer Facts and Figures 2008. American Cancer Society Inc, 2008. [Available from: http://www.cancer.org].
4. Cancer Research UK Cancer Stats 2008. [Available from: http://www.cancerresearchuk.org].
5. Preston DL, Kusumi S, Tomonaga M, et al. Cancer incidence in atomic bomb survivors. Part III. Leukemia, lymphoma and multiple myeloma, 1950–1987. Radiat Res 1994; 137: S68–97.
6. Sandler DP. Recent studies in leukemia epidemiology. Curr Opin Oncol 1995; 7: 12–18.
7. Arseneau JC, Sponzo RW, Levin DL, et al. Nonlymphomatous malignant tumors complicating Hodgkin's disease. Possible association with intensive therapy. N Engl J Med 1972; 287: 1119–22.
8. Aisenberg AC. Acute nonlymphocytic leukemia after treatment for Hodgkin's disease. Am J Med 1983; 75: 449–54.
9. Curtis RE, Boice JD Jr, Stovall M, et al. Risk of leukemia after chemotherapy and radiation treatment for breast cancer. N Engl J Med 1992; 326: 1745–51.
10. Kaldor JM, Day NE, Pettersson F, et al. Leukemia following chemotherapy for ovarian cancer. N Engl J Med 1990; 322: 1–6.
11. Robert-Guroff M, Reitz MS Jr, Robey WG, et al. In vitro generation of an HTLV-III variant by neutralizing antibody. J Immunol 1986; 137: 3306–9.
12. Kalyanaraman VS, Sarngadharan MG, Nakao Y, et al. Natural antibodies to the structural core protein (p24) of the human T-cell leukemia (lymphoma) retrovirus found in sera of leukemia patients in Japan. Proc Natl Acad Sci USA 1982; 79: 1653–57.
13. Weber J. HTLV-I infection in Britain. Br Med J 1990; 301: 71–2.
14. Anonymous. HTLV-1 comes of age. Lancet 1988; 1: 217–19.
15. Barcos M, Lane W, Gomez GA, et al. An autopsy study of 1206 acute and chronic leukemias (1958–1982). Cancer 1987; 60: 827–37.
16. Henderson ES, Afshani E. Clinical manifestation and diagnosis. In: Henderson ES, Lister TA, eds. Leukaemia, 5th edn. Philadelphia: W B Saunders, 1990; 291–359.
17. Graus F, Rogers LR, Posner JB. Cerebrovascular complications in patients with cancer. Medicine (Baltimore) 1985; 64: 16–35.
18. Freireich EJ, Thomas LB, Frei E, et al. A distinctive type of intracerebral haemorrhage associated with "blastic crisis" in patients with leukaemia. Cancer 1960; 13: 146–54.
19. Fernbach DJ. Natural history of acute leukemia. In: Sutow W, Vietti TJ, Fernbach DJ, eds. Pediatric Oncology, 2nd edn. St Louis: Mosby, 1977; 291–333.
20. Thomas LG, Forkner CEJ, Frei E. The skeletal lesions of acute leukemia. Cancer 1961; 14: 608.
21. Hann IM, Gupta S, Palmer MK, et al. The prognostic significance of radiological and symptomatic bone involvement in childhood acute lymphoblastic leukaemia. Med Pediatr Oncol 1979; 6: 51–5.
22. Nies BA, Kundel DW, Thomas LB, et al. Leucopenia, bone pain, and bone necrosis in patients with acute leukemia. A clinicopathological complex. Ann Intern Med 1965; 62: 698.
23. Neiman RS, Barcos M, Berard C, et al. Granulocytic sarcoma: a clinicopathologic study of 61 biopsied cases. Cancer 1981; 48: 1426–37.
24. Pui MH, Fletcher BD, Langston JW. Granulocytic sarcoma in childhood leukemia: imaging features. Radiology 1994; 190: 698–702.
25. Muss HB, Moloney WC. Chloroma and other myeloblastic tumors. Blood 1973; 42: 721–8.
26. Liu PI, Ishimaru T, McGregor DH, et al. Autopsy study of granulocytic sarcoma (chloroma) in patients with myelogenous leukemia, Hiroshima-Nagasaki 1949–1969. Cancer 1973; 31: 948–55.
27. Krause JR. Granulocytic sarcoma preceding acute leukemia: a report of six cases. Cancer 1979; 44: 1017–21.
28. Burns A. Observation of the Surgical Anatomy of the Head and Neck. Edinburgh, Scotland: Thomas Bryce, 1811.
29. King A. A case of chloroma. Monthly J Med Soc 1853; 17: 97.
30. Henderson ES, Hoelzer D, Freeman AI. The treatment of acute lymphoblastic leukaemia. In: Henderson ES, Lister TA, eds. Leukaemia, 5th edn. Philadelphia: W B Saunders, 1990; 443–82.
31. Ortega JA, Nesbit ME, Sather HN, et al. Long-term evaluation of a CNS prophylaxis trial–treatment comparisons and outcome after CNS relapse in childhood ALL: a report from the Children's Cancer Study Group. J Clin Oncol 1987; 5: 1646–54.

32. de Vries EG, Mulder NH, Houwen B, et al. Combination chemotherapy for acute lymphocytic leukaemia in 25 adults. Blut 1982; 44: 151–8.

33. Veerman AJ, Hahlen K, Kamps WA, et al. High cure rate with a moderately intensive treatment regimen in non-high-risk childhood acute lymphoblastic leukemia. Results of protocol ALL VI from the Dutch Childhood Leukemia Study Group. J Clin Oncol 1996; 14: 911–18.

34. Thomas X, Le QH. Central nervous system involvement in adult acute lymphoblastic leukemia. Hematology 2008; 13: 293–302.

35. Bleyer WA. Central nervous system leukemia. In: Henderson ES, Lister TA, eds. Leukaemia, 5th edn. Philadelphia: W B Saunders, 1990; 733–68.

36. Price RA, Johnson WW. The central nervous system in childhood leukemia. I. The arachnoid. Cancer 1973; 31: 520–33.

37. Azzarelli V, Roessmann U. Pathogenesis of central nervous system infiltration in acute leukemia. Arch Pathol Lab Med 1977; 101: 203–5.

38. Brant-Zawadzki M, Enzmann DR. Computed tomographic brain scanning in patients with lymphoma. Radiology 1978; 129: 67–71.

39. Enzmann DR, Krikorian J, Yorke C, et al. Computed tomography in leptomeningeal spread of tumor. J Comput Assist Tomogr 1978; 2: 448–55.

40. Pagani JJ, Libshitz HI, Wallace S, et al. Central nervous system leukemia and lymphoma: computed tomographic manifestations. Am J Roentgenol 1981; 137: 1195–201.

41. Ginsberg LE, Leeds NE. Neuroradiology of leukemia. Am J Roentgenol 1995; 165: 525–34.

42. Paakko E, Patronas NJ, Schellinger D. Meningeal Gd-DTPA enhancement in patients with malignancies. J Comput Assist Tomogr 1990; 14: 542–6.

43. Sze G, Abramson A, Krol G et al. Gadolinium-DTPA in the evaluation of intradural extramedullary spinal disease. AJR Am J Roentgenol 1988; 150: 911–21.

44. Kao SC, Yuh WT, Sato Y et al. Intracranial granulocytic sarcoma (chloroma): MR findings. J Comput Assist Tomogr 1987; 11: 938–41.

45. Pomeranz S J, Hawkins H H, Towbin R et al. Granulocytic sarcoma (chloroma): CT manifestations. Radiology 1985; 155: 167–70.

46. Moudden M, El-Moutawakil B, Boulajaj F L, Slassi I, Azhar A. Granulocytic sarcoma of the brain revealed on vascular mode. Rev Neurol 2005; 161: 1191–6.

47. Ahn JY, Kwon SO, Shin MS, et al. Meningeal chloroma (granulocytic sarcoma) in acute lymphoblastic leukemia mimicking a falx meningioma. J Neurooncol 2002; 60: 31–5.

48. Barnett MJ, Zussman WV. Granulocytic sarcoma of the brain: a case report and review of the literature. Radiology 1986; 160: 223–5.

49. Williams MP, Olliff JF, Rowley MR. CT and MR findings in parameningeal leukaemic masses. J Comput Assist Tomogr 1990; 14: 736–42.

50. Ho CL, Chen CY, Chen YC, et al. Cerebral dural sinus thrombosis in acute lymphoblastic leukemia with early diagnosis by fast fluid-attenuated inversion recovery (FLAIR) MR image: a case report and review of the literature. Ann Hematol 2000; 79: 90–4.

51. Henderson ES. Complications of leukaemia: a selective overview. In: Henderson ES, Lister TA, eds. Leukaemia, 5th edn. Philadelphia: W B Saunders, 1990; 671–85.

52. Mulrooney DA, Dover DC, Li S, et al. Twenty years of follow-up among survivors of childhood and young adult acute myeloid leukemia: a report from the Childhood Cancer Survivor Study. Cancer 2008; 112: 2071–9.

53. Bleyer WA. Neurologic sequelae of methotrexate and ionizing radiation: a new classification. Cancer Treat Rep 1981; 65(Suppl 1): 89–98.

54. Jager HR, Williams EJ, Savage DG, et al. Assessment of brain changes with registered MR before and after bone marrow transplantation for chronic myeloid leukemia. Am J Neuroradiol 1996; 17: 1275–82.

55. Packer RJ, Zimmerman RA, Bilaniuk LT. Magnetic resonance imaging in the evaluation of treatment-related central nervous system damage. Cancer 1986; 58: 635–40.

56. Duffner PK, Cohen ME, Brecher ML, et al. CT abnormalities and altered methotrexate clearance in children with CNS leukemia. Neurology 1984; 34: 229–33.

57. Laitt RD, Chambers EJ, Goddard PR, et al. Magnetic resonance imaging and magnetic resonance angiography in long term survivors of acute lymphoblastic leukemia treated with cranial irradiation. Cancer 1995; 76: 1846–52.

58. Chan YL, Roebuck DJ, Yuen MP, et al. Long-term cerebral metabolite changes on proton magnetic resonance spectroscopy in patients cured of acute lymphoblastic leukemia with previous intrathecal methotrexate and cranial irradiation prophylaxis. Int J Radiat Oncol Biol Phys 2001; 50: 759–63.

59. Rubinstein LJ, Herman MM, Long TF, et al. Disseminated necrotizing leukoencephalopathy: a complication of treated central nervous system leukemia and lymphoma. Cancer 1975; 35: 291–305.

60. Pande AR, Ando K, Ishikura R, et al. Disseminated necrotizing leukoencephalopathy following chemoradiation therapy for acute lymphoblastic leukemia. Radiat Med 2006; 24: 515–19.

61. Matsubayashi J, Tsuchiya K, Matsunaga T, Mukai K. Methotrexate-related leukoencephalopathy without radiation therapy: distribution of brain lesions and pathological heterogeneity on two autopsy cases. Neuropathology 2009; 29: 105–15.

62. Price RA, Birdwell DA. The central nervous system in childhood leukemia. III. Mineralizing microangiopathy and dystrophic calcification. Cancer 1978; 42: 717–28.

63. Ito M, Akiyama Y, Asato R, et al. Early diagnosis of leukoencephalopathy of acute lymphocytic leukemia by MRI. Pediatr Neurol 1991; 7: 436–9.

64. Bjorgen JE, Gold LH. Computed tomographic appearance of methotrexate-induced necrotizing leukoencephalopathy. Radiology 1977; 122: 377–8.

65. Vera P, Rohrlich P, Stievenart JL, et al. Contribution of single-photon emission computed tomography in the diagnosis and follow-up of CNS toxicity of a cytarabine-containing regimen in pediatric leukemia. J Clin Oncol 1999; 17: 2804–10.

66. Buizer AI, de Sonneville LM, Veerman AJ. Effects of chemotherapy on neurocognitive function in children with acute lymphoblastic leukemia: A critical review of the literature. Pediatr Blood Cancer 2009; 52: 447–54.

67. Harila-Saari AH, Paakko EL, Vainionpaa LK, et al. A longitudinal magnetic resonance imaging study of the brain in survivors in childhood acute lymphoblastic leukemia. Cancer 1998; 83: 2608–17.

68. Iuvone L, Mariotti P, Colosimo C, et al. Long-term cognitive outcome, brain computed tomography scan, and magnetic resonance imaging in children cured for acute lymphoblastic leukemia. Cancer 2002; 95: 2562–70.

69. Mabbott DJ, Noseworthy MD, Bouffet E, Rockel C, Laughlin S. Diffusion tensor imaging of white matter after cranial radiation in children for medulloblastoma: correlation with IQ. Neuro-oncol. 2006 ; 8: 244–52.

70. Khong P-L, Leung LH, Fung AA, et al. White matter anisotropy in post-treatment childhood cancer survivors: preliminary evidence of association with neurocognitive function. J Clinical Oncol 2006; 24: 884–90.

71. Kumar J, Seith A, Bakhshi S, et al. Isolated granulocytic sarcoma of the orbit. Eur J Haematol 2007; 78: 456.

72. Manabe Y, Hamakawa Y, Sunami K, et al. Granulocytic sarcoma with orbit, cauda equina, muscle and peripheral nerve extension but without bone marrow involvement. Intern Med 2007; 46: 633–5.

73. Lackner H, Sovinz P, Benesch M, et al. Management of brain abscesses in children treated for acute lymphoblastic leukemia. Pediatr Blood Cancer 2009; 52: 408–11.

74. Lee WA, Hruban RH, Kuhlman JE, et al. High resolution computed tomography of inflation-fixed lungs: pathologic–radiologic correlation of pulmonary lesions in patients with leukemia, lymphoma, or other hematopoietic proliferative disorders. Clin Imaging 1992; 16: 15–24.

75. George CD, Wilson AG, Philpott NJ, et al. The radiological features of adult T-cell leukaemia/lymphoma. Clin Radiol 1994; 49: 83–8.

76. Armstrong P, Dyer R, Alford BA, et al. Leukemic pulmonary infiltrates: rapid development mimicking pulmonary edema. Am J Roentgenol 1980; 135: 373–4.

77. Berkman N, Polliack A, Breuer R, et al. Pulmonary involvement as the major manifestation of chronic lymphocytic leukemia. Leuk Lymphoma 1992; 8: 495–9.

78. Green RA, Nichols NJ. Pulmonary involvment in leukemia. Am Rev Resp Dis 1959; 80: 833–44.

79. Kakihana K, Ohashi K, Sakai F, et al. Leukemic infiltration of the lung following allogenic hematopoietic stem cell transplantation. Int J Hematol 2009; 89: 118–22.

80. Schimpff SC. Infection in the leukaemia patient: diagnosis, therapy and prevention. In: Henderson ES, Lister TA, eds. Leukaemia, 5th edn. Philadelphia: W B Saunders, 1990; 687–709.

81. DeGregorio MW, Lee WM, Linker CA, et al. Fungal infections in patients with acute leukemia. Am J Med 1982; 73: 543–8.

82. Olliff JF, Williams MP. Radiological appearances of cytomegalovirus infections. Clin Radiol 1989; 40: 463–7.

83. Crassard N, Hadden H, Pondarré C, et al. Invasive aspergillosis and allogeneic hematopoietic stem cell transplantation in children: a 15-year experience. Transpl Infect Dis 2008; 10: 177–83.

84. Dee P. Drug- and radiation-induced lung disease. In: Armstrong P, Wilson AG, Hansell DM, eds. Imaging Diseases of the Chest, 2nd edn. St Louis: Mosby, 1995; 461–84.

85. Chan CK, Hyland RH, Hutcheon MA, et al. Small-airways disease in recipients of allogeneic bone marrow transplants. An analysis of 11 cases and a review of the literature. Medicine 1987; 66: 327–40.

86. Graham NJ, Muller NL, Miller RR, et al. Intrathoracic complications following allogeneic bone marrow transplantation: CT findings. Radiology 1991; 181: 153–6.

87. Da'as N, Polliack A, Cohen Y, et al. Kidney involvement and renal manifestations in non-Hodgkin's lymphoma and lymphocytic leukemia: a retrospective study in 700 patients. Eur J Haematol 2001; 67: 158–64.

88. Gore RM, Shkolnik A. Abdominal manifestations of pediatric leukemias: sonographic assessment. Radiology 1982; 143: 207–10.

89. Boggs DA, Wintrobe MM, Cartwright GE. The acute leukaemias. Analysis of 322 cases and review of the literature. Medicine 1962; 41: 163.

90. Epstein RJ, McDonald GB, Sale GE, et al. The diagnostic accuracy of the rectal biopsy in acute graft-versus-host disease: a prospective study of thirteen patients. Gastroenterology 1980; 78: 764–71.

91. Slavin RE, Woodruff JM. The pathology of bone marrow transplantation. In: Somers SC, ed. Pathology Annual. New York: Appleton-Century Crofts, 1974; 291.

92. Kalantari BN, Mortelé KJ, Cantisani V, et al. CT features with pathologic correlation of acute gastrointestinal graft-versus-host disease after bone marrow transplantation in adults. AJR Am J Roentgenol 2003; 181: 1621–5.

93. Belli AM, Williams MP. Graft-versus-host disease: findings on plain abdominal radiography. Clin Radiol 1988; 39: 262–4.

94. Fisk JD, Shulman HM, Greening RR, et al. Gastrointestinal radiographic features of human graft-versus-host disease. Am J Roentgenol 1981; 136: 329–36.

95. Maile CW, Frick MP, Crass JR, et al. The plain abdominal radiograph in acute gastrointestinal graft-versus-host disease. Am J Roentgenol 1985; 145: 289–92.

96. Jones B, Fishman EK, Kramer SS, et al. Computed tomography of gastrointestinal inflammation after bone marrow transplantation. Am J Roentgenol 1986; 146: 691–5.

97. Cartoni C, Dragoni F, Micozzi A, et al. Neutropenic enterocolitis in patients with acute leukemia: prognostic significance of bowel wall thickening detected by ultrasonography. J Clin Oncol 2001; 19: 756–61.

98. deCastro LA, Kuhn JP, Freeman AI, et al. Complete remodeling of the vertebrae in a child successfully treated for acute lymphocytic leukemia (ALL). Cancer 1977; 40: 398–401.

99. Tricot G, Boogaerts MA, Broeckaert-Van Orshoven A, et al. Hypercalcemia and diffuse osteolytic lesions in the acute phase of chronic myelogenous leukemia. A possible relation between lymphoid transformation and hypercalcemia. Cancer 1983; 52: 841–5.

100. Van Slyck EJ. The bony changes in malignant hematologic disease. Orthop Clin North Am 1972; 3: 733–4.

101. Goergen TG, Alazraki NP, Halpern SE, et al. "Cold" bone lesions: a newly recognized phenomenon of bone imaging. J Nucl Med 1974; 15: 1120–4.

102. Parker BR, Marglin S, Castellino RA. Skeletal manifestations of leukemia, Hodgkin disease, and non-Hodgkin's lymphoma. Semin Roentgenol 1980; 15: 302–15.

103. Porter BA, Shields AF, Olson DO. Magnetic resonance imaging of bone marrow disorders. Radiol Clin North Am 1986; 24: 269–89.

104. Jones RJ. The role of bone marrow imaging. Radiology 1992; 183: 321–2.

105. Moore SG, Gooding CA, Brasch RC, et al. Bone marrow in children with acute lymphocytic leukemia: MR relaxation times Radiology 1986; 160: 237–40.

106. McKinstry CS, Steiner RE, Young AT, et al. Bone marrow in leukemia and aplastic anemia: MR imaging before, during, and after treatment. Radiology 1987; 162: 701–7.

107. Van de Berg BC, Michaux L, Scheiff JM, et al. Sequential quantitative MR analysis of bone marrow: differences during treatment of lymphoid versus myeloid leukemia. Radiology 1996; 201: 519–23.

108. Lecouvet FE, van de Berg BC, Michaux L, et al. Chronic lymphocytic leukemia: changes in bone marrow composition and distribution assessed with quantitative MRI. J Magn Reson Imaging 1998; 8: 733–9.

109. Ballon D, Dyke J, Schwartz LH, et al. Bone marrow segmentation in leukemia using diffusion and T(2)-weighted echo planar magnetic resonance imaging. NMR Biomed 2000; 13: 321–8.

110. Shih TT, Hou HA, Liu CY, et al. Bone marrow angiogenesis MR imaging in patients with acute myeloid leukemia: peak enhancement ratio is an independent predictor for overall survival. Blood 2009; 113: 3161–7.

111. Stevens SK, Moore SG, Amylon MD. Repopulation of marrow after transplantation: MR imaging with pathologic correlation. Radiology 1990; 175: 213–18.

112. Tanner SF, Clarke J, Leach MO, et al. MRI in the evaluation of late bone marrow changes following bone marrow transplantation. Br J Radiol 1996; 69: 1145–51.

36 General Principles in Pediatric Oncology
David Stringer and Harvey Teo

INTRODUCTION

Children with cancer are a relatively small group within a typical pediatric-imaging department. However they place the greatest demand on staff and services. This is because they are often very ill and have enormous anxieties concerning all medical interactions, not least radiological. Understandably, the parents are also likely to be under considerable stress and expect urgent, immediate, safe radiological investigation with rapid, correct diagnosis. The radiologist needs to be particularly sensitive to these needs, giving objective, decisive, and diagnostically accurate reports. Close rapport with the oncologist is required, not least because he will be under considerable pressure from the parents to expedite treatment.

It is essential that all modalities are available in the hospital where investigation and treatment are being undertaken, including:

- Plain radiography
- Ultrasound (US)
- Nuclear medicine
- Computed tomography (CT)
- Magnetic resonance (MR) imaging
- Angiography/interventional facilities
- PET-CT

THE DEPARTMENT

Children with cancer ideally should be investigated and treated in a department that deals extensively or exclusively with children. In a busy general hospital it is difficult to give the same attention to detail and for staff inexperienced in dealing with sick children, the situation can be very stressful . Hence pediatric hospitals or women's and children hospitals with fully trained pediatric staff in all disciplines (radiologists, radiographers, sonographers, and nurses) will undoubtedly give the most comfortable and supportive service.

Special attention should be given to the facilities provided by the department in order to obtain optimum results from imaging.

General Ambience
The general ambience of a pediatric imaging facility should be designed to make the child feel secure in what is otherwise a frightening environment. Hence murals, toys, and other decorations, which can be adequately cleaned, should be readily available. For older children suitable reading materials should be made available. It is important to cater to all age groups.

Some manufacturers of major radiology equipment offer special ambience programs that can be purchased along with their major pieces of equipment. Examples of this are mood videos and electronic wall decorations that can be programmed into the MR suite which are individually chosen by each child. Multiple television sets in strategic locations are also useful for keeping children entertained whilst waiting for or during studies. A ceiling mounted television with low sound can help keep a very fretful child quiet and motionless during US studies. During MR imaging music should be provided either using earplugs or headphones and if a CD player is available children can be encouraged to bring their own music to play during the examination.

Injections
Many radiological examinations require an intravenous (IV) injection, either for administration of contrast medium or for sedation. Children with cancer frequently undergo multiple IV injections during the course of treatment and investigation and many of these injections consist of cytotoxic materials which make them feel extremely unwell. Hence these children may develop needle phobia which renders the whole diagnostic examination more difficult than in adults. However, with the assistance of staff experienced in gaining IV access in children, the procedure can be performed in a calm and controlled environment. Nevertheless some children are terrified at the prospect of having an injection, usually having had multiple painful injections in the past and therefore these injections should be given in a private room with relative sound proofing as the sound of crying is likely to make other children apprehensive.

The use of a local anesthetic cream prior to an injection may help to reduce discomfort of needle puncture and in some departments acupuncture has been reported to be effective in reducing chemotherapy side effects (1). A butterfly needle system should be used because the flexible tube reduces the risk of displacement of the needle as a result of sudden movement. If injection speed is not important for the particular study, a very small needle of 23 to 27 French Gauge can be used.

By working closely with the pediatric oncology team a schedule of procedures can be planned for the day and in order to avoid multiple injections on the same day, it may be appropriate to insert an IV cannula instead of a butterfly needle.

Cancer treatment reduces children's immunity and hence great care should be taken to avoid any possible risk of infection. In particular if an IV access long line has been inserted and is to be used for IV contrast administration or sedation then strict adherence to hospital protocols must be maintained.

Sedation and General Anesthesia for Imaging
Some children are uncooperative either due to their young age or sometimes due to medical or developmental factors. General anesthesia (GA) is most often required for MR imaging examinations between the ages of one and seven years, because the long claustrophobic tube is frightening, the examination takes a long time and the procedure is noisy. Furthermore diagnostic quality is impaired because movement degrades the images. Multidetector CT (MDCT) is much less of a problem than MR imaging studies and using 64-slice MDCT sedation is only required occasionally. Nuclear medicine studies also sometimes require sedation.

If sedation or GA is to be performed for an investigation it is imperative to check with the referring physicians whether any other

tests need to be performed so that these can be combined with the radiological investigation and carried out under the same anesthetic procedure. These other tests could include insertion of a long-line, biopsy, bone marrow aspiration, lumbar puncture, or even just a venepuncture. GA will require close co-operation between the pediatric anesthetist and MR imaging scheduler. It is best to organize dedicated general anesthesia days. This makes scheduling for both the anesthetist and for radiologists much simpler and safer.

In the design of an MR imaging or CT suite an induction and recovery area should be incorporated so that dedicated nurses or doctors can easily monitor these patients. Radiographers should not be responsible for monitoring sedation, firstly because they are unlikely to be specifically trained in resuscitation of children and secondly because their expertise should be dedicated to achieving a high quality diagnostic imaging study.

Sedation generally works well for infants under one year of age and for selected children of an older age. There are three stages of sedation—mild, moderate, and deep.

- Mild sedation that does not depress respiratory function, like Chloral
- A typical moderate sedation agent is Midazolam
- Deep sedation should only be performed by an anesthetist

Mild and moderate sedation should be performed only by those who are fully trained to give these agents. Pediatric anesthetists with input from radiologists and nursing staff should develop strict hospital protocols for sedation during radiology procedures. There should be an accreditation process for those staff (doctors and nurses) who are given the responsibility to give and monitor sedation.

Heat Loss

Young children, particularly infants, lose heat very quickly and significant medical problems can arise if they are not kept warm. Blankets and commercially available heating devices should be used. There are special MR imaging coils which mimic an incubator that should be used if available.

Equipment and Radiation

Imaging equipment is manufactured by a relatively small number of companies and is primarily designed for adults. Hence when purchasing any equipment, it is particularly important to consider pediatric applications.

X-rays are more harmful to children than adults because they are rapidly growing and dividing cells are the most sensitive to radiation damage (2,3). Radiation should be avoided unless absolutely necessary; therefore equipment such as US and MR imaging are the preferred modalities.

Ultrasound

US is a safe modality using high frequency sound only. It is excellent for the initial evaluation of a palpable mass in the soft tissues or abdomen and can also be used for routine screening of the abdomen. Follow-up of some tumors is also possible with US but the technique is not as reproducible as CT or MR imaging. In the chest, US has limited value. Also, since most brain tumors arise after fontanelles have closed the technique is of little value in children with suspected intracranial malignancy. US equipment, when purchased, should include pediatric transducers. These include very high frequency linear and sector transducers. These achieve the best spatial and contrast resolution for the small anatomical structures in children. Color Doppler and spectral Doppler are essential. All equipment should be cleaned scrupulously between patients to prevent cross infection, which is particularly important in these children who are often immunodepressed.

Plain Radiography

Plain radiography gives a low dose of radiation, lower than any other x-ray modality, but is only of value in musculoskeletal, chest, and abdominal tumors. It is important to keep the radiation dose for each study as low as possible, tailoring the dosage to the size of the child. Adult doses should never be used. Using computed radiography (CR) it is possible to reduce dosage significantly for some examinations, for example a scoliosis series, as image quality to assess fine detail is less important in such examinations.

Nuclear Medicine

Nuclear medicine, particularly utilizing bone scans, is very useful for the investigation, staging, and follow-up of many tumors (Fig. 36.1). Acquisition time is relatively long so some patients will need sedation and providing television programs or music can decrease the need for sedation. High-resolution collimation must be available. Radiation doses should be tailored to the size of the child.

Positron emission tomography (FDG PET) is increasingly being used in pediatric oncology, and is especially useful in detecting

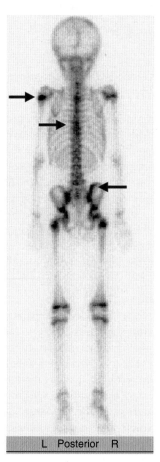

Figure 36.1 Seven-year-old boy with neuroblastoma. Posterior image taken during Tc-99m methylenediphosphonate bone scan shows the presence of multiple hot spots in the spine, left upper humerus, and medial aspect of the right iliac wing (arrows) due to bone metastases.

occult disease in a variety of tumors. This equipment is the most expensive of all radiology equipment and a high radiation dose is given. The cost of studies and limited availability make this a less used modality than CT or MR imaging, but in selected cases, it can be extremely useful, providing unique information.

Computed Tomography

The need for sedation and general anesthesia is considerably reduced using CT scanners with a fast acquisition time and therefore these are recommended for all pediatric examinations.

There is increased concern in the literature of the risks of CT radiation in children (2–5). Children, as explained above, are much more sensitive to radiation and cancer induction and/or cancer mortality in later life. Hence the benefit of the examination must always be compared to the risks. In cancer patients requiring multiple examinations, the risk increases in a linear fashion to the radiation dose. Estimates of carcinogenesis resulting in death are possibly as high as one in 1000 CTs. Dose reduction can be achieved by all of the above methods as well as changing the scan parameters, reducing mAs and kVp according to patient weight and altering slice thickness or scan pitch (4,5).

Adult radiation doses and settings should never be used in children and each study should be tailored to get the maximum information with the least radiation, the ALARA principle (as low as reasonably achievable) (4,5). Detector systems and scan protocols should be chosen to minimize radiation dose (4,5). Ideally a multidetector 64-slice CT scanner with dose modulation technology should be used as this can give the lowest doses. To screen sensitive areas such as breast and thyroids, shields can be used. Taking the scout view with the x-ray tube underneath the patient will reduce the radiation dose to exposed organs as well.

Magnetic Resonance Imaging

MR imaging is increasingly used for diagnosis and follow-up of cancer as there is no ionizing radiation, but the cost of studies and general availability of MR imaging remain important considerations. MR imaging is especially good for some specific tumors, particularly brain, spinal, bone and soft tissue tumours (Fig. 36.2).

Of all imaging equipment MR is one of the most daunting for a child. Hence many younger children (usually aged between one and seven years) will require GA or moderate sedation. To reduce the need for sedation or GA, a thorough age appropriate discussion is necessary and a mock-up of the scanner demonstrated on a teddy bear or similar toy can be most helpful in alleviating fears. Tapes of the very loud tapping noise that occurs during the scan process will significantly improve acceptance by the child. Scan sequences should be chosen for the shortest time possible that will provide the necessary information. Cardiac and respiratory gating may be necessary.

Fluoroscopy

Fluoroscopy is a rarely required. If needed for any purpose, low dose techniques, including using the last image hold, pulsed fluoroscopy, rare earth filters, and short fluoroscopy time without a grid, will very significantly reduce radiation dose. The tabletop should be covered with lead except for the area to be examined. This reduces radiation to the patient and reduces scatter radiation to the operators. Preferably, a nurse should be in the room with the patient and the radiologist in addition to a radiographer.

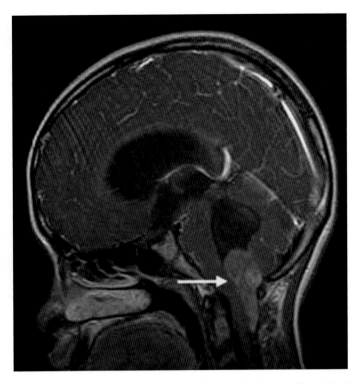

Figure 36.2 Ten-year-old boy presenting with headache. Sagittal T1-weighted post-contrast MR image shows the presence of a tumor (arrow) in the fourth ventricle causing hydrocephalus. Histologically this was an ependymoma.

Staff

Training and motivation of all staff is extremely important. Empathetic radiographers, nurses, reception staff, and radiologists can reduce anxiety of the patient and parents tremendously thus enabling optimum image quality to be obtained during subsequent imaging studies. To successfully image a child requires special commitment and those who show aptitude should be selected to be part of the team who perform all pediatric studies in a mixed adult and children's department.

Key Points: General Considerations

■ Radiological work-up is best performed in pediatric departments that deal exclusively or extensively with children and staff are experienced in cancer imaging

■ Fully trained pediatric imaging staff are essential for achieving successful imaging studies

■ Facilities for pediatric imaging should be designed to provide a homely child-friendly ambience

■ Strict protocols for sedation should be in place, prepared in conjunction with the anesthesia department

■ US is an excellent modality for initial investigation of suspected malignancy

■ Dose reduction techniques are critically important, particularly for examining children with CT who will require multiple studies during follow-up. 64-slice MDCT offers the most effective dose reduction technology

■ MR imaging is indicated for brain and spinal tumors as well as for bone and soft tissue tumors

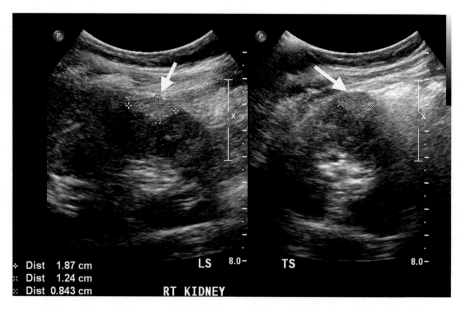

Figure 36.3 Ten-year-old girl with Beckwith-Weidemann syndrome on six-monthly ultrasound follow-up for nephroblastomatosis of the right (RT) kidney (arrows) shown on longitudinal (LS) and transverse (TS) sections. This echogenic lesion in the right kidney has been stable for several years.

ROLE OF IMAGING

The role of imaging in pediatric cancer management includes:

- Screening
- Diagnosis
- Staging
- Follow-up

Screening

There are a few conditions in children that predispose or are associated with higher risks of cancer. Examples include:

- Genitourinary malformations (renal ectopia, ureteral duplication, renal hypoplasia, horseshoe kidney, and cryptorchidism), sporadic aniridia (Wilms' tumors)
- Denys-Drash syndrome (male pseudohermaphroditism and nephritis) (Wilms' tumor)
- Beckwith-Weidemann syndrome (Fig. 36.3) (embryonal tumors such as Wilms' tumor, hepatoblastoma, neuroblastoma, rhabdomyosarcoma)

There are also some other rare syndromes, such as Perlman syndrome (fetal gigantism, hypotonia, and multiple congenital abnormalities) and overgrowth syndromes such as congenital hypertrophy and WAGR syndrome (Wilms' tumor, sporadic aniridia, genital malformations, and retardation) which all have a significantly increased incidence of Wilms' tumors (6). Hence regular three- to six-monthly US studies can be used to screen the kidneys. Unless there is such a predisposing risk, screening is not otherwise indicated.

Diagnosis

In most instances the radiologist is among the first to diagnose a tumor. Although the final diagnosis will be histological, many pediatric tumors have sufficiently characteristic appearances to allow a preliminary diagnosis to be made. In the initial investigation plain films followed by US and/or CT can be very helpful. A plain film of the musculoskeletal system is useful if the suspected tumor is peripheral (Fig. 36.4). A chest radiograph should be performed in all patients suspected of having a malignant tumor.

US is the second modality of choice to investigate the abdomen and soft tissues. Once a malignant tumor is suspected on initial investigation, a CT or MR imaging study is essential. CT is most useful in the thorax. In the abdomen both CT and MR imaging can be used, depending on location and type of tumor suspected. The aim of the diagnostic work-up is to obtain the maximum amount of information with the minimum number of tests and the least radiation dosage.

MR imaging is the modality of choice for examination of:

- Brain
- Spine
- Pelvis
- Bone
- Soft tissues

Investigation is best performed in the center where the tumor is to be treated. Biopsies should never be performed before the full imaging work-up has been obtained. For example, if a biopsy of a suspected osteogenic sarcoma of the knee is performed prior to an MR imaging examination it will not be possible to determine whether the lesion is operable or inoperable because the biopsy will have disturbed the tumor margins.

Some tumors have a characteristic appearance. For example, the two most common tumors in the abdomen, neuroblastoma, and Wilms' tumor can usually be differentiated on imaging alone (see chaps. 37 and 38). For example, a neuroblastoma surrounds blood

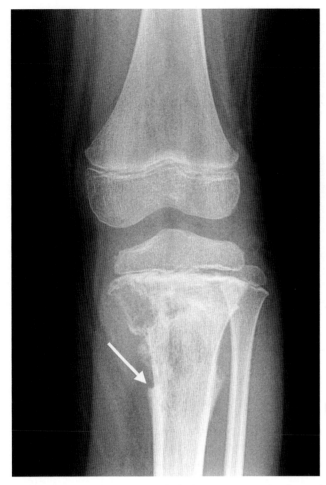

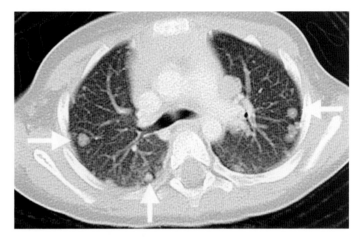

Figure 36.5 One-year-old girl with lung metastases from hepatoblastoma. Axial CT of the chest, at the level of the carina, shows multiple lung metastases in both lungs (arrows).

Figure 36.4 Six-year-old boy with a left tibial osteosarcoma. The plain radiograph of the left tibia shows the presence of an ill-defined destructive lesion in the metaphysis of the tibia. There is periosteal new bone formation with lifting of the periosteum giving the typical appearance of "Codman's triangle" (arrow). These features are highly suggestive of osteosarcoma, which was proven histologically.

vessels whereas a Wilms' tumor displaces them. This is readily demonstrated on US, CT, and MR imaging.

Biopsy

Biopsy is required for almost all tumors, except some inaccessible brain tumors. The surgeon often performs the biopsy, but increasingly radiologists are involved in image guidance or undertake the entire procedure.

If there is more than one tumor, then the most accessible is biopsied. It is essential that the specimens obtained are of sufficient size and quality for the pathologist to undertake accurate cytogenetic and immuno-histochemistry studies, that appropriate storage medium is used and that arrangements are in place for rapid transport of tissue samples to the pathology department. Thus close liaison with the pathology department is essential.

If the radiologist is performing the biopsy then close liaison with the surgeon is essential to ensure that the region biopsied and the path of the biopsy needle will not interfere with subsequent

surgical management. Imaging should be performed prior to biopsy when possible in order to demarcate the tumor as accurately as possible and to define its local extent.

Staging

The order of frequency of pediatric tumors is as follows:

- Leukemia
- Central nervous system
- Lymphoma
- Neuroblastoma
- Renal tumor
- Soft tissue sarcoma
- Bone tumors
- Others

Once a tumor has been detected, localized, and delineated, local and distant spread needs to be assessed. CT is the modality of choice for detecting lung metastases (e.g., Wilms' tumor) (Fig. 36.5) but is unnecessary for some tumors as lung metastases are very rare, for example, neuroblastoma.

Follow-up

Imaging is an essential part of follow-up and should be performed on a regular basis, working closely with the team providing the patient's care which includes the oncologist, surgeon, pathologist, and the patient's family. Co-ordination by this team approach gives the best healthcare delivery to the child.

The imaging modality used should be the one which provides the necessary information with the least discomfort and risk to the child. This will vary according to the type and location of each tumor. Ideally the examination should be performed in the same hospital for each study and where treatment is being given, as this will facilitate good reproducible comparison between studies to be made by the team that knows the patient well (Fig. 36.6).

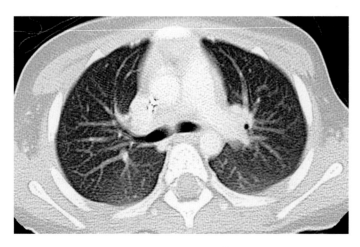

Figure 36.6 Same patient as in Figure 36.5 (hepatoblastoma with lung metastases). Axial CT of the chest, at the level of the carina, performed one year later after resection of the primary tumor, and chemotherapy shows complete resolution of the lung metastases.

Key Points: Role of Imaging

- Screening should only be performed for children with congenital syndromes which predispose to malignancy such as genitourinary malformations
- Plain films and US provide initial imaging modalities of choice in a child with suspected malignancy
- Most pediatric tumors have sufficient characteristic appearances to permit an initial diagnosis although histological diagnosis is essential
- CT and MR imaging are required for further evaluation of suspected malignancy and for staging
- Imaging should be performed prior to biopsy when possible in order to demarcate the tumor as accurately as possible
- The modality used for follow-up should be the one which will provide the necessary information with the lowest risk to the child and the least discomfort

INVESTIGATION OF THERAPEUTIC COMPLICATIONS

The short-term effect of chemotherapy and long-term effects of radiation can result in a number of serious and significant life-threatening complications which may be acute or chronic. Both radiation and chemotherapeutic agents can cause acute complications. These are related to depression of the hematological system, particularly with respect to the production of platelets and white blood cells. Thus hemorrhage and infection as well as other immunological abnormalities can occur. Strict attention to hygiene while imaging, cleaning of patient areas and separating those who are most at risk from others, is essential to prevent cross infections.

Acute Complications

Infection

Immunosuppression associated with both chemotherapy and radiation renders these children susceptible to all types of infection,

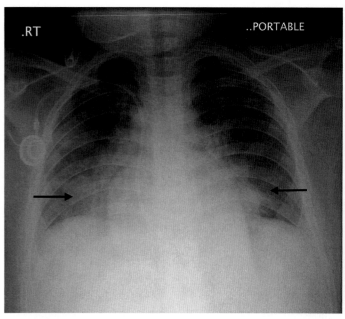

Figure 36.7 Eight-year-old girl with acute myeloid leukemia and shortness of breath. The chest radiograph shows the presence of bilateral lower lobe infiltrates (arrows). A porta-cath is noted in situ. Microbiological studies revealed infection due to cytomegalovirus. *Abbreviations*: RT, right side

but especially to opportunistic infections. Common sense hygiene and meticulous attention to detail, such as well-rehearsed hand washing routines between each patient, can lead to a significant reduction in this complication. As far as possible during this period they should be kept away from other patients with known infections, including staff that have common colds or other minor ailments.

Various types of infection can occur with the commonest being pneumonia (Fig. 36.7). The most frequent pneumonias are viral or bacterial but opportunistic infection also commonly occurs. The opportunistic infections most frequently seen include fungal disease, tuberculosis, mycoplasma, and pneumocystis carinii pneumonia (7–12). Although, their imaging features have been described elsewhere, the causative organism cannot be accurately diagnosed by imaging alone (7–12). In children with AIDS, atypical tuberculosis may occur giving rise to lymphadenopathy (11). In the early stages the diagnosis is difficult to make but later pulmonary infiltrates develop and these are best visualized by high resolution CT (HRCT) (10,13,14). Pulmonary infiltrates may appear as mass-like lesions and therefore may be confused with metastases and furthermore lymphadenopathy due to tuberculosis may be ascribed to metastatic disease. Clinical correlation and comparison with previous CT studies will help to distinguish infection from relapsing or progressive cancer. The diagnosis of tuberculosis should be confirmed by bronchial lavage or biopsy.

Fungal infection should be suspected in the febrile neutropenic patient (7–10). Fungal infection often gives rise to unusual radiological appearances which may resemble lung metastases. Correlation with previous chest radiographs or CT as well as clinical correlation usually make this an easy differentiation due to the typical appearance and speed of change of infective processes. A common fungus is

aspergillus, which can give arise to mycetoma (fungus ball) or may be frankly invasive, especially in the severely immunocompromised. Wedge-shaped areas of consolidation may be seen.

Infection resulting from long intravenous lines is a frequent cause of pyrexia in neutropenic children. When an infusion is given through an infected line, clumps of bacteria can become septic emboli which carry the risk of causing bacterial endocarditis. The emboli can also cause foci of infection in other organs, such as the liver, kidneys, and brain.

Other Complications of Intravenous Lines

Intravenous lines may be misplaced, may migrate to the wrong position, become thrombosed or blocked by debris or even fracture. Great care should be taken in assessing all lines. A single frontal radiograph may be misleading. Where the line appears in perfect position on one projection, for example often overlying the region of the superior vena cava, a lateral view may show that it is significantly displaced. The radiologist is often the first to realize there is a line problem either on reporting a follow-up chest radiograph (if the line is significantly displaced), or when infusing the line by discovering a resistance to flow. Such an occurrence should be treated extremely seriously and immediate investigation should be undertaken with radiography and, if necessary, linography (injection of a small amount of contrast fluoroscopically). If some contrast can be injected then a linogram is the most useful test, as it will accurately show the correct site of the problem. If the line is completely blocked then a decision, based on the radiographic findings, needs to be made as to whether it can be safely removed. If there is any question that it has perforated a blood vessel or the heart then further evaluation, usually by CT, is necessary to accurately localize the tip to determine whether it is safe to withdraw the line blindly or whether an operation is indicated.

Occasionally a thrombosis develops which extends beyond the line itself into the superior vena cava. Depending on the exact site of the obstruction, superior vena cava syndrome may ensue with associated edema of the upper limb and neck. A Doppler study may exclude this serious complication or occasionally venography, MR venography (MRV), and/or MR angiography (MRA) is necessary to demonstrate the anatomy of the vessels, as well as the site and extent of obstruction (15,16).

Hemorrhagic Complications

Hemorrhage is a rare complication of treatment even though the platelet count during treatment is often low. Plain films are useful for determining the presence of hemorrhage in the chest. US, CT, and MR imaging are the modalities of choice for investigating suspected hemorrhage in the abdomen, pelvis, soft tissues, and brain. Unenhanced studies should be performed because acute hemorrhage, which has a high attenuation on CT and a high signal intensity on T1-weighted MR imaging, may be masked by parenchymal enhancement.

Gastrointestinal Complications

The three main complications of the gastrointestinal tract are:

- Neutropenic enterocolitis
- Pseudomembranous colitis
- Systemic disease - graft versus host disease

Neutropenic Enterocolitis

Neutropenic enterocolitis primarily affects the cecum. In Greek the cecum is called the typhlos and hence neutropenic enterocolitis is often referred to as typhlitis. It occurs in children who are immunosuppressed, irrespective of the cause, but is most commonly seen in children who have been treated with chemotherapy for leukemia (17). The classical presentation is that of abdominal pain, pyrexia, and bloody diarrhea. However the presentation may be variable with one or more of these symptoms.

Plain radiography is the initial investigation of choice. In children over one year of age there should always be some fecal shadowing in the right lower quadrant. Lack of fecal shadowing in a patient, who is eating normally and is not taking aperients, is abnormal. Hence in the correct clinical setting, absence of any fecal shadowing in the right lower quadrant should alert the radiologist to the possibility of neutropenic enterocolitis. Lack of right iliac fecal bowel gas, thickened bowel, thumb-printing, or evidence of pneumatosis coli are diagnostic. There may be evidence of generalized paralytic ileus secondary to the inflammation. Perforation is rare.

US is a very useful modality, especially as these very sick patients may need portable studies (18). The US findings include bowel wall thickening and rigidity with increased blood flow on color Doppler. Free fluid is often present. US may identify a localized perforation or an abscess. CT is occasionally indicated for further evaluation of complex cases (Fig. 36.8) (19,20). Rarely intussusceptions can occur.

Pseudomembranous Colitis

Pseudomembranous colitis is less common than neutropenic enterocolitis. It is due to overgrowth with *Clostridium difficile* and its toxin and is secondary to antibiotic therapy (21). The radiographic, US, and CT findings are similar to neutropenic enterocolitis, although with a higher risk of pneumatosis intestinalis and perforation (21–23).

Systemic Disease—Graft Versus Host Disease

Children who have bone marrow transplantation and who become profoundly neutropenic can suffer an unusual multisystem abnormality, *graft verses host disease (GVHD)*. Usually the

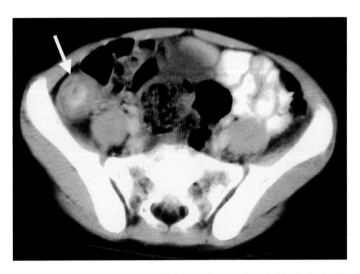

Figure 36.8 Neutropenic 10-year-old boy with acute lymphoblastic leukemia undergoing chemotherapy presenting with right-sided abdominal pain. CT shows a circumferentially thick-walled cecum consistent with neutropenic colitis (arrow).

901

gastrointestinal tract is the most affected region but the liver and skin can also be affected. Treatment is conservative unless perforation or abscess formation occurs. Plain radiography shows a non-specific dilatation and generalized bowel wall thickening, confirmed on sonography (24). Pneumatosis intestinalis can also occur (25,26).

Sonography may show the pneumatosis as a circle of increased echogenicity within the bowel wall (27), and color Doppler may show increased blood flow to the bowel. CT or MR imaging are indicated only for investigating complications and will also show bowel wall thickening associated with abnormal contrast enhancement due to increased vascularity of the bowel wall (28–30).

Lung GVHD, presenting with cough, and bronchospasm gives an obstructive pattern with hyperinflation. Very high infiltration leads to a diffuse interstitial pattern and is best confirmed on HRCT (31). Definite diagnosis is made by biopsy.

Key Points: Acute Complications

- Acute complications of chemotherapy and radiotherapy include infection, hemorrhage, and gastrointestinal disorders
- Immunosuppression renders children susceptible to viral, bacterial, and opportunistic infections
- Opportunistic infections are usually due to tuberculosis, fungal, or *Pneumocystis carinii*
- Long IV lines may become infected, misplaced, may migrate, or become thrombosed. Occasionally a line may fracture
- Hemorrhage is a rare complication of therapy
- Neutropenic enterocolitis most commonly occurs in immunosuppressed children with leukemia
- Pseudomembranous colitis is secondary to *C. difficile*
- Graft versus host disease most commonly affects the gastrointestinal tract but is a multisystem disorder

---

Chronic Complications

Increasingly children are being cured of their primary cancer and more long-term complications are appearing (32–34). Complications are secondary to irradiation radiotherapy or from chemotherapy (32,35). Following radiotherapy the anatomical site of treatment will determine the complication which in turn will determine the imaging to be performed.

Chronic complications from therapy affect primarily the following regions:

- Central nervous system
- Musculoskeletal system
- Heart
- Lungs
- Gonads
- Thyroid
- Kidneys

Central Nervous System

Generalized long-term damage to the brain can be caused by radiotherapy and chemotherapy, even in the absence of treatment of a primary brain tumor. This occurs particularly in children with leukemia and leads to cerebral atrophy with loss of cerebral

tissue. There is a compensatory non-obstructive dilatation of the ventricles (see chap. 31).

Sometimes functional neuroendocrine defects can occur following treatment of a primary brain tumor, especially if the tumor originated close to the pituitary gland. Cranial MR imaging is the modality of choice for assessing these complications.

Musculoskeletal System

Therapeutic doses of radiation in the primary beam cause damage to a growing skeleton. Thus unless the whole spine is irradiated, a short segment scoliosis will occur due to the lack of growth of the irradiated side of the spine. The face may also become asymmetrical following radiotherapy for craniofacial tumors.

Plain films should be undertaken initially and these will demonstrate most abnormalities. Limb length can be measured by a scanogram of the hips, knees, and the ankles using a low dose technique or by three-foot plain film images.

Bone age assessments can be useful when there are growth abnormalities (36). If surgery or further detail of any osseous deformity is required, 3D reconstructions from an unenhanced CT are necessary.

Heart

Radiotherapy can result in a constrictive pericarditis (32). This only occurs following mediastinal radiation, but this type of therapy is rarely used today. Cardiac function can be disturbed by chemotherapy with impairment of left ventricular function. Echocardiography is the best initial investigation.

Lungs

Both radiotherapy and chemotherapy can cause pneumonitis and fibrosis which is best demonstrated on HRCT.

Gonadal Effects

Generalized growth failure can also be a result of radiation of the gonads or as a result of chemotherapy. Bone age assessments can be useful for assessment of gonadal failure (36). Infertility and early menopause may result (37). Boys appear to be more likely to be affected than girls and may present with small testes and elevated gonadotrophins.

Thyroid

The thyroid is sensitive to irradiation and hence can be damaged with resulting dysfunction. In the long term, this can lead to palpable nodularity that is best evaluated by US.

Kidneys

Acute or chronic nephrotoxicity can occur and may result in deteriorating renal function or hypertension. Hypertension should be investigated initially with Doppler sonography to exclude renal artery stenosis. Further evaluation is done with Captopril reno-graphy, MRA or angiography. If a major vessel stenosis is diagnosed then angioplasty can be performed. Radiotherapy and some chemotherapy agents can cause radiation cystitis resulting in bladder wall thickening and a small volume bladder, best evaluated by US.

Key Points: Chronic Complications

- Long-term brain injury can result from both radiotherapy to the brain and from systemic chemotherapy, especially in leukemia
- Skeletal growth failure following radiotherapy leads to asymmetric growth. This complication should be taken into account when treating areas of the skeleton
- Radiotherapy and chemotherapy may cause lung pneumonitis and fibrosis
- Gonadal failure is more common in boys than girls and may result from radiotherapy or chemotherapy
- Renal impairment may result from chemotherapy, and radiation cystitis may result in a small fibrosed bladder

Summary

- Ideally children with cancer should be investigated and treated in a specialist department or unit
- Special equipment which improves the ambience of the surroundings should be available for pediatric examinations
- Cancer treatment reduces a child's immunity and therefore great care should be taken to avoid unnecessary infection when administering IV contrast medium
- General anesthesia is usually required for MR examinations between the ages of one and seven years
- Children are more sensitive to the harmful effects of radiation than adults
- US is an excellent method for the initial investigation of a palpable mass
- Using CT techniques to reduce radiation dose is critically important for those children who will expect to undergo multiple follow-up studies
- MR imaging is the modality of choice for investigation of tumors of the brain and spine, and for bone and soft tissue tumors
- The imaging modality used for follow-up should be the one which will provide the necessary information with the lowest risk to the child and the least discomfort
- Acute complications of cancer therapy include infection, hemorrhage, and neutropenic enterocolitis
- Chronic complications of radiotherapy depend on the anatomical area irradiated and the disturbed function of adjacent structures and organs

REFERENCES

1. Reindl TK , Geilen W, Hartmann R, et al. Acupuncture against chemotherapy-induced nausea and vomiting in pediatric oncology. Interim results of a multicenter crossover study. Supportive Care Cancer 2006; 14: 172–6.
2. Brenner DJ, Elliston CD, Hall EJ, Berdon WE. Estimated risks of radiation induced fatal cancer from pediatric CT. AJR Am J Roentgenol 2002; 176: 289–96.
3. Paterson A, Frush DP, Donnelly LF. Helical CT of the body: are settings adjusted for paediatric patients? AJR Am J Roentgenol 2002; 176: 297–301.
4. Donnelly LF, Emery KH, Body AS, et al. Minimising radiation dose for pediatric body applications of single-detector helical CT: Strategies at a large children's hospital. AJR Am J Roentgenol 2002; 176: 303–6.
5. Frush DP. Pediatric CT: practical approach to diminish the radiation dose. Pediatr Radiol 2002; 32: 714–17.
6. Babyn PS, Seigel MJ. Chapter 9: The kidney and ureter. In: Seigel MJ, ed. Pediatric Body CT, 2nd edn. Philadelphia: Lippincott Williams & Wilkins, 2007, 297.
7. Markowitz RI, Kramer SS. The spectrum of pulmonary infection in the immunocompromised child. Sem Roentgenol 2000; 2: 171–80.
8. Jeanes AC, Owens CM. Chest imaging in the immunocompromised child. Pediatr Respir Rev 2002; 3: 59–69.
9. Donnelly LF. CT of Acute pulmonary infection/trauma. In: Lucaya J, Strife JL, eds. Pediatric Chest Imaging. Chest Imaging in Infants and Children. Berlin Heidelberg: Springer-Verlag, 2002: 113–27.
10. Hiorns MP, Screaton NJ, Müller NL. Acute lung disease in the immunocompromised host. Radiol Clin North Am 2001; 39: 1137–51.
11. Pursner M, Hallet JO, Berdon WE. Imaging features of Mycobacterium avium-intracellulae complex (MAC) in children. Pediatr Radiol 2000; 30: 426–9.
12. John SD, Ramanathan J, Swischuk LE. Spectrum of clinical and radiographic findings in pediatric Mycoplasma pneumonia. Radiographics 2001; 21: 121–31.
13. Kim CK, Chung CY, Kim JS, et al. Late abnormal findings on high resolution computed tomography after Mycoplasma pneumonia. Pediatrics 2000; 105: 372–8.
14. Leong MA, Nachajon R, Ruchelli E, Allen JL. Bronchiolitis obliterans due to Mycoplasma pneumonia. Pediatr Pulmonol 1997; 23: 375–81.
15. Shinde TS, Lee VS, Rofsky NM, et al. Three-dimensional Gadolinium enhanced MR venographic evaluation of patency of central veins in the thorax: initial experience. Radiology 1999; 213: 555–60.
16. Rose SC, Gomes AS, Yoon HC. MR angiography for mapping potential central venous access sites in patients with advanced venous occlusive disease. AJR Am J Roentgenol 1996; 166: 1181–7.
17. Baerg J, Murphy JJ, Anderson R, Magee JF. Neutropenic enteropathy: a 10-year review. J Pediatr Surg 1999; 34: 1068–71.
18. Cartoni C, Dragoni F, Micozzi A, et al. Neutropenic enterocolitis in patients with acute leukaemia: prognostic significance of bowel wall thickening detected by ultrasonography. J Clin Oncol 2001; 19: 756–61.
19. Donnelly LF. CT Imaging of immunocompromised children with acute abdominal symptoms. AJR Am J Roentgenol 1996; 167: 909–13.
20. Horton KM, Corl FM, Fishman EK. CT evaluation of the colon: inflammatory disease. Radiographics 2000;20: 399–418.
21. Gillett PM, Russell RK, Wilson DC, Thomas AE. C. difficile induced pneumatosis intestinalis in a neutropenic child. Archives Dis Child 2002; 87: 85.
22. Ros PR, Buetow PC, Pantograg-Brown L, et al. Pseudomembranous colitis. Radiology 1996; 198: 1–9.

23. Zamora S, Coppes MJ, Scott RB, Mueller DL. Clostridium difficile, Pseudomembranous enterocolitis: striking CT and sonographic features in a pediatric patient. Eur J Radiol 1996; 23: 104–6.

24. Haber HP, Schlegel PG, Dette S, et al. Intestinal acute graft-versus-host disease: findings on sonography. AJR Am J Roentgenol 2000; 174: 118–20.

25. Jones B, Wall SD. Gastrointestinal disease in the immunocompromised host. Radiol Clin North Am 1992; 30: 555–77.

26. Yeager AM, Kanof ME, Kramer SS, et al. Pneumatosis intestinalis in children after allogenic bone marrow transplantation. Pediatr Radiol 1987; 17: 18–22.

27. Goske MJ, Goldblum JR, Applegate KE, et al. The "circle sign": a new sonographic sign of Pneumatosis intestinalis—clinical, pathologic and experimental findings. Pediatr Radiol 1999; 29: 530–5.

28. Donnelly LF, Morris CL. Acute graft-versus-host disease in children: abdominal CT findings. Radiology 1996; 199: 265–8.

29. Donnelly LF. CT imaging of immunocompromised children with acute symptoms. AJR Am J Roentgenol 1996; 167: 909–13.

30. Mentzel H-J, Kentouche K, Kosmehl H, et al. US and MRI of gastrointestinal graft-versus-host disease. Pediatr Radiol 2002; 32: 195–8.

31. Armstrong P, Dee P. AIDS and other forms of immunocompromise. In: Armstrong P, Wilson AG, Dee P, Hansell DM, eds. Imaging of Diseases of the Chest. London: Mosby, 2000: 255–304.

32. Malpas JS. Clinical review: long-term effects of treatment of childhood malignancy. Clin Radiol 1996; 51: 466–74.

33. Schwartz CL. Long-term survivors of childhood cancer: the late effects of therapy. The Oncologist 1999; 4: 45–54.

34. Friedman DL, Meadows AT. Late effects of childhood cancer therapy. Pediatr Clin North Am 2002; 49: 1083–106.

35. Lipscultz SE, Colan SD, Gelber RD, et al. Late cardiac effects of doxorubicin therapy. New Engl J Med 1991; 324: 808–15.

36. Tanner JM, Whitehouse RH, Marshall WA, et al. In: Assessment of Skeletal Maturity and Prediction of Adult Height (TW2 Method). London: Academic Press, 1975.

37. Byrne J. Infertility and premature menopause in childhood cancer survivors. Medical Pediatric Oncology 1999; 33: 24–28.

37 Wilms' Tumor and Associated Neoplasms of the Kidney
Rebecca Leung and Kieran McHugh

WILMS' TUMOR

Incidence and Epidemiology

Wilms' tumor is one of the most common primary malignant tumors of childhood and also the most common renal tumor, accounting for 6% of all pediatric malignancy (1,2). It occurs mainly in young children with a mean age at diagnosis of three to four years (2) and 95% are diagnosed by the age of 10 years (1). There is an equal distribution between the sexes (3). In Europe the incidence is 10/1,000,000 per year with approximately 900 cases diagnosed each year (2). The incidence has remained relatively constant and therefore was once considered an "index" tumor of childhood. However, there are variations according to ethnicity, with higher rates reported in the Afro-Caribbean population (9–12/1,000,000) than in Caucasians (6–10/1,000,000) and the lowest rates reported among East-Asians (3/1,000,000) (4). These variations are ethnic rather than geographical, suggesting that environmental factors do not play an important role. The role of environmental exposures *in utero* as a cause of early onset of Wilms' tumor in infancy remains unproven (5).

Genetics and Associated Conditions

Only 2% of patients have a family history of Wilms' tumor (5,6), while 15% of those with Wilms' tumor have associated congenital anomalies (7). The remainder are sporadic. A review of 1905 cases from the National Wilms Tumor Study (NWTS) carried out between 1969 and 1981 (8) revealed that the most common anomalies are cryptorchidism (2.8%), hemihypertrophy (2.5%), and hypospadias (1.8%). Other conditions include horseshoe kidney (9), Fanconi anemia (10,11), Beckwith-Wiedemann syndrome (9,12) (visceromegaly, macroglossia, omphalocele, and hyperinsulinemic hypoglycemia), Denys-Drash syndrome (10,13) (nephropathy, renal failure, and male pseudohermaphrodism), Soto's (8) (cerebral gigantism), Bloom's (8) (immunodeficiency and facial telangiectasia), Perlman (8,10,14) (autosomal recessive overgrowth), and Simpson-Golabi-Behmel (10) (X-linked overgrowth) syndromes. Wilms' tumor is also associated with the sporadic form of aniridia (8,15) (absence of ophthalmic iris), with one-third of patients with sporadic aniridia having Wilms' tumor and 1% of Wilms' tumor patients having aniridia (16). A related condition is the WAGR complex (10,13) (Wilms' tumor, aniridia, genitourinary abnormalities, and mental retardation). Patients with WAGR have a deletion within the short arm of chromosome 11 at band p13 (11p13 deletion) (17). This chromosome was subsequently found to be the location of the WT-suppressor gene (WT1) (18–20). This gene encodes a transcription factor which regulates the expression of growth factors critical to renal and gonadal development. Inactivation of the WT-1 gene gives rise to the unregulated growth of Wilms' tumor. Inactivating point mutations in the WT1 gene occur in the Denys-Drash syndrome (21,22).

Based on tumor specific loss of heterozygosity (LOH), a further WT locus, called WT2 was mapped to chromosome 11p15, which is also shared by Beckwith-Wiedemann syndrome (23,24). Loss of heterozygosity has also been found at chromosomes 1p and 16q (25). LOH at these sites has been associated with anaplastic Wilms' tumor (26) i.e., unfavorable histology, an increased rate of relapse and greater risk of mortality. Results from the fifth National Wilms Tumor Study (NWTS-5) have shown that even in children with favorable histology tumors, LOH on both chromosomes 1p and 16q was correlated with a greater risk of relapse and death (26). Thus LOH at 1p and 16q has been introduced in the United States Children's Oncology Group (COG) protocols as a risk-stratifying molecular marker and affected children will receive augmented therapy (25,26).

Pathology

Macroscopic

The majority of Wilms' tumors are solitary with 7% to 12% occurring multifocally within one kidney and 5% to 7% bilaterally (5,27). Most bilateral tumors present synchronously but 1% to 1.9% present metachronously (5), usually in infants of less than one year who have already been successfully treated for a unilateral tumor and whose resected kidney contained nephrogenic rests.

Typically the tumor is a solid spherical mass that is sharply demarcated from surrounding renal parenchyma by a fibrous pseudocapsule (27). On histological sections they have a gray-white appearance and may have foci of hemorrhage, necrosis, cysts, and rarely calcifications. Wilms' tumor can arise anywhere in the cortex or medulla and may protrude into the calyces and ureter.

Microscopic

Wilms' tumor, or nephroblastoma, is derived from the primitive metanephric blastema and classically consists of three different cell types: blastemal (small round cells), stromal (spindle, myxoid), and epithelial (tubular, glomerular), reflecting different stages of normal renal development. This coexistence of all three cell lines is described as a "triphasic" pattern. The proportion of each cell type may vary between different tumors; some may even be biphasic or monomorphous. The histological pattern is defined by the predominant component, which comprises more than two-thirds of the tumor sample. The histological diversity of these tumors has led to correlations between different histological subtypes and prognosis. For example, triphasic tumors, which lack anaplasia, are regarded as "favorable histology" (28). Approximately 90% of patients have favorable histology (16). Conversely the anaplastic type (hyperchromatic cells with large nuclei and irregular mitotic figures), which accounts for approximately 5% of Wilms' tumor (27) and usually occurs in children over two years (5), defines "unfavorable histology" and is associated with an

increased rate of hematogenous metastasis, poor outcome, and increased rate of recurrence (16,27,29). The presence of anaplasia is so far the strongest indicator of adverse outcome (30) and is judged to be a marker of chemotherapy resistance (29,30). Thus, even when present in low stage tumors, intensive chemotherapy is required. Focal anaplasia carries a better prognosis than diffuse anaplasia (29,30). Clear-cell sarcoma of the kidney and malignant rhabdoid tumor of the kidney were originally believed to be variants of Wilms' tumor and were defined as unfavorable histology. They are now considered to be distinct tumors in their own right and will be discussed below.

Clinical Presentation

The clinical presentation of Wilms' tumor is not tumor specific. The most common presentation is of the incidental discovery of an asymptomatic abdominal mass (83%) (31) typically found by parents whilst bathing or clothing the child. By the time it is discovered therefore, the mass is large. In one series of 130 patients, detection occurred after coincidental minor trauma in 10% of cases (32). Up to about one-third of patients present with a combination of abdominal pain, pyrexia of unknown origin, anorexia, malaise, and vomiting (30). Abdominal pain may be secondary to local distension, intratumoral hemorrhage, or peritoneal rupture. Other presentations include hypertension (seen in up to 25%) (30,33) gross or microscopic hematuria (reported in 10–30%) (7,30,31) which may signify tumor invasion of the renal pelvis (34), coagulopathy (less than 10%) (30,35), and spontaneous intratumoral hemorrhage (8%) (31) which manifests as rapid abdominal enlargement, anemia, hypotension, and fever. Although tumor extends into the renal vein and inferior vena cava in 6% of patients, this is manifest symptomatically in only 50% of these cases (36), typically as hepatomegaly, ascites, or congestive heart failure (37). Invasion of the renal vein or inferior vena cava may also manifest as a varicocele, secondary to obstruction of the spermatic vein (5,37). Paraneoplastic manifestations of Wilms' tumor include acquired von Willebrand disease (reported in up to 8%) (35,38), tumor-induced glomerulonephritis (3), and erythropoietin and hyaluronidase secretion (3,39).

Key Points: General Features

- Wilms' tumor is one of the most common childhood malignancies
- Wilms' tumor is the most common renal tumor of childhood
- Wilms' tumor is predominantly sporadic but is associated with congenital syndromes in 15% of cases
- The most common anomalies associated with Wilms' are cryptorchidism and hemihypertrophy
- The majority of Wilms' tumors are solitary
- Wilms' tumor arises from primitive metanephric blastema and consists of three different cell types
- Over 90% of patients have favorable histology
- The most common presentation is of an asymptomatic abdominal mass
- Some patients present with non specific abdominal pain, pyrexia, and malaise

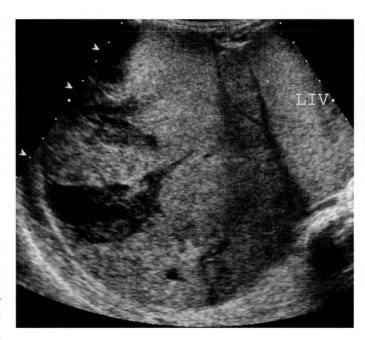

Figure 37.1 Wilms' tumor. Abdominal US shows a large heterogeneous solid mass in the right flank, with a mixture of hyperechoic, hypoechoic, and cystic areas. This is abutting the undersurface of the liver (LIV) and on other images the mass was seen to arise from the right kidney.

Role of Imaging in Diagnosis

Initial investigations include biochemical tests such as a full blood count and differential renal function tests, liver function tests, coagulation tests, and urinalysis. Radiological investigations play a crucial role in diagnosis, staging, surgical planning, and assessment of response to treatment. Due to differences in approach to treatment between the United States and Europe, there are differences in the approach to imaging, particularly in the choice of imaging modality at diagnosis. For example, as the International Society of Paediatric Oncology (SIOP) protocol, mainly used in Europe, is based on pre-operative chemotherapy, imaging is primarily used for diagnosis and initial presumptive staging. Chemotherapy is commenced on this basis only and not on a biopsy result, although biopsy is performed routinely in the United Kingdom. In the National Wilms' Tumor Study (NWTS) protocol primarily used in the United States, surgery precedes radiotherapy and chemotherapy; the role of imaging here is to provide anatomical information to aid surgical planning.

Ultrasound

Ultrasound (US) is first line investigation of an abdominal mass. At US, the renal origin of a Wilms' tumor can be confirmed by distortion of the adjacent renal parenchyma. A large (5–10 cm) predominantly solid spherical mass with heterogeneous echotexture is seen (Fig. 37.1). There are often anechoic areas reflecting hemorrhage, necrosis, or cyst formation (Fig. 37.2). The mass is well demarcated from the adjacent renal parenchyma. Invasion of the renal vein and inferior vena cava occurs in 4% to 10% of cases (40,41); extension into the right atrium occurs rarely. Color Doppler US is able to visualize thrombus within the renal vein and inferior vena cava better than CT and therefore is regarded as the most reliable method of assessment (Fig. 37.2C) (36). On US,

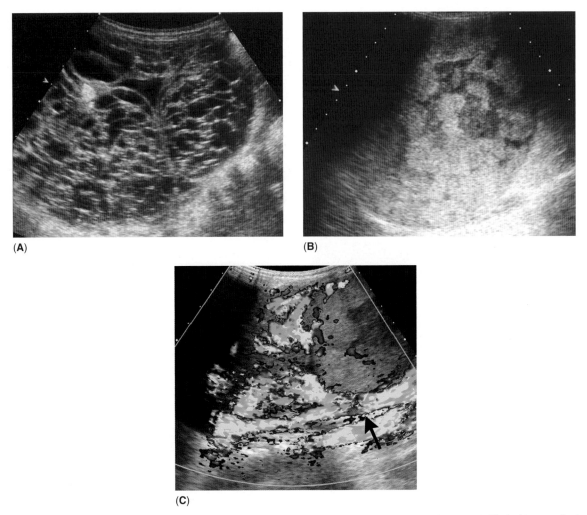

Figure 37.2 (**A**) Abdominal US shows a predominantly cystic Wilms' tumor. The marked cystic nature of this mass makes it unsuitable for biopsy and primary nephrectomy is indicated. (**B**) Wilms' tumor in another patient which appears predominantly hyperechoic with a few hypoechoic foci. These may represent areas of necrosis or hemorrhage. (**C**) Longitudinal color Doppler US in the same patient demonstrates a patent inferior vena cava (arrow) with no evidence of tumor thrombus.

careful evaluation must also be made of the contralateral kidney, liver for metastases, and retroperitoneum for lymphadenopathy (Fig. 37.3B and C).

Computed Tomography and Magnetic Resonance Imaging

Computed tomography (CT) or magnetic resonance (MR) imaging is usually performed to confirm the US findings and to provide additional information about local anatomical relationships between the tumor, the great vessels, and retroperitoneal structures. It also identifies associated anatomical malformations such as a horseshoe kidney (Fig. 37.4). However, it is notable that some European centers only perform US, both for diagnosis and follow-up of these tumors (7).

Metastases occur most commonly in the lungs (10%) (41) followed by local para-aortic lymph nodes and liver (2%) (41). It is extremely rare for brain or bone metastases to occur. CT tends to be used for the initial evaluation of regional invasion, metastases, and lymphadenopathy (Fig. 37.3D) since it is more readily available than MR imaging. Assessment of the lungs for the presence of pulmonary metastases is also better with CT (Fig. 37.5B).

On CT, the primary tumor is usually well-circumscribed with a beak or claw of surrounding renal parenchyma (Fig. 37.6A). It is typically of heterogeneous attenuation, demonstrating a mixture of hemorrhage, necrosis, cysts, and calcification. Fat is rarely seen at diagnosis but may develop within the tumor after treatment. Enhancement following injection of intravenous (IV) contrast medium is seen but the degree of enhancement is much less than that of the adjacent normal renal parenchyma.

If US is deemed inadequate for assessment of treatment response, MR imaging is the preferred imaging modality since CT exposes the child to ionizing radiation; the rationale of this being the ALARA principle, i.e., keeping the radiation dose to the child "as low as reasonably achievable" (42). On MR imaging, the tumor is a well-circumscribed mass demonstrating low signal intensity on T1-weighted sequences and usually a high signal intensity on T2-weighted sequences (Fig. 37.6B and C). The mass enhances heterogeneously but as with CT, much less than normal renal parenchyma. Assessment of vascular invasion may also be made on MR imaging, particularly through the use of magnetic resonance angiography (MRA).

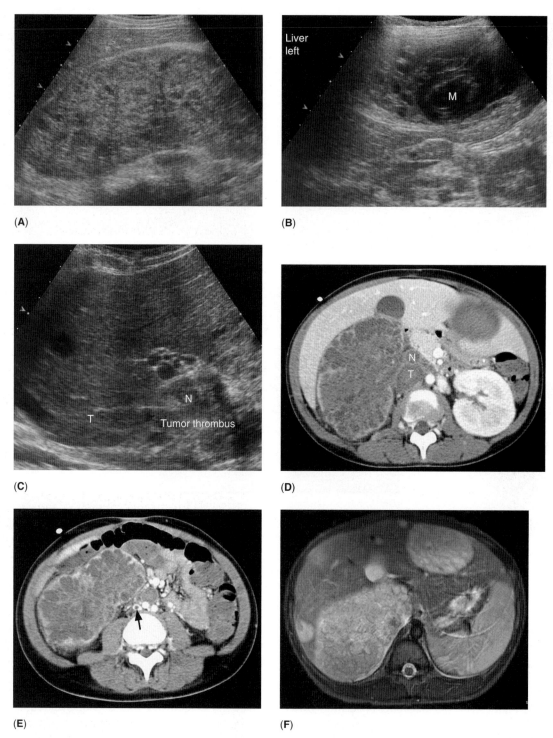

Figure 37.3 Metastatic Wilms' tumor. (**A**) Abdominal US shows a large right sided tumor of heterogeneous echotexture. (**B**) A hepatic metastasis in the same patient (M). (**C**) A para-aortic nodal mass (N) with tumor thrombus (T) in the inferior vena cava. (**D**) Contrast-enhanced CT in the same patient shows the large right-sided Wilms' tumor with adjacent para-aortic lymph node mass (N), tumor thrombus in the IVC (T), and multiple hepatic metastases. (**E**) Same CT at a more inferior level shows the thrombus in the IVC (arrow). (**F**) Axial fat-suppressed T2-weighted MR image demonstrates the hyperintense Wilms' tumor and multiple hepatic metastases.

Differential Diagnoses

Encasement and anterior displacement of the great vessels, the presence of a paravertebral mass or invasion of the spinal canal, and the presence of calcification on CT are more suggestive of neuroblastoma than Wilms' tumor (43).

Other primary renal neoplasms, which may be indistinguishable from Wilms' tumor on imaging, include mesoblastic nephroma (in infants less than one year of age), rhabdoid tumors, clear cell sarcomas of the kidney, and renal cell carcinomas (44). On CT, classically rhabdoid tumors are reported to display a peripheral fluid crescent sign (45) but this is not pathognomonic and is seldom seen. Cases of predominantly cystic Wilms' tumor can be sonographically indistinguishable from multilocular cystic nephroma, a benign tumor.

In infants less than six months of age a renal mass is most likely to be a mesoblastic nephroma (45). In children over seven years of age other renal malignancies start to predominate.

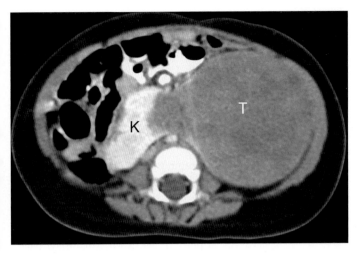

Figure 37.4 Contrast-enhanced CT demonstrating a Wilms' tumor (T) arising from a horseshoe kidney (K).

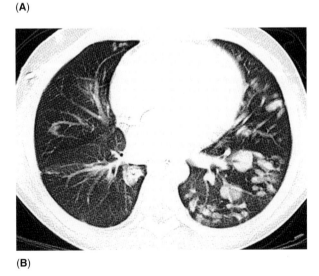

Figure 37.5 Lung metastases in a Wilms' tumor patient. (A) PA chest radiograph shows multiple ill defined opacities, predominantly in the left lower zone. (B) Chest CT in the same patient more clearly demonstrates multiple bilateral lung metastases.

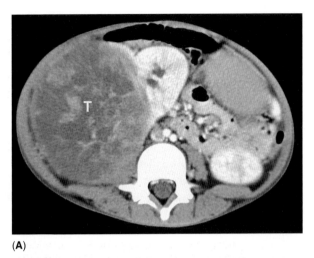

(A)

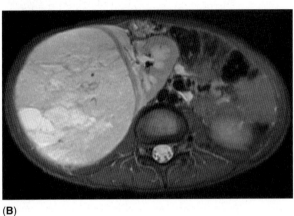

(B)

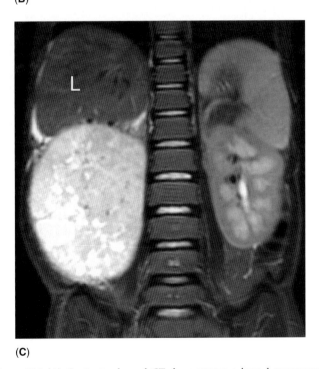

(C)

Figure 37.6 (**A**) Contrast-enhanced CT demonstrates a large heterogeneous mass (T) arising from the right kidney, which is displaced anteromedially with a beak or claw of renal parenchyma surrounding the mass. The mass shows little enhancement compared with the adjacent renal parenchyma. (**B**) Axial fat suppressed T2-weighted MR image at the same level as (**A**) demonstrating a well-circumscribed hyperintense mass with displacement of adjacent renal parenchyma. (**C**) Coronal fat-suppressed T2-weighted MR image shows that the mass is separate from the liver (L). The left kidney is normal in appearance.

909

Chest Imaging in Wilms' Tumor

There has been controversy for many years regarding the best way to image the chest in Wilms' tumor. The traditional method of screening for lung metastases has been a postero-anterior and lateral plain chest radiograph (CXR) (Fig. 37.5A) (46,47). However, chest CT is more sensitive than CXR (48–51) and can detect small volume lesions, termed "CT-only lesions," or "CXR-negative, CT-positive disease," that are not visible on plain films in a small group of patients (48). Chest CT has become the routine method of assessing the lungs for pulmonary lesions in North America. However, since clinical outcomes have traditionally been based on lesions detected by plain radiography (47), there is some uncertainty as to how patients with CT-only lesions should be treated, since not all pulmonary nodules are necessarily metastases (47,48,52). There have been two approaches to treatment of these lesions: one has been to treat by local stage of the primary tumor and "ignore" the pulmonary lesions, the rationale being that small volume lung metastases have a lower tumor burden and require less intensive chemotherapy (51). For a Stage I or II patient this typically involves two-drug chemotherapy and no radiotherapy. The other approach has been to treat as if there were metastases detected by CXR, resulting in the addition of doxorubicin, which is cardiotoxic, and whole lung irradiation. This is based on the premise that the small-volume pulmonary metastases identified on CT lie at the lower end of a continuum and will eventually develop into the much larger lesions visible on plain film (53). Making the assumption that they are metastases may lead to overtreatment in some cases; conversely, there is potential danger in disregarding these CT-only lesions. The general consensus from the NWTS, SIOP, and UKW3 studies has been to advise treatment of CXR-negative, CT-positive lesions as if lung metastases did not exist, on the premise that small volume lung metastases respond well to less chemotherapy. However, there is some limited evidence to suggest that these patients have a higher relapse rate (47,54). Thus, in the latest SIOP study, chest CT is also now recommended (7), but a lesion must measure more than 10 mm to be considered a metastasis, with biopsy confirmation of smaller nodules being usually impractical.

Key Points: Radiological Diagnosis

- US is the first line investigation of an abdominal mass
- US can distinguish between a cystic and a solid mass, assess vascular invasion, and examine the contralateral kidney
- Invasion of the renal vein and inferior vena cava occurs in 4% to 10% of cases
- Color Doppler is the most reliable method of detecting vascular invasion
- CT and MR imaging give additional information about local anatomical relationships between the tumor and adjacent structures and can assess distant spread
- Magnetic resonance angiography (MRA) is useful for surgical planning
- A wide variety of primary renal neoplasms may have identical imaging characteristics to Wilms' tumor
- Chest CT is more sensitive than plain chest radiography in detecting small pulmonary nodules and is now recommended by SIOP

Staging

The most important prognostic factors in Wilms' tumor are the histological grade and stage of the tumor (29). Staging criteria are based on the anatomical extent of the tumor on imaging studies and on both surgical and pathological findings at nephrectomy; biological, genetic, or molecular markers are currently not generally taken into account, although they are expected to be included in the future (30). The staging system has been progressively updated as adverse prognostic features have been identified. There are currently two major staging systems in use: a pre-chemotherapy, surgery based system developed by the National Wilms Tumor Study Group (NWTS), now called the Children's Oncology Group (COG), in the United States, and a post-chemotherapy based system developed by the International Society of Pediatric Oncology (SIOP). The staging protocols are summarized in Tables 37.1 and 37.2. Due to differences in surgical timing, the histological classification and formal staging given by these two protocols is not

Table 37.1 Staging According to SIOP

Stage	Criteria
I	Tumor limited to kidney or surrounded by fibrous pseudocapsule if outside the normal contours of the kidney; tumor does not breach outer surface of renal capsule. Tumor is completely resected
	Tumor may protrude into pelvic system but does not infiltrate their walls
	No involvement of vessels of renal sinus
	Intrarenal vessels may be involved
II	Tumor extends beyond kidney or penetrates through renal capsule and/or through fibrous pseudocapsule into perirenal fat, but is completely resected
	Tumor infiltrates renal sinus and/or invades blood and lymphatics outside renal parenchyma, but is completely resected
	Tumor infiltrates adjacent organs or vena cava, but is completely resected
	Surgical (wedge) biopsy has been performed prior to preoperative chemotherapy or surgery
III	Incomplete excision of tumor, which extends beyond resection margins
	Abdominal lymph node involvement
	Tumor rupture before or during surgery (irrespective of other criteria for staging)
	Tumor has penetrated the peritoneal surface
	Tumor thrombi evident at resection; margins of vessels or ureter transected or removed at surgery
IV	Hematogenous metastases (to lung, liver, brain, etc.) or lymph node metastases outside the abdomen or pelvis
V	Bilateral renal tumors at diagnosis. Each side is substaged using the above classification

Table 37.2 Staging According to NWTS/COG

Stage	% of pts	Criteria
I	43%	Tumor limited to kidney or surrounded by fibrous pseudocapsule if outside the normal contours of the kidney; tumor does not breach outer surface of renal capsule. Tumor is completely resected
		Tumor may protrude into pelvic system but does not infiltrate their walls
		No involvement of vessels of renal sinus
		Intrarenal vessels may be involved
II	23%	Tumor extends beyond kidney or penetrates through renal capsule and/or through fibrous pseudocapsule into perirenal fat, but is completed resected
		Tumor infiltrates renal sinus and/or invades blood and lymphatics outside renal parenchyma, but is completely resected
		Tumor infiltrates adjacent organs or vena cava, but is completely resected
		Surgical (wedge) biopsy has been performed or there was tumor spillage before or during surgery that is confined to the flank and does not involve the peritoneal surface
III	23%	Residual tumor is present and confined to the abdomen
		Any one of: Abdominal lymph node involvement
		Tumor has penetrated through the peritoneal surface
		Tumor implants found on the peritoneal surface
		Gross or microscopic tumor remains postoperatively
		Tumor is nonresectable due to local infiltration into vital structures
		Tumor spill before or during surgery
IV	10%	Hematogenous metastases (lung, liver, bone, brain, etc.) or lymph node metastases outside the abdomen or pelvis
V	5%	Bilateral renal tumors at diagnosis. Each side is substaged using the above classification

directly comparable. The NWTS/COG classification is based on favorable and unfavorable histology and the presence or absence of anaplasia. The SIOP classification, which has recently been revised as a result of the SIOP 9 and 93-01 trials and studies, stratifies patients who have undergone pre-operative chemotherapy into low, intermediate, and high-risk histology on the basis of their nephrectomy pathological findings (55,56). According to this classification, the "blastemal" type is defined as the survival of large amounts of blastema following pre-operative chemotherapy and is believed to confer an adverse outcome. Conversely, tumors with epithelial or stromal predominance after pre-operative chemotherapy have a favorable outcome. Anaplasia, whether focal or diffuse, is regarded as "unfavorable" and "high-risk" by both NWTS and SIOP classification schemes.

Treatment

Primary surgical resection followed by adjuvant chemotherapy and radiotherapy as indicated, based on the extent of disease defined at surgery remains the mainstay of treatment for Wilms' tumor in North America (NWTS/COG). This approach enables as much information as possible about prognostic factors to be gathered at the time of surgery, in order to tailor an individual's therapy. Due to the large size and central location of Wilms' tumors, total nephrectomy is performed. Biopsy of adjacent or regional lymph nodes is important because nodal involvement upstages from II to III, although radical lymph node dissection is unnecessary (29,30), as there is no evidence that it alters the outcome (5). Biopsy of nodes at the level of the renal vessels is obligatory, regardless of size (29,57). Extension of tumor into the renal vein must be determined before vessel ligation (37). Surgical exploration of the contralateral kidney is no longer recommended (57,58), as CT or MR imaging now provides sufficient sensitivity in excluding contralateral disease (37). The only indications for pre-operative chemotherapy under NWTS are for patients with bilateral tumors, tumors in a solitary kidney, tumors with inferior vena caval extension above the hepatic veins, and tumors found to be unresectable at surgery (3).

Nephron-sparing surgery such as polar hemi-nephrectomy, wedge resection or enucleation is controversial, as it carries the risk of leaving nephrogenic rests in the unresected portion of the kidney (30). At present, such procedures are only indicated for those patients with a solitary kidney, bilateral Wilms' tumor, renal insufficiency, disorders affecting the contralateral kidney, and those at risk of multiple neoplasms such as Beckwith-Wiedemann syndrome (30). According to the SIOP 2001 protocol (July 2004) the contraindications to partial nephrectomy are: pre-operative tumor rupture or biopsy, tumor-infiltrating extrarenal structures, intra-abdominal metastases or lymph nodes on pre-operative imaging, renal vein or IVC thrombus, tumor involving more than one-third of the kidney, multifocal tumor, central location, calyceal involvement, hematuria, and little experience with the surgical procedure (59).

In Europe (SIOP and UKW3 trials), staging and histological diagnosis are delayed until surgery, which occurs several weeks after clinical and imaging diagnosis. Pre-operative chemotherapy is used to shrink the size of the tumor to facilitate surgery and improve the chance of resectability. It has also been shown to reduce the incidence of per-operative tumor rupture or spillage [from 20% in primary surgical resection to 6% with pre-operative chemotherapy in the NWTS-4 trial (60)] by inducing fibrosis, thereby rendering the capsule less friable. Reducing the size also downstages the tumor which then requires less intensive adjuvant chemotherapy and avoids radiotherapy in the majority of patients. The recent UKW3 trial carried out by the United Kingdom Children's Cancer Study Group (UKCCSG) shows a more favorable stage distribution, reduction in surgical complications and reduced overall treatment burden in patients who undergo neoadjuvant chemotherapy as opposed to immediate nephrectomy (61). Prospective data gave a morbidity rate of 7% in the groups treated by the SIOP approach compared with 10% in the NWTS groups (61). The pre-operative chemotherapy approach also allows for *in vivo* assessment of histological response to chemotherapy.

One disadvantage of the delayed surgical approach is that if a tumor demonstrates the typical imaging and clinical features of

Wilms' tumor, neoadjuvant chemotherapy may be commenced without a histological diagnosis. This may result in the alteration of the tumor histology and the loss of accurate staging information. Of particular concern is the risk of missing diffuse anaplasia. The approach of omitting pre-operative biopsy also results in 1% of children with a benign renal lesion, such as mesoblastic nephroma, receiving chemotherapy, including actinomycin D, which carries a 3% risk of hepatotoxicity (62). Conversely, patients with highly malignant tumors such as rhabdoid tumor or clear cell sarcoma, which respond to intensive chemotherapy, go unrecognized and are therefore under-treated. Thus, during the UKW3 trial, immediate biopsy was recommended prior to treatment with pre-operative chemotherapy. The results of this study show that 12% of "Wilms' tumors" diagnosed on the basis of imaging studies were found to have other diagnoses on biopsy, with 1% of children having a non-malignant lesion (62). There was also no evidence from the trial to suggest that percutaneous biopsy increases the risk of needle track tumor recurrence (62), although biopsy in COG trials is actually considered local spill and automatically upstages a tumor to Stage III disease.

Current chemotherapy regimens are based on three first line drugs: dactinomycin (actinomycin-D), vincristine, and doxorubicin (37). Four second line drugs: cyclophoshamide, ifosfamide, carboplatin, and etoposide are used in patients who have relapsed or have a poor response to first line chemotherapy (37). Different treatment algorithms depend on the stage and grade of the tumor.

Studies on the relationship between chemotherapy and radiotherapy have enabled both dose reduction and narrowing of the indications for radiotherapy without compromising the survival rates. The current indications for radiotherapy are therefore:

- Stage III—positive lymph nodes and/or diffuse peritoneal spillage
- Stage II–IV—diffuse anaplasia
- Stage IV—metastatic disease (usually pulmonary) according to NWTS protocol
- Residual lung metastases after chemotherapy and metastatectomy in SIOP (3)

Key Points: Staging and Therapy

- The most important prognostic factors in Wilms' tumor are the histological grade and stage of the tumor
- Staging criteria are based on the anatomical extent of the tumor on imaging and on both surgical, and pathological findings at nephrectomy
- There are two major staging systems in use: a pre-chemotherapy, surgery based system (NWTS/COG), and a pre-operative chemotherapy based system (SIOP)
- Surgical resection of the primary tumor (usually total nephrectomy) is performed either before or after treatment with chemotherapy and radiotherapy depending upon local protocols
- Nephron-sparing surgery is considered in patients with a solitary kidney, abnormalities of the contralateral kidney, or risk of multiple tumors
- Different chemotherapy and radiotherapy treatment algorithms depend on the stage and grade of the tumor

Role of Imaging in Biopsy

In the SIOP protocol, diagnosis has been traditionally based on the characteristic imaging features of a Wilms' tumor. Biopsy was not recommended as it was generally believed to increase the risk of flank relapse; possibly upstaging the tumor to Stage III. As mentioned previously, however, there are dangers to treating a child without a histological diagnosis and as a result of the UKW3 study (62), pre-chemotherapy biopsy has been routinely adopted. During this study, patients amenable to primary nephrectomy were randomly assigned to either immediate surgery then chemotherapy, or immediate biopsy followed by six weeks of pre-operative chemotherapy. The results of the study showed that there was complete concordance between biopsy and nephrectomy diagnoses in 99.5% of cases (62). Of 182 children who underwent percutaneous cutting needle biopsy, 20% had a subsequent fall in hemoglobin and 19% had local pain. One child required emergency nephrectomy due to massive intra-tumoral bleeding, one had tumor rupture which was not thought to be biopsy related, and one developed a needle track recurrence eight months following biopsy (62).

The traditional method of obtaining histology has been through open surgical biopsy. Percutaneous US or CT-guided biopsy, however, improves the diagnostic yield compared to blind biopsy (63), and is technically safer as it is able to direct the operator away from large tumor vessels. It also enables sampling of appropriate areas within the tumor mass (63): viable tumor is present peripherally whilst necrotic areas are often centrally located, thus there is more potential for sampling error in blind biopsies. A posterior approach is preferred thereby avoiding peritoneal dissemination. The morbidity associated with percutaneous biopsy is small. Microscopic hematuria and mild flank pain are relatively common occurrences after percutaneous biopsy, and are generally not considered to be significant complications (62). There is a 20% risk of bleeding post-core-needle biopsy, but the incidence of massive tumor bleeding or lethal tumor rupture is rare (62,63). Arterio-venous fistula has been reported in 2% to 8% of renal biopsies but only in one case of biopsied Wilms' tumor (64). Needle-track recurrence has been reported in only three Wilms' tumor cases in the literature, including the one reported from the UKW3 trial (62,65,66). Thus the concern with tumor recurrence by this procedure is likely to be unfounded, given the large number of percutaneous biopsies now performed in many centers.

Role of Imaging in Treatment

Radiological follow-up during neo-adjuvant chemotherapy for localized disease consists of abdominal sonography and plain chest radiograph every three months (67). For patients with lung metastases (Stage IV disease), a chest radiograph is performed at six weeks and then at 12 weeks to confirm response to treatment. Thereafter three-monthly chest radiographs and abdominal sonography is recommended during treatment (67).

In the SIOP protocol, since Response Evaluation Criteria In Solid Tumors (RECIST) has not been validated for pediatric Wilms' tumors, the response to treatment is assessed by measuring the tumor size at diagnosis, usually by the largest diameter in three planes, and using that as a comparison during subsequent

follow-up studies (68). The guidelines for tumor measurement according to the NWTS/COG also include maximal tumor dimensions in three planes (41). These measurements must be made on the same imaging modality throughout treatment and follow-up, be it with CT or MR imaging. In addition to reduction in size, change in tumor characteristics such as necrosis may indicate response.

Role of Imaging in Follow-up

Most Wilms' tumor recurrences arise in the lung (58%) and abdomen (29%) and rarely in bone, brain, and mediastinum (46). Ninety percent of relapses occur during the first four years after diagnosis (47). The overall relapse rates for all patients enrolled on NWTS and SIOP studies is 17% to 24% (3). The use of multi-agent intensive salvage regimes has improved the survival from relapsed Wilms' from less than 30% (69) just 20 years ago to 50% to 60% (70). Local relapse is defined as recurrence in the original tumor bed, retroperitoneum, abdomen, or pelvis.

A higher risk of local recurrence is seen in patients with:

- Lymph node involvement
- Unfavorable histology
- Tumor spillage
- Incomplete tumor removal
- Absence of lymph node sampling during surgery (57)

Good prognostic factors for relapse include an initial diagnosis of Stage I or II, initial two chemotherapy agent treatment, no radiotherapy, favorable histology, and longer time from diagnosis to relapse (30). The recommended imaging protocol under SIOP for post-treatment surveillance is summarized in Table 37.3. Those patients who survive relapse-free for more than three years after diagnosis are unlikely to develop recurrent disease (71). Therefore the main aim of long-term follow-up is to monitor the growth of the remaining kidney, blood pressure, and renal function well into adulthood.

Table 37.3 Recommended Imaging Follow-up After Treatment for Wilms' Tumor

Region	Imaging modality	Frequency
Chest	X-ray	1st year every 3 months
		2nd year every 6 months
		3rd to 5th years every 12 months
		If initally stage IV lung:
		1st and 2nd years every 2–3 months
		3rd and 4th years every 6 months
		5th year every 12 months
Abdomen/pelvis	US	At end of treatment
		1st and 2nd years every 6 months
		3rd to 5th years every 12 months
		If nephrogenic rests, local Stage
		III and/or high risk histology:
		1st and 2nd years every 3 months
		3rd to 5th years every 6 months
		6th to 10th years every 12 months

Source: Adapted from Nephroblastoma Clinical Trial and Study Protocol, SIOP 2001.

Bilateral Disease

Wilms' tumors are bilateral in 5% to 7% of patients (5,72), with 5% to 6% occurring synchronously (30,73). Bilateral Wilms' tumor are classified as Stage V disease. They are more frequent in girls and children of a younger mean age of 2.5 years than those with unilateral disease (73). They are associated with nephrogenic rests (in 90% of synchronous and 94% of metachronous bilateral Wilms' tumors) (33,74), congenital anomalies, and predisposing syndromes (5). Patients with unilateral tumors who subsequently develop contralateral disease share the same associations as synchronous bilateral disease, but the risk is higher in infants younger than one year of age at the time of diagnosis (73). The 10-year survival rate in patients with bilateral synchronous disease is approximately 70% (37,75), and 50% for bilateral metachronous disease (75). However, there is a high incidence of renal failure (76). The overriding aim, therefore, is to preserve renal function without compromising the cancer therapy. Bilateral synchronous disease is one group of patients in whom there is a consensus between both SIOP and NWTS regarding optimum management: pre-operative chemotherapy after biopsy confirmation to decrease the tumor volume, then reassessment of tumor to evaluate feasibility of nephron-sparing surgery (76). A useful imaging modality in this situation may be positron emission tomography (PET) to detect viable post-chemotherapy tumor (73). As a minimum, multiplanar MR imaging or CT should be performed to assess to extent of the bilateral tumors and proximity to the surrounding anatomy (77). Surgeons find that contrast-enhanced CT with good definition of the arterial anatomy is particularly useful for bilateral tumors (Fig. 37.7). The imaging of bilateral disease is similar to that of unilateral disease, although each kidney is staged separately. Intraoperative sonography may also be helpful to determine the intrarenal extent of the tumor (78).

Nephroblastomatosis and Nephrogenic Rests

Nephrogenic rests are remnants of renal embryonal tissue which arise from incomplete induction of the metanephric blastema into mature renal parenchyma. They are regarded as precursor lesions to Wilms' tumor and were found to co-exist with 41% of Wilms' tumors in the National Wilms Tumor Study (79), although it is estimated that only 1% undergo malignant transformation (35,80). Two distinct

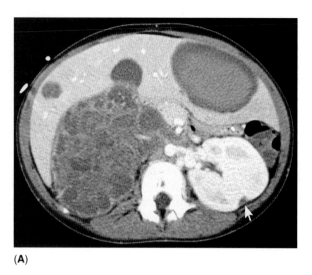

(A)

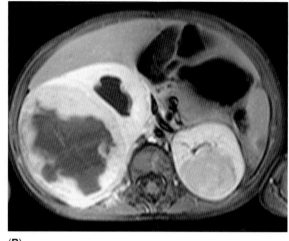

(B)

Figure 37.7 Bilateral Wilms' tumors. (**A**) Contrast-enhanced CT of the same patient as in Figure 37.3 shows a synchronous lesion in the posterior aspect of the contralateral kidney (arrow), in addition to hepatic metastases. This lesion could be either another Wilms' tumor or a focus of nephroblastomatosis—only a biopsy could establish the pathological diagnosis. (**B**) Axial T1-weighted post-gadolinium enhanced MR image in another patient shows bilateral synchronous tumors.

categories of nephrogenic rests have been identified: perilobar nephrogenic rests (PLNR), which occur later on in nephrogenesis at the periphery of the renal lobe and are associated with an older age at diagnosis, hemihypertrophy and Beckwith-Wiedemann syndrome, and intralobar nephrogenic rests (ILNR) which occur early in nephrogenesis and are associated with a younger age at diagnosis, WAGR, Denys-Drash syndrome, and bilateral disease (34). Multifocal or diffuse nephrogenic rests are termed "nephroblastomatosis."

The clinical course of nephroblastomatosis is highly variable; lesions may remain stable over many years or proliferate. Imaging plays an important role in recognizing these lesions due to the risk of developing Wilms' tumor. Microscopic nephrogenic rests are not visible on imaging. In one study, macroscopic nephrogenic rests were found to be better resolved by MR imaging and CT (to 0.5 cm) than by US (to 0.8 cm), although this was not by high-resolution US (81).

On US, diffuse nephroblastomatosis is shown as a homogeneous and hypoechoic rim in the periphery of the kidney, which preserves its renal shape but causes an increase in its size. The appearances on sonography may be similar to those of leukemia or lymphoma (Fig. 37.8A). Isolated macroscopic nephrogenic rests appear on US as isoechoic or slightly hypoechoic nodules which cause a local bulge or lobulated renal contour.

On unenhanced CT and MR imaging nephroblastomatosis is very similar in attenuation and intensity to normal renal parenchyma and is only made conspicuous after contrast enhancement, where normally enhancing renal parenchyma is clearly different from non-enhancing nephroblastomatosis (Fig. 37.8B and C). On CT, isolated nephrogenic rests are iso- or slightly hyperdense to renal cortex and do not enhance. On MR imaging, so-called dormant, sclerotic nephrogenic rests are typically homogeneously hypointense on T1-weighted, and T2-weighted or STIR sequences, and do not enhance post-Gadolinium (Fig. 37.8C). These are thought to have a low malignant potential (81,82). Hyperplastic rests are hyperintense on T2-weighted and STIR sequences and are considered to have a higher malignant risk (81,82).

Differentiation of nephroblastomatosis from Wilms' tumor on percutaneous biopsy is often inconclusive as they have similar histological characteristics and there are potential sampling errors.

Imaging characteristics are also very similar, although nephrogenic rests tend to be less than 2 cm in size and of ovoid or lenticular shape, while Wilms' tumors are usually greater than 3 cm and spherical (83). However, any criteria based on these observations is unreliable (83).

The management of nephroblastomatosis and nephrogenic rests remains controversial. There is currently no specific treatment for nephrogenic rests apart from close radiological surveillance for the development of Wilms' tumor. The role of chemotherapy in attempting to halt or slow the progression of nephroblastomatosis is unclear. It has been suggested that there may be some benefit in treating diffuse nephroblastomatosis for up to one year with vincristine and actinomycin-D (84). Small focal areas of nephroblastomatosis still present at the end of chemotherapy require surveillance with MR imaging for at least one year.

Key Points: Bilateral Disease and Nephroblastomatosis

- Wilms' tumors are bilateral in 5% to 7% of patients and are classified as Stage V disease
- Bilateral tumors are associated with nephrogenic rests, congenital anomalies, and predisposing syndromes
- There is a high incidence of eventual renal failure with bilateral disease, therefore nephron-sparing procedures are indicated
- Nephrogenic rests are regarded as precursor lesions to Wilms' tumor
- Nephroblastomatosis may have similar imaging and histological characteristics to Wilms' tumor
- Foci of nephroblastomatosis show homogeneous non-enhancement with contrast administration on CT and MR imaging, while Wilms' tumors show heterogeneous enhancement
- There is no specific treatment for nephroblastomatosis
- Small focal areas of nephroblastomatosis still present at the end of chemotherapy require initial surveillance with MR imaging for at least one year

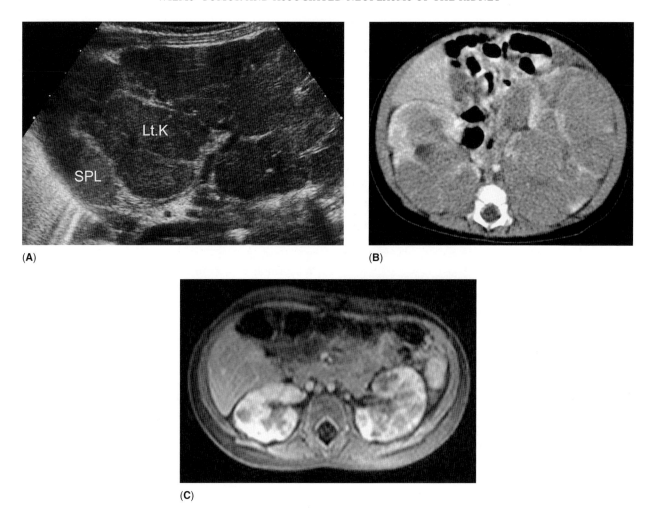

Figure 37.8 Nephroblastomatosis. (**A**) US shows an enlarged left kidney (Lt.K) with complete distortion of the normal architecture and replacement by multiple soft tissue masses. [Spleen (SPL)] The right kidney showed similar appearances. (**B**) Contrast-enhanced CT demonstrates bilaterally enlarged kidneys containing multiple non-enhancing soft tissue masses. There is a thin rim of normal enhancing renal parenchyma. (**C**) Axial T1-weighted post-gadolinium MR image, performed one year later after chemotherapy treatment, demonstrates improved appearances with multiple small residual non-enhancing lesions in both kidneys.

Complications and Late Effects of Treatment

The success of Wilms' tumor treatment has improved patients' long-term survival into adulthood and this has enabled the late effects of treatment to be studied. These effects are defined as those absent or unrecognized at the end of therapy. Acute toxicity is usually caused by the immunosuppression induced by chemotherapy.

Following unilateral nephrectomy in childhood the remaining kidney shows compensatory hypertrophy, and one year later the glomerular filtration rate (GFR) and effective renal plasma flow are 90% of normal (85). Children who receive both surgery and chemotherapy also have close to normal renal function. The addition of radiation significantly reduces renal function to about 73% of normal GFR. Renal failure is rare among unilateral Wilms' tumor survivors (85), although the incidence appears to be increased in those with Wilms' tumor and aniridia, and also in those with intralobar nephrogenic rests on long-term follow-up (86). Adjuvant chemotherapy and radiotherapy may also cause both acute and chronic damage to organs such as the heart, lungs, liver, bones, and gonads. The cardiotoxicity of doxorubicin can cause cardiac failure even many years following treatment. Whole lung irradiation can cause pneumonitis, and restrictive lung disease and can also affect cardiac function. Abdominal irradiation

and the chemotherapeutic agent actinomycin-D are hepatotoxic and can cause hepatic veno-occlusive disease (VOD) which consists clinically of the triad of hepatomegaly, ascites, and icterus. VOD can be fatal, and is usually treated with supportive measures and the withholding of chemotherapy until the patient has clinically recovered. Trunk irradiation can cause the late effects of scoliosis and soft tissue underdevelopment but asymmetric skeletal effects are now largely preventable by symmetric radiotherapy doses across the midline. Osteochondromas are common in the ribs or scapulae in patients who have had chest irradiation (87). A high incidence of infertility, spontaneous miscarriages, and intra-uterine growth retardation has been found in girls where the uterus and ovaries were within the radiation field (88). Along with an inherent predisposition towards developing other malignancies, both chemotherapy and radiotherapy can induce secondary malignant neoplasms (SMNs). Types of SMNs encountered include bone and soft tissue sarcomas, lymphoma, breast carcinoma, gastro-intestinal tumors, melanoma and acute leukemias (89).

Role of Imaging in Surveillance

US is the preferred modality for the purposes of surveillance (90), as CT carries the risk of ionizing radiation and MR imaging the need

Table 37.4 Conditions with Risk of Developing Wilms' Tumor in Excess of 5%

Gene	Phenotype	WT risk
WT1	WAGR syndrome	High >20%
	Denys-Drash syndrome	
	Frasier syndrome	
	Familial WT	
	Aniridia	
	Isolated WT	
BRCA2	Fanconi anemia	High >20%
	Some childhood cancers	
BUB1B	Mosaic variegated aneuploidy	High >20%
Unknown	Perlman syndrome	High >20%
11p15	Beckwith-Wiedemann syndrome	Moderate 5–20%
	Some hemihypertrophy cases	
GPC3	Simpson-Golabi-Behmel syndrome	Moderate 5–20%

Source: Adapted from Ref. 90 on behalf of the Wilms' Tumor Surveillance Working Group.

83% for Stage IV, and 70% for Stage V (7). However, the four-year survival rate for diffuse anaplastic disease is 45% for Stage III and only 7% for Stage IV tumors (7). The two-, five-, and ten-year survival rates for bilateral synchronous Wilms' tumor are 83%, 73%, and 70% respectively (91). The long-term survival of patients with relapse/recurrence is about 50% to 60% (70).

Key Points: Late effects, Surveillance, and Prognosis

- Adjuvant chemotherapy and radiotherapy may cause both acute and chronic damage to organs such as the heart, lungs, liver, bones, and gonads
- Long-term survivors are prone to developing secondary malignant neoplasms
- US is the preferred modality for the purposes of surveillance
- Screening is recommended in individuals who have a >5% risk of developing Wilms' tumor
- The prognosis for most children diagnosed with Wilms' tumor is excellent

for sedation in young children. Regular surveillance of children thought to be at increased risk (in the order of 10–30%) of developing Wilms' tumor, for example, those with Wilms' tumor-related congenital syndromes, has become widespread practice (91). Recommendations for such surveillance approved by the Children's Cancer and Leukaemia Group (CCLG) include offering screening to those at greater than 5% risk of developing Wilms' tumor via three to four-monthly renal sonography up to the age of five to seven years (90). Specifically, surveillance should continue until five years of age for all those conditions except for proven Beckwith-Wiedemann syndrome, Simpson-Golabi-Behmel syndrome, and some familial Wilms' tumors where it should continue until seven years of age as the risk of developing Wilms' tumor is considered to be high (>20%) (90). Table 37.4 summarizes the conditions and syndromes associated with a greater than 5% risk of Wilms' tumor.

Long term follow-up is also important in patients with known nephrogenic rests or nephroblastomatosis due to the risk of developing Wilms' tumor. Attention should also be paid to the contralateral kidney in patients with previous unilateral nephrectomy for Wilms' tumor. Even though the risk of contralateral, metachronous relapse is low, the risk is increased if nephrogenic rests were identified at initial diagnosis or if the patient was less than one year of age at the time of diagnosis (74). Early detection of primary or metachronous tumor occurring in pre-existing nephroblastomatosis will facilitate nephron-sparing surgery. Clues to the malignant transformation of a lesion include rapid increase in size, the appearance of a nodular lesion or heterogeneity within a lesion (73). In such cases the patient should proceed to surgery, as percutaneous biopsy is unhelpful.

Prognosis

The treatment of Wilms' tumor is one of the most significant success stories in pediatric oncology. The prognosis for most children diagnosed with Wilms' tumor is excellent, with no significant difference in relapse-free survival between the two treatment approaches of primary surgical resection and pre-operative chemotherapy (38). The four-year survival rate is 86% to 96% for Stages I to III, up to

OTHER RENAL NEOPLASMS OF CHILDHOOD

Clear Cell Sarcoma of the Kidney

Clear cell sarcoma of the kidney (CCSK) is a primitive mesenchymal tumor which comprises 4% of all renal tumors of childhood (7,45). The peak age of incidence is similar to that of Wilms' tumor and there is a male preponderance (7). CCSK has not been reported with Wilms' tumor associated conditions nor have there been any reports of bilateral tumors (16,45). The clinical presentation is most often of an abdominal mass and the imaging appearances are very similar to those of Wilms' tumor (Fig. 37.9). CCSK has a propensity to metastasize to bone, with 23% developing bone metastases compared to 0.3% of all other patients enrolled in the UKW3 study. Hence, once the diagnosis is made, 99mTc-MDP bone scintigraphy is indicated to stage the tumor. Appearances may be either of reduced (osteolytic) or increased (osteoblastic) isotope uptake (16). However, relapse is more commonly seen in the lungs or central nervous system (7). The relapse and mortality rates in CCSK are higher than in Wilms' tumor. The four-year relapse-free survival rate in CCSK treated with a combination of vincristine, adriamycin, and actinomycin-D on the NWTS-3 trial was 71%. The current long-term survival is about 60% to 70% (45).

Rhabdoid Tumor of the Kidney

Rhabdoid tumor is the most aggressive malignant pediatric renal tumor with the worst prognosis of all the primary childhood renal tumors. The tumor is unrelated to rhabdomyosarcoma or Wilms' tumor and may be of neural crest origin. It occurs almost exclusively in young children, accounting for 1% to 2% of all childhood renal neoplasms, with most cases diagnosed in infancy (7). Clinical presentation may be that of hematuria, but due to the aggressive nature of the tumor, symptoms are often related to metastatic disease.

There is a known association between rhabdoid tumors and synchronous, or metachronous primary central nervous system neoplasms (7,16,45). Hence cranial CT or MR imaging is recommended

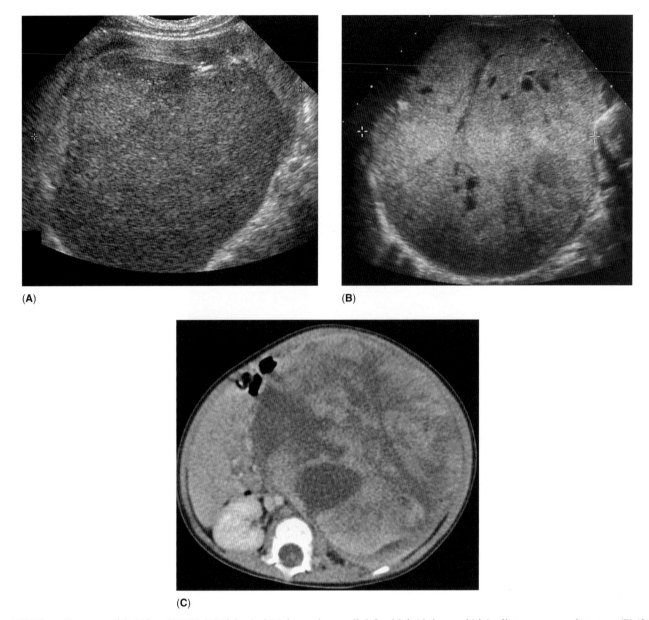

(A)

(B)

(C)

Figure 37.9 Clear cell sarcoma of the kidney (CCSK). (A) Abdominal US shows a large, well-defined, left sided mass which is of heterogeneous echotexture. (B) Abdominal US in another patient with CCSK demonstrating small hypoechoic areas within a mass which may represent necrosis or hemorrhage. (C) Contrast-enhanced CT in the same patient demonstrates imaging characteristics that are indistinguishable from those of Wilms' tumor.

in all patients. Brain lesions have a propensity for the posterior fossa, and include primitive neuroectodermal tumor (PNET), ependymoma, and cerebellar and brainstem astrocytomas. On imaging, rhabdoid tumors are indistinguishable from Wilms' tumors (Fig. 37.10). However, if present, the characteristic feature of subcapsular fluid collections manifest as the peripheral fluid crescent sign can point to the correct diagnosis (7,16,45).

Rhabdoid tumors require more intensive chemotherapy, but despite this, the prognosis is poor and the tumor metastasizes early to lungs, liver, brain, and bone. The four-year relapse-free survival on a combination of vincristine, adriamycin, and actinomycin-D was 23.1% in the NWTS-3, with four-year overall survival of only 25%.

Renal Cell Carcinoma

Renal cell carcinoma is rare in the first two decades of life, with less than 1% of all cases occurring in pediatric patients (7).

However, there are increasing numbers of cases reported in children (92), some of whom are associated with hereditary cancer syndromes, such as von Hippel-Lindau disease (93). In this syndrome tumors tend to be multiple and present at a younger age (93). The mean age at presentation is nine years (7), which is the main differentiating feature between renal cell carcinoma and Wilms' tumor. Clinical presentation is typically of a palpable mass or flank pain, with hematuria occurring less frequently.

The gross morphology can be indistinguishable from that of Wilms' tumor: both are solid intrarenal masses with variable amounts of necrosis, hemorrhage, calcification, and cystic degeneration. Renal cell carcinomas have a higher frequency of calcification (25%) than Wilms' tumor (9%) (33). In addition, the calcifications in renal cell carcinoma tend to be ring-like (7), which are unusual in Wilms' tumor. Both tumors distort the adjacent renal architecture and form a pseudocapsule. However, renal

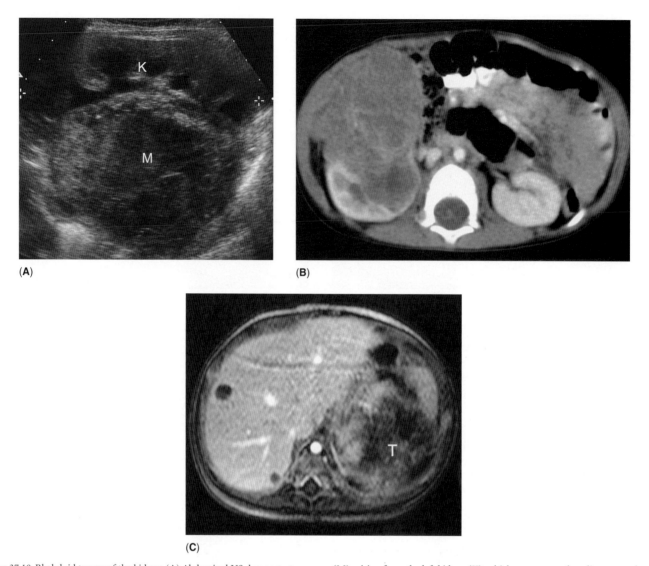

Figure 37.10 Rhabdoid tumor of the kidney. (A) Abdominal US demonstrates a mass (M) arising from the left kidney (K), which compresses the adjacent renal parenchyma. (B) Contrast-enhanced CT shows imaging characteristics that are typical for a renal neoplasm and thus essentially similar to those of a Wilms' tumor. Note the unfused neural arch indicating that this is an infant or young toddler. (C) Axial T1-weighted post-gadolinium MR image shows a left sided rhabdoid tumor (T) with multiple hepatic metastases.

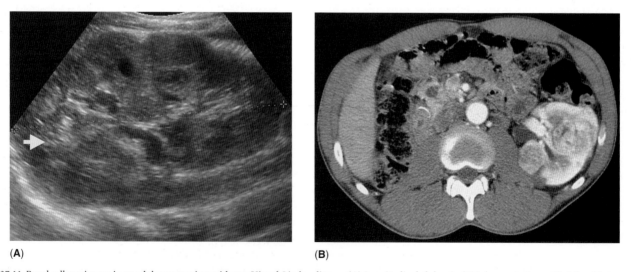

Figure 37.11 Renal cell carcinoma in an adolescent patient with von Hippel-Lindau disease. (A) Longitudinal abdominal US demonstrates an ill-defined heterogeneous mass in the upper pole of the left kidney (arrow) (B) Contrast-enhanced CT reveals multiple ill-defined and heterogeneously enhancing lesions in the left kidney. Note a previous right sided nephrectomy has been performed for contralateral renal cell carcinoma.

cell tumors tend to be smaller in size than Wilms' at diagnosis and therefore less easily identifiable at US and better detected on CT or MR imaging, where they show similar imaging characteristics to Wilms' tumor (Fig. 37.11) (45). Local and regional lymph node spread, in the absence of distant metastases, does not appear to be a poor prognostic factor in children, unlike in adults. Metastases to the lungs, liver, bone, or brain occur in 20% of patients at diagnosis (45). Renal cell carcinoma is more likely than Wilms' tumor to manifest bilaterally and metastasize to bone. The overall survival rate is approximately 64% (45). The tumor is not particularly chemosensitive and the best results have been obtained from radical nephrectomy and regional lymphadenectomy, with nephron-sparing surgery for bilateral disease.

Mesoblastic Nephroma

So-called congenital mesoblastic nephroma (CMN) is the most common solid renal tumor presenting in the neonatal period. It was historically thought to represent a congenital Wilms' tumor, but was recognized as a distinct entity in 1967 (16,45). Ninety percent of cases present within the first year of life, most frequently as a large, palpable abdominal mass (45). Other symptoms may include hematuria, hypertension, vomiting, and jaundice. The mass is infiltrative with ill-defined margins and no capsule, but is histologically benign. Imaging appearances may be indistinguishable from a Wilms' tumor. As CMN is the most likely renal mass in the first six months of life, most collaborative oncology groups advise against biopsy before six months and advocate primary nephrectomy in this setting. The tumor is usually successfully treated by nephrectomy alone. However, metastases are rare but can occur to lungs, brain, and bone. Therefore close monitoring for one year after surgery is recommended (45).

Key Points: Other Renal Neoplasms of Childhood

- Clear cell sarcoma of the kidney (CCSK) is a primitive mesenchymal tumor which comprises 4% of all renal tumors of childhood
- Imaging appearances of CCSK are similar to Wilms' tumors
- CCSK has a propensity to spread to bone
- Rhabdoid tumor is the most aggressive childhood renal tumor and accounts for 1% to 2% of all renal tumors of childhood
- Renal cell carcinoma is rare and may be associated with hereditary cancer disorders
- Mesoblastic nephroma is the most common renal tumor presenting in the neonatal period
- Mesoblastic nephroma is histologically benign but metastases can occur

FUTURE DIRECTIONS IN IMAGING

FDG PET

The experience of [18]FDG PET-CT in childhood cancers is limited, being used in Hodgkin's lymphoma and sarcomas but untried in Wilms' tumor (73). Since Wilms' tumor, particularly the more aggressive anaplastic type, is presumed to be FDG-avid (94), there is a theoretical role for this technique in, for example, the targeted

biopsy of viable and biologically aggressive tissue. Monitoring of the biological treatment response of the primary tumor as well as of FDG-positive lung metastases might also be possible.

Quantitative MR Imaging

Diffusion-weighted imaging (DWI) is being increasingly used in body MR imaging, particularly in the detection, characterization, and subsequent monitoring of neoplastic disease. Studies have shown that there is a correlation between cellularity and apparent diffusion coefficient (ADC) values with high cellularity associated with low ADC and low cellularity with high ADC values (95) (see chap. 65). Thus quantitative MR imaging has the potential to evaluate treatment response and has the advantage over other methods of not utilizing ionizing radiation.

Contrast-Enhanced Ultrasound

US evaluation of renal and other tumors following the administration of IV contrast medium has been shown to improve the accuracy of their detection and characterization in adults (96). The role of this imaging technique in children is as yet unproven because these contrast media are unlicensed for use in children.

Summary

- Wilms' tumor is one of the most common renal tumors of childhood
- Wilms' tumor is associated with congenital syndromes in 15% of cases
- The majority of Wilms' tumors are solitary; bilateral tumors occuring in 5% to 7% of patients
- The most common presentation is of an asymptomatic abdominal mass and over 90% of patients have favorable histology
- US can distinguish between a cystic and a solid mass, assess vascular invasion, and examine the contralateral kidney
- CT and MR imaging give additional information and chest CT is now recommended by SIOP for detecting pulmonary metastases
- There are two major staging systems in use: a pre-chemotherapy, surgery based system (NWTS/COG), and a preoperative chemotherapy based system (SIOP).
- Ninety percent of relapses occur during the first four years after diagnosis
- Nephroblastomatosis may have similar imaging and histological characteristics to Wilms' tumor
- The prognosis for most children diagnosed with Wilms' tumor is excellent
- US is the preferred modality for the purposes of surveillance and screening is recommended in individuals who have a >5% risk of developing Wilms' tumor
- Clear cell sarcoma of the kidney comprises 4% of renal tumors of childhood, rhabdoid tumors account for about 1% and renal cell carcinomas are very rare
- Mesoblastic nephroma tumors usually present during the first year of life and are histologically benign

REFERENCES

1. Kaste SC, Dome JS, Babyn PS, et al. Wilms tumour: prognostic factors, staging, therapy, and late effects. Pediatr Radiol 2008; 38: 2–17.
2. Mitry E, Ciccolallo L, Coleman MP, Gatta G, Pritchard-Jones K. EUROCARE Working Group. Incidence of and survival from Wilms' tumour in adults in Europe: data from the EUROCARE study. Eur J Cancer 2006; 42: 2363–8.
3. de Camargo B, Pritchard-Jones K. Nephroblastoma. In: Voute PA, Barrett A, Stevens MCG, and Caron HN, eds. Cancer in Children: Clinical Management, 5th edn. Oxford University Press, 2005: 321–36.
4. Fukuzawa R, Reeve AE. Molecular pathology and epidemiology of nephrogenic rests and Wilms tumors. J Pediatr Hematol Oncol 2007; 29: 589–94.
5. Grundy PE, Green DM, Coppes MJ, et al. Renal tumors. In: Pizzo PA, Poplack DG, eds. Principles and Practice of Paediatric Oncology. Philadelphia: Lippincott Williams and Wilkins, 2003: 865–93.
6. Hartman DJ, MacLennan GT. Wilms tumor. J Urol 2005; 173: 2147.
7. McHugh K. Renal and adrenal tumours in children. Cancer Imaging 2007; 7: 41–51.
8. Breslow NE, Beckwith JB. Epidemiological features of Wilms' tumor: results of the National Wilms' Tumor Study. J Natl Cancer Inst 1982; 68: 429–36.
9. Mesrobian HG, Kelalis PP, Hrabovsky E, et al. Wilms tumor in horseshoe kidneys: a report from the National Wilms Tumour Study. J Urol 1985; 133: 1002–3.
10. Scott RH, Stiller CA, Walker L, Rahman N. Syndromes and constitutional chromosomal abnormalities associated with Wilms tumour. J Med Genet 2006; 43: 705–15.
11. Reid S, Renwick A, Seal S, et al. Biallelic BRCA2 mutations are associated with multiple malignancies in childhood including familial Wilms tumour. J Med Genet 2005; 42: 147–51.
12. Weksberg R, Shuman C, Smith AC. Beckwith-Wiedemann syndrome. Am J Med Genet C Semin Med Genet 2005; 137: 12–23.
13. Royer-Pokora B, Beier M, Henzler M, et al. Twenty-four new cases of WT1 germline mutations and review of the literature: genotype-phenotype correlations for Wilms tumor development. Am J Med Genet A 2004; 127A: 249–57.
14. Henneveld HT, van Lingen RA, Hamel BC, Stolte-Dijkstra I, van Essen AJ. Perlman syndrome: four additional cases and review. Am J Med Genet 1999; 86: 439–46.
15. Francois J, Coucke D, Coppieters R. Aniridia-Wilms' tumour syndrome. Ophthalmology 1977; 174: 35–9.
16. White KS, Grossman H. Wilms' and associated renal tumors of childhood. Pediatr Radiol 1991; 21: 81–8.
17. Riccardi VM, Sujansky E, Smith AC, Francke U. Chromosomal imbalance in the Aniridia-Wilms' tumor association: 11p interstitial deletion. Pediatrics 1978; 61: 604–10.
18. Call KM, Glaser T, Ito CY, et al. Isolation and characterization of a zinc finger polypeptide gene at the human chromosome 11 Wilms' tumor locus. Cell 1990; 60: 509–20.
19. Gessler M, Poutska A, Cavenee W, et al. Homozygous deletion in Wilms tumours of a zinc-finger gene identified by chromosome jumping. Nature 1990; 343: 774–8.
20. Bonetta L, Kuehn SE, Huang A, et al. Wilms tumor locus on 11p13 defined by multiple CpG island-associated transcripts. Science 1990; 250: 994–7.
21. Coppes MJ, Huff V, Pelletier J. Denys-Drash syndrome: relating a clinical disorder to genetic alterations in the tumor suppression gene WT1. J Pediatr 1993; 123: 673–8.
22. Pelletier J, Bruening W, Kashtan CE, et al. Germline mutations in the Wilms' tumour suppressor gene are associated with abnormal urogenital development in Denys-Drash syndrome. Cell 1991; 67: 437–47.
23. Koufos A, Grundy P, Morgan K, et al. Familial Wiedemann-Beckwith syndrome and a second Wilms' tumor locus both map to 11p15.5. Am J Human Genet 1989; 44: 711–19.
24. Ping AJ, Reeve AE, Law DJ, et al. Genetic linkage of Beckwith-Wiedemann syndrome to 11p15. Am J Hum Genet 1989; 44: 720–3.
25. Driscoll K, Isakoff M, Ferrer F. Update on pediatric genitourinary oncology. Curr Opin Urol 2007; 17: 281–6.
26. Grundy PE, Breslow NE, Li S, et al. Loss of heterozygosity for chromosomes 1p and 16q is an adverse prognostic factor in favourable-histology Wilms tumor: a report from the National Wilms Tumor Study Group. J Clin Oncol 2005; 23: 7312–21.
27. Hartman DJ, MacLennan GT. Wilms tumor. J Urol 2005; 173: 2147.
28. Beckwith JB, Palmer NF. Histopathology and prognosis of Wilms' tumor. Cancer 1978; 41: 1937–48.
29. Kaste SC, Dome JS, Babyn PS, et al. Wilms tumour: prognostic factors, staging, therapy, and late effects. Pediatr Radiol 2008; 38: 2–17.
30. Kalapurakal JA, Dome JS, Perlman EJ, et al. Management of Wilms' tumour: current practice and future goals. Lancet Oncol 2004; 5: 37–46.
31. Halperin EC. Wilms' tumor. In: Halperin EC, Constine LS, Tarbell NJ, and Kun LE, eds. Pediatric Radiation Oncology, 4th edn. Philadelphia: Lippincott Williams & Wilkins, 2005: 379–421.
32. Miller RC, Sterioff S, Jr, Drucker WR, et al. The incidental discovery of occult abdominal tumors in children following blunt abdominal trauma. J Trauma 1996; 6: 99–106.
33. Lonergan GJ, Martinez-Leon MI, Agrons GA, Montemarano H, Suarez ES. Nephrogenic rests, nephroblastomatosis, and associated lesions of the kidney. Radiographics 1998; 18: 947–68.
34. Niu CK, Chen WF, Chuang JH, et al. Intrapelvic Wilms' tumor: report of 2 cases and review of the literature. J Urol 1993; 150: 936–9.
35. Leung RS, Liesner R, Brock P. Coagulopathy as a presenting feature of Wilms tumour. Eur J Pediatr 2004; 163: 369–73.
36. Ritchey ML, Kelalis PP, Breslow N, et al. Intracaval and atrial involvement with nephroblastoma: review of National Wilms Tumor Study-3. J Urol 1988; 140: 1113–18.
37. Gommersall LM, Arya M, Mushtaq I, Duffy P. Current challenges in Wilms' tumor management. Nat Clin Pract Oncol 2005; 2: 298–304.
38. Coppes MJ, Zandvoort SW, Sparling CR, et al. Acquired von Willebrand disease in Wilms' tumor patients. J Clin Oncol 1992; 10: 422–7.

39. Lin RY, Argenta PA, Sullivan KM, Stern R, Adzick NS. Urinary hyaluronic acid is a Wilm's tumor marker. J Pediatr Surg 1995; 30: 304–8.

40. Lall A, Pritchard-Jones K, Walker J, et al. Wilms' tumor with intracaval thrombus in the UK Children's Cancer Study Group UKW3 trial. J Pediatr Surg 2006; 41: 382–7.

41. Brisse HJ, Smets AM, Kaste SC, Owens CM. Imaging in unilateral Wilms tumour. Pediatr Radiol 2008; 38: 18–29.

42. Slovis TL, ed. The ALARA (as low as reasonably achievable) concept in pediatric CT intelligent dose reduction. Multidisciplinary conference organized by the Society of Pediatric Radiology 2001. Pediatr Radiol 2002; 32: 217–313.

43. Scott DJ, Wallace WH, Hendry GM. With advances in medical imaging can the radiologist reliably diagnose Wilms' tumours? Clin Radiol 1999; 54: 321–7.

44. Panuel M, Bourliere-Najean B, Gentet JC, et al. Aggressive neuroblastoma with initial pulmonary metastases and kidney involvement simulating Wilms' tumor. Eur J Radiol 1992; 14: 201–3.

45. Lowe LH, Isuani BH, Heller RM, et al. Pediatric renal masses: Wilms' tumor and beyond. Radiographics 2000; 20: 1585–603.

46. Grundy P, Breslow N, Green DM, et al. Prognostic factors for children with recurrent Wilms' tumor: results from the Second and Third National Wilms' Tumor Study. J Clin Oncol 1989; 7: 638–47.

47. Grundy P, Perlman E, Rosen NS, et al. Current issues in Wilms' tumor management. Curr Probl Cancer 2005; 29: 221–60.

48. Owens CM, Veys PA, Pritchard J, et al. Role of chest computed tomography at diagnosis in the management of Wilms' tumor: a study by the United Kingdom Children's Cancer Study Group. J Clin Oncol 2002; 20: 2768–73.

49. Wootton-Gorges SL, Albano EA, Riggs JM, et al. Chest radiography versus chest CT in the evaluation for pulmonary metastases in patients with Wilms' tumor: a retrospective review. Pediatr Radiol 2000; 30: 533–7.

50. Ditchfield MR, De Campo JF, Waters KD, Nolan TM. Wilms' tumor: a rational use of preoperative imaging. Med Pediatr Oncol 1995; 24: 93–6.

51. D'Angio GJ, Rosenberg H, Sharples K, et al. Position paper: imaging methods for primary renal tumors of childhood: costs versus benefits. Med Pediatr Oncol 1993; 21: 205–12.

52. Ehrlich PF, Hamilton TE, Grundy P, et al. The value of surgery in directing therapy for patients with Wilm's tumor with pulmonary disease. A report from the National Wilms' Tumor Study Group (National Wilms' Tumor Study 5). J Pediatr Surg 2006; 41: 162–7.

53. Attard-Montalto SP, Kingston JE, Eden OB, Plowman PN. Late follow-up of lung function after whole lung irradiation for Wilms' tumour. Br J Radiol 1992; 65: 1114–18.

54. McHugh K, Pritchard J. Problems in the imaging of three common pediatric solid tumours. Eur J Radiol 2001; 37: 72–8.

55. Delemarre JF, Sandstedt B, Harms D, Boccon-Gibod L, Vujanić GM. The new SIOP (Stockholm) working classification of renal tumours of childhood. International Society of Paediatric Oncology. Med Pediatr Oncol 1996; 26: 145–6.

56. Vujanić GM, Sandstedt B, Harms D, et al. Revised International Society of Paediatric Oncology (SIOP) working classification of renal tumors of childhood. Med Pediatr Oncol 2002; 38: 79–82.

57. Shamberger RC, Guthrie KA, Ritchey ML, et al. Surgery-related factors and local recurrence of Wilms tumor in National Wilms Tumor Study 4. Ann Surg 1999; 229: 292–7.

58. Ritchey ML, Shamberger RC, Hamilton T, et al. Fate of bilateral renal lesions missed on preoperative imaging: a report from the National Wilms Tumor Study Group. J Urol 2005; 174: 1519–21.

59. de Kraker J, Graf N, van Tinteren H, et al. Reduction of postoperative chemotherapy in children with stage I intermediate-risk and anaplastic Wilms' tumour (SIOP 93-01 trial): a randomised controlled trial. Lancet 2004; 364; 1229–35.

60. Ritchey ML, Shamberger RC, Haase G, et al. Surgical complications after primary nephrectomy for Wilms' tumour: report from the National Wilms' Tumor Study Group. J Am Coll Surg 2001; 192: 63–8.

61. Mitchell C, Pritchard-Jones KP, Shannon R, et al. and for the United Kingdom Cancer Study Group. Immediate nephrectomy versus preoperative chemotherapy in the management of non-metastatic Wilms' tumour: results of a randomised trial (UKW3) by the UK Children's Cancer Study Group. Eur J Cancer 2006; 42: 2554–62.

62. Vujanić GM, Kelsey A, Mitchell C, Shannon RS, Gornall P. The role of biopsy in the diagnosis of renal tumours of childhood: results of the UKCCSG Wilms tumor study 3. Med Pediatr Oncol 2003; 40: 18–22.

63. Dykes EH, Marwaha RK, Dicks-Mireaux C, et al. Risks and benefits of percutaneous biopsy and primary chemotherapy in advanced Wilms' tumour. J Pediatr Surg 1991; 26: 610–12.

64. Coppes MJ, Anderson RA, Mueller DL, et al. Arteriovenous fistula: a complication following renal biopsy of suspected bilateral Wilms' tumor. Med Pediatr Oncol 1997; 28: 455–61.

65. Lee IS, Nguyen S, Shanberg AM. Needle tract seeding after percutaneous biopsy of Wilms tumor. J Urol 1995; 153: 1074–6.

66. Aslam A, Foot AB, Spicer RD. Needle track recurrence after biopsy of non-metastatic Wilms tumour. Pediatr Surg Int 1996; 11: 416–17.

67. Duncan A, on behalf of the United Kingdom Children's Cancer Study Group. UKCCSG Radiology Imaging Guidelines, June 2001.

68. Barnacle AM, McHugh K. Limitations with the response evaluation criteria in solid tumours (RECIST) guidance in disseminated pediatric malignancy. Pediatr Blood Cancer 2006; 46: 127–34.

69. Miser JS, Tournade MF. The management of relapsed Wilms tumour. Hematol Oncol Clin North Am 1995; 9: 1287–302.

70. Dome JS, Liu T, Krasin M, et al. Improved survival for patients with recurrent Wilms tumour: the experience at St Jude Children's Research Hospital. J Pediatr Hematol Oncol 2002; 24: 192–8.

71. Pritchard-Jones K. Controversies and advances in the management of Wilms' tumour. Arch Dis Child 2002; 87: 241–4.

72. Petruzzi MJ, Green DM. Wilms tumour. Pediatr Clin North Am 1997; 44: 939–52.

73. Owens CM, Brisse HJ, Olsen OE, Begent J, Smets AM. Bilateral disease and new trends in Wilms tumour. Pediatr Radiol 2008; 38: 30–9.

74. Merchant SA, Badhe PB. Nephroblastomatosis—pathological and imaging characteristics. J Postgrad Med 1995; 41: 72–80.

75. Ahmed HU, Arya M, Tsiouris A, et al. An update on the management of Wilms' tumour. Eur J Surg Oncol 2007; 33: 824–31.

76. Montgomery BT, Kelalis PP, Blute ML, et al. Extended followup of bilateral Wilms tumor: results of the National Wilms Tumor Study. J Urol 1991; 146: 514–18.

77. Hoffer FA. Magnetic resonance imaging of abdominal masses in the pediatric patient. Semin Ultrasound CT MR 2005; 26: 212–23.

78. Berenyi P, Pinter J, Szokoly V. Intraoperative sonography in organ preserving operations of kidney tumours. Z Urol Nephrol 1990; 83: 419–24.

79. Beckwith JB, Kiviat NB, Bonadio JF. Nephrogenic rests, nephroblastomatosis, and the pathogenesis of Wilms' tumor. Pediatr Pathol 1990; 10: 1–36.

80. Perlman E, Dijoud F, Boccon-Gibod L. Nephrogenic rests and nephroblastomatosis. Ann Pathol 2004; 24: 510–15.

81. Rohrschneider WK, Weirich A, Rieden K, et al. US, CT and MR imaging characteristics of nephroblastomatosis. Pediatr Radiol 1998; 28: 435–43.

82. Gylys-Morin V, Hoffer FA, Kozakewich H, Shamberger RC. Wilms tumour and nephroblastomatosis: imaging characteristics at gadolinium-enhanced MR imaging. Radiology 1993; 188: 517–21.

83. Subhas N, Argani P, Gearhart JP, Siegelman SS. Nephrogenic rests mimicking Wilms' tumour on CT. Pediatr Radiol 2004; 34: 152–5.

84. Beckwith JB. New developments in the pathology of Wilms tumour. Cancer Invest 1997; 15: 153–62.

85. Bailey S, Roberts A, Brock C, et al. Nephrotoxicity in survivors of Wilms' tumours in the North of England. Br J Cancer 2002; 87: 1092–8.

86. Breslow NE, Takashima JR, Ritchey ML, Strong LC, Green DM. Renal failure in the Deny-Drash and Wilms' tumor-aniridia syndromes. Cancer Res 2000; 60: 4030–2.

87. Walker DA, Dillon M, Levitt G, et al. Multiple exostosis (osteochondroma) and Wilms' tumour—a possible association. Med Pediatr Oncol 1992; 20: 360–1.

88. Green DM, Whitton JA, Stovall M, et al. Pregnancy outcome of female survivors of childhood cancer: a report from the Childhood Cancer Survivor Study. Am J Obstet Gynecol 2002; 187: 1070–80.

89. Carli M, Frascella E, Tournade MF, et al. Second malignant neoplasms in patients treated on SIOP Wilms tumour studies and trials 1, 2, 5 and 6. Med Pediatr Oncol 1997; 29: 239–44.

90. Scott RH, Walker L, Olsen OE, et al. Surveillance for Wilms tumour in at-risk children: pragmatic recommendations for best practice. Arch Dis Child 2006; 91: 995–9.

91. Metzger ML, Dome JS. Current therapy for Wilms' tumor. Oncologist 2005; 10: 815–26.

92. Kawashima A, Glockner JF, King BF Jr. CT urography and MR urography. Radiol Clin North Am 2003; 41: 945–61.

93. Leung RS, Biswas SV, Duncan M, Rankin S. Imaging features of von Hippel-Lindau disease. Radiographics 2008; 28: 65–79.

94. Wegner EA, Barrington SF, Kingston JE, et al. The impact of PET scanning on management of paediatric oncology patients. Eur J Nucl Med Mol Imaging 2005; 32: 23–30.

95. Humphries PD, Sebire NJ, Siegel MJ, Olsen OE. Tumors in pediatric patients at diffusion-weighted MR imaging: apparent diffusion coefficient and tumor cellularity. Radiology 2007; 245: 848–54.

96. Ascenti G, Mazziotti S, Zimbaro G, et al. Complex cystic renal masses: characterization with contrast-enhanced US. Radiology 2007; 243: 158–65.

38 Neuroblastoma
Marilyn J Siegel

INTRODUCTION

Neuroblastoma is the most common extracranial solid malignant tumor of childhood. It has a spectrum of locations and degrees of histopathologic differentiation resulting in a diversity of clinical and biologic features (1–3). With the exception of infants under the age of one year, the prognosis of children with neuroblastoma is generally poor. Tumor stage is an extremely important indicator of patient outcome and imaging therefore plays a crucial role in the determination of stage prior to treatment.

EPIDEMIOLOGY

Neuroblastoma accounts for 8% to 10% of all childhood cancers (1). The prevalence is about one case per 7000 live births and there are approximately 800 newly diagnosed cases of neuroblastoma in the United States annually (1–3). In the United Kingdom, recent data indicates a rate of 8.4 per million for all ages 0 to 14 years (4). Thus in the United Kingdom, the expected annual number of new cases of neuroblastoma is between 75 and 80. Neuroblastoma is the most common cancer of infancy. The median age at diagnosis of children with neuroblastoma is approximately 19 months (1). Approximately 36% of patients are infants; 89% are under five years; and 98% are under 10 years of age. Boys are affected slightly more often than girls with a male-to-female ratio of 1.1:1 (1).

GENETICS OF NEUROBLASTOMA

In a subgroup of patients, neuroblastoma exhibits an autosomal dominant pattern of inheritance, possibly related to an abnormality in the short arm of chromosome 16 (16p12-13) (5,6). In this subset, the median age at diagnosis is nine months and there is an increased prevalence of bilateral adrenal or multifocal primary tumors. In addition, there are data suggesting that genes associated with the genesis of other tumors of neural crest origin, such as neurofibromatosis type 1 and Hirschsprung disease, may be involved in the initiation or progression of neuroblastoma (1).

PROGNOSTIC FACTORS

Certain biochemical, biologic, and histologic markers are predicators of outcome in children with neuroblastoma (Table 38.1). These markers help to define specific subgroups of patients with widely divergent natural histories and survival rates (Table 38.2).

Biochemical markers include serum levels of lactate dehydrogenase, ferritin, and neuron-specific enolases (1,7,8). In general, low levels of any of these serum markers predict a good outcome, whereas high serum levels are associated with a poorer prognosis. Urinary catecholamine levels are not predictive of outcome. However, high homovanillic acid (HVA) and low vanillylmandelic acid (VMA) serum levels have been associated with shortened survival (1).

Biologic markers with prognostic value include amplification of the N-myc oncogene (9–12), the amount of tumor cell DNA (11,12) and karyotype (1,13–15). Up to 30% of children with neuroblastoma present with N-myc amplification in tumor cells (greater than 10 copies of a segment of DNA termed N-myc oncogene). N-myc amplification and diploid karyotype (normal or near-normal DNA content) are associated with aggressive tumor behavior and poor prognosis, regardless of tumors stage. Partial deletions of chromosome 1 and 11 and gains of chromosome 17 are other poor prognostic signs.

Histopathologic prognostic factors include tumor stromal content, degree of mitosis (16–18), and level of nerve growth factor tyrosine kinase receptors (Trk) expression (11,19). A stroma-rich tumor matrix, low mitotic activity, and a high level of expression of nerve growth factor TrkA correlate highly with favorable outcome. High expression of TrkB is seen with unfavorable neuroblastoma (11). Selected prognostic factors are summarized in Table 38.1.

PATHOLOGY

Neuroblastoma arises from primitive sympathetic cells, which are derived from the embryonic neural crest, and is one of the small, round blue-cell tumors of childhood. There are three histopathologic patterns of neuroblastoma, which correlate with the degree of tumor differentiation: neuroblastoma, ganglioneuroblastoma, and ganglioneuroma (1–3). Neuroblastoma is composed of small round cells with scant cytoplasm and hyperchromatic nuclei, often arranged in clusters resembling rosettes. Ganglioneuroblastoma contains rests of neuroblasts along with mature or maturing ganglion cells. Ganglioneuroma is fully differentiated and is composed of mature ganglion cells and Schwann cells. Neuroblastoma and ganglioneuroblastoma are usually grouped together (and referred to as neuroblastoma) for purposes of staging and reporting survival statistics as well as imaging features.

Macroscopically, neuroblastomas average 6 to 8 cm in size and often are hemorrhagic. Areas of stroma are often interposed between areas of hemorrhagic tissue, giving the tumor a lobular appearance. Areas of hemorrhage, necrosis and calcification are common on cut section (3). Distinguishing neuroblastoma from other small, round blue-cell tumors of childhood, including Ewing sarcoma, primitive neuro-ectodermal tumor, rhabdomyosarcoma, leukemia, and lymphoma, can be difficult on routine light microscopy and often requires the adjunctive use of electron microscopy or immunohistochemistry.

Table 38.1 Selected Biologic Prognostic Factors

Biologic parameter	Adverse finding
Tumor cell features	
N-myc oncogene	>10 copies
Chromosomal ploidy	Near diploid
Chromosome 17 q	Gain
Chromosome 1p36	Deletion
Chromosome 11q14–22	Deletion
Histopathologic markers	
TrkA	Absent or low expression
TrkB	High expression
Shimada histopathology	Unfavorable
Biochemical marker	
Serum lactate dehydrogenase	>1500 U/L
Serum neuron-specific enolase	>100 ng/mL
Serum ferritin	>142 ng/mL
Urine VMA:HVA ratio	<1

Abbreviations: HVA, homovanillic acid; VMA, vanillylmandelic acid.
Source: From Refs. 1, 44.

Table 38.2 Biologic and Clinical Subtypes of Neuroblastoma

Feature	Type 1	Type 2	Type 3
N-myc oncogene	Normal	Normal	Amplified
DNA ploidy	Hyperdiploid/triploid	Near diploid	Near diploid
Chromosome 17q gain	Rare	Common	Common
Chromosome 1p loss	Rare	±Present	Common
Chromosome 11q loss	Rare	Common	Rare
TrkA expression	High	Low or absent	Low or absent
TrkB expression	Truncated	Low or absent	High (full length)
Age (yr)	Usually <1	Usually ≥1	Usually 1–5
Stage	Usually 1, 2, 4S	Usually 3, 4	Usually 3, 4
5-yr survival (%)	95	40–50	25

Source: From Refs. 1, 44.

Key Points: Incidence, Prognosis, Pathology

- Neuroblastoma is the most common extracranial malignant tumor of childhood
- Eighty-nine percent of tumors occur under five years of age and the prognosis is generally poor
- Approximately two-thirds of tumors occur in the abdomen, 50% to 75% in the adrenal medulla
- Prognosis depends on multiple variables: clinical (patient age, tumor stage), biochemical (lactate dehydrogenase, ferritin, neuron-specific enolase), biologic (tumor cell DNA, loss of chromosome 1p, N-myc oncogene amplification), and histopathologic (stromal content, degree of mitosis, level of nerve growth factor expression)
- Urinary catecholamine levels are not predictive of patient outcome
- There are three histopathologic types of neuroblastoma: neuroblastoma, ganglioneuroblastoma, and ganglioneuroma

CLINICAL PRESENTATION

Most children with neuroblastoma are symptomatic. The tumor, however, can be detected incidentally on antenatal ultrasonography (20), post-natal screening programs (1,21–25), physical examination, or imaging studies obtained for other indications.

Screening Programmes

Neuroblastoma in situ has been described in fetuses (21–23). Postnatal clinical and radiological follow-up has demonstrated spontaneous resolution in virtually all cases, confirming the benign nature of these antenatal tumors.

Post-natal screening programs have been introduced in Canada, Europe, and Japan (24–28). The basis of urine catecholamine population screening programs is that early detection of neuroblastoma will decrease the prevalence of advanced stage disease in children older than one year of age. These screening studies increased detection of neuroblastoma in infants less than one year of age without decreasing the incidence of advanced stage disease and the mortality from neuroblastoma in older children. Those patients in whom neuroblastomas were identified generally had lower stages of disease and virtually all of the tumors were biologically favorable.

Symptoms due to Primary Tumor

Neuroblastoma can arise anywhere along the sympathetic chain, from the neck to the pelvis. Approximately two-thirds occur in the abdomen and 50% to 75% of these arise in the adrenal medulla. The remaining abdominal tumors arise from sympathetic paraspinal ganglia. Less common sites of origin are the posterior mediastinum (10–15%), neck (5%), and pelvis (5%). In approximately 1% of children, a primary tumor cannot be found. The sites of origin also vary with patient age. Infants have more cervical and thoracic tumors, whereas older children have more primary adrenal tumors (3).

The clinical presentation varies depending on the site of tumor and extent of disease (1–3,29). Tumors occurring in the abdomen are more likely to be symptomatic than those arising in the chest. Abdominal disease is likely to result in a palpable abdominal mass or abdominal pain. Sudden increase in abdominal size can result from spontaneous hemorrhage into the tumor. Large abdominal tumors can compress the kidney or encase or stretch the renal artery, activating the renin-angiotensin system and causing hypertension. Pelvic tumors can result in sciatic nerve palsy, urinary and fecal incontinence, neuropathic bladder, leg weakness or nerve root injury, and lower extremity edema resulting from compression of venous and lymphatic drainage (30).

Primary posterior mediastinal tumors often are an incidental finding on chest radiographs obtained to evaluate respiratory symptoms or trauma. High thoracic and cervical neuroblastomas can be associated with dysphagia, stridor, or Horner syndrome (unilateral ptosis, pupillary constriction, and anhydrosis) (31). Occasionally, thoracic tumors result in superior vena cava syndrome.

Paraspinal tumors can result in scoliosis, back pain, urinary or fecal retention, and peripheral neurologic deficits due to neural foraminal invasion and nerve root or cord compression. The neurologic manifestations are usually related to the level and extent of tumor invasion in the spinal canal and include radicular pain and subacute or acute paraplegia as well as bladder or bowel dysfunction (1).

Symptoms due to Distant Disease

At least 70% of patients with neuroblastoma will have disseminated disease at the time of diagnosis, including 70% of infants and 85% of children older than one year of age (1). Metastatic

extension occurs via lymphatic and hematogenous routes. In infants under 12 months of age, metastases are predominantly to the skin, liver, bone marrow, and lymph nodes. Metastases to the skin or subcutaneous tissue cause non-tender, bluish, mobile nodules ("blueberry muffin baby"), while metastases to the liver can present as hepatomegaly. In neonates the enlarging liver can cause severe respiratory compromise and compression of the inferior vena cava with resultant ascites, anasarca, and renal failure.

In children older than one year of age, metastases are to cortical bone, bone marrow, lymph nodes, and liver. Long bone and bone marrow metastases may cause migratory or recurrent bone pain or a palpable mass. These symptoms are often confused with leukemia, juvenile rheumatoid arthritis, or osteomyelitis (32). Metastatic disease to the sphenoid bone or retrobulbar soft tissues can result in proptosis and ecchymosis, creating a characteristic "raccoon eye" appearance. Metastatic lesions to the dura or brain can present with findings of increased intracranial pressure, such as widened cranial sutures, or focal neurologic signs. Non-specific signs and symptoms, including fever, irritability, weight loss, and anemia, are also common findings.

Paraneoplastic Syndromes

Several paraneoplastic syndromes have been associated with localized and disseminated neuroblastoma, including opsoclonus-myoclonus syndrome, intractable diarrhea, and flushing associated with hypertension. These findings have been attributed to metabolic and immunological disturbances associated with the tumor. The opsoclonus-myoclonus syndrome, also referred to as myoclonic encephalopathy of infants, is characterized by acute cerebellar and truncal ataxia and random eye movements ("dancing eyes") (33,34). It occurs in up to 4% of patients with newly diagnosed neuroblastoma. Conversely, up to 50% of children with this syndrome may have neuroblastoma (1). The primary tumor is most commonly found in the posterior mediastinum (50% of cases), but it may be found anywhere along the sympathetic chain. The majority of patients with opsoclonus-myoclonus syndrome have favorable outcomes with respect to their tumor. However, most have long term neurologic deficits that can progress even after removal of the tumor (33,34). These deficits are presumably due to antineural antibodies against the primary tumor that cross-react with neural cells in the cerebellum or elsewhere in the brain (34).

Intractable watery diarrhea associated with hypokalemia and dehydration is a result of tumor secretion of vasoactive intestinal peptide (VIP). Flushing in combination with hypertension is thought to be a manifestation of very high levels of catecholamines. Most patients with tumor-related diarrhea and hypertension have histologically mature tumors (either ganglioneuroma or ganglioneuroblastoma) and favorable outcomes (35,36). Surgical resection of the tumor leads to resolution of symptoms.

METHODS OF DIAGNOSIS

An unequivocal pathological diagnosis can be made based on tissue sampling and light microscopy, electron microscopy, or immunohistology. A diagnosis can also be established by the combination of a bone marrow aspirate or biopsy that shows unequivocal tumor cells and increased serum or urinary catecholamines

Table 38.3 INSS Staging System for Neuroblastoma

Stage	Definition
1	Localized tumor with complete resection, with or without microscopic residual disease; representative ipsilateral lymph nodes negative for tumor microscopically
2A	Localized tumor with incomplete gross excision; representative ipsilateral nonadherent lymph nodes negative for tumor microscopically
2B	Localized tumor with or without complete gross excision, with representative ipsilateral non-adherent lymph nodes positive for tumor. Enlarged contralateral lymph nodes must be negative microscopically.
3	Unresectable unilateral tumor infiltrating across the midline, with or without regional lymph node involvement; or localized unilateral tumor with contralateral regional lymph node involvement; or midline tumor with bilateral extension by infiltration (unresectable) or by lymph node involvement.
4	Any primary tumor with dissemination to distant lymph nodes, bone, bone marrow, liver, skin, and/or other organs (except as defined for stage 4S)
4S	Localized primary tumor (as defined for Stage 1, 2A, or 2B), with dissemination limited to skin, liver, and/or bone marrow. Bone marrow involvement should be minimal (<10% of total nucleated cells identified as malignant on bone marrow biopsy or on marrow aspirate). Limited to infants less than one year of age.

or metabolites. Percutaneous biopsy of the primary tumor or liver metastases in children with advanced disease (Stages 3, 4, or 4S) is an alternative to open biopsy for diagnosis and determination of prognostic information (37).

STAGING

The most widely used staging system for neuroblastoma is the International Neuroblastoma Staging System (INSS) (Table 38.3) (38,39). This classification takes into account radiological findings, surgical resectability and lymph node and bone marrow involvement. Regional disease is divided into Stages 1, 2, and 3, based on whether the tumor extends across the midline or is resectable, and on regional lymph node status. Distant disease in all patients ≥12 months is Stage 4 disease. In infants <12 months, widespread disease is characterized as Stage 4S ("special"), which is defined as a small tumor (Stage 1 or 2), rare (<10%) tumor cells in bone marrow, and no distant osseous metastases.

TREATMENT

Based on clinical factors of patient age at diagnosis, INSS stage and selected biologic factors (tumor histopathology, chromosomal ploidy, and N-myc amplification status), patients are grouped into low-, intermediate-, and high-risk categories for treatment planning (1). The goal is to reduce chemotherapy treatment in low- and intermediate-risk patients and to increase the intensity of chemotherapy in high-risk patients.

Treatment of Low-Risk Disease

Patients included in this group are: all patients with INSS Stage 1 disease; patients with INSS Stage 2 disease (except patients older

than one year at diagnosis with N-myc amplification and unfavorable Shimada pathology); and infants with 4S disease that have tumors with hyperdiploidy, favorable Shimada and no N-myc amplification (1). Treatment of low-risk neuroblastoma consists of surgical resection of the primary tumor (40,41).

Treatment of Intermediate-Risk Disease

Included in this group are: INSS stage 3 patients younger than one year with no N-myc amplification; INSS stage 3 patients older than one year with no N-myc amplification and favorable Shimada pathology; Stage 4 infants with no N-myc amplification; and nonamplified stage 4S patients with either unfavorable Shimada histopathology or tumor diploidy (or both) (1). Treatment of intermediate-risk disease consists of combination chemotherapy including carboplatin, etoposide, cyclophosphamide, and doxorubicin. Once the tumor decreases sufficiently in volume, delayed surgical resection may be performed.

Treatment of High-Risk Disease

Patients included in this group are: INSS Stage 4 patients older than one year at diagnosis; any INSS Stage 3 patients with N-myc amplification; INSS Stage 3 patients older than one year at diagnosis with unfavorable Shimada pathology; INSS Stage 2 patients with N-myc amplification and unfavorable Shimada pathology; and INSS Stage 4S patients with N-myc amplification (1). Treatment of high-risk disease has included intensive induction and consolidation chemotherapy, local radiotherapy to prevent relapse in primary tumor sites, 13-cis retinoic acid, and targeted radiotherapy with ^{131}I-metaiodobenzylguanidine (MIBG) or ^{131}I-labelled monoclonal antibodies (1,30,42–44). Surgical resection following treatment may also have an important place in management.

Occasionally, neuroblastoma will spontaneously regress. Spontaneous regression occurs most commonly in infants. Neuroblastoma cells also may differentiate into more benign ganglion cells, either spontaneously or after chemotherapy (1).

When disease recurs, it may be in the primary tumor site with extension into surrounding tissues or in other areas of the body. Bone and bone marrow relapses are common sites of relapse.

Key Points: Clinical Features, Staging, Treatment

■ The majority of tumors arise in the abdomen and 50% to 75% of these occur in the adrenal gland. Most children are symptomatic at presentation with abdominal pain and/or a palpable mass

■ At least 70% of patients have disseminated disease at the time of diagnosis. Metastases are predominantly to the skin, liver, bone marrow, and lymph nodes

■ Paraneoplastic syndromes are associated with neuroblastoma

■ Pathological diagnosis is made on tissue sampling and light microscopy, electron microscopy, and immunohistology

■ The International Neuroblastoma Staging System (INSS) is now the most widely used staging classification

■ Treatment is based on an assessment of risk and includes surgery, combination chemotherapy and radiotherapy

PRIMARY NEUROBLASTOMA: IMAGING CHARACTERISTICS

Imaging of neuroblastoma requires diagnosis of the primary tumor along with evaluation of the extent of local and distant disease. The multiple sites of origin and varying patterns of metastases make assessment of disease dependent on a multitude of imaging studies (44).

Imaging Studies

Plain Radiographs

Plain radiography is an insensitive method of diagnosing neuroblastoma. However plain radiographs undertaken to investigate unrelated clinical features may reveal unsuspected tumor in the neck, chest, or abdomen, or evidence of metastatic disease. Occasionally plain radiographs are obtained to further evaluate an abnormality shown on other imaging studies.

Plain radiographic findings include a posterior retroperitoneal, thoracic, or cervical mass (Fig. 38.1) and enlargement of the intervertebral foramina or erosion of the pedicles due to intraspinal extension of tumor. The tumor may contain calcifications.

Ultrasonography

The evaluation of patients with palpable abdominal masses, including neuroblastoma, usually begins with sonography.

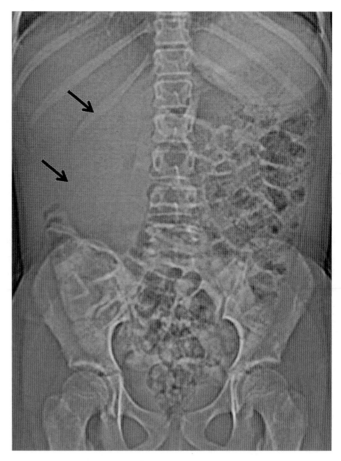

Figure 38.1 Right adrenal neuroblastoma in a two-year-old girl. Abdominal radiograph shows a large right paraspinal mass (arrows) displacing bowel gas to the left.

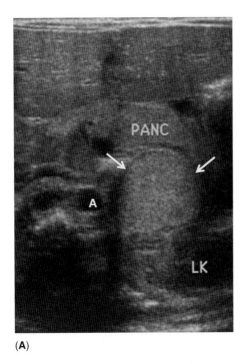

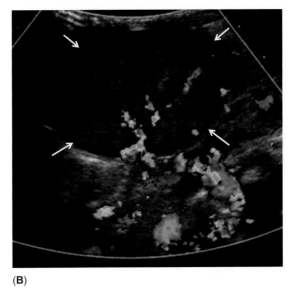

(A)   **(B)**

Figure 38.2 Suprarenal neuroblastoma in a 15-month-old girl. (**A**) Transverse longitudinal sonogram of the left upper quadrant shows a homogeneous echogenic left suprarenal mass (arrows) anterior to the left kidney (LK), posterior to the pancreas (PANC), and lateral to the aorta (A). (**B**) Color Doppler sonogram shows minimal vascularity within the tumor (arrows).

Sonography is an excellent study to confirm the presence of an abdominal or pelvic mass and its site of origin. Neuroblastoma appears either as a suprarenal or paraspinal mass (Fig. 38.2). The tumors are echogenic. They may be homogeneous or heterogeneous, containing focal echogenic areas secondary to calcification and hypoechoic areas, secondary to hemorrhage, necrosis, cystic change, or some combination thereof (45–47). Doppler sonography may show increased peripheral or central tumor vascularity.

In newborns, neuroblastomas may appear predominantly cystic or anechoic, corresponding to hemorrhage, degenerative change in the tumor or, in some cases, clusters of microcysts in the tumor cells (Fig. 38.3) (48,49). Unfortunately, this imaging appearance is non-specific and can mimic adrenal hematoma, another common lesion of the neonate. Differentiation requires demonstration of metastatic disease or positive laboratory studies (i.e., urinary catecholamine analysis) or serial sonographic examination. The generally excellent prognosis of neuroblastoma in this age group makes observation rather than surgery a reasonable alternative.

Computed Tomography

After the presence of a mass has been confirmed by sonography or plain radiography, patients undergo further imaging with either computed tomography (CT) or magnetic resonance (MR) imaging to determine the extent of disease and guide staging. On CT, neuroblastoma appears as a homogeneous or heterogeneous soft-tissue mass in a suprarenal or paraspinal location (Figs. 38.4 and 38.5) (44,49–51). The tumor enhances less than that of surrounding tissues after administration of IV contrast material. At CT, approximately 85% of abdominal and 50% of thoracic neuroblastomas demonstrate calcification (Fig. 38.6).

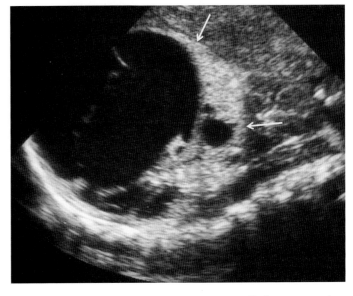

Figure 38.3 Neonatal adrenal neuroblastoma. Longitudinal sonogram views through the left upper quadrant of a one-week-old boy show a complex suprarenal mass (arrows), with hypoechoic areas, representing hemorrhage and cystic change.

Magnetic Resonance Imaging

On MR imaging, neuroblastoma appears as an extrarenal or paraspinal mass which is iso-, hypo-, or hyperintense to surrounding soft tissues on T1-weighted spin-echo images and hyperintense on fat-suppressed T2-weighted or STIR sequences (52,53). The margins may be smooth, irregular, or lobulated. Heterogeneity is common due to hemorrhage, necrosis, or calcification. Hemorrhage results in variable signal intensity, dependent on the

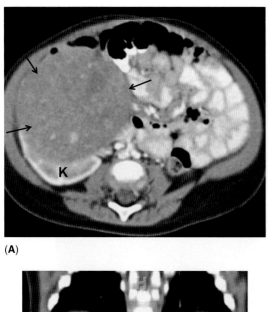

(A)

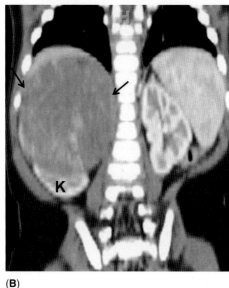

(B)

Figure 38.4 Adrenal neuroblastoma. (A) Axial CT and (B) coronal reformation in a three-year-old girl shows a large soft-tissue mass (arrows) with calcifications in the right suprarenal area. The tumor displaces the right kidney (K) posteriorly and inferiorly. There is no midline extension.

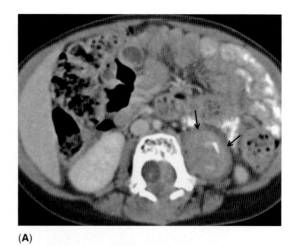

(A)

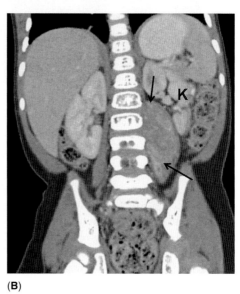

(B)

Figure 38.5 Sympathetic ganglion neuroblastoma. (A) Axial CT and (B) coronal reformation in a two-year-old girl shows a soft-tissue mass (arrows) with coarse calcifications in the paraspinal location. The tumor displaces the left kidney (K) superiorly and laterally.

age of the blood. Necrotic foci usually appear hypointense on T1-weighted sequences and hyperintense on T2-weighted sequences, while tumor calcification has low signal intensity on both pulse sequences. Most neuroblastomas enhance after administration of IV gadolinium chelate agents (Fig. 38.7).

Additional Findings of Primary Abdominal Tumors
Adrenal masses commonly displace the kidney inferiorly and laterally (Fig. 38.4). Neuroblastomas originating from ganglion cells displace the kidney superiorly and laterally (Fig. 38.5). Occasionally, the kidney is displaced anteriorly and medially. Aggressive neuroblastoma may invade the kidney and simulate Wilms' tumor (54,55). Renal atrophy can be the result of infarction due to encasement or compression of the renal vessels by the primary tumor, surgical trauma, chemotherapy, or radiation therapy.

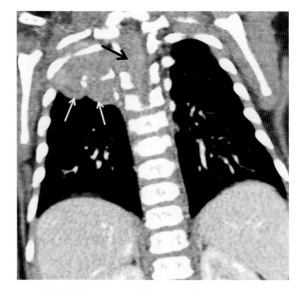

Figure 38.6 Calcified thoracic neuroblastoma, eight-month-old girl. Coronal CT shows a well circumscribed mass in the right paraspinal region (white arrows) with calcification. The tumor invades the spinal canal (black arrow).

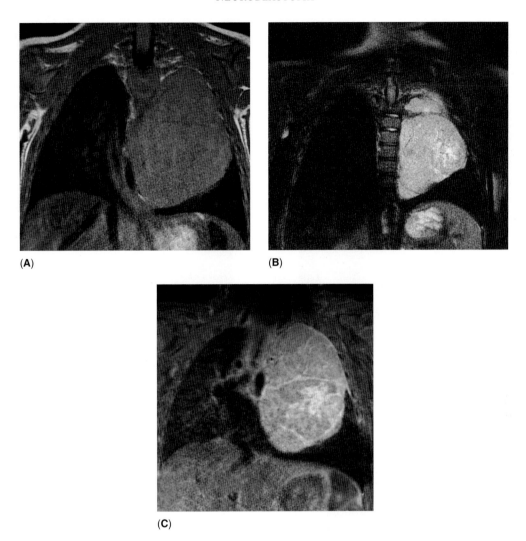

(A)

(B)

(C)

Figure 38.7 Thoracic neuroblastoma, 14-month-old girl. (**A**) Coronal T1-weighted MR image of the chest demonstrates a large left paraspinal neuroblastoma that is isointense with soft tissues. (**B**) On the fat-suppressed T2-weighted MR image, the tumor is hyperintense compared with subcutaneous fat. (**C**) Heterogeneous enhancement is noted on the fat-suppressed T1-weighted MR image following administration of gadolinium chelate.

Additional Findings of Extra-abdominal Neuroblastomas

Pelvic Neuroblastoma

Pelvic tumors are typically presacral in location and are situated behind the rectum and bladder. Erosion of the sacrum and bony pelvis and extension of tumor into the lateral pelvic sidewalls, sacral foramina, and sciatic notches may be commonly observed (Fig. 38.8).

Thoracic Neuroblastoma

Thoracic neuroblastoma is almost always paravertebral and may be associated with rib and vertebral body erosion and scoliosis.

Cervical Neuroblastoma

The mass seen in cervical neuroblastoma is usually well demarcated in the parapharyngeal space, displacing the carotid and jugular anteriorly (Fig. 38.9) (56–59). Extension through the skull base into the infratemporal fossa may be seen on CT and MR imaging.

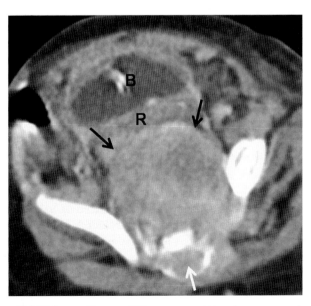

Figure 38.8 Pelvic neuroblastoma. CT in a two-year-old boy shows a presacral mass (black arrows) displacing the rectum (R) and bladder (B) anteriorly. The tumor invades the obturator muscles bilaterally and the spinal canal (white arrow).

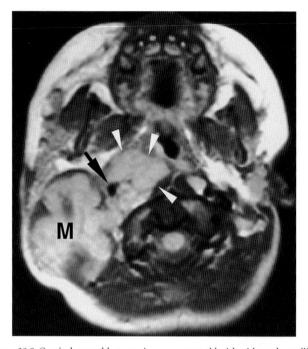

Figure 38.9 Cervical neuroblastoma in a one-year-old girl with neck swelling. Axial proton-density MR image shows a large right neck mass (M) surrounds the common carotid artery (arrow) and extends into the right parapharyngeal space (arrowheads). The right internal jugular vein is compressed and not seen. *Source:* From Ref. 59.

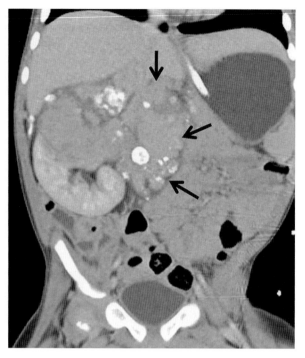

Figure 38.10 Midline extension. Coronal CT shows a large mass with calcification arising in the right suprarenal area and crossing the midline (arrows).

Key Points: Primary Neuroblastoma, Imaging Characteristics

- Ultrasonography is used predominantly to confirm the presence of a mass lesion; CT and MR imaging are used to stage the disease
- In newborns, neuroblastomas are often cystic
- On CT approximately 85% of abdominal tumors and 50% of thoracic tumors show calcification
- Most neuroblastomas enhance on CT and MR imaging after administration of IV contrast material
- Aggressive neuroblastomas may invade the kidney and simulate Wilms' tumor
- Pelvic tumors are usually presacral and thoracic tumors are almost always paravertebral in location

Local Disease Extent: Imaging Characteristics

The presence or absence of midline extension, vascular encasement, regional lymph node enlargement, and intraspinal extension need to be determined since these factors can affect surgical planning, staging, and prognosis.

Midline extension is defined as tumor extending to or beyond the pedicle contralateral to the primary tumor. Midline extension is important because it alters staging and upgrades the disease to Stage 3 (Fig. 38.10).

Vascular encasement is defined as tumor surrounding at least three-fourths of the circumference of one or more major abdominal arteries or veins, including the aorta, superior mesenteric artery and vein, inferior vena cava, or right or left renal artery and vein (Fig. 38.11). Vascular encasement can be

a contraindication to total surgical resection because of the risk of loss of vital structures or significant postoperative morbidity. Complications have been reported in 5% to 25% of patients with neuroblastoma related to surgical resection of the primary abdominal tumor at diagnosis (60). Commonly encountered complications related to vascular encasement include nephrectomy, operative hemorrhage, and injury to renal or mesenteric vessels.

Lymph node involvement is defined as discrete masses separate from the main tumor mass. The extent of nodal disease is important because it alters stage. Ipsilateral nodes correspond to a Stage 2 disease. Contralateral nodal disease indicates Stage 3 disease (Fig. 38.12).

Intraspinal extension of neuroblastoma is defined as a mass within the spinal canal (with or without cord displacement) that is contiguous with the main tumor mass (Fig. 38.13) (61). Intraspinal extension of neuroblastoma associated with spinal symptoms requires either urgent treatment with chemotherapy and steroids or a laminectomy alone or in combination with radiation therapy to reduce cord compression prior to tumor resection or debulking.

Ultrasonography has limited value in demonstrating involvement of retroperitoneal and retrocrural nodes and extension into the spinal canal. The choice of CT versus MR imaging for determining local extent has been the subject of continuing debate. Unfortunately, there are no large prospective series that compare MR imaging and CT in neuroblastoma for staging accuracy. CT with contrast enhancement can reliably demonstrate the primary tumor and it is superior to MR imaging in demonstrating calcification. A prospective multicenter study of children with newly diagnosed neuroblastoma found that overall,

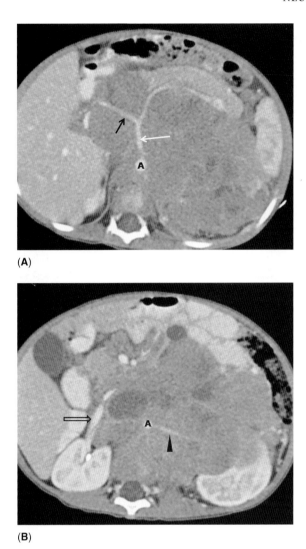

(A)

(B)

Figure 38.11 Midline extension. (**A**) CT in a 12-month-old boy shows a mass arising in the left adrenal gland, crossing the midline and encasing the aorta (A), superior mesenteric artery (white arrow), and hepatic artery (black arrow). (**B**) At a lower level, the tumor encases the left renal artery (arrowhead) and the aorta (A). The right renal artery and vein (open arrow) and the left kidney are pushed laterally. The renal arteries may be sufficiently compressed to cause hypertension. Extensive vascular encasement can be a contraindication to early surgical resection.

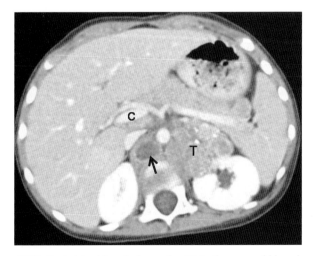

Figure 38.12 Contralateral lymphadenopathy. CT in three-year-old boy shows a left adrenal tumor (T) with calcification and an enlarged contralateral necrotic lymph node (arrow) displacing the inferior vena cava anteriorly (C).

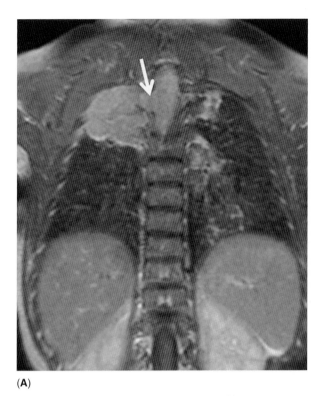

(A)

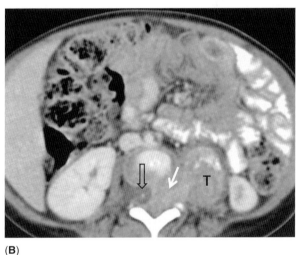

(B)

Figure 38.13 Intraspinal extension. (**A**) Coronal T1-weighted gadolinium-enhanced MR image in an eight-month-old girl (same patient as Fig. 38.6) shows an enhancing mass within the right lateral aspect of the chest cavity with tumor extension through the neural foramina (arrow) into the spinal canal of the upper thoracic spine. (**B**) CT in a two-year-old girl shows a left paravertebral tumor (T) with neural foraminal invasion (arrow), with marked thecal sac (open arrow) displacement toward the right.

CT and MR had statistically similar, but relatively poor performance for assessing features of local disease (62). However a major limitation of the study was that it was designed to evaluate distant not local disease and the prevalence of local disease was relatively low. The positive predictive values (PPV) and negative predictive values (NPV) for CT in detection of tumor extension across the midline were 73% and 83%, respectively. For MR imaging, corresponding PPV and NPV were 81% and 79%. PPV and NPV for CT in detection of local nodes were 20% and 95%, respectively. For MR imaging, corresponding PPV and NPV were 19% and 99%, respectively.

- Midline tumor extension, vascular encasement, regional lymph node enlargement, and intraspinal extension are important features of local tumor spread
- Midline extension is defined as tumor extending to or beyond the pedicle contralateral to the primary tumor. This feature upstages the tumor
- Vascular encasement and intraspinal extension affect surgical management but do not affect stage
- Lymphadenopathy is defined as a tumor mass separate from the primary mass and upstages disease
- Intraspinal tumor is defined as a mass within the spinal canal (with or without cord displacement) that is contiguous with the main tumor mass
- CT and MR imaging are both useful for determining extent of local tumor spread and appear to provide similar accuracy

Distant Disease: Imaging Characteristics

Detection of distant metastases upstages the tumor to a Stage 4 or 4S. Neuroblastoma metastasizes to liver, distant nodes, cortical bone, and bone marrow. Lung and intracranial metastases are rare.

Hepatic Metastases

Hepatic metastases occur in 5% to 10% of children with neuroblastoma. Two common patterns of hepatic metastases have been described; focal metastases, typically seen in older children, and diffuse infiltration, usually occurring in infants with Stage 4S disease. Focal lesions tend to be well-defined and they may be single or multiple (Fig. 38.14). They are equally well recognized on CT and MR imaging. Diffuse infiltration can be difficult to detect on CT and may be easier to recognize on MR imaging, especially on T2-weighted sequences, where hyperintense masses can be seen throughout the liver.

Distant Nodal Metastases

Distant nodes are those that are outside the cavity of origin of the tumor. Evaluation of the chest, abdomen, and pelvis, regardless of the site of primary disease, is performed in all patients with neuroblastomas to increase detection of distant nodal involvement. A common site of distant nodal spread is the supraclavicular region (63).

Skeletal and Bone Marrow Metastases

Skeletal metastases occur in 50% to 60% of patients at diagnosis, mostly in patients older than one year of age. These can involve cortical bone or bone marrow.

Plain Radiographs

While plain radiographs are not routinely used in the detection of bony metastases, the initial presentation in some patients may be bone pain, prompting skeletal radiographs. Thus, recognition of the conventional radiographic features is important. Skull radiographic findings include sutural diastasis secondary to dural involvement, focal lytic defects, periosteal reaction ("sunburst" appearance), and foci of sclerosis (Fig. 38.15). Metastatic disease to long bones may manifest as metaphyseal lucencies, periosteal

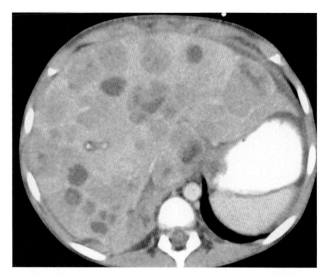

Figure 38.14 Hepatic metastases. Five-year-old boy with Stage 4 neuroblastoma who presented with an enlarging abdomen and worsening abdominal pain. CT shows multiple low attenuation hepatic metastases.

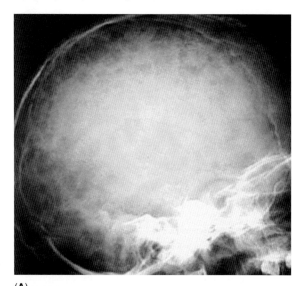

(A)

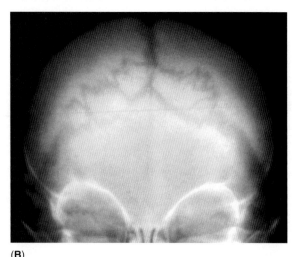

(B)

Figure 38.15 Metastatic neuroblastoma. (A) Lateral skull radiograph shows diffuse poorly defined lytic lucencies throughout the calvarium, consistent with diffuse metastatic disease. (B) Frontal radiograph in another patient shows cranial sutural widening due to dural metastases.

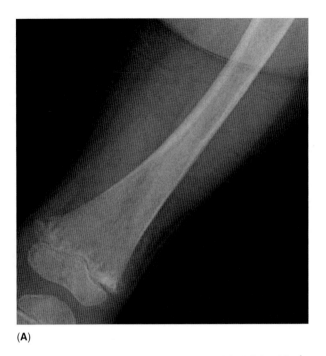
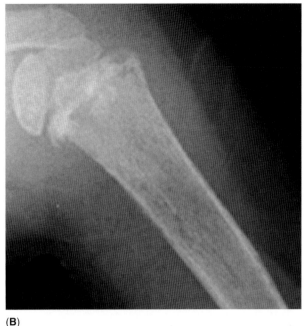

(A)   **(B)**

Figure 38.16 Osseous metastases. (A) Frontal radiograph of the left distal femur in a two-year-old boy shows multiple lytic areas in the femoral metaphysis. (B) Frontal radiograph of the left humerus shows metaphyseal lucencies and a permeative appearance in the diaphysis, representing diffuse marrow infiltration.

reaction, or sclerotic foci (Fig. 38.16). In both appendicular and axial skeleton, there may be a generalized reduction in bone density and a mottled trabecular or permeative pattern due to diffuse marrow infiltration (Fig. 38.16B).

Computed Tomography

CT is not a primary study for confirming skeletal metastases. However, metastases may be seen on CT when the primary tumor is evaluated and in some instances, there may be unsuspected findings on scans obtained for evaluation of other clinical problems. Metastases are most frequently destructive lesions (Fig. 38.17) but occasionally sclerotic lesions may be seen. Associated findings include periosteal new bone and a soft-tissue mass.

Skeletal Scintigraphy

Scintigraphy with ^{99m}Tc-dimercaptophosphonate (MDP) is known to be superior to the conventional skeletal survey in the detection of cortical bone metastases. MDP is taken up by cells active in bone metabolism. The sensitivity of ^{99m}Tc-MDP is about 90%, compared to a sensitivity of 35% to 70% for the radiographic skeletal survey (64,65). Metastases appear either as focal areas of increased radiopharmaceutical accumulation (Fig. 38.18) or rarely, as photopenic or cold lesions. Asymmetrical metaphyseal uptake is typical. Common sites of metastases are the skull, facial bones, orbits, ribs, and vertebral bodies. Increased tracer activity can also be seen in the primary tumor, but this has no clinical significance.

MIBG Scintigraphy

Metaiodobenzylguanidine (MIBG) has become the study of choice for imaging skeletal metastases (66–72). MIBG, an analogue of catecholamine precursors, is taken up by catecholamine-producing tumors. MIBG can be labeled with ^{123}I or ^{131}I. ^{123}I MIBG is preferable

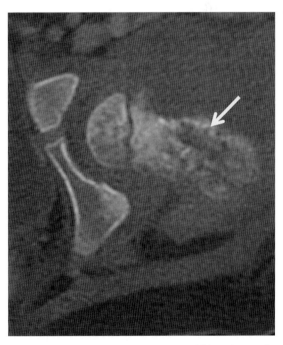

Figure 38.17 Osseous metastasis. CT in a two-year-old boy shows a destructive lesion in the left femoral metaphysis (arrow).

to ^{131}I MIBG because of lower radiation dose to the patient, better image resolution, greater sensitivity for disease detection, and shorter time to scanning following tracer administration. In patients with neuroblastoma, abnormal activity can be seen in the primary tumor and in bone, bone marrow, and soft tissue metastases (Fig. 38.19). The sensitivity of ^{123}I MIBG for tumor detection in bone, bone marrow, and lymph nodes is 90% to 95% (69,71). Absence of MIBG activity has been reported in more

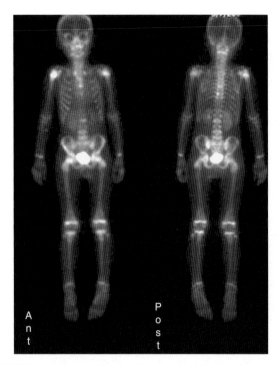

Figure 38.18 Metastatic neuroblastoma, bone scintigraphy. Anterior and posterior bone scintigrams after injection of Tc-99m MDP in a three-year-old girl show abnormal osseous uptake in multiple vertebral bodies, several ribs, right humeral head and proximal diaphysis, and bilateral proximal femoral and tibial metaphyses.

mature tumors and also in very poorly differentiated tumors. Causes of false-negative MIBG scans include non-visualization of lesions due to intense radiotracer uptake in normal liver, myocardium, salivary glands, intestines, and thyroid (44). Several rare tumors may also show MIBG uptake, potentially resulting in false-positive scans. These include neuroendocrine tumors, pancreatico-blastomas, neuro-ectodermal tumors, pheochromocytomas, carcinoid tumors, and medullary thyroid carcinomas (69). However, these lesions are extremely uncommon in the pediatric population and MIBG activity in a child is virtually specific for neuroblastoma (69,71,73). The specificity of MIBG for neuroblastoma in the appropriate clinical context is greater than 95% (74).

Magnetic Resonance Imaging

MR imaging can be performed as a dedicated study for evaluation of localized bone pain or as whole-body imaging for detection of distant metastases (62,75–82). Typically, metastatic disease produces low signal intensity on T1-weighted sequences and high signal intensity on T2-weighted and fat suppressed images (Fig. 38.20). The sensitivity of MR imaging for detecting marrow involvement is between 85% and 100% (62,77,79,82). MR imaging can show abnormalities not detected by bone marrow biopsy (62).

Two morphologic patterns of bone marrow involvement have been described: focal and diffuse (82). The diffuse form of marrow infiltration is invariably associated with cortical destruction (84% of cases) and commonly (>75% of cases) leaves residual signal

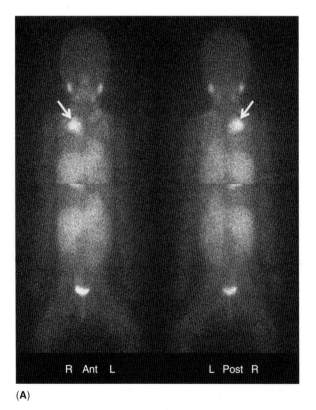

(A)

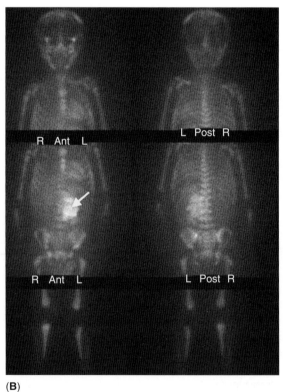

(B)

Figure 38.19 Metastatic neuroblastoma, I-123 MIBG. (**A**) Anterior and posterior scintigrams obtained 24 hours after injection of I-123 MIBG demonstrate increased uptake in a right posterior mediastinal neuroblastoma (arrows). There is expected I-123 MIBG activity in the salivary glands, liver, myocardium, and urinary bladder. Normal skeleton/marrow does not demonstrate MIBG activity. (**B**) I-123 MIBG in another patient shows increased tracer uptake throughout the skeleton consistent with diffuse osseous/marrow metastases. There also is uptake in the left adrenal primary (arrow).

934

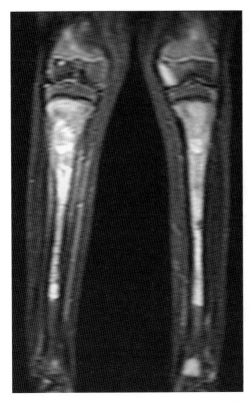

Figure 38.20 In this patient with metastatic neuroblastoma, coronal fat-suppressed T2-weighted MR image shows abnormally bright signal indicative of diffuse marrow infiltration. By comparison, normal red marrow would have signal intensity similar to that of muscle on fat-suppressed images.

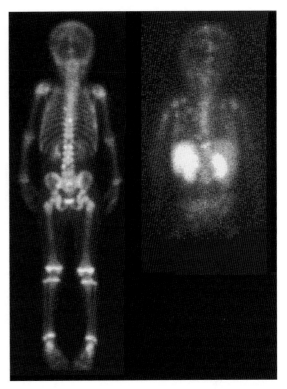

Figure 38.21 Metastatic neuroblastoma, octreotide scan. Posterior bone scintigram (left panel) and Indium-111 pentetreotide scintigram (right panel) demonstrate multifocal osseous metastases from neuroblastoma. Normal activity seen in the spleen, kidneys, and liver on the octreotide study.

abnormalities after chemotherapy. The focal form of disease is rarely associated with cortical involvement (16% of cases), but if present it virtually always disappears after chemotherapy.

Indium-111 Pentetreotide Scintigraphy

Indium-111 pentetreotide (octreotide), a radiolabeled somatostatin analogue, has an affinity for binding to the somatostatin receptors in neuroblastomas (Fig. 38.21) (83–85). Scans are more frequently positive in undifferentiated tumors and in tumors associated with elevated urinary catecholamines. Pentetreotide may be picked up in MIBG-negative tumors (86,87) and vice versa. The sensitivity of pentetreotide for detection of the primary tumor varies from 65% to 100% (88–90). In small series, patients with receptor-positive tumors had 100% one-year survival, while those with receptor-negative tumors had less than 60% one-year survival (88,89). The usefulness of octreotide for staging distant disease is still to be determined.

Positron Emission Tomography

In contrast to the dependence primarily on anatomic imaging features, positron emission tomography (PET) exploits the metabolic characteristics of tissue for the detection of disease. The metabolic activity of neuroblastoma is usually evaluated by utilizing 2-[fluorine-2418]-fluoro-2-deoxy-D-glucose (FDG) (Fig. 38.22) (91–93), or less commonly 11Chydioxyephedrine (HED) (94). FDG uptake is directly proportional to tumor burden and to tumor-cell proliferation. Most neuroblastomas and their metastases avidly concentrate FDG prior to chemotherapy or radiation therapy. The uptake after therapy is variable. These agents may also be useful for imaging tumors that do not concentrate MIBG. A limitation of PET scanning is the poor visualization of lesions in the cranial vault, because of the normally high physiologic FDG activity in the brain. Causes of false-positive scans include physiologic uptake in bowel, thymus, urinary tract, normal adrenal gland, hyperactive bone marrow, and sites of inflammation.

Intracranial Metastases

Intracranial involvement is generally confined to the dura and leptomeninges. Parenchymal disease is usually attributed to direct extension from adjacent skull or dural disease (95,96). Isolated parenchymal brain metastases from extracranial neuroblastoma without associated calvarial or dural involvement are rare. When present these lesions are generally solid and show heterogeneous contrast enhancement on CT and MR imaging; on occasion, hemorrhagic and cystic metastases may also been seen (97). Cerebral metastatic disease is usually seen at the time of relapse, rather than at the time of diagnosis.

Metastases to the skull and orbit have been reported in up to 25% of cases of neuroblastoma, often being the first evidence of the primary tumor (98). CT or MR imaging can show sutural widening, calvarial new bone formation, and tumor extension into the soft tissues of the scalp or through the inner table of the

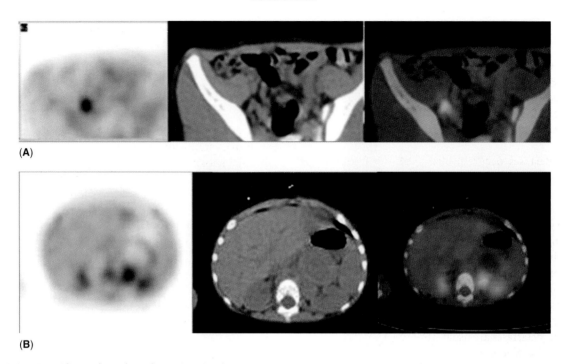

(A)

(B)

Figure 38.22 PET imaging with F-18 fluorodeoxyglucose (FDG). (**A**) Metastatic neuroblastoma in an eight-year-old boy. FDG-PET with corrected attenuation image (*left*), unenhanced CT (*middle*) and CT fusion image (*right*) show focus of increased FDG uptake within the right internal iliac chain, consistent with metastatic disease. (**B**) In another patient FDG-PET with corrected attenuation image (*left*), unenhanced CT (*middle*) and CT fusion image (*right*) show increased FDG uptake within a left adrenal neuroblastoma, representing the primary tumor. There was no evidence of metastatic disease.

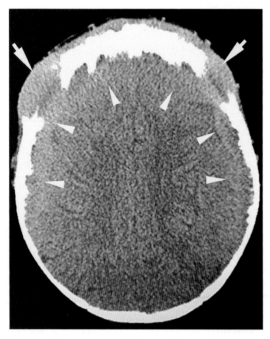

Figure 38.23 Calvarial metastases. CT shows widening of the coronal sutures (arrows), irregular calvarial new bone formation, and epidural spread of tumor (arrowheads). *Source*: From Ref. 99.

skull (Fig. 38.23). When there is sphenoid bone involvement, the tumor can extend into the orbits and cause proptosis.

Thoracic Metastases

Pulmonary and/or pleural involvement are rare initial complications of neuroblastoma, occurring in less than 3% of

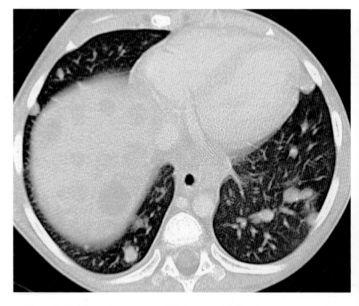

Figure 38.24 Thoracic metastases. CT shows multiple pulmonary metastases.

children (54). More commonly, thoracic disease is seen at the time of relapse. Pulmonary involvement can result from hematogenous or lymphatic spread or from direct extension. On CT, parenchymal metastases appear as either single or multiple small nodules (Fig. 38.24) or large parenchymal masses. Pleural disease may manifest as either an effusion or as pleural masses.

Key Points: Distant Disease

- Distant metastases upstages disease to Stage 4 or 4S
- Hepatic metastases occur in up to 5% to 10% of children
- Distant nodal metastases are defined as those occurring outside the body cavity of the origin of the primary tumor
- Supraclavicular node involvement is a common site of nodal spread
- Skeletal metastases occur in 50% to 60% of children at diagnosis
- MIBG ^{123}I is the method of choice for detecting skeletal metastases and distant metastases can also be identified in the primary tumor, bone marrow, and soft tissue sites
- MR imaging is useful for assessing localized skeletal pain or as a screening study for skeletal metastases
- The role of Indium-111 pentetreotide (octreotide) in the detection of metastases has not yet been established
- Most primary neuroblastomas and their metastases take up FDG avidly on PET scanning
- Intracranial metastases are usually the result of direct spread from skull or dural lesions
- Pulmonary disease is most frequently seen at the time of relapse

RESPONSE TO TREATMENT

The International Neuroblastoma Response Criteria (INRC) were established in 1988 and subsequently modified in 1993 (38,39). Response to treatment consists of response of the primary tumor and also of the metastatic sites. The INRC requires that the primary tumor lymph nodes, and liver metastases be evaluated by CT and/or MR imaging and that distant metastases be evaluated using MIBG scans, Tc-99m bone scans, and bilateral iliac crest marrow aspirates and trephine biopsies. Because of the difficulties in making accurate measurements of a tumor with an irregular shape, volume (three-dimensions rather than the product of the two largest diameters) has been suggested to assess response.

A complete response (CR) indicates complete disappearance of all primary and metastatic disease. A very good partial response (VGPR) indicates a 90% to 99% volume reduction in the primary tumor with resolution of pre-existing metastatic disease and no new bone lesions. The only exception to this is that there can be residual abnormality on technetium bone scintigraphy attributable to incomplete healing of the bone at sites of previous metastases. The MIBG scan should be negative at all metastatic sites. A partial response (PR) indicates a 50% to 90% reduction in both the primary tumor and all measurable metastatic sites. No response (NR) indicates a less than 50% reduction of some or all measurable lesions, but no increase of greater than 25% in any existing lesion and no new lesions. Progressive disease (PD) indicates the presence of a new lesion; increase of any measurable lesion by greater than 25%; or conversion of marrow from negative to positive (38,39).

Most tumors that are going to respond to treatment do so by three to four months and therefore, it is recommended that evaluations for response be performed at approximately four months from the initiation of chemotherapy. Further evaluation is

recommended at the end of treatment, before and after surgical procedures, before stem cell transplantation, and as clinically indicated (1).

Key Points: Follow-up

- Measurement of response requires monitoring change in the primary tumor and in the metastases
- The International Neuroblastoma Response Criteria (1993) require that the primary tumor, lymph nodes, and liver metastases are monitored using CT and/or MR imaging, and distant metastases are assessed using MIBG, Tc-99m bone scans, and bone marrow biopsies
- Complete response indicates disappearance of all disease sites. A very good partial response indicates a 90% to 99% volume reduction of primary tumor and resolution of all metastases
- Response is assessed at approximately four months after initiation of chemotherapy
- Further evaluation is recommended at the end of treatment, before and after surgical procedures, before stem cell transplantation, and as clinically indicated

Summary

- Neuroblastoma is the most common extracranial malignant tumor of childhood, accounting for 8% to 10% of all childhood cancers
- Serum markets (lactate dehydrogenase, ferritin, and neuron-specific enolases) provide important prognostic information. Urinary catecholamine levels are not predictive of outcome
- The majority of children present with clinical symptoms or signs, most commonly an abdominal mass or abdominal pain
- Paraneoplastic syndromes are associated with both local and disseminated disease
- The International Neuroblastoma Staging System is now the most widely used for staging
- Treatment is based on an assessment of risk and includes surgery, combination chemotherapy, and radiotherapy
- There are no large prospective series comparing CT with MR imaging for local staging accuracy. However, MR imaging is the preferred technique for showing intraspinal extension
- Ultrasonography is an excellent screening tool for detection of abdominal tumor, but it is seldom used to demonstrate the full extent of a large tumor
- Imaging is vital in the detection of distant metastases. These are chiefly to bone and/or bone marrow, occurring in over half the children with neuroblastoma
- Tc99m-labelled MDP and MIBG remain the techniques of choice for the detection of bone metastases
- The International Neuroblastoma Response Criteria (1993) require that the volume of the primary tumor, the liver and lymph nodes are evaluated by CT and/or MR imaging, and that metastases are evaluated with MIBG scans and Tc99m MDP bone scans., and that the bone marrow is assessed by bilateral iliac crest marrow aspirates and trephine biopsies

REFERENCES

1. Brodeur GM, Maris JM. Neuroblastoma. In: Pizzo PA, Poplack DG, eds. Principles and Practice of Pediatric Oncology, 5th edn. Philadelphia: Lippincott Williams & Wilkins, 2006; 933–70.

2. Gurney JG, Davis, Severson RK, Fang JY, Ross JA, Robison LL. Trends in cancer incidence among children in the U.S. Cancer 1996; 78: 532–41.

3. Lonergan GJ, Schwab CM, Suarez ES, Carlson CL. Neuroblastoma, ganglioneuroblastoma and ganglioneuroma: radiologic-pathologic correlation. Radiographics 2002; 22: 911–34.

4. Spix C, Pastore G, Sankila R, Stiller CA, Steliarova-Foucher E. Neuroblastoma incidence and survival in European children (1978-1997): Report from the Automatic Childhood Cancer Information System project. Eur J Cancer 2006; 42: 2081–91.

5. Maris JM, Weiss MJ, Mosse Y, et al. Evidence for a hereditary neuroblastoma predisposition locus at chromosome 16p12-13. Cancer Res 2002; 62: 6651–8.

6. Maris JM, Matthay KK. Molecular biology of neuroblastoma. J Clin Oncol 1999; 17: 2264–79.

7. Berthold F, Trechow R, Utsch S, Zieschang J. Prognostic factors in metastatic neuroblastoma. A multivariate analysis of 182 cases. Am J Pediatr Hematol Oncol 1992; 14: 207–15.

8. Zeltzer PM, Marangos PJ, Evans AE, Schneider SL. Serum neuron-specific enolase in children with neuroblastoma: relationship to stage and disease course. Cancer 1986; 57: 1230–4.

9. Bordow SB, Norris MD, Haber PS, Marshall GM, Haber M. Prognostic significance of MYCN oncogene expression in childhood neuroblastoma. J Clin Oncol 1998; 16: 3286–94.

10. Brodeur GM, Seeger RC, Schwab M, Varmus HE, Bishop JM. Amplification of N-myc in untreated human neuroblastomas correlates with advanced disease stage. Science 1984; 224: 1121–4.

11. Brodeur GM. Neuroblastoma: biologic insights into a clinical enigma. Nat Rev Cancer 2003; 3: 203–16.

12. Look AT, Hayes FA, Shuster JJ, et al. Clinical relevance of tumour cell ploidy and N-myc gene amplification in childhood neuroblastoma: A Pediatric Oncology Group study. J Clin Oncol 1991; 9: 581–91.

13. Attiyeh EF, London WB, Mosse YP, et al. Chromosome 1p and 11q deletions and outcome in neuroblastoma. N Engl J Med 2005; 353: 2243–53.

14. Caron H, van Sluis P, de Kraker J, et al. Allelic loss of chromosome 1p as a predictor of unfavourable outcome in patients with neuroblastoma. N Engl J Med 1996; 334: 225–30.

15. Maris JM, White PS, Beltinger CP, et al. Significance of chromosome 1p loss of heterozygosity in neuroblastoma. Cancer Res 1995; 55: 4664–9.

16. Joshi VV, Cantor AB, Altshuler G, et al. Recommendations for modification of terminology of neuroblastic tumours and prognostic significance of Shimada classification. A clinicopathologic study of 213 cases from the Pediatric Oncology Group. Cancer 1992; 69: 2183–96.

17. Shimada H, Ambros IM, Dehner LP, et al The International Neuroblastoma Pathology Classification (the Shimada system). Cancer 1999; 86: 364–72.

18. Shimada H, Stram DO, Chatten J, et al. Identification of subsets of neuroblastomas by combined histopathologic and N-myc analysis. J Natl Cancer Inst 1995; 87: 1470–6.

19. Nakagawara A, Arima-Nakagawara M, Scavarda NJ, et al. Association between high levels of expression of the TRK gene and favourable outcome in human neuroblastoma. New Engl J Med 1993; 328: 847–54.

20. Lukens JN. Neuroblastoma in the neonate. Semin Perinatol 1999; 22: 263–73.

21. Granata C, Fagnani AM, Gambini C, et al. Features and outcome of neuroblastoma detected before birth. J Pediatr Surg 2000; 35: 88–91.

22. Ho PT, Estroff JA, Kozakewich H, et al. Prenatal detection of neuroblastoma: a ten-year experience from the Dana-Farber Cancer Institute and Children's Hospital. Pediatrics 1993; 92: 358–64.

23. Erttmann R, Tafese T, Berthold F, et al. 10 years' neuroblastoma screening in Europe: preliminary results of a clinical and biological review from the Study Group for Evaluation of Neuroblastoma Screening in Europe (SENSE). Eur J Cancer 1998; 34: 1391–7.

24. Nishi M, Miyake H, Takeda T, et al. Mass screening of neuroblastoma in Sapporo City, Japan. Am J Pediatr Hematol Oncol 1992; 14: 327–31.

25. Nishihira H, Toyoda Y, Tanaka Y, et al: Natural course of neuroblastoma detected by mass screening: a 5-year prospective study at a single institution. J Clin Oncol 2000; 18: 3012–17.

26. Woods WG, Tuchman M, Robison LL, et al. Screening for neuroblastoma is ineffective in reducing the incidence of unfavourable advanced stage disease in older children. Eur J Cancer 1997; 33: 2106–12.

27. Woods WG, Tuchman M, Robison LL, et al. A population-based study of the usefulness of screening for neuroblastoma. Lancet 1996; 348: 1682–7.

28. Yamamoto K, Hayashi Y, Hanada R, et al. Mass screening and age-specific incidence of neuroblastoma in Saitame Prefecture, Japan. J Clin Oncol 1995; 13: 2033–8.

29. Abramson SJ. Adrenal neoplasms in children. Radiol Clin North Am 1997; 35: 1415–53.

30. Cruccetti A, Kiely EM, Spitz L, et al. Pelvic neuroblastoma: low mortality and high morbidity. J Pediatr Surg 2000; 35: 724–8.

31. Abramson SJ, Berdon WE, Ruzal–Shapiro C, Stolar C, Garvin J. Cervical neuroblastoma in eleven infants – a tumour with favourable prognosis. Clinical and radiologic (US, CT, MRI) findings. Pediatr Radiol 1993; 23: 253–7.

32. Applegate K, Connolly LP, Treves ST. Neuroblastoma presenting clinically as hip osteomyelitis: a "signature" diagnosis on skeletal scintigraphy. Pediatr Radiol 1995; 25: S93–S96.

33. Koh PS, Raffensperger JG, Berry S, et al. Long-term outcome in children with opsoclonus-myoclonus and ataxia and coincident neuroblastoma. J Pediatr 1994; 125: 712–16.

34. Mitchell WG, Snodgrass SR. Opsoclonus-ataxia due to childhood neural crest tumours: a chronic neurologic syndrome. J Child Neurol 1990; 5: 153–8.

35. Tiedemann K, Pritchard J, Long R, Bloom SR. Intractable diarrhoea in a patient with vasoactive intestinal peptide-secreting

neuroblastoma. Attempted control by somatostatin. Eur J Pediatr 1981; 137: 217–19.

36. Mendelsohn G, Eggleston JC, Olson JL, et al. Vasoactive intestinal peptide and its relationship to ganglion cell differentiation in neuroblastoma. Lab Invest 1979; 41: 144–9.

37. Hoffer FA, Chung T, Diller L, et al. Percutaneous biopsy for prognostic testing of neuroblastoma. Radiology 1996; 200: 213–16.

38. Brodeur GM, Seeger RC, Barrett A, et al. International criteria for diagnosis, staging and response to treatment in patients with neuroblastoma. J Clin Oncol 1988; 6: 1874–81.

39. Brodeur GM, Pritchard J, Berthold F, et al. Revisions of the international criteria for neuroblastoma diagnosis, staging and response to treatment. J Clin Oncol 1993; 11: 1466–77.

40. Perez CA, Matthay KK, Atkinson JB, et al. Biologic variables in the outcome of stages I and II neuroblastoma treated with surgery as primary therapy: a children's cancer group study. J Clin Oncol 2000; 18: 18–26.

41. Weinstein JL, Katzenstein HM, Cohn SL. Advances in the diagnosis and treatment of neuroblastoma. Oncologist 2003; 8: 278–92.

42. Matthay KK, Villablanca JG, Seeger RC, et al. Treatment of high-risk neuroblastoma with intensive chemotherapy, radiotherapy, autologous bone marrow transplantation, and 13-cis retinoic acid. N Engl J Med 1999; 341: 1165–73.

43. Pashankar FD, O'Dorisio MS, Menda Y. MIBG and somatostatin receptor analogs in children: current concepts on diagnostic and therapeutic use. J Nucl Med 2005; 46: 55S–61S.

44. Kushner BH. Neuroblastoma: a disease requiring a multitude of imaging studies. J Nucl Med 2004; 45: 1172–88.

45. Berdon WE, Ruzal-Shapiro C, Abramson SJ, Garvin J. The diagnosis of abdominal neuroblastoma: relative roles of ultrasonography, CT and MRI. Urol Radiol 1992; 14: 252–62.

46. Siegel MJ. Adrenal glands, pancreas and retroperitoneum. In: Siegel MJ, ed. Pediatric Sonography, 3rd edn. Philadelphia: Lippincott Williams & Wilkins, 2002; 476–527.

47. Cassady C, Winters WD. Bilateral cystic neuroblastoma: imaging features and differential diagnosis. Pediatr Radiol 1997; 27: 758–9.

48. Hugosson C, Nyman R, Jorulf H, et al. Imaging of abdominal neuroblastoma in children. Acta Radiol 1999; 40: 534–42.

49. Teoh SK, Whitman GJ, Chew FS. Neonatal neuroblastoma. AJR Am J Roentgenol 1997; 168: 54.

50. Siegel MJ. Adrenal glands, pancreas, and other retroperitoneal structures. In: Siegel MJ, ed. Pediatric Body CT, 2nd edn. Philadelphia: Lippincott Williams & Wilkins, 2008; 323–60.

51. Slovis TL, Meza MP, Cushing B, et al. Thoracic neuroblastoma: what is the best imaging modality for evaluating extent of disease? Pediatr Radiol 1997; 27: 273–5.

52. Meyer JS. Retroperitoneal MR imaging in children. Magn Reson Imaging Clin N Am 1996; 4: 657–78.

53. Siegel MJ. MR imaging of pediatric abdominal neoplasms. Magn Reson Imaging Clin N Am 2000; 8: 837–51.

54. Panuel M, Bourliere-Najean B, Gentet JC, et al. Aggressive neuroblastoma with initial pulmonary metastases and kidney involvement simulating Wilms' tumour. Eur J Radiol 1992; 14: 201–3.

55. Rosenfield NS, Leonidas JC, Barwick KW. Aggressive neuroblastoma simulating Wilms tumour. Radiology 1988; 166: 165–7.

56. Casselman JW, Smet MH, Van Damme B, Lemahieu SF. Primary cervical neuroblastoma: CT and MR findings. J Comput Assist Tomogr 1988; 12: 684–6.

57. Herman TE, Siegel MJ. Cervical neuroblastoma, stage IV-S. J Perinatol 2001; 21: 470–2.

58. Goldberg RM, Keller IA, Schonfeld SM, Mezrich RS, Rosenfeld DL. Intracranial route of a cervical neuroblastoma through skull base foramina. Pediatr Radiol 1996; 26: 715–16.

59. Siegel MJ, Coley BD. Neck. In: Siegel MJ, Coley BD, eds. The Core Curriculum: Pediatric Imaging. Philadelphia: Lippincott Williams & Wilkins, 2006: 12.

60. Nitschke R, Smith EI, Shochat S, et al. Localized neuroblastoma treated by surgery: a Pediatric Oncology Group study. J Clin Oncol 1988; 6: 1271–9.

61. Siegel MJ, Jamroz GA, Glazer HS, Abramson CL. MR imaging of intraspinal extension of neuroblastoma. J Comput Assist Tomogr 1986; 10: 593–5.

62. Siegel MJ, Ishwaran H, Fletcher BD, et al. Staging of neuroblastoma by imaging: report of the Radiology Diagnostic Oncology Group. Radiology 2002; 223: 168–75.

63. Abramson SJ, Berdon WE, Stolar C, Ruzal-Shapiro C, Garvin J. Stage IVN neuroblastoma: MRI diagnosis of left supraclavicular "Virchow's" nodal spread. Pediatr Radiol 1996; 26: 717–19.

64. Heisel MA, Miller JH, Reid BS, Siegel SE. Radionuclide bone scan in neuroblastoma. Pediatrics 1983; 71: 206–9.

65. Howman-Giles RB, Gilday DL, Ash JM. Radionuclide skeletal survey in neuroblastoma. Radiology 1979; 131: 497–502.

66. Gelfand MJ. Meta-iodobenzylguanidine in children. Semin Nucl Med 1993; 23: 231–42.

67. Gelfand MJ, Elgazzar AH, Kriss VM, Masters PR, Golsch GJ. Iodine-123-MIBG SPECT versus planar imaging in children with neural crest tumours. J Nucl Med 1994; 35: 1753–7.

68. Gordon I, Peters AM, Gutman A, et al. Skeletal assessment in neuroblastoma. The pitfalls of iodine-123-MIBG scans. J Nucl Med 1990; 31: 129–34.

69. Howman Giles R, Shaw PJ, Uren RF, Chung DK. Neuroblastoma and other neuroendocrine tumours. Semin Nucl Med 2007; 37: 286–302.

70. Parisi MT, Greene MK, Dykes TM, et al. Efficacy of metaiodobenzylguanidine as a scintigraphic agent for detection of neuroblastoma. Invest Radiol 1992; 27: 768–73.

71. Paltiel HJ, Gelfand MJ, Elgazzar AH, et al. Neural crest tumours: I-123 MIBG imaging in children. Pediatr Radiol 1994; 190: 117–21.

72. Shulkin BL, Shapiro B, Hutchinson RJ. Iodine-131-metaiodobenzylguanidine and bone scintigraphy for the detection of neuroblastoma. J Nucl Med 1992; 33: 1735–40.

73. Pfluger T, Schmied C, Porn U, et al. Integrated imaging using MRI and ^{123}I metaiodobenzylguanidine scintigraphy to improve sensitivity and specificity in the diagnosis of pediatric neuroblastoma. AJR Am J Roentgenol 2003; 181: 1115–24.

74. Leung A, Shapiro B, Hattner R, et al. Specificity of radioiodinated MIBG for neural crest tumours in childhood. J Nucl Med 1997; 38: 1352–7.

75. Couanet D, Geoffray A, Hartmann O, Leclere JG, Lumbroso JD. Bone marrow metastases in children's neuroblastoma studied by magnetic resonance imaging. Prog Clin Biol Res 1988; 271: 547–55.

76. Daldrup-Link HE, Franzius C, Link TM. Whole-body MR imaging for detection of bone metastases in children and young adults: comparison with skeletal scintigraphy and FDG PET. AJR Am J Roentgenol 2001; 177: 229–36.

77. Goo HW, Choi SH, Ghim T, Moon HN, Seo JJ. Whole-body MRI of paediatric malignant tumours: comparison with conventional oncological imaging methods. Pediatr Radiol 2005; 35: 766–73.

78. Kellenberger CJ, Epelman M, Miller SF, Babyn PS. Fast STIR whole-body MR imaging in children. Radiographics 2004; 24: 1317–30.

79. Mazumdar A, Siegel MJ, Narra V, Luchtman-Jones L. Whole-body fast inversion recovery MR imaging of small cell neoplasms in pediatric patients: a pilot study. AJR Am J Roentgenol 2002; 179: 1261–6.

80. Ruzal-Shapiro C, Berdon WE, Cohen MD, Abramson SJ. MR imaging of diffuse bone marrow replacement in pediatric patients with cancer. Radiology 1991; 181: 587–9.

81. Sofka CM, Semelka RC, Kelekis NL, et al. Magnetic resonance imaging of neuroblastoma using current techniques. Magn Reson Imaging 1999; 17: 193–8.

82. Tanabe M, Ohnuma N, Iwai J, et al. Bone marrow metastasis of neuroblastoma analyzed by MRI and its influence on prognosis. Med Pediatr Oncol 1995; 24: 292–9.

83. Dorr U, Sautter-Bihl ML, Schilling FH, et al. Somatostatin receptor scintigraphy: a new diagnostic test in neuroblastoma. Prog Clin Biol Res 1994; 385: 355–61.

84. Maggi M, Baldi E, Finetti G, et al. Identification, characterization and biological activity of somatostatin receptors in human neuroblastoma cell lines. Cancer Res 1994; 54: 124–33.

85. Sautter-Bihl ML, Dorr U, Schilling F, Treuner J, Bihl H. Somatostatin receptor imaging: a new horizon in the diagnostic management of neuroblastoma. Semin Oncol 1994; 21: 38–41.

86. Lauriero F, Rubini G, D'Addabbo F, et al. I-131 MIBG scintigraphy of neuroectodermal tumours. Comparison between I-131 MIBG and In-111 DTPA octreotide. Clin Nucl Med 1995; 20: 243–9.

87. Manil L, Edeline V, Lumbroso J, Lequen H, Zucker JM. Indium-111-pentetreotide scintigraphy in children with neuroblast-derived tumours. J Nucl Med 1996; 37: 893–6.

88. Moertel CL, Reubi JC, Scheithauer BS, Schaid DJ, Kvols LK. Expression of somatostatin receptors in childhood neuroblastoma. Am J Clin Pathol 1994; 102: 752–6.

89. O'Dorisio MS, Hauger M, Cecalupo AJ. Somatostatin receptors in neuroblastoma: diagnostic and therapeutic implications. Semin Oncol 1994; 21: 33–7.

90. Schilling FH, Bihl H, Jacobsson H, et al. Combined ^{111}In-pentetreotide scintigraphy and ^{123}I-MIBG scintigraphy in neuroblastoma provides prognostic information. Med Pediatr Oncol 2000; 35: 688–91.

91. Kushner BH, Yeung HW, Larson SM, Kramer K, Cheung NK. Extending positron emission tomography scan utility to high-risk neuroblastoma: fluorine-18 fluorodeoxyglucose positron emission tomography as sole imaging modality in follow-up patients. J Clin Oncol 2001; 19: 3397–405.

92. Rigo P, Paulus P, Kaschten BJ, et al. Oncological applications of positron emission tomography with fluorine-18-fluorodeoxyglucose. Eur J Nucl Med 1996; 23: 1641–74.

93. Shulkin BL, Hutchinson RJ, Castle VP, et al. Neuroblastoma: positron emission tomography with 2-[Fluorine-18]-Fluoro-2-deoxy-D-glucose compared with metaiodobenzylguanidine scintigraphy. Radiology 1996; 199: 743–50.

94. Shulkin BL, Wieland DM, Baro ME, et al. PET hydroxyephedrine imaging of neuroblastoma. J Nucl Med 1996; 37: 16–21.

95. Aronson MR, Smoker WR, Oetting GM. Haemorrhagic intracranial parenchymal metastases from primary retroperitoneal neuroblastoma. Pediatr Radiol 1995; 25: 284–5.

96. Sener RN. CT of diffuse leptomeningeal metastasis from primary extracerebral neuroblastoma. Pediatr Radiol 1993; 23: 402–3.

97. Kenny BJ, Pizer BL, Duncan AW, Foreman NK. Cystic metastatic cerebral neuroblastoma. Pediatr Radiol 1995; 25: S97–S98.

98. Egelhoff JC, Zalles C. Unusual CNS presentation of neuroblastoma. Pediatr Radiol 1996; 26: 51–4.

Uncommon Pediatric Neoplasms
Kieran McHugh

INTRODUCTION

All solid tumors are rare in childhood. One in 600 children develops cancer before 16 years of age, 33% of these are leukemias and 25% brain tumors. After the more common pediatric malignancies discussed in chapters 37 and 38, notably Wilms' tumor, neuroblastoma and the lymphomas, the following tumors are the most prevalent pediatric malignancies:

- Rhabdomyosarcoma
- Liver tumors, including hepatoblastoma and hepatocellular carcinoma
- Germ cell tumors—extragonadal and gonadal
- Non-rhabdomyomatous soft tissue tumors

Collectively these tumors account for up to 15% of pediatric malignancies although individually they are all very uncommon. Because of their rarity, they present a diagnostic challenge to the radiologist who encounters only an occasional case. This chapter reviews the clinical and imaging features of uncommon tumors in children and adolescents.

RHABDOMYOSARCOMA

Rhabdomyosarcoma (RMS) is the third most common extracranial solid childhood tumor, after neuroblastoma and Wilms' tumor, accounting for at least 4% of malignancies in childhood. RMS is the most common soft tissue sarcoma in children under the age of 15 years (1). Almost two-thirds of cases are diagnosed in children aged six years or younger with a smaller incidence peak in early to mid adolescence (2).

Histology

RMS arises from immature mesenchymal cells committed to skeletal cell lineage but may arise anywhere in the body, often in sites lacking striated muscle such as the bladder. It is a typical small, round, blue-cell tumor on conventional histology, and is classified histologically using the International Classification of RMS which is based on the relationship between prognosis and histology (3). Histologically, the presence of myofibrils and cross striations and/or a positive immunohistochemical staining for markers of muscle differentiation, like desmin and myoD1, is essential in the diagnosis of RMS.

There are four subtypes of tumor: undifferentiated sarcoma and alveolar RMS, both of which have the worst prognoses, embryonal RMS which has an intermediate prognosis and other botryoid and spindle-cell RMS which have the best prognosis. Botryoid RMS is seen almost exclusively in the bladder or vagina of infants or young girls, or the nasopharynx of slightly older children (Fig. 39.1). Botryoid RMS has a particularly favorable prognosis, rarely metastasizing and responding favorably to chemotherapy. Of newly diagnosed RMS, 60% are of the embryonal subtype and 20% are of the alveolar subtype (1). Alveolar RMS is more aggressive than its embryonal counterpart and has a worse prognosis. For example, results from the Intergroup Rhabdomyosarcoma Study (IRS) I-III studies gave a 94% five-year survival for orbital embryonal RMS versus a 74% five-year survival for orbital alveolar RMS (4).

The genetic changes associated with RMS vary with histiotype (2). Alveolar RMS (aRMS) is associated with t(2;13)(q35) or t(1;13)(p36;q14) chromosomal translocations which cause rearrangement of transcription factors (generating PAX3-FKHR and PAX7-FKHR fusion products) and ultimately result in modification of cell growth, differentiation and apoptotic pathways. In contrast, most embryonal RMS (eRMS) tumors have allelic loss at chromosome 11p15.5. Studies demonstrate repression of tumor growth from this chromosome region, suggesting the presence of a tumor suppressor gene. In both eRMS and aRMS some common targets are affected, such as the p53 and RB pathways. The majority of cases are sporadic but there is an association with certain familial syndromes such as the Li Fraumeni syndrome, RMS as well as other soft tissue sarcomas which have been associated with germline mutations of the p53 tumor suppressor gene (5).

Clinical Presentation and Location

In the majority of patients presentation comprises a mass lesion or disturbance of body function caused by the large tumor and/or associated enlarged lymph nodes. RMS in childhood differs from adult soft tissue sarcomas in that only a minority occur in the limbs; 40% of tumors occur in the head and neck region, 30% occur in the genitourinary tract, 10% are truncal, and 20% arise in the extremities (2).

Of the head and neck tumors, 50% occur in a parameningeal location, 25% are orbital and 25% arise in other head and neck sites, with embryonal histological type being the most common subtype. Orbital primaries present with proptosis or less commonly with ophthalmoplegia and are usually diagnosed before distant dissemination (Fig. 39.2). Non-orbital parameningeal primaries present with nasal, aural or sinus obstruction or discharge, or with cranial nerve palsy suggesting infiltration of the skull base. Superficial head and neck tumors may simply present as a painless lump (Fig. 39.3). Metastases occur to lungs and bones.

RMS in the male genitourinary tract is seen most commonly in the bladder and prostate. Embryonal and botryoid histological type are the most common subtypes, and alveolar histological type is uncommon in this location (2). Bladder RMS is often polypoid and tends to grow intraluminally in or near the trigone, typically presenting with hematuria or acute retention. Vaginal RMS is almost invariably botryoid and affects very young girls. Cervical and uterine RMS are seen more commonly in older girls and present with a mass or discharge. Regional lymph node involvement is uncommon but should be excluded on imaging (Fig. 39.4). Paratesticular RMS presents as painless unilateral

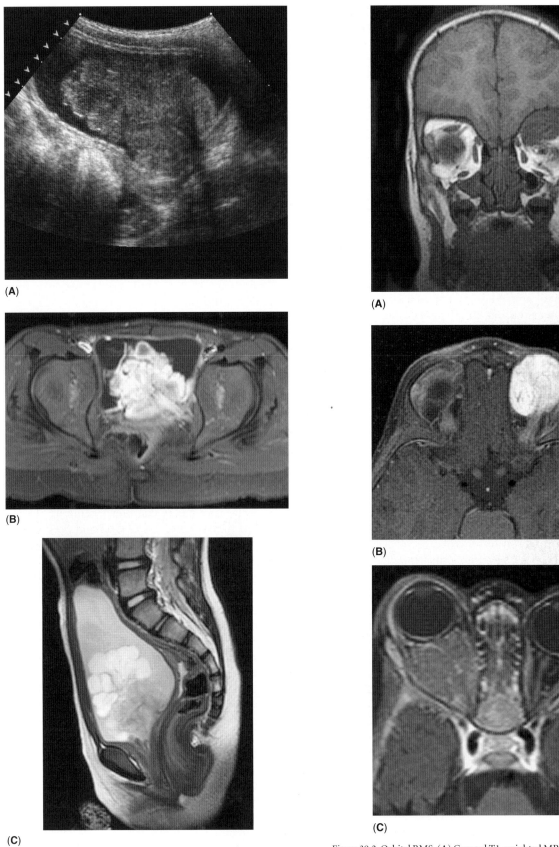

Figure 39.1 Botryoid rhabdomyosarcoma (RMS) of the bladder. (**A**) Longitudinal ultrasound showing a large intravesical solid tumor. (**B**) Axial fat-suppressed T1-weighted MR image after gadolinium administration showing avid enhancement by the tumor mass. (**C**) On a sagittal T2-weighted MR image the mass can be seen protruding into the urethral orifice without obvious bladder base invasion.

Figure 39.2 Orbital RMS. (**A**) Coronal T1-weighted MR image shows a mass lesion in the superior aspect of the left orbit in a four year old boy who presented with proptosis. (**B**) The anteriorly positioned mass demonstrates vivid enhancement on a fat-suppressed T1-weighted MR image after gadolinium administration. (**C**) Fat-suppressed T1-weighted axial MR image after gadolinium administration in a different patient shows a poorly enhancing right-sided intraconal mass lesion.

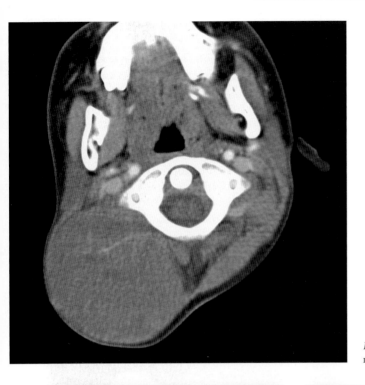

Figure 39.3 Neck RMS. Contrast-enhanced CT demonstrating a solid non-descript mass, proven on biopsy to be embryonal RMS. No bone erosion was evident.

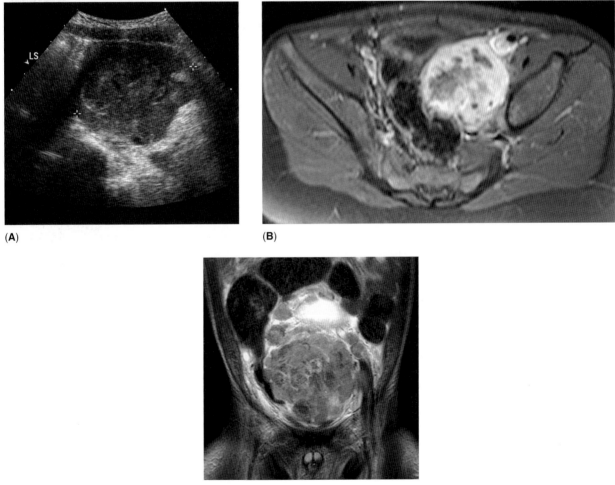

(A)

(B)

(C)

Figure 39.4 Nodal involvement in pelvic RMS. (A) Solid mass seen on routine surveillance ultrasound in a boy previously treated for a bladder/prostate RMS. (B) An enhancing mass is seen on a T1-weighted MR image after gadolinium administration, to the left of an underfilled bladder. This nodal recurrence was outside the initial radiotherapy field. (C) Coronal T2-weighted MR image at initial presentation, in another patient, of a large pelvic RMS. Nodules of tissue are seen superolateral to the mass on both sides which have similar signal characteristics to the primary tumor, indicating locoregional spread of disease.

943

scrotal or inguinal enlargement and is seen in both pre- and postpubertal boys. Under 10 years old, retroperitoneal lymph node involvement is rare, but occurs in up to 50% of older boys.

RMS in the limbs presents primarily as a non-tender swelling. Occasionally the primary mass is impalpable but clinical presentation is with painless regional adenopathy, underscoring the importance of examining the whole limb both clinically and with imaging in this context. 50% to 75% of cases are of the alveolar histological type. Regional lymph node enlargement is present in up to 50% at presentation, being more common with alveolar RMS. Despite wide local excision local recurrence remains a risk.

Thoracic, abdominal, and pelvic tumors are often large at diagnosis with complete surgical resection being difficult due to widespread tumor infiltration and vascular encasement.

Biliary tract RMS is very rare and classically manifests as obstructive jaundice. Spread occurs locally, within the liver and then to the retroperitoneum or lungs. Other unusual primary sites include liver, brain, trachea, heart, breast, and ovary. Metastatic RMS with unknown primary is also well recognized and in this scenario, in addition to the trunk, all four limbs should be examined thoroughly.

Staging and Prognosis

A number of different staging systems have been used by various cooperative pediatric oncology groups worldwide, the majority being postsurgical systems based on tumor resectability (Table 39.1) (6). The following is a brief synopsis of current staging methods.

An initial staging system, adopted in the first three Intergroup Rhabdomyosarcoma Study Group (IRSG) trials, categorized patients on the basis of the extent of disease and the completeness of their surgical resection. Investigators in IRS-IV attempted to use the tumor, node, and metastasis (TNM) system to standardize the staging system in the United States with those in other parts of the world. Unlike the first system, TNM staging does not take the extent of surgery into account, though it does take size and location into consideration.

The two staging systems have been combined, and children with rhabdomyosarcoma are now given one of three risk classifications: low, intermediate, or high. Treatment options are tailored for these risk classifications.

Risk Classification
- Low risk: Patients have embryonal rhabdomyosarcoma at a favorable site (Stage I), at an unfavorable site with complete resection (Group I), or at an unfavorable site with microscopic residual disease (Group II).
- Intermediate risk: Patients have embryonal rhabdomyosarcoma at an unfavorable site with gross residual disease (Group III), or non-metastatic alveolar rhabdomyosarcoma at any site.
- High risk: Includes any patient with metastatic disease.

Group Staging System
- Group I: This group is defined by localized disease with complete surgical resection and no evidence of regional nodal involvement.

- Group II: 20% of patients with rhabdomyosarcoma are in Group II.
  - Group IIA patients have grossly resected disease with microscopic residual disease and no regional involvement.
  - Group IIB patients have had complete resection with no residual disease, but they also have regional disease with involved nodes.
- Group III: Approximately 50% of patients with rhabdomyosarcoma are in Group III. This group is marked by incomplete resection or biopsy only; therefore, they have gross residual disease.
- Group IV: Distant metastases at diagnosis.

TNM Staging System
- Stage I: Disease is localized and involves the orbit, the head, and neck region (excluding parameningeal sites), or the non-bladder and/or non-prostate genitourinary region.
- Stage II: Includes any localized disease of any unfavorable primary site not included in the Stage I category. The primary tumor must be less than or equal to 5 cm in diameter.
- Stage III: The criteria are the same as in Stage II except the primary tumor is larger than 5 cm in diameter and/or it involves regional lymph nodes.
- Stage IV: Like Group IV, Stage IV implies metastatic disease at diagnosis.

Both stage and group have been shown to be highly predictive of outcome and were correlated (7,8). The International Society of Pediatric Oncology (SIOP) now also uses this staging system for RMS. As a consequence there is an increasing use of, and reliance on, imaging techniques, in particular computed tomography (CT) and magnetic resonance (MR) imaging for staging RMS. This in turn should facilitate a better assessment of tumor extent at diagnosis, including the demonstration of enlarged regional lymph nodes which are presumed to harbor metastases.

Table 39.1 Intergroup Rhabdomyosarcoma Study Group Staging: Surgical–Pathologic Grouping System (6)

Stage	Extent of disease
I	Localized tumor, completely resected
A	Confined to the organ of origin
B	Infiltration outside organ; regional nodes not involved
II	Compromised or regional resection of three types:
A	Grossly resected tumor with microscopic residual
B	Regional disease, completely resected, in which lymph nodes may be involved and/or tumor extension into adjacent organ may be present
C	Regional disease or involved lymph nodes, macroscopically resected but with evidence of microscopic residual
III	Incomplete resection or biopsy with macroscopic residual tumor
A	Localized or locally extensive tumor, gross residual disease after biopsy
B	Localized or locally extensive tumor, gross residual disease after major resection
IV	Distant metastases

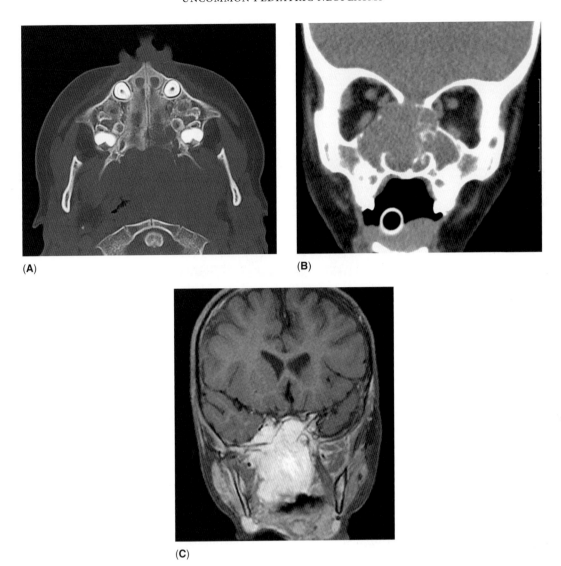

(A)

(B)

(C)

Figure 39.5 Parameningeal RMS. (A) CT at bone window settings reveals a large soft tissue mass in the nasopharyngeal region. The left medial pterygoid plate is indistinct as is the posterior aspect of the hard palate due to tumor erosion. Note the left lateral pterygoid plate is slightly displaced laterally compared to the normal right side. (B) Coronal CT in another patient showing a nasopharyngeal tumor causing widespread bone destruction. Both medial orbital walls and floor of the anterior cranial fossa have been eroded in addition to destruction of the nasal cavity. (C) Coronal T1-weighted MR image after gadolinium administration showing a large enhancing mass lesion. Enhancing tumor extension into the right cavernous sinus and along the dura in the floor of the right middle cranial fossa is seen.

Favorable prognosis factors for RMS are: (9)

- The absence of metastases at diagnosis
- Favorable tumor site
- Grossly complete surgical removal of tumor at the time of diagnosis
- Embryonal or botryoid histology
- Tumor size less than 5 cm
- Age younger than 10 years at diagnosis

Currently the reported cure rate for RMS is approximately 70%. In general the five-year overall survival for low risk patients is between 85% and 90%, for intermediate risk patients is 70%, and for those with metastatic disease is 25%.

Imaging
Head and Neck
RMS of the head and neck grows insidiously and often invades the intracranial space through the foramina (Fig. 39.5). MR imaging is mandatory because of its capability of assessing both local and intracranial extension. Frequently CT of the skull base is also needed to fully evaluate the presence or absence of osseous destruction. RMS masses are typically isointense or near isointense to muscle on T1-weighted MR images. Consequently, they are generally easily distinguished from benign lesions in the head and neck of children, such as a branchial cleft cyst, which are generally of lower intensity than muscle on T1-weighted images. Variable hyperintense T2-weighted signal intensity is seen again with variable enhancement on T1 weighting following administration of IV contrast medium. As surgery is often not feasible, all parameningeal tumors merit radiotherapy. Orbital tumors with intracranial invasion or bone destruction are also treated with radiotherapy.

Orbital RMS is usually non-invasive and confined to the bony orbit. Tumor mass at presentation is commonly of similar size to the globe and the mass may be intra- or extraconal (10). Regional lymph node extension is rare, believed to be due to a paucity of

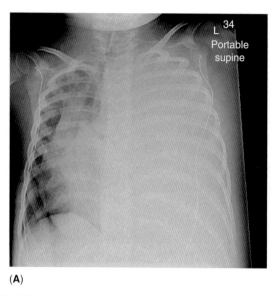 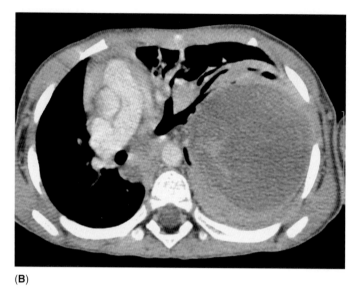

(A) (B)

Figure 39.6 Thoracic RMS. (A) Chest radiograph shows complete white-out of the left lung with mediastinal shift to the right. Note no rib erosion is evident. (B) An earlier contrast-enhanced CT in the same child, when some left lung aeration was still present, demonstrates a very large heterogeneous mass and anterior displacement of the left main bronchus.

orbital lymphatics. Excellent survival rates in excess of 90% have been reported (11). When performing MR imaging of the orbit, fat saturation techniques are recommended to reduce signal from normal orbital fat. Despite being a favorable site, chemotherapy alone is generally not sufficient to achieve local control for orbital disease (11). Despite varied long-term sequelae of local irradiation, combined radiation therapy, and chemotherapy provide an excellent outcome and good quality of life.

Thorax and Abdomen

Approximately 10% of RMS is truncal (Fig. 39.6). A few reports exist of RMS arising from congenital cystic lesions of the lungs including cystic adenomatoid malformation but it is likely these alleged RMS tumors were actually pleuropulmonary blastomas rather than thoracic RMS (12).

RMS is the most common pediatric tumor of the biliary tree, but is still very rare, accounting for only 1% of all RMS. Biliary RMS is the commonest cause of malignant obstructive jaundice in childhood and US typically reveals biliary dilatation and a hilar mass. However, a biliary origin in a large hepatic tumor may be hard to prove as intraductal growth may not be obvious. The tumor may, in fact, arise from the intra or extrahepatic bile ducts, the gallbladder or cystic duct, a choledocal cyst or the liver parenchyma (10). Extension into the duodenum or the liver parenchyma is common. US, as well as CT or MR imaging, would be required to show the full tumor extent. Metastases to the liver or peritoneal surfaces, including the omentum, are also common. Intraperitoneal metastatic disease is seen in 11% of children with RMS either at presentation or later at relapse (10).

Genitourinary

Genitourinary (GU) RMS accounts for approximately one-third of all childhood RMS cases and RMS is the most common malignant neoplasm of the pelvis in children.

Tumors in the bladder and prostate have a worse prognosis as compared to other GU RMS. Prostatic tumors commonly spread laterally to the periurethral tissues and posteriorly to the perivesical tissues often invading the bladder base, hence the commonly used term bladder/prostate tumor. Tumor extension can also occur superiorly and anteriorly to the bladder into the retropubic space of Retzius. Fat-saturated T1-weighted images after intravenous (IV) gadolinium-DTPA administration can usually define tumor extent initially. At the end of treatment however, residual bladder wall thickening due to fibrosis can be extremely difficult to differentiate from residual tumor. Biopsy is often necessary and the role of positron emission tomography—computed tomography (PET-CT) in this context is as yet unproven. The goal of therapy in bladder or bladder/prostate RMS is long-term survival with an intact and functioning bladder.

Paratesticular RMS is applied to primary tumors arising in the spermatic cord, testis, epididymis or penis. Paratesticular RMS accounts for 7% of RMS and 12% of childhood scrotal tumors. The initial imaging investigation for any scrotal abnormality is US. Paratesticular RMS has variable echogenicity with a heterogeneous appearance due to hemorrhage and necrosis. The tumor may show increased flow on color Doppler and mimic infection. Abdominal CT imaging with both oral and IV contrast medium is merited in all these patients due to the high incidence of lymph node involvement (10). There has been a trend away from routine retroperitoneal dissection in recent years resulting in an increased reliance on CT to detect involved abdominal nodes. Reliance on CT with the omission of nodal sampling has however resulted in a higher relapse rate for paratesticular primaries, such that sampling of ipsilateral lymph nodes is again being advocated in North America.

Limbs

MR imaging is particularly good for evaluating tumors arising in the limbs. Neurovascular encasement and bone marrow involvement are best evaluated with MR imaging. Multiplanar imaging for assessment of tumor extent is ideal. Fat-suppressed sequences

can readily demonstrate tumor cranio-caudal extent and regional lymphadenopathy.

Key Points: Rhabdomyosarcoma

- Rhabdomyosarcomas (RMS) are the most common soft tissue tumors of childhood and the third most common malignancy of childhood after neuroblastoma and Wilms' tumors
- There are four histological subtypes of tumor: alveolar sarcoma, embryonal, botryoid, and spindle cell
- RMS usually present with a mass lesion (either the primary tumor or lymph node mass) or symptoms due to compression of an organ or structure
- Forty percent of RMS occur in the head and neck region, 30% in the GU tract, 10% in the trunk, and 20% in the extremities
- The most common sites for head and neck tumors are parameningeal (50%) and orbits (25%)
- RMS of the GU tract may arise in the bladder, prostate, vagina, or in the paratesticular structures
- The predominant histological subtypes in the GU tract are embryonal and botryoid tumors
- Favorable prognostic factors include embryonal or botryoid histology, tumor <5 cm diameter and age less than 10 years at diagnosis
- Cure rates for RMS are of the order of 70%
- Ultrasonography is useful for diagnosis but CT and MR imaging are the preferred methods for staging local spread and lymph node metastases
- Lymph node and distant metastases occur at presentation in 10% to 20% of patients with RMS
- Regional lymphadenopathy must always be sought with US and CT or MR imaging
- CT is needed to screen for pulmonary metastases

HEPATIC TUMORS

Primary hepatic tumors account for 1% to 4% of all pediatric tumors, with an approximate annual incidence rate of 1.5 per million children. The vast majority of malignant hepatic tumors are either hepatoblastomas or hepatocellular carcinomas.

In the United States, approximately 100 to 150 new cases of liver cancer develop in children each year (13). Between 60% and 70% of all primary liver tumors in children are malignant, with hepatoblastoma and hepatocellular carcinoma constituting the vast majority of these malignancies. The remaining hepatic malignancies are usually either undifferentiated embryonal sarcoma or rhabdomyosarcoma. Hemangioendothelioma/hemangioma lesions and mesenchymal hamartoma account for nearly all the non-malignant tumors in children.

Hepatoblastoma

Hepatoblastoma is the most common malignant liver tumor in childhood. Typically, it is diagnosed in young children less than four years of age, with a median age at diagnosis of one year. It is more common than hepatocellular carcinoma, occurring at an annual rate of 1.3 cases per 1 million children under 15 years of age (14). In contrast, hepatocellular carcinoma is typically diagnosed in older children, between 5 and 15 years with a median age of 12 years (14). Both tumors show a male predominance, with a male to female ratio of 1.4–2.0:1.0.

Clinical Presentation

Infants and children with hepatoblastoma usually present with an abdominal mass or distension. Abdominal pain, anorexia, weight loss, or vomiting are common while precocious puberty (related to the secretion of chorionic gonadotrophins) may rarely be seen in some cases. Hepatoblastoma has been associated with Beckwith–Wiedemann syndrome, hemi-hypertrophy, fetal alcohol syndrome, familial polyposis coli and Gardner's syndrome, and more recently with low birth weight (15). The incidence of this tumor in children less than five years of age doubled between 1979 and 1999, and survival of very low birth weight infants is at least part of the reason for this increase (15). The serum level of alpha-fetoprotein (AFP) is elevated in over 90% of patients with hepatoblastomas and over 60% of those with hepatocellular carcinoma. Rarely serum AFP is not raised in a proven hepatoblastoma and this is now regarded as a poor prognostic indicator.

Pathology

Hepatoblastoma tends to be a solitary mass (Fig. 39.7). The right lobe is involved more often than the left. Multifocal widespread tumors are also possible but localized growth beyond the liver is very uncommon. Histologically, hepatoblastoma contains small, primitive epithelial cells, resembling fetal liver at six to eight weeks of gestation. These may be mixed with mesenchymal elements (osteoid, cartilaginous, and fibrous tissue), embryonal cells, or small undifferentiated cells resembling neuroblastoma cells. Numerous histological sub-types of hepatoblastoma are described. The pure fetal sub-type has a very good prognosis. The small cell undifferentiated sub-type and tumors with a macrotrabecular growth pattern appear to have a worse outcome.

Staging

Metastatic disease occurs in 10% to 15% of patients with hepatoblastomas at initial presentation. The most common sites of distant spread, in order of decreasing frequency, are the lungs, bone, and brain.

The pre-treatment extent (PRETEXT) staging system used by the International Childhood Liver Tumor Strategy Group (SIOPEL) is gaining widespread acceptance. The PRETEXT pre-operative staging system is the basis for risk stratification in current SIOPEL studies (Table 39.2) (16,17). PRETEXT is used to describe tumor extent before any therapy, thus allowing more effective comparison between studies conducted by different collaborative groups. The system has good interobserver variability and good prognostic value (16). Most pediatric oncology groups now utilize the PRETEXT system to describe the imaging findings at diagnosis even if it is not their main staging system (17). PRETEXT staging is based on Couinaud's system of liver segmentation. Involvement of only one section by a hepatoblastoma mass is denoted as a PRETEXT I tumor (Fig. 39.8), more

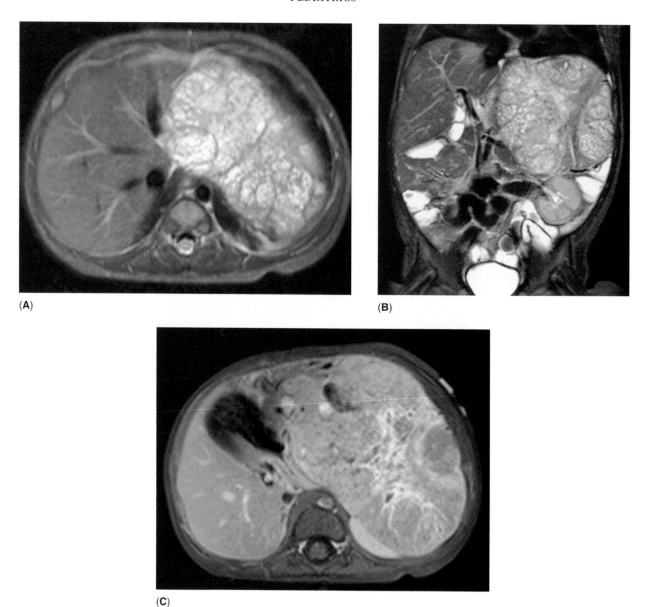

(A)

(B)

(C)

Figure 39.7 Hepatoblastoma. (**A**) Axial T2-weighted MR image in an 18 month old boy showing a mass lesion lateral to the left hepatic vein. (**B**) Coronal T2-weighted MR image of the same lesion. (**C**) Fat-suppressed axial T1-weighted MR image after gadolinium administration shows heterogeneous tumor enhancement, and confirmed the lesion was confined to segments 2 and 3 (PRETEXT I).

Table 39.2 Risk Stratification for Current SIOPEL Hepatoblastoma Studies (17)

High risk	Standard risk
Serum AFP <100 µg/ml	All other patients
PRETEXT IV	
Tumor rupture	
Extrahepatic spread, portal or hepatic vein tumor involvement	
Metastases	

involvement by a tumor to involve two, three or all four sections is classified as PRETEXT II, III or IV respectively (Fig. 39.9). Increasing PRETEXT number gives, very roughly, an estimate of the difficulty of the planned surgical procedure. Further refinements of the system include assessment for extrahepatic disease, tumor rupture, portal or hepatic vein involvement, lymph node spread, and distant metastases (17). The caudate lobe, previously ignored, is now also incorporated into the current system. PRETEXT I-III tumors are generally amenable to surgical resection whilst PRETEXT IV tumors typically require liver transplantation.

Imaging

US with Doppler interrogation is the preferred initial examination to screen for a possible intrahepatic mass and to differentiate solid and cystic masses. US is also particularly useful for identifying the presence and extent of vascular involvement by a tumor. On US, hepatoblastoma appears as a predominantly solid mass but there may be more cystic areas due to necrosis or hemorrhage. The solid components may be hypo-, iso-, or hyperechoic relative to the normal parenchyma. Central calcification is present in up to 20%

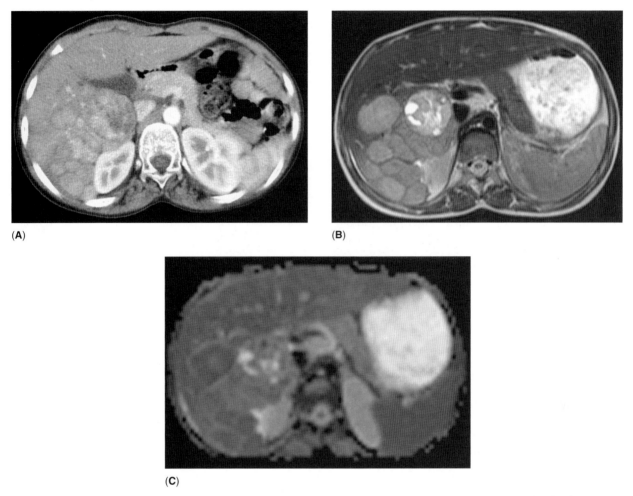

(A)

(B)

(C)

Figure 39.8 Hepatoblastoma. (**A**) CT after intravenous contrast enhancement and (**B**) axial T2-weighted MR image showed a lesion confined to the posterior segments of the right lobe of the liver (limited to segments 6 and 7, i.e., PRETEXT I). (**C**) ADC map shows the tumor has restricted diffusion, reflecting dense cellularity.

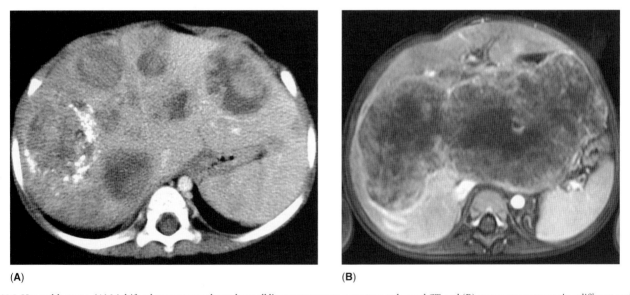

(A)

(B)

Figure 39.9 Hepatoblastoma. (**A**) Multifocal tumors seen throughout all liver segments on a contrast-enhanced CT, and (**B**) an enormous tumor in a different patient on a contrast-enhanced T1-weighted MR image spanning all liver sections. Both tumors would be classified as PRETEXT IV.

to 30% of tumors and appears as small hyperechoic foci with acoustic shadowing. With Doppler evaluation, prominent internal vascularity or areas of arteriovenous shunting may be identified.

CT or ideally MR imaging is needed to fully assess tumor extent. CT findings of hepatoblastoma include an intrahepatic soft tissue mass, which may have well-demarcated or ill-defined margins, with or without calcification. These tumors tend to be hypo- or isodense to liver on pre-contrast images but it is important to note that in the evaluation of most pediatric masses non-contrast-enhanced CT images are seldom helpful and can generally be avoided. Liver masses are an exception as multiphase studies can show lesions with varying conspicuity depending on the timing of the contrast enhancement. As multiphase CT studies carry the additional burden of radiation, MR imaging is preferred in this setting (always after an initial US examination). The periphery of the mass is frequently hypervascular during the arterial phase of enhancement and usually hypodense to liver during the portal venous phase. On MR imaging, hepatoblastoma is typically hypointense to normal liver on T1-weighted sequences, although it may have foci of high signal intensity within it, due to the presence of fat or hemorrhage. On T2-weighted sequences, these tumors are generally heterogeneous and hyperintense. Similar to CT, early arterial enhancement with rapid wash-out is typical after administration of Gadolinium-DTPA.

The crucial factors in assessing resectability of hepatic neoplasms are the extent of the primary tumor, most importantly the presence of tumor in surgically critical areas such as the porta hepatis, portal vein and IVC, and the presence of regional extrahepatic lymph node spread or distant metastases. The PRETEXT system requires an initial evaluation regarding potential resectability, which is frequently difficult at diagnosis (this is the reason for the SIOPEL group recommending central review of all new liver tumors at diagnosis). Tumor thrombus appears as an echogenic focus on US, a low attenuation filling defect on CT, a high signal intensity area on T2-weighted MR imaging, and typically a signal void on contrast-enhanced MR images. Lymph node metastases may have soft tissue attenuation on CT, low signal intensity (similar to liver) on T1-weighted images, and intermediate or high signal intensity on T2-weighted images. However they are seldom identified on imaging. With the advent of CT and MR imaging, conventional angiography is no longer performed in the initial staging evaluation of children with hepatic malignancy. Occasionally CT or MR angiography may be useful for vascular assessment and for tumor mapping prior to surgery.

Because the vast majority of metastases present at diagnosis are in the lungs, plain chest radiographs and chest CT are routinely obtained as part of initial staging. Skeletal involvement may be assessed by scintigraphy but is not a routine requirement in most studies. Cerebral metastases are very rare and therefore brain CT or MR imaging are usually reserved for patients with relevant clinical symptoms.

Most recurrences occur in the first two post-operative years, hence US of the liver and abdomen is obtained at regular intervals for at least two years after surgery. The exact timing of the follow-up examinations is determined by the specific treatment protocol used by each collaborative oncology group.

Treatment

The treatment of hepatoblastoma is based on a combination of chemotherapy and surgery. The North American Children's Oncology Group (COG) favors primary surgery followed by chemotherapy if deemed necessary, whereas the SIOPEL Group advocate pre-operative chemotherapy, usually with prior biopsy confirmation, followed by post-operative chemotherapy. Surgical complete resection is ultimately essential for cure. Features that may limit surgical resection are:

- Involvement of both lobes
- Bulky tumor
- Adenopathy in the porta hepatis
- Extension into the inferior vena cava (IVC)
- Involvement of the main hepatic artery or branches of the hepatic veins

Only 30% to 50% of hepatoblastomas are resectable at the time of diagnosis (18–21). With preoperative chemotherapy, the resectability rate for hepatoblastoma increases to almost 90% (20). Radiation therapy has only a limited role in the treatment of hepatoblastoma, as an adjunct in children with residual tumor following chemotherapy or for localized relapse.

Hepatoblastoma treatment is one of the great success stories for pediatric oncology over the past few years. Survival rates have increased from 25% to over 80% in the past two decades (22). Platinum-based chemotherapy has become the gold standard for hepatoblastoma but does have long-term sequelae, notably ototoxicity, and nephrotoxicity. At least 60% of children, cured of their tumor, suffer high frequency hearing loss. Survival rates approach 100% for Stage I tumors within COG studies or PRETEXT I disease within SIOPEL studies (although these two staging systems are not directly comparable).

Key Points: Hepatoblastoma

- Hepatoblastoma is the most common liver tumor of childhood
- The median age at diagnosis is one year
- Most children present with an abdominal mass or distension
- Hepatoblastoma may be associated with other genetic abnormalities
- Hepatoblastoma consists of primitive epithelial cells
- AFP is elevated for the child's age in over 90% of patients with hepatoblastoma
- Crucial criteria for determining resectability include the presence of spread into the portal vein, IVC, porta hepatis, or regional lymphadenopathy
- The PRETEXT system is used to assess tumor extent prior to any therapy
- PRETEXT has been shown to be a useful predictor of five-year survival
- Tumors are usually solitary but may be multifocal
- Hepatoblastoma and hepatocellular carcinoma have similar imaging features on US, CT, and MR imaging
- Either CT or MR imaging suffices for staging local tumor extent (after initial US evaluation)

Hepatocellular Carcinoma

Hepatocellular carcinoma is more prevalent and outnumbers hepatoblastoma in areas where hepatitis B infection is endemic. The tumor occurs in children older than five years, often on a background of pre-existing cirrhosis. According to the SIOPEL 1 study, 39% of tumors were associated with cirrhosis and >50% of tumors were multifocal (23). The disease is often advanced at diagnosis with 31% having metastatic disease, and extrahepatic spread or vascular invasion is seen in up to 40% of cases. Hepatocellular carcinoma has also been associated with Type I glycogen storage disease, cystinosis, tyrosinemia, Wilson's disease, extrahepatic biliary atresia, and giant cell hepatitis (14).

Fibrolamellar hepatocellular carcinoma is a histological subtype of hepatocellular carcinoma that occurs in non-cirrhotic livers. It is seen predominantly in adolescents and younger adults. Histologically, it contains eosinophilic-laden hepatocytes separated by thin, fibrous bands arranged in a lamellar pattern, hence the term "fibrolamellar". A central scar and calcification are common. Hepatomegaly and abdominal pain are common presenting features. Serum AFP levels are usually normal. Fibrolamellar hepatocellular carcinoma is less aggressive than hepatocellular carcinoma in general and has a more favorable prognosis (24).

Only 30% of hepatocellular carcinomas are resectable at the time of diagnosis (14). Fibrolamellar carcinoma is typically a large well-demarcated tumor (mean diameter, 12 cm). On US it may be hyper- or isoechoic to liver. At CT, the tumor is either hypo- or isodense to liver on pre-contrast scans and it often shows heterogeneous enhancement during the arterial phase of

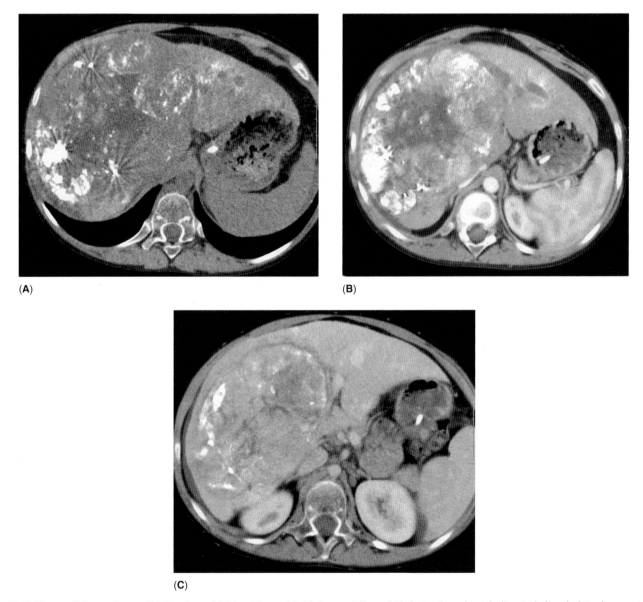

(A) (B)

(C)

Figure 39.10 Hepatocellular carcinoma. (A) Unenhanced CT in a 12 year old girl shows a diffuse calcific lesion throughout the liver including the lateral segment of the left lobe (segment 2). (B) Contrast-enhanced CT, arterial phase, shows the heterogeneous lesion in the right lobe but the abnormality in segment 2 is less easy to visualize. (C) In the portal venous phase the left lobe lesion is even more inconspicuous emphasizing the possible varied enhancement characteristics of liver tumors and the need for multiphase studies.

enhancement. During the portal venous phase of enhancement, it may become isodense to liver (Fig. 39.10). The central scar is typically hypodense during both the arterial and portal venous phases of enhancement. On MR imaging, fibrolamellar carcinoma is typically hypointense to liver on T1-weighted images and hyperintense on T2-weighted images. The central scar is hypointense on both sequences. As is the case on CT, the tumor parenchyma, but not the central scar, enhances after administration of gadolinium. Central calcifications are common (up to 68% of cases). Associated findings include intrahepatic biliary obstruction (42%), portal or hepatic vein invasion (87%), lymphadenopathy (65%), and extrahepatic tumor spread (42%) (24).

Complete surgical resection offers the only hope of cure but tumors are often too far advanced at diagnosis. Despite aggressive chemotherapy and surgical management, only a 13% five-year survival rate has been reported in children with hepatocellular carcinoma (14). Fibrolamellar carcinomas have an increased chance of resectability compared to hepatocellular carcinomas.

Undifferentiated Embryonal Sarcoma

Undifferentiated embryonal sarcoma is a highly aggressive tumor of the liver and is the third most common hepatic malignancy in the pediatric population (25). The tumor usually affects children between 6 and 10 years of age and it also has a slight male predominance. Clinical findings include right upper quadrant pain and/or palpable mass. The serum AFP levels are normal. Association with other conditions is rare. Gross anatomical section reveals a soft lesion with solid, gelatinous or cystic areas, and areas of hemorrhage and necrosis. Histologically, the tumor contains undifferentiated spindle cells in an abundant myxoid matrix. Prognosis is poor, with a median

survival of approximately one year (25). Metastases are to lung and bone.

On US, embryonal sarcomas typically have a predominantly solid appearance, usually related to the presence of gelatinous material. The solid components are iso- or hyperechoic to the surrounding hepatic parenchyma. CT shows a large intrahepatic mass with solid and cystic areas. The solid components may enhance on dynamic CT examinations. On T1-weighted MR imaging, most embryonal sarcomas are hypointense to liver and very hyperintense on T2-weighted sequences. A fluid–debris level or areas of high attenuation on CT and high signal intensity on T1-weighted images, due to hemorrhage, may also be seen.

Benign Hepatic Tumors

Between 30% and 40% of hepatic tumors in children are benign, with *hemangioendothelioma and multilocular cystic hamartoma* accounting for the vast majority of these masses. *Hepatic adenomas* and *nodular hyperplasia* account for less than 5% of benign hepatic tumors in childhood. Their imaging features are similar to those seen in adults and they will not be discussed here further.

Hemangioendothelioma is seen almost exclusively in the first six months of life. Although still slightly controversial, most pathologists now view hemangioendotheliomas of the liver and hemangiomas elsewhere in infancy as essentially the same lesion (26). This tumor is rarely seen in children over two years of age (Fig. 39.11). Hepatic hemangiomas, though histologically benign, may be associated with significant morbidity and mortality in afflicted infants. The literature presents much confusion regarding the natural history and treatment options for hepatic hemangiomas. Clinical manifestations range from asymptomatic self-limiting lesions to congestive heart failure

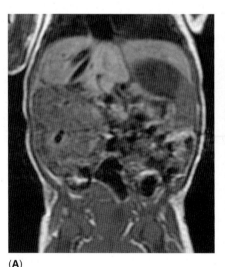 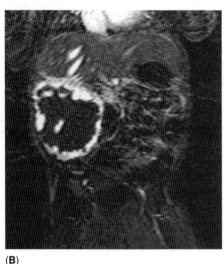 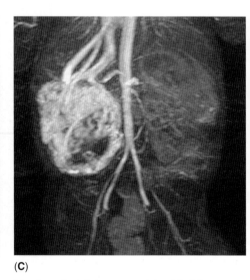

(A)   (B)   (C)

Figure 39.11 Hepatic hemangioma. (A) Coronal T1-weighted MR image showing an ill-defined liver mass arising from the inferior aspect of the right lobe in a two month old baby. There is a signal void centrally due to a vessel within the lesion. (B) T1-weighted fat-suppressed image after gadolinium administration shows early peripheral enhancement by the mass. (C) Delayed MIP image demonstrates diffuse enhancement and also clearly shows enlarged draining veins, indicating arteriovenous shunting within the hemangioma.

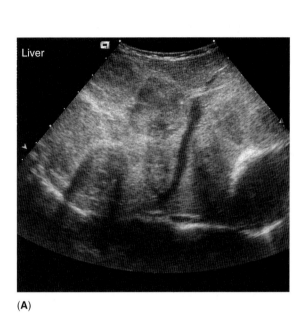
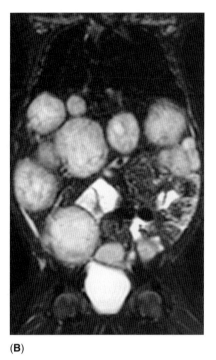

(A)   **(B)**

Figure 39.12 Hepatic hemangiomatosis. (**A**) Transverse liver ultrasound, in a baby who presented with asymptomatic hepatomegaly, shows multiple hypoechoic solid lesions which were moderately vascular on Doppler evaluation. (**B**) Coronal T2-weighted MR image shows multifocal homogeneous hyperintense lesions.

associated with high-volume vascular shunting to fulminant hepatic failure with hypothyroidism, abdominal compartment syndrome, and death. Histologically, hemangioendotheliomas contain thin-walled, endothelial-lined vascular spaces. They may be solitary or multifocal (Fig. 39.12) (26). On US, hemangioendotheliomas are characteristically well-defined and hypoechoic. Doppler US usually demonstrates internal vascularity to a variable degree.

The classic appearance on CT is of a low attenuation mass or masses on pre-contrast images, which demonstrate early nodular peripheral enhancement and progressive centripetal fill-in on delayed images. Small lesions may show early uniform enhancement, whereas large lesions may demonstrate persistent central low density due to the presence of fibrosis, thrombosis, or degeneration. On MR imaging, these lesions are hypointense to normal liver on T1-weighted images and hyperintense on T2-weighted sequences, with signal intensity equal to that of cerebrospinal fluid. The enhancement pattern after administration of intravenous contrast medium is similar to that seen on CT. If the typical findings of centripetal enhancement and fill-in are present, hemangioendothelioma can be diagnosed with certainty. The tumor, whether solitary or multifocal, may appear similar on all imaging modalities to hepatoblastoma. However, the serum AFP is not raised. In younger infants, particularly with vascular shunting, biopsy is seldom necessary. The clinical outcome is usually favorable. When treatment is deemed necessary, there has been little rationale to choose between the various treatment options; namely observation, corticosteroids, other pharmacologic agents, arterial embolization, hepatic artery ligation, resection, or liver transplantation for any given patient (26).

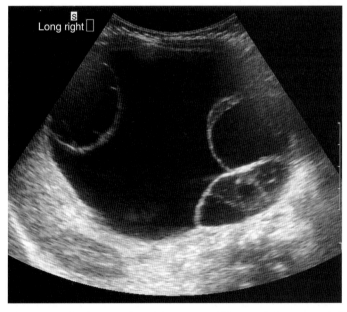

Figure 39.13 Cystic mesenchymal hamartoma. Ultrasound shows a typical multicystic liver lesion in a 15 month old boy, which had no discernible solid components on US or MR imaging.

Hepatic mesenchymal hamartoma is an uncommon benign tumor in childhood. A cystic mesenchymal hamartoma is a benign lesion composed of cysts of varying size, surrounded by fibrous septations which contain a disorganized mixture of mesenchyme, abnormal bile ducts and hepatocytes (Fig. 39.13). Nearly all lesions are seen in children under two years of age with only 5% occurring

after five years of age. Median patient age at diagnosis is approximately 10 months. Affected patients usually present with a palpable mass or painless abdominal enlargement. It is typically a single tumor (27). On CT or US, a multi-septated cystic tumor, a mixed solid and cystic tumor, or even a relatively solid tumor may be seen, although the mass typically has few, if any, solid parts (27). On US, the septa may be thin in multi-septated cystic tumors or irregularly thick in mixed solid and cystic tumors. On a post-contrast CT scan, solid portions or thick septa of the tumors show heterogeneous enhancement.

Key Points: Hepatic Neoplasms—General Points

- Primary hepatic tumors are the third most common pediatric cancer in the abdomen
- The majority of hepatic tumors are hepatoblastomas, hepatocellular carcinomas, and rarely undifferentiated embryonal sarcomas
- Hepatoblastoma occurs in infants and young children, whereas hepatocellular carcinoma is seen in older children
- Pathological differentiation between hepatoblastoma and hepatocellular carcinoma is based on cellular maturity
- Fibrolamellar carcinoma is rare and occurs in older children and young adults, in a non-cirrhotic liver
- Between 30% and 40% of hepatic tumors in children are benign
- Hemangioendothelioma and multilocular cystic hamartoma account for the vast majority of benign tumors

Hepatic Metastases

The malignant tumors of childhood that most frequently metastasize to the liver are:

- Wilms' tumor
- Neuroblastoma
- Rhabdomyosarcoma
- Lymphoma

Neuroblastoma may affect the liver in either Stage IV or IV-S disease. Stage IV disease is generally characterized by the presence of a retroperitoneal mass and distant metastases to skeleton, liver, or lymph nodes. The liver metastases are usually well defined focal lesions. Stage IV-S neuroblastoma occurs in patients under one year of age, who typically have small tumors (not crossing the midline) and metastases to liver, skin, and bone marrow, but not to cortical bone. The liver metastatic spread in IV-S disease is usually so widespread that the whole liver is infiltrated and enlarged, and no focal masses as such are seen. The liver involvement in this setting may be best visualized with a linear high resolution US probe.

Clinically, patients with hepatic metastases present with hepatomegaly, jaundice, abdominal pain or mass, or abnormal hepatic function tests. In general, hepatic metastases are often multiple and well-circumscribed. They can be hypo- or hyper-echoic relative to normal liver on US, low attenuation on contrast-enhanced CT, hypointense on T1-weighted MR imaging and hyperintense on T2-weighted images. Although the signal intensity is high on T2-weighted MR imaging, it is not usually as high as that seen with hemangiomas or cysts. Most metastases in children are hypovascular on both the arterial and portal venous phases of enhancement. Occasionally, internal or peripheral (ring) enhancement may be seen after contrast administration.

GERM CELL TUMORS

Germ cell tumors are believed to arise from primordial germ cells which migrate to the urogenital ridges in the retroperitoneal region where they are incorporated into the gonads. Tumors arise in the gonads or along both normal or aberrant migration paths, and are often midline in location. Common sites for these tumors are in the sacrococcygeal region, retroperitoneum, anterior mediastinum, and the pineal and hypophyseal regions. CNS tumors are dealt with elsewhere in this text. The primordial cell may form a monophasic tumor (dysgerminoma, seminoma, endodermal sinus tumor) or a more complex neoplasm (teratoma) which incorporates two or three of the embryonic germ layers (ecto-, endo-, or mesoderm). A mature teratoma is benign. An immature teratoma has immature embryonic tissue within it, typically neural tissue. Immature teratomas are potentially malignant but in patients less than 15 years of age these tumors demonstrate a biological and clinical behavior similar to mature teratomas (28). They are usually localized and curable by surgery alone despite not being, strictly speaking, benign. A truly malignant teratoma contains frankly malignant cells of germ cell origin (germinoma, choriocarcinoma).

Germ cell tumors (GCT) arising in gonadal or extragonadal sites account for approximately 3% of all pediatric malignancies. Sacrococcygeal tumors are most common at birth, with yolk sac gonadal tumors becoming the more frequent type in early childhood. Seminomas and dysgerminomas are seen in adolescence. Extragonadal tumors represent nearly two thirds of all germ cell tumors in childhood. The sacrococcygeal region is the most common site of origin overall for germ cell tumors in children, accounting for approximately 40% of all germ cell tumors and between 70% and 80% of extragonadal germ cell tumors (14,29). The majority of extragonadal tumors are teratomas.

Pathology

The benign teratoma consists of well-differentiated tissues that are foreign to the anatomic site. The tumors are commonly cystic as they contain secretory structures such as choroid plexus in neural tissue, respiratory or gastrointestinal epithelia. The septa between cysts may contain any type of tissue and it is in the septa that immature elements are found. The immature teratoma contains an admixture of mature and primitive neuroectodermal tissues (29). Approximately 65% of sacrococcygeal tumors are mature teratomas; the remaining tumors have either immature or malignant histologies. As a general rule, the more solid the tumors, the more likely they are to contain immature or malignant tissues. Endodermal sinus cells (and hepatocytes) are the only sources of alpha-fetoprotein. If this marker is elevated in the absence of a primary liver tumor,

an endodermal sinus tumor component within a germ cell tumor is the most likely explanation.

It has recently become clear that the location of a GCT is a major determinant of outcome (30). Stage III and IV tumors originating in the gonad had excellent overall survival (OS) (95% OS) whereas Stages III/IV extragonadal GCTs had worse OS in the region of 80% (30). A new risk stratification for pediatric GCTs has been suggested (30). Low risk tumors include gonadal Stage I, intermediate risk are extragonadal Stages I/II or gonadal Stages II-IV, and high risk are Stage III/IV extragonadal tumors which emphasizes the greater risk with advanced stage extragonadal GCTs.

Extragonadal Germ Cell Tumors

Sacrococcygeal Teratomas

Sacrococcygeal teratomas are usually non-familial and affect females and males in a 3:1 ratio. Most are diagnosed in neonates because the large exophytic component produces a visible mass in the perineal or gluteal region (Fig. 39.14). The diagnosis may be delayed if the tumors are small and confined to the presacral area. Tumors located solely in the presacral area present in later childhood or in adolescence, producing chronic constipation, and are more likely to be malignant (Fig. 39.14C).

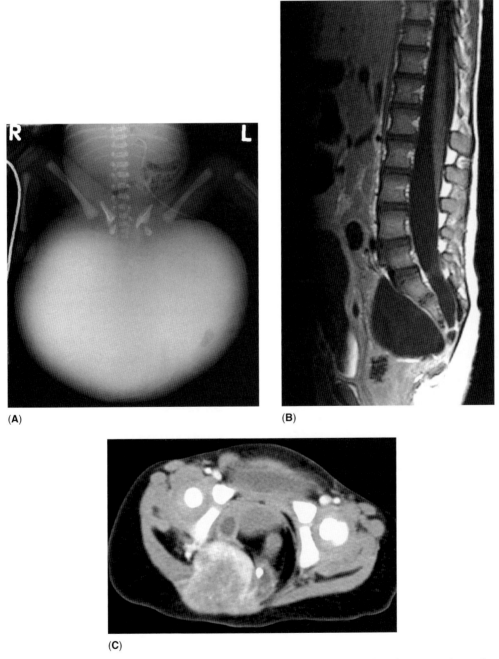

(A)

(B)

(C)

Figure 39.14 Sacrococcygeal teratomas. (A) Abdominal radiograph shows a very large exophytic mass protruding from the perineum in a newborn baby. (B) T1-weighted sagittal MR image after gadolinium enhancement in a child who previously had a sacrococcygeal teratoma removed. The lower sacrum had also been excised but the cystic pre-sacral mass visible here is recurrent tumor. (C) Contrast-enhanced CT in another child, aged three years, showed a mixed solid and cystic mass. The solid enhancing component in the right gluteal area proved on biopsy to be a malignant yolk sac tumor.

Four types of sacrococcygeal teratomas have been described based on the relative amounts of internal and external tumor.

- Type I—predominantly external; limited extension into the presacral space (47%)
- Type II—similar external and intrapelvic components (34%)
- Type III—minimal external tumor; large pelvic and abdominal components (9%)
- Type IV—purely presacral tumor without an external component (10%)

The frequency of malignancy varies with the type of teratoma and age of the patient at diagnosis. Overall, about 17% of all sacrococcygeal teratomas have malignant elements. The frequency of malignant elements varies from approximately 8% for Type I, 21% for Type II, 34% for Type III, and 38% for Type IV sacrococcygeal tumors (29). In addition, only 2% of sacrococcygeal teratomas diagnosed in infants under six months of age are malignant compared to up to 65% of teratomas diagnosed after six months of age. The most common sites of metastases are the lungs, inguinal and retroperitoneal lymph nodes, followed in frequency by liver, bone, and brain. Raised AFP is a useful serum marker for malignant disease at diagnosis, for tumor surveillance and early relapse detection.

Benign mature sacrococcygeal tumors are mainly cystic masses, whilst malignant tumors are typically more complex with large areas of solid tissue easily depicted with US. Malignant sacrococcygeal teratomas appear as soft tissue masses on CT with or without fat or calcification, although MR imaging is, of course, preferred due to the radiation burden from CT. The tumor displays intermediate signal intensity masses on T1-weighted images and intermediate or high signal intensity masses on T2-weighted images and contrast-enhanced images. Tumor margins are often poorly defined, infiltration of adjacent soft tissues and intraspinal tumor extension are commonly seen.

Although both CT and MR imaging can demonstrate the extent of intrapelvic and intra-abdominal tumor, MR is better for the detection of soft tissue extension, such as the relationship of tumor to the gluteal muscles, and for the detection of intraspinal involvement. It is debated whether MR imaging is needed in neonates because most lesions are benign. Some surgeons advocate only plain radiographs and US. After two to three months of age, however, when the frequency of malignant change increases, cross-sectional imaging is recommended.

Primary excision is the mainstay of treatment. Operative management includes complete resection of the tumor and the coccyx. Of note is the fact that an increased recurrence rate is seen if the coccyx is not resected. Complete resection suffices for benign mature teratomas. In general, tumors with a lot of immature tissues are more likely to harbor foci of malignant GCTs and are thus more likely to recur. Malignant tumors are treated surgically together with multi-agent chemotherapy. The long-term survival rates of children with malignant sacrococcygeal teratomas are more than 80% (29,30).

Retroperitoneal Teratomas

Primary abdominal and retroperitoneal teratomas are extremely rare and represent only 4% to 6% of all teratomas (31). The majority (85%) are benign. Although benign, abdominal teratomas in infants are often large and have a particular tendency to infiltrate widely. Thus a description of these tumors as retroperitoneal masses is often anatomically too simplistic and ascribing a definite organ or anatomical compartment of origin is difficult. They have a propensity to expand anteriorly and frequently occupy virtually the entire abdomen (Fig. 39.15); for example, contact with the anterior abdominal wall is common. Thus, whilst these masses are frequently described as pancreatic, gastric, mesenteric or gallbladder lesions, such a presumed location may simply reflect the largest

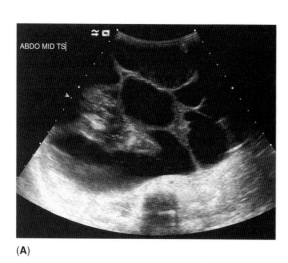

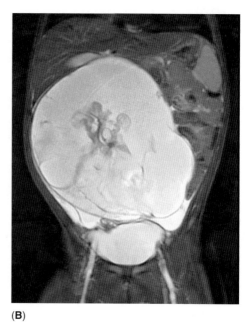

(A)   (B)

Figure 39.15 Abdominal teratoma. (**A**) Transverse abdominal ultrasound demonstrates a mainly cystic mass with some thick stranding in an otherwise well infant. (**B**) Coronal T2-weighted MR image shows the large mass occupying much of the abdomen inferior to the liver, with some central low signal solid components. There is some additional ascites in both paracolic gutters.

component of a tumor originating in the retroperitoneum or within the root of the mesentery.

The typical radiological features of a retroperitoneal teratoma is that of a large, complex mass, usually with well-circumscribed cystic components, containing fat and areas of calcification (32). The sonographic appearances of mature retroperitoneal teratoma are usually those of a mixed tumor with cystic and solid components. Calcification and characteristic adipose content or fat-fluid levels (sebum) are better demonstrated on CT or MR imaging. Contrast enhancement of an intra-cystic solid component has been suggested as a criterion to distinguish benign from rarer malignant lesions in adults (with a sensitivity and specificity of approximately 80%) (33). This is also likely to be true for pediatric GCTs.

It is noteworthy, that vascular displacement seems to occur in a different pattern in abdominal teratomas to that seen with other infiltrative pediatric tumors such as neuroblastoma. Mass-effect can cause marked distortion of normal anatomical relationships and compression or complete effacement of the inferior vena cava. In addition, marked anterior displacement of the IVC away from the aorta may be seen occasionally. This is an important surgical risk and is an important factor to consider pre-operatively. These masses may also prove difficult to remove at surgery because they are often densely adherent to adjacent structures. Current CT angiographic techniques should be adequate to assess the arterial anatomy, but the optimum technique for delineation of the compressed abdominal veins remains to be established.

Mediastinal Teratomas
Primary germ cell tumors account for up to 10% of mediastinal masses in children. They are second only to lymphoma as a cause of a thymic mass. Germ cell tumors are most often located in the anterior mediastinum (28). Only 2% to 3% of mediastinal GCTs occur in the posterior mediastinum. There is an association between Kleinfelter's syndrome (XXY) and mediastinal germ cell tumors (GCT). Up to a half of all patients are asymptomatic at the time of diagnosis (34). Conversely, large tumors causing tracheal compression or superior vena caval obstruction are also well recognized (Fig. 39.16). Occasionally, ectopic production of sex hormones or insulin may lead to presentation with pseudoprecocious puberty or hypoglycemia before the onset of respiratory symptoms. As with malignant GCTs elsewhere they are frequently associated with elevated serum levels of human chorionic gonadotropin or AFP. Teratomas account for the vast majority of mediastinal germ cell lesions in children and they may contain varied amounts of mature and immature somatic tissues.

CT attenuation values and MR signal intensity for all these tumors are highly variable depending on the amount of fat, calcium, or soft tissue in the mass. Most teratomas have well-defined margins, thick walls and some fatty tissue or calcification, or both. Approximately 25% of teratomas contain calcification (35). Fatty tissue plus calcification in an anterior mediastinal mass almost invariably indicates a germ cell origin. Seminomas typically are more homogeneous, with soft-tissue attenuation while the more malignant lesions frequently contain large necrotic components. However, there is wide spectrum of appearances of all these tumors.

Teratomas may rupture into adjacent structures such as the pleural space, pericardium, lung parenchyma, or tracheobronchial

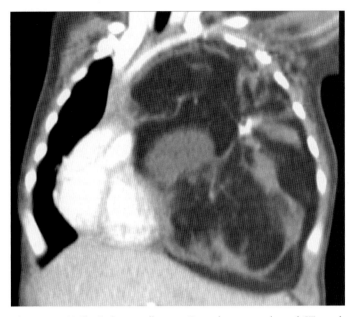

Figure 39.16 Mediastinal germ cell tumor. Coronal contrast-enhanced CT reveals a large left chest lesion which has cystic, solid, and calcific components.

tree. Up to one-third of mature benign mediastinal teratomas are reported to rupture, while malignant lesions have a significantly lower tendency to leak their contents (34). Severe symptoms such as chest pain or hemoptysis are more commonly found in ruptured tumors than those that remain intact. Proteolytic or digestive enzymes and sebaceous materials within these teratomas are thought to play a role in the tendency to rupture and in causing adjacent non-infectious inflammation. High amylase levels have been found in pleural effusions and within the tumor contents (34). Additional findings in ruptured tumors depend on the space into which the rupture occurs. Rupture into the lung or through the tracheobronchial tree may cause a chemical pneumonitis or fat-containing masses in the adjacent lung parenchyma. Hemoptysis with expectoration of hair or sebaceous material indicates a fistula between the tumor and the tracheobronchial tree and is said to be pathognomonic of a mature teratoma. Rupture into the pleura or pericardium results in pleural or pericardial effusions. Adjacent consolidation or atelectasis should be regarded as suspicious for rupture but can also, of course, be seen with simple atelectasis caused by compression from any large mass. It is important to recognize rupture as inflammatory changes and adhesions secondary to extravasation of tumor contents may result in more hazardous surgery than might have been anticipated.

Key Points: Extragonadal Germ Cell Tumors

- Sacrococcygeal tumors account for 40% of all germ cell tumors
- Most sacrococcygeal tumors are benign with only 17% having malignant elements
- Retroperitoneal teratomas may displace the IVC anteriorly, presenting a risk to operative removal
- Rupture of a mediastinal teratoma may result in a pleural or pericardial effusion

Gonadal Germ Cell Tumors

Testicular Germ Cell Tumors

With an annual incidence of 0.5–2 cases per 100,000 children, testicular tumors account for 2% to 3% of solid cancers in prepubertal boys (29,36). The majority of pediatric testicular tumors are of germ cell origin and most of these tumors are malignant (80%) (14). Testicular tumors have a bimodal distribution, affecting very young children and adolescent boys. The median age at diagnosis of prepubertal children with malignant tumors is two years (36).

Most patients with testicular tumors present with painless testicular or scrotal enlargement. With metastatic disease, children may however present with nodal enlargement or malignant ascites. Serum AFP and Human gonadotrophin (HCG) levels are often elevated in patients with malignant testicular germ cell tumors (90% of cases) (36). In prepubertal boys, testicular germ cell tumors of the testes are nearly always yolk sac tumors (endodermal sinus tumors) or benign teratomas. In adolescent boys, testicular tumors typically have histologies similar to those seen in adults including embryonal carcinomas or seminomas. The majority of testicular tumors are non-metastatic and localized to the scrotum at presentation (36). In the remaining patients, the tumor may spread to retroperitoneal lymph nodes, lungs, and liver or rarely, to bone or brain.

US is the technique of choice for the diagnosis of any testicular lesion. US can define the cystic or solid nature of a mass and its relationship to the testes. The distinction between intra- and extratesticular masses is important because the majority of intratesticular lesions are malignant, whereas most extratesticular lesions are benign (with the exception of paratesticular rhabdomyosarcoma). At US, CT and MR imaging testicular tumors usually appear as discrete solid masses, but occasionally they present as diffuse testicular enlargement. On sonography, they may be hypo- or isoechoic to normal testicular tissue. They also may be homogeneous or contain calcifications or hypoechoic areas, which may be due to the presence of hemorrhage or necrosis. Findings of extratesticular extension include irregularity of the tunica albuginea and reactive hydroceles. Scrotal skin thickening is rare. In practice, the combination of scrotal skin thickening and an intra-testicular mass is more characteristic of an inflammatory process than a neoplasm. Imaging of the chest, abdomen and pelvis are routinely performed to search for metastases. The abdomen and pelvis can be further evaluated by CT or MR imaging. CT is necessary to evaluate the lungs. After tumor resection, US usually suffices for defining local scrotal recurrence, as well as assessing the status of the contralateral testis and abdomen.

The most widely utilized staging system for testicular germ cell tumors is the one from the Children's Oncology Group (Table 39.3). Approximately 80% to 90% of children with malignant germ cell tumors have Stage I disease; the remainder usually have Stage II or III disease. In comparison, adolescent patients with testicular tumors are more likely to have advanced stage tumor at the time of diagnosis (29).

Needle biopsy and scrotal incision are contraindicated for testicular tumors due to the risk of tumor seeding. Stage I disease is cured by radical orchidectomy alone. Chemotherapy is reserved for patients with advanced disease (e.g., metastases) and those whose tumor markers fail to decline after orchidectomy. Survival rates exceed 90% (30).

Table 39.3 Staging of Testicular Germ Cell Tumors (29)

Stage I	Limited to testis, tumor markers normal after appropriate half-life decline
Stage II	Transscrotal orchidectomy, microscopic disease in scrotum or high in spermatic cord (<5 cm from proximal end), retroperitoneal lymph node involvement (<2 cm), increased tumor marker levels after appropriate half-life decline
Stage III	Retroperitoneal lymph node involvement (>2 cm), no visceral or extra-abdominal involvement
Stage IV	Distant metastases

Differential Diagnosis of Primary Testicular Neoplasms

Approximately 10% of primary testicular neoplasms in children are stromal tumors and the vast majority of these are benign (>90%) (36). The histologies of these tumors include Leydig cell, Sertoli cell, and granulosa cell tumors. Gonadoblastoma is a rare stromal tumor (1% of all testicular tumors) that nearly always occurs in phenotypic females with streak gonads or testes and a male karyotype. Non-neoplastic intratesticular masses are rarer than primary malignant testicular tumors. These lesions include: lipoma, hemangioma, Leydig cell hyperplasia, adrenal rests, epidermoid cysts, and hematomas. On US, the stromal and non-neoplastic testicular lesions may appear as solid, complex, or cystic masses. They cannot be differentiated on the basis of imaging, and final diagnosis requires tissue sampling.

Secondary Neoplasms

Leukemia and lymphoma are causes of secondary testicular neoplasms. Leukemic infiltrates are found in 60% to 90% of children at autopsy who die from complications of leukemia, but are clinically apparent only in about 8% of children (37). US may show either a diffusely enlarged testis or a focal hypoechoic lesion. Testicular involvement is usually bilateral, but it can be unilateral or asymmetric.

> ## Key Points: Testicular Tumors
>
> - Testicular tumors account for 1% of all childhood malignancy
> - The majority of testicular neoplasms in childhood are germ cell tumors, most being yolk sac (endodermal sinus) tumors
> - Most boys with a malignant testicular germ cell tumor have elevated serum AFP levels
> - Ninety percent of testicular tumors are localized at diagnosis
> - Metastatic disease occurs in approximately 10% of patients and is usually to lymph nodes and lungs
> - US is reliable in detecting testicular tumors and in distinguishing between intra- and extratesticular masses
> - CT is the technique of choice for staging testicular cancer spread to lymph nodes and lungs

Ovarian Germ Cell Tumors

Ovarian tumors account for about 25% of all pediatric germ cell tumors. Most ovarian germ cell tumors are diagnosed late in the first decade of life, with a peak age incidence at diagnosis of 10 years (14). Approximately two-thirds are benign and one-third are malignant (14). Most patients with ovarian tumors present with a palpable abdominal or pelvic mass or pain, which may be severe if there is associated torsion of the ovarian pedicle. Other presentations include constipation, amenorrhea and vaginal

bleeding. In cases of metastatic disease, patients may present with abdominal swelling due to ascites. The serum levels of AFP and HCG levels usually are elevated in patients with malignant tumors.

Dysgerminoma and *endodermal sinus tumor* account for almost 90% of malignant ovarian neoplasms in girls. Immature teratomas (containing embryonic elements, mostly prominent neural tissue) account for approximately 10% of ovarian malignancies. Tumors of stromal cell origin (Sertoli-Leydig cell, granulose-theca cell and undifferentiated neoplasms) and epithelial carcinomas are extremely rare in children (29).

The diagnosis of an ovarian mass is established usually by US (Fig. 39.17). US findings of ovarian malignancy include a solid mass with central necrosis and thickened irregular septa or papillary projections. Ancillary signs of malignancy include ascites, typically containing echogenic material, and liver metastases. CT findings of malignant ovarian lesions include: a cystic soft tissue mass with thick, irregular walls, low-attenuation areas due to necrosis or hemorrhage, and thickened septa. Irregular, coarse calcifications are common in both

dysgerminomas and immature or malignant teratomas. On MR imaging, malignant ovarian tumors commonly have low to intermediate signal intensity on T1-weighted images and intermediate or high signal intensity on T2-weighted images, with the solid areas showing variable enhancement after gadolinium administration. Fibrovascular septa may be noted. These are hypo- or isointense on T1-weighted images and typically show marked enhancement after administration of IV gadolinium-DTPA. The staging evaluation should include CT of the chest, and CT or MR imaging of the abdomen.

Peritoneal tumor implants appear as soft tissue nodules on the lateral peritoneal surfaces or in the ligaments and mesenteries of the abdomen. Omental implants appear as nodules or conglomerate masses ("omental cake") beneath the anterior abdominal wall. They may enhance after IV administration of iodinated contrast agents or gadolinium. Peritoneal seeding is more common with immature teratomas than with the other germ cell neoplasms.

Malignant ovarian neoplasms spread by contiguous extension, lymphatic spread, or hematogenous dissemination. Ovarian germ

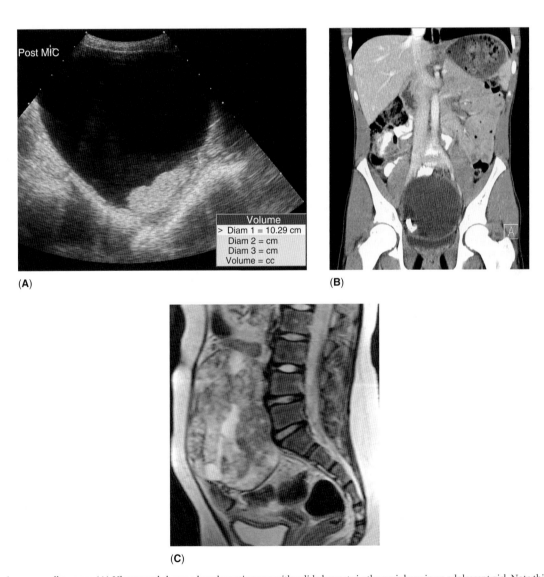

(A)

(B)

(C)

Figure 39.17 Ovarian germ cell tumors. (A) Ultrasound shows a largely cystic mass with solid elements in the periphery in an adolescent girl. Note this image was taken after bladder emptying as it is easy to mistake a cystic ovarian mass for the bladder. (B) Coronal contrast-enhanced CT image shows a cystic mass arising out of the pelvis in an 11 year old girl, which has a calcified area on the right side. (C) Sagittal T2-weighted MR image in another adolescent girl shows a heterogeneous mass superior to the bladder.

Table 39.4 Staging of Ovarian Germ Cell Tumors (29)

Stage I	Tumor is limited to one or both ovaries. Tumor marker levels return to the reference range after an appropriate post-surgical half-life decline
Stage II	Microscopic residual or positive lymph nodes (<2 cm as measured by pathologist) are present
Stage III	Lymph node or nodes with malignant metastatic nodule (>2 cm as measured by pathologist) are present. Gross residual disease or biopsy only. Contiguous visceral involvement (omentum, intestine, or bladder) is observed
Stage IV	Distant metastases

cell tumors usually metastasize to the liver, lungs, or lymph nodes; metastases to bone and peritoneal surfaces are rare. Ovarian germ cell tumors can be staged using the Children's Oncology Group system (Table 39.4).

Treatment is complete resection of the primary tumor whenever possible. Benign tumors require no further treatment. In unusually difficult cases, surgical debulking or biopsy may be all that is possible. Malignant GCTs are then treated with multi-agent chemotherapy. Approximately 75% of patients with malignant ovarian neoplasms have Stage I disease at diagnosis. Survival rates exceed 90% for both localized and more advanced stage disease (29,30).

Key Points: Ovarian Tumors

- Ovarian germ cell tumors account for 25% of all pediatric germ cell tumors
- Approximately 30% are malignant
- Dysgerminoma and yolk sac tumors are the most common malignant ovarian tumors
- Stromal cell and epithelial tumors are extremely rare ovarian tumors in childhood
- AFP and HCG levels are elevated in children with malignant germ cell tumors
- Ovarian tumors spread typically to the peritoneum, lymph nodes, and lungs
- CT of the chest is required to detect pulmonary metastases
- Surgery offers the best chance of cure and approximately 70% of children have Stage I disease at diagnosis

NON-RHABDOMYOSARCOMATOUS SOFT TISSUE TUMORS

Epidemiology and Histology

Approximately half of pediatric soft tissue tumors are non-rhabdomyomatous soft tissue sarcomas (NRSTS), which account for about 3% of childhood malignancies. They are a heterogeneous group of tumors, all of mesenchymal origin, that share some biological characteristics but differ histologically. The most common NRSTS are:

- synovial cell sarcoma (17–42%)
- fibrosarcoma (13–15%)
- malignant fibrous histiocytoma (12–13%)
- malignant peripheral nerve sheath tumors (10%) (38,39)

There are numerous other histological types which include malignant neurogenic tumors, hemangiopericytomas, alveolar soft part sarcomas, epitheloid sarcoma, leiomyosarcomas, liposarcomas, and desmoplastic small cell tumors.

The frequency of most of these tumors is age dependent. Fibrosarcomas occur more commonly in children under one year of age, with synovial sarcomas and malignant peripheral nerve sheath tumors (MPNST) being more common in children over 10 years. The clinical behavior and outcomes of NRSTS in children are often very different to those in adults and particularly in infants and young children prognosis is generally better. An example of this different natural history is infantile fibrosarcoma which, unlike the adult tumor, rarely metastasizes and is generally cured if complete surgical removal is achieved. Adolescent NRSTS, however, tend to behave more like those seen in adults (40,41).

The vast majority of cases of NRSTS are sporadic and, as with RMS, many have been shown to have specific chromosomal translocations, for example, t(X;18)(p11;q11) occurs in more than 90% of synovial sarcomas. There are familial associations, with NRSTS occurring in patients with Li-Fraumeni syndrome as well as in neurofibromatosis Type 1. The latter is strongly associated with the development of MPNSTs. Genetic studies suggest loss of heterozygosity of a tumor suppressor gene or genes within the tumor cells.

Clinical Presentation

NRSTS can arise anywhere in the body but are most common in the extremities and trunk (38). Presentation is usually with a painless mass but symptoms may occur secondary to local invasion or mass effect. Systemic symptoms such as fever, night sweats, or weight loss are rare but may be observed with widespread metastatic disease. MPNST can present with motor and sensory involvement. Rarely patients may present with metabolic disturbances. Dillon et al. looked at the anatomical location of a cohort of 75 pediatric NRSTS and found 65% in the extremities, 28% in the trunk, and 7% in the head and neck (38). Metastases at time of presentation were more common with truncal tumors than those in the extremities. All upper limb tumors were localized at the time of presentation, whereas 78% of abdominal tumors had metastatic disease at diagnosis. It is noteworthy that although one can suspect a NRSTS from the clinical presentation and age of the child, all these masses have similar imaging features and some form of biopsy confirmation is mandatory.

The role of image-guided percutaneous core biopsy, usually with US, is a well-established method for diagnosis of malignancy in adults but is a more controversial area in the pediatric setting. The histopathologist requires an adequate tissue sample to make the diagnosis, which increasingly relies on complex immunohistochemical testing. This need for plentiful tissue must be balanced against a desire to be as minimally invasive as possible for the child's benefit. It is however usually possible to obtain adequate diagnostic tissue using needle biopsy. Difficulties arise if the tumor is cystic or an insufficient sample is obtained. Biopsies in younger children are usually performed under general anesthesia, and clinicians are reluctant to subject the child to another anesthetic episode should the percutaneous biopsy fail to yield a diagnosis. For

these reasons, many centers favor open surgical biopsy. However, in our center image-guided biopsy with a 14G or 16G cutting needle virtually always gives adequate cores of tissue, with only a rare need to repeat the biopsy. US or CT guidance is used to avoid large vessels, cystic or necrotic areas of tumor which improves diagnostic yield and decreases risk of hemorrhage. Close co-operation between the radiology and local histopathology department is required. It should be noted, however, that fine needle aspiration cytology is unreliable for most pediatric tumors, particularly at initial diagnosis and therefore the technique is not recommended.

Staging

There are a number of different staging systems in use for pediatric NRSTS but traditionally staging has been according to the Intergroup Rhabdomyosarcoma Study Group surgicopathological system, as used for rhabdomyosarcomas (Table 39.1). Histological grade is also used in clinical staging as it is highly predictive of clinical outcome (42). Assessments of percentage of cases presenting with metastatic disease vary widely from as little as 5% to as much as 30% (38). Pulmonary metastases are the most common site, followed by bone, liver, and mesenteric metastases. Lymphatic spread is rare, particularly in tumors in the extremities where it is approximately 4% but is seen more commonly with high grade lesions such as synovial sarcoma, angiosarcoma, and epithelioid sarcoma. Risk factors for local recurrence differ from those for distant recurrence (43). Local recurrence is predicted by positive surgical margins, intra-abdominal primary tumor site and the omission of radiotherapy. Distant recurrence is predicted by tumor size (5 cm or more), invasiveness, and high grade.

The most important prognostic factor seems to be complete surgical removal of the tumor with five-year survival rates of 84% to 90% with complete resection, and only 30% to 50% with incomplete resection or metastases at presentation. Children in whom complete

resection was achieved had a local recurrence rate of 12.8% and a distant recurrence rate of 11.8% at five years (43). Several reports have shown prolonged survival after surgical treatment of pulmonary metastases from soft tissue sarcoma. Prognosis is better in Grade I and II tumors and if complete resection of the metastases is achieved.

Key Points: Non-Rhabdomyosarcomatous Soft Tissue Sarcomas (NRSTS)

- Almost 50% of pediatric soft tissue tumors are non-rhabdomyomatous sarcomas
- The majority of NRSTS are synovial sarcomas; others include fibrosarcoma, malignant histiocytoma, and malignant peripheral nerve sheath tumors
- Most NRSTS arise in the extremities and the trunk
- Metastases at presentation are more common in truncal tumors
- Fine needle aspiration cytology is unreliable for diagnosis
- Metastases are most commonly to the lungs, liver, bone, and mesentery
- Local recurrence is predicted by positive surgical margins and distant relapse by the size of the primary tumor

Synovial Cell Sarcoma

Synovial sarcoma is the most common NRSTS in adolescents and young adults. Synovial cell sarcomas arise *de novo* from mesenchymal tissue, which differentiates sufficiently to resemble the histological appearance of synovium. Presentation occurs at a mean age of 13 years and 60% to 75% are seen in the lower extremity, often around the thigh or knee with the upper extremity being the next most common site of occurrence (44). The tumors usually arise remote from normal synovial tissues (Fig. 39.18) and 5% to 12% have metastases at presentation, of which 94% are in the lungs (37). Five-year survival

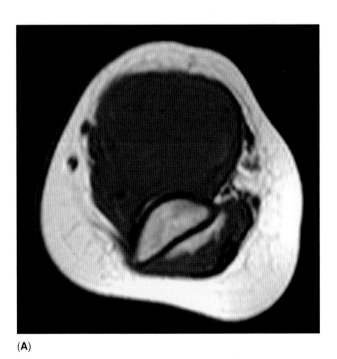

(A)

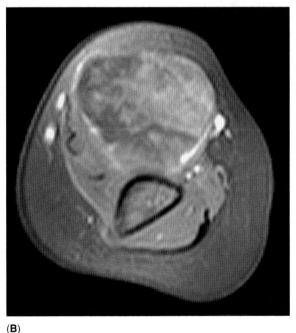

(B)

Figure 39.18 Synovial cell soft tissue sarcoma. (A) Axial T1-weighted MR image shows a solid mass on the anterior arm, without any adjacent osseous or bone marrow change. (B) The mass shows heterogeneous enhancement on an axial fat-suppressed T1-weighted MR image after gadolinium administration.

rates are of the order of 80% with Grade I and II tumors but only 17% with Grades III and IV (45). Treatment is with wide local excision with or without radiotherapy. The role of chemotherapy is uncertain.

MR imaging is the modality of choice when evaluating synovial cell sarcoma, providing greater contrast resolution between tumor and normal tissue than CT. The tumors tend to be sharply marginated on MR imaging and may appear cystic which can lead to misdiagnosis as a hematoma, ganglion cyst, Baker's cyst, or other benign cystic mass. A contemporaneous US study should easily clarify the solid nature of the mass. US should also be used, as with all suspected malignancies in children, to check for regional lymphadenopathy and for hepatic metastases. A mixed pattern of signal intensity is recognized on MR imaging, known as the triple signal (46). This is seen in about one third of synovial sarcomas with high signal intensity similar to that of fluid, intermediate signal intensity which can be iso- or slightly hyperintense to fat and slightly lower signal intensity that resembles fibrous tissue. Fluid-fluid levels are seen in around 18%. Tumors smaller than 5 cm typically have homogeneously low signal intensity on T1-weighted sequence and marked heterogeneity on T2-weighted sequences. There may be a variable degree of internal septation. About three-quarters of the tumors are intimately related to bone, with 50% abutting bone and 21% showing cortical thinning or medullary invasion. Approximately 30% of synovial sarcomas contain calcification, best seen with CT (47). Peripheral calcification with or without osseous invasion may be seen with plain radiographs or CT (46).

Key Points: Synovial Sarcomas

- Synovial sarcomas present at a mean age of 13 years
- Sixty to seventy percent are in the lower extremity
- The tumor usually arises remote from the synovium
- MR imaging is the modality of choice for evaluating these tumors

Fibrosarcoma

Fibrosarcoma makes up 13% to 15% of childhood NRSTS and is the most common sarcoma in the first 12 months of life (infantile fibrosarcoma) (39). A second peak is seen in the 10–15 year old age group. The infantile form, despite looking identical histologically, has a more benign course than that in older children and rarely metastasizes, even in cases with repeated local recurrence (Fig. 39.19). Treatment is therefore often confined to wide local excision without recourse to radiotherapy or chemotherapy. Spontaneous regression is also recognized, albeit difficult to predict. With large masses, preoperative chemotherapy has been shown to reduce tumor size allowing more conservative surgery (48). Retroperitoneal and head and neck lesions have a worse prognosis than extremity lesions with metastases developing in 26% of cases as compared to 10% in the extremities (40). Metastases, mostly of the lung, are more frequent in post-pubertal children.

Congenital fibrosarcoma has non-specific imaging appearances which reflect the non-aggressive behavior of the lesion. Initially, mistaken diagnoses such as a hemangioma or vascular

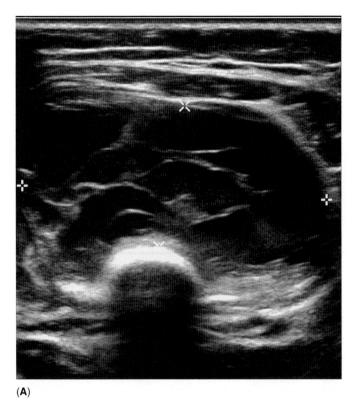

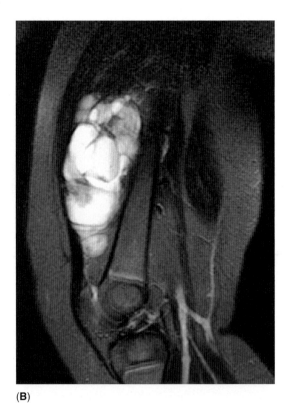

(A)

(B)

Figure 39.19 Fibrosarcoma. (A) Transverse ultrasound shows a very cystic mass in the anterior right thigh in a six month old baby. Initially this was thought to be a venous malformation but as no flow was demonstrable on Doppler evaluation, a biopsy was performed which confirmed an infantile fibrosarcoma. (B) Sagittal fat-saturated T2-weighted MR image shows the full extent of the large mass, which contains fluid-fluid levels. Note the small epiphyses and unfused physes.

malformation are commonly made. The most common radiographic finding is of a soft tissue mass, which may cause a mass effect leading to deformity of adjacent bony structures. Bone destruction is unusual but can occur. Bone changes are easily assessed in infancy simply with plain radiographs and musculoskeletal US which can easily identify periosteal new bone formation and/or a soft tissue mass. In the older adolescent, bone involvement is best assessed with CT. Overall the full extent of a fibrosarcoma, particularly in relation to the presence or absence of local invasion is best demonstrated with MR imaging, the nondescript mass typically showing medium signal intensity on T1-weighted and high signal intensity on T2-weighted sequences. The signal intensity resembles that of muscle on T1-weighted images, and like so many other tumors, there is commonly a heterogeneous pattern of variable enhancement after the administration of IV contrast medium. Areas of heterogeneity representing necrosis may be seen within the tumor although homogeneous appearances may occasionally be demonstrated, particularly in tumors of infancy. On US, the mass often appears vascular and solid.

Key Points: Fibrosarcoma

- Fibrosarcomas account for 13% to 15% of all childhood NRSTS
- The most common age of presentation is during the first year of life
- A second peak incidence is seen at 10 to 15 years
- Treatment is surgical, chemotherapy is useful for large tumors
- Metastases occur most commonly in truncal tumors (26%) compared with 10% in children with extremity tumors

Malignant Fibrous Histiocytoma

Malignant fibrous histiocytoma (MFH) can occur anywhere in the body but, like many NRSTS, is more common in the extremities. It makes up 12% to 13% of childhood NRSTS. It is rarely seen in infancy unlike fibrosarcoma. MFH is known to be one of the radiation-induced sarcomas, although radiation-induced tumors are seldom seen in a young population. Microscopically, MFH resembles fibrosarcoma but has a number of distinctive features which include the presence of marked cellular pleomorphism, the presence of multiple cell types and a generally more malignant appearance. However, distinguishing MFH from fibrosarcoma recurrence can be difficult.

Angiomatoid MFH is the only relatively common form of MFH occurring as a primary tumor in childhood (under 15 years of age) and ongoing work suggests that it should be differentiated from adult-type MFH. Angiomatoid MFH has a very favorable prognosis with only 1% of tumors developing metastases. The most common site of metastasis is the lung, although metastases to the brain and other sites are also seen. Patients with tumors in the extremities have a better three-year survival (81%) than those of the trunk, or head and neck (54%) (49). Initial management is with wide local excision alone, particularly with angiomatoid MFH. The tumor does appear to be chemosensitive and the role of chemotherapy is currently under investigation.

MR imaging typically reveals a well-defined intramuscular mass with heterogeneous signal intensity on all sequences. The signal intensity pattern is non-specific but usually low to intermediate on T1-weighted images and intermediate to high on T2-weighted. Regions of fibrous tissue and calcification may be seen and solid components of the tumor typically reveal nodular and peripheral enhancement (37).

Key Points: Malignant Fibrous Histiocytoma

- MFH is most common in the extremities but may occur anywhere in the body
- MFH accounts for 12% to 13% of childhood NRSTS
- Angiomatoid MFH has a favorable prognosis and only 1% metastasize

Malignant Peripheral Nerve Sheath Tumor

Malignant peripheral nerve sheath tumor (MPNST) accounts for approximately 5% to 10% of childhood NRSTS. There is a strong association with neurofibromatosis type 1 (NF1), with approximately 5% to 16% of patients with NF1 developing MPNST. Furthermore, MPNST contributes significantly to the reduced life-span of NF1-patients. Genetic data suggests the loss of a tumor suppressor gene on chromosome 17 is important in the pathogenesis of this tumor. The tumor has a variety of histological appearances and a superficial resemblance to fibrosarcoma. MPNST constitutes a heterogeneous group of malignant tumors that probably arise from cells of the peripheral nerve sheath. MPNST may arise from plexiform neurofibromas with an invasive or displacing growth pattern on MR imaging. Many patients report pain and neurological deficits at the time of presentation. Diagnosis of MPNST in this age group often takes longer compared to adults. The overall survival time in a small cohort was 30.5 months (50). Those children who died showed a median survival time after diagnosis of only 20 months. (50). The NF1 mutation analysis in that MPNST pediatric age group revealed the same mutational spectrum as the adult group (50).

The most common primary sites are extremities (42%), retroperitoneum (25%), and trunk (21%). Metastases are seen in about 12% of patients at diagnosis. Surgical excision plays a key role in management. If gross surgical resection is possible, up to three-quarters of patients remain disease-free at three years with less than one third of patients, in whom gross surgical resection is not possible, remaining disease-free at three years. Patients treated with gross resection and irradiation to microscopic residual disease had a similar good outcome to those with complete excision with disease-free margins. The role of chemotherapy in MPNST has not yet been established. It has been shown to produce tumor regression in metastatic disease and, results for disease-free survival in patients with advanced disease are not good (39).

Nerve sheath tumors have a low attenuation on unenhanced CT images and on MR imaging are isointense to muscle on T1-weighted images and hyperintense on T2 with moderate to marked contrast enhancement (51). Unfortunately, the imaging features are not specific enough to distinguish benign nerve tumors from malignant. It is important not to assume an MPNST is simply a plexiform neurofibroma and a low threshold for biopsy is always warranted. On T2-weighted MR images, a "target sign"

with central hypointensity and a hyperintense rim may be helpful as it is much more common in neurofibromas than MPNSTs (52). PET-CT may prove useful in that context but large series will be necessary to clarify this.

Key Points: Malignant Peripheral Nerve Sheath Tumor

■ MPNST accounts for 5% to 10% of childhood NRSTS
■ There is a strong association with neurofibromatosis type1 (NF1)
■ Many patients have pain and neurological deficit at the time of diagnosis
■ Most common sites are the extremities, the retroperitoneum, and the trunk
■ MPNST are well shown on MR imaging and are low signal intensity on T1-weighted and hyperintense on T2-weighted images

Summary

■ Rhabdomyosarcoma is the third most common extracranial tumor of childhood accouning for 4% of all childhood malignancies
■ Most cases of rhabdomyosarcoma present under the age of six years
■ There are four histological subtypes of RMS. Sixty percent are embryonal and 20% are alveolar. Botryoid subtype has the best prognosis
■ RMS most commonly occurs in the head and neck region. Other sites in order of frequency are the genitourinary tract, the trunk, and the extremities
■ CT and MR imaging are the key modalities for staging and follow-up of RMS
■ Lymph node metastases occur in 20% of patients with RMS at presentation
■ Hepatoblastoma presents under the age of four years (median age one year)
■ Hepatoblastoma usually presents with an abdominal mass or distension
■ In hepatoblastoma, metastatic disease is seen at presentation in 20% of cases
■ Imaging is required to assess resectability, particularly in relation to the presence of tumor in critical areas such as the porta hepatis, portal vein, and IVC
■ Between 30% and 40% of hepatic tumors in children are benign (e.g., hemangioendothelioma, multilocular cystic hamartoma)
■ Malignant tumors of childhood which most frequently metastasize to the liver are Wilms', neuroblastoma, rhabdomyosarcoma, and lymphoma
■ Sacrococcygeal teratomas affect females more frequently than males and account for 40% of all germ cell tumors. They are usually benign
■ Testicular germ cell tumors account for 1% of all childhood malignancies and 90% are Stage I at presentation
■ Ovarian germ cell tumors of childhood have a peak age incidence of 10 years

■ Ovarian tumors spread typically to the peritoneum, lymph nodes, and lungs
■ Non-rhabdomyomatous soft tissue tumors account for 3% of all malignancies in children
■ The majority of NRSTS are synovial sarcomas; others include fibrosarcoma, malignant histiocytoma, and malignant peripheral nerve sheath tumors

REFERENCES

1. Pappo AS, Shapiro DN, Crist WM. Rhabdomyosarcoma. Biology and treatment. Pediatr Clin North Am 1997; 44: 953–72.
2. Van Rijn RR, Wilde J, Bras J, et al. Imaging findings in non-craniofacial childhood rhabdomyosarcoma. Pediatr Radiol 2008; 38: 617–34.
3. Newton WA Jr, Gehan EA, Webber BL, et al. Classification of rhabdomyosarcomas and related sarcomas. Pathologic aspects and proposal for a new classification—an Intergroup Rhabdomyosarcoma Study. Cancer 1995; 76: 1073–85.
4. Kodet R, Newton WA Jr, Hamoudi AB, et al. Orbital rhabdomyosarcomas and related tumors in childhood: relationship of morphology to prognosis—an Intergroup Rhabdomyosarcoma study. Med Pediatr Oncol 1997; 29: 51–60.
5. Malkin D, Li FP, Strong LC, et al. Germ line p53 mutations in a familial syndrome of breast cancer, sarcomas, and other neoplasms. Science 1990; 250: 1233–8.
6. Wexler LH, Crist WM, Helman LJ. Rhabdomyosarcoma and the undifferentiated sarcomas. In: Pizzo PA, Poplack DG, eds. Principles and Practice of Pediatric Oncology, 4th edn. Philadelphia: Lippincott Williams & Wilkins, 2002; 943–71.
7. Lawrence W Jr, Anderson JR, Gehan EA, Maurer H. Pretreatment TNM staging of childhood rhabdomyosarcoma: a report of the Intergroup Rhabdomyosarcoma Study Group. Children's Cancer Study Group. Pediatric Oncology Group. Cancer 1997; 80: 1165–70.
8. Heyn R, Beltangady M, Hays D, et al. Results of intensive therapy in children with localized alveolar extremity rhabdomyosarcoma: a report from the Intergroup Rhabdomyosarcoma Study. J Clin Oncol 1989; 7: 200–7.
9. Bisogno GB, Jenney M, Kazanowska B, et al. EpSSG RMS 2005; a protocol for non metatatic rhabdomyosarcoma. Sarcoma Meeting Stuttgart 2005. Sarcoma 2005; 9: 43–118.
10. McHugh K, Boothroyd AE. The role of radiology in childhood rhabdomyosarcoma. Clin Radiol 1999; 54: 2–10.
11. Donaldson SS, Anderson J. Factors that influence treatment decisions in childhood rhabdomyosarcoma. Intergroup Rhabdomyosarcoma Study Group of the Children's Cancer Group, the Pediatric Oncology Group, and the Intergroup Rhabdomyosarcoma Study Group Statistical Center. Radiology 1997; 203: 17–22.
12. Priest JR, Hill DA, Williams GM, et al. Type I pleuropulmonary blastoma: a report from the International Pleuropulmonary Blastoma Registry. J Clin Oncol 2006; 24: 4492–8.

13. Tomlinson GE, Finegold MJ. Tumors of the liver. In: Pizzo PA, Poplack DC, eds. Principles and Practice of Pediatric Oncology, 4th edn. Philadelphia: Lippincott Williams & Wilkins, 2002; 847–64.

14. Ebb DH, Green DM, Shamberger RC, Tarbell NJ. Solid tumors of childhood. In: DeVita VT Jr, Hellman S, Rosenberg SA, eds. Cancer: Principles and Practice of Oncology, 6th edn. Philadelphia: Lippincott Williams & Wilkins, 2001; 2169–214.

15. Slovis TL, Roebuck DJ. Hepatoblastoma: why so many low-birth-weight infants? Pediatr Radiol 2006; 36: 173–4.

16. Roebuck DJ, Olsen O, Pariente D. Radiological staging in children with hepatoblastoma. Pediatr Radiol 2006; 36: 176–82.

17. Roebuck DJ, Aronson D, Clapuyt P, et al. 2005 PRETEXT: a revised staging system for primary malignant liver tumours of childhood developed by the SIOPEL group. Pediatr Radiol 2007; 37: 123–32.

18. Finegold MJ. Tumors of the liver. Semin Liver Dis 1994; 14: 270–81.

19. Chen JC, Chen CC, Chen WJ, et al. Hepatocellular carcinoma in children: clinical review and comparison with adult cases. J Pediatr Surg 1998; 33: 1350–4.

20. Stringer MD, Hennayake S, Howard ER, et al. Improved outcome for children with hepatoblastoma. Br J Surg 1995; 82: 386–91.

21. Reynolds M. Conversion of unresectable to resectable hepatoblastoma and long term follow-up study. World J Surg 1995; 19: 814–16.

22. Morland B. Commentary on hepatoblastoma minisymposium. Pediatr Radiol 2006; 36: 175.

23. Czauderna P, Mackinlay G, Perilongo G, et al. Hepatocellular carcinoma in children: results of the first prospective study of the International Society of Pediatric Oncology group. J Clin Oncol 2002: 20; 2798–804.

24. Ichikawa T, Federle MP, Grazioli L, Marsh W. Fibrolamellar hepatocellular carcinoma: pre- and post-therapy evaluation with CT and MR imaging. Radiology 2000; 217: 145–51.

25. Baron PW, Majlessipour F, Bedros AA, et al. Undifferentiated embryonal sarcoma of the liver successfully treated with chemotherapy and liver resection. J Gastrointest Surg 2007; 11: 73–5.

26. Christison-Lagay ER, Burrows PE, Alomari A, et al. Hepatic hemangiomas: subtype classification and development of a clinical practice algorithm and registry. J Pediatr Surg 2007; 42: 62–7.

27. Kim SH, Kim WS, Cheon JE, et al. Radiological spectrum of hepatic mesenchymal hamartoma in children. Korean J Radiol. 2007; 8: 498–505.

28. Dulmet EM, Macchiarini P, Suc B, Verley JM. Germ cell tumours of the mediastinum: a 30 year experience. Cancer 1993: 72; 1894–901.

29. Cushing B, Perlman EJ, Marina NM, Castleberry RP. Germ cell tumors. In: Pizzo PA, Poplack DG, eds. Principles and Practice of Pediatric Oncology, 4th edn. Philadelphia: Lippincott Williams and Wilkins, 2002; 1091–113.

30. Frazier AL, Rumcheva P, Olson T, et al. Application of the adult international germ cell classification system to pediatric malignant non-seminomatous germ cell tumors: a report from the Children's Oncology Group. Pediatr Blood Cancer 2008; 50: 746–51.

31. De Backer A, Madern GC, Hazebroek FW. Retroperitoneal germ cell tumours: a clinical study of 12 patients. J Pediat Surg 2005; 40: 1475–81.

32. Hayasaka K, Yamada T, Saitoh Y, et al. CT evaluation of primary benign retroperitoneal tumor. Radiat Med 1994; 12: 115–20.

33. Nobusawa H, Hashimoto T, Munechika H, et al. CT findings of primary retroperitoneal cystic tumors; special emphasis on the distinction of benignancy from malignancy. Nippon Igaku Hoshasen Gakkai Zasshi 1995; 55: 861–6.

34. Sasaka K, Kurihara Y, Nakajima Y, et al. Spontaneous rupture: a complication of benign mature teratomas of the mediastinum. AJR Am J Roentgenol 1998; 170: 323–8.

35. Alper F, Kaynar H, Kantarci M, et al. Trichoptysis caused by intrapulmonary teratoma: computed tomography and magnetic resonance imaging findings. Australas Radiol 2005; 49: 53–6.

36. Skoog SJ. Benign and malignant pediatric scrotal masses. Pediatr Clin North Am 1997; 44: 1229–50.

37. Kransdorf M. Imaging of Soft Tissue Tumors. Philadelphia: W Saunders Co., 1997.

38. Dillon P, Maurer H, Jenkins J, et al. A prospective study of nonrhabdomyosarcoma soft tissue sarcomas in the pediatric age group. J Pediatr Surg 1992; 27: 241–4.

39. McGrory JE, Pritchard DJ, Arndt CA, et al. Nonrhabdomyosarcoma soft tissue sarcomas in children. The Mayo Clinic experience. Clin Orthop Relat Res 2000; 374: 247–58.

40. Blocker S, Koenig J, Ternberg J. Congenital fibrosarcoma. J Pediatr Surg 1987; 22: 665–70.

41. Enzinger FM, Smith BH. Hemangiopericytoma. An analysis of 106 cases. Hum Pathol 1976; 7: 61–82.

42. Guillou L, Coindre JM, Bonichon F, et al. Comparative study of the National Cancer Institute and French Federation of Cancer Centers Sarcoma Group grading systems in a population of 410 adult patients with soft tissue sarcoma. J Clin Oncol 1997; 15: 350–62.

43. Spunt SL, Poquette CA, Hurt YS, et al. Prognostic factors for children and adolescents with surgically resected nonrhabdomyosarcoma soft tissue sarcoma: an analysis of 121 patients treated at St Jude Children's Research Hospital. J Clin Oncol 1999; 17: 3697–705.

44. Schmidt D, Thum P, Harms D, Treuner J. Synovial sarcoma in children and adolescents. A report from the Kiel Pediatric Tumor Registry. Cancer 1991; 67: 1667–72.

45. Pappo AS, Fontanesi J, Luo X, et al. Synovial sarcoma in children and adolescents: the St Jude Children's Research Hospital experience. J Clin Oncol 1994; 12: 2360–6.

46. O'Sullivan PJ, Harris AC, Munk PL. Radiological features of synovial cell sarcoma. Br J Radiol 2008; 81: 346–56.

47. McCarville MB, Spunt SL, Skapek SX, Pappo AS. Synovial sarcoma in pediatric patients. AJR Am J Roentgenol 2002; 179: 797–801.

48. Kurkchubasche AG, Halvorson EG, Forman EN, Terek RM, Ferguson WS. The role of preoperative chemotherapy in the treatment of infantile fibrosarcoma. J Pediatr Surg 2000; 35: 880–3.

49. Shinjo K. Analysis of prognostic factors and chemotherapy of malignant fibrous histiocytoma of soft tissue: a preliminary report. Jpn J Clin Oncol 1994; 24: 154–9.

50. Friedrich RE, Hartmann M, Mautner VF. Malignant peripheral nerve sheath tumors (MPNST) in NF1-affected children. Anticancer Res 2007; 7: 1957–60.

51. Verstraete KL, Achten E, De Schepper A, et al. Nerve sheath tumors: evaluation with CT and MR imaging. J Belge Radiol 1992; 75: 311–20.

52. Bhargava R, Parham DM, Lasater OE, et al. MR imaging differentiation of benign and malignant peripheral nerve sheath tumors: use of the target sign. Pediatr Radiol 1997; 27: 124–9.

40 Lymph Node Metastases
Dow-Mu Koh and Janet E Husband

INTRODUCTION

The unregulated growth of tumors results not only in local infiltration, but also in the spread of disease via lymphatics to lymph nodes. Although tumor dissemination to lymph nodes is common, the prevalence of nodal disease differs according to the site of the primary tumor and the underlying histopathology. For example, lymph node metastases are relatively frequent in patients with colorectal cancers but are rarely encountered in patients with soft tissue sarcomas (1).

In the majority of cancers, a definitive diagnosis of nodal disease can only be made after careful histopathological analysis of lymph nodes in the surgically excised tumor specimen or by lymph node biopsy. Identification of nodal involvement is important because it influences the choice of treatment. Thus the ability to diagnose the presence and extent of nodal involvement non-invasively with imaging is a critical factor in optimizing patient management. For example, in a patient diagnosed with surgically resectable uterine cancer, a confident diagnosis of nodal disease may support the decision to perform radical nodal dissection along the pelvic sidewall. Likewise, in patients with squamous cell carcinoma of the anus, where the tumor treatment is primarily non-surgical, knowledge of the extent of nodal involvement in the mesorectum, pelvic sidewall, and inguinal areas contributes to radiotherapy planning.

Prior to the advent of ultrasound (US), computed tomography (CT), and magnetic resonance (MR) imaging, the assessment of lymph node spread could only be made using lymphography and although the technique is now obsolete it remains the only established clinical tool that is capable of demonstrating both the lymphatic vessels and the architecture of lymph nodes. Today CT remains the most widely used imaging modality for nodal assessment but positron emission tomography (PET) and lymphoscintigraphy are utilized with increasing frequency to detect nodal metastases.

In this chapter, the classification systems used to stage nodal disease are reviewed and a brief resume of the current understanding of the lymphatic system and the mechanism of nodal metastasis is presented. The use of conventional US, CT, and MR imaging to evaluate nodal disease is discussed, highlighting the radiological features which can aid in the differentiation of malignant from non-malignant lymph nodes. Recent advances in nodal imaging are also considered.

CLASSIFICATION OF NODAL STATUS AND NODAL STAGING

Nodal disease is most frequently staged using the TNM staging system, which classifies tumors according to the local Tumor extent (T), Nodal involvement (N), and the presence or absence of Metastatic disease (M) (2). N0 signifies no detected nodal metastases, Nx indicates that nodal involvement is unknown and the presence of nodal disease may be further categorized into N1, N2, and N3 disease depending on the tumor type. These subcategories relate to the number of involved nodes, for example in colorectal, gastric, urinary bladder, melanoma, breast, and renal tumors. In other tumors, for example, the lung, esophagus, prostate, cervix, ovary, and anus, the site of nodal involvement influences the category of nodal staging. Nodal involvement beyond the immediate areas of tumor drainage is considered to be metastatic disease. Thus, to ensure accurate nodal assessment, the radiologist should be familiar with the full staging classification of the primary tumor being studied.

In addition to the TNM system, other nodal staging classifications are used that are specific to certain cancers. These systems also provide useful prognostic information that informs treatment decisions. For example, in patients with lymphoma, where the disease primarily affects the lymph nodes, the Ann Arbor Classification system (Stage I to Stage IV, depending on the extent of nodal involvement) is frequently used. Although this system was initially devised for the classification of Hodgkin's disease, it has been expanded to include the non-Hodgkin's lymphomas.

In colorectal cancer, the Dukes' staging system is still widely used but has no major advantage over the TNM system (3). It combines the depth of tumor invasion through the colonic wall and regional lymph node involvement to define three tumor stages: A, B, and C. Stage C denotes the presence of lymph node metastases.

Micro-metastases are generally defined as foci of metastases measuring less than 2 mm in diameter in lymph nodes. These small clusters of tumor deposits are beyond the spatial resolution of conventional imaging techniques but as imaging technology continues to advance, their detection may become more important in the overall management of patients with malignant disease. However it is still unclear whether the presence of micro-metastases in lymph nodes is associated with an adverse patient outcome across different tumor types, and further research in this area is required.

Key Points: General Considerations

- Nodal involvement is an adverse prognostic feature in the majority of cancers
- Nodal stage is confirmed by histopathological examination
- US, CT, and MR imaging are frequently employed to evaluate nodal stage prior to treatment but CT remains the most widely used imaging modality
- The TNM staging system is the most widely used classification
- Staging is based on the number of involved nodes or the presence and site of nodal involvement.
- Cancer specific nodal staging classifications are also used in certain tumor types

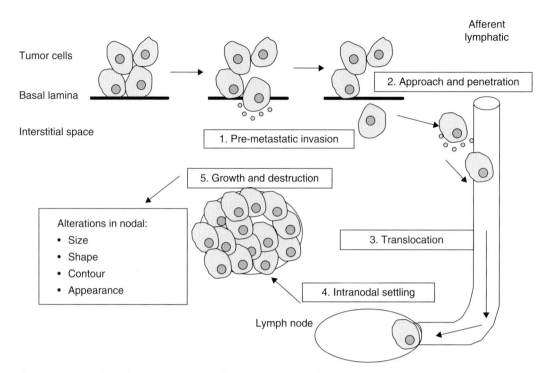

Figure 40.1 Steps in the pathogenesis of nodal metastases. Tumor cells arising in an epithelial surface can invade the basal lamina by the production of cytokines (Pre-metastatic invasion) to lie within the interstitial spaces of the submucosa or subcutaneous tissue. By a chemically mediated process, a cancer cell lying adjacent to a small afferent lymphatic vessel can penetrate through the wall of the lymphatic (approach and penetration). Once within the lymphatic lumen, the cancer cell is transported into the lymph node (translocation), where it frequently settles in the subcapsular sinus (intranodal settling). Proliferation of tumor cells within the node leads to destruction of the nodal architecture and potential nodal enlargement. This is reflected by alterations in the size, shape, contour, and appearance of the node on imaging.

PATHOGENESIS OF NODAL METASTASES

The earliest recorded reference of lymph node and lymphatics was made by Hippocrates (460–360 BC) who described axillary nodes and associated "white blood" (4). However, little significance was attached to these observations and it was not until the late 17th century that Henri Francos LeDran (1685–1770) described the spread of cancer along lymphatic channels, and thus made one of the earliest observations relating to the mechanism of tumor spread to lymph nodes.

The lymphatic system is a complex network of lymphoid organs, lymph nodes, and lymph vessels that produce and transport lymph fluid from the tissue to the circulatory system. Lymphatic fluid originates as blood plasma that leaks from the capillaries of the circulatory system, becoming interstitial fluid, and filling the space between individual cells within the body tissues. Excess interstitial fluid is collected by diffusion into lymph capillaries, and is filtered by lymph nodes prior to being returned to the circulatory system. Once the fluid is within the lymphatic system it is called lymph.

Our understanding of the mechanism of cancer spread to lymph nodes is derived from the pioneering work of Zeidman and Buss (5). The following stages (Fig. 40.1) have been described in the pathway of lymphatic metastasis (6–8):

Pre-Metastatic Invasion. At this stage, proliferating cancer cells penetrate the basal lamina of an epithelial lining of the organ or tissue in which the tumor originates. The basal lamina and surrounding tissue matrix are broken down by enzymes (cyto-kines) released by the tumor cells or by lymphoreticular cells (9). As the

interstitial pressure of the tumor is usually elevated, the hydrostatic pressure of the fluid may play a role in driving cancer cells towards the lymphatic capillaries located in the interstitial space.

Approach. The tumor cells come to lie in close proximity to the lymphatic endothelium.

Penetration. The tumor cells penetrate the endothelial barrier of the lymphatic vessel and enter the lymphatic capillary lumen. This may occur through a small number of open inter-endothelial gaps or through the opening up of spaces which result from the release of soluble chemical mediators.

Translocation. Tumor cells migrate through lymphatic vessels towards the draining lymph nodes. The division of cancer cells behind the head of a column may push the whole column forwards. However, single cells or clusters of cancer cells can move passively up the lymphatics to the draining node (6).

Intranodal Settling. Tumor cells settle within the sinusoids of the lymph node where they proliferate. Clumps of the tumor cells frequently settle in the subcapsular sinus (6,8).

Growth and Destruction of the Lymph Node. Tumor cells grow and destroy the sinusoidal endothelium and continue to proliferate within the parenchyma of the node. Eventually, the entire node may be replaced by tumor.

Further Seeding to Secondary Nodes. Tumor cells migrate along the sinusoids towards the efferent lymphatics at the nodal hilum. Penetration into the efferent lymphatics may lead to further metastases in adjacent lymph nodes.

The pathological appearance of a malignant node is variable depending on the size of the metastasis, the site of the initial focus

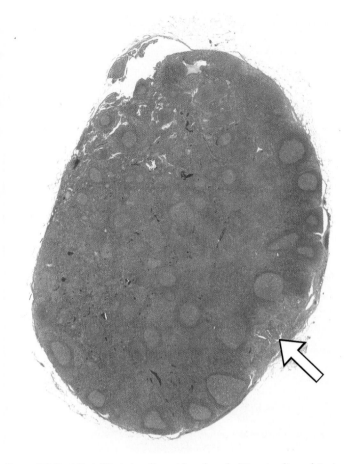

Figure 40.2 Partially infiltrated malignant lymph node (Hematoxylin and Eosin stain, 5×). Histological section through this node shows a small focus of metastasis (arrow) in the subcapsular area of the lymph node. However, there is considerable reactive nodal hyperplasia, which accounts for nodal enlargement.

within the lymph node, and the reaction of the node to tumor invasion. Thus the tumor deposit may stimulate the production of a stroma (fibrotic, vascular, calcified or necrotic) similar to that encountered in the primary tumor, or a small nidus of metastasis may provoke marked reactive changes within the node, resulting in nodal enlargement due to the reactive change rather than the growth of tumor cells (Fig. 40.2). Occasionally tumor cells may block afferent lymphatics resulting in an extracapsular mass. When a node is entirely replaced by tumor, further growth may lead to breach of the nodal cortex, leading to extracapsular extension of disease (10).

In summary, the development of lymph node metastases and the associated nodal response are complex processes which account for the diverse imaging appearances of metastatic lymph nodes and explain some of the difficulties encountered in the accurate diagnosis of nodal spread.

Key Points: Pathogenesis of Nodal Metastases

- Tumor spread to lymph nodes is a complex multi-step process
- The pathological features of a malignant node depend on the size of the metastasis and the associated nodal response

IMAGING LYMPH NODES IN ONCOLOGY

Ultrasound
Lymph nodes in superficial locations such as in the neck, axilla, and inguinal region are particularly amenable to US evaluation. Imaging at these sites can be performed using a high frequency transducer probe (e.g., 10–12.5 MHz), which allows real-time high-resolution assessment of nodal size, nodal contour, and internal nodal echo-texture.

On US, a normal lymph node is usually ovoid in shape, appears mildly hypoechoeic compared with muscle, and frequently contains an echogenic fatty hilum (Fig. 40.3A). The hilum is a linear, echogenic, non-shadowing structure containing nodal vessels, and it appears continuous with fat around the node. One of the key advantages of using US is the ability to obtain cytological or biopsy sampling of indeterminate nodes quickly and effectively under imaging guidance (11). However, US is also a technique with significant intra- and inter-operator variability, which can make it difficult to compare results between studies. In addition, deep-seated lymph nodes in the body are poorly visualized.

Endoscopic ultrasound (EUS) probes are frequently used to evaluate disease that cannot be satisfactorily assessed by conventional transabdominal techniques. EUS can also be combined with cytological sampling and is widely used to assess nodal disease associated with esophageal, gastric, pancreatic, anorectal, and gynecological malignancies. EUS may be highly specific, for example in esophageal cancer the technique has been reported to have a specificity of 98% but a lower sensitivity of 67% in the detection of nodal disease in the upper abdomen (12).

The following criteria have been used to discriminate between normal and malignant nodes on US evaluation.

Nodal Size
Generally, lymph nodes measuring greater than 1 cm in the maximum short axis diameter are considered to be malignant. However, the size threshold applied to define nodal disease varies with the anatomical site, underlying tumor type and individual clinical practices. For example, in rectal cancer lymph nodes larger than 5 mm are regarded as pathological.

Nodal Shape and Ratio of Long and Short Axis Diameters
In US literature, round (spherical) nodes have been found to be more likely to be malignant compared to ovoid nodes (Fig. 40.3B). Nodes showing a long axis versus short axis diameter of less than two are more likely to be malignant (13).

Nodal Appearance
The sonographic features of malignant nodes include loss of the echogenic nodal hilum, marked hypoechogenicity, internal nodal heterogeneity, irregular nodal contour, and matting of lymph nodes. Heterogeneity of nodal echogenicity may result also from intranodal calcifications, cystic necrosis, or coagulative necrosis.

Vascularity on Doppler Ultrasound
The pattern of vascularity on color Doppler US has been used to discriminate between benign and malignant lymph nodes. Normal and benign reactive nodes have been reported to show central hilar vascularity and central symmetric vascularity.

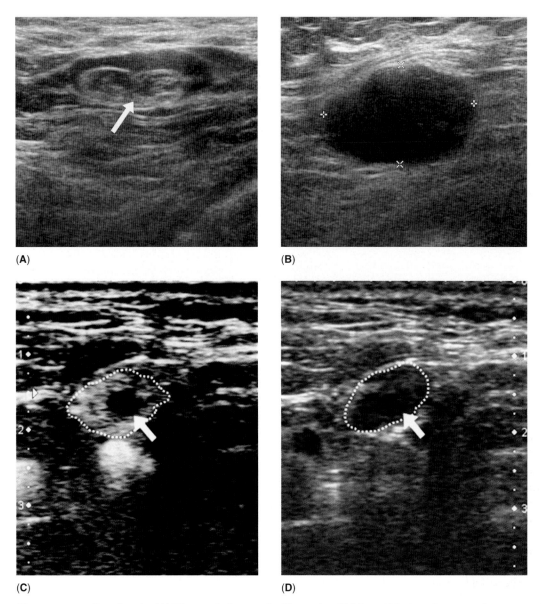

Figure 40.3 Sonographic appearances of lymph nodes. (**A**) Ultrasound of a normal axillary node, which is ovoid in shape, has a smooth contour, and demonstrates an echogenic hilum (arrow). (**B**) By contrast, ultrasound of a malignant axillary node in a patient with breast cancer shows a rounded appearance to the lymph node. The ratio of the long (++) to short (××) axis of the node is less than two. (**C**) and (**D**) Imaging using ultrasound contrast medium reveals smaller foci of disease in a partially replaced lymph node. In this example, imaging was performed using a 6.2-MHz probe and a low MI (0.03) using a phase and amplitude non-linear contrast mode and 4.8 mL of SonoVue (Bracco, Milan). The contrast-enhanced image (**C**) shows a filling defect that represents metastatic disease (arrow), which is difficult to discern on the grey-scale ultrasound image (arrow) (**D**). The lymph node is outlined by dotted lines in (**C**) and (**D**). *Source*: Courtesy of Prof. David Cosgrove, Hammersmith Hospital, London, U.K.

In contrast, eccentric or absent hilar vascularity, multi-focal aberrant vascularity, focal perfusion defects, and peripheral subcapsular vascularity are more frequently observed in malignant nodes (14,15). Metastatic nodes often reveal peripheral perfusion or diffuse aberrant vascularity. On quantitative measurement, malignant nodes have been reported to return a high resistive index (>1.0) and a high pulsatility index (>1.5) (16,17). However, other studies have reported contrary results (17). Hence, the usefulness of quantitative analysis is yet to be established (18,19). The administration of sonographic contrast medium can help to identify foci of metastases within lymph nodes (Fig. 40.3C). It has been shown that sonographic contrast increases the perception of nodal blood vessels but this does not necessarily improve the accuracy of detection of malignant nodal deposits (19,20).

Computed Tomography and Magnetic Resonance Imaging

CT and MR imaging are now the most widely used imaging modalities for nodal assessment. On CT, normal nodes are ovoid in shape and are of soft tissue density. These can be visualized clearly using thin-section or multi-detector CT, and viewing the images on a workstation. Slice section thickness of 2 to 3 mm is ideal for nodal assessment and allows multiplanar reformats to be obtained in any appropriate plane.

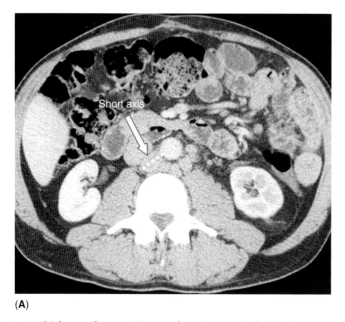

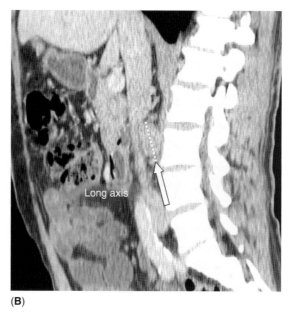

(A)   (B)

Figure 40.4 Multiplanar reformats. Viewing of a node in multiple CT planes may aid in determining the long and short axes of lymph nodes. Enlarged lymph node shown on (A) axial, and (B) reformatted sagittal images (arrows). The maximum short and long axis diameters of this aortocaval lymph node are shown by the dotted lines.

On MR imaging, nodes are typically isointense to muscle on T1-weighting and are isointense or mildly hyperintense on T2-weighting (Fig. 40.2). On short-tau inversion recovery (STIR) sequence, nodes have a very high signal intensity which facilitates their identification. However, the choice of the MR sequence for nodal identification and assessment varies with the anatomical region being examined as well as on individual preference. A combination of high spatial resolution T1- and T2-weighted sequences is usually employed. High spatial resolution turbo spin-echo T2-weighted (21) and 3D T1-weighted MP-RAGE (22) sequences have been found to be useful for visualiing nodes in oblique planes.

The CT and MR imaging findings of malignant lymph nodes are frequently non-specific. The most widely used CT and MR criteria to determine whether a node is benign or malignant is nodal size. However, a substantial proportion of nodes harboring metastases from pelvic and abdominal cancers are not enlarged beyond the accepted size for normality. Furthermore, nodal enlargement can result from reactive nodal hyperplasia or coincidental diseases. Hence, when using cross-sectional imaging to evaluate nodal disease, the following parameters should be considered:

Size

The maximum short axis nodal diameter is usually ascertained. The maximum short axis diameter may not be always apparent on the axial imaging, and multiplanar reformats may be useful in this regard (Fig. 40.4). In the abdomen, the upper limit of the maximum short axis diameter of normal nodes varies between 6 and 10 mm, increasing in size caudally (23,24). For example, it is generally accepted that the upper limit in the maximum short axis diameter of a normal retrocrural node is 6 mm and of a retroperitoneal abdominal node is 10 mm (25). In the pelvis, normal nodes are usually smaller than 8 to 10 mm in diameter (25,26). The mean maximum short axis diameter of normal inguinal

Table 40.1 The Upper Limit of Normal of Nodal Size According to Anatomical Regions in the Abdomen and Pelvis

Site	Nodal Size (mm)[a]
Retrocrural	6
Paracardiac	12
Gastrohepatic	8
Porta hepatis	7
Portacaval	10 (13[b])
Upper Paraortic	9
Lower Paraortic	11
Mesenteric	5
Pelvic	10
Inguinal	15

[a]Based on Refs. 23–26, 28–30.
[b]Refer to Ref. 30.

nodes varies between 4 and 6 mm, but can measure up to 15 mm (23,27). The upper limit of the mean maximum short axis diameters of nodes according to anatomical regions in the abdomen and pelvis is summarized in Table 40.1 (23–26,28–30). It should be noted that these criteria are for guidance only and their application shows some variation depending on tumor type and individual clinical practice.

In testicular cancer, a study evaluating different size criteria (4, 6, 8, 10 mm) (31) showed that using a size threshold of 10 mm resulted in a sensitivity of 37% and a specificity of 100% for the detection of malignant nodes. However, with a 4 mm criterion, the sensitivity was 93% and the specificity was 58%. Using a smaller size criterion increased sensitivity, but was accompanied by diminished specificity (31). In our clinical practice, a retroperitoneal node measuring greater than 10 mm in the maximum short axis diameter in a patient with testicular cancer is considered to be

definitely malignant, whereas a node that is between 8 and 10 mm in diameter is considered suspicious.

Shape and Contour

Using multidetector CT, assessment of the shape and contour of nodes can be enhanced by multiplanar reformats. However, the usefulness of nodal shape on CT or MR imaging is less certain compared to reports in US literature. One CT study in gastric cancer found that malignant nodes were round and had a significantly higher short-to-long axis ratio compared with benign nodes (0.81 vs. 0.57) (32). However in a study of early stage non-seminomatous testicular cancer, Lien et al. (33) found that a rounded node less than 20 mm on CT was a poor predictor of malignancy. Nodal shape has also been shown to be unhelpful in the assessment of pancreatic cancer (34). By comparison, the nodal contour on CT and MR imaging can be of greater discriminatory value. An irregular border of a lymph node has been shown to represent extracapsular extension of disease. In rectal cancer, irregular nodal contour is more accurate than nodal size in determining involvement of mesorectal nodes using MR imaging (Fig. 40.5) (21).

Number of Nodes

A cluster of otherwise normal appearing nodes on CT and MR imaging can suggest malignancy. For example, in patients with non-Hodgkin lymphoma, a cluster of non-enlarged nodes may be seen at the root of the small bowel mesentery or the retroperitoneum (Fig. 40.6). However, the specificity of the sign is low and can lead to false positive interpretation, particularly in the pelvis where nodal asymmetry in not uncommon (35).

Internal Nodal Morphology

A number of internal nodal features on CT and MR imaging can help to determine metastatic involvement. Some of these features are associated with specific tumor histology, while others are related to therapy.

Calcification

Calcification may be observed on CT within metastatic nodes arising from ovarian, colorectal, breast, and bladder cancers. Malignant nodes may also show calcifications following successful treatment, such as in lymphoma and seminomatous germ cell tumors (Fig. 40.7).

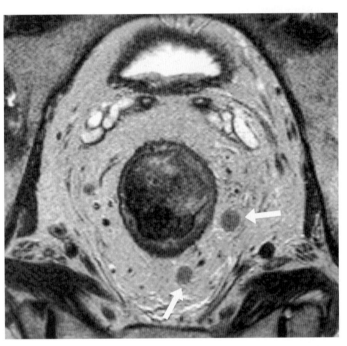

Figure 40.5 Nodal contour. In this patient with a polypoidal tumor arising from the anterior wall of the rectum, there are two nodes (<5 mm in maximum short axis diameters) in the left mesorectum (arrows) which demonstrate ill-defined and irregular contours.

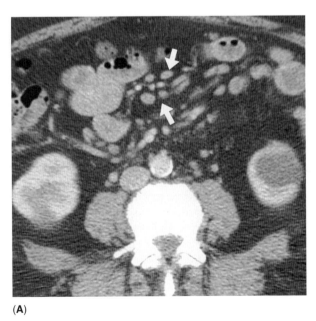

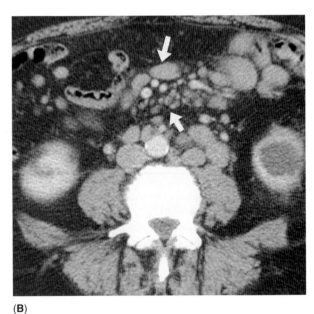

(A) **(B)**

Figure 40.6 Clustering of lymph nodes. In this 56-year-old female patient with chronic lymphocytic leukemia, initial CT (A) revealed multiple normal sized nodes clustered within the mesentery (arrows) and in the retroperitoneum. (B) Repeat CT six months later showed that these nodes (arrows) have all increased in size in keeping with disease infiltration. (Note left renal cyst).

Heterogeneous Appearance

Large metastatic nodes frequently appear heterogeneous in density on contrast-enhanced CT and MR imaging. A relatively lower density nodal center on CT can result from necrosis, a feature commonly seen in squamous cell carcinoma (e.g., head and neck, cervical, and anal carcinomas). On MR imaging, the detection of central necrosis, which typically returns a high T2-signal, has been found to have a very high positive predictive value in patients with cervical cancer (Fig. 40.8) (36). In patients with rectal cancer, nodal signal heterogeneity is also a feature of malignant mesorectal lymph nodes on high spatial resolution T2-weighted MR imaging (21).

Low-Density "Cystic" Appearance

Metastatic nodes arising from non-seminomatous germ cell tumor of the testes (NSGCT) frequently exhibit foci of low-density within the metastatic lymph node mass on CT (37). Typically these nodes are of high signal intensity on T2-weighted MR imaging. In patients with NSGCT it is also well documented that solid to cystic change occurring within a nodal mass treated with chemotherapy represents mature differentiation of teratoma (Fig. 40.9) (38). Furthermore in colorectal, ovarian, and pancreatic cancers, mucinous histological subtypes can result in low density "cystic" appearing metastatic lymph nodes on CT and high signal intensity on T2-weighted MR imaging (Fig. 40.10). However, it should be noted that low density / high signal nodes are not pathognomonic of malignant infiltration, as they may also be observed in tuberculosis and fungal infections.

Contrast Enhancement

On both CT and MR imaging inhomogeneous enhancement of an enlarged node is more likely to indicate malignant infiltration than benign pathology (39,40). However uniform homogeneous nodal enhancement may result from both benign and malignant conditions (39,40). The degree and pattern of enhancement mimics that of the primary tumor and may also reflect its biological aggressiveness (41). It may be possible to discriminate benign from malignant nodes based on semi-quantitative or quantitative analysis of the rate of nodal contrast enhancement on CT or MR imaging (39). Nevertheless, such evaluation is still largely used for research and is not yet widely applied clinically.

Nodal Signal Characteristics on MR Imaging

In general it is not possible to distinguish between malignant and benign lymph nodes by measuring the T1 and T2 relaxation times of the nodes on unenhanced MR imaging (42).

Fat Density

The presence of a focus of fat within a node usually indicates benignity particularly if the node is replaced by fat. However it should be noted that small foci of metastases may exist in a node with just a fatty hilum (Fig. 40.11).

Potential Pitfalls in Nodal Assessment

Normal structures and pathological processes can mimic nodal disease. Whilst many of these pitfalls can now be overcome by the use of thin section multi-channel CT with multiplanar reformats, there remains potential for errors in interpretation. The common pitfalls in the diagnosis of nodal disease in the abdomen and pelvis are:

Loops of Bowel

Small bowel loops in close proximity to the retroperitoneum can simulate nodal disease.

Normal Ovaries

The normal ovaries can simulate external iliac nodal enlargement. However, demonstration of the position of the ureter should avoid this pitfall: the ureter lies lateral to the normal ovary and medial to the external iliac nodal chain.

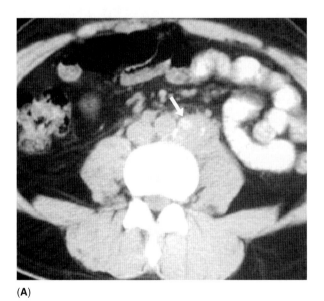

(A)

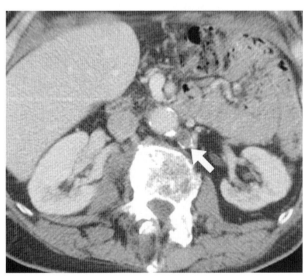

(B)

Figure 40.7 Nodal calcifications. (**A**) In this 24-year-old man with testicular seminoma, post-treatment CT revealed calcifications within a residual left paraortic nodal mass (arrow). In another example (**B**), rim calcification (arrow) is observed in a small residual left paraortic node in a 60-year-old man treated for non-Hodgkin's lymphoma.

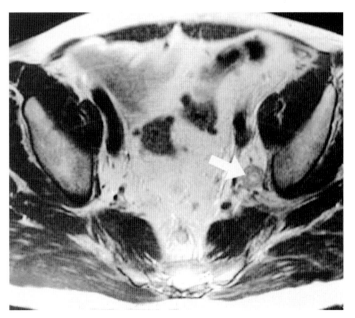

Figure 40.8 Internal nodal heterogeneity. T2-weighted axial image through the mid-pelvis in a lady with cervical cancer reveals a left 1.5 cm internal iliac node (arrow) demonstrating central high T2 signal intensity diagnostic of metastatic nodal disease.

Vessels and Aneurysms

Blood vessels can be mistaken for lymph node, especially on non-contrast-enhanced CT scans. Within the pelvis, imaging should not be performed in the arterial phase of enhancement since unopacified veins can simulate nodal disease (43). For example in the abdomen, unopacified small lumbar veins can simulate nodal disease. Normal anatomical variants such as left sided inferior vena cava or duplicated vena cava can mimic nodal enlargement on unenhanced images. On occasion a prominent cisterna chyli may simulate retrocrural nodal enlargement (Fig. 40.12) (44). However, it should be noted that this normal variant is low in density (similar to CSF or fluid containing structures) and is continuous with the thoracic duct. The relationship with the thoracic duct can be confirmed using multiplanar reformatting. Unusually, the cisternal chyli may be located in the left retrocrural space.

Lymphocoele

Following surgery, lymphocoeles may simulate low density nodal disease (Fig. 40.13). However, knowledge of the site of surgical dissection may be helpful in making a confident diagnosis.

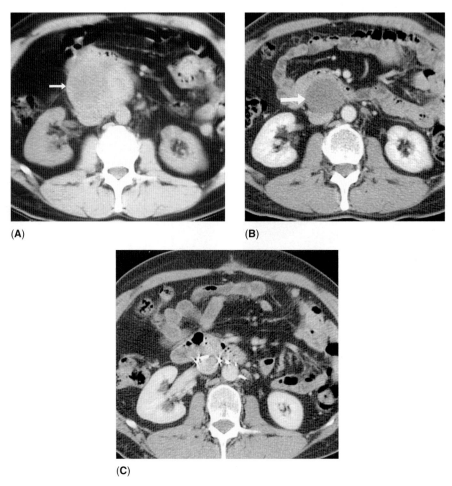

Figure 40.9 Cystic change in lymph node following treatment. (**A**) In this 28-year-old man with non-seminomatous germ cell tumor of the right testes, staging CT revealed a large 6.5 cm aortocaval nodal metastasis of soft tissue attenuation (arrow). (**B**) Following chemotherapy, there was reduction in size of the mass (arrow), associated with reduction in density of the node in keeping with cystic change and treatment response. (**C**) The residual mass was surgically removed and found to contain mature teratoma only. Follow-up CT showed no evidence of recurrence.

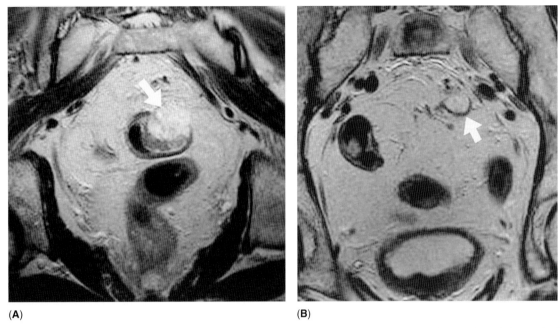

(A)   **(B)**

Figure 40.10 Mucinous tumor and nodal metastasis. (**A**) Oblique coronal T2-weighted MR image shows a mucinous rectal tumor (arrow) characterized by the very high T2 signal intensity. (**B**) A metastatic node in the left mesorectum (arrow) demonstrates similar T2 signal intensity as the primary tumor.

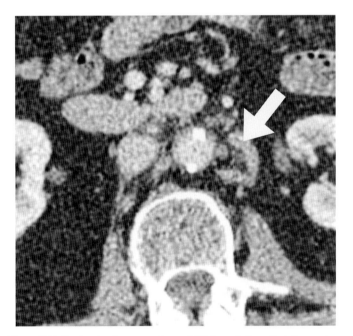

Figure 40.11 Fat density. Contrast-enhanced CT through the mid-abdomen demonstrates a left paraortic node with a fatty nodal hilum (arrow).

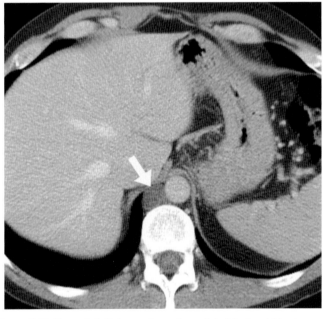

Figure 40.12 Cisternal chyli. A prominent cisternal chyli in the right retrocrural space can mimic nodal disease (arrow).

Hematoma and Abscess

Post-operative hematomas or fluid collections can also simulate nodal disease (Fig. 40.14). These usually resolve over time and the diagnosis can be confirmed on follow-up imaging.

Nerves

The nerves arising from the hypogastric plexus may simulate nodal disease. In addition, neurogenic tumors, such as neurofibromas, may also be confused with enlarged nodes.

Peritoneal Disease

Peritoneal nodules may simulate mesenteric or pelvic sidewall lymphadenopathy.

Diagnostic Accuracy

The diagnostic accuracy of CT and MR imaging for nodal staging of cancer in the abdomen and pelvis varies widely. For pelvic malignancies, the accuracy of CT and MR imaging is similar (45–47). The reported sensitivities range from 40% to 87% and the specificities

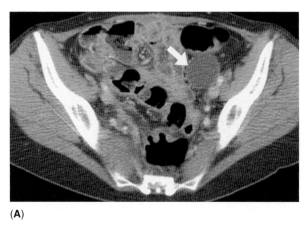
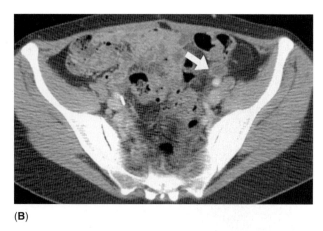

(A)   **(B)**

Figure 40.13 Lymphocoele. Following pelvic surgery (**A**) contrast-enhanced CT shows a thin-walled cystic structure in the left pelvic sidewall (arrow) consistent with a lymphocoele. (**B**) Repeat CT imaging at six months shows that the lymphocoele has reduced in size. However, on this scan the lymphocoele mimics a necrotic lymph node (arrow).

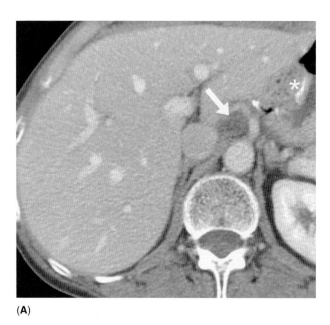
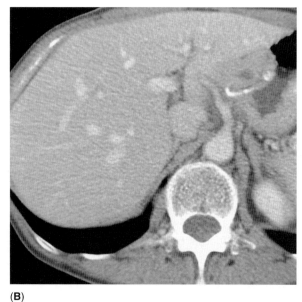

(A)   **(B)**

Figure 40.14 Hematoma/seroma. (**A**) Contrast-enhanced CT performed one month after partial gastrectomy (*) revealed a low density area to the right celiac axis (arrow). This abnormality was not present on the pre-surgical CT. (**B**) Follow-up CT at three months confirmed that the post-surgical collection has resolved.

from 64% to 100% (45–52). The diagnostic performance of CT and MR imaging in the upper abdomen for nodal staging is also limited. In one study of gastric cancer, the accuracy of nodal staging using CT and MR imaging was 58% and 55% respectively (53). In another study of pancreatic cancer, a sensitivity of 14%, specificity of 85%, and accuracy of 73% was achieved for nodal staging (34).

Both conventional CT and MR imaging are limited by their ability to detect metastases in normal or minimally enlarged lymph nodes. The ability to detect nodes has to be tempered against the clinical importance of detection. For example, in patients undergoing radical prostatectomy and nodal dissection for prostate cancer, the diagnosis of metastatic nodal involvement may preclude surgery and a high specificity is therefore required. By comparison, precise nodal staging may be less critical in a patient with locally advanced prostate cancer who would be treated with local radiotherapy.

Positron Emission Tomography (PET) and PET-CT

PET imaging can detect malignancy in non-enlarged nodes leading to a change in patient management (Fig. 40.15). The fusion of the metabolic information from PET imaging with the anatomical detail of CT has been shown to further improve nodal staging. For example, in esophageal cancer, a recent study showed that using fusion PET-CT images improved nodal staging by 30% compared with reading PET and CT images side-by-side (54).

In a study of patients with non small cell lung cancer (NSCLC), ^{18}F-fluorodeoxyglucose positron emission tomography ([18]FDG PET) was found to have an overall accuracy of 76% in the identification of malignant mediastinal lymph nodes. Furthermore FDG PET has been shown to be more accurate than CT for the differentiation of TNM stage N0 or N1 from N2 disease in patients with NSCLC. Nevertheless, PET imaging does not appear to be

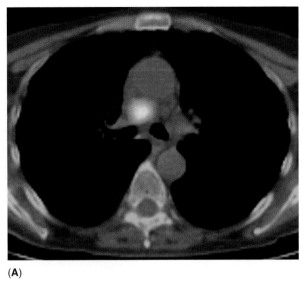 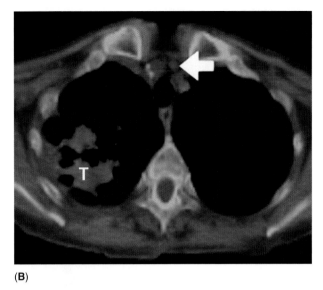

(A)   **(B)**

Figure 40.15 ¹⁸FDG-PET-CT imaging. (**A**) A focus of intense tracer uptake in a malignant right paratracheal node in a 61-year-old patient with lung cancer. (**B**) Note the primary tumor (T). PET-CT revealed a further subcentimeter node in the superior mediastinum (arrow) which was metabolically active but not visible on the initial diagnostic CT. The stage of disease of disease was changed from N2 to N3 resulting in a change in patient management.

sufficiently specific to replace mediastinoscopy, especially in parts of the world where granulomatous and inflammatory mediastinal diseases are prevalent (55).

In patients newly diagnosed with lymphoma, FDG PET has been found to be superior to Ga-67 imaging, and equal or superior to CT for the detection of nodal and extranodal lymphoma at initial staging (56). Following chemotherapy in lymphoma, persistent ¹⁸FDG tracer uptake during and after chemotherapy has a high sensitivity and specificity for the prediction of subsequent disease relapse.

Overall there is gathering evidence for the effective use of ¹⁸FDG PET for the evaluation of nodal disease in a range of tumor types, including esophageal, cervical, head and neck, and melanoma. However, the following potential pitfalls of FDG PET for nodal staging also need to be noted:

- Although nodal size should not directly influence disease detectability, the tracer activity emanating from small nodes (less than 1 cm) may be insufficient to allow detection by the PET camera
- Tumors with low FDG metabolism (e.g., bronchoalveolar cell carcinoma, mucinous carcinoma, prostate carcinoma, low grade lymphoma) can lead to false negative results due to low tracer activity
- Inflammatory processes may cause false positive findings due to increased tracer activity

Key Points: Imaging Features

- Nodal size, nodal echogenicity, the ratio of long versus short axis nodal diameters and nodal vascularity on Doppler studies are used to evaluate lymph nodes on US
- On CT and MR imaging, nodal size is the most widely used criterion to discriminate between malignant and non-malignant nodes

- Other criteria used for nodal assessment on CT and MR imaging include shape, contour, and clustering of normal sized nodes
- Presence of calcification, heterogeneous appearance, cystic change, contrast enhancement, fat density on CT and MR imaging can help to identify malignant nodes
- Normal anatomical structures can mimic nodal enlargement, e.g., normal ovary
- ¹⁸FDG PET imaging detects malignancy based on increased metabolism in infiltrated nodes. However, false negatives can occur in tumors with low metabolic activity or small volume disease; inflammatory conditions can lead to false positives

OPTIMIZATION OF NODAL ASSESSMENT BY IMAGING

The key to successful interpretation of imaging for nodal diseases requires a good understanding of the normal nodal anatomy, pathways of nodal dissemination, the clinical, biochemical and pathological features of the disease, and the details of previous treatment.

Nodal Anatomy

In the pelvis, lymph nodes along the pelvic sidewall are divided into the following groups in relation to the pelvic vessels: common iliac, external iliac (including obturator), hypogastric (along the internal iliac vessels), and pre-sacral (Fig. 40.16). Lymphatics associated with these nodal groups drain upwards into the retroperitoneum. Lymphatics associated with some pelvic viscera can also drain externally into the inguinal nodes.

In the abdomen, lymph nodes within the retroperitoneum are named and grouped according to their relation to the inferior vena cava and the abdominal aorta. These include the paracaval, precaval, retrocaval, aortocaval, preaortic, and paraortic nodes.

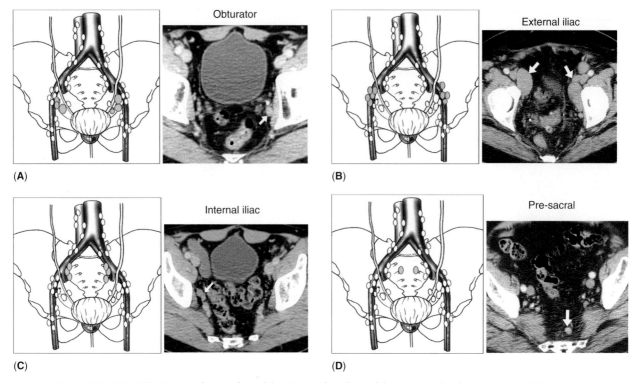

Figure 40.16 (A) to (D) Diagrams showing the nodal stations in the pelvis and the corresponding locations on axial CT imaging.

These nodes lie along the major lumbar lymphatic trunks, which receive lymphatic drainage from the lower limbs and the pelvis. In testicular cancers, the pathway of spread to retroperitoneal nodes occurs in a predictable fashion based on the nodal anatomy (see chap. 20).

There are also lymph nodes associated with abdominal viscera. These are found distributed along the celiac axis, superior mesenteric artery, and inferior mesenteric artery. Celiac axis nodes include those along the greater and lesser curvatures of the stomach, at the portal hepatis and pancreatico-duodenal region. Mesenteric nodes are found between the layers of the small bowel mesentery at the root of the superior mesenteric artery. Using multi-detector CT, normal mesenteric nodes smaller than 5 mm in diameter can be visualized readily, especially when the images are scrolled on a workstation (57). The majority of these are found at the mesenteric root, but some may be seen in the mesenteric periphery or within the right iliac fossa (57). Lymph nodes can also be identified in the distribution of the inferior mesenteric artery, within the sigmoid mesentery and along the superior rectal vessels. Lymphatics from the abdominal viscera ultimately drain into the retroperitoneum and via the cisterna chyli into the thorax.

Within the thorax, pulmonary and mediastinal lymph nodes are described and classified by a system derived by the American Joint Committee on Cancer (AJCC) and the Union Internationale Contre le Cancer (UICC) using surgically recognizable anatomical landmarks. This classification was introduced to facilitate meaningful pathological staging and analysis of treatment outcomes in lung cancer. While such detailed assessment is deemed mandatory in patients with lung cancer who are being considered

for surgery, a simpler approach of classifying nodes according to anatomical location is considered sufficient for staging patients with other malignancies, such as lymphoma. Thus nodes are classified as follows:

- Chest wall (axillary, supraclavicular, internal mammary, and posterior intercostal)
- Anterior mediastinal (prevascular and paraortic)
- Paratracheal and tracheobronchial (paratracheal, retrotracheal, aortopulmonary, azygos, and subcarinal)
- Posterior mediastinal (para-esophageal and pulmonary ligament)
- Hilar
- Intrapulmonary lymph nodes
- Nodes close to the diaphragm or to the chest wall (diaphragmatic nodes)
- Nodes adjacent to the heart (paracardiac)

In the neck, a specialized nomenclature has been devised for the description of cervical lymph nodes in patients with head and neck cancers (Fig. 40.17) (58). The system provides nodal mapping to guide the selection of the most appropriate surgical procedure and is based on identifying the nodal "levels" rather than anatomical descriptions. Typically, lymph nodes in the neck are grouped into seven levels (I to VII) according to their relation to the mandible, hyoid bone, and cricoid cartilage; as well as the sternocledomastoid muscle, trapezius muscle, carotid artery, and the internal jugular vein. The approximate anatomical counterparts of these nodal levels are shown in Table 40.2. This nodal classification has been recommended by the American Joint Committee on Cancer and the American Academy of Otolaryngology–Head and

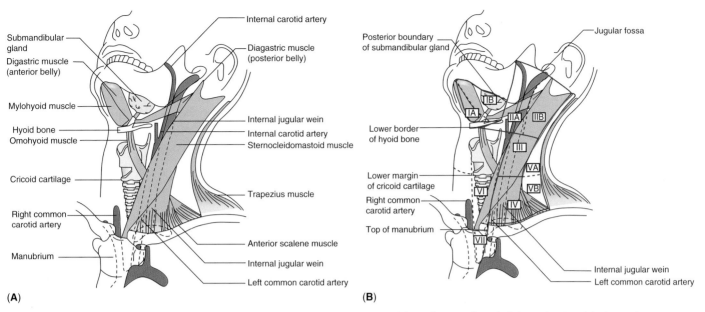

Figure 40.17 Nodal stations of the neck. Level system of lymph node classification. Diagram of the neck as seen from the left anterior view. (**A**) The pertinent anatomy that relates to the nodal classification. (**B**) An outline of the levels of the classification. Note that the line of separation between levels I and II is the posterior margin of the submandibular gland. The separation between levels II and III and level V is the posterior edge of the sternocleidomastoid muscle. However, the line of separation between levels IV and V is an oblique line extending from the posterior edge of the sternocleidomastoid muscle to the posterolateral edge of the anterior scalene muscle. The posterior edge of the internal jugular vein separates level IIA and IIB nodes. The top of the manubrium separates levels VI and VII.

Table 40.2 Nodal Levels for the Assessment of Head and Neck Tumors and Their Approximate Anatomical Counterparts

I	Submandibular and submental
II	Jugulodigastric (base of skull to hyoid)
III	Deep cervical (hyoid to cricoid)
IV	Virchow (cricoid to clavicle)
V	Accessory spinal (posterior triangle)
VI	Prelaryngeal/pretracheal/Delphian node
VII	Superior mediastinal

Neck Surgery. A detailed description of this is beyond the scope of this chapter, but the reader should be acquainted with this system and adopt it for the reporting of head and neck tumors (58).

Patterns of Tumor Spread

A clear understanding of the pathway of tumor spread allows close scrutiny of the most likely sites of nodal involvement.

In the pelvis, the most common site of nodal dissemination in patients with vulval, penile, and anal cancer is to the inguinal nodes.

Typically *prostate carcinoma* spreads via lymphatics in the neurovascular bundles to the obturator, presacral, hypogastric, and external iliac lymph nodes. Further spread is to the common iliac and paraortic nodes. The obturator and external iliac nodes are commonly involved in up to 50% to 60% of cases (Fig. 40.18) (59). However, the pre-sacral or lateral sacral nodes are the sole sites of nodal disease in 10% to 30% of cases.

Bladder cancer spreads to the paravesical nodes, which drain into obturator (59) and external iliac nodes. Disease can also spread into the hypogastric and presacral nodes. These pathways eventually drain into the common iliac and paraortic chain of lymph nodes.

The pathway of nodal dissemination in gynecological malignancies (cervical, ovarian, and uterine) follows a similar pattern, most frequently to the obturator nodes, which is part of the medial chain of the external iliac nodes. From here, further spread occurs along the common iliac vessels into the retroperitoneum. Nodal spread can also involve the hypogastric nodes along the internal iliac vessels. Less commonly, tumor tracks along the uterosacral ligament into the lymphatic plexus anterior to the sacrum and coccyx, which in turn drains into the common iliac nodes located between the common iliac arteries (60).

In colorectal cancer, right-sided tumors disseminate along lymph nodes following ileocolic vessels and the superior mesenteric vein. Left-sided colonic tumors spread to lymph nodes along the inferior mesenteric vessels. Rectal cancers most commonly involve mesorectal nodes and nodes along the superior rectal vessels. However, in advanced disease, there may be lateral spread of disease by lymphovascular invasion to the pelvic sidewall (Fig. 40.19). Lymph nodes are more frequently detected in colon cancer compared with diverticulitis and their presence is therefore a useful factor in the differential diagnosis of these two conditions (61).

In patients with testicular cancer, lymphatic spread occurs along lymphatic channels that accompany the spermatic cord. These lymphatic vessels drain into nodes within the retroperitoneum. Typically, right-sided testicular tumors disseminate to the retroperitoneal nodes on the right (the precaval, paracaval, aortocaval, and retrocaval nodes). Left-sided testicular tumors spread to nodes on the left (preaortic and paraortic nodes), usually at or just below the level of the left renal vein (see Fig. 20.1). Cross-over of nodal involvement sometimes occurs, more frequently from the right to the left. More unusually, disease may spread to the so-called "echelon node," which lies anterior to the iliopsoas muscle (Fig. 40.20).

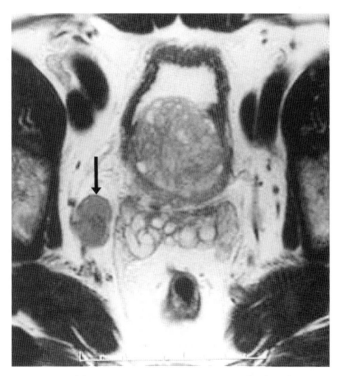

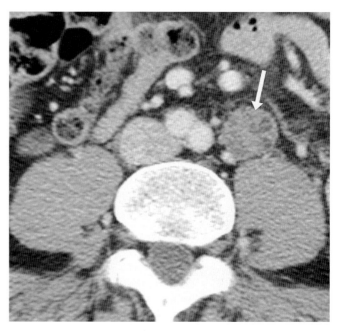

Figure 40.18 Nodal metastasis in prostate cancer. T2-weighted axial MR image through the lower pelvis reveals an enlarged and heterogeneous right obturator node (arrow) in a patient with prostate carcinoma.

Figure 40.20 Echelon node. Contrast-enhanced CT shows an enlarged node (arrow) lying anterior to the left psoas muscle.

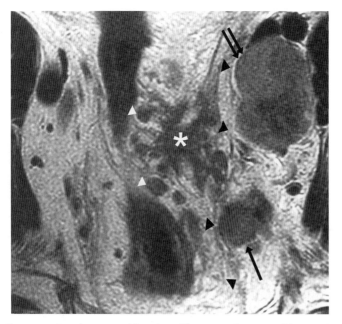

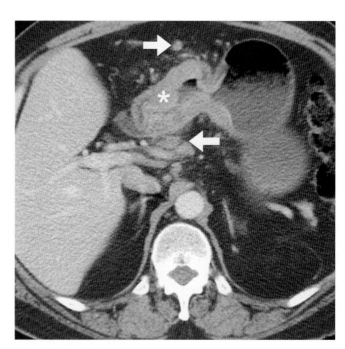

Figure 40.19 Rectal cancer. In this patient with an aggressive tumor of the rectosigmoid colon (not shown), T2-weighted oblique axial MR imaging demonstrates the presence of serpigenous structures in the sigmoid mesentery (*) due to extramural venous invasion by tumor. A number of malignant irregular and heterogeneous nodes are visible in the sigmoid mesentery (white arrowheads). However, there is also metastatic disease to left external iliac (double black arrows) and internal iliac nodes (black arrow). These nodes lie lateral to the fascial plane which divides the pelvic sidewall from the peritoneal compartment (black arrowheads).

Figure 40.21 Gastric cancer. Contrast-enhanced CT demonstrates annular thickening of the gastric antrum (*) in a 56-year-old female patient. Nodal enlargement is present in the left gastric and celiac artery territories (arrows).

The nodal pathway for upper gastrointestinal malignancy (gastric, pancreatic, liver, gallbladder, and bile ducts) is usually into the hepatoduodenal, peri-pancreatic, and aortocaval nodes (Fig. 40.21) (62). These may be involved singly or in combination, representing the flow of lymphatics from the lesser omentum into the retroperitoneum. The lymphatic drainage for the kidneys is variable, but generally follows the ipsilateral renal vein to the paraortic/paracaval lymph nodes.

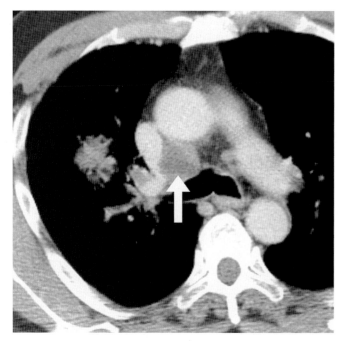

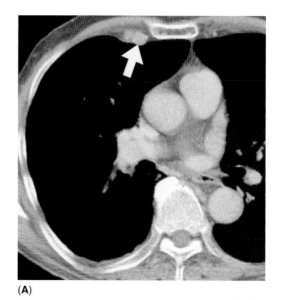

(A)

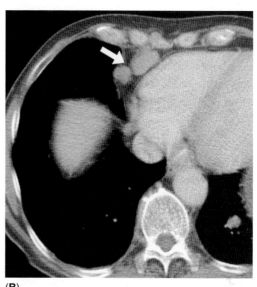

(B)

Figure 40.22 Non-small cell lung cancer. In this 45-year-old male patient with non-small lung cancer of the right lung, there is an enlarged right paratracheal lymph node indicating stage N2 disease (arrow).

In the thorax, lung carcinoma typically involves ipsilateral hilar lymph nodes, which drain into the mediastinal lymph nodes (Fig. 40.22) with the paratracheal and tracheobronchial nodes being most commonly involved. Further spread is to nodes in the anterior and superior mediastinum. In advanced disease, contralateral hilar nodes may be affected as well. In contrast, pleurally-based malignancy, such as malignant mesothelioma, most frequently spreads to nodes along the chest wall, including the posterior intercostal, internal mammary, and diaphragmatic nodes (Fig. 40.23).

In breast cancer, nodal dissemination is most often to the axillary nodes, from where further nodal dissemination to subpectoral and supraclavicular lymph nodes can occur. It has been shown that tumors within the breast tend to spread to one particular node first, before draining through the rest of the lymph nodes in the axilla. That first lymph node is called the sentinel lymph node. The sentinel node is identified pre-operatively by injection of a radioactive tracer (technetium-labeled sulfur colloid) or by a blue dye (isosulfan blue) and is sampled at breast surgery (Fig. 40.24). A negative result reduces the need for a full axillary nodal dissection, a procedure which is associated with significant morbidity.

Tumors in the head and neck region most frequently disseminate to the node that is most proximal to the primary tumor on the ipsilateral side. From here, disease spreads to other nodal levels. Bilateral nodal involvement usually indicates advanced disease.

Clinical Features, Tumor Markers, and Histopathological Information

In most abdominal and pelvic cancers, the incidence of nodal disease increases with the stage of the primary tumor. For example, prostate cancer patients with organ-confined disease (TNM stage T1/T2) have a less than 5% incidence of nodal metastasis compared with an incidence of 30% in patients with extracapsular spread of

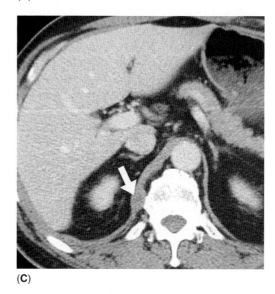

(C)

Figure 40.23 Nodal involvement in mesothelioma and chest wall diseases. (A) Internal mammary nodes (arrow), (B) diaphragmatic nodes (arrow), and (C) posterior intercostal nodes (arrow) are more frequently involved in malignant diseases of the pleural space and chest wall due to the pattern of lymphatic drainage.

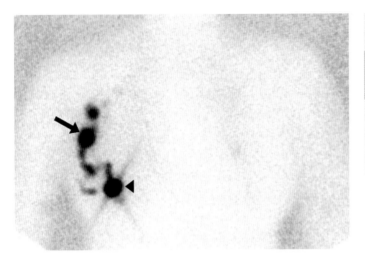

Table 40.3 Examples of the Increasing Incidence of Nodal Disease with Increasing Local Tumor Stage (63–68)

	Incidence of nodal disease			
	T1	T2	T3	T4
Prostate	<5%	<5%	15% (Early) 30% (T3)	>40%
Bladder	<5%	10–15% (T2a) 15–20% (T2b)	30–50%	40–45%
Colorectal	3–10%	10–30%	>50%	>50%

Figure 40.24 Sentinel node. Technetium sulfur colloid tracer is injected into the breast near the site of tumor (arrowhead) and the distribution of tracer into the axilla is monitored. The first node showing increased tracer activity in the axilla (arrow) is the sentinel node. The node can be located at surgery using a radioactive probe. *Source*: Courtesy of Dr. Sue Chua, Royal Marsden Hospital, Sutton, U.K.

disease (Stage T3) (63–65). The relationship between the stage of the tumor and the likelihood of nodal metastasis in prostate, bladder, and colorectal cancers is illustrated in Table 40.3 (63–68).

The grade of malignancy and other histological characteristics of tumors also have a bearing on the likelihood of nodal metastasis. In cervical cancer, the presence of parametrial invasion, lymphovascular invasion, and depth of tumor invasion are linked to the development of nodal disease (69). In early gastric cancer, the presence of submucosal and vascular invasion predicts for the likelihood of nodal disease (53). Lymphovascular invasion also increases the risk of nodal disease in patients with colorectal cancer (70) and testicular tumors (71,72).

Other biological indices can help to alert the radiologist to the likelihood of nodal metastases. Patients with prostate tumors that express high levels of prostate specific antigen (PSA) in the serum (>20 ng/ml) and have a high Gleason score (>7) on prostate biopsy have a higher risk of extracapsular prostatic disease and nodal disease than patients with lower levels of PSA or lower Gleason scores. Nomograms are based on the pre-operative serum prostate specific antigen, clinical TNM stage and the biopsy Gleason score, which are predictive of the histopathological staging at radical prostatectomy and the likelihood of nodal disease.

Thus in patients with prostate cancer, reference to the Partin nomograms can be useful to determine the risk of nodal disease thus aiding image interpretation (73).

Details of Previous Therapy (Surgery, Chemotherapy, or Radiotherapy)

Knowledge of previous treatment is important since therapy can modify the pattern of nodal disease encountered.

In prostate cancer, nodal relapse usually occurs outside the pelvis following radiotherapy or radical prostatectomy which includes pelvic lymph node dissection (65). Similarly, following radical cystectomy for bladder cancer, nodal relapse is more frequently encountered within the hypogastric (internal iliac), presacral, and paraortic nodes (74). These represent nodal sites that are not usually removed at nodal dissection (Fig. 40.25).

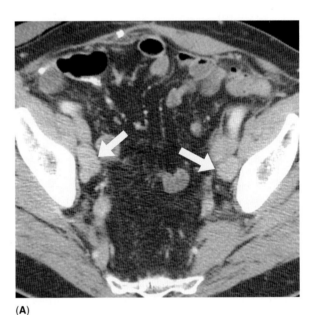

(A)

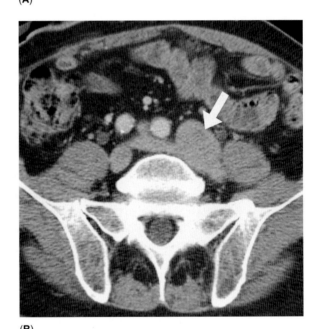

(B)

Figure 40.25 Pattern of nodal recurrence following total cystectomy. (A) Nodal relapse in the hypogastric nodes bilaterally (arrows), (B) nodal relapse in the left common iliac nodes (arrow).

In patients with germ cell tumor of the testes, pelvic nodes are not usually involved. Exceptions include:

- Previous scrotal surgery
- Tumor arising in an undescended testis
- Retrograde lymphatic spread due to bulky retroperitoneal nodal disease
- Previous retroperitoneal nodal dissection (75)

Following total mesorectal excision surgery for rectal cancer, nodal recurrence may develop within the obturator chain along the pelvic sidewall or more cranially within the retroperitoneum.

Key Points: Optimization of Nodal Assessment

- Imaging assessment of nodes can be optimized by having a clear understanding of nodal anatomy and the pathway of nodal spread in different cancers
- Tumor stage, tumor grade, and serum tumor markers can indicate the likelihood of nodal disease. Knowledge of the pre-test probability of nodal disease can facilitate accurate image interpretation
- Details of previous therapy should always be sought since this may have a bearing on the site of nodal relapse

ADVANCES IN NODAL STAGING

There are clear limitations to the morphological assessment of nodal diseases but the wider availability of [18]FDG PET and PET-CT has significantly improved nodal staging in several different cancers during recent years. In addition new imaging techniques are in development which are anticipated to further improve the accuracy of nodal staging.

MR Lymphography

MR lymphography permits discrimination between malignant and non-malignant nodes based on the pattern and degree of contrast enhancement independent of nodal size or morphology. MR lymphography is performed after the administration of a lymphotrophic MR contrast medium, and the most widely evaluated is USPIO (ultrasmall iron oxide particles).

Following IV contrast infusion, the USPIO particles escape into the interstitial space and are transported by lymphatics into lymph nodes. Within the lymph node, the USPIO particles are phagocytosed by nodal macrophages, which results in signal loss in normal nodes on T2*-weighted MR imaging. Malignant nodes, being macrophage depleted, retain high signal intensity on the post-contrast T2*-weighted imaging (Fig. 40.26). USPIO-enhanced MR lymphography has been applied to characterize breast, lung, and pelvic malignancies, with reported improvement in diagnostic accuracy (76–80). In particular in prostate cancer, the technique has shown encouraging results for the detection of malignant nodes less than 1 cm in size, with a high diagnostic sensitivity and specificity compared to conventional imaging (78). The potential advantages of the technique are the ability to detect foci of metastatic disease in non-enlarged lymph nodes and to characterize the nature of nodal enlargement due to benign reactive hyperplasia.

PET Imaging with Novel Tracers

The perceived limitations of [18]FDG-PET for nodal staging have led to the development of novel tracers which can provide information on a wide range of pathophysiological processes. These include markers for protein synthesis (C-11 methionine), cellular proliferation [(F-18)-fluoro-3′-deoxy-3′-L-fluorothymidine], hypoxia [copper-60 or copper-64 labelled diacetyl-bis N(4)-ethyl-thiosemicarbazone], and specific receptor-binding (16beta-^{18}F-fluoro-5alpha-dihydrotestosterone). It is hoped that the use of

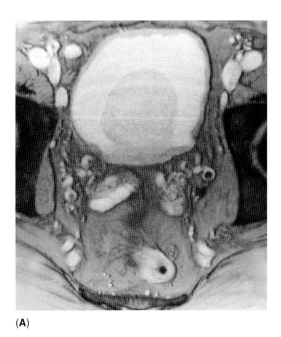

(A)

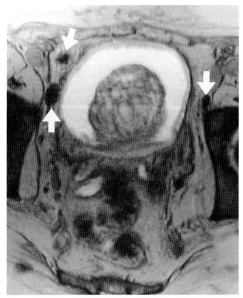

(B)

Figure 40.26 USPIO enhanced MR imaging in an elderly man with prostate cancer. T2*-weighted axial image (**A**) before and (**B**) after the administration USPIO contrast demonstrates uniform signal reduction in several external iliac nodes (arrows) indicating that they are benign.

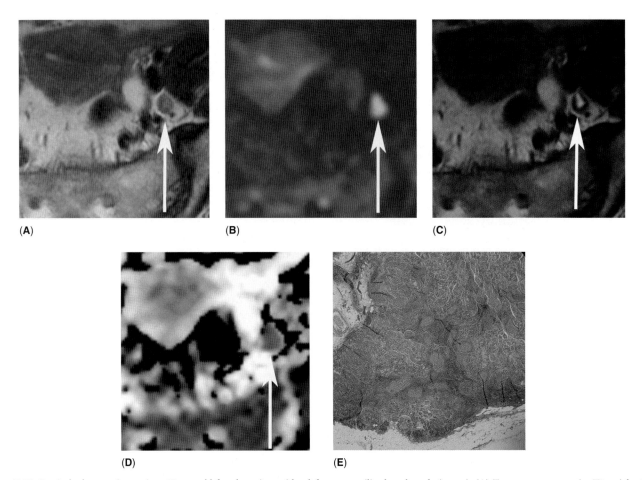

Figure 40.27 Cervical adenocarcinoma in a 46-year-old female patient with a left common iliac lymph node (arrow). (**A**) Transverse preoperative T2-weighted MR image, (**B**) diffusion-weighted MR image, (**C**) fused T2-weighted and colourized diffusion-weighted MR image, (**D**) apparent diffusion coefficient (ADC) map (b = 0,1000 sec/mm^2). The left common iliac lymph node measures 8 × 7 mm in size and is determined to be a metastatic node because its ADC value of 0.94 × 10^{-3} mm^2/sec is similar to that of the primary tumor (0.96 × 10^{-3} mm^2/sec). (**E**) Histopathological examination (hematoxylin and eosin, magnification, ×200) showed tumor deposit within the node. *Source*: Courtesy of Dr. Gigin Lin, Department of Radiology, Chang Gung Memorial Hospital and Chang Gung University College of Medicine, Taiwan.

these novel tracers, either singly or in combination, will be introduced into the clinical arena soon and will yield highly accurate diagnostic and prognostic information.

Diffusion-Weighted MR Imaging

There is considerable interest in the application of diffusion-weighted imaging in oncology for the detection and characterization of different tumors. The technique can be performed quickly (within a few minutes) without the need for IV contrast administration, and yields both qualitative and quantitative information.

The image contrast on diffusion-weighted imaging is based on differences in the mobility of water protons between tissues, and reflects tissue cellularity and the integrity of cellular membranes. Tumor tissues are generally more cellular compared with the native tissues they originate from, and thus show high signal restricted diffusion on diffusion-weighted MR imaging. The degree of tissue diffusion can be quantified using the apparent diffusion coefficient which is typically lower in tumor tissues.

Diffusion-weighted MR imaging has been shown to improve the detection of lymph nodes. Fusion images created by the addition of a diffusion-weighted image to a conventional T1- or T2-weighted image can increase the perception of small nodes throughout the body. There have also been encouraging reports of the use of diffusion-weighted imaging to identify malignant nodes in patients with head and neck, as well as squamous cell carcinoma of the cervix (Fig. 40.27). The technique can be extended to the whole body to obtain maps of nodal disease in patients with lymphoma.

Summary

- Nodal disease is an independent adverse prognostic factor
- US, CT, MR, and PET imaging are used to detect malignant nodes, although CT and MR imaging are still the most widely used
- The application of size criteria on imaging has a moderate diagnostic accuracy, but nodal assessment can potentially be improved by having a clear knowledge and understanding of the underlying disease entities, and by applying ancillary criteria in the interpretation of the images
- New imaging methods such as dynamic contrast-enhanced imaging, the application of novel PET tracers and diffusion-weighted MR imaging are likely to significantly impact on nodal staging in the future

REFERENCES

1. Fong Y, Coit DG, Woodruff JM, Brennan MF. Lymph node metastasis from soft tissue sarcoma in adults. Analysis of data from a prospective database of 1772 sarcoma patients. Ann Surg 1993; 217: 72–7.

2. Sobin LH, Wittekind Ch, eds. International Union Against Cancer (UICC): TNM Classification of Malignant Tumours, 6th edn. New York: Wiley-Liss, 2002.

3. Dukes CE. The classification of cancer of the rectum. J Pathol Bacteriol 1932; 35: 323–32.

4. Kanter MA. The lymphatic system: an historical perspective. Plast Reconstr Surg 1987; 79: 131–9.

5. Zeidman I, Buss JM. Experimental studies on the spread of cancer in the lymphatic system. I. Effectiveness of the lymph node as a barrier to the passage of embolic tumour cells. Cancer Res 1954; 14: 403–5.

6. Carr I. Lymphatic metastasis. Cancer Metastasis Rev 1983; 2: 307–17.

7. Van de Velde CJ, Carr I. Lymphatic invasion and metastasis. Experimentia 1977; 33: 37–884.

8. Carr I, Carr J. Experimental models of lymphatic metastasis. In: Liotta LA, Hart IR, eds. Tumour invasion and metastasis. The Hague: Martinus Nijhoff, 1982; 189–205.

9. Liotta LA, Tryggvason K, Garbisa S, et al. Metastatic potential correlateds with enzymatic degradation of basement membrane collagen. Nature 1980; 284: 67–8.

10. Heide J, Krull A, Berger J. Extracapsular spread of nodal metastasis as a prognostic factor in rectal cancer. Int J Radiat Oncol Biol Phys 2004; 58: 773–8.

11. van den Brekel MW, Stel HV, Castelijns JA, Croll GJ, Snow GB. Lymph node staging in patients with clinically negative neck examinations by ultrasound and ultrasound-guided aspiration cytology. Am J Surg 1991; 162: 362–6.

12. Puli SR, Reddy JB, Bechtold ML, Antillon MR, Ibdah JA. Accuracy of endoscopic ultrasound in the diagnosis of distal and celiac axis lymph node metastasis in esophageal cancer: a meta-analysis and systematic review. Dig Dis Sci 2008; 53: 2405–14.

13. Steinkamp HJ, Cornehl M, Hosten N, et al. Cervical lymphadenopathy: ratio of long- to short-axis diameter as a predictor of malignancy. Br J Radiol 1995; 68: 266–70.

14. Na DG, Lim HK, Byun HS, et al. Differential diagnosis of cervical lymphadenopathy: usefulness of color Doppler sonography. AJR Am J Roentgenol 1997; 168: 1311–16.

15. Steinkamp HJ, Mueffelmann M, Bock JC, et al. Differential diagnosis of lymph node lesions: a semiquantitative approach with colour Doppler ultrasound. Br J Radiol 1998; 71: 828–33.

16. Choi MY, Lee JW, Jang KJ. Distinction between benign and malignant causes of cervical, axillary, and inguinal lymphadenopathy: value of Doppler spectral waveform analysis. AJR Am J Roentgenol 1995; 165: 981–4.

17. Magarelli N, Guglielmi G, Savastano M, et al. Superficial inflammatory and primary neoplastic lymphadenopathy: diagnostic accuracy of power-doppler sonography. Eur J Radiol 2004; 52: 257–63.

18. Adibelli ZH, Unal G, Gul E, et al. Differentiation of benign and malignant cervical lymph nodes: value of B-mode and color Doppler sonography. Eur J Radiol 1998; 28: 230–4.

19. Schroeder RJ, Maeurer J, Gath HJ, Willam C, Hidajat N. Vascularization of reactively enlarged lymph nodes analyzed by color duplex sonography. J Oral Maxillofac Surg 1999; 57: 1090–5.

20. Schulte-Altedorneburg G, Demharter J, Linne R, et al. Does ultrasound contrast agent improve the diagnostic value of colour and power Doppler sonography in superficial lymph node enlargement? Eur J Radiol 2003; 48: 252–7.

21. Brown G, Richards CJ, Bourne MW, et al. Morphologic predictors of lymph node status in rectal cancer with use of high-spatial-resolution MR imaging with histopathologic comparison. Radiology 2003; 227: 371–7.

22. Jager GJ, Barentsz JO, Oosterhof GO, Witjes JA, Ruijs SJ. Pelvic adenopathy in2prostatic and urinary bladder carcinoma: MR imaging with a three-dimensional TI-weighted magnetization-prepared-rapid gradient-echo sequence. AJR Am J Roentgenol 1996; 167: 1503–7.

23. Dorfman RE, Alpern MB, Gross BH, Sandler MA. Upper abdominal lymph nodes: criteria for normal size determined with CT. Radiology 1991; 180: 319–22.

24. Magnusson A. Size of normal retroperitoneal lymph nodes. Acta Radiol Diagn (Stockh) 1983; 24: 315–18.

25. Einstein DM, Singer AA, Chilcote WA, Desai RK. Abdominal lymphadenopathy: spectrum of CT findings. Radiographics 1991; 11: 457–72.

26. Vinnicombe SJ, Norman AR, Nicolson V, Husband JE. Normal pelvic lymph nodes: evaluation with CT after bipedal lymphangiography. Radiology 1995; 194: 349–55.

27. Peters PE, Beyer K. [Normal lymph node cross sections in different anatomic regions and their significance for computed tomographic diagnosis]. Radiologe 1985; 25: 193–8.

28. Balfe DM, Mauro MA, Koehler RE, et al. Gastrohepatic ligament: normal and pathologic CT anatomy. Radiology 1984; 150: 485–90.

29. Grey AC, Carrington BM, Hulse PA, Swindell R, Yates W. Magnetic resonance appearance of normal inguinal nodes. Clin Radiol 2000; 55: 124–30.

30. Zirinsky K, Auh YH, Rubenstein WA, et al. The portacaval space: CT with MR correlation. Radiology 1985; 156: 453–60.

31. Hilton S, Herr HW, Teitcher JB, Begg CB, Castellino RA. CT detection of retroperitoneal lymph node metastases in patients with clinical stage I testicular nonseminomatous germ cell cancer: assessment of size and distribution criteria. AJR Am J Roentgenol 1997; 169: 521–5.

32. Fukuya T, Honda H, Hayashi T, et al. Lymph-node metastases: efficacy for detection with helical CT in patients with gastric cancer. Radiology 1995; 197: 705–11.

33. Lien HH, Lindskold L, Stenwig AE, Ous S, Fossa SD. Shape of retroperitoneal lymph nodes at computed tomography does not correlate to metastatic disease in early stage non-seminomatous testicular tumors. Acta Radiol 1987; 28: 271–3.

34. Roche CJ, Hughes ML, Garvey CJ, et al. CT and pathologic assessment of prospective nodal staging in patients with

ductal adenocarcinoma of the head of the pancreas. AJR Am J Roentgenol 2003; 180: 475–80.

35. Matsukuma K, Tsukamoto N, Matsuyama T, Ono M, Nakano H. Preoperative CT study of lymph nodes in cervical cancer—its correlation with histological findings. Gynecol Oncol 1989; 33: 168–71.

36. Yang WT, Lam WW, Yu MY, Cheung TH, Metreweli C. Comparison of dynamic helical CT and dynamic MR imaging in the evaluation of pelvic lymph nodes in cervical carcinoma. AJR Am J Roentgenol 2000; 175: 759–66.

37. Scatarige JC, Fishman EK, Kuhajda FP, Taylor GA, Siegelman SS. Low attenuation nodal metastases in testicular carcinoma. J Comput Assist Tomogr 1983; 7: 682–7.

38. Husband JE, Hawkes DJ, Peckham MJ. CT estimations of mean attenuation values and volume in testicular tumors: a comparison with surgical and histologic findings. Radiology 1982; 144: 553–8.

39. Barentsz JO, Jager GJ, van Vierzen PB, et al. Staging urinary bladder cancer after transurethral biopsy: value of fast dynamic contrast-enhanced MR imaging. Radiology 1996; 201: 185–93.

40. Noworolski SM, Fischbein NJ, Kaplan MJ, et al. Challenges in dynamic contrast-enhanced MRI imaging of cervical lymph nodes to detect metastatic disease. J Magn Reson Imaging 2003; 17: 455–62.

41. Husband JE, Koh DM. Bladder cancer. In: Husband JE, Reznek RH, eds. Imaging in Oncology, 2nd ed. London: Taylor and Francis, 2004; 343–74.

42. Dooms GC, Hricak H, Moseley ME, et al. Characterization of lymphadenopathy by magnetic resonance relaxation times: preliminary results. Radiology 1985; 155: 691–7.

43. Teefey SA, Baron RL, Schulte SJ, Shuman WP. Differentiating pelvic veins and enlarged lymph nodes: optimal CT techniques. Radiology 1990; 175: 683–5.

44. Gollub MJ, Castellino RA. The cisterna chyli: a potential mimic of retrocrural lymphadenopathy on CT scans. Radiology 1996; 199: 477–80.

45. Kim SH, Choi BI, Lee HP, et al. Uterine cervical carcinoma: comparison of CT and MR findings. Radiology 1990; 175: 45–51.

46. Kim SH, Kim SC, Choi BI, Han MC. Uterine cervical carcinoma: evaluation of pelvic lymph node metastasis with MR imaging. Radiology 1994; 190: 807–11.

47. Williams AD, Cousins C, Soutter WP, et al. Detection of pelvic lymph node metastases in gynecologic malignancy: a comparison of CT, MR imaging, and positron emission tomography. AJR Am J Roentgenol 2001; 177: 343–8.

48. Fukuda H, Nakagawa T, Shibuya H. Metastases to pelvic lymph nodes from carcinoma in the pelvic cavity: diagnosis using thin-section CT. Clin Radiol 1999; 54: 237–42.

49. Oyen RH, Van Poppel HP, Ameye FE, et al. Lymph node staging of localized prostatic carcinoma with CT and CT-guided fine-needle aspiration biopsy: prospective study of 285 patients. Radiology 1994; 190: 315–22.

50. Salo JO, Kivisaari L, Rannikko S, Lehtonen T. The value of CT in detecting pelvic lymph node metastases in cases of bladder and prostate carcinoma. Scand J Urol Nephrol 1986; 20: 261–5.

51. Subak LL, Hricak H, Powell CB, Azizi L, Stern JL. Cervical carcinoma: computed tomography and magnetic resonance imaging for preoperative staging. Obstet Gynecol 1995; 86: 43–50.

52. Sugiyama T, Nishida T, Ushijima K, et al. Detection of lymph node metastasis in ovarian carcinoma and uterine corpus carcinoma by preoperative computerized tomography or magnetic resonance imaging. J Obstet Gynaecol 1995; 21: 551–6.

53. Sohn KM, Lee JM, Lee SY, et al. Comparing MR imaging and CT in the staging of gastric carcinoma. AJR Am J Roentgenol 2000; 174: 1551–7.

54. Schreurs LM, Pultrum BB, Koopmans KP, et al. Better assessment of nodal metastases by PET/CT fusion compared to side-by-side PET/CT in oesophageal cancer. Anticancer Res 2008; 28: 1867–73.

55. Turkmen C, Sonmezoglu K, Toker A, et al. The additional value of FDG PET imaging for distinguishing N0 or N1 from N2 stage in preoperative staging of non-small cell lung cancer in region where the prevalence of inflammatory lung disease is high. Clin Nucl Med 2007; 32: 607–12.

56. Kostakoglu L, Leonard JP, Coleman M, Goldsmith SJ. The role of FDG-PET imaging in the management of lymphoma. Clin Adv Hematol Oncol 2004; 2: 115–21.

57. Lucey BC, Stuhlfaut JW, Soto JA. Mesenteric lymph nodes: detection and significance on MDCT. AJR Am J Roentgenol 2005; 184: 41–4.

58. Som PM, Curtin HD, Mancuso AA. An imaging-based classification for the cervical nodes designed as an adjunct to recent clinically based nodal classifications. Arch Otolaryngol Head Neck Surg 1999; 125: 388–96.

59. Golimbu M, Morales P, Al-Askari S, Brown J. Extended pelvic lymphadenectomy for prostatic cancer. J Urol 1979; 121: 617–20.

60. Park JM, Charnsangavej C, Yoshimitsu K, et al. Pathways of nodal metastasis from pelvic tumors: CT demonstration. Radiographics 1994; 14: 1309–21.

61. Chintapalli KN, Esola CC, Chopra S, Ghiatas AA, Dodd GD 3rd. Pericolic mesenteric lymph nodes: an aid in distinguishing diverticulitis from cancer of the colon. AJR Am J Roentgenol 1997; 169: 1253–5.

62. Efremidis SC, Vougiouklis N, Zafiriadou E, et al. Pathways of lymph node involvement in upper abdominal malignancies: evaluation with high-resolution CT. Eur Radiol 1999; 9: 868–74.

63. Bundrick WS, Culkin DJ, Mata JA, Zitman RI, Venable DD. Evaluation of the current incidence of nodal metastasis from prostate cancer. J Surg Oncol 1993; 52: 269–71.

64. Neal AJ, Dearnaley DP. Prostate cancer: pelvic nodes revisited—sites, incidence and prospects for treatment with radiotherapy. Clin Oncol (R Coll Radiol) 1993; 5: 309–12.

65. Spencer J, Golding S. CT evaluation of lymph node status at presentation of prostatic carcinoma. Br J Radiol 1992; 65: 199–201.

66. Herr HW. Bladder cancer: pelvic lymphadenectomy revisited. J Surg Oncol 1988; 37: 242–5

67. Lerner SP, Skinner DG, Liesovsky G, et al. The rationale for en bloc pelvic lymph node dissection for bladder cancer patients with nodal metastases: long-term results. J Urol 1993; 149: 758–64.

68. Graham RA, Garnsey L, Jessup JM. Local excision of rectal carcinoma. Am J Surg 1990; 160: 306–12.

69. Sakuragi N, Satoh C, Takeda N, et al. Incidence and distribution pattern of pelvic and paraaortic lymph node metastasis in patients with Stages IB, IIA, and IIB cervical carcinoma treated with radical hysterectomy. Cancer 1999; 85: 1547–54.

70. Brown G, Radcliffe AG, Newcombe RG, et al. Preoperative assessment of prognostic factors in rectal cancer using high-resolution magnetic resonance imaging. Br J Surg 2003; 90: 355–64.

71. Nicolai N, Miceli R, Artusi R, et al. A simple model for predicting nodal metastasis in patients with clinical stage I nonseminomatous germ cell testicular tumors undergoing retroperitoneal lymph node dissection only. J Urol 2004; 171: 172–6.

72. Marks LB, Rutgers JL, Shipley WU, et al. Testicular seminoma: clinical and pathological features that may predict para-aortic lymph node metastases. J Urol 1990; 143: 524–7.

73. Partin AW, Mangold LA, Lamm DM, et al. Contemporary update of prostate cancer staging nomograms (Partin Tables) for the new millennium. Urology 2001; 58: 843–8.

74. Koh DM, Husband JE. Pattern of disease recurrence of bladder carcinoma following radical cystectomy. Cancer Imaging 2003; 3: 96–100.

75. Husband JE, MacVicar D. Testicular germ cell tumour. In: Husband JE, Reznek RH, eds. Imaging in Oncology. Oxford: ISIS Medical Media, 1998; 259–76.

76. Koh DM, Brown G, Temple L, et al. Rectal cancer: mesorectal lymph nodes at MR imaging with USPIO versus histopathologic findings–initial observations. Radiology 2004; 231: 91–9.

77. Bellin MF, Lebleu L, Meric JB. Evaluation of retroperitoneal and pelvic lymph node metastases with MRI and MR lymphangiography. Abdom Imaging 2003; 28: 155–63.

78. Harisinghani MG, Barentsz J, Hahn PF, et al. Noninvasive detection of clinically occult lymph-node metastases in prostate cancer. N Engl J Med 2003; 348: 2491–9.

79. Deserno WM, Harisinghani MG, Taupitz M, et al. Urinary bladder cancer: preoperative nodal staging with ferumoxtran-10-enhanced MR imaging. Radiology 2004; 233: 449–56.

80. Harisinghani MG, Saini S, Slater GJ, Schnall MD, Rifkin MD. MR imaging of pelvic lymph nodes in primary pelvic carcinoma with ultrasmall superparamagnetic iron oxide (Combidex): preliminary observations. J Magn Reson Imaging 1997; 7: 161–3.

41 Lung and Pleural Metastases
Matthew Gilman and Amita Sharma

INTRODUCTION

Understanding the patterns of involvement of various tumors that metastasize to the lungs and pleura helps to establish a specific differential diagnosis. The purpose of this chapter is to review metastatic disease to the lungs and pleura and to identify tumors based on the patterns found on computed tomography (CT). High-resolution CT (HRCT) provides better resolution of the interstitial architecture and therefore improves localization of tumor involvement. This can be particularly useful in detecting the lymphangitic spread of tumor.

Historically, conventional radiologic screening for thoracic metastases relied on chest radiographs for the detection of lung nodules. Over the past decade, helical CT has replaced plain film radiography as the preferred imaging modality for surveying patients with malignancy for thoracic metastases. Helical CT provides rapid scanning of the body with minimal motion artefacts. This technology introduced interslice reconstruction in which helical data can be reconstructed into three-dimensional or volumetric data sets by overlapping image slices (1). Small nodules lost on conventional non-helical CT due to interslice gaps were potentially retrievable (2,3). Single detector helical CT had its limitations in slice thickness and pitch. In order to scan an entire thorax at a single breath-hold, slice thickness, and pitch had to be prolonged. As a trade off, resolution was compromised and small metastases could potentially still be missed. Multidetector helical CT revolutionized thoracic imaging by providing near isocubic volumetric scanning. A patient's entire thorax can be scanned in less than 10 seconds, resulting in minimal respiratory motion artefact. Slice reconstruction capabilities provided thinner slices without loss of resolution. In essence, with volumetric imaging, and the elimination of interscan gaps and respiratory motion, multidetector CT allowed for greater sensitivity in the detection of pulmonary metastases (4,5).

Despite improved detection of lung metastases, there are still significant limitations, particularly with nodules smaller than 5 mm (7). Sensitivity rates of 53% to 84% have been reported for these small nodules (6–9). Computer aided diagnosis (CAD) is a method used to enhance detection and analysis of CT and radiographic images by means of computer image analysis. The use of CAD for pulmonary nodule detection has the potential to improve a radiologist's performance in the detection of pulmonary nodules that may indicate metastatic disease. The reported sensitivity of CAD for the detection of pulmonary nodules ranges between 35% to 95% (10–18). The moderate sensitivity of CAD for detection of pulmonary nodules precludes its use as a stand-alone technique and mandates its use as a second reader only. However, the use of CAD as a second reader has been shown to improve radiologist sensitivity for nodule detection (19). This may be important for patients in whom the detection of small pulmonary metastases would alter the therapeutic approach (such as young patients with sarcoma).

2-[F-18]fluoro-2-deoxy-D-glucose positron emission tomography (¹⁸FDG PET) imaging for the diagnosis and staging of cancer has become well established in recent years. Many studies have reported the significance of ¹⁸FDG PET for the detection of metastases in lung, colon, head and neck tumors, melanoma, breast, and lymphoma (20,21). Results on lung cancer patients have shown that ¹⁸FDG PET has the additional advantage of detecting extrathoracic metastases that conventional diagnostic tests have missed and can indicate whether indeterminate nodules show ¹⁸FDG uptake (21,22).

Surgical resection is useful in patients with limited metastatic lung disease for the treatment of many solid tumors of epithelial, sarcomatous, and germ cell origin (23–25). Pulmonary metastatectomy is indicated if there is complete control of the primary tumor and the patient can tolerate the loss of pulmonary function. Nodules can be resected through median sternotomy or thoracotomy. The use of video-assisted thoracoscopic surgery (VATS) is limited due to the relative poor sensitivity of CT and this necessitates manual surgical palpation to completely resect lung metastases (7,8,26).

Key Points: General

- Multidetector CT allows for greater detection of pulmonary metastases but, as most metastases are <5 mm, maximum overall sensitivity is 53% to 84%
- CAD may increase sensitivity of CT for nodule detection
- HRCT improves localization of tumor involvement within the lung parenchyma
- ¹⁸FDG PET has become useful in differentiating benign from malignant nodules

---

PATTERNS OF METASTASES IN THE LUNGS

Nodules

Nodular metastases are the most common pattern found in the lungs. Metastatic nodules can range from miliary in size to several centimeters (Figs. 41.1 and 41.2). Miliary nodules are more likely to be seen in tumors such as thyroid carcinoma, renal cell carcinoma, and melanoma. Their distribution with respect to the interstitial compartments is random (27,28).

Ground Glass Nodules

Ground glass nodules can be seen in metastases as a result of focal interstitial infiltration, as seen with lymphoma (Fig. 41.3) or filling of the airspaces with tumor, or its by-products. Ground glass nodules or nodules with surrounding ground glass are seen with hemorrhagic metastases. Metastases such as choriocarcinoma, melanoma, renal cell carcinoma, and angiosarcoma tend to be hypervascular, and bleed into the adjacent lungs to give this pattern (Fig. 41.4) (29,30). Mucin-producing tumors, such as adenocarcinoma from the

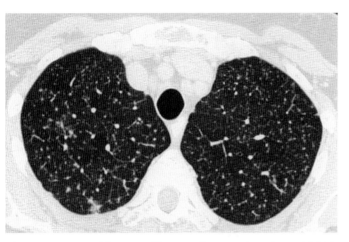

Figure 41.1 A 60-year-old woman with metastatic pancreatic carcinoma. Multiple pulmonary nodules are present that range from miliary size, 2–3 to 5 mm. This patient also had lymphangitic spread to her lungs (shown in Figure 41.19).

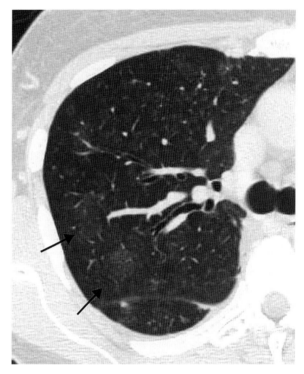

Figure 41.3 CT scan of a 45-year-old woman with non- Hodgkin's lymphoma showing new ground glass nodules (arrows).

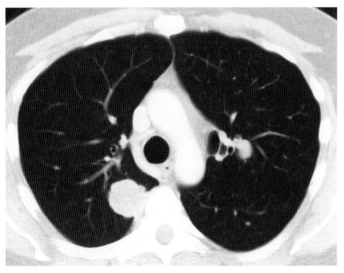

Figure 41.2 A 49-year-old man with metastatic renal cell carcinoma. CT scan shows a 3 cm nodule in the superior segment of the right lower lobe.

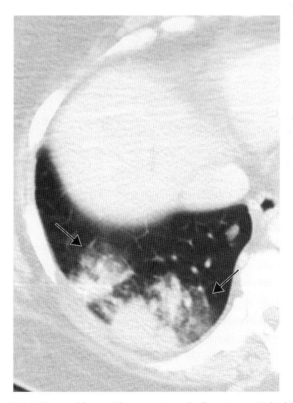

Figure 41.4 A 53-year-old man with metastatic renal cell carcinoma. Multiple nodules show surrounding ground glass consistent with hemorrhage (arrows).

pancreas or colon, show ground glass metastases (Fig. 41.5). In the early stages of involvement this appears as ground glass. As the disease progresses, however, areas of ground glass become consolidated and may resemble pneumonia (Fig. 41.6).

Ground glass nodules or solid nodules with surrounding ground glass are also found in diffuse bronchioloalveolar cell carcinoma. This pattern is due to both direct tumor scaffolding of the alveolar walls, termed lipidic growth, and filling of the airspaces with mucinous material.

Non-malignant lung diseases such as invasive aspergillosis or arteriovenous malformation may also develop multiple nodules with surrounding ground glass (30). In both these disorders, the ground glass is due to surrounding hemorrhage. The distinction between invasive aspergillosis and metastases may be difficult in an immunosuppressed oncology patient who has received chemotherapy or bone marrow transplantation. In such instances, clinical information is necessary to distinguish whether the patient is febrile and more likely to have infection rather than recurrent disease.

Pulmonary epithelioid hemangio-endothelioma or intravascular bronchoalveolar tumor is a low-grade endothelial sarcoma that can arise in the lung, skeleton, or soft tissues. The radiographic appearance varies and includes multiple interstitial nodules, interstitial thickening, calcified nodules, pleural thickening, effusion

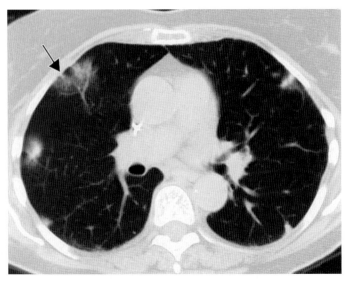

Figure 41.5 A 73-year-old woman with metastatic mucin-producing pancreatic carcinoma. The lungs show multiple pulmonary nodules including a ground glass nodule in the right upper lobe (arrow).

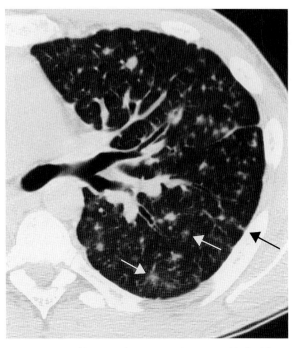

Figure 41.7 A 23-year-old man with primary pulmonary epithelioid hemangio-endotheliosis. CT scan shows multiple ill-defined nodules (white arrows), many of which appear as ground glass. There are subpleural nodules and thickened interlobular septa (black arrow) consistent with tumor deposition along the interstitium.

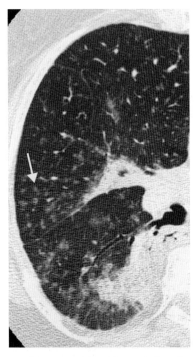

Figure 41.6 A 70-year-old woman with mucin-producing adenocarcinoma of the cecum. Right lung shows both airspace opacities and ground glass nodules (arrow) consistent with diffuse mucinous metastases.

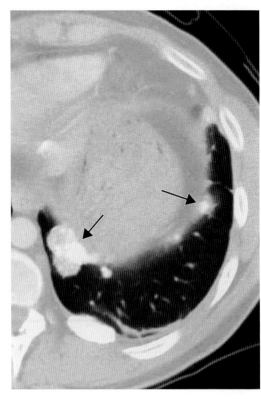

Figure 41.8 A 26-year-old man with osteosarcoma of the femur. CT scan of the lower thorax shows multiple subpleural calcified nodules consistent with metastatic osteosarcoma (arrows).

that tends to be a hemorrhagic or mediastinal mass. The multinodular pulmonary form is similar to metastatic angiosarcoma to the lungs. On HRCT, ill-defined ground glass nodules lie in a perivascular or centrilobular distribution (Fig. 41.7). Thickening of the interstitium resembles lymphangitic spread of tumor (31). These CT scan findings along with a presentation of hemoptysis may hint at the diagnosis of this unusual disease.

Nodules with Calcifications

The diagnosis of a calcified metastasis is straightforward in a patient with new nodules and a history of osteosarcoma or chondrosarcoma (Fig. 41.8) (32). Without prior radiographs available to show

that a nodule is new, other considerations for a calcified nodule would include a granuloma, amyloid, or a hamartoma. Metastatic mucinous adenocarcinoma may also manifest as multiple pulmonary nodules containing calcification (Fig. 41.9). Dystrophic calcification can be

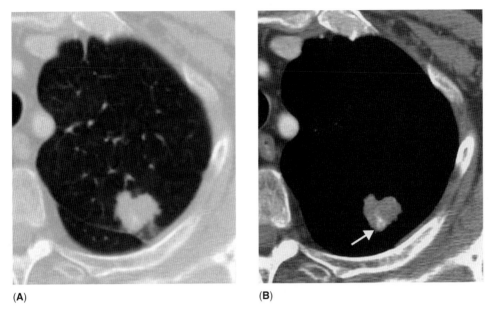

(A) (B)

Figure 41.9 An 80-year-old man with metastatic papillary adenocarcinoma of the colon. (**A**) CT scan of the thorax shows a left upper lobe nodule. (**B**) Soft tissue windows demonstrate calcification within the nodule (arrow).

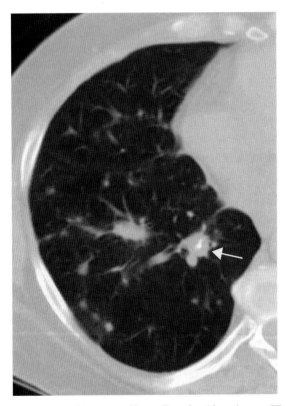

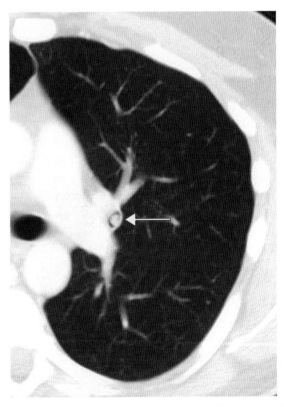

Figure 41.10 A 40-year-old woman with papillary thyroid carcinoma. CT scan shows multiple irregular pulmonary nodules. Intermediate windows show a focus of calcification within a nodule in the right lower lobe (arrow).

Figure 41.11 A 49-year-old man with metastatic renal cell carcinoma. CT scan through the apical posterior segmental bronchus of the left upper lobe shows a filling defect from an endobronchial metastasis (arrow).

seen in metastases from papillary thyroid carcinoma, synovial cell sarcoma and, rarely, in treated metastases (Fig. 41.10) (33).

Branching Nodules

Airway metastases tend to involve the airways from the trachea to the segmental bronchi. Metastases from breast, kidney, colon, lymphoma, and melanoma are the most common sources for this process (34–37). Endobronchial metastases with complete

obstruction of an airway may lead to complete collapse of the involved lung or resultant air trapping. An airway-filling defect or mass with mucus filling of a distal occluded airway is best seen on CT (Fig. 41.11). An occluded airway will appear as an arborizing opaque structure that parallels the adjacent vasculature on CT lung windows (Fig. 41.12). This has been called the "finger-in-glove" sign on chest radiograph because the branching plugged airways

resemble white-gloved fingers. If airway plugging extends to the respiratory and terminal bronchioles on CT, branching centrilobular opacities, or "tree-in-bud" opacities will be seen (Fig. 41.13). These will be optimally seen in the subpleural regions (38).

Tumor emboli are the result of hematogenous metastases occluding and proliferating within the small- and intermediate-sized

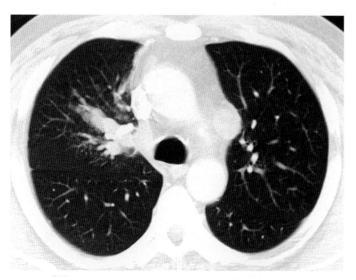

Figure 41.12 A 47-year-old man with renal cell carcinoma and an endobronchial metastasis in the right upper lobe bronchus. Large arborizing opacity in right upper lobe correlates with an obstructed bronchus filled with tumor and mucus.

pulmonary arteries (39). On chest radiograph, this pattern is indistinguishable from other nodular metastases. On CT, tumor emboli appear as branching lobulated enlargements or smooth symmetric beading of the small- and medium-sized pulmonary arteries (Fig. 41.14) (40). With helical CT, this pattern is now more readily detected due to thinner sequential images in which symmetric focal enlargement of a small artery is seen. Tumor emboli are associated with tumors such as soft tissue sarcomas, renal cell carcinoma, hepatoma, and melanoma that spread hematogenously via the venous system. Distal infarction may occur with distal parenchymal ground glass or consolidation.

Nodular lymphangitic spread of tumor along the vascular interstitium may resemble tumor emboli. CT features, which help to identify tumor involving the interstitium rather than within the vasculature, include asymmetric and irregular nodularity along vessels, coexisting signs of lymphangitic spread in other interstitial compartments, as well as lymphadenopathy.

Branching opacities may also occur with localized dilated veins and, in the presence of metastatic disease, this can be seen with tumor venous thrombosis. This rare process is seen if tumor invades the venous system or the left atrium (41). This has been reported with squamous cell carcinoma and sarcoma. If pulmonary infarction results, patients may present with pleuritic chest pain, cough, and hemoptysis. CT findings include dilated pulmonary veins (Fig. 41.15), a filling defect in the pulmonary vein, particularly the proximal veins, and/or a filling defect in the left atrium.

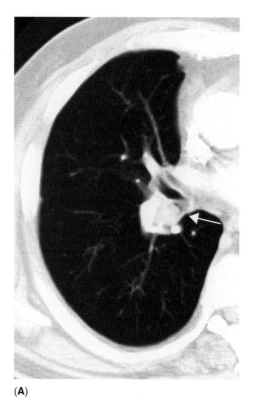

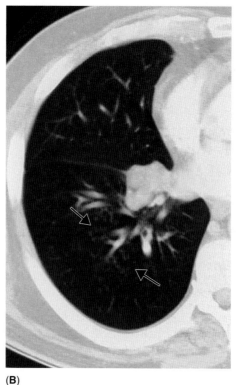

(A)   **(B)**

Figure 41.13 A 47-year-old man with renal cell carcinoma. (**A**) CT scan of the right lower lobe shows a filling defect in the right lower lobe bronchus consistent with an endobronchial metastasis (white arrow). (**B**) Computed tomography scan through the right lower lobe shows clusters of centrilobular nodules and plugged small airways consistent with a "tree-in-bud" pattern (black arrows).

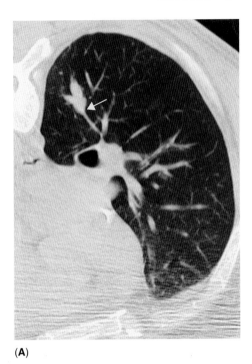

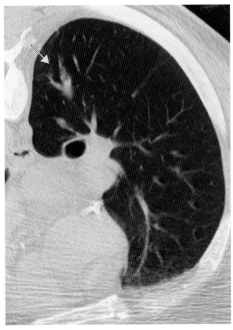

(A)   (B)

Figure 41.14 A 48-year-old man with renal cell carcinoma and new pulmonary nodules. (A) CT scan of the thorax in the prone position shows dilatation of a small pulmonary artery in the right lower lobe consistent with a tumor embolus (arrow). (B) Sequential CT scan slice shows branching of the dilated artery (arrow).

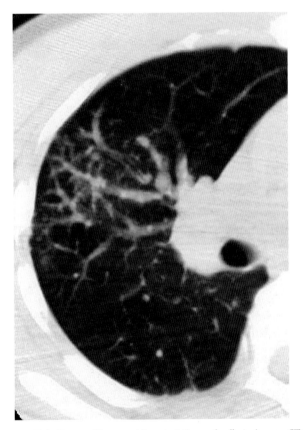

Figure 41.15 A 45-year-old man with metastatic renal cell carcinoma. CT scan shows multiple pulmonary metastases. Scattered pulmonary veins are dilated consistent with tumor thrombosis of the pulmonary veins.

Key Points: Nodular Metastases

- Nodular metastases are the most common pattern found in the lungs
- Ground glass nodules occur as a result of partial filling of the airspaces or the interstitium with tumor or hemorrhage
- Calcified nodules can be seen in metastases from osteo- or chondrosarcoma, mucin-producing adenocarcinoma and due to dystrophic calcification in metastases from thyroid carcinoma and synovial cell sarcoma
- Branching nodules may be secondary to endobronchial metastases and mucus filling of the distal airway, or due to tumor embolus in the pulmonary artery or, rarely, pulmonary vein

Cystic or Cavitary Nodules

Cavitary metastases are most likely from metastatic squamous cell carcinoma of the cervix, head, and neck (Fig. 41.16) but are also seen with colorectal carcinoma, sarcoma, transitional cell carcinoma, and lymphoma (42–44).

Non-malignant disorders such as Wegener's granulomatosis, Churg–Strauss disease, rheumatoid arthritis, and amyloidosis may also present with numerous cavitary nodules (45). Cavitary nodules associated with Langerhans' cell histiocytosis usually measure 3 to 4 mm and have irregular thin walls. Distribution tends to be in the upper lungs and interstitial fibrosis may coexist. Fungal infection, mycobacterial infection, septic emboli, and tracheobronchial papillomatosis may also cause multiple pulmonary cavities and cysts. In the appropriate clinical setting, where infection is suspected, they should be included in the differential diagnosis. Pulmonary involvement of tracheobronchial papillomatosis manifests as multiple thin- or thick-walled cavities and may contain air–fluid levels. Transmission to the lungs is through the airways and, therefore, these cavities and cysts tend to distribute centrally in the lungs. This

993

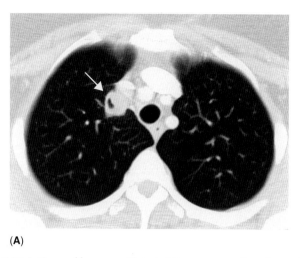
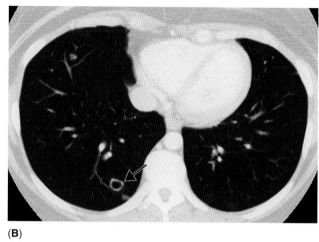

(A)   **(B)**

Figure 41.16 A 48-year-old woman with metastatic squamous cell carcinoma. (A) CT scan of the upper thorax shows a cavitary nodule (white arrow) with an asymmetric thickened wall in the right upper lobe. (B) Computed tomography scan in lower thorax shows a thinner-walled nodule in the right lower lobe (black arrow). Other nodules in the lungs were solid.

disease is associated with malignant degeneration to squamous cell carcinoma. Any change in cyst formation (to solid) or lymphadenopathy on CT may indicate malignant transformation.

The CT pattern of multiple nodules associated with complex cystic changes is often attributed to Langerhans' cell histiocytosis of the lungs. However, nodular metastases such as transitional cell carcinoma, lymphoma, renal cell carcinoma, squamous cell carcinoma can also cavitate in a similar pattern in a background of coexisting small nodules (Fig. 41.17) (46,47). Additional findings in the thorax, including lymphadenopathy, pleural effusion, bone lesions, as well as intra-abdominal metastases, may help to define the presence of metastases over a non-malignant process. Metastatic nodules may cavitate prior to chemotherapy. Cavitation and decrease in nodule size may indicate a tumor's response to therapy. Although rare, spontaneous pneumothorax may develop if a cavitary nodule is subpleural and ruptures into the pleural space.

Spontaneous pneumothorax is a well-described complication of metastatic sarcoma. The mechanism of this complication is attributed to extension of the pulmonary tumor into the pleural space, creating a communication between the airspaces, and the pleura. The sarcomas associated with this complication include osteosarcoma, synovial cell sarcoma, angiosarcoma, and leiomyosarcoma. Smevik and Klepp reported an increased risk for pneumothorax after the induction of chemotherapy (48).

Key Points: Cystic Metastases

- Cystic metastases should be differentiated from infection causing cavitary nodules
- Cystic metastases are most likely from squamous carcinoma of cervix, head, and neck, but also sarcomas and transitional cell carcinoma

Reticular Disease

Reticular opacities in the lungs from metastases primarily result from infiltration of tumor into the interstitial compartments. These compartments include the perihilar axial interstitium, the centrilobular interstitium, subpleural interstitium, and interlobular septa (49,50). Usually, all compartments or regions of an

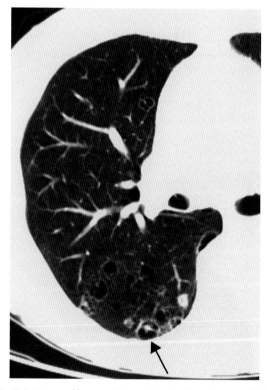

Figure 41.17 A 63-year-old man with transitional cell carcinoma of the bladder. CT scan of the thorax shows multiple nodules and cysts. Some of the cysts are complex with central nodules and septations (arrow).

involved lung will be infiltrated. The key feature in distinguishing lymphangitic spread from other causes of interstitial lung disease on HRCT is the preservation of lung architecture. Associated findings on CT such as lymphadenopathy, a unilateral pleural effusion, an asymmetric distribution in the lungs and lung nodules will help confirm its presence. Malignancies that commonly involve the interstitium by lymphangitic spread include lung, breast, gastro-intestinal tract, melanoma, and lymphoma (49).

Tumor spread through the lymphatics and surrounding interstitium may initially originate either from pulmonary arterial metastases or by direct extension from hilar lymphadenopathy

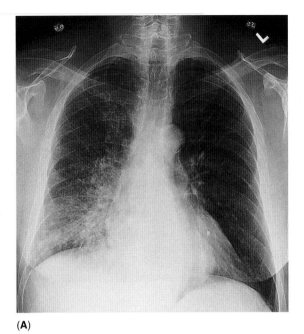

(A)

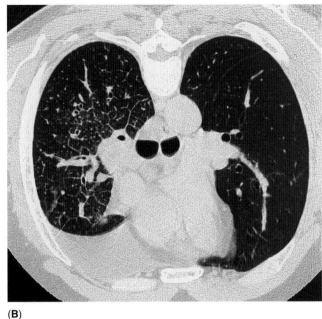

(B)

Figure 41.18 A 50-year-old man with non-small cell lung carcinoma. (**A**) Chest radiograph shows asymmetric right hilar fullness with ground glass and reticular opacities in the right lung. (**B**) High-resolution CT in the prone position shows smooth thickened interlobular septa with preserved lung architecture.

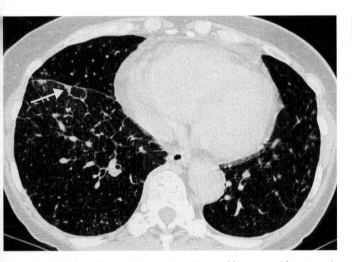

Figure 41.19 High-resolution CT scan in a 60-year-old woman with metastatic pancreatic carcinoma. The interlobular septa show nodular thickening (arrow) consistent with tumor deposition in the interstitium.

along the axial interstitium. The former route is most commonly seen in malignancies from the breast, gastro-intestinal tract, and melanoma. Direct extension from the hilum is more likely to be seen in primary lung cancer with hilar disease, lymphoma (especially Hodgkin's disease) and, on rare occasions, leukemia (51).

The pattern of lymphangitic spread in the interstitium can be smooth (Fig. 41.18) or nodular (Fig. 41.19) and is best seen with thin section images. A smooth pattern may be the result of direct tumor deposit in the interstitium. Alternatively, this pattern may be the result of obstructed lymphatics from extensive lymphadenopathy with subsequent interstitial edema. Imaging should display a proximal tumor mass or extensive hilar and mediastinal lymphadenopathy in the thorax to suggest this disease process. Nodular lymphangitic disease is easier to recognize and is indicative of tumor deposits in the interstitium or lymphatics.

Key Points: Reticular Disease

- Malignancies which commonly involve the interstitium by lymphatic spread include lung, breast, gastro-intestinal tract, melanoma, and lymphoma
- Lymphangitic spread can be nodular or smooth, and is best seen on HRCT

Reticular and Nodular Disease

As mentioned above, lymphangitic tumor will cause a combined nodular and reticular pattern. Tumors to be considered by this pattern, which can involve the lung, are breast, gastro-intestinal tract, melanoma, and lymphoma.

Lymphocytic interstitial pneumonia (LIP), a benign disease caused by the deposit of numerous benign lymphocytes and plasma cells in the interstitium of the lung, resembles metastatic disease or diffuse lymphoma. Patients at risk for acquiring this disorder, such as those with immune deficiency disorders, are also at risk for lymphoma. Distinction between the two on a clinical and radiological basis can be difficult. A chest radiograph commonly shows reticular and/or nodular opacities in the lungs. On CT, nodules may be seen that are interstitial, including centrilobular, in distribution. These nodules may contain an air bronchogram, may be ground glass or solid, and range in size from a few millimeters to 1 cm (Fig. 41.3). Although uncommon, associated parenchymal cysts may help distinguish LIP from low-grade lymphoma of the lungs (Fig. 41.20) (52). These cysts result from cellular infiltration into the walls of small airways, endoluminal obstruction, and subsequent air-trapping in the distal airspaces (53). Specific patient populations are at risk for LIP, which may help associate the CT findings with the disease. These include those with acquired immuno deficiency syndrome (AIDS), Sjögren's syndrome, and primary immunodeficiency disorders (54).

995

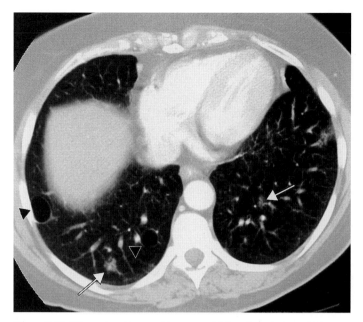

Figure 41.20 CT scan in a 52-year-old woman with lymphocytic interstitial pneumonia. The lungs show a mixture of soft tissue nodules (arrows) and parenchymal cysts (arrowheads).

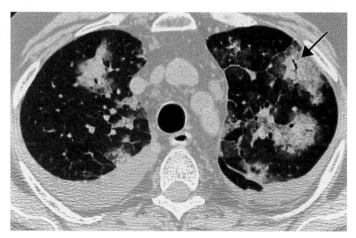

Figure 41.21 A 54-year-old man with diffuse pulmonary non-Hodgkin's lymphoma. CT scan shows bilateral large consolidative masses (arrow) that contain air bronchograms, and have surrounding ground glass. Some of the interlobular septa are also thickened. The patient also had pleural effusions.

TUMORS WITH MIXED NODULES, AIRSPACE, AND INTERSTITIAL DISEASE

Lymphoma involvement of the lungs may manifest as a mixture of consolidation, nodules, and interstitial disease (Fig. 41.21) (see also chap. 33). The latter form is commonly seen as an extension of tumor along the axial bronchovascular interstitium from hilar nodal disease. The consolidative and nodular forms often have an air bronchogram that may be confused with infection. Cavitation of nodules may occur, which may be equally confusing if the clinical differential diagnosis includes infections such as invasive aspergillosis (Fig. 41.22) (55). The presence of lymphadenopathy may help, especially with Hodgkin's disease, but will not necessarily be present in primary non-Hodgkin's involvement of the lungs (56–58).

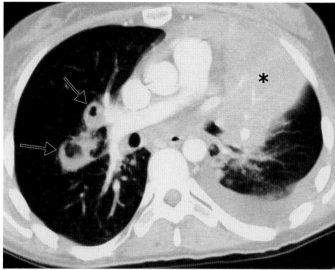

Figure 41.22 A 21-year-old woman with progressive Hodgkin's lymphoma. CT scan of the thorax shows dense consolidative tumor in the left upper lobe (*) and cavitary nodules in the right perihilar region (arrows). There is a left pleural effusion.

The consolidative form of bronchoalveolar carcinoma (BAC) or adenocarcinoma with bronchoalveolar cell type is often mistakenly diagnosed as lobar pneumonia on initial chest radiographs. Many patients present with fever, cough, and systemic symptoms that are consistent with infection (they can be superimposed on the tumor). Coexisting pulmonary findings on CT scan, such as associated subcentimeter nodules (which can be ground glass and cavitary) or scattered areas of ground glass in other regions of the lung, should raise suspicion for this disease (Fig. 41.23) (59,60). On rare occasions, cyst-like changes in the consolidation may develop which can be mistaken for cavitary pneumonia or bronchiectasis. Lymphadenopathy is unusual and is, therefore, not helpful in distinguishing tumor from infection. Ground glass with septal thickening, sometimes called "'crazy paving'" on HRCT, is an unusual pattern for BAC, but is well described (Fig. 41.24) (61,62). This pattern, along with other features described above, may raise the suspicion for this disease if found.

Kaposi's sarcoma involvement of the lungs commonly includes mediastinal and hilar lymphadenopathy (see chap. 59). This tumor tends to spread from hilar nodal disease and infiltrate along the interstitial compartment of the axial bronchovasculature. Multiple flame-shaped lesions or nodules with ill-defined borders arise in the thickened interstitium (Fig. 41.25). These nodules commonly surround the bronchus and thus contain an air bronchogram. High-resolution CT better displays the relationship of tumor with the bronchovasculature. Other possible patterns of Kaposi's sarcoma involvement in the thorax include a single pulmonary nodule, unilateral pleural effusion that can be bloody on thoracocentesis, or endoluminal tracheal and bronchial lesions that are best seen on bronchoscopy rather than CT scan (63).

ASSESSING TREATMENT RESPONSE

Measurement of the response to chemotherapy at each time point requires accurate and reproducible assessment of the number and

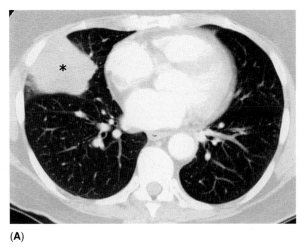

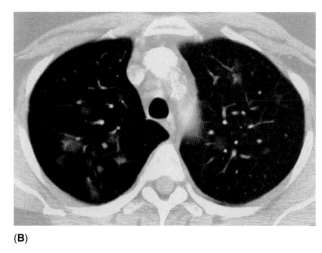

(A) (B)

Figure 41.23 A 55-year-old woman with bronchoalveolar cell carcinoma. (A) CT scan of the mid thorax shows a dominant mass in the middle lobe (*). (B) Computed tomography scan through the upper lobes shows multiple ground glass nodules consistent with metastases.

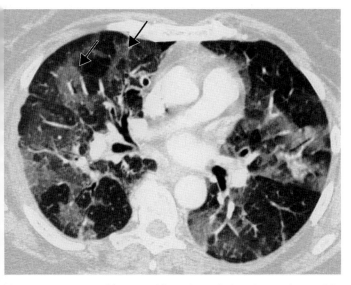

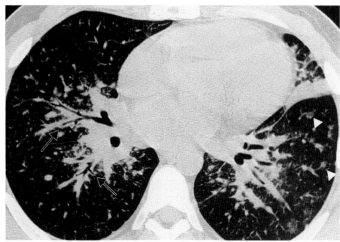

Figure 41.25 A 40-year-old man with AIDS and Kaposi's sarcoma. Tumor extends from hilar nodal involvement along the bronchovascular bundles (arrows). Scattered nodules in the left lower lobe (arrowheads) are consistent with metastatic disease.

Figure 41.24 A 50-year-old woman with mucin-producing adenocarcinoma of the lung. CT scan of the lungs shows diffuse ground glass opacities (arrows) and scattered thickened interlobular septa. Although this is not a bronchioloalveolar cell carcinoma by histopathology, its pattern is indistinguishable.

size of lung metastases. Lung metastases can grow at different rates in an individual, even when they are of identical histology. They can also show a variable response to chemotherapy (64,65). Radiologists often vary in the number or sites of nodules that they evaluate. This inter-observer variation can significantly alter the assessment of treatment change. If too few nodules are remeasured at follow-up CT, the therapeutic response may not be accurately reflected (64). Nodules can be measured on CT in three ways: unidirectional, bidirectional, and volumetric analysis. Use of unidirectional (RECIST criteria) or bidirectional measurements (WHO criteria) are comparable (64). CAD allows automated volumetric assessment. Automated CT volumetry potentially offers the opportunity for earlier and more accurate detection of lesion growth or regression when compared to 2D measurements (66,67). Additional studies will be required before CT volumetry becomes widely accepted as a basis for clinical decision making in all pulmonary nodules.

As a result of chemotherapy, pulmonary metastases may develop cavitation or calcification, especially in colon and bladder cancer. Radiofrequency ablation has recently been introduced as a minimally invasive treatment for lung tumors (see chap. 51). Metastases that are treated by radiofrequency ablation (RFA) have characteristic appearances on follow-up CT (Fig. 41.26) (68–73). During RFA, the lung around the tumor must also be ablated to create a safety margin of necrosis. The inflammation, hemorrhage, and necrosis of the metastasis and adjacent lung will result in a postablation lesion that is larger than the baseline nodule (69,70). This increase in size is seen immediately after RFA as surrounding ground-glass opacity. The opacity changes from ground-glass to dense consolidation within a few days and reaches maximum dimensions at one month. There may be associated cavitation and pleural thickening (70–72). Such changes should not be interpreted by the unwary as progressive disease or secondary infection. The postablation lesion subsequently decreases in size as resorption and fibrosis occur between three and six months (70,71,73).

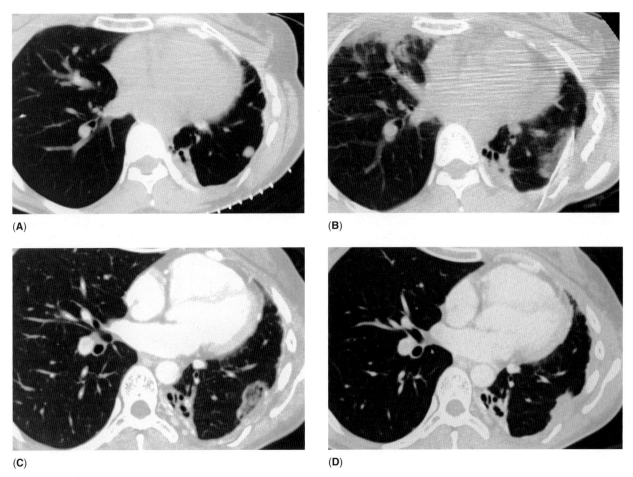

(A) (B)

(C) (D)

Figure 41.26 CT scans of a 30-year-old woman with metastatic sarcoma in the left lower lobe (A) treated with radiofrequency ablation (RFA). (B) Ground-glass opacity is from RFA of the surrounding lung. (C) At one-month follow-up there is peripheral consolidation of the post-RFA lesion and pleural thickening. (D) The lesion becomes dense and contracts to form a peripheral scar by 12 months.

Key Points: Assessing Treatment Response

- An adequate number of nodules should be measured at each time-point as metastases can grow and shrink at different rates
- Unidirectional and bidirectional measurement of nodules are comparable
- Radiofrequency ablation (RFA) treatment causes an initial increase in lesion size, possible cavitation, and pleural thickening that should not be misinterpreted as progressive disease

PLEURAL METASTATIC DISEASE

The pleural space is involved in metastatic disease in three main ways:

- Effusions
- Thickening
- Nodules or masses

The presence of metastatic pleural disease is an ominous sign. The average time until death following the diagnosis of a malignant effusion is approximately 5 to 16 months (74–76). Most malignant effusions are exudative and unilateral. In adult patients, 25% of newly diagnosed pleural effusions identified by chest radiograph are due to malignancy. The likelihood of a unilateral effusion being malignant increases with the patient's age and with the size of the effusion (77,78). Bilateral pleural effusions with a normal heart size are reported to be secondary to malignancy in 50% of patients (79).

Almost every tumor has been reported to metastasize to the pleura but, histologically, adenocarcinoma is responsible for over 80% of malignant effusions (80). In 6% to 13% of patients who present with a malignant effusion, the primary site of disease is unknown (81,82). The most common malignancy associated with pleural metastatic disease is lung cancer, which is responsible for up to half of malignant pleural effusions (82–84). Breast cancer is the second most common cause and accounts for one quarter of malignant effusions. (74,75,82). Lymphoma is responsible for 13% to 16% of all malignant effusions (75,83). Approximately one in seven of patients with either Hodgkin's or non-Hodgkin's lymphoma will have an effusion at initial presentation (84,85).

Metastatic pleural disease may also manifest with pleural thickening or nodules. Tumors most likely to demonstrate this pattern are metastatic adenocarcinoma, lymphoma, and invasive thymoma (Fig. 41.27).

The role of radiology is to identify patients with pleural disease and provide aids to diagnosis and treatment, such as image-guided thoracocentesis, biopsy, and pleurodesis (86). More than 300 ml of pleural fluid is necessary for visualization on an erect chest radiograph (Fig. 41.28), but lateral decubitus films can detect as little as

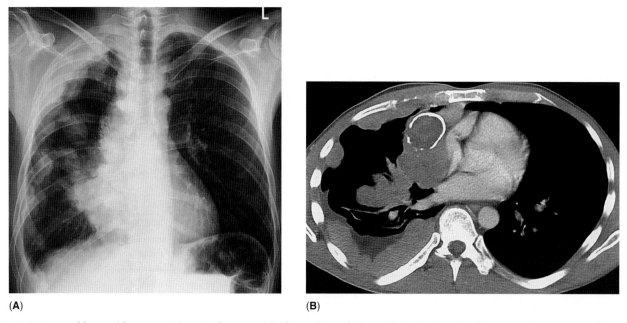

(A)　　　　　　　　　　　　　　　**(B)**

Figure 41.27 A 23-year-old man with metastatic invasive thymoma. (**A**) Chest radiograph shows lobulated right pleural masses and an anterior mediastinal mass. (**B**) CT scan shows a heterogeneous mediastinal mass that contains curvilinear calcification. There are multiple enhancing pleural nodules and a small right pleural effusion.

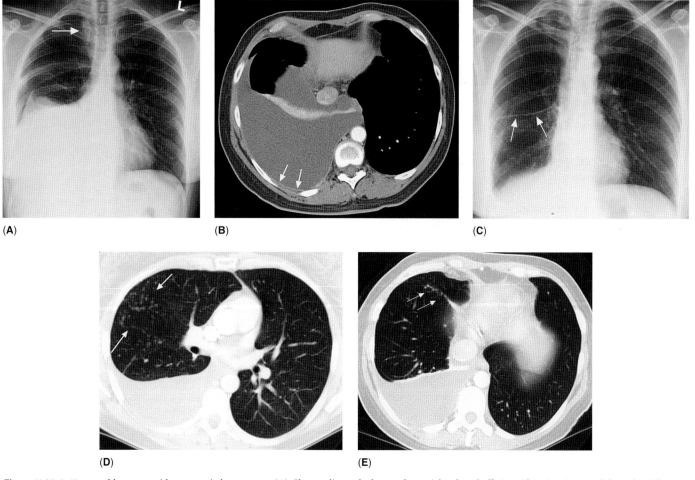

(A)　　　　　　　　　　　**(B)**　　　　　　　　　　　**(C)**

(D)　　　　　　　　　　　**(E)**

Figure 41.28 A 47-year-old woman with metastatic lung cancer. (**A**) Chest radiograph shows a large right pleural effusion. There is a 2 cm nodule at the right apex (arrow). (**B**) CT scan in the same patient confirms a large right pleural effusion with linear pleural thickening and enhancement (arrows). (**C**) Following thoracocentesis of 2 L of fluid, the second chest radiograph shows nodular pleural thickening involving the horizontal fissure (arrows). CT scan in the same patient with selected images on lung windows confirms multiple pleural metastases involving the (**D**) horizontal and (**E**) oblique fissures (arrows).

5 ml of fluid (87). US is more sensitive in the detection and quantification of an effusion (88). This modality also will display the presence of fluid echogenicity, which suggests exudates, pleural nodules, and thickening (Fig. 41.29) (89).

In many instances, tumor deposits within the pleura and pleural space are below the resolution of CT and US (90). The majority of malignant exudative effusions do not demonstrate pleural changes on contrast-enhanced CT (91,92). Several studies have evaluated the use of CT in establishing criteria for detecting malignant pleural disease (91–93). The features that are most helpful are pleural nodules and nodular pleural thickening (Fig. 41.28) (92). In

patients with diffuse pleural thickening, the presence of mediastinal pleural involvement, circumferential distribution, or parietal thickening greater than 1 cm are all suggestive of malignant disease (93) (Fig. 41.30). However, metastatic pleural disease (in particular, adenocarcinoma) and malignant mesothelioma are frequently indistinguishable radiologically, and histologic confirmation is necessary.

MR has also been evaluated in the diagnosis of metastatic pleural disease (94). High-signal intensity in relation to intercostal muscle on T2-weighted or contrast-enhanced T1-weighted sections was found to be suggestive for malignant disease (Fig. 41.31).

There have been reports of the clinical role of [18]FDG PET in differentiating malignant from benign pleural disease. Gupta et al. (95) reported a sensitivity and specificity of 88.8% and 94.1%, respectively, of [18]FDG PET in correctly separating benign pleural disease from malignant pleural disease in patients with lung cancer (Fig. 41.32). Further studies are warranted to assess the role of [18]FDG PET in the assessment of pleural disease.

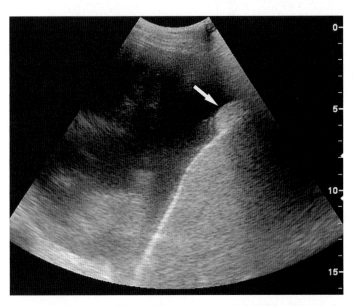

Figure 41.29 An 82-year-old man with recurrent non-Hodgkin's lymphoma in the right pleural cavity. Ultrasound of the right hemithorax demonstrates an echogenic effusion and a diaphragmatic nodule (arrow).

Key Points: Pleural Metastases

- Pleural metastases can manifest as effusions, pleural thickening, nodules, or masses
- The most common malignancies that spread to the pleura are lung, breast, and lymphoma
- More than 300 ml of pleural fluid is necessary for detection on an erect chest radiograph
- The majority of malignant exudative effusions are not associated with pleural thickening on CT
- Pleural nodules and circumferential or mediastinal pleural thickening are the most helpful CT features in distinguishing benign from malignant disease

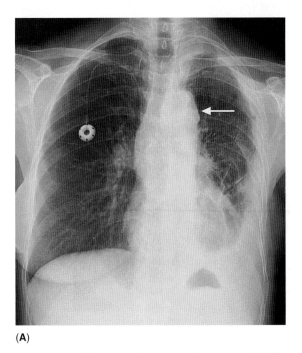

(A)

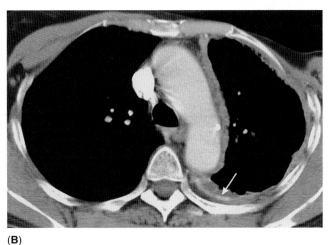

(B)

Figure 41.30 A 46-year-old woman with metastatic breast cancer. (A) Chest radiograph shows lobulated left pleural thickening which extends along the mediastinal border and distorts the outline of the aortic arch (arrow). (B) CT scan shows mediastinal pleural thickening along the aortic arch. There is high-density material (arrow) within the left pleural cavity, which is consistent with talc from prior pleurodesis.

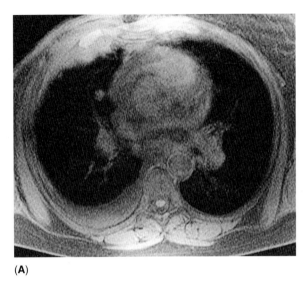 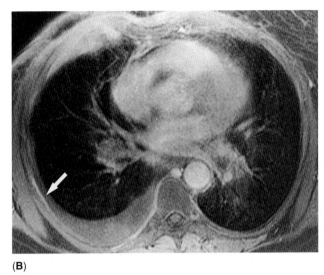

(A) **(B)**

Figure 41.31 A 41-year-old woman with metastatic breast cancer to the right chest wall and a malignant right pleural effusion. Fatsaturated pre- and postcontrast T1-weighted images (A and B) demonstrate high signal intensity in the right chest wall and pleural fluid. Postcontrast (B) image show enhancement of the pleura (arrow).

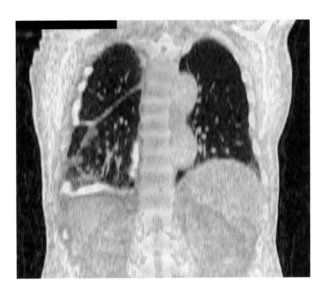

Figure 41.32 [18]FDG PET/CT scan of a 67-year-old man with pleural metastases from adenocarcinoma of the lung showing intense nodular [18]FDG activity in the right pleural cavity.

Summary

- CT scanning is now routinely used in the screening and follow-up of patients with pulmonary metastatic disease; helical CT offers advantages over chest radiography in the detection of lung nodules
- HRCT gives exquisite detail of the lung parenchyma and enables the radiologist to localize tumor involvement more accurately and establish a more specific differential diagnosis based on the lung compartments involved
- The patterns of metastatic pulmonary disease vary between tumors, but solid nodules are most common. Other patterns, such as ground glass attenuation, branching configuration, calcification, or cavitation, are identifiable on CT and can be specific for tumor types:

- Reticular disease or involvement of the interstitium suggests lymphangitic and interstitial spread of tumor. A mixed parenchymal pattern including consolidation may also be seen with metastatic disease, most commonly in patients with bronchioloalveolar cell carcinoma or lymphoma
- Metastatic disease within the pleural space can manifest as effusions, pleural thickening, or pleural nodules. The most common malignancies are adenocarcinomas from the lung, breast or from lymphoma
- US and CT are more sensitive than chest radiography in identifying pleural effusions. Most malignant effusions show no other CT abnormality
- The presence of pleural nodules or circumferential pleural involvement is more indicative of malignancy

REFERENCES

1. Vock P, Soucek M, Daepp M, Kalender WA. Lung: spiral volumetric CT with single-breath-hold technique. Radiology 1990; 176: 864–7.
2. Remy-Jardin M, Remy J, Giraud F, Marquette CH. Pulmonary nodules: detection with thick-section spiral CT versus conventional CT. Radiology 1993; 187: 513–20.
3. Diederich S, Lentschig MG, Winter F, Roos N, Bongartz G. Detection of pulmonary nodules with overlapping vs. non-overlapping image reconstruction at spiral CT. Eur Radiol 1999; 9: 281–6.
4. Rydberg J, Buckwalter KA, Caldemeyer KS, et al. Multisection CT: scanning techniques and clinical applications. Radiographics 2000; 20: 1787–806.
5. Berland LL, Smith JK. Multidetector-array CT: once again, technology creates new opportunities. Radiology 1998; 209: 327–9.
6. Waters DJ, Coakley FV, Cohen MD, et al. The detection of pulmonary metastases by helical CT: a clinicopathologic study in dogs. J Comput Assist Tomogr 1998; 22: 235–40.

7. Ambrogi V, Paci M, Pompeo E, Mineo TC. Transxiphoid video-assisted pulmonary metastasectomy: relevance of helical computed tomography occult lesions. Ann Thorac Surg 2000; 70: 1847–52.

8. Margaritora S, Porziella V, D'Andrilli A, et al. Pulmonary metastases: can accurate radiological evaluation avoid thoracotomic approach? Eur J Cardiothorac Surg 2002; 21: 1111–14.

9. Picci P, Vanel D, Briccoli A, et al. Computed tomography of pulmonary metastases from osteosarcoma: the less poor technique. A study of 51 patients with histological correlation. Ann Oncol 2001; 12: 1601–4.

10. Giger ML, Bae KT, MacMahon H. Computerized detection of pulmonary nodules in computed tomography images. Invest Radiol 1994; 29: 459–65.

11. Kanazawa K, Kawata Y, Niki N, et al. Computer-aided diagnosis for pulmonary nodules based on helical CT images. Comput Med Imaging Graph 1998; 22: 157–67.

12. Armato SG 3rd, Giger ML, MacMahon H. Automated detection of lung nodules in CT scans: preliminary results. Med Phys 2001; 28: 1552–61.

13. Ko JP, Betke M. Chest CT: automated nodule detection and assessment of change over time--preliminary experience. Radiology 2001; 218: 267–73.

14. Gurcan MN, Sahiner B, Petrick N, et al. Lung nodule detection on thoracic computed tomography images: preliminary evaluation of a computer-aided diagnosis system. Med Phys 2002; 29: 2552–8.

15. Wormanns D, Fiebich M, Saidi M, Diederich S, Heindel W. Automatic detection of pulmonary nodules at spiral CT: clinical application of a computer-aided diagnosis system. Eur Radiol 2002; 12: 1052–7.

16. Awai K, Murao K, Ozawa A, et al. Pulmonary nodules at chest CT: effect of computer-aided diagnosis on radiologists' detection performance. Radiology 2004; 230: 347–52.

17. Bae KT, Kim JS, Na YH, Kim KG, Kim JH. Pulmonary nodules: automated detection on CT images with morphologic matching algorithm–preliminary results. Radiology 2005; 236: 286–93.

18. Armato SG 3rd, Li F, Giger ML, et al. Lung cancer: performance of automated lung nodule detection applied to cancers missed in a CT screening program. Radiology 2002; 225: 685–92.

19. Beyer F, Zierott L, Fallenberg EM, et al. Comparison of sensitivity and reading time for the use of computer-aided detection (CAD) of pulmonary nodules at MDCT as concurrent or second reader. Eur Radiol 2007; 17: 2941–7.

20. Patz EF, Lowe VJ, Hoffman JM, et al. Focal pulmonary abnormalities: evaluation with F-18 fluorodeoxyglucose PET scanning. Radiology 1993; 188: 487–90.

21. Sazon DA, Santiago SM, Soo Hoo GW, et al. Fluorodeoxyglucose-positron emission tomography in the detection and staging of lung cancer. Am J Respir Crit Care Med 1996; 153: 417–21.

22. Pieterman RM, van Putten JW, Meuzelaar JJ, et al. Preoperative staging of non-small-cell lung cancer with positron-emission tomography. N Engl J Med 2000; 343: 254–61.

23. Mawatari T, Watanabe A, Ohsawa H, et al. Surgery for metastatic lung tumors at our department during the last 10 years. Kyobu Geka 2003; 56: 28–31 (in Japanese).

24. Watanabe M, Deguchi H, Sato M, et al. Midterm results of thoracoscopic surgery for pulmonary metastases especially from colorectal cancers. J Laparoendosc Adv Surg Tech A 1998; 8: 195–200.

25. Karnak I, Emin Senocak M, Kutluk T, Tanyel FC, Büyükpamukçu N. Pulmonary metastases in children: an analysis of surgical spectrum. Eur J Pediatr Surg 2002; 12: 151–8.

26. McCormack PM, Bains MS, Begg CB, et al. Role of video-assisted thoracic surgery in the treatment of pulmonary metastases: results of a prospective trial. Ann Thorac Surg 1996; 62: 213–17.

27. Benditt JO, Farber HW, Wright J, Karnad AB. Pulmonary hemorrhage with diffuse alveolar infiltrates in men with high-volume choriocarcinoma. Ann Intern Med 1988; 109: 674–5.

28. Patel AM, Ryu JH. Angiosarcoma in the lung. Chest 1993; 103: 1531–5.

29. Hirakata K, Nakata H, Haratake J. Appearance of pulmonary metastases on high-resolution CT scans: comparison with histopathologic findings from autopsy specimens. Am J Roentgenol 1993; 161: 37–43.

30. Kim Y, Lee KS, Jung KJ, et al. Halo sign on high-resolution CT: findings in spectrum of pulmonary diseases with pathologic correlation. J Comput Assist Tomogr 1999; 23: 622–6.

31. Bhagavan BS, Dorfman HD, Murthy MS, Eggleston JC. Intravascular bronchiolo-alveolar tumor (IVBAT): a low-grade sclerosing epithelioid angiosarcoma of lung. Am J Surg Pathol 1982; 6: 41–52.

32. Johnson GL, Askin FB, Fishman EK. Thoracic involvement from osteosarcoma: typical and atypical CT manifestations. Am J Roentgenol 1997; 168: 347–9.

33. Maile CW, Rodan BA, Godwin JD, Chen JT, Ravin CE. Calcification in pulmonary metastases. Br J Radiol 1982; 55: 108–13.

34. Ikezoe J, Johkoh T, Takeuchi N, et al. CT findings of endobronchial metastasis. Acta Radiol 1991; 32: 455–60.

35. Baumgartner WA, Mark JB. Metastatic malignancies from distant sites to the tracheobronchial tree. J Thorac Cardiovasc Surg 1980; 79: 499–503.

36. Berg HK, Petrelli NJ, Herrera L, Lopez C, Mittelman A. Endobronchial metastasis from colorectal carcinoma. Dis Colon Rectum 1984; 27: 745–8.

37. Mason AC, White CS. CT appearance of endobronchial non-Hodgkin lymphoma. J Comput Assist Tomogr 1994; 18: 559–61.

38. Aquino SL, Gamsu G, Webb WR, Kee ST. Tree-in-bud pattern: frequency and significance on thin section CT. J Comput Assist Tomogr 1996; 20: 594–9.

39. Shepard JA, Moore EH, Templeton PA, McLoud TC. Pulmonary intravascular tumor emboli: dilated and beaded peripheral pulmonary arteries at CT. Radiology 1993; 187: 797–801.

40. Kang CH, Choi JA, Kim HR, et al. Lung metastases manifesting as pulmonary infarction by mucin and tumor embolization: radiographic, high-resolution CT, and pathologic findings. J Comput Assist Tomogr 1999; 23: 644–6.

41. Nelson E, Klein JS. Pulmonary infarction resulting from metastatic osteogenic sarcoma with pulmonary venous tumor thrombus. Am J Roentgenol 2000; 174: 531–3.

42. Dodd GD, Boyle JJ. Excavating pulmonary metasteses. Am J Roentgenol 1961; 85: 277–93.

43. Chaudhuri MR. Cavitary pulmonary metastases. Thorax 1970; 25: 375–81.

44. Shin MS, Shingleton HM, Partridge EE, Nicolson VM, Ho KJ. Squamous cell carcinoma of the uterine cervix. Patterns of thoracic metastases. Invest Radiol 1995; 30: 724–9.

45. Ohdama S, Akagawa S, Matsubara O, Yoshizawa Y. Primary diffuse alveolar septal amyloidosis with multiple cysts and calcification. Eur Respir J 1996; 9: 1569–71.

46. Essadki O, Chartrand-Lefebvre C, Finet JF, Grenier P. Cystic pulmonary metastasis simulating a diagnosis of histiocytosis X. J Radiol 1998; 79: 886–8.

47. Thalinger AR, Rosenthal SN, Borg S, Arseneau JC. Cavitation of pulmonary metastases as a response to chemotherapy. Cancer 1980; 46: 1329–32.

48. Smevik B, Klepp O. The risk of spontaneous pneumothorax in patients with osteogenic sarcoma and testicular cancer. Cancer 1982; 49: 1734–7.

49. Stein MG, Mayo J, Müller N, et al. Pulmonary lymphangitic spread of carcinoma: appearance on CT scans. Radiology 1987; 162: 371–5.

50. Mathieson JR, Mayo JR, Staples CA, Muller NL. Chronic diffuse infiltrative lung disease: comparison of diagnostic accuracy of CT and chest radiography. Radiology 1989; 171: 111–16.

51. Heyneman LE, Johkoh T, Ward S, et al. Pulmonary leukemic infiltrates: high-resolution CT findings in 10 patients. Am J Roentgenol 2000; 174: 517–21.

52. Dodd GD, Ledesma-Medina J, Baron RL, Fuhrman CR. Post-transplant lymphoproliferative disorder: intrathoracic manifestations. Radiology 1992; 184: 65–9.

53. Ichikawa Y, Kinoshita M, Koga T, et al. Lung cyst formation in lymphocytic interstitial pneumonia: CT features. J Comput Assist Tomogr 1994; 18: 745–8.

54. Carignan S, Staples CA, Muller NL. Intrathoracic lymphoproliferative disorders in the immunocompromised patient: CT findings. Radiology 1995; 197: 53–8.

55. Shahar J, Angelillo VA, Katz D, Moore JA. Recurrent cavitary nodules secondary to Hodgkin's disease. Chest 1987; 91: 273–4.

56. Lee KS, Kim Y, Primack SL. Imaging of pulmonary lymphomas. Am J Roentgenol 1997; 168: 339–45.

57. Berkman N, Breuer R, Kramer MR, Polliack A. Pulmonary involvement in lymphoma. Leuk Lymph 1996; 20: 229–37.

58. Lewis ER, Caskey CI, Fishman EK. Lymphoma of the lung: CT findings in 31 patients. Am J Roentgenol 1991; 156: 711–14.

59. Jang HJ, Lee KS, Kwon OJ, et al. Bronchioloalveolar carcinoma: focal area of ground-glass attenuation at thin-section CT as an early sign. Radiology 1996; 199: 485–8.

60. Aquino SL, Chiles C, Halford P. Distinction of consolidative bronchioloalveolar carcinoma from pneumonia: do CT criteria work? Am J Roentgenol 1998; 171: 359–63.

61. Akira M, Atagi S, Kawahara M, Iuchi K, Johkoh T. High-resolution CT findings of diffuse bronchioloalveolar carcinoma in 38 patients. Am J Roentgenol 1999; 173: 1623–9.

62. Tan RT, Kuzo RS. High-resolution CT findings of mucinous bronchioloalveolar carcinoma: a case of pseudopulmonary alveolar proteinosis. Am J Roentgenol 1997; 168: 99–100.

63. Wolff SD, Kuhlman JE, Fishman EK. Thoracic Kaposi sarcoma in AIDS: CT findings. J Comput Assist Tomogr 1993; 17: 60–2.

64. Chojniak R, Yu LS, Younes RN. Response to chemotherapy in patients with lung metastases: how many nodules should be measured? Cancer Imaging 2006; 13: 107–12.

65. Chojniak R, Younes RN. Pulmonary metastases tumor doubling time: assessment by computed tomography. Am J Clin Oncol 2003; 26: 373–7.

66. Ko JP, Naidich DP. Computer-aided diagnosis and the evaluation of lung disease. J Thorac Imaging 2004; 19: 136–55.

67. Marten K, Engelke C. Computer-aided detection and automated CT volumetry of pulmonary nodules. Eur Radiol 2007; 17: 888–901.

68. Goldberg SN, Gazelle GS, Compton CC, Mueller PR, McLoud TC. Radio-frequency tissue ablation of VX2 tumour nodules in the rabbit lung. Acad Radiol 1996; 3: 929–35.

69. Tominaga J, Miyachi H, Takase K, et al. Time-related changes in computed tomographic appearance and pathological findings after radiofrequency ablation of the rabbit lung: preliminary experimental study. J Vasc Interv Radiol 2005; 16: 1719–26.

70. Steinke K, King J, Glenn D, Morris DL. Radiologic appearance and complications of percutaneous computed tomography-guided radiofrequency-ablated pulmonary metastases from colorectal carcinoma. J Comput Assist Tomogr 2003; 27: 750–7.

71. Bojarski JD, Dupuy DE, Mayo-Smith WW. CT imaging findings of pulmonary neoplasms after treatment with radiofrequency ablation: results in 32 tumours. Am J Roentgenol 2005; 185: 466–71.

72. Marchand B, Perol M, De La Roche E, et al. Percutaneous radiofrequency ablation of a lung metastasis: delayed cavitation with no infection. J Comput Assist Tomogr 2002; 26: 1032–4.

73. Jin GY, Lee JM, Lee YC, Han YM, Lim YS. Primary and secondary lung malignancies treated with percutaneous radiofrequency ablation: evaluation with follow-up helical CT. Am J Roentgenol 2004; 183: 1013–20.

74. Fentiman IS, Millis R, Sexton S, Hayward JL. Pleural effusion in breast cancer: a review of 105 cases. Cancer 1981; 47: 2087–92.

75. Sears D, Hajdu SI. The cytologic diagnosis of malignant neoplasms in pleural and peritoneal effusions. Acta Cytol 1987; 31: 85–97.

76. van de Molengraft FJ, Vooijs GP. Survival of patients with malignancy-associated effusions. Acta Cytol 1989; 33: 911–16.

77. Marel M, Zrustova M, Stasny B, Light RW. The incidence of pleural effusion in a well-defined region. Epidemiologic study in central Bohemia. Chest 1993; 104: 1486–9.

78. Salyer WR, Eggleston JC, Erozan YS. Efficacy of pleural needle biopsy and pleural fluid cytopathology in the diagnosis of malignant neoplasm involving the pleura. Chest 1975; 67: 536–9.

79. Rabin CB, Coleman NS. Bilateral pleural effusion and significance in association with a heart of normal size. J Mt Sinai Hosp 1957; 24: 45–53.

80. Monte SA, Ehya H, Lang WR. Positive effusion cytology as the initial presentation of malignancy. Acta Cytol 1987; 31: 448–52.

81. Sahn SA. Pleural diseases related to metastatic malignancies. Eur Respir J 1997; 10: 1907–13.

82. Chernow B, Sahn SA. Carcinomatous involvement of the pleura: an analysis of 96 patients. Am J Med 1977; 63: 695–702.

83. Rodriguez-Panadero F, Borderas Naranjo F, Lopez Mejias J. Pleural metastatic tumours and effusions. Frequency and pathogenic mechanisms in a post-mortem series. Eur Respir J 1989; 2: 366–9.

84. Xaubet A, Diumenjo MC, Marin A, et al. Characteristics and prognostic value of pleural effusions in non-Hodgkin's lymphomas. Eur J Respir Dis 1985; 66: 135–40.

85. Castellino RA, Blank N, Hoppe RT, Cho C. Hodgkin disease: contributions of chest CT in the initial staging evaluation. Radiology 1986; 160: 603–5.

86. McLoud TC, Flower CD. Imaging the pleura: sonography, CT, and MR imaging. Am J Roentgenol 1991; 156: 1145–53.

87. Moskowitz H, Platt RT, Schachar R, Mellins H. Roentgen visualization of minute pleural effusion. An experimental study to determine the minimum amount of pleural fluid visible on a radiograph. Radiology 1973; 109: 33–5.

88. Eibenberger KL, Dock WI, Ammann ME, et al. Quantification of pleural effusions: sonography versus radiography. Radiology 1994; 191: 681–4.

89. Yang PC, Luh KT, Chang DB, et al. Value of sonography in determining the nature of pleural effusion: analysis of 320 cases. Am J Roentgenol 1992; 159: 29–33.

90. Akaogi E, Mitsui K, Onizuka M, et al. Pleural dissemination in non-small cell lung cancer: results of radiological evaluation and surgical treatment. J Surg Oncol 1994; 57: 33–9.

91. Aquino SL, Webb WR, Gushiken BJ. Pleural exudates and transudates: diagnosis with contrast-enhanced CT. Radiology 1994; 192: 803–8.

92. Arenas-Jiménez J, Alonso-Charterina S, Sánchez-Payá J, et al. Evaluation of CT findings for diagnosis of pleural effusions. Eur Radiol 2000; 10: 681–90.

93. Leung AN, Muller NL, Miller RR. CT in differential diagnosis of diffuse pleural disease. Am J Roentgenol 1990; 154: 487–92.

94. Hierholzer J, Luo L, Bittner RC, et al. MRI and CT in the differential diagnosis of pleural disease. Chest 2000; 118: 604–9.

95. Gupta NC, Rogers JS, Graeber GM, et al. Clinical role of F-18 fluorodeoxyglucose positron emission tomography imaging in patients with lung cancer and suspected malignant pleural effusion. Chest 2002; 122: 1918–24.

42 Bone Metastases
David Wilson and Gina Allen

INTRODUCTION

Metastatic deposits are the hallmark of disseminated malignancy. They are in one sense diagnostic of advanced malignancy but at the same time a diagnostic conundrum. Perhaps the most common presentation of a malignant disease is pain or dysfunction resulting from metastases. As they may develop in many locations the effects on the patient are extremely variable. As a result patients may present to almost any medical or paramedical practice and metastases are often confused with other diseases.

The key clinical decisions are:

- Are the symptoms due to a metastasis?
- What other disease could cause these symptoms?
- Will the lesion cause mechanical risk to the integrity of the skeleton?
- What is the cell type?
- Is it safe to biopsy the lesion?
- Are there any safer locations for biopsy?
- Where is the primary?
- Have the metastases responded to therapy?

Imaging and image-guided biopsy have clear and important roles in responding to these questions.

All imaging techniques may be employed in this process and often more than one. Each method has its strengths, weaknesses, and potential pitfalls, or traps. In this chapter we present a pragmatic and practical approach to the management of a soft tissue mass or a bone lesion with an emphasis on metastases.

The diagnosis of metastatic malignancy is serious but the prognosis varies from under a third of patients alive six months later to almost 90% alive at one year. The difference between these groups is the result of many factors but most important of these is the tumor type (1).

MECHANISMS OF METASTATIC SPREAD

The appearance and presentation of metastatic malignancy depends on the origin of the tumor, the cell type, the degree of differentiation, the physical location of the primary lesion, and the predilection of spread via each of the following routes:

- Hematogenous
- Lymphatic
- Cavity
- Direct invasion
- Within the structure (skip lesions)

Strictly direct invasion might be regarded as expansion of the primary lesion but there are occasions when lobulation makes direct spread appear like separate deposits.

Hematogenous spread is thought to be via venous plexi and this mechanism explains deposits that center on the drainage region of the primary tumor. However remote deposits and widespread

lesions must have developed from clusters of cancer cells which have passed through the arterial system.

Lymphatic spread to the spinal column is seen more frequently on the left side of the spine due to imbalance of lymph channels between the left and right sides. However metastases in the spinal column may occur on either side (Fig. 42.1). Metastases are found more commonly in the spine (2) than in the extremities although certain tumor types predispose to extremity bone deposits (e.g., squamous cell carcinoma of the lung).

Skip lesions are deposits that occur in the same bone as the primary lesion but are physically separate. They may be regarded as intracavity spread within the marrow of one bone.

There is debate as to the mechanisms whereby tumor cells may remain quiescent for years and then appear as bone metastases. This topic has great potential for further research (3–5).

One of the main roles of histological diagnosis is to predict the likelihood and pattern of tumor spread based on knowledge of the natural history of each malignancy. Ewing sarcoma may spread via lymphatic channels to the regional lymph nodes while osteosarcoma is more likely to spread by hematogenous routes. Computed tomography (CT) of the lungs may show deposits in cases of osteosarcoma. In Ewing sarcoma, an abdominal CT is a wise supplement to lung CT as part of the routine staging.

Bone metastases are most likely to arise from malignancies of the:

- Breast
- Prostate
- Lung
- Kidney
- Gastrointestinal tract
- Primary bone sarcoma

TYPES OF METASTASES

Depending on the cell type metastases may be:

- Solid
- Glandular
- Partly cystic
- Vascularized
- Lytic
- Sclerotic
- Calcified
- Ossified

Each type of metastasis has a different imaging characteristic which can be used to predict the origin of the primary tumor or at least create a shortlist. However the essence of accurate diagnosis is histological examination and there is little practical value in spending too much effort on predicting the primary tumor from imaging alone.

Metastases will change with treatment and time. Radiotherapy may shrink sensitive deposits and they may become calcified or fibrosed. Sclerosis is common after effective chemotherapy. Necrosis, internal cavitation, and hemorrhage may occur simply because of the size of

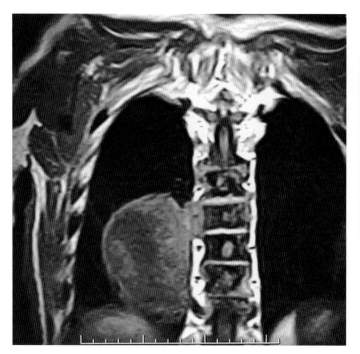

Figure 42.1 MR image of paravertebral extension of a spinal metastasis.

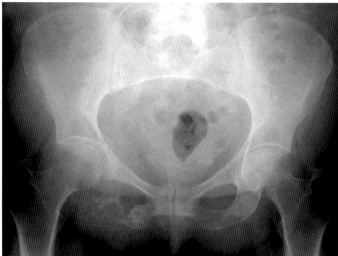

Figure 42.2 Conventional radiograph of treated metastases from carcinoma of the breast—mixed lytic and sclerotic lesions are seen.

the lesion and poor blood supply or as the result of treatment. Therapies that might lead to this change include radiation, chemotherapy, embolization, high frequency ultrasound (US), and cryotherapy.

Above all the radiologist must be aware that patients with metastatic malignancy have a poor prognosis. There is a mean survival of five years. In one study only four out of 578 patients with metastatic malignancy were disease-free after 10 years (6).

CLINICAL FEATURES OF METASTASES

As metastases have a finite size when detected, the vast majority must have been clinically silent for a considerable period of time. However with the increased use of imaging for many purposes the accidental detection of lesions by imaging is an increasingly common presentation. Symptomatic presentation depends on the location. Symptoms that may occur include:

- Pain
- Fracture through the metastasis (pathological fracture)
- Paralysis (or progressive neurological deficit) in cases of spine metastases
- Palpable mass
- Restriction of movement

Pain

Pain may be mediated by increased pressure within the bone marrow, physical pressure on adjacent structures including nerves, microfractures, or overt fractures.

Bone pain tends to be worse or more noticeable at night. It is not related to motion and has a low gnawing quality.

Neuralgic pain due to pressure or invasion of a nerve will radiate to the areas innervated and may be associated with motor and sensory loss. If nerve roots are compressed the symptoms may mimic nerve root compression due to a prolapsed intervertebral disc.

However, the compression tends to be progressive and unremitting. Neural compression due to disc prolapse fluctuates and tends to be worse after rising in the morning when the disc protrudes more.

Fractures

Fractures may be mistaken for those due to osteoporosis or straightforward trauma. The differential diagnosis of spinal fractures is covered below. In other bones the features that suggest a malignant origin as opposed to trauma alone are:

- Too little bone remaining—the holes are larger than expected for the type of fracture (Fig. 42.2)
- Unusual fracture directions—particularly transverse or "banana" fractures (Fig. 42.3) (1)
- History of insufficient trauma to cause the fracture observed (Fig. 42.4)

Paralysis (and Neural Deficit)

Compression of the spinal cord will eventually lead to paralysis (Fig. 42.5). Long tract signs present first with brisk reflexes and progressive neurological deficit. Later in the condition a sensory level may be identified where there is loss of feeling and power below the affected level. However, these signs are rarely seen at the onset and neurological clinical examination is very unreliable in determining the level of the lesion. With the advent of newer magnetic resonance (MR) systems that can achieve wide fields of view in reasonable examination times, it is prudent to examine a wide area beyond the level suspected because metastases are frequently widespread and it is therefore appropriate to examine the spine for multiple lesions. There are also occasions when the compression is at more than one level and sometimes the compression is worse at a higher level than that suggested by the symptoms. Many institutions will examine the whole spine.

Non-metastatic effects of malignancy may give symptoms of neuritis, mimic cord compression, or cause a myasthenic syndrome (e.g., Eaton Lambert syndrome in small cell carcinoma of the lung). Similarly Landry-Guillain-Barré Syndrome and demyelinating diseases are potential mimics of metastatic disease. In all these conditions imaging is important to exclude spinal cord or root compression.

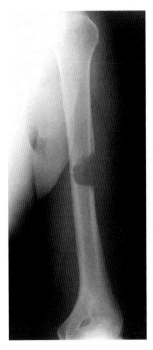

Figure 42.3 Radiograph of the humerus showing a metastasis from adenocarcinoma.

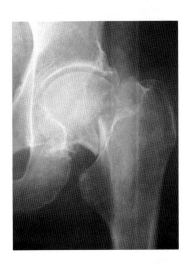

(A)

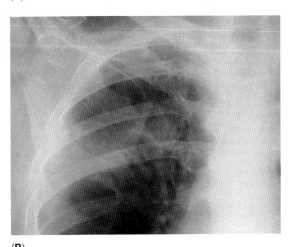

(B)

Figure 42.4 (**A**) Radiograph showing a fracture of the femoral neck. There appears to be some bone missing. (**B**) Chest radiograph in the same patient demonstrating a primary squamous cell carcinoma in the upper right zone.

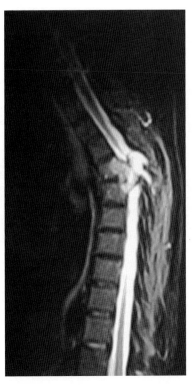

Figure 42.5 Metastases from carcinoma of the breast presenting with spinal cord paralysis due to spinal cord compression.

Although paresis is a strong indication of an overall poor prognosis the tumor type has a greater impact (7). Even in cases of paralysis there is value in determining the type of metastatic tumor.

Mass

Bone metastases occasionally present as a mass lesion. The more superficial bones in the forearm and lower leg are easily palpable and expansion will be clinically apparent (Figs. 42.6 and 42.7). The peripheral skeleton is a less common site for metastases than the axial skeleton so this presentation is relatively uncommon.

Restriction of Movement

On rare occasions the mass effect of a metastatic deposit impinges on a joint or adjacent bone and prevents a full range of motion. Joints with a wide range of excursion such as the shoulder or hip are more often affected.

Key Points: General Features

- Pain or dysfunction are the most frequent presenting manifestation of bone metastases
- Hematogenous spread is probably via the venous plexi, explaining the location of deposits in the center of the drainage area of the primary tumor
- Lymphatic spread to the spine is more common on the left side reflecting the imbalance in lymphatic channels
- Most metastases have been present for a considerable length of time before the development of symptoms declare their presence

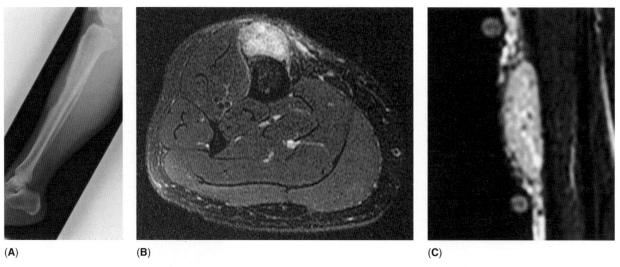

Figure 42.6 (A) Renal cell carcinoma metastasis to the tibia showing cortical destruction. (B) Axial and (C) coronal fast STIR MR images in the same patient showing low signal dots which indicate flow voids.

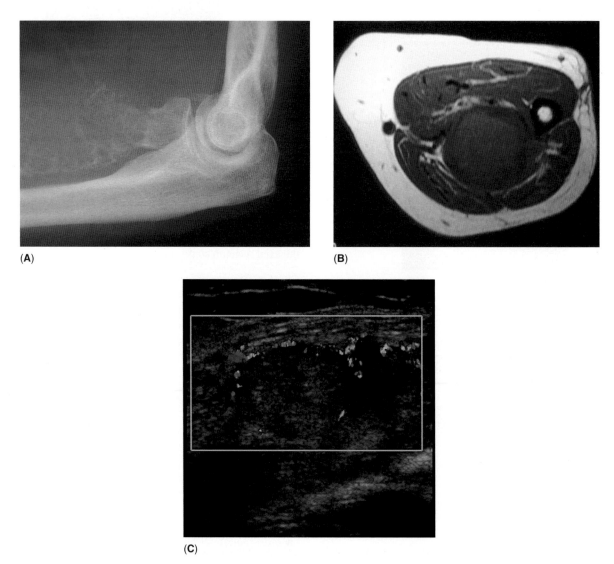

Figure 42.7 (A) Conventional radiograph of the radius showing an aggressive destructive metastasis from adenocarcinoma. (B) Axial T1-weighted MR image defines the extent of the lesion. (C) US with Doppler of this patient shows peripheral vascularization assisting in planning and guiding the biopsy route.

IMAGING METHODS

All imaging methods may detect or delineate metastases. In order of effectiveness for detection of lesions they are:

- Magnetic resonance (MR) imaging
- Bone scintigraphy (nuclear medicine) NM
- Positron emission tomography with computed tomography (PET-CT)
- Positron emission tomography (PET)
- Computed tomography (CT)
- Conventional radiography (CR)
- Ultrasound (US)

In order of their value in defining the nature of a known lesion they are:

- MR imaging
- PET-CT
- CT
- CR
- PET
- NM
- US

The logic that results in this ranking is explained below under the sections describing each method of imaging.

Magnetic Resonance Imaging

Tumors, and especially metastases, tend to contain more water than normal bone or muscle. Therefore images that are weighted to show water as white will show metastases as white (high signal intensity lesions). As fat also shows high signal intensity and marrow of bone contains a great deal of fat in the adult, there is considerable advantage in suppressing the signal from fat to make the metastases more obvious. Tumors will appear dark on conventional T1-weighted images as they replace the normal fatty marrow (Fig. 42.8).

Fat Suppression

There are two methods commonly used for fat suppression:

- STIR (short Tau inversion recovery)
- RF Fat Sat (Radiofrequency fat suppression)

Conventional STIR sequences take far too long to acquire for practical use so a variant using Fast Spin-Echo (FSE) protocols is employed—Fast STIR (FSTIR).

FSTIR sequences give uniform suppression of fat and are very sensitive to fluid. Indeed they are so sensitive that minor fluid changes in bone are observed. A long distance runner will show normal increase in the fluid in bone around joints for a few hours after a race. FSTIR images are rather grainy and of poorer resolution compared to other sequences, but remain the best way of showing early bone disease.

RF Fat Sat images utilize fast spin-echo protocols to acquire data quickly. The images will have the fine resolution of FSE but inhomogeneity effects of the magnetic field may result in areas of inadequate fat suppression within the bone marrow. Such foci may be misinterpreted as metastases. Inhomogeneity artefacts are a particular problem in the extremities: the shoulder and the hip.

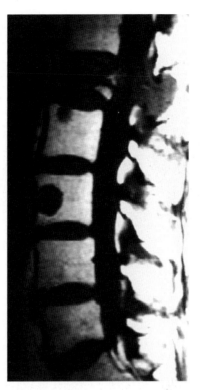

Figure 42.8 T1-weighted spin-echo MR image of the lumbar spine showing metastases as low signal intensity focal lesions replacing white fatty marrow.

MR machines vary in their ability to provide good FSTIR and good RF Fat Sat without artefact. The choice of sequence will depend on the area to be examined, the size of the patient (larger means nearer to the edge of the magnetic field), and the apparatus used. Local protocols should be drawn up as appropriate.

Sclerosis

If the metastasis is sclerotic, calcified, ossified, or fibrosed the water content will be lower or even very low. This means that the water signal will fall and on FSTIR of RF Fat Sat images deposits may be overlooked (Fig. 42.9A). However, metastases replace the normal fatty marrow with material that has low signal and any sequence that shows fat as bright will show the metastases as dark and therefore they will be obvious. The most effective sequence for fat imaging is a T1-weighted conventional spin-echo (CSE) protocol. The short TE (time-to-excitation) means that these sequences can be achieved in a reasonable time (below four minutes at 1.5T). Unfortunately many operators who wisely use fast spin-echo (FSE) to achieve good quality T2-weighted images imagine that T1-weighted FSE images are as good as CSE in detecting bone lesions. This is not the case; sclerotic metastases may disappear when switching from CSE to FSE (Fig. 42.9).

The worst sequences for bone marrow conspicuity are gradient-echo (GE). Chemical shift results from the slightly different resonant frequency of fat, water, and trabecular bone. This is exaggerated in gradient-echo imaging as the refocusing process that is uniquely used in GE increases the impact of chemical shift. This in effect blurs the images inside trabeculae and will cause areas of bone edema to disappear.

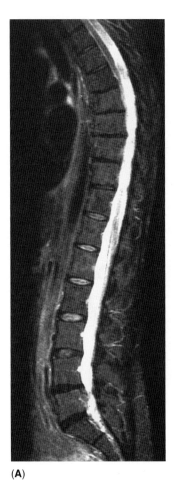
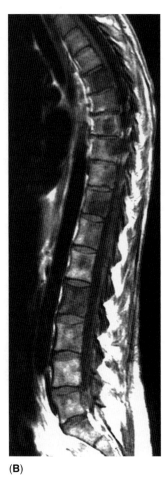

(A)   **(B)**

Figure 42.9 (A) Fast STIR sagittal MR image shows only minor low signal abnormalities—an equivocal study. (B) T1-weighted sagittal spin-echo MR image of the same patient shows multiple low signal intensity lesions due to sclerotic metastases; this appearance is seen in breast and prostate metastases.

Table 42.1 Signal Characteristics of Metastases

	FSTIR	T1SE
Most metastasis	High	Low
Sclerotic (e.g., prostate)	Low	Low
Melanoma	High	High

In summary the following guidance provides a standard optimum approach to detection of bone metastases:

- To detect fluid containing metastases—FSTIR or second best RF Fat Sat
- To detect sclerotic or fibrotic metastases—T1 conventional spin-echo (CSE)

Low Signal Intensity Areas

Malignant melanoma metastases show features that are highly characteristic, frequently permitting a definitive diagnosis to be made. They are often fluid containing metastases with high signal on the FSTIR images but, unusually, also a high signal on the T1-weighted SE images. This is due to the paramagnetic qualities of melanin. Signal intensity characteristics of metastases are shown in Table 42.1.

A rich vascular supply to a metastasis is seen as low signal "voids" within the lesion on all sequences. The vessels contain flowing blood which produces a pattern of black dots (8). This sign is highly suggestive of a renal cell carcinoma metastasis but is also seen in cases of metastasizing hemanogiopericytoma.

Increased Sensitivity

While a combination of CSE and FSTIR is a routine and practical means of detecting metastases, other sequences are required occasionally. This most frequently occurs in cases where the presence of metastases would significantly change surgical or chemotherapy decisions and all other imaging is negative. Considerable efforts have been made to improve MR imaging techniques to increase the detection of metastases (9) and current options include diffusion-weighted imaging and gadolinium-DTPA contrast agent enhancement.

Whole Body MR Imaging

Whole body MR imaging as a means of screening for metastatic disease is a recent advancement in MR which promises to be a valuable adjunct (10). The technique requires a wide field of view to encompass most of the skeleton and a series of smaller field of view images patched together electronically. A series of surface coils linked electronically may be employed (phased array). Some devices use a moving motorized table to move the area of imaging along the body.

Results of recent studies are very encouraging with respect to the sensitivity and specificity of detecting bone metastases (11).

Key Points: Magnetic Resonance Imaging

- Fat saturation techniques are the most sensitive sequences for detecting bone metastases
- Sclerotic, calcified, or osseous deposits are likely to be overlooked on fat saturation sequences but will be clearly shown on T1-weighted conventional spin-echo sequences
- Melanoma metastases frequently show a high signal on T1-weighted images
- A rich vascular supply to a metastasis is seen as signal "voids" within the lesion
- Whole body MR imaging is a recent advancement which is likely to be a useful adjunct to staging metastatic disease
- Diffusion-weighted imaging and gadolinium enhancement are evolving techniques

Bone Scintigraphy

Radiopharmaceutical agents linked to phosphate molecules equilibrate with bone. The uptake of the injected compound depends on the bone turnover and provides a map of bone metabolism. The agents most often used are Monodiphosphonate linked to Technetium 99m (Tc99m MTP), a metastable isotope with an emission at 149 KeV. This energy level is well suited to imaging using a gamma camera and may be studied by a series of images taken in different directions or by rotating the camera around the patient to acquire tomographic images (ECAT—emission computed tomography). The gamma ray emission of Tc99m MDP is absorbed and therefore attenuated by tissue. Scintillation arising from the front of the body will be difficult to detect by posterior views using conventional gamma camera imaging. Several views

overcome some of these problems but ECAT allows detailed and more precise examination of deep and complex regions. This particularly applies to the sacroiliac region and the base of the skull.

Most, but not all, metastases have different metabolic activity to normal bone and usually appear as areas of increased scintillation (hot) at the bone imaging interval of around four hours after injection (Fig. 42.10). Necrotic areas will produce scintillation voids (cold) areas. Fibrotic or calcified metastases after treatment may also create cold areas. Occasionally metastases may have the same metabolic turnover as normal bone and are therefore very hard to detect using nuclear medicine techniques.

A major advantage of bone scintigraphy is that it can easily and reliably produce images of the whole skeleton, and in general is a very sensitive technique. However, areas affected by recent trauma, infection, degeneration and in the immature skeleton, active bone growth plates will all be active (hot) and may mimic metastatic disease. This means that the technique is not specific and metastatic disease tends to be overcalled. Thus an area of abnormal activity will require additional imaging to determine the cause. Most often this will be conventional radiographs, with CT, MR imaging, or biopsy being required in certain cases.

Studies comparing whole body MR imaging with bone scintigraphy show that MR is more specific in most cases and arguably more sensitive (12) (Figs. 42.10 and 42.11). MR imaging does not carry a radiation burden and does not normally require an IV injection. MR imaging is however more difficult to interpret and has the added disadvantage that it is more likely to lead to claustrophobic intolerance of the examination.

Positron Emission Tomography

Although relatively specific for lytic metastatic deposits compared to conventional nuclear medicine, studies have shown that PET is less sensitive than bone scintigraphy for the detection of sclerotic bony metastasis typically encountered in prostate carcinoma but also in breast (13–15). The expense of PET-CT may limit its uses as a screening test but it may be employed in equivocal cases and has a role in follow-up of treated metastases.

Simultaneous acquisition of CT images allow precise anatomical placement of lesions that are active on PET and also permits electronic adjustment of the PET images to account for different tissue density and likelihood of differential photon attenuation(16). PET-CT is more accurate and more sensitive than

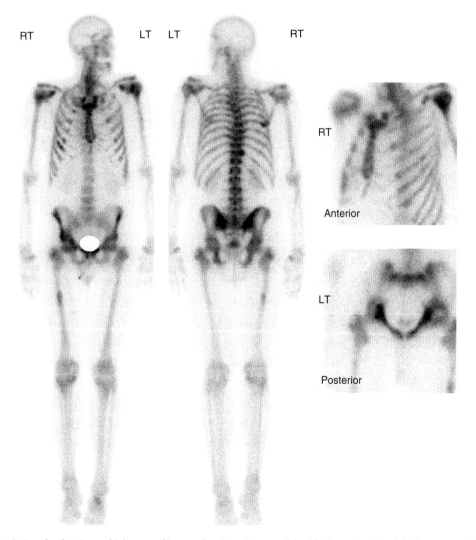

Figure 42.10 Tc99m MDP scintigraphy showing multiple areas of increased activity. Compare this with Figure 42.11C and E. The extent and severity of the metastases are probably underestimated. The renal images are low activity which is a sign that the bone has taken up a disproportionately high level of scintillations. This is termed a "superscan" and is a sign of very extensive marrow involvement.

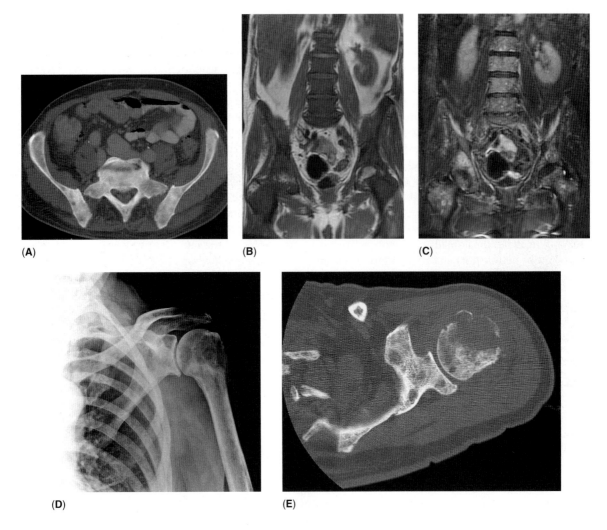

Figure 42.11 (**A**) CT of the pelvis of a patient with advanced metastatic adenocarcinoma. (**B**) T1-weighted MR image of the same patient shows extensive fatty (bright) marrow replacement by tumor. (**C**) The FSTIR images show the multiple deposits in fine detail and provide the best impression of the extent and the severity of the disease. (**D**) Conventional radiograph of the shoulder in the same patient. (**E**) CT of the same patient demonstrates the extent of bone destruction. This image allows pain relieving procedures to be considered and planned.

conventional PET but is still less accurate than bone scintigraphy or whole body MR imaging (Fig. 42.12).

Key Points: Bone Scintigraphy and Positron Emission Tomography

- Tc99mMTP bone scanning is a reliable and easily reproducible technique producing images of the whole skeleton
- In general Tc99mMTP bone scanning is a sensitive technique but arguably less sensitive than MR imaging
- False positive examinations result from degeneration, infection and recent trauma
- PET is less sensitive than conventional bone scanning in the detection of sclerotic metastases
- PET-CT is more accurate than PET in the detection of bone metastases

Computed Tomography

Before the advent of MR imaging, CT was used for the detection of metastases more frequently than it is today, but with modern multidetector CT (MDCT) scanners fast reconstruction can create images virtually instantaneously. The latest 256 detector devices can image large areas of the body at speeds fast enough to freeze motion from bowel movement or even breathing.

The technique best detects destruction of ossified areas of bone. Lytic deposits are seen as grey voids in white bone (Fig. 42.13). Sclerotic (blastic) deposits appear as whiter areas of bone. Many lesions exhibit a mixed lytic and blastic nature. Defects in the cortex are well-delineated and this is especially important for detecting lesions that may extend into dangerous areas such as the spinal canal. This is of particular relevance prior to certain interventional radiology therapies.

CT has a particular use in determining the nature of vertebral fractures and can demonstrate whether the affected bone is at risk of pathological fracture (Fig. 42.14).

IV non-ionic iodinated contrast agents may be used to enhance CT images. The margins of tumors and metastases are arguably better delineated than on unenhanced CT and the vascularity of the lesion can be judged.

CT is often used to determine whether equivocal lytic areas seen on conventional radiographs are areas of true destruction of bone. If CT of the bone is normal, metastases are very unlikely.

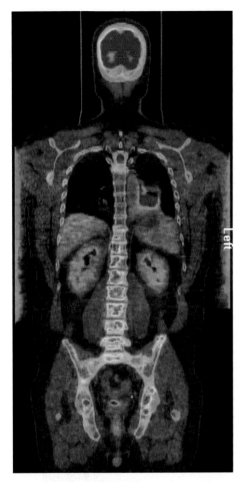

Figure 42.12 ^{18}FDG PET-CT image of a 38-year-old male. This shows a recurrent lung carcinoma with extensive metastatic disease; note radiotherapy change (hypometabolism) to the thoracic spine. *Source*: Courtesy of Dr. Kevin Bradley.

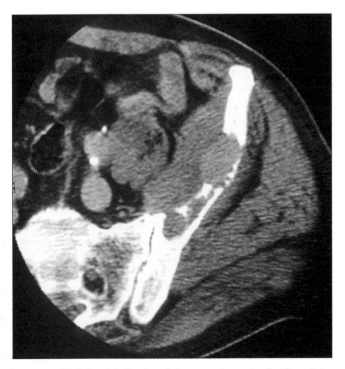

Figure 42.13 CT of the pelvis showing a lytic metastasis associated with a soft tissue mass. CT enables biopsy to be planned using a safe route.

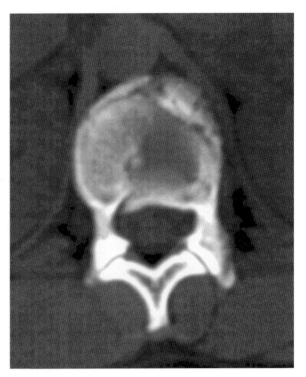

Figure 42.14 CT of the vertebral body of T12 showing cortical destruction strongly suggesting malignancy.

Conventional Radiography

Many metastases are detected using conventional radiographs, sometimes as a serendipitous (accidental) finding. Most deposits are lytic and appear as a hole in the bone (Figs. 42.2 and 42.3). Some exhibit bone expansion (Fig. 42.7A). Others are sclerotic or mixed sclerotic and lytic in appearance. The following describes the commonest conventional radiographic appearances of metastases from specific primary lesions (17).

Commonly lytic and expanded (e)
- Lung
- Renal (e)
- Thyroid (e)
- Adrenal
- Uterus
- Melanoma (e)

Commonly blastic
- Prostate
- Bladder with prostate
- Bronchial Carcinoid

Commonly mixed
- Breast
- Lung
- Ovary
- Testis
- Cervix

Conventional radiographs depend on a shadow cast by multiple overlapping trabeculae. The image is created by composite shadows and the lines seen in bone marrow represent an "interference

pattern" where the overlapping trabecular wall intersects. The lines do not represent the individual trabeculae. CT images are a more accurate assessment of individual trabeculae. This means that destructive (lytic) lesions in bone will be visible using CT or MR imaging long before the conventional radiograph is abnormal. This is especially true when there is no or minimal cortical destruction. Estimates are that a lesion must destroy over 90% of the trabeculae before it is easily seen using conventional radiographs (Fig. 42.15).

Therefore conventional radiographs are poor at screening for early disease. They will overlook many metastases that would readily be seen using other imaging methods. This is especially true in the spine so that a conventional radiograph of the spine does not exclude metastatic disease. Sacral metastases are also commonly missed due to overlying bowel gas.

Ultrasound

US examination is especially useful for the examination of soft tissues. Bone surfaces reflect all sounds and the internal structure of bone is normally not visible with this method. Therefore US examination has only a supplementary role in the examination of bone metastases. However holes in the bone are easily and accurately detected and soft tissue extension is well-visualized. Periosteal reaction will be visible using US as lamination and elevation of the normal periosteum. There may be a specific role in determining the nature of areas of activity found with bone scintigraphy, as US examination helps to distinguish metastases from fractures (18).

Unlike MR imaging and CT, US allows accurate and detailed delineation of blood vessels within soft tissue lesions by means of Doppler imaging (Fig. 42.7C). Knowledge of the degree of vascularity may assist in the differential diagnosis and will allow biopsy to be made avoiding larger vessels. US guidance is also useful when performing a biopsy of the soft tissue extension of bone metastases; this would be relatively difficult using fluoroscopy guidance.

Key Points: CT and Ultrasound

- MDCT with reconstructed images has improved the visualization of bone metastases
- Contrast enhancement may delineate deposits better than unenhanced images
- Plain radiographs only reveal metastases when approximately 90% of the trabeculae are destroyed by tumor
- US using Doppler imaging may be useful for determining the vascularity of a soft tissue mass extension of a bone metastasis and for guiding biopsy

DIFFERENTIAL DIAGNOSIS

Imaging is particularly important in determining the nature of a lesion in bone. The possible diagnoses are broadly:

- Trauma
- Multiple benign lesions
- Infection
- Infiltrations
- Focal marrow lesions

Trauma

Fractures have a cortical breach usually in linear pattern. The adjacent marrow and soft tissues are edematous. Microfractures due to bone impaction (bone bruise) may not show cortical breaches and are a particular problem when using MR imaging or scintigraphy as the primary investigation.

Options include:

- Review or performance of conventional radiographs to look for fracture lines
- CT examination—metastases will show holes in the trabecular pattern, fractures will show line defects or no change in trabecular pattern in microfracture
- Wait for several weeks and repeat the examination— fractures heal, metastases enlarge
- In exceptional cases biopsy may be indicated

Fracture through a deposit will confuse all these features. A hole that is larger than expected or unusual fracture directions are useful pointers. Biopsy may be indicated when there is doubt.

Multiple Benign Lesions

Multiple osteomata, osteopoikilosis, melorheostosis, granulomatosis, and lymphangiomatosis are examples of rare conditions that may cause confusion with metastases. If there is doubt the conventional radiographs should be reviewed first. In difficult cases CT may be helpful and if doubt persists CT should be repeated in a few weeks.

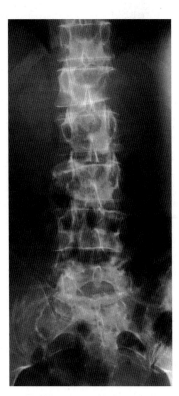

Figure 42.15 Conventional radiograph showing lytic metastases in the spine. Note the missing pedicles at L1 on the left and L3 on the right.

Sclerosing osteitis and chronic multifocal (non-infective) osteo-myelitis may affect several bones but they have typical conventional radiographic and CT appearances.

Infection

Lesions of bone caused by infection (osteomyelitis) are most often solitary. Unlike metastases the center of the lesion tends to be close to the joint (metaphyseal) or at a disc space. Both sides of the joint and disc are involved. Rare indolent infections, such as fungal infection or tuberculosis, may mimic tumor. Miliary infection is very difficult to distinguish from metastatic disease and this is more common in immunosuppressed patients. Particular care should be taken to eliminate infection in patients who are taking immunosuppressive drugs or who are suffering from acquired immune deficiency syndrome (AIDS).

Infection tends to show a variable pattern with areas of fast and slow development. Metastases contain tissue that is usually uniform and at the same stage of development. Thus a heterogeneous pattern is suspicious of infection but necrosis in metastases may look the same.

Only 30% of cases of bone infection are culture positive and histological examination is frequently more reliable. A tumor should always be cultured and histological examination performed on material deemed to be infection.

Infiltrations

Marrow replacement by any infiltrative disorder may mimic metastases.

The commonest focal lesion in the spine to mimic metastases is residual red marrow in young patients or reactivation of red marrow in debilitated or anemic patients or heavy smokers. Geographic or patchy involvement of several bones with fluid containing tissue is the typical appearance. If there is real doubt, a limited CT examination of an affected area will show no evidence of bone destruction.

Similarly leukemic and lymphomatous infiltration may mimic metastases and these conditions are also probably best investigated with CT.

Rare infiltrations such as macroglobulinemia (Fig. 42.16), Gaucher's disease, lysosome storage diseases, amyloid disease, and myelofibrosis may also appear similar to metastatic disease. Again there is no bone destruction in these cases.

Focal Marrow Lesions

Benign hemangiomata are very common in the spine (Figs. 42.17 and 42.18). They typically contain fat and vessels. MR imaging appearances are typical and are diagnostic in most cases. Thus hemangiomas are of high signal intensity on fat specific sequences (T1-SE or T1-FSE) and of low signal intensity on water specific sequences (T2-FS or T2-FSE Fat Sat or FSTIR). There are internal striae of low signal on all sequences. Atypical hemangiomata may have water content (high signal on water specific sequence (T2-SE or T2-FSE Fat Sat or FSTIR) (Fig. 42.17). In these cases CT examination will reveal no destruction of bone and sometimes "dot-like" calcified areas.

Radiotherapy may cause areas of bone necrosis and repair that can present many years after treatment. Radiotherapy damage

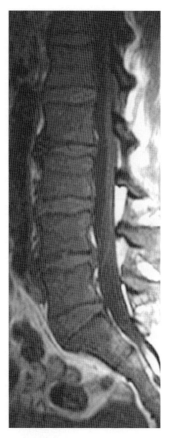

Figure 42.16 Sagittal T1-weighted MR image in a patient with macroglobulinemia resulting in diffuse replacement of fatty marrow.

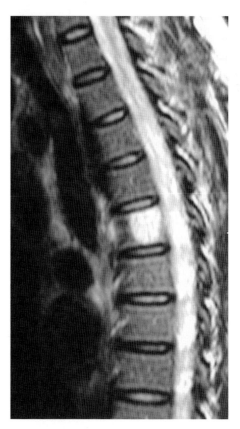

Figure 42.17 T2-weighted MR image showing a hemangioma demonstrating atypical high signal intensity.

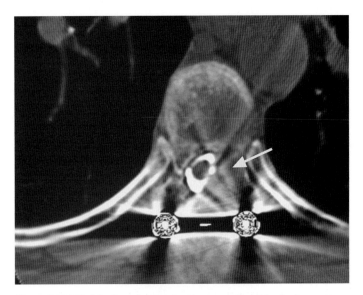

Figure 42.18 CT of the thoracic spine showing a complicated benign hemangioma with soft tissue extension into the spinal canal (arrow). This lesion has been treated by surgical decompression.

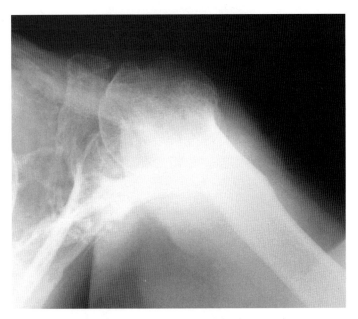

Figure 42.19 Conventional radiograph of the shoulder showing radiation necrosis. There are mixed lytic and sclerotic lesions mimicking metastases.

may also present as a progressive lesion (Fig. 42.19). As most of these patients must have been treated for malignancy there is likely to be a strong suspicion of recurrence. The mixed sclerotic and lytic pattern and the localization of the abnormal area to that of the radiation field are helpful signs. MR imaging may show fatty replacement of marrow in the treated bone area. Involvement of the soft tissues with the presence of a mass is more in keeping with recurrent disease.

On MR imaging, an acute radiation effect in the bone may be observed within the radiation field, for example, in the treatment of the axilla in patients with breast cancer the humerus may show typical appearances or in the treatment of prostate cancer acute radiotherapy changes may be seen in the pelvic bones. MR imaging shows soft tissue edema as well as bone edema. These changes

may persist for several months following treatment and should not be mistaken for "new" disease within bone.

Key Points: Differential Diagnosis

- Fractures in unusual directions cause suspicion for underlying metastasis
- Multiple benign lesions may cause confusion with metastatic disease
- Foci of infection tend to be heterogeneous whereas metastatic deposits are usually homogeneous unless they are necrotic
- Normal bone marrow in young adults can mimic metastases
- Acute radiotherapy change appears as edema within the bone marrow of the irradiated area
- Long-term effects of radiotherapy include bone necrosis with areas of repair producing a mixed sclerotic and lytic appearance on imaging

BIOPSY

Bone biopsy will provide the definitive diagnosis in most cases. As systemic therapy varies with tumor type in all but the most advanced disease, biopsy should be considered as a key step in planning treatment.

The majority of bone lesions will be accessible to image-guided bone biopsy. Key phases in the process are:

Planning
Surgeon
It is prudent to discuss the route of biopsy, especially in solitary lesions that may be excised. Seeding of tumor along the needle tract has been observed and it is therefore prudent to use a biopsy route that will be excised during surgical removal in cases where immediate excision is planned (19). Since most cases of metastatic bone disease will not be treated surgically this remains an important consideration only in a minority of cases.

Pathologist
The type of specimen required and its handling should be agreed with the pathologist in advance of the procedure. Some histopathologists prefer imprint slides taken from the fresh specimen and others ask for core biopsy. Depending on whether the pathology department is open, fresh or fixed specimens may be preferred. Some histopathology departments provide a frozen section service even for bone-containing specimens.

Imaging
In planning a bone biopsy:

- The safest site should always be sought
- The safest route of approach should be sought
- Necrotic areas should be avoided; these are usually central within the tumor
- Fractures should be avoided as the repair process of fractures may mimic mitotic activity of malignancy

Guidance

There are several alternatives for guidance of the biopsy. The preferred method will depend on the location of the lesion, the method showing the structure(s) that should be avoided (lung, vessels, nerves, bowel, bladder, spinal cord, etc.) and which the operator feels most confident using.

Fluoroscopy guidance is most often employed for bone lesions (Fig. 42.20). It allows real-time visualization of the needle and does not interfere with larger and longer needles. It does not show bowel, vessels, or lung sufficiently well to safely avoid these structures and other imaging methods will be required when the route of approach places these in the path of the needle.

CT guidance is precise and helps to avoid important structures. However, radiation dose to both the patient and the operator may be higher, the needles may protrude too far from the patient to enable a rescan to show the needle position, and the technique is limited to the axial plane. When oblique approaches are necessary, for example in the thoracic spine, it may prevent safe access.

MR imaging guidance is of limited availability but has potential advantages in that the needle track can be watched in real time and the method has other advantages similar to those of CT guidance. The open architecture scanners allow easy access with long needles.

US guidance is best for biopsy of soft tissue tumor masses as it demonstrates structures which should be avoided, shows the areas of maximum vascularity and gives real-time views of the needle as it advances. However it is not a good method for biopsy through cortical bone.

Specimens should be as large as possible. Bone cutting needles may be used but softer lesions will require side cutting soft tissue needles. Drilling devices are often required to penetrate bone. As indicated above, material should always be sent for culture and histological examination.

Preparation should cover control of coagulation defects and warnings of potential complications (allergy, infection, damage to adjacent structures, hematoma, and pain). Many biopsies can be undertaken using local anesthesia. It is important to anesthetize the periosteum, as well as the soft tissues. Some patients will require neuroleptic anesthesia and occasionally others will need full general anesthesia. It may be necessary to halt a local anesthetic procedure and recall the patient for sedation or general anesthesia.

Key Points: Biopsy

■ Fluoroscopy guidance is most commonly used for biopsy of bone lesions
■ CT guidance is accurate but limited to the axial plane
■ US guidance is frequently the best method for biopsy of soft tissue components of bone lesions

IMAGING PROTOCOLS

Screening for Metastases

Methods that are used to screen a patient for metastases must be judged by their sensitivity and specificity. The risks are of:

- Overdiagnosis
  - Degenerative disease
  - Osteoporotic collapse
  - Infection

- Omission
  - Six percent detection at best using any imaging method
  - Sclerotic metastases

Given the strengths and weaknesses of each method described above it is becoming apparent that whole body MR imaging (Fig. 42.11B and C) is likely to be the preferred method for the exclusion of metastatic deposits. However this is expensive and is rather more observer-dependent than bone scintigraphy (Fig. 42.10) which currently remains the commonest method employed in many centers.

In malignant disease where CT is used to search for organ involvement this is also an effective means of examining the bones (20). Care should be taken to review the images on bone window settings as well as for soft tissue abnormalities.

Conventional radiographs supplemented by CT or MR imaging in selected cases should be used to examine suspicious areas when abnormal activity is found on bone scintigraphy.

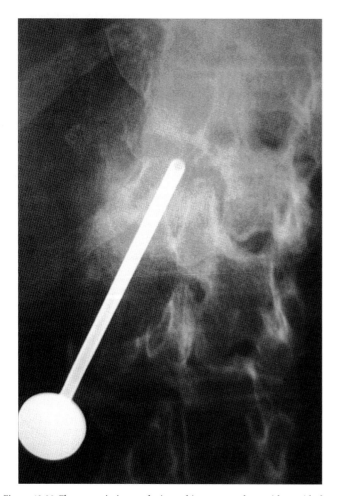

Figure 42.20 Fluoroscopic image during a biopsy procedure with a wide bore needle to obtain diagnostic specimens.

ECAT, PET, PET-CT, and US are unlikely to be used as screening methods.

After Treatment

When judging the response of a bone metastasis to local or systemic therapy it is best to employ the same modality that was used for the baseline examination prior to treatment. Ideally the study will be performed using the same machine, the same protocol and the same operator.

Occasionally if there is doubt on MR imaging or CT, IV contrast enhancement may provide additional information on disease activity.

VERTEBRAL FRACTURES

The commonest cause of spontaneous vertebral fractures is osteoporosis. As this condition affects the same age group as is affected by metastatic disease, the differentiation is important. Initially the treatment of vertebral compression fractures is symptomatic at first (analgesia and time) followed by intervention including vertebroplasty, kyphoplasty, and in rare cases surgery if there is no objective response. Both radiotherapy and systemic treatment have a place in the management of vertebral fractures. Analgesia, vertebroplasty, kyphoplasty, and surgery may also be employed in selected cases.

Signs that suggest osteoporotic fractures are:

- Different aged lesions
- Pedicles spared
- Minimal soft tissue mass
- No expansion
- Healing with time

In osteoporotic lesions recovery of the marrow to a normal fatty signal in the affected vertebra(e) is a good sign of a benign lesion. However edema and hemorrhage from an acute fracture has identical appearances to a metastatic lesion.

CT is a useful means of detecting bone destruction. Holes without a sclerotic margin are typical of metastases.

Problem cases may be resolved by waiting and rescanning after an interval. Most osteoporotic fractures heal whilst metastases progress. If delay is impractical then a biopsy may be indicated.

Multiple myeloma deserves special mention. In a small proportion of cases discrete multiple plasmacytomas appear exactly like metastases. These will be positive on nuclear medicine studies and MR imaging, and are managed the same way as metastases from other sources. However the majority of fractures in myeloma arise from tumor-induced severe osteoporosis. These fractures are treated in the same way as those from osteoporosis but the disease must also be addressed systemically. The osteoporotic type fracture is positive on nuclear medicine studies but diffuse marrow disease may be negative to bone scintigraphy. Diffuse marrow replacement showing low signal in marrow on T1-weighted studies in the older population should be investigated by serum electrophoresis, urine analysis for Bence Jones proteins and in equivocal cases by marrow aspirate.

Key Points: Vertebral Fractures

- Osteoporosis is the commonest cause of vertebral fractures
- Edema and hemorrhage resulting from fracture of an osteoporotic vertebra may mimic a metastasis
- Discrete multiple plasmacytomas may appear identical to metastases

CURRENT THERAPIES FOR BONE METASTASES

Radiotherapy

Perhaps the longest standing intervention to treat pain from metastases is radiotherapy. This often takes a few weeks to work. The method is less appropriate if there are associated fractures although sometimes there is response even in these cases (21).

Bisphosphonates

There is evidence that oral or IV bisphosphonates may reduce pain from osseous metastases (21,22).

Vertebroplasty

Currently over 250,000 patients a year in the United States and over 4000 patients in the United Kingdom are treated for painful vertebral fractures by vertebroplasty or its variants. This includes a substantial proportion of patients with metastatic malignancy or tumor-induced osteoporosis. The method is broadly the percutaneous injection of a cement to fill fracture lines and harden the affected bone (23). Pain relief of more than five points on a 10-point pain score is reported in 75% to 85% of cases. Kyphoplasty and a variety of other forms of distraction vertebroplasty are intended to decompress the fracture before cement insertion. Risks include infection, nerve root compression, paralysis, and cement embolus. However, recent large series show less than 1% overall complication rates with the serious risks being rare (see chap. 50).

Cementoplasty

Metastatic cavities in bone can be treated by percutaneous cement injection outside the spine. Sites commonly treated include the acetabular roof and the sacrum. Treating lesions in long bones by this method carries serious risk of fracture and surgical collaboration is mandatory in such cases (24).

Cryotherapy

Large lesions in bone may be treated by cryoprobe cooling to alleviate pain. Under local anesthesia two broad gauge needles are placed to bracket the deposit and are cooled by an Argon/Helium system that refrigerates the soft tissue between. Ovoids of several centimeters diameter can be frozen and the area which is being treated can be monitored by CT during the therapy. Two 10-minute cycles are typical. This method may be combined with coblation and cementoplasty to repair the structural defect (25).

Coblation

Coblation utilizes radiofrequency generated plasma in saline around the tip of a probe (called a coblation wand) which is passed percutaneously under local anesthesia through a needle into the

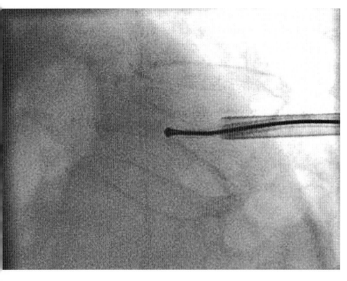

Figure 42.21 Coblation of a spinal metastasis prior to vertebroplasty in a 75-year-old patient. The primary tumor was an undifferentiated sarcoma of unknown origin. Coblation was undertaken to create a cavity within the vertebral body because there was a posterior wall defect. This reduced the risk of pushing tumor into the spinal canal. The procedure was without complication and at follow-up the patient's pain had resolved.

metastasis. Tissue for 1 mm around the wand is vaporized. Multiple passes allow the creation of a cavity which can then be filled with cement in the same way as for cementoplasty or vertebroplasty. This procedure allows treatment of lesions that could not be treated by cement injection for fear of pushing tumor tissue into the spinal canal or into a joint space. It is also argued that coblation prior to cement injection will reduce the risk of pushing tumor cells into the venous circulation (Fig. 42.21).

Key Points: Current Therapies for Bone Metastases

- Vertebroplasty involves the percutaneous injection of cement into the fracture line to harden the affected bone
- Vertebroplasty results in pain relief in 75% to 80% of patients
- The complication rate of vertebroplasty is as low as 1%
- Risks of vertebroplasty include infection and neurological deficit
- Cementoplasty, cryotherapy, and coblation are all evolving techniques for the treatment of bone metastases

Surgery

Depending on the extent, prognosis, and symptoms, excision of metastases may be considered (26,27) More commonly, reinforcement of affected long bones by intramedullary nails may be undertaken. These techniques may be combined with the percutaneous methods described above.

SEARCH FOR THE PRIMARY TUMOR

There is debate as to the advantage of searching for the primary tumor when the diagnosis of metastatic bone deposits is confirmed. In a study by Katagiri et al. (28) 64 patients with unknown primary tumors underwent clinical and laboratory tests, chest x-ray, and CT of the thorax and the abdomen. A primary

malignancy was identified in 88%. They concluded from their data and a literature review that:

- Pelvic and gastrointestinal imaging is not recommended
- Markers help with hematological and primary bone tumors
- Early skeletal biopsy is not recommended
  - Deposits may be myeloma
  - Spine deposits are common and "difficult" to biopsy
  - Histology is unhelpful

This and similar studies provide conflicting evidence (6). For example, many would argue that spine deposits are not difficult to biopsy and the histological advice depends on the team involved.

A pragmatic approach is to look for the primary tumor in cases where there is evidence that removal might lead to regression of metastases. This supposes that there is hormonally-mediated control of tumor deposits or non-metastatic effects.

Summary

- Hematogenous spread of bone metastases is thought to be via venous plexi
- Breast, prostate, lung, kidney, gastrointestinal tract, and primary bone sarcomas are the most frequent primary sites associated with bone metastases
- The majority of metastases have been present for a considerable length of time before the development of symptoms declare their presence
- Pain or dysfunction is the most frequent presenting manifestation of bone metastases. Pain is usually worse at night
- Non-spinal fractures due to metastases may show suspicious features such as too little bone remaining or unusual fracture directions particularly transverse or "banana" fractures
- Metastases may present with a mass lesion
- Fat saturation techniques are the most sensitive sequences for detecting bone metastases. T1-weighted sequences are required to visualize sclerotic, calcified, or osseous metastases
- Tc99mMTP bone scanning is a reliable and easily reproducible technique producing images of the whole skeleton
- Plain films only reveal metastases when 90% of the trabecular bone is destroyed
- MDCT with reconstructed images has improved identification of metastases
- Whole body MR imaging is a useful recent advance in the detection of bone metastases
- PET is less sensitive than conventional bone scanning in the detection of sclerotic metastases
- PET-CT is more accurate than PET in the detection of bone metastases
- Acute radiotherapy change appears as edema within the bone marrow within the irradiated area
- US guidance is frequently the best method for biopsy of soft tissue components of bone lesions
- Edema and hemorrhage resulting from fracture of an osteoporotic vertebra may mimic a metastasis
- Vertebroplasty results in pain relief in 75% to 80% of patients and the complication rate is as low as 1%

ACKNOWLEDGMENTS

We offer our thanks to Dr. Kevin Bradley, Consultant Radiologist in PET-CT, Oxford Radcliffe Hospital for his technical advice.

REFERENCES

1. Katagiri H, Takahashi M, Wakai K, et al. Prognostic factors and a scoring system for patients with skeletal metastasis. J Bone Joint Surg Br 2005; 87: 698–703.
2. Guillevin R, Vallee JN, Lafitte F, et al. Spine metastasis imaging: review of the literature. J Neuroradiol 2007; 34: 311–21.
3. Ye L, Kynaston HG, Jiang WG. Bone metastasis in prostate cancer: molecular and cellular mechanisms (Review). Int J Mol Med 2007; 20: 103–11.
4. Clezardin P, Teti A. Bone metastasis: pathogenesis and therapeutic implications. Clin Exp Metastasis 2007; 24: 599–608.
5. Clines GA, Guise TA. Molecular mechanisms and treatment of bone metastasis. Expert Rev Mol Med 2008; 10: e7.
6. Alcalay M, Azais I, Brigeon B, et al. Strategy for identifying primary malignancies with inaugural bone metastases. Rev Rhum Engl Ed 1995; 62: 632–42.
7. Hosono N, Ueda T, Tamura D, Aoki Y, Yoshikawa H. Prognostic relevance of clinical symptoms in patients with spinal metastases. Clin Orthop Relat Res 2005; 436: 196–201.
8. Choi JA, Lee KH, Jun WS, et al. Osseous metastasis from renal cell carcinoma: "flow-void" sign at MR imaging. Radiology 2003; 228: 629–34.
9. Söderlund V. Radiological diagnosis of skeletal metastases. Eur Radiol 1996; 6: 587–95.
10. Steinborn MM, Heuck AF, Tiling R, et al. Whole-body bone marrow MRI in patients with metastatic disease to the skeletal system. J Comput Assist Tomogr 1999; 23: 123–9.
11. Schmidt GP, Reiser MF, Baur-Melnyk A. Whole-body imaging of the musculoskeletal system: the value of MR imaging. Skeletal Radiol 2007; 36: 1109–19.
12. Kosuda S, Kaji T, Yokoyama H, et al. Does bone SPECT actually have lower sensitivity for detecting vertebral metastasis than MRI? J Nucl Med 1996; 37: 975–8.
13. Peterson JJ, Kransdorf MJ, O'Connor MI. Diagnosis of occult bone metastases: positron emission tomography. Clin Orthop Relat Res 2003; 415(Suppl): S120–8.
14. Schirrmeister H. Detection of bone metastases in breast cancer by positron emission tomography. Radiol Clin North Am 2007; 45: 669–76, vi.
15. Cook GJ, Houston S, Rubens R, Maisey MN, Fogelman I. Detection of bone metastases in breast cancer by 18FDG PET: differing metabolic activity in osteoblastic and osteolytic lesions. J Clin Oncol 1998; 16: 3375–9.
16. Nakamoto Y, Cohade C, Tatsumi M, Hammoud D, Wahl RL. CT appearance of bone metastases detected with FDG PET as part of the same PET/CT examination. Radiology 2005; 237: 627–34.
17. Rosenthal DI. Radiologic diagnosis of bone metastases. Cancer 1997; 80(8 Suppl): 1595–607.
18. Paik SH, Chung MJ, Park JS, Goo JM, Im JG. High-resolution sonography of the rib: can fracture and metastasis be differentiated? AJR Am J Roentgenol 2005; 184: 969–74.
19. Chen YJ, Chang GC, Chen WH, Hsu HC, Lee TS. Local metastases along the tract of needle: a rare complication of vertebroplasty in treating spinal metastases. Spine 2007; 32: E615–E618.
20. Akin O, Hricak H. Imaging of prostate cancer. Radiol Clin North Am 2007; 45: 207–22.
21. Ural AU, Avcu F, Baran Y. Bisphosphonate treatment and radiotherapy in metastatic breast cancer. Med Oncol 2008; 25: 350–5.
22. Riccio AI, Wodajo FM, Malawer M. Metastatic carcinoma of the long bones. Am Fam Physician 2007; 76: 1489–94.
23. Burton AW, Hamid B. Kyphoplasty and vertebroplasty. Curr Pain Headache Rep 2008; 12: 22–7.
24. Basile A, Giuliano G, Scuderi V, et al. Cementoplasty in the management of painful extraspinal bone metastases: our experience. Radiol Med 2008; 113: 1018–28.
25. Gillams A. Tumor ablation: current role in the liver, kidney, lung and bone. Cancer Imaging 2008; 8(Suppl A): S1–S5.
26. Lin PP, Mirza AN, Lewis VO, et al. Patient survival after surgery for osseous metastases from renal cell carcinoma. J Bone Joint Surg Am 2007; 89: 1794–801.
27. Talbot M, Turcotte RE, Isler M, et al. Function and health status in surgically treated bone metastases. Clin Orthop Relat Res 2005; 438: 215–20.
28. Katagiri H, Takahashi M, Inagaki J, Sugiura H, Iwata H. Determining the site of the primary cancer in patients with skeletal metastasis of unknown origin: a retrospective study. Cancer 1999; 86: 533–37.

43 Liver Metastases
Claus Koelblinger, Gerald Lesnik, Ahmed Ba-Ssalamah, and Wolfgang Schima

INTRODUCTION

The liver is the most common site of metastatic disease of epithelial tumors, the primary sites being predominantly in the colon, the breast, the lung, the pancreas, and the stomach (1). Only infiltration of regional lymph nodes occur more frequently. The true prevalence of metastatic liver disease is unknown, but in autopsy series liver metastases are detected in up to 70% of cancer patients (1,2).

Early detection and correct characterization of liver metastases is of utmost importance in patients with malignancies, particularly with regard to prognosis and further management. In general, the presence of liver metastases indicates non-resectability of the primary tumor and chemotherapy becomes the treatment of choice. In the majority of cases, however, surgery of the primary tumor is still performed for palliation of local complications (e.g., to relieve obstruction of the gastrointestinal tract). Nonetheless, resection of liver metastases has been shown to improve patient survival for a few malignancies (3). In patients with colorectal cancer with isolated liver metastases, which are present in roughly 25% of cases at the time of diagnosis of the primary tumor, partial liver resection offers the only chance of cure. The five-year survival rates following surgery typically range between 25% and 40% compared to 0% to 10% in patients from the same group treated conservatively (3–6). In patients with solitary colorectal liver metastases five-year survival rates of more than 70% have been reported after resection (7). However, only a minority of patients (10–15%) with colorectal liver metastases are amenable for resection due to the number, location, and size of the metastases or other clinical parameters. Therefore, accurate imaging plays a crucial role in identifying patients who may benefit from surgery, and also in preventing unnecessary surgery by identifying features like vessel invasion or extrahepatic disease which contraindicate surgery.

In patients with suspected liver metastases treated with chemotherapy high quality imaging is also crucial. It is essential to assess therapy response by providing reproducible results, which allows accurate measurement of tumor burden. Therefore an ideal radiologic examination in patients with suspected liver metastases should provide:

- High sensitivity and specificity
- Should be of low cost, non-invasive, and able to detect extrahepatic disease

With the advent of antiangiogenesis agents in chemotherapy, imaging should provide not only morphological but also functional information about metastatic liver disease in the future.

This chapter will discuss imaging options and their appropriate use in patients with liver metastases, the appearance of liver metastases and their differential diagnoses on different imaging modalities. It will also provide an overview of the pathophysiological background and future trends.

PATHOPHYSIOLOGY, MORPHOLOGY, AND CONTRAST MEDIA ENHANCEMENT OF LIVER METASTASES

The liver is extremely vulnerable to metastatic invasion, not only because of the high blood flow out of both the systemic arterial and the portal venous system but also local growth factors, preferential tumor cell adherence to the endothelium, and the specific configuration of the endothelial lining of the hepatic sinusoids, which allows communication with the extracellular matrix (2). Detection of focal liver lesions with imaging methods depends on the demonstration of morphological or physiological differences between the lesion and the liver parenchyma. Differences in the microscopic structure, which produce an increased or decreased number of reflective surfaces result in hyper- or hypoechogenicity of the lesion, which can be detected with ultrasound (US). In general, compared to normal liver parenchyma, liver metastases possess a lower amount of glycogen and a greater water content, which are responsible for the hypoattenuating appearance (Fig. 43.1) of most larger liver metastases on unenhanced CT scans and the typically decreased signal intensity on T1-weighted and increased signal intensity on T2-weighted MR images (8,9). Metastatic lesions may calcify, contain melanin (seen in metastases from melanoma) or mucin (produced by metastases from mucinous carcinomas of the pancreas or the ovaries) or, rarely, show intralesional hemorrhage. Tumor necrosis is quite common in liver metastases, especially after successful chemotherapy treatment and in rapidly growing lesions.

In the normal liver 20% to 25% of the total blood flow is supplied by the hepatic artery and the remainder by the portal vein (10–12). Clinically detectable liver metastases receive a blood supply almost exclusively from the hepatic artery (13,14). Animal models have shown that in micrometastases (0–2 mm) there is a stepwise change from direct diffusion over portal perfusion, to mixed portal and arterial perfusion, and finally to arterial perfusion in accordance with a stepwise tumor neovascularization (15). Consequently the proportion of portal blood flow in patients with liver metastases is decreased which can be detected experimentally in overt as well as occult metastases (16,17). Assessment of the hepatic blood flow *in vivo* using CT or MRI may play a role in the future especially in the treatment response assessment of liver metastases in patient receiving antiangiogenesis chemotherapy (18).

Following intravenous (IV) injection of a bolus of contrast medium, three different phases of enhancement are distinguished in hepatic imaging: (*i*) arterial, (*ii*) portal-venous, and (*iii*) equilibrium phase. The onset and duration of the different phases varies among patients and is dependent on the cardiac output, the patient's weight, volume of extracellular space, and the concentration, volume, and flow rate of the contrast medium. Typically arterial-phase images are produced between 25 and 30 seconds after the start of contrast medium injection; the time ranges for the portal venous, equilibrium, and the delayed phases are at 60 to

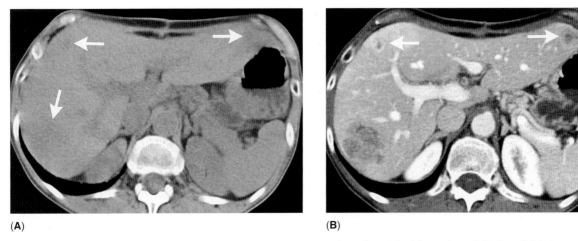

(A)   **(B)**

Figure 43.1 Hypovascular colorectal liver metastases: improved delineation at contrast-enhanced CT. (A) With unenhanced CT three slightly hypoattenuating lesions in the right and left liver lobe (arrows) are vaguely depicted. (B) In the portal venous phase image these lesions are predominantly hypovascular with rim enhancement, typical for colorectal metastases (arrows).

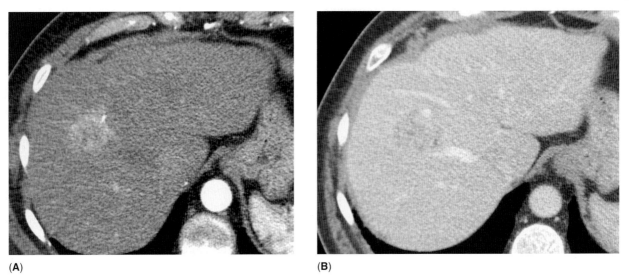

(A)   **(B)**

Figure 43.2 Hypervascular liver metastasis in a patient with renal cell carcinoma. (A) Arterial phase CT scan shows a hypervascular inhomogeneous lesion suspicious for a hypervascular metastasis. (B) Due to rapid CM-washout the lesion becomes iso- to slightly hypoattenuating in the portal-venous phase and is less conspicuous.

Table 43.1 Vascularization of Liver Metastases

Hypervascular lesions
Neuroendocrine tumors (carcinoid, insulinoma, pheochromocytoma, etc.)
Thyroid carcinoma
Renal cell carcinoma (RCC)
Breast carcinoma (small lesions, rarely)
Melanoma
Sarcomas

Hypovascular lesions
Adenocarcinoma (GI tract, pancreas, lung)
Breast carcinoma
Squamous cell carcinoma (ENT, lung, anus)
Lymphomas

70 seconds, 120 to 180 seconds, and at 5 to 10 minutes after starting contrast media injection, respectively.

In the arterial phase, strong enhancement of the hepatic artery but only slight enhancement of the liver parenchyma is visible due to the dilution effect of unopacified portal venous blood. *Hypervascular lesions* are hepatic tumors that receive a greater arterial blood supply than normal liver parenchyma, so called hypervascular lesions, show significant enhancement and are therefore best depicted in this phase (Fig. 43.2). Metastases from hepatocellular carcinoma, renal cell carcinoma, breast cancer, neuroendocrine tumors, and sarcomas typically show this enhancement pattern (Table 43.1). The flow rate of the contrast medium injection is an important factor in the production of arterial-phase images and should be at least 4 mL/sec in CT scanning to achieve optimum image quality.

The portal venous phase is reached as contrast medium enhancement via the portal vein becomes dominant and the liver parenchyma shows maximal enhancement. To obtain optimal contrast medium enhancement in this phase the contrast medium volume (and therefore the total iodine load) is more important than the flow rate. The majority of liver metastases are less vascular (hypovascular lesions, i.e., receive less portal venous blood) than the normal liver parenchyma and are delineated best in the portal venous-phase (Fig. 43.1).

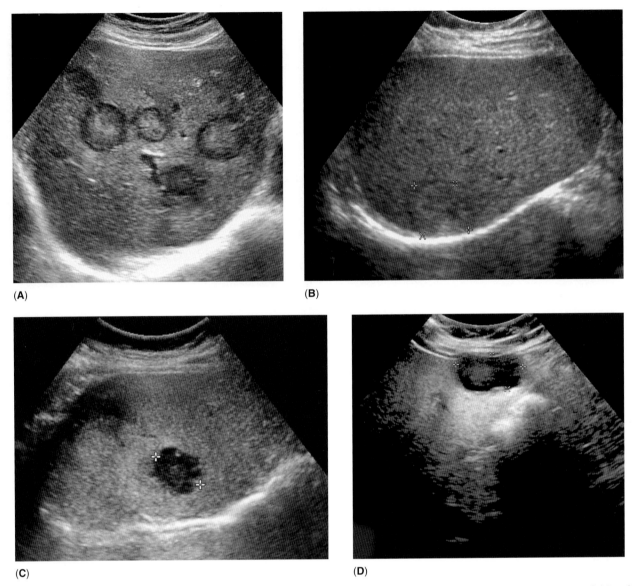

Figure 43.3 Different echogenity of liver metastases in US. Metastases may present as (**A**) hyperechogenic, sometimes with a hypoechogenic rim, (**B**) isoechogenic, (**C**) hypoechogenic, or (**D**) anechoic/cystic lesions on grey-scale US.

Hypervascular lesions, however, may become less conspicuous or even be obscured in the portal venous-phase due to washout of contrast material received in the arterial phase (Fig. 43.2).

The equilibrium or interstitial phase is dominated by diffusion of contrast material into the interstitium. Contrast enhancement is present in almost all solid lesions at this point, which is better used for lesion characterization than for lesion detection.

Key Points: Pathophysiology, Morphology, and Contrast Media Enhancement of Liver Metastases

- Blood supply of the liver parenchyma is predominantly by the portal vein, whereas clinically detectable metastases are almost exclusively fed by the arterial system
- Liver metastases can be detected by imaging due to differences in the microscopic structure and blood supply

- Contrast-enhanced imaging is characterized by different phases: arterial, portal-venous, equilibrium and delayed phases
- Most liver metastases are "hypovascular"; "hypervascular" metastases are quite typical for specific primary tumors (e.g., RCC, thyroid, NET, melanoma)

SONOGRAPHY

Grey-Scale, Doppler, and Tissue Harmonic Ultrasound

Real-time ultrasound (US) provides a rapid and non-invasive method to examine patients with suspected right upper quadrant disease. Hepatic metastases may be hypoechogenic, hyperechogenic, isoechogenic, anechogenic (cystic), or of mixed echogenicity (Fig. 43.3) (19). They usually do not exhibit distal shadowing or enhancement. The hypoechoic pattern is the most common

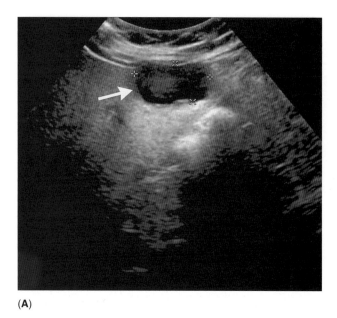

(A)

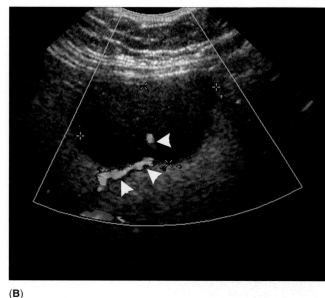

(B)

Figure 43.4 Color-coded US may be helpful for lesion characterization. (A) Grey-scale US shows a cystic lesion (arrow) with slightly irregular margins in a patient with ovarian cancer (arrow). (B) Doppler US demonstrates lesion vascularization (arrowheads), which allows the confident diagnosis of a cystic liver metastasis.

and it is observed in any type of primary tumor. Hyperechoic metastases are typically found in metastases of GI tract and vascular primary tumors where numerous vessel interfaces account for hyperechogenicity. Sensitivity of standard grey scale US for detecting liver metastases is generally quite low (between 53% and 66%) and may drop to 20% for lesions smaller than 10 mm (20–22). Therefore, several technical efforts to increase the diagnostic power of US have been made.

Color flow Doppler imaging is used to assess vessel patency, the direction of the blood flow, and the discrimination of vessels and dilated bile ducts. It does not improve lesion detection but can be helpful in differentiation of cystic and solid lesions (Fig. 43.4). Typical US enhancement patterns for large focal nodular hyperplasia (FNH) and hepatocellular carcinoma (HCC) have also been described (23).

Tissue harmonic imaging detects the reflected harmonic response (usually the second harmonic) of a transmitted pulse and, depending on the used technique, allows a reduction of the artefacts from the body wall, improved signal-to-noise ratio, and better axial resolution due to the higher receiver frequency (24,25). Compared with standard grey-scale US it provides better image quality and increases the detection rate of focal liver lesions (24).

Contrast-Enhanced Ultrasound

Clinically useful US contrast agents, which consist of gas-filled microbubbles typically smaller than 8 μm surrounded by a stabilizing layer and dissolved in water, were introduced in the mid 1990s (26,27). After IV injection, depending on the sound pressure, different mechanisms augment the grey-scale and Doppler signals of up to 30 dB in the vascular system for several minutes as the microbubbles do not leave the intravascular space as they are blood pool agents (28). Moreover, some contrast agents additionally show a hepatosplenic uptake, probably due to uptake in the reticuloendothelial system or pooling in the sinusoids after the vascular enhancement has faded (= liver-specific agents) (29–31).

Contrast-enhanced ultrasound (CEUS) allows dynamic imaging not only as a single acquisition in the arterial, portal-venous, and delayed-phases but also with a very high temporal resolution. Similar to contrast-enhanced dynamic CT and MR, different focal liver lesions show characteristic enhancement features. Metastases are either hypoechogenic or hyperechogenic in the arterial-phase and usually hypoechogenic in the portal venous and the delayed vascular-phase due to contrast agent washout (Fig. 43.5) (31,32). Benign lesions like hemangiomas (Fig. 43.6) typically show sustained enhancement in the portal-venous and delayed vascular-phases (31,32).

Compared to standard grey-scale US, CEUS allows better detection (Fig. 43.7) and characterization of focal liver lesions. In the study by von Herbay et al. the use of CEUS improved the sensitivity and specificity of US in the differentiation of malignant versus benign lesions from 78% to 100% and from 23% to 92%, respectively (33). In a large multicenter study the addition of contrast-enhanced US increased the sensitivity of detection of metastases on a per lesion basis from 71% with standard US to 87% with CEUS (34). However, intraoperative US, the accepted standard-of-reference in comparative imaging studies, was available in only a small number of patients or not at all in these studies (34,35). According to these data the European guidelines for the use of contrast agents in US recommend their use in oncologic patients to clarify a questionable lesion detected at baseline examination (36). Moreover, CEUS is recommended in every oncology patient referred for liver US unless clearly disseminated disease is present at baseline examination. CEUS has the same limitations as conventional US. It is user-dependent, has limitations in the visualization of segmental distribution and 3D-shape of metastases, and is particularly problematic in obese patients and those with severe steatosis due to limited sound penetration into the liver.

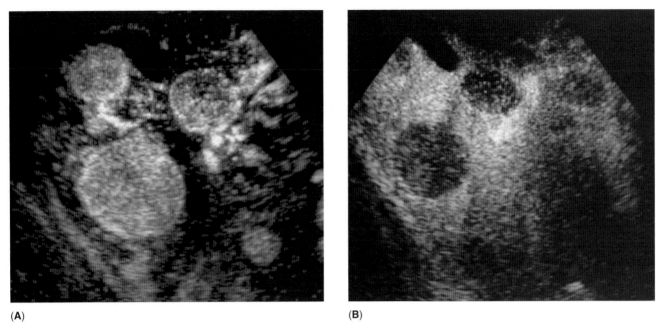

(A)   **(B)**

Figure 43.5 US contrast-media enhancement is different. (**A**) Even hypoechoic metastases appear hyperechoic in the arterial phase due their arterial blood supply. (**B**) There is rapid contrast material wash-out in the portal-venous phase.

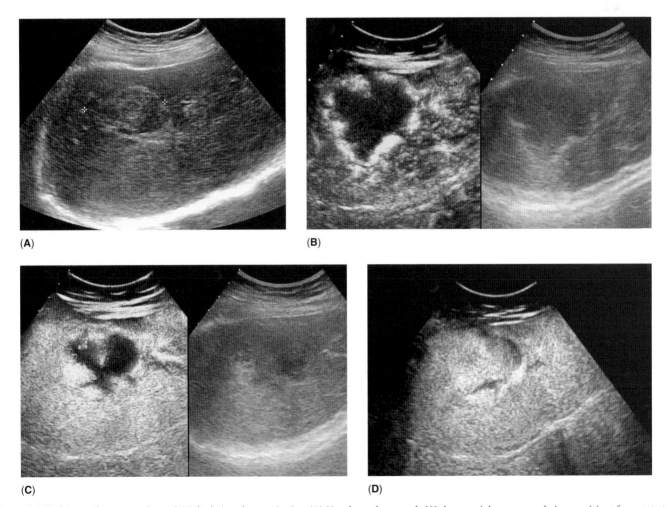

(A)   **(B)**

(C)   **(D)**

Figure 43.6 Usefulness of contrast-enhanced US for lesion characterization. (**A**) Unenhanced grey-scale US shows an inhomogenous lesion suspicious for a metastasis in a patient with known cancer. After CM injection (**B**) the lesion demonstrates peripheral, nodular enhancement in the arterial phase. (**C**) The portal venous and (**D**) delayed phase images demonstrate a progressive centripetal fill in, typical of a hemangioma.

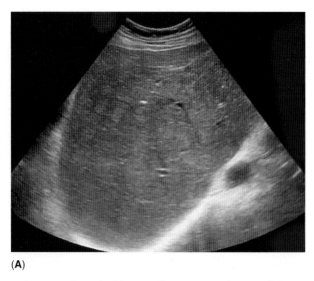 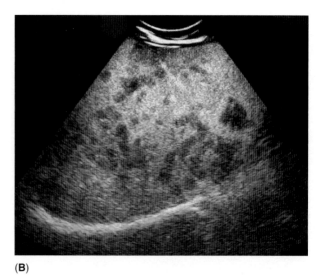

(A)   (B)

Figure 43.7 Contrast-enhanced US improves liver metastases detection. (A) On unenhanced US metastases are hardly visible. (B) Contrast-enhanced US in the portal-venous phase shows the lesions much better and allows the detection of multiple additional metastases.

Key Points: Sonography

- Most liver metastases are hypoechoic on grey-scale sonography
- CEUS markedly improves the specificity and sensitivity of grey-scale sonography
- In every patient with cancer referred for liver US contrast media injection is recommended unless disseminated disease is obvious

MULTIDETECTOR-ROW CT (MDCT)

Computed tomography (CT) is the most widely used imaging modality for detection and characterization of hepatic metastases. With the advent of four-row detector scanners in 1998 it became possible to scan the entire liver within one breath-hold of 10 to 14 seconds. Nowadays scanners with up to 320 detector rows are available and most institutions use MDCT technique for CT imaging. Therefore the focus of this paragraph is on MDCT and single-detector CT is not discussed.

How Many Scans Are Necessary?

There is an ongoing debate whether an unenhanced-phase in CT imaging of the liver is necessary (37–39). Unenhanced-phase images may be very helpful for the detection of calcified metastases, which are present in up to 11% of patients with colorectal liver metastases, and the differentiation of small simple cysts (40). Arterial-phase imaging improves the detection of hypervascular liver metastases and is helpful for differentiation of benign (FNH or hemangioma) and malignant (metastases) focal liver lesions (41–44). The portal-venous-phase has to be included in each CT examination of the liver as detection of hypovascular metastases, which represent the large majority of hepatic metastases, is best in this phase (41–44). Interstitial-phase imaging may help in the differentiation between small cysts and solid tumors. Solid tumors show some contrast enhancement in this phase, which renders the margin of these lesions blurred in contrast to the clear margin of the non-enhancing cyst. It can also aid in the

differentiation between small hypervascular metastases and hemangiomas which show pooling in this phase (44).

Therefore, in our institution the imaging protocol of the first CT scan of patients with suspected liver metastases includes unenhanced, arterial, and portal-venous phase images. For follow-up studies only arterial-dominant and portal-venous phase scans are required. Equilibrium-phase images in the delayed-phase are not routinely acquired because of the additional scanner time and increased radiation exposure. In principle, detection of focal liver lesions is dependent on the lesion-parenchyma contrast and image noise. Thinner sections provide a better contrast between small liver lesions and liver parenchyma due to a smaller partial-volume effect (45). On the other hand, the image noise increases with the reconstruction of thinner sections. The value of using thin slices to improve the detection of liver metastases has been evaluated in several studies. Weg et al. showed that the use of 2.5 mm thick sections results in a significant increase (22–86%) in the detection rate of small (<1 cm) liver lesions compared to 5, 7.5 and 10 mm thick sections (46). In the study of Kopka and Grabbe a slice thickness of 3.75 mm proved to be superior to 5 mm in terms of lesion detection, and superior to 7.5 mm in terms of lesion detection and characterization (47). Decreasing the section thickness to 1 mm does not further improve lesion detection because of the deterioration of image quality due to the increase of image noise (45). Therefore a slice thickness of 2–4 mm is recommended for axial viewing. However, with the newer MDCT scanners (from 40 rows and up) the acquisition of isotropic voxels and the reconstruction of multiplanar reformations (MPR) with excellent spatial resolution are possible. To benefit from these capabilities, all CT scans need to be acquired with thin sections to be reconstructed as high quality MPRs.

Invasive CT Techniques

CT During Arterial Portography

CT during arterial portography (CTAP) is performed by a selective injection of contrast material in the superior mesenteric and/or splenic artery some 30s before CT scanning is started. This creates a purely portal venous contrast enhancement and metastases,

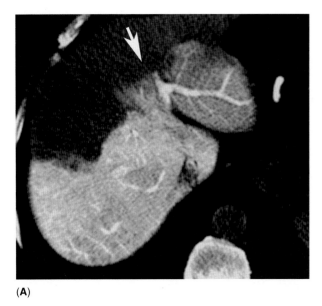

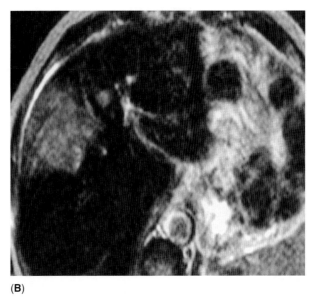

(A) (B)

Figure 43.8 CTAP: false-positive diagnosis (A) CTAP shows a large confluent hypoattenuating area affecting the liver segments VIII and IV (arrow) suspicious for a large metastasis. (B) Ferucarbotran-enhanced T2w-MRI demonstrates one large metastasis with a small satellite lesion at the border between segments VIII and IV, but shows normal liver parenchyma in segment IV, which was confirmed at surgery. Therefore a normal right instead of an extended right hepatectomy was performed.

due to their lack of portal venous blood supply, appear hypoattenuating during CTAP. Combined with thin-section helical imaging, CTAP is extremely sensitive for the detection of even small hepatic lesions. Due to the fact that nearly all lesions including benign tumors will be hypoattenuating, the specificity of CTAP is quite low. This can be improved with biphasic scanning. The presence of tiny pseudolesions, caused by perfusion anomalies like portal perfusion defects, arterio-portal shunting, portal venule obstruction or compression effect, are other drawbacks of CTAP which are responsible for high false-positive rates of up to 25% (48,49). Furthermore, contrast-enhanced new CT techniques and MR almost reach the sensitivity of CTAP and offer similar accuracy due to the lower rate of false-positives (Fig. 43.8) (48–51). Additionally, CTAP is not routinely performed anymore because of its invasive character.

CT During Hepatic Arteriography
CT during hepatic arteriography (CTHA) is performed by a selective injection of contrast material in the hepatic artery during CT scanning. Due to their mainly arterial blood supply, hepatic metastases appear hyperattenuating during CTHA. This technique is occasionally still performed for the detection of small hepatocellular carcinomas; for all other indications it has been replaced by CT scanning after administration of IV contrast medium.

Key points: MDCT

- The baseline examination requires an unenhanced, arterial-phase and portal-venous-phase CT scan; protocols for follow-up scans may be tailored according to the primary tumor
- A slice thickness of 2 to 4 mm is optimal for axial viewing
- Additional thin sections (1 mm or less) allow the reconstruction of multiplanar reformation with excellent spatial resolution

MAGNETIC RESONANCE IMAGING (MRI)

With its inherent high soft tissue contrast, provision of biochemical (e.g., fat content) and anatomical information, multiplanar imaging and sensitivity to blood flow, and blood-breakdown products, MR imaging represents a powerful tool in liver imaging. Moreover gadolinium-enhanced MR minimizes the risk of contrast-induced nephropathy inherent to iodinated contrast material used for CT scanning (52). However, the decreased risk of contrast-induced nephropathy is to some extent being counterbalanced by a higher risk of developing nephrogenic systemic fibrosis in patients with renal insufficiency (53,54). Therefore, in this patient group (glomerular filtration rate, GFR < 30 mL/min/1.73m^2), the use of gadolinium-based MR contrast agents should be avoided and non-gadolinium-based, liver-specific contrast agents such as mangafodipir, or ferumoxide (see section "Liver-Specific Contrast Agents") should be administered instead. Although several studies showed that MR is superior to CT regarding detection and classification of focal liver lesions, its use lags far behind that of CT, mainly because of cost and availability problems (55–60).

MR Imaging Technique

One of the major challenges of MR imaging of the abdomen and especially of the liver is to overcome motion artifacts secondary to respiration, peristalsis, and cardiac and aortic pulsation. Therefore, imaging is either performed with navigator-triggered or with breath-hold sequences. In breath-hold technique, periods of up to 20 seconds are possible in relatively healthy patients. However, in patients in a worse general condition shorter breath-hold periods have to be sought, either by reducing the number of slices (i.e., using thicker slices) or by decreasing the matrix (i.e., using lower spatial resolution). Phased-array torso coils are now standard in body MR imaging and field strength of 1.5 T or more is preferable.

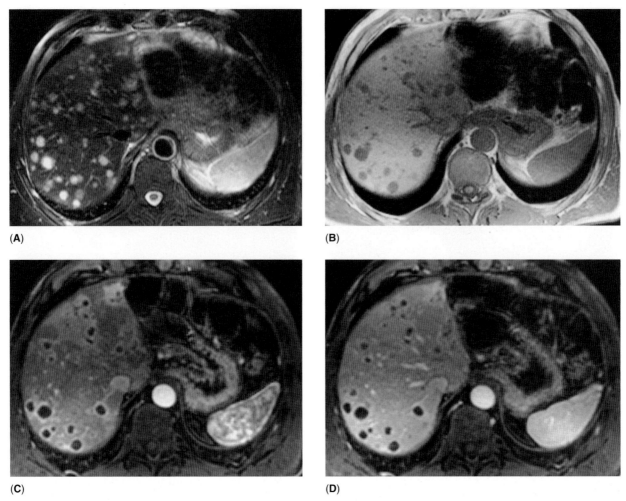

Figure 43.9 Multiple liver metastases from pancreatic adenocarcinoma. (**A**) Axial T2-w images show multiple hyperintense metastases, (**B**) which are hypointense on unenhanced T1-w in-phase images. (**C**) The lesions show marked rim enhancement in the arterial phase, which (**D**) fades in the portal-venous phase. Wegde-shaped hyperperfusion areas in the arterial phase are caused by tumor stenosis/occlusion of portal vein branches.

The standard MR imaging protocol should always include unenhanced T1- and T2-weighted and contrast-enhanced sequences. To assess the fat content of the liver parenchyma and to show focal steatosis or fatty sparing in diffuse steatosis, unenhanced T1 weighted in- and opposed-phased GRE sequences are necessary. Turbo-spin echo (TSE) or fast-spin echo (FSE) with fat saturation is preferred for T2-weighted imaging. They show better tissue contrast than single-shot TSE sequences, which on the other hand are less susceptible to artefacts and, therefore, may be used instead in patients with limited breath-hold capability. For detection of focal lesions a TE of approximately 80 to 100 msec is chosen. In addition, heavily T2-weighted pulse sequences with a long TE or single-shot TSE (HASTE) may be of help in the differentiation between solid (e.g., metastases) and non-solid (e.g., hemangioma, cysts) lesions (61,62). For dynamic imaging after contrast media, T1-weighted GRE sequences, preferably a 3D GRE fat sat technique is employed with better spatial resolution.

T1- and T2-weighted MR
Typically liver metastases are hypointense on T1-weighted images and slightly hyperintense on T2-weighted images because of their extracellular matrices that harbor abundant free water. However,

the signal intensities of hepatic metastases can vary. Whenever liquefactive necrosis or high amounts of mucin are present within the metastasis the signal intensity increases on T2-weighted images (Fig. 43.9). Also, cystic hepatic metastases, for example, from ovarian cystadenocarcinoma, will present with similar high signal intensity on T2-weighted images. For small metastases of this kind only dynamic gadolinium-enhanced imaging may help to differentiate from small cysts or hemangiomas. In metastases with coagulation necrosis, fibrous matrix or calcifications, the signal intensity on T2-weighted images decreases and these lesions may appear isointense or even hypointense. Finally, blood-breakdown products, after subacute intralesional hemorrhage or melanin (in metastases from melanomas), typically increase the signal intensity of the lesion in T1-weighted images (Fig. 43.10) (8).

Diffusion-Weighted MRI
Due to increased cellularity and complex intratumoral matrices, water molecule diffusion is restricted in most types of liver metastases which can be utilized by diffusion-weighted MR imaging (DWI). Several studies have shown that the use of DWI can improve the detection of focal liver lesions (Fig. 43.11) (63–65). Even as an adjunct to MR with liver-specific contrast agents, DWI

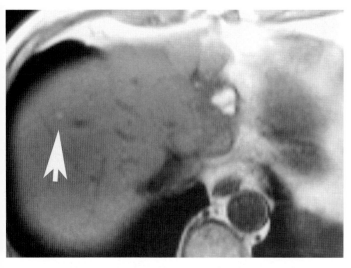

Figure 43.10 Melanoma metastases: The T1-w in-phase GRE image shows a large hyperintense lesion adjacent to the resection plane after left segmentectomy. There is another tiny lesion seen in the right lobe (arrow).

may improve lesion detection (64,66). DWI may also help in the characterization of focal hepatic lesions using the apparent diffusion coefficient (ADC) (67–70). Moreover, quantitative DWI has been shown to be a useful tool to assess early treatment response in animal studies (71–73).

ADC values in liver metastases are reported to range from 0.85 to 2.85 [$\times 10^{-3}$ mm²/sec], which may partly reflect the influence of the used b factor (sec/mm²) (63,67,69,70,74,75). Low b factors (50–100 sec/mm²) lead to an overestimation of the ADC value as the capillary lesion perfusion is not excluded, whereas high b factors (800–100 sec/mm²) cause underestimation (69,74,76). The commonly used EPI sequences are very sensitive for image artifacts, especially at higher field strengths (3.0 T). DWI of the liver is therefore preferably performed at 1.5 T. To compensate for breathing, these sequences are either obtained in a single shot breath-hold or navigator triggered technique. Nevertheless, pulsation of the heart and the aorta still influences the ADC value, which is reflected by a different value in the right and the left lobes (67,69). Moreover, large, centrally necrotic metastases may show different ADC values within a single lesion with a high diffusivity in the necrotic center and restricted diffusion in the viable tumor rim (Fig. 43.12). In these

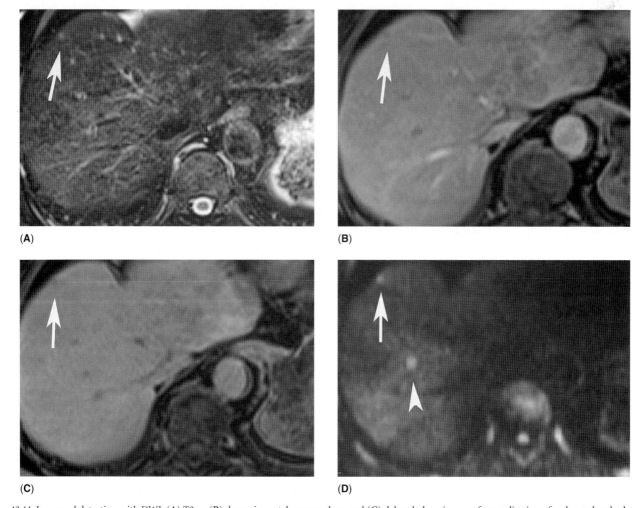

(A)

(B)

(C)

(D)

Figure 43.11 Improved detection with DWI. (A) T2-w, (B) dynamic portal venous phase and (C) delayed phase images after application of gadoxate barely show a subcapsular lesion in segment 4 (arrows), which can easily be missed. (D) DW image (b = 800) clearly depicts the surgery proven subcapsular metastasis (arrow). The second, centrally located lesion (arrowhead) is also delineated with higher conspicuity than on the other pulse sequences.

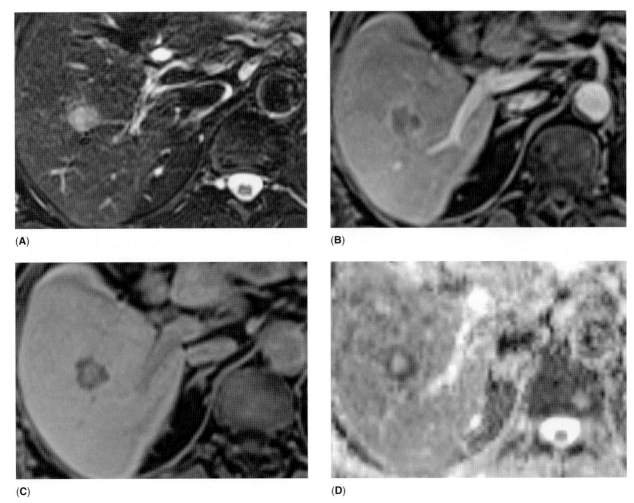

(A)

(B)

(C)

(D)

Figure 43.12 Different diffusion within one metastasis due to central necrosis. (A) After chemotherapy the colorectal metastasis is still hyperintense on T2-w. (B) Dynamic Gd-enhanced arterial phase image shows early peripheral enhancement, with (C) delayed central enhancement and peripheral wash-out in the equilibrium phase. (D) ADC map shows restricted diffusion in the periphery and increased diffusion in the necrotic, central part which is consistent with the dynamic imaging properties.

lesions the average ADC value of the lesion is misleading. The extent of necrosis itself is probably the reason why ADC values of hepatic metastases can be slightly higher and not significantly different to or lower than that of normal liver parenchyma, and that smaller hepatic metastases show lower ADC values than larger ones because they are less necrotic (67–70). To obtain a deeper insight into the correlation between ADC values and morphology/pathophysiology of liver metastases, and the possible applications in routine liver MR imaging, however, further research is necessary.

Gadolinium Chelate-Enhanced MRI

Non-specific gadolinium chelates (extracellular contrast agents) are distributed rapidly in blood vessels and extracellular spaces after an IV bolus injection, and liver lesion enhancement patterns are similar to those obtained with iodinated contrast-enhanced CT. Several agents are available and are injected intravenously as a bolus at a standard dosage of 0.1 mmol/kg body weight. Routinely dynamic axial T1W GRE images are obtained at least in the arterial (approximately 20 seconds post-injection), the portal venous (approximately 60 seconds post-injection) and the equilibrium phase (three to five minutes post-injection). Most liver metastases are hypovascular and similar to CT, and can be best delineated in

the portal venous phase. Some metastases, especially from renal and neuroendocrine primaries, are hypervascular (Table 43.1) and therefore best seen in the arterial phase. The equilibrium phase is important for lesion characterization. Hemangioma typically show persistent contrast material pooling at this time-point, whereas most metastases appear hypointense or centrally isointense with peripheral washout (61). Cystic metastases can appear smaller with a blurred edge in the equilibrium phase compared to the non-enhanced images (due to contrast material wash-in into the tumor periphery), which helps in the differentiation of metastases from simple cysts and biliary hamartomas. According to Danet and colleagues, the two most common patterns of enhancement of both hypo- and hypervascular metastatic lesions in the arterial phase are peripheral ring enhancement (72%) and heterogeneous enhancement (17%) (77). Homogeneous arterial enhancement was typically found in small (<1.5 cm) hypervascular lesions, whereas larger metastases (>3 cm) tend to appear heterogeneous. In the portal-venous and the delayed-phase images, 64% of the metastases showed an incomplete central progression of lesion enhancement, 13% appeared isointense, and 21% showed progression to central hyperintensity not always accompanied by peripheral washout, which makes differentiation

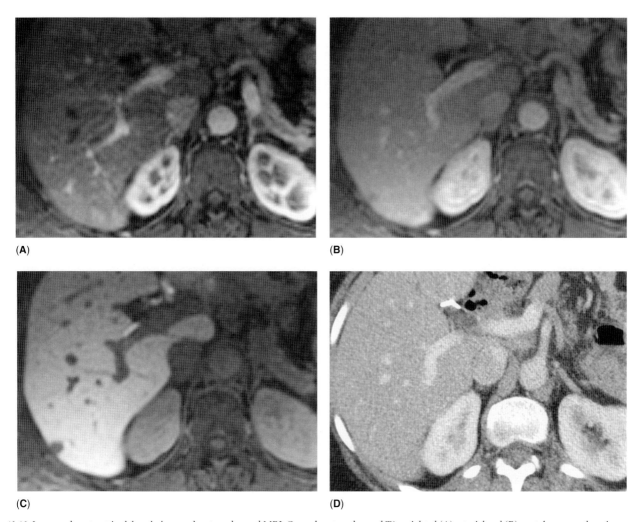

(A)

(B)

(C)

(D)

Figure 43.13 Improved contrast in delayed phase gadoxate-enhanced MRI. On gadoxate-enhanced T1-weighted (A) arterial and (B) portal-venous phase images a small subcapsular metastasis is barely visible. (C) On delayed phase (20 min p.i.) T1-W image the lesion can be depicted easily due to a much better lesion-parenchyma contrast. (D) On the portal-venous phase CT scan the metastasis is not visible.

from a hemangioma by gadolinium-enhanced images alone diffi- cult. Perilesional enhancement is typically found in hypovascular metastases either with a wedge-shaped pattern, probably resulting from portal venous obstruction (Fig. 43.9), or a circumferential perilesional pattern, which is thought to result from sinusoidal compression of adjacent tissue (78).

Liver-Specific Contrast Agents

In contrast to the non-specific gadolinium chelates, which are distributed into the extracellular space, liver-specific contrast agents are taken up intracellularly either by hepatocytes (hepa- tobiliary contrast agents) or by Kupffer cells, for example, cells of the reticuloendothelial system of the liver [superparamag- netic iron oxide-based contrast agents (SPIO)]. Some contrast agents combine extracellular and hepatobiliary properties (hybrid contrast agents).

Hepatobiliary Agents

Hepatobiliary agents represent a group of different paramagnetic molecules of which a fraction is taken up by hepatocytes and excreted into the bile. Mangafodipir trisodium (Teslascan®, GE Healthcare) is a manganese-based T1-shortening contrast agent.

Most of it is taken up by hepatocytes but smaller fractions are also taken up by the pancreas and the adrenal glands (79,80). After a short IV infusion of over 10 to 20 minutes, an enhancement pla- teau in liver signal intensity is reached within 20 minutes from the start of the infusion and persists for several hours. Overall about 50% of mangafodipir is excreted via the bile (81). In general, focal non-hepatocellular lesions (i.e., metastases) do not enhance post- contrast, resulting in a better lesion to parenchyma contrast and improved lesion conspicuity. Mangafodipir-enhanced MR has been shown to be superior to unenhanced MR and helical CT for detection of liver metastases (80,82).

Gadobenate dimeglumine (MultiHance®, Bracco, formerly known as Gd-BOPTA), and gadoxate acid (Primovist®, Bayer-Schering, formerly known as Gd-EOB-DTPA), are hybrid gadolinium-based contrast agents carrying a lipophilic ligand (81). After IV bolus injection these agents show rapid biphasic liver enhancement similar to that of non-specific gadolinium chelates. Due to their ligand a fraction is taken up by the hepatocytes, which leads to a rise in hepatic signal intensity. Meanwhile the interstitial contrast agent component is washed out, which results in increasing contrast between the liver and non-hepatocellular lesions (i.e., metastases) on delayed-phase images (Fig. 43.13). Gadoxate with

Table 43.2 Metastasis Detection Rates: CT and MR with Liver-Specific Contrast Agents from Selected Publications

Author, year	Number of lesions	Type of lesions	CT	Plain MRI	Enhanced MRI	
			Sensitivity	Sensitivity	Contrast agent	Sensitivity
Bluemke et al., 2005 (129)	189	Metastases	65%	68%	Gadoxate	77%
Hammerstingl et al., 2008 (130)	302	Metastases, mixed[a]	70%	–	Gadoxate	73%
Bartolozzi et al., 2004 (55)	128	Metastases	71%	72%	Mangafodipir	90%
Koh, 2008 (66)	83	Metastases	–	–	Mangafodipir	81%
Kim et al., 2006 (57)	55	Metastases	80%	–	Ferucarbotran	95%
Ward et al., 2005 (60)	215	Metastases	76%	–	Ferucarbotran	87%
del Frate et al., 2002 (83)	37	Metastases	–	–	Ferucarbotran	97%
del Frate et al., 2002 (83)	37	Metastases	–	–	Gadobenate	81%
Pirovano et al., 2000 (87)	94	Metastases	–	54%	Gadobenate	73%

[a]Of the overall 302 lesions 172 were metastatic lesions.

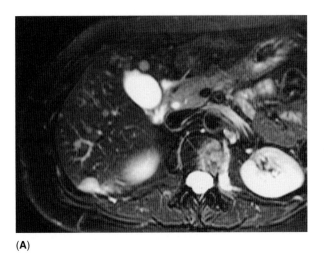
(A)

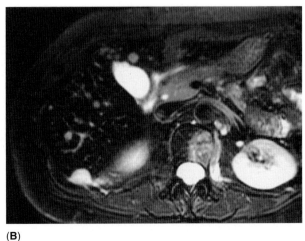
(B)

Figure 43.14 Improved visualization of metastases on SPIO-enhanced images. (A) Unenhanced T2-TSE FS image shows several hyperintense metastases. (B) On ferucarbotran-enhanced image the liver parenchyma shows considerable signal loss which improves delineation of small metastases. Incidental note is made of a bone metastasis.

a biliary excretion rate of about 50% is taken up by the hepatocytes relatively rapidly and, therefore, imaging in the delayed or liver-specific phase can be started as soon as 20 minutes after injection of contrast medium. Only about 4% of gadobenate is excreted via the bile. Therefore the signal intensity of hepatocytes continues to rise for 60 to 90 minutes after gadobenate injection and delayed-phase imaging should not be started before 60 minutes after injection. In contrast to gadobenate, which has only very limited uptake into the liver parenchyma and is thus administered at the standard dose of 0.1 mmol/kg bodyweight, gadoxate with its strong hepato-biliary uptake is approved at a dose of 0.025 mmol/kg bodyweight, which limits its usefulness for dynamic liver imaging. It has been shown that the detection of liver metastases is improved through additional delayed-phase imaging compared to dynamic imaging for gadobenate and compared to non-enhanced MR for gadoxate (Table 43.2) (83–87).

Reticuloendothelial Agents

All reticuloendothelial system (RES) agents are superparamagnetic iron oxide-based contrast agents (SPIO). They are predominantly phagocytosed by the Kupffer cells in the liver and in the spleen and cause local field inhomogeneities, which in turn shorten T2 relaxation times and thus decrease SI of the liver and spleen on T2-weighted pulse sequences. Currently, two SPIO agents [ferumoxide, Endorem®, Guerbet (Europe) or Feridex, Berlex (United States); ferucarbotran, Resovist®, Bayer Schering] are available for liver imaging. Ferucarbotran, which has fewer side effects than ferumoxide, is administered as an IV bolus and dynamic T1-weighted images can be obtained to assess lesion vascularization similarly to non-specific gadolinium chelates (88). However, ferucarbotran has been withdrawn from the market in 2009. Different T2-weighted sequences including a TSE fat sat and a T2* GRE sequence, which most pronounces the susceptibility effect of the SPIO agents, are obtained before and at least 10 minutes after contrast media injection. The liver parenchyma, containing Kupffer cells, shows a marked decrease in signal intensity after SPIO administration, whereas metastases and other tumors lacking Kupffer cells do not change their signal intensity. Therefore, metastases appear more hyperintense compared to the black background liver parenchyma on the postcontrast T2-weighted images (Fig. 43.14) (89). It has been shown that the detection of liver metastases is improved with SPIO-enhanced MR compared to non-specific gadolinium-enhanced and to gadobenate-enhanced MR (Table 43.2) (60,83).

Key Points: MR Imaging

- Contrast media administration is essential for identification of liver deposits on MRI
- The administration of liver-specific contrast agents improves the detection of liver metastases and is useful for lesion characterization
- Diffusion-weighted imaging may further improve detection (at least at 1.5 T)

RADIOLOGICAL ASSESSMENT OF TREATMENT RESPONSE

Chemotherapy and the RECIST Criteria

Imaging plays a major role in the evaluation of treatment response of liver metastases in patients who receive chemotherapy. Due to its availability, diagnostic accuracy, and reproducibility, CT is the method of choice to assess treatment response of liver metastases during chemotherapeutic regimens. MR is also a valuable method for tumor monitoring, for example, if there are contraindications to the use of iodine contrast media, but special care has to be taken that the different examinations are performed at the same magnetic field strength and, if possible, also with the same MR device (90). Tumor staging or follow-up with US is not valid because of operator-dependency and the low reproducibility of this method.

So far, in most cases, a change in size is still the main criterion in radiological tumor response evaluation. The WHO definitions have been the criteria most commonly used by investigators all over the world (91). However various modifications and clarifications to the WHO criteria led to a situation where response criteria were no longer comparable among research organizations. Therefore in 2000 new guidelines to evaluate the response to treatment in solid tumors and response evaluation criteria in solid tumors (RECIST) were implemented (90). Primarily, these guidelines were developed to compare different clinical trials and not for use in daily clinical practice, because outside the context of a clinical trial it might be appropriate to make a distinction between "clinical improvement" and "objective tumor response." According to the RECIST criteria, at the baseline scan tumor lesions are categorized into measurable ("target") and non-measurable ("non-target") lesions. At CT the images should be reconstructed with a slice thickness of 5 mm and measurable lesions are defined as lesions that can be accurately measured in at least one dimension with the longest diameter more than 10 mm (twice the CT slice thickness). All other lesions are non-target lesions, including lesions smaller than 10 mm, ascites, pleural/pericardial effusion, leptomeningeal disease, and cystic lesions. On the baseline image, the sum of the longest diameter of all target lesions, representing the tumor burden, is calculated. Up to a maximum of two target lesions per organ and five target lesions in total, representative of all involved organs, are assessed. All other lesions should be identified and recorded as non-target lesions.

In contrast to the WHO criteria, which relied on two perpendicular dimensional measurements, the RECIST criteria requires only one dimensional measurement. The criteria for target lesions are as follows:

- Complete response (CR)—disappearance of all target lesions
- Partial response (PR)—at least a 30% decrease in the sum of the longest diameter of target lesions compared with the baseline image (Fig. 43.15)
- Progressive disease (PD)—at least a 20% increase in the sum of the longest diameter of target lesions, with the baseline measurement as a reference, or any new lesion (Fig. 43.16)
- Stable disease (SD)—change in size too small to qualify for partial response or progressive disease (Fig. 43.17)

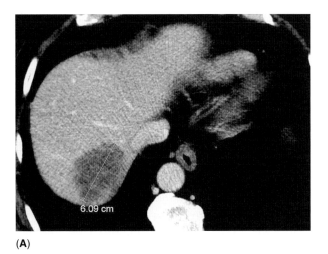

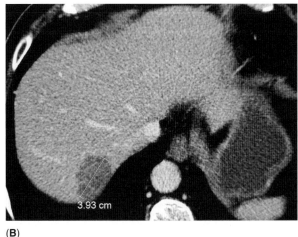

(A)   (B)

Figure 43.15 Partial response after neoadjuvant chemotherapy in a patient with a solitary colorectal liver metastasis. (**A**) Baseline CT scan shows a large liver metastasis in segment 7. (**B**) Preoperative three-month follow-up scan shows a significant decrease in size (–36%), which is defined as a partial response according to RECIST.

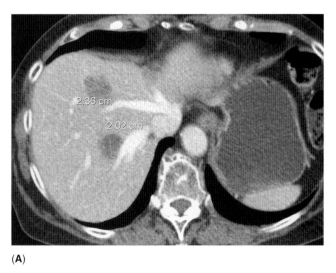

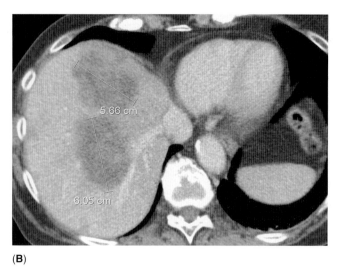

(A)   **(B)**

Figure 43.16 Progressive disease-RECIST. (**A**) CT-scan after chemotherapy and (**B**) six-month follow-up scan. There is an increase of the sum of the longest diameter from 4.4 to 11.7 cm (more than 20%) indicating progressive disease using RECIST.

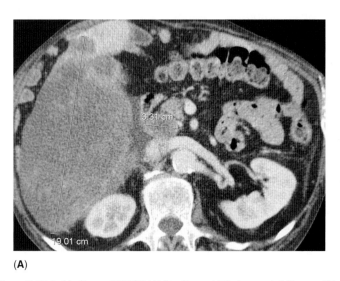

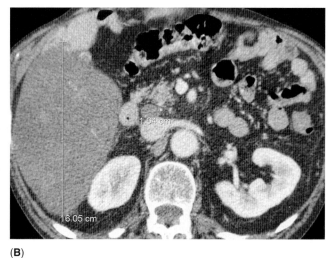

(A)   **(B)**

Figure 43.17 Stable disease-RECIST. (**A**) Baseline and (**B**) six-month follow-up CT-scans. Although there is a substantial decrease of the sum of the longest diameter of the target lesions (liver metastasis and metastatic lymph node) from 22.3 to 19.7cm (= −12%) it is stable disease (less than 30% decrease) according to RECIST.

The evaluation criteria for non-target lesions are as follows

- Complete response (CR)—disappearance of all target lesions and normalization of tumor marker levels
- Stable disease (SD)—persistence of one or more non-target lesions and/or the maintenance or raised tumor marker levels
- Progressive disease (PD)—appearance of new lesions and/or unequivocal progression of existing non-target lesions

For a complete radiological tumor response assessment, both target and non-target lesions have to be evaluated. If discrepancies in different treatment responses are measured in both groups the worse response determines the overall assessment.

These criteria raise the question as to whether the radiological disappearance of liver metastases means that there are no viable tumor cells persisting at these sites. This has been investigated for patients with liver metastases from colorectal cancer and although a complete response has been shown to be a good prognostic factor with a survival advantage compared to patients with partial

response, in about 80% of patients with complete response seen on imaging, viable cancer cells are present in resected specimens or *in situ* recurrence can be observed after one year (92,93). Sometimes, however, the converse applies: a partial response at imaging with lesions still being visible may yield total necrosis at evaluation of the surgical specimen (i.e., a complete response at histology) (Fig. 43.18).

For the evaluation of response in metastastic gastro-intestinal stroma tumors (GISTs) under imatinib therapy, size criteria are unreliable as these tumors are unlikely to shrink even after successful chemotherapy. As Benjamin et al. stated, "We should desist using RECIST, at least in GIST" (94). Choi et al. have proposed an adaptation of the RECIST criteria which takes the change of CT density of liver metastases under therapy into account (94,95). According to the Choi criteria, a partial response is defined by a decrease in CT density of more than 15% (reflecting tumor necrosis upon chemotherapy) independent of size changes or a decrease in size (sum of longest diameter of target lesions) of at least 10% (Fig. 43.19). These criteria are promising in early response

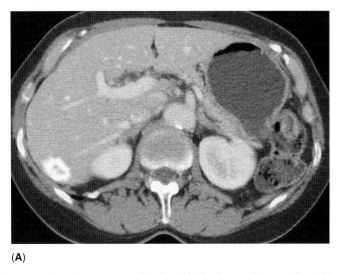

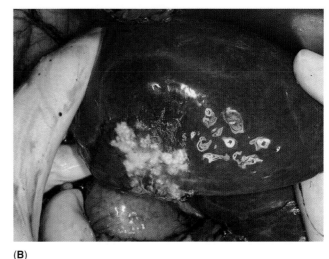

(A) **(B)**

Figure 43.18 Complete response at histology. (A) On the portal-venous phase CT-scan a residual calcified mass is seen after chemotherapy. (B) However, at histological assessment of the surgical specimen complete tumor necrosis was found.

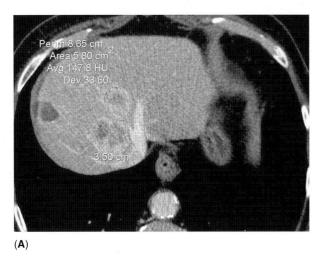

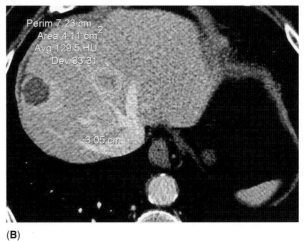

(A) **(B)**

Figure 43.19 Choi criteria for treatment response evaluation of GIST under imatinib therapy. (A) Axial portal-venous phase CT scan shows two liver metastases from a GIST with marked rim enhancement. (B) Three-month follow up scan shows a decrease in size of one lesion of more than 10%. The other lesion demonstrates a decrease in CT density (HU) of more than 10%. Therefore both lesions show partial response according to the Choi criteria. After RECIST the lesions would have been rated as stable disease.

evaluation and have excellent prognostic value in this special patient population, superior to RECIST criteria and comparable to FDG-PET evaluation.

Key Points: Radiological Assessment of Treatment Response

■ RECIST criteria using unidimensional measurements of target lesions are generally used for radiological assessment of treatment response

■ Even in patients with complete response by imaging (no malignant lesion visible any more) viable tumor cells are still present in up to 80% of patients

■ For response evaluation of gastrointestinal stromal tumors (GIST), the Choi criteria, which rely more on contrast enhancement than on lesion size, should be used instead of RECIST

Imaging After Surgery, Radiofrequency Ablation (RFA), and Radiation

For patients with resectable colorectal liver metastases (CRCLM) hepatic resection is the treatment of choice associated with low morbidity and mortality, and has reported five-year survival rates of up to 70% (7). Radiofrequency ablation (RFA) is an alternative treatment option in patients who refuse surgery or in whom surgical resection is contraindicated for medical reasons. Even in small metastases, local recurrence rates are significantly higher after RFA when compared to surgery (3% vs. 31%, for metastases smaller than 3 cm). Combined with other factors such as promotion of intrahepatic proliferation of residual metastatic cells and heat-sink effects next to vessels, surgery results in significantly better survival rates for patients (7,96–98). Therefore, despite proposals to the contrary, RFA has to be considered as a palliative rather than a curative treatment option, and the indications have to be chosen carefully (99,100).

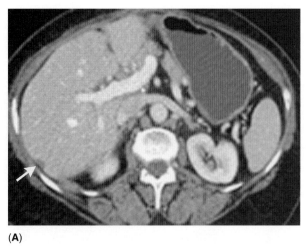
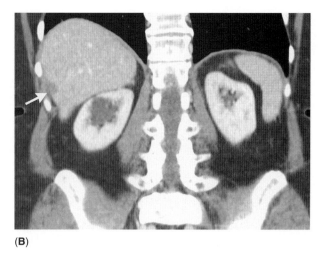

(A)   **(B)**

Figure 43.20 Typical defect after atypical liver metastasis resection. (**A**) Axial and (**B**) coronal contrast-enhanced CT scans show a subcapsular hypodense liver lesion (arrows), which is typical for a postoperative defect because of its cone shape.

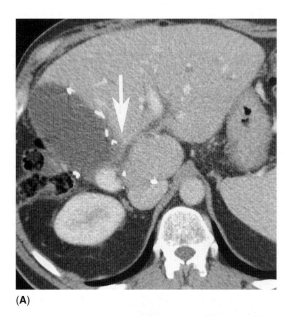
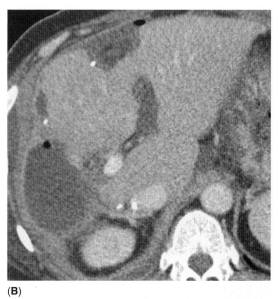

(A)   **(B)**

Figure 43.21 Post-operative complications: biloma vs. abscess. (**A**) On the CT-scan a large circumscribed fluid collection, suspicious for a biloma next to the resection margin is visible on the three month follow-up CT scan. The lesion compresses the left hepatic bile duct (arrow), which leads to mild intrahepatic bile duct dilatation. (**B**) The large fluid collection next to the resection margin demonstrates rim enhancement on the contrast-enhanced CT scan. Moreover air collections within the lesion are still present (on the 10th post-operative day). The patient had a recent onset of fever, which makes the lesion highly suspicious for a post-operative abscess.

The detection of tumor recurrence and treatment complications following RFA and surgery relies almost exclusively on imaging. CT is the method of choice because it may detect treatment complications, incomplete tumor ablation, local tumor recurrence, and remote tumor progression. After hepatic lobe resection (typically either left or right lobe hepatectomy) the anatomic situation of the remnant liver may be quite different to the presurgical situation because of compensatory growing of the liver tissue left *in situ*. Following resection there is a hypodense, wedge-shaped subcapsular region with water-like CT density (Fig. 43.20), which usually shrinks over time. Without prior imaging studies, however, it might be impossible to differentiate small postsurgical defects from simple liver cysts. Fluid collections in the resection bed are a typical finding immediately after hemihepatectomy. If they don't resolve on follow-up scans or show a distinct round shape the presence of a biloma has to be suspected (Fig. 43.21).

In rare cases, abscesses, which present as circumscribed fluid collections with an enhancing rim (sometimes containing air collections within the lesion) and typical clinical features, may be observed postoperatively (Fig. 43.21). Tumor recurrence is typically detected as an enhancing hypodense mass inside the surgical clips (Fig. 43.22). As the enhancement may be very subtle, the comparison with prior imaging studies is mandatory for early recurrence detection. On the initial CT scan after RFA, metastases typically are seen as a nonenhancing hypodense area corresponding to coagulation necrosis. For the ablation to be considered complete, the ablative margin should at least reach a thickness of 0.5 cm. Frequently, a rim enhancement around the ablation zone is found immediately after RFA. It is considered to be a physiologic reaction of normal liver parenchyma to heat damage and usually disappears at one month. If the enhancement pattern is eccentric (Fig. 43.23) rather than rim-like or the ablation area is

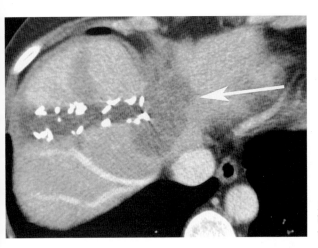

Figure 43.22 Local tumor recurrence after surgery. Next to the resection margin (marked by the surgical clips) a large hypodense lesion indicative for local tumor recurrence is visible (arrow).

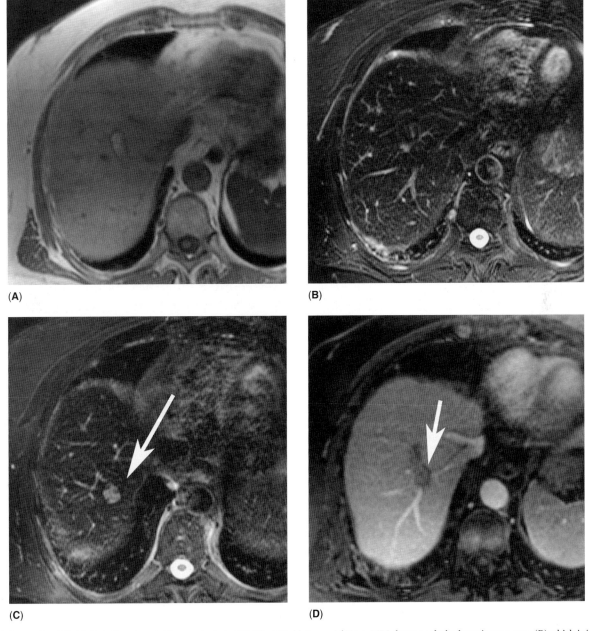

(A)

(B)

(C)

(D)

Figure 43.23 Incomplete RF ablation of a colorectal liver metastasis. (A) After RF ablation axial T1-w MRI shows a tubular hyperintense area, (B) which is isointense on the T2-w sequences and corresponds to the coagulation necrosis along the path and the tip of the RF device. (C, D) Adjacent to the end of the necrosis there is a T2-weighted hyperintense, nodular, enhancing lesion (arrows). The lesion corresponds to the area of the pre-existing metastasis, indicative of incomplete ablation.

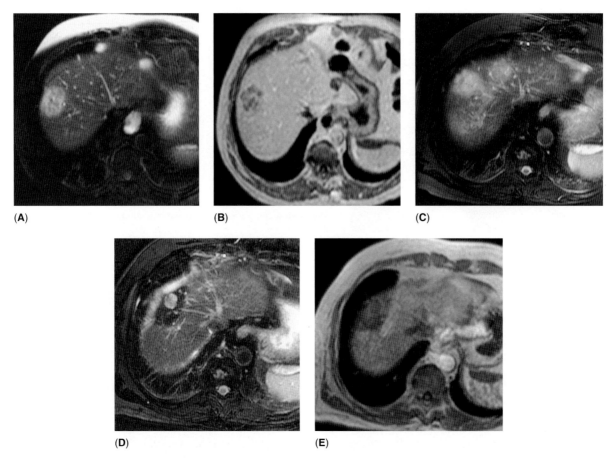

Figure 43.24 Typical MR appearance of the liver after radiation therapy. (**A, B**) T2-w and gadolinium-enhanced T1-w GRE sequences of a metastasis pre radiotherapy. (**C**) On the T2-weighted image three months after radiation therapy a T2-hyperintense edema according to the radiation field can be delineated next to the metastasis. (**D, E**) On the follow-up scan at eight months the edema has changed to fibrosis, which is markedly hypointense on T2-w and gadolinium-enhanced sequences. Within the fibrotic area the shrunken tumor is still seen.

smaller than the index lesion, residual tumor has to be suspected and another intervention is indicated. The ablation zone typically gradually decreases in size over time. Therefore any increase in size or newly detectable areas of enhancement within or next to the ablated area in follow-up scans are indicative of tumor recurrence (101). Bile duct injuries after RFA are reported in up to 1% of cases (102,103). Mostly they appear as dilatation of peripheral bile ducts but greater heat damage may also cause the formation of bilomas. Although the hepatic vessels are protected from heat damage due to their cooling effect they may still be damaged sometimes. This may result in the formation of pseudoaneuryms or hepatic infarctions, which typically present as wedge-shaped subcapsular hypoattenuating areas (102,104). MR may also be performed for imaging follow-up. Compared to CT it offers a better soft tissue contrast. It is mainly performed as an initial follow-up scan for detection of residual tumor tissue after RFA (105). CT also allows the detection of extrahepatic tumor progression and is therefore the preferred modality for long-term disease surveillance.

After radiation therapy, a wedge-shaped edema in the radiation field is found in the first months, which is typically slightly hyperintense on T2W and hypointense on T1W images. The lesion may present a residual rim like enhancement which is thought to represent an inflammatory reaction. About six months after treatment the radiated field becomes fibrotic which yields to a shrinkage with capsular retraction and T2 hypointensity (Fig. 43.24).

Key Points: Radiological Assessment of Treatment Response

- In the first weeks following REA, rim enhancement around the ablated area corresponds to physiological hyperemia. An eccentric peripheral enhancement, however, is suspicious for local recurrence
- Cone shaped subcapsular defects represent atypical resection areas. These should not be confused with subcapsular metastases

DIFFERENTIAL DIAGNOSIS

Metastases Vs. Focal Nodular Hyperplasia (FNH)

FNH is the second most common benign liver tumor and is typically found in women between 20 to 50 years of age. The typical imaging feature of this hypervascular tumor is the central scar, which shows enhancement in the equilibrium phases in gadolinium enhanced MR and contrast-enhanced CT imaging and is typically hyperintense on T2-weighted sequences. However, especially small FNHs may not show these typical imaging features and, furthermore, some FNHs show atypical dynamic contrast characteristics such as a pronounced washout in the

portal-venous phase. In patients with known breast cancer these FNHs cannot be reliably differentiated from small hypervascular liver metastases with CT and gadolinium-enhanced MR. In this case, however, hepatobiliary liver-specific contrast agents represent an optimal problem-solving tool to avoid biopsy. After application of mangafodipir, gadobenate, or gadoxate, FNHs show a contrast medium uptake in the delayed-phase and therefore appear iso- or hyperintense in the delayed-phase T1-weighted sequences, whereas metastases are hypointense in this phase (86,106–108). Contrast medium uptake of FNH has also been shown for liver-specific RES agents, but hepatobiliary agents are probably superior to RES agents for the identification and characterization of FNH (109,110).

Metastases Vs. Hemangiomas

Hemangiomas are primarily diagnosed on the basis of their typical dynamic enhancement pattern and their marked T2 hyperintensity. However, atypical small hemangiomas with homogeneous arterial enhancement and only intermediate T2 hyperintensity may be difficult to differentiate from hypervascular metastases because the typical peripheral washout of the metastasis in the portal-venous and the equilibrium phase may not be visible due to the small lesion size. Hepatobiliary contrast agents are not helpful for differentiation because both meatastases and hemangiomas do not show hepatobiliary contrast medium uptake in the delayed phase. Hemangiomas typically show contrast medium pooling in the equilibrium phase after the application of RES agents (Resovist®, ferucarbotran, Bayer-Schering; Endorem®, ferumoxide, Guerbet), which may further improve diagnostic confidence. Hemangiomas do not contain Kupffer cells and therefore do not take up SPIO contrast agents into the RES. However, hemangiomas show intravascular pooling of SPIO in the delayed-phase imaging (10 minutes after injection), which leads to a slight decrease in signal intensity in T2-weighted sequences compared to precontrast sequences not observed in metastases (111,112).

Metastases Vs. Cysts

Simple liver cysts typically show no enhancement and clear cut margins on contrast-enhanced CT, MR with water equivalent CT density and MR intensity values. They are enechoic on US images. For small cysts, however, CT density measurements may not be reliable due to partial-volume effects and also the margins sometimes do not appear unequivocally sharp. In these cases stability over a period of six months will give diagnostic confidence. MR is a problem-solving tool if immediate answers are being sought.

Key Points: Differential Diagnosis

- Hepatobiliary contrast agents are useful for the differentiation between FNH and metastases
- RES contrast agents and non-specific gadolinium chelates are useful for the differentiation between hemangiomas and metastases
- Small cysts can be diagnosed confidently with MR if the CT appearance is equivocal

PET AND PET-CT

By far the most commonly used radiotracer for PET-imaging of liver metastases is 2-[^{18}F] fluoro-2-deoxy-D-glucose (FDG). Tumor imaging with this tracer is based on the principle that cancer cells possess an increased glucose uptake and an altered intracellular glucose metabolism, which traps ^{18}F-FDG intracellular (Fig. 43.25). The metabolic activity of the tumor can be assessed semiquantitatively by calculating the standardized uptake value (SUV). Respiratory movement during the PET scan, which typically lasts several minutes, and the fact that ^{18}F-FDG also accumulates in normal liver tissue, limits the detection of liver metastases with PET. Moreover, not all tumors are FDG-avid and false-positive findings may occur in the presence of chronic inflammation and following surgery or chemotherapy.

FDG-PET is a valuable tool in the detection of hepatic metastases (56,113–117) and in patients with equivocal CT and MR findings, and for the detection of recurrent disease, FDG-PET has proven to be especially helpful (115). PET-CT scanners combine the functional information obtained from a PET scan with the

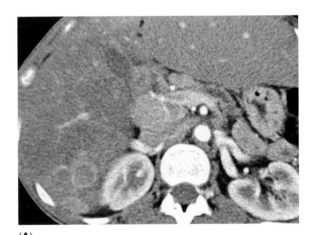

(A)

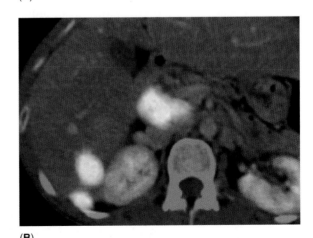

(B)

Figure 43.25 PET-CT of a patient with a neuroendocrine tumor of the pancreatic head and liver metastases. (A) Arterial phase CT scan demonstrates a large hypervascular tumor in the pancreatic head and two liver metastases in segment 6. (B) Fused FDG-PET-CT image demonstrates high tracer uptake in both the pancreatic primary and liver metastases. Physiological renal tracer uptake can also be seen.

anatomical details of a CT scan; the combination provides superior information and is proposed as the imaging modality of choice using adequate contrast-enhanced CT scanning parameters (118–120). Therefore, it may be implemented in the routine preoperative assessment of patients with colorectal liver metastases undergoing metasectomy (115,118,121).

Whether PET-CT is superior to a combined reading of PET and CT in patients with hepatic metastases, however, has not yet been investigated. In general, PET will probably be used more and more in routine clinical practice as a problem-solving tool complementary to CT and MR in patients with liver metastases. Moreover, it has been shown to be an excellent tool for early therapy assessment in patients with liver metastases from gastrointestinal stromal tumors receiving imatinib (122,123). Whether this applies to liver metastases from other primaries is still being investigated.

EVALUATION OF LIVER METASTASES: WHICH MODALITY?

There is an ongoing debate as to which imaging modality offers the best non-invasive, cost-effective assessment of the liver in oncologic patients. The use of multiple imaging modalities should be avoided as far as possible as it is both costly and time-consuming.

A meta-analysis from Bipat et al. has compared the diagnostic value of CT, MR, and PET in the evaluation of colorectal liver metastases derived from studies published between 1990 and 2003 (56). The authors found that FDG-PET is the most sensitive method for detection of metastases on a per lesion basis with a mean sensitivity of 75.9% compared to 52.3%, 63.8%, 66.1%, and 64.4% for nonhelical CT, helical CT, 1.0-T MR imaging, and 1.5-T MR imaging, respectively. However, these data were derived from very different imaging protocols. The use of MDCT scanners with an appropriate amount of contrast medium (120–150 ml) and MR scanners with high gradients combined with gadolinium-based non-specific or liver-specific contrast agents has markedly improved the image quality for both CT and MR. Therefore, these data do not reflect current state-of-the-art imaging of the liver. Another major problem in studies comparing the different sensitivities and specifities in detection of liver metastases is the use of different standard of references which makes comparison between different studies difficult and also leads to an underestimation of the true prevalence of liver metastases (124). Therefore, the interpretation of results from different studies is critical and the most reliable comparison between different modalities is when state-of-the-art modalities are compared within the same patients with surgical correlation as the standard-of-reference (124,125).

Generally, MDCT scanning is used as a "screening" examination of the liver in most instituitions as it is a robust, widely available, and valuable imaging technique, and moreover allows the assessment of extrahepatic disease. PET scanning is not used routinely in the initial assessment of oncologic patients because of its expense and poor anatomic resolution. Moreover, it has not been shown to be superior to MDCT in the initial staging of primary colorectal cancer (126).

Depending on local availability and user experience, contrast-enhanced US may be an option for initial liver assessment with a sensitivity for the detection of liver metastasis comparable to that of MDCT (34,35,127). Unenhanced US, however, is now regarded obsolete for liver evaluation in oncologic patients due to its low sensitivity for lesion detection (36). To date only a few studies have compared MDCT and MR regarding liver evaluation. These show that MR, either gadolinium-enhanced or with liver-specific SPIO contrast agents, demonstrates a higher diagnostic accuracy than MDCT for detection and characterization of focal liver lesions (57,60). Compared to helical CT, multiple studies have shown that MR with different contrast agents is superior regarding lesion detection and characterization (55,58,59,89,128–130). MR is routinely used in patients with unequivocal CT scans or with contraindications to a CT examination. It should also be used in patients with severe liver steatosis as this condition markedly decreases the diagnostic performance of US and CT in liver evaluation (Fig. 43.26) (131). Moreover, it plays a major role in the assessment of patients who are eligible for resection of liver metastases.

Key Points: Which Modality?

- MDCT is the standard imaging modality for oncologic staging and follow-up
- MR is superior to CT for lesion detection and characterization, and is therefore indicated in patients with equivocal CT scans and in patients amenable to liver surgery
- Contrast-enhanced US outperforms grey-scale US for detection of lesions and is an adjunct for characterization of specific lesions

PREOPERATIVE EVALUATION

In patients with colorectal liver metastases (CRCLM), who are possibly amenable to liver surgery, preoperative imaging has to address two major questions: (*i*) the extent of metastatic liver involvement, and (*ii*) the presence of extrahepatic disease.

Assessment of the Extent of Metastastic Liver Involvement

Intraoperative Ultrasound

Intraoperative ultrasound (IOUS) has been shown to be the most sensitive imaging method for detecting small focal liver lesions and it is a standard routine in hepatic surgery (132,133). Combined with intraoperative inspection and palpation, it is considered as the standard of reference for comparative studies of different imaging modalities. It helps to clarify equivocal lesions detected with preoperative imaging and should only add 10 to 15 minutes in operating room time in expert hands. Because of its already high detection rate IOUS is usually performed without contrast agents. Current studies have shown that contrast-enhanced IOUS may find additional metastases in 5% to 19% of patients in comparison to grey-scale IOUS (134–136). However, it did not improve the diagnostic accuracy compared to preoperative CT combined with grey-scale IOUS and, therefore, the debate as to whether contrast media application should be routinely used for IOUS is still ongoing (134).

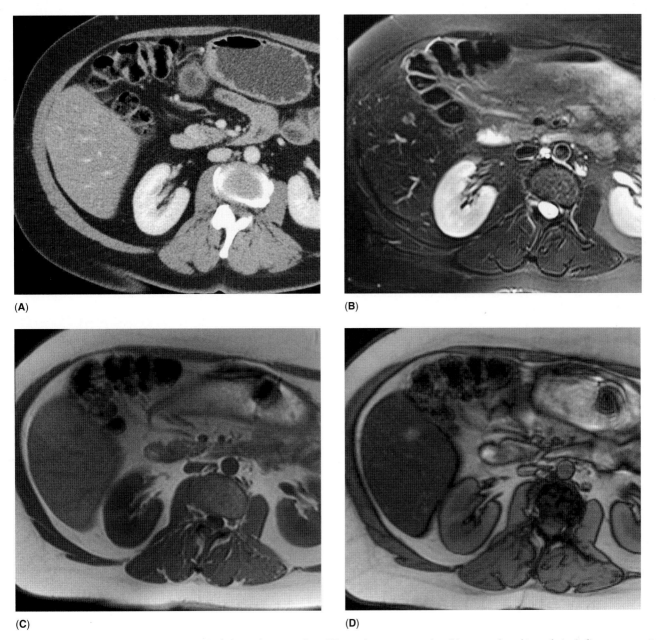

Figure 43.26 Improved detection with MRI in steatosis. (**A**) Portal-venous phase CT scan demonstrates only a faint parenchymal irregularity in liver segment 5 in a patient with severe liver steatosis. (**B**) T2w, (**C**) T1w in- and (**D**) opposed phase images clearly demonstrate a suspicious lesion. Be aware of the large signal drop of the liver parenchyma in the opposed phase images indicative of severe steatosis.

The Diagnostic Value of Preoperative CT, MR, PET, and PET/CT
Preoperative imaging capabilities with CT and MR in patients with colorectal liver metastases have dramatically improved in the last decade. While older studies report the detection of additional liver metastases during surgery with palpation and IOUS in up to 50% of patients, it has been shown that with the use of state-of-the-art MDCT and/or MR with appropriate protocols combined with a specialist multidisciplinary preoperative evaluation, additional liver metastases are only found in 8% of patients during metastasectomy (132,133,137). Gadolinium- or SPIO-enhanced MR have been shown to be superior to MDCT for detection of liver metastases (60). This is probably also true for other liver-specific contrast agents like mangafodipir (Teslascan®, GE Healthcare) and gadoxate acid (Primovist®, Bayer-Schering)

although no studies have compared this yet. Compared to gadobenate dimeglumine, however, SPIO has been shown to be superior for detection of liver metastases (83). SPIO-enhanced MR was also shown to be at least equal to CTAP for preoperative liver evaluation (138). Because of its invasiveness and higher costs this technique is not used routinely for preoperative evaluation anymore. The distinction between small solid lesions and cysts remain a challenge on MDCT and sometimes is even impossible. Because of the higher sensitivity regarding the detection of liver metastases, and the better differentiation between small solid and cystic lesions, we therefore recommend an MR study with a liver-specific contrast agent in all patients undergoing metastasectomy.

In all studies with surgical confirmation that compared the sensitivities of PET with CT for detection of liver metastases,

single-slice helical CT and not MDCT was used, which does not represent state-of-the art imaging. In two newer studies with the slice thicknesses of 5.5 and 7 mm, single-slice helical CT showed an equivalent sensitivity to PET for the detection of all metastases and performed better than PET in detecting small (<1.5 cm) liver metastases (116,139). In a study by Sahani and colleagues, mangafodipir-enhanced MR detected 33 subcentimeter metastases, whereas PET only showed 12 of these small lesions (140). Therefore, PET must be considered to be less sensitive when compared to state-of-the-art contrast-enhanced MDCT or MR, and has only a limited role for preoperative liver evaluation.

As the detection of hypermetabolic areas in the liver is impaired due to the high metabolism rate of the liver itself and by breathing motion, a combined PET/CT will probably not improve the detection rate of this imaging technique. Therefore, it has to be stressed that if a PET/CT is performed for preoperative liver evaluation, a full diagnostic MDCT with optimal CT parameters regarding as slice thickness, contrast media amount and flow rate, and scan delay has to be included.

Assessment of Extrahepatic Tumor

Contrast-enhanced MDCT of the thorax and abdomen is the standard staging technique in patients with colorectal cancer. There seems to be good evidence that FDG-PET is superior to CT (mostly single slice) for the detection of extrahepatic disease (116,121,139,141). According to a meta-analysis on this subject, this results in a change of clinical management in 31.6% of cases (142). However, in most of the included studies, chest CT was rarely used routinely (143–145). Some authors even considered it as a positive impact of PET if lung metastases, not seen on a chest X-ray, were detected with PET, even if they were visible on a subsequent chest CT scan (144,146). Therefore, the true added value of PET as defined by a change of clinical managment is probably much lower. One recent study with a relatively small number of patients (n = 44) even showed that PET alone is not superior to MDCT in the preoperative staging of colorectal cancer (126). Tumor staging with combined PET/CT has been shown to be more accurate than CT alone, PET alone, and side-by-side PET plus CT (116,119).

Therefore, we would recommend that patients with colorectal liver metastases should undergo PET/CT before surgery including a diagnostic state-of-the-art MDCT study evaluated by an experienced abdominal radiologist. This is especially true for patients with a high clinical risk score [more than one lymph node metastasis (LM), LM > 5 cm, CEA >200 ng/mL, node-positive primary, disease-free interval from primary to metastases >12 months] because the probability that PET will find extrahepatic tumor manifestations in this patient group is higher compared to patients with a low clinical risk score (147). In patients who recently underwent chemotherapy, PET/CT probably is not indicated as the sensitivity of PET is reduced in this patient group. The lack of availability of appropriate PET/CT devices and a lack of financial resources combined with an absence of cost benefit analyses, however, may delay a wide-spread use of PET/CT in clinical practice.

Cost Effectiveness

Only few data regarding the cost effectiveness of different preoperative imaging strategies are available. Mann and colleagues showed that for preoperative liver evaluation the use of mangafodipir-enhanced MR instead of helical or incremental contrast-enhanced CT can save US $2758 per patient as unnecessary non-therapeutic operations can be spared (82). Annemans et al. showed savings of about €1400 per patient if the preoperative liver evaluation is performed with SPIO-enhanced MR instead of contrast-enhanced spiral CT (148). However, cost savings are definitely lower if state-of-the art MDCT is compared with MR. Studies dealing with this topic or comparing PET-(CT) with other imaging modalities are needed considering worldwide concern regarding healthcare costs.

Conclusion

In conclusion, both contrast-enhanced chest and (at least biphasic) abdomen MDCT and liver MR with liver-specific contrast agents are recommended for an optimal preoperative evaluation of patients undergoing a metastasectomy. If possible a PET/CT including a state-of-the-art MDCT scan should be performed for extrahepatic tumor staging.

Summary

- In patients with known malignancy, contrast-enhanced US or, preferably, MDCT are the modalities of choice for evaluation of the liver
- The baseline CT examination has to include two contrast-enhanced scans (i.e., arterial and a portal-venous phase); follow-up scans may be tailored according to the primary tumor
- In MR imaging contrast agent administration is essential
- MR is helpful if CT or sonography demonstrate equivocal lesions and in preoperative assessment
- In surgical candidates, the use of liver-specific MR contrast agents is recommended. If available, an additional PET/CT scan for the assessment of extrahepatic tumor spread is reasonable
- Follow-up after chemotherapy is monitored by CT to assess treatment response
- RECIST criteria using unidimensional measurements of target lesions are generally used for radiological assessment of treatment response

REFERENCES

1. Abrams HL, Spiro R, Goldstein N. Metastases in carcinoma; analysis of 1000 autopsied cases. Cancer 1950; 3: 74–85.
2. Baker ME, Pelley R. Hepatic metastases: basic principles and implications for radiologists. Radiology 1995; 197: 329–37.
3. Lodge JP. Modern surgery for liver metastases. Cancer Imaging 2000; 1: 77–85.
4. Nordlinger B, Van Cutsem E, Rougier P, et al. Does chemotherapy prior to liver resection increase the potential for cure in patients with metastatic colorectal cancer? A report from the European Colorectal Metastases Treatment Group. Eur J Cancer 2007; 43: 2037–45.
5. Rees M, John TG. Current status of surgery in colorectal metastases to the liver. Hepatogastroenterology 2001; 48: 341–4.

6. Simmonds PC, Primrose JN, Colquitt JL, et al. Surgical resection of hepatic metastases from colorectal cancer: a systematic review of published studies. Br J Cancer 2006; 94: 982–99.

7. Aloia TA, Vauthey JN, Loyer EM, et al. Solitary colorectal liver metastasis: resection determines outcome. Arch Surg 2006; 141: 460–6; discussion 6–7.

8. Bartolozzi C, Cioni D, Donati F, Lencioni R. Focal liver lesions: MR imaging-pathologic correlation. Eur Radiol 2001; 11: 1374–88.

9. Kanematsu M, Kondo H, Goshima S, et al. Imaging liver metastases: review and update. Eur J Radiol 2006; 58: 217–28.

10. Bader TR, Grabenwoger F, Prokesch RW, Krause W. Measurement of hepatic perfusion with dynamic computed tomography: assessment of normal values and comparison of two methods to compensate for motion artifacts. Invest Radiol 2000; 35: 539–47.

11. Greenway CV, Stark RD. Hepatic vascular bed. Physiol Rev 1971; 51: 23–65.

12. Hashimoto K, Murakami T, Dono K, et al. Quantitative tissue blood flow measurement of the liver parenchyma: comparison between xenon CT and perfusion CT. Dig Dis Sci 2007; 52: 943–9.

13. Ridge JA, Bading JR, Gelbard AS, Benua RS, Daly JM. Perfusion of colorectal hepatic metastases. Relative distribution of flow from the hepatic artery and portal vein. Cancer 1987; 59: 1547–53.

14. Taniguchi H, Daidoh T, Shioaki Y, Takahashi T. Blood supply and drug delivery to primary and secondary human liver cancers studied with in vivo bromodeoxyuridine labeling. Cancer 1993; 71: 50–5.

15. Liu Y, Matsui O. Changes of intratumoral microvessels and blood perfusion during establishment of hepatic metastases in mice. Radiology 2007; 243: 386–95.

16. Cuenod C, Leconte I, Siauve N, et al. Early changes in liver perfusion caused by occult metastases in rats: detection with quantitative CT. Radiology 2001; 218: 556–61.

17. Nott DM, Grime SJ, Yates J, et al. Changes in the hepatic perfusion index during the development of experimental hepatic tumours. Br J Surg 1989; 76: 259–63.

18. Miyazaki K, Collins DJ, Walker-Samuel S, et al. Quantitative mapping of hepatic perfusion index using MR imaging: a potential reproducible tool for assessing tumour response to treatment with the antiangiogenic compound BIBF 1120, a potent triple angiokinase inhibitor. Eur Radiol 2008; 18: 1414–21.

19. Viscomi GN, Gonzalez R, Taylor KJ. Histopathological correlation of ultrasound appearances of liver metastases. J Clin Gastroenterol 1981; 3: 395–400.

20. Albrecht T, Hoffmann CW, Schmitz SA, et al. Phase-inversion sonography during the liver-specific late phase of contrast enhancement: improved detection of liver metastases. AJR Am J Roentgenol 2001; 176: 1191–8.

21. Kinkel K, Lu Y, Both M, Warren RS, Thoeni RF. Detection of hepatic metastases from cancers of the gastrointestinal tract by using noninvasive imaging methods (US, CT, MR imaging, PET): a meta-analysis. Radiology 2002; 224: 748–56.

22. Wernecke K, Rummeny E, Bongartz G, et al. Detection of hepatic masses in patients with carcinoma: comparative sensitivities of sonography, CT, and MR imaging. Am J Roentgenol 1991; 157: 731–9.

23. Harvey CJ, Albrecht T. Ultrasound of focal liver lesions. Eur Radiol 2001; 11: 1578–93.

24. Hann LE, Bach AM, Cramer LD, et al. Hepatic sonography: comparison of tissue harmonic and standard sonography techniques. Am J Roentgenol 1999; 173: 201–6.

25. Shapiro RS, Wagreich J, Parsons RB, et al. Tissue harmonic imaging sonography: evaluation of image quality compared with conventional sonography. Am J Roentgenol 1998; 171: 1203–6.

26. Angeli E, Carpanelli R, Crespi G, et al. Efficacy of SH U 508 A (Levovist) in color Doppler ultrasonography of hepatocellular carcinoma vascularization. Radiol Med (Torino) 1994; 87: 24–31.

27. Ernst H, Hahn EG, Balzer T, Schlief R, Heyder N. Color doppler ultrasound of liver lesions: signal enhancement after intravenous injection of the ultrasound contrast agent Levovist. J Clin Ultrasound 1996; 24: 31–5.

28. Schlief R. Developments in echo-enhancing agents. Clin Radiol 1996; 51(Suppl 1): 5–7.

29. Bauer A, Blomley M, Leen E, Cosgrove D, Schlief R. Liver-specific imaging with SHU 563A: diagnostic potential of a new class of ultrasound contrast media. Eur Radiol 1999; 9(Suppl 3): S349–52.

30. Hauff P, Fritzsch T, Reinhardt M, et al. Delineation of experimental liver tumors in rabbits by a new ultrasound contrast agent and stimulated acoustic emission. Invest Radiol 1997; 32: 94–9.

31. Hohmann J, Albrecht T, Oldenburg A, Skrok J, Wolf KJ. Liver metastases in cancer: detection with contrast-enhanced ultrasonography. Abdom Imaging 2004; 29: 669–81.

32. Brannigan M, Burns PN, Wilson SR. Blood flow patterns in focal liver lesions at microbubble-enhanced US. Radiographics 2004; 24: 921–35.

33. von Herbay A, Vogt C, Willers R, Haussinger D. Real-time imaging with the sonographic contrast agent SonoVue: differentiation between benign and malignant hepatic lesions. J Ultrasound Med 2004; 23: 1557–68.

34. Albrecht T, Blomley MJ, Burns PN, et al. Improved detection of hepatic metastases with pulse-inversion US during the liver-specific phase of SHU 508A: multicenter study. Radiology 2003; 227: 361–70.

35. Oldenburg A, Hohmann J, Foert E, et al. Detection of hepatic metastases with low MI real time contrast enhanced sonography and SonoVue. Ultraschall Med 2005; 26: 277–84.

36. Albrecht T, Blomley M, Bolondi L, et al. Guidelines for the use of contrast agents in ultrasound. Ultraschall Med 2004; 25: 249–56.

37. Oliver JH 3rd, Baron RL, Federle MP, Jones BC, Sheng R. Hypervascular liver metastases: do unenhanced and hepatic arterial phase CT images affect tumor detection? Radiology 1997; 205: 709–15.

38. Patten RM, Byun JY, Freeny PC. CT of hypervascular hepatic tumors: are unenhanced scans necessary for diagnosis? Am J Roentgenol 1993; 161: 979–84.

39. Sica GT, Ji H, Ros PR. CT and MR imaging of hepatic metastases. Am J Roentgenol 2000; 174: 691–8.

40. Hale HL, Husband JE, Gossios K, Norman AR, Cunningham D. CT of calcified liver metastases in colorectal carcinoma. Clin Radiol 1998; 53: 735–41.

41. Bonaldi VM, Bret PM, Reinhold C, Atri M. Helical CT of the liver: value of an early hepatic arterial phase. Radiology 1995; 197: 357–63.

42. Paulson EK, McDermott VG, Keogan MT, et al. Carcinoid metastases to the liver: role of triple-phase helical CT. Radiology 1998; 206: 143–50.

43. Scott DJ, Guthrie JA, Arnold P, et al. Dual phase helical CT versus portal venous phase CT for the detection of colorectal liver metastases: correlation with intra-operative sonography, surgical and pathological findings. Clin Radiol 2001; 56: 235–42.

44. van Leeuwen MS, Noordzij J, Feldberg MA, Hennipman AH, Doornewaard H. Focal liver lesions: characterization with triphasic spiral CT. Radiology 1996; 201: 327–36.

45. Kulinna C, Helmberger T, Kessler M, Reiser M. [Improvement in diagnosis of liver metastases with the multi-detector CT]. Radiologe 2001; 41: 16–23.

46. Weg N, Scheer MR, Gabor MP. Liver lesions: improved detection with dual-detector-array CT and routine 2.5-mm thin collimation. Radiology 1998; 209: 417–26.

47. Kopka L, Grabbe E. [Biphasic liver diagnosis with multiplanar-detector spiral CT]. Radiologe 1999; 39: 971–8.

48. Ba-Ssalamah A, Heinz-Peer G, Schima W, et al. Detection of focal hepatic lesions: comparison of unenhanced and SHU 555 A-enhanced MR imaging versus biphasic helical CTAP. J Magn Reson Imaging 2000; 11: 665–72.

49. Valls C, Andia E, Sanchez A, et al. Hepatic metastases from colorectal cancer: preoperative detection and assessment of resectability with helical CT. Radiology 2001; 218: 55–60.

50. Semelka RC, Cance WG, Marcos HB, Mauro MA. Liver metastases: comparison of current MR techniques and spiral CT during arterial portography for detection in 20 surgically staged cases. Radiology 1999; 213: 86–91.

51. Valls C, Lopez E, Guma A, et al. Helical CT versus CT arterial portography in the detection of hepatic metastasis of colorectal carcinoma. Am J Roentgenol 1998; 170: 1341–7.

52. Gleeson TG, Bulugahapitiya S. Contrast-induced nephropathy. Am J Roentgenol 2004; 183: 1673–89.

53. Broome DR. Nephrogenic systemic fibrosis associated with gadolinium based contrast agents: a summary of the medical literature reporting. Eur J Radiol 2008; 66: 230–4.

54. Sadowski EA, Bennett LK, Chan MR, et al. Nephrogenic systemic fibrosis: risk factors and incidence estimation. Radiology 2007; 243: 148–57.

55. Bartolozzi C, Donati F, Cioni D, et al. Detection of colorectal liver metastases: a prospective multicenter trial comparing unenhanced MRI, MnDPDP-enhanced MRI, and spiral CT. Eur Radiol 2004; 14: 14–20.

56. Bipat S, van Leeuwen MS, Comans EF, et al. Colorectal liver metastases: CT, MR imaging, and PET for diagnosis – meta-analysis. Radiology 2005; 237: 123–31.

57. Kim YK, Ko SW, Hwang SB, Kim CS, Yu HC. Detection and characterization of liver metastases: 16-slice multidetector computed tomography versus superparamagnetic iron oxide-enhanced magnetic resonance imaging. Eur Radiol 2006; 16: 1337–45.

58. Semelka RC, Martin DR, Balci C, Lance T. Focal liver lesions: comparison of dual-phase CT and multisequence multiplanar MR imaging including dynamic gadolinium enhancement. J Magn Reson Imaging 2001; 13: 397–401.

59. Ward J, Naik KS, Guthrie JA, Wilson D, Robinson PJ. Hepatic lesion detection: comparison of MR imaging after the administration of superparamagnetic iron oxide with dual-phase CT by using alternative-free response receiver operating characteristic analysis. Radiology 1999; 210: 459–66.

60. Ward J, Robinson PJ, Guthrie JA, et al. Liver metastases in candidates for hepatic resection: comparison of helical CT and gadolinium- and SPIO-enhanced MR imaging. Radiology 2005; 237: 170–80.

61. Bennett GL, Petersein A, Mayo-Smith WW, et al. Addition of gadolinium chelates to heavily T2-weighted MR imaging: limited role in differentiating hepatic hemangiomas from metastases. Am J Roentgenol 2000; 174: 477–85.

62. Schima W, Saini S, Echeverri JA, et al. Focal liver lesions: characterization with conventional spin-echo versus fast spin-echo T2-weighted MR imaging. Radiology 1997; 202: 389–93.

63. Ichikawa T, Haradome H, Hachiya J, Nitatori T, Araki T. Diffusion-weighted MR imaging with a single-shot echo-planar sequence: detection and characterization of focal hepatic lesions. Am J Roentgenol 1998; 170: 397–402.

64. Nasu K, Kuroki Y, Nawano S, et al. Hepatic metastases: diffusion-weighted sensitivity-encoding versus SPIO-enhanced MR imaging. Radiology 2006; 239: 122–30.

65. Okada Y, Ohtomo K, Kiryu S, Sasaki Y. Breath-hold T2-weighted MRI of hepatic tumors: value of echo planar imaging with diffusion-sensitizing gradient. J Comput Assist Tomogr 1998; 22: 364–71.

66. Koh DM, Brown G, Riddell AM, et al. Detection of colorectal hepatic metastases using MnDPDP MR imaging and diffusion-weighted imaging (DWI) alone and in combination. Eur Radiol 2008; 18: 903–10.

67. Bruegel M, Holzapfel K, Gaa J, et al. Characterization of focal liver lesions by ADC measurements using a respiratory triggered diffusion-weighted single-shot echo-planar MR imaging technique. Eur Radiol 2008; 18: 477–85.

68. Gourtsoyianni S, Papanikolaou N, Yarmenitis S, et al. Respiratory gated diffusion-weighted imaging of the liver: value of apparent diffusion coefficient measurements in the differentiation between most commonly encountered benign and malignant focal liver lesions. Eur Radiol 2008; 18: 486–92.

69. Koh DM, Scurr E, Collins DJ, et al. Colorectal hepatic metastases: quantitative measurements using single-shot echo-planar diffusion-weighted MR imaging. Eur Radiol 2006; 16: 1898–905.

70. Taouli B, Vilgrain V, Dumont E, et al. Evaluation of liver diffusion isotropy and characterization of focal hepatic lesions with two single-shot echo-planar MR imaging sequences: prospective study in 66 patients. Radiology 2003; 226: 71–8.

71. Roth Y, Tichler T, Kostenich G, et al. High-b-value diffusion-weighted MR imaging for pretreatment prediction and early

monitoring of tumor response to therapy in mice. Radiology 2004; 232: 685–92.

72. Thoeny HC, De Keyzer F, Chen F, et al. Diffusion-weighted MR imaging in monitoring the effect of a vascular targeting agent on rhabdomyosarcoma in rats. Radiology 2005; 234: 756–64.

73. Thoeny HC, De Keyzer F, Vandecaveye V, et al. Effect of vascular targeting agent in rat tumor model: dynamic contrast-enhanced versus diffusion-weighted MR imaging. Radiology 2005; 237: 492–9.

74. Kim T, Murakami T, Takahashi S, et al. Diffusion-weighted single-shot echoplanar MR imaging for liver disease. Am J Roentgenol 1999; 173: 393–8.

75. Namimoto T, Yamashita Y, Sumi S, Tang Y, Takahashi M. Focal liver masses: characterization with diffusion-weighted echo-planar MR imaging. Radiology 1997; 204: 739–44.

76. Le Bihan D, Breton E, Lallemand D, et al. Separation of diffusion and perfusion in intravoxel incoherent motion MR imaging. Radiology 1988; 168: 497–505.

77. Danet IM, Semelka RC, Leonardou P, et al. Spectrum of MRI appearances of untreated metastases of the liver. Am J Roentgenol 2003; 181: 809–17.

78. Lin G, Gustafson T, Hagerstrand I, Lunderquist A. CT demonstration of low density ring in liver metastases. J Comput Assist Tomogr 1984; 8: 450–2.

79. Mitchell DG, Outwater EK, Matteucci T, et al. Adrenal gland enhancement at MR imaging with Mn-DPDP. Radiology 1995; 194: 783–7.

80. Schima W, Fugger R, Schober E, et al. Diagnosis and staging of pancreatic cancer: comparison of mangafodipir trisodium-enhanced MR imaging and contrast-enhanced helical hydro-CT. Am J Roentgenol 2002; 179: 717–24.

81. Reimer P, Schneider G, Schima W. Hepatobiliary contrast agents for contrast-enhanced MRI of the liver: properties, clinical development and applications. Eur Radiol 2004; 14: 559–78.

82. Mann GN, Marx HF, Lai LL, Wagman LD. Clinical and cost effectiveness of a new hepatocellular MRI contrast agent, mangafodipir trisodium, in the preoperative assessment of liver resectability. Ann Surg Oncol 2001; 8: 573–9.

83. del Frate C, Bazzocchi M, Mortele KJ, et al. Detection of liver metastases: comparison of gadobenate dimeglumine-enhanced and ferumoxides-enhanced MR imaging examinations. Radiology 2002; 225: 766–72.

84. Huppertz A, Balzer T, Blakeborough A, et al. Improved detection of focal liver lesions at MR imaging: multicenter comparison of gadoxetic acid-enhanced MR images with intraoperative findings. Radiology 2004; 230: 266–75.

85. Kim YK, Lee JM, Kim CS, et al. Detection of liver metastases: gadobenate dimeglumine-enhanced three-dimensional dynamic phases and one-hour delayed phase MR imaging versus superparamagnetic iron oxide-enhanced MR imaging. Eur Radiol 2005; 15: 220–8.

86. Zech CJ, Herrmann KA, Reiser MF, Schoenberg SO. MR imaging in patients with suspected liver metastases: value of liver-specific contrast agent Gd-EOB-DTPA. Magn Reson Med Sci 2007; 6: 43–52.

87. Pirovano G, Vanzulli A, Marti-Bonmati L, et al. Evaluation of the accuracy of gadobenate dimeglumine-enhanced MR imaging in the detection and characterization of focal liver lesions. Am J Roentgenol 2000; 175: 1111–20.

88. Wersebe A, Wiskirchen J, Decker U, et al. Comparison of Gadolinium-BOPTA and Ferucarbotran-enhanced three-dimensional T1-weighted dynamic liver magnetic resonance imaging in the same patient. Invest Radiol 2006; 41: 264–71.

89. Reimer P, Jahnke N, Fiebich M, et al. Hepatic lesion detection and characterization: value of nonenhanced MR imaging, superparamagnetic iron oxide-enhanced MR imaging, and spiral CT-ROC analysis. Radiology 2000; 217: 152–8.

90. Therasse P, Arbuck SG, Eisenhauer EA, et al. New guidelines to evaluate the response to treatment in solid tumors. European Organization for Research and Treatment of Cancer, National Cancer Institute of the United States, National Cancer Institute of Canada. J Natl Cancer Inst 2000; 92: 205–16.

91. Miller AB, Hoogstraten B, Staquet M, Winkler A. Reporting results of cancer treatment. Cancer 1981; 47: 207–14.

92. Benoist S, Brouquet A, Penna C, et al. Complete response of colorectal liver metastases after chemotherapy: does it mean cure? J Clin Oncol 2006; 24: 3939–45.

93. Dy GK, Krook JE, Green EM, et al. Impact of complete response to chemotherapy on overall survival in advanced colorectal cancer: results from Intergroup N9741. J Clin Oncol 2007; 25: 3469–74.

94. Benjamin RS, Choi H, Macapinlac HA, et al. We should desist using RECIST, at least in GIST. J Clin Oncol 2007; 25: 1760–4.

95. Choi H, Charnsangavej C, Faria SC, et al. Correlation of computed tomography and positron emission tomography in patients with metastatic gastrointestinal stromal tumor treated at a single institution with imatinib mesylate: proposal of new computed tomography response criteria. J Clin Oncol 2007; 25: 1753–9.

96. Mahvi DM, Lee FT, Jr. Radiofrequency ablation of hepatic malignancies: is heat better than cold? Ann Surg 1999; 230: 9–11.

97. von Breitenbuch P, Kohl G, Guba M, et al. Thermoablation of colorectal liver metastases promotes proliferation of residual intrahepatic neoplastic cells. Surgery 2005; 138: 882–7.

98. White RR, Avital I, Sofocleous CT, et al. Rates and patterns of recurrence for percutaneous radiofrequency ablation and open wedge resection for solitary colorectal liver metastasis. J Gastrointest Surg 2007; 11: 256–63.

99. Lencioni R, Crocetti L, Cioni D, Della Pina C, Bartolozzi C. Percutaneous radiofrequency ablation of hepatic colorectal metastases: technique, indications, results, and new promises. Invest Radiol 2004; 39: 689–97.

100. Oshowo A, Gillams A, Harrison E, Lees WR, Taylor I. Comparison of resection and radiofrequency ablation for treatment of solitary colorectal liver metastases. Br J Surg 2003; 90: 1240–3.

101. Park MH, Rhim H, Kim YS, et al. Spectrum of CT findings after radiofrequency ablation of hepatic tumors. Radiographics 2008; 28: 379–92.

102. Akahane M, Koga H, Kato N, et al. Complications of percutaneous radiofrequency ablation for hepato-cellular carcinoma: imaging spectrum and management. Radiographics 2005; 25(Suppl 1): S57–68.

103. Livraghi T, Solbiati L, Meloni MF, et al. Treatment of focal liver tumors with percutaneous radio-frequency ablation: complications encountered in a multicenter study. Radiology 2003; 226: 441–51.

104. Tamai F, Furuse J, Maru Y, Yoshino M. Intrahepatic pseudo-aneurysm: a complication following radio-frequency ablation therapy for hepatocellular carcinoma. Eur J Radiol 2002; 44: 40–3.

105. Clasen S, Boss A, Schmidt D, et al. Magnetic resonance imaging for hepatic radiofrequency ablation. Eur J Radiol 2006; 59: 140–8.

106. Grazioli L, Morana G, Kirchin MA, Schneider G. Accurate differentiation of focal nodular hyperplasia from hepatic adenoma at gadobenate dimeglumine-enhanced MR imaging: prospective study. Radiology 2005; 236: 166–77.

107. Scharitzer M, Schima W, Schober E, et al. Characterization of hepatocellular tumors: value of mangafodipir-enhanced magnetic resonance imaging. J Comput Assist Tomogr 2005; 29: 181–90.

108. Zech CJ, Grazioli L, Breuer J, Reiser MF, Schoenberg SO. Diagnostic performance and description of morphological features of focal nodular hyperplasia in Gd-EOB-DTPA-enhanced liver magnetic resonance imaging: results of a multicenter trial. Invest Radiol 2008; 43: 504–11.

109. Grazioli L, Morana G, Kirchin MA, et al. MRI of focal nodular hyperplasia (FNH) with gadobenate dimeglumine (Gd-BOPTA) and SPIO (ferumoxides): an intra-individual comparison. J Magn Reson Imaging 2003; 17: 593–602.

110. Terkivatan T, van den Bos IC, Hussain SM, et al. Focal nodular hyperplasia: lesion characteristics on state-of-the-art MRI including dynamic gadolinium-enhanced and superparamagnetic iron-oxide-uptake sequences in a prospective study. J Magn Reson Imaging 2006; 24: 864–72.

111. Paley MR, Mergo PJ, Torres GM, Ros PR. Characterization of focal hepatic lesions with ferumoxides-enhanced T2-weighted MR imaging. Am J Roentgenol 2000; 175: 159–63.

112. Schmitz SA, Nikolova A, O'Regan D, et al. Quantitative assessment of iron-oxide-enhanced magnetic resonance imaging of the liver: Vessel isointensity is a potential characteristic of liver hemangiomas on late T1-weighted images. Acta Radiol 2006; 47: 634–42.

113. Bohm B, Voth M, Geoghegan J, et al. Impact of positron emission tomography on strategy in liver resection for primary and secondary liver tumors. J Cancer Res Clin Oncol 2004; 130: 266–72.

114. Delbeke D, Martin WH, Sandler MP, et al. Evaluation of benign vs malignant hepatic lesions with positron emission tomography. Arch Surg 1998; 133: 510–6.

115. Herbertson RA, Lee ST, Tebbutt N, Scott AM. The expanding role of PET technology in the management of patients with colorectal cancer. Ann Oncol 2007; 18: 1774–81.

116. Ruers TJ, Langenhoff BS, Neeleman N, et al. Value of positron emission tomography with [F-18]fluorodeoxyglucose in patients with colorectal liver metastases: a prospective study. J Clin Oncol 2002; 20: 388–95.

117. Vitola JV, Delbeke D, Sandler MP, et al. Positron emission tomography to stage suspected metastatic colorectal carcinoma to the liver. Am J Surg 1996; 171: 21–6.

118. Antoch G, Saoudi N, Kuehl H, et al. Accuracy of whole-body dual-modality fluorine-18-2-fluoro-2-deoxy-D-glucose positron emission tomography and computed tomography (FDG-PET/CT) for tumor staging in solid tumors: comparison with CT and PET. J Clin Oncol 2004; 22: 4357–68.

119. Bar-Shalom R, Yefremov N, Guralnik L, et al. Clinical performance of PET/CT in evaluation of cancer: additional value for diagnostic imaging and patient management. J Nucl Med 2003; 44: 1200–9.

120. Hany TF, Steinert HC, Goerres GW, Buck A, von Schulthess GK. PET diagnostic accuracy: improvement with in-line PET-CT system: initial results. Radiology 2002; 225: 575–81.

121. Selzner M, Hany TF, Wildbrett P, et al. Does the novel PET/CT imaging modality impact on the treatment of patients with metastatic colorectal cancer of the liver? Ann Surg 2004; 240: 1027–36.

122. Antoch G, Kanja J, Bauer S, et al. Comparison of PET, CT and dual-modality PET/CT imaging for monitoring of imatinib (STI571) therapy in patients with gastrointestinal stromal tumors. J Nucl Med 2004; 45: 357–65.

123. Van den Abbeele AD, Badawi RD. Use of positron emission tomography in oncology and its potential role to assess response to imatinib mesylate therapy in gastrointestinal stromal tumors (GISTs). Eur J Cancer 2002; 38(Suppl 5): S60–S65.

124. van Erkel AR, Pijl ME, van den Berg-Huysmans AA, et al. Hepatic metastases in patients with colorectal cancer: relationship between size of metastases, standard of reference, and detection rates. Radiology 2002; 224: 404–9.

125. Rappeport ED, Loft A. Liver metastases from colorectal cancer: imaging with superparamagnetic iron oxide (SPIO)-enhanced MR imaging, computed tomography and positron emission tomography. Abdom Imaging 2007; 32: 624–34.

126. Furukawa H, Ikuma H, Seki A, et al. Positron emission tomography scanning is not superior to whole body multidetector helical computed tomography in the preoperative staging of colorectal cancer. Gut 2006; 55: 1007–11.

127. Dietrich CF, Kratzer W, Strobe D, et al. Assessment of metastatic liver disease in patients with primary extrahepatic tumors by contrast-enhanced sonography versus CT and MRI. World J Gastroenterol 2006; 12: 1699–705.

128. Lencioni R, Donati F, Cioni D, et al. Detection of colorectal liver metastases: prospective comparison of unenhanced and ferumoxides-enhanced magnetic resonance imaging at 1.5 T, dual-phase spiral CT, and spiral CT during arterial portography. MAGMA 1998; 7: 76–87.

129. Bluemke DA, Sahani D, Amendola M, et al. Efficacy and safety of MR imaging with liver-specific contrast agent: U.S. multicenter phase III study. Radiology 2005; 237: 89–98.

130. Hammerstingl R, Huppertz A, Breuer J, et al. Diagnostic efficacy of gadoxetic acid (Primovist)-enhanced MRI and spiral CT for a therapeutic strategy: comparison with intraoperative and histopathologic findings in focal liver lesions. Eur Radiol 2008; 18: 457–67.

131. Oliva MR, Saini S. Liver cancer imaging: role of CT, MRI, US and PET. Cancer Imaging 2004; 4 Spec No A: S42–S46.

132. Cervone A, Sardi A, Conaway GL. Intraoperative ultrasound (IOUS) is essential in the management of metastatic colorectal liver lesions. Am Surg 2000; 66: 611–15.

133. Zacherl J, Scheuba C, Imhof M, et al. Current value of intra-operative sonography during surgery for hepatic neoplasms. World J Surg 2002; 26: 550–4.

134. Fioole B, de Haas RJ, Wicherts DA, et al. Additional value of contrast enhanced intraoperative ultrasound for colorectal liver metastases. Eur J Radiol 2008; 67: 169–76.

135. Leen E, Ceccotti P, Moug SJ, et al. Potential value of contrast-enhanced intraoperative ultrasonography during partial hepatectomy for metastases: an essential investigation before resection? Ann Surg 2006; 243: 236–40.

136. Torzilli G, Del Fabbro D, Palmisano A, et al. Contrast-enhanced intraoperative ultrasonography during hepatectomies for colorectal cancer liver metastases. J Gastrointest Surg 2005; 9: 1148–53; discussion 53–4.

137. Tamandl D, Herberger B, Gruenberger B, et al. Adequate preoperative staging rarely leads to a change of intraopera-tive strategy in patients undergoing surgery for colorectal cancer liver metastases. Surgery 2008; 143: 648–57.

138. van Etten B, van der Sijp J, Kruyt R, et al. Ferumoxide-enhanced magnetic resonance imaging techniques in pre-operative assessment for colorectal liver metastases. Eur J Surg Oncol 2002; 28: 645–51.

139. Truant S, Huglo D, Hebbar M, et al. Prospective evaluation of the impact of [18F]fluoro-2-deoxy-D-glucose positron emission tomography of resectable colorectal liver metasta-ses. Br J Surg 2005; 92: 362–9.

140. Sahani DV, Kalva SP, Fischman AJ, et al. Detection of liver metastases from adenocarcinoma of the colon and pancreas: comparison of mangafodipir trisodium-enhanced liver MRI and whole-body FDG PET. Am J Roentgenol 2005; 185: 239–46.

141. Strasberg SM, Dehdashti F, Siegel BA, Drebin JA, Linehan D. Survival of patients evaluated by FDG-PET before hepatic resection for metastatic colorectal carcinoma: a prospective database study. Ann Surg 2001; 233: 293–9.

142. Wiering B, Krabbe PF, Jager GJ, Oyen WJ, Ruers TJ. The impact of fluor-18-deoxyglucose-positron emission tomog-raphy in the management of colorectal liver metastases. Cancer 2005; 104: 2658–70.

143. Flamen P, Stroobants S, Van Cutsem E, et al. Additional value of whole-body positron emission tomography with fluorine-18-2-fluoro-2-deoxy-D-glucose in recurrent colorectal cancer. J Clin Oncol 1999; 17: 894–901.

144. Lai DT, Fulham M, Stephen MS, et al. The role of whole-body positron emission tomography with [18F]fluorodeoxyglucose in identifying operable colorectal cancer metastases to the liver. Arch Surg 1996; 131: 703–7.

145. Staib L, Schirrmeister H, Reske SN, Beger HG. Is (18) F-fluorodeoxyglucose positron emission tomography in recurrent colorectal cancer a contribution to surgical decision making? Am J Surg 2000; 180: 1–5.

146. Topal B, Flamen P, Aerts R, et al. Clinical value of whole-body emission tomography in potentially curable colorectal liver metastases. Eur J Surg Oncol 2001; 27: 175–9.

147. Schussler-Fiorenza CM, Mahvi DM, Niederhuber J, Rikkers LF, Weber SM. Clinical risk score correlates with yield of PET scan in patients with colorectal hepatic metasta-ses. J Gastrointest Surg 2004; 8: 150–7; discussion 7–8.

148. Annemans L, Lencioni R, Warie H, et al. Health economic evaluation of ferucarbotran-enhanced MRI in the diagnosis of liver metastases in colorectal cancer patients. Int J Col-orectal Dis 2008; 23: 77–83.

44 Metastatic Effects on the Nervous System
David MacVicar

INTRODUCTION

Neurological complications in the cancer patient are an increasingly common problem. A simplistic explanation for this is that patients survive longer with their tumor and therefore develop more metastases at all sites, but it is also possible that the central nervous system (CNS) is a genuine "sanctuary site" for malignant cells from common solid tumors treated with systemic chemotherapy, just as it is in leukemia. A study of nearly 12,000 patients identified neurological complaints including altered mental state, headache, back pain, and leg weakness in 15% of patients with a variety of tumors (1). In small cell lung cancer, the incidence of neurological disorder caused by the disease is 29% (2), and a report from the Johns Hopkins Cancer Center identified neurological problems as the cause of 50% of unplanned hospital admissions, with changes in mental status, brain metastases and epidural spinal cord compression being the major problems (3). The effects of metastatic disease on the nervous system can be severely disabling, with a catastrophic effect on the quality of life of a patient whose tumor may be eminently treatable. This is partly because the brain and spinal cord are enclosed in bone, and thus relatively small-volume disease can cause disproportionately severe symptoms. In addition, the CNS lacks lymphatics, making removal of edema and biological detritus difficult and the capacity for regeneration of nervous tissue after damage is very limited.

A further difficulty is the sometimes bewildering clinical presentation of neurological problems in the cancer patient. An apparently simple symptom such as leg weakness has a wide differential diagnosis in a patient with systemic cancer, including:

- Cerebral deposits
- Compression of the spinal cord or cauda equina
- Leptomeningeal metastatic disease
- The effects of therapy such as cytotoxic drugs or steroids
- General debility

The effects of cancer on the nervous system may be classified into:

- Metastatic or direct effects of cancer
- Mass lesions compressing or infiltrating nervous tissues
- Indirect effects—non-metastatic or paraneoplastic syndromes

Paraneoplastic phenomena include vascular disorders, infections, metabolic effects, sequelae of treatment and the unusual but fascinating paraneoplastic syndromes. For the radiologist, a more useful approach is to classify by site in an attempt to narrow the area to be examined.

Once the area of greatest clinical suspicion has been identified, the majority of important differential diagnoses can be addressed using the most appropriate technique. The principal causes of neurological presentation in cancer patients according to site are listed in Table 44.1.

BRAIN

Clinical Presentation

Brain metastases may arise from any primary systemic cancer, but the majority of brain metastases originate from:

- Carcinoma of lung
- Carcinoma of breast
- Melanoma

Less common primary sites include renal and gastro-intestinal tumors and non-seminomatous testicular tumors; a significant number of brain metastases develop from a primary source that remains unknown even at autopsy (4). The following tumors rarely metastasize to the brain:

- Prostate
- Ovary
- Osteosarcoma
- Hodgkin's lymphoma

Most brain metastases, particularly those which arise from primary neoplasms other than the lung, occur at a late stage in dissemination of malignancy, and the presence of brain deposits is commonly associated with more widespread disease. Autopsy series have shown that asymptomatic brain metastases are present in patients dying of disseminated cancer in as many as 30% of cases.

The commonest presenting symptoms are:

- Headache
- Focal weakness
- Mental disturbance
- Seizures

Unsteadiness of gait is a prominent presenting complaint when the tumor lies in the cerebellum or brain stem but may occasionally occur as a result of a large frontal lobe metastasis or hydrocephalus caused by obstruction of cerebrospinal fluid (CSF) pathways. Less common presenting symptoms are:

- Difficulty with speech
- Visual disturbance
- Sensory disturbance

Signs of visual field loss and sensory abnormalities may be elicited by neurological examination. Some physical signs are present in most, but not all, patients with brain metastases. The onset of symptoms is frequently insidious.

Pathophysiology of Brain Metastases

Metastasis is a complicated pathophysiological process which is not completely understood. For malignant cells to metastasize from, for example, breast to brain, they must first enter the bloodstream, then cross the pulmonary capillary bed to enter the

Table 44.1 Major Neurological Problems (Classified by Site)

Site	Differential diagnosis
Brain	Parenchymal metastasis
	Leptomeningeal metastasis
	Infection (meningitis, brain abscess)
	Radiation encephalopathy
	Cerebral hemorrhage or infarction
	Metabolic and toxic encephalopathy (e.g., following cytotoxic chemotherapy)
	Primary brain tumors
Cranial neuropathy	Parenchymal deposits (false localizing signs)
	Leptomeningeal metastases
	Bony lesions of skull base
Spinal cord and cauda equina	Epidural compression
	Leptomeningeal metastasis
	Intramedullary metastasis
	Epidural abscess or hematoma
	Radiation myelopathy
	Myelopathy following intrathecal chemotherapy
	Paraneoplastic myelopathy
Peripheral nerves and plexuses	Extrinsic compression by tumor mass
	Direct infiltration by tumor
	Drug toxicity
	Varicella zoster infection
	Radiation plexopathy
	Paraneoplastic neuropathy
Neuromuscular junction and muscle	Drugs
	Paraneoplastic disorders (Eaton–Lambert myasthenic syndrome, myasthenia gravis)
	Corticosteroid-induced myopathy
	Cachectic myopathy
	Paraneoplastic polymyositis or dermatomyositis

arterial blood supply of the brain. The tumor embolus, if large enough, is likely to lodge in the watershed areas of the brain at the terminations of the major end-arteries and also in the grey/white junction where penetrating arterioles separate into capillary beds. This simple hemodynamic model should result in a predictable distribution of metastases within the brain, but there is clearly some variation in the distribution of metastases from certain tumors. The fertile soil hypothesis proposes that the host organ may synthesize and secrete factors which attract certain clones of circulating tumor cells and promote their growth (5). Delattre et al. have drawn attention to the preferential distribution of metastatic lesions to watershed areas, but also noted that in patients with gastro-intestinal and pelvic tumors there was predominant involvement of the posterior fossa, whereas with other tumors the cerebral hemispheres were more likely to be involved (6). It appears that infiltrating ductal carcinoma of the breast has a predilection to cause parenchymal brain metastases, whereas infiltrating lobular carcinoma is said to affect meningeal surfaces preferentially (7). Melanoma frequently metastasizes to the grey matter and experimental mouse melanoma lines have been developed which have specific predilection for brain parenchyma or the leptomeninges (8). Although these preferential distributions are fascinating, in practice virtually any tumor can metastasize to any part of the brain or meninges and variance with the expected pattern of distribution should not discourage the diagnosis of metastatic disease.

Imaging Techniques

In 1972, the introduction of computed tomography (CT) by Hounsfield and Ambrose revolutionized the diagnosis of brain tumors. Nearly 40 years later it remains a viable method of establishing the presence of brain deposits. Ideally, CT scans should be performed before and after intravenous (IV) contrast administration, but if a patient has a known primary tumor and a clinical presentation strongly supporting a diagnosis of metastasis, little is lost by performing postcontrast scans only.

Although CT is sufficient for diagnosis in many cases, there is no doubt that magnetic resonance (MR) imaging is a more sensitive technique than contrast-enhanced CT scanning for the detection of metastases to the brain parenchyma and remains the gold standard (Fig. 44.1) (9,10). A suitable protocol would include axial T2-weighted spin-echo and T1-weighted spin-echo images supplemented by gadolinium (Gd)-enhanced T1-weighted spin-echo sequences. A fluid attenuation inversion recovery (FLAIR) sequence is also useful for detecting metastatic edema and small focal areas of ischemic change. The use of the coronal plane should be considered, particularly if surgery is being contemplated, but the key factor is to ensure that the entire brain is covered. There is controversy over the dosage of gadolinium, particularly in the United States. Some authorities consider a dosage of 0.1 ml/kg body weight to be adequate, while others recommend a high-dose technique using three times this dose. Advocates of the high-dose technique point out the increased sensitivity as its chief advantage; in practical terms this is only important if local therapy is being considered for an ostensibly solitary metastasis and the cost implications of trebling the dose prevent routine use of this technique. Most European centers routinely administer an intermediate dose of gadolinium of 0.2 mg/kg body weight (11–13).

As MR imaging equipment evolves, there is constant reappraisal of the technical capabilities of the machinery. Magnetization transfer sequences have been tried, but have not entered the diagnostic mainstream (14). FLAIR sequences have been more durable (15), and more recently FLAIR with contrast enhancement has been advocated by Terae and colleagues (16). The authors conclude that addition of postcontrast FLAIR imaging to pre- and postcontrast T1-weighted imaging improves diagnostic confidence in the evaluation of brain metastases. Technical evaluation of 3T magnets in detection of brain metastases is underway. Kakeda et al. found that a contrast-enhanced three-dimensional gradient-echo sequence allowing reconstruction with 1.4 mm isotropic voxels was clinically more valuable for detecting small brain metastases than spin-echo and inversion recovery fast spin-echo sequences with a wider section thickness (17). Furutani et al. performed a similar comparison using a three-dimensional fast gradient-recalled acquisition in steady state and spin-echo T1-weighted imaging at 3T. They found that the enhancement following contrast medium injection was less on the three-dimensional images than on spin-echo images under the same conditions, but considered the 3D acquisition to be useful for detecting small lesions when a high dose of contrast medium was given and a suitable delay time was applied (18). In scientific literature, it is noticeable that few efforts are made to reduce the use of contrast agents. Considerable effort is put into detecting very small lesions, using high doses of contrast medium and thin slice reconstructions. While individual small lesions

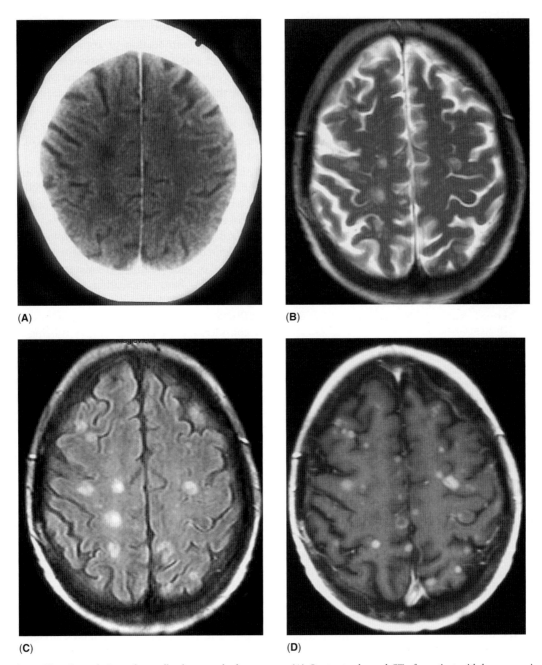

Figure 44.1 Comparison of imaging techniques for small volume cerebral metastases. (A) Contrast-enhanced CT of a patient with known carcinoma of breast with clinical suspicion of brain metastases. The deep cerebral white matter shows possible abnormality of attenuation, but no focal mass lesion was identified and the investigation was reported as clear of cerebral deposits. (B) T2-weighted spin-echo MR sequence obtained two days later owing to persisting clinical suspicion of cerebral metastatic disease shows abnormal signal intensity in white matter and at grey/white junction. (C) A FLAIR sequence shows multiple areas of abnormal signal intensity. (D) Gadolinium-enhanced T1-weighted spin-echo sequence at the same slice shows multiple enhancing lesions characteristic of cerebral deposits in white and grey matter of both hemispheres.

might be suitable for stereotactic radiotherapy or focal use of gamma radiation ("gamma knife" therapy), it should be remembered that discovery of brain metastases puts the patient into a position where treatment is essentially palliative and false positive diagnoses of brain metastases are potentially more damaging than a delay in diagnosis. The vast majority of MR imaging for brain metastases in oncological practice is done on machines operating at 1.5T, and in practice, gadolinium-enhanced T1-weighted spin-echo or fast spin-echo sequences remain the single most reliable sequence. It is also worth noting that detecting

brain metastases when clinically occult does not appear to have a survival advantage (19).

The role of ^{18}F-fluoro-deoxyglucose positron emission tomography (^{18}FDG PET) remains under evaluation. Compared with other organ systems, ^{18}FDG PET imaging of the brain is at a disadvantage because of high background glucose uptake and metabolism by normal grey matter. Although tumors may exhibit an increased uptake of glucose, this is difficult to detect. Co-registration with CT, or preferably MR imaging, is essential for accurate evaluation (20). However, it has been reported that metastatic brain lesions may

demonstrate photopenia on [18]FDG PET (21). Isotope studies, including [18]FDG PET and single photon emission computed tomography (SPECT) lack the necessary diagnostic accuracy and spatial resolution to challenge MR imaging as the investigation of choice for brain tumors.

Cerebral angiography retains a limited role in diagnostic evaluation and surgical planning of some primary brain tumors but does not have a role in management of metastatic disease. Plain radiographs, air-encephalography, and electro-encephalography are obsolete in the diagnosis of metastases.

Screening for Asymptomatic Brain Metastases

Cranial CT and MR imaging are only occasionally used as staging techniques at initial presentation of malignant disease in a patient with no neurological symptoms.

A specific clinical situation where brain imaging is performed in patients with no neurological symptoms is when thoracotomy is being considered with curative intent for non-small cell lung cancer. For many years, CT had been the mainstay of staging of the chest prior to thoracotomy, but PET-CT has recently become the investigation of choice (22,23). Lung cancer has a propensity to metastasize to the brain relatively early in the natural history of the disease compared with other common malignancies. For many years, cranial CT was added on to presurgical staging of thoracic disease with CT. With the move to more frequent use of PET-CT in local staging of lung cancer, there is a dilemma over which further imaging technique should be used. PET-CT is hampered by the high background uptake of FDG by the grey matter. MR imaging is established as a more sensitive technique, and its use as a staging procedure is likely to cause "stage migration". Seute et al., in a retrospective review demonstrated this "Will Rogers phenomenon". Between 1980 and 1991, their institution used CT as a staging investigation for brain metastases. From 1991 they changed to MR imaging. The prevalence of brain metastases in newly diagnosed small cell lung cancer was 10% in the CT era and 24% in the MR imaging era. In the CT era all detected brain metastases were symptomatic whereas in the MR imaging era, 11% were asymptomatic. The use of MR imaging made fewer patients eligible for prophylactic cranial irradiation (24). Yokoi et al. showed a similar tendency for MR imaging to detect more brain metastases than CT in a preoperative group of potentially operable non-small cell lung cancer. They noted that the mean maximum diameter of brain metastases was significantly smaller in the MR imaging group. However, the median survival time after treatment of detected brain metastases was 10 months in the CT group and 17 months in the MR imaging group. More significantly, the two-year survival rate after treatment of brain metastases was 27% in the CT group and 28% in the MR imaging group (25).

Tumor histology and local stage appear to have some influence on the incidence of brain metastases. In patients with Stage I and Stage II squamous cell lung carcinoma, no brain metastases were found, but in potentially resectable Stage III disease the incidence was 8%. For Stage III localized adenocarcinoma, the incidence was 23%; for Stage III large cell carcinoma, 57%. For Stage III non-small cell tumors of all histological types, the overall incidence of asymptomatic brain deposits was 17.5%, which is clearly relevant when considering such patients for surgery. In patients with small cell lung carcinoma and apparently limited disease, the incidence of asymptomatic brain deposits was 14% (26). Although very few patients with small cell lung cancer are suitable for surgery, cranial irradiation can palliate, and some centers include brain scanning as a staging investigation for this disease. If a policy of screening for asymptomatic brain metastases is to be pursued with any primary tumor, MR remains the most sensitive investigation. [18]FDG PET used as a "whole-body" staging method has been demonstrated to be less sensitive and specific for demonstration of brain metastases (27).

Computed tomography (CT) or MR imaging of the brain is included as a staging investigation in selected patients with non-seminomatous germ cell tumors of the testis (NSGCT). Asymptomatic brain metastases may be seen at presentation in patients with aggressive disseminated disease and are more common in patients with trophoblastic teratoma than with any other histological type (28). Those patients considered at high risk will have grossly elevated serum tumor markers [human chorionic gonadotrophin (HCG) greater than 20,000 IU] or multiple pulmonary metastases (more than 50). Asymptomatic brain deposits may also be seen at the time of large-volume pulmonary relapse following chemotherapy, and any patient being put forward for high-dose salvage chemotherapy for multiple relapses of non-seminomatous germ cell tumor should have a brain scan. If cerebral deposits are present, any residual mass following treatment is likely to contain differentiated tumor, and will be resected if accessible.

Notwithstanding these exceptions, and acknowledging that brain lesions may be the presenting symptom of unknown primaries, the majority of brain metastases present late in the natural history of the disease, and are usually associated with some symptomatology, however vague. Early diagnosis of asymptomatic brain lesions rarely influences the outcome of disease, and brain imaging is not recommended as a staging investigation in most clinical circumstances (29).

General Imaging Features

The majority of metastases in the brain grow as spherical masses, displacing rather than destroying brain tissue. Some metastases are more irregular, and all create edema in the surrounding brain. The amount of edema is extremely variable, and its extent is not a reliable sign in differential diagnosis of metastasis from other pathological entities. Brain metastases are usually solid, but if they grow rapidly, they may undergo central necrosis. "Cystic" lesions occasionally occur, particularly from primary breast carcinoma and squamous cell carcinoma from any site. At a pathological level, metastatic brain tumors usually show extensive neovascularization, and are accompanied by breakdown of the blood–brain barrier. Some tumors, for example melanoma and NSGCT, have a tendency to be hemorrhagic. The typical appearance of a metastasis from a primary carcinoma on CT is a mass of similar attenuation to normal brain, associated with surrounding edema and brisk enhancement following IV contrast injection. On MR, most metastatic lesions are masses with a signal intensity higher than that of normal brain on T2-weighted sequences and surrounded by very high signal intensity edema. On T1-weighted sequences they are isointense with brain and show enhancement with Gd-DTPA (Fig. 44.2). Metastases are usually discrete masses but are not necessarily multiple. The maxim that not all metastases are multiple, and not all multiple lesions are metastases remains valid in clinical practice.

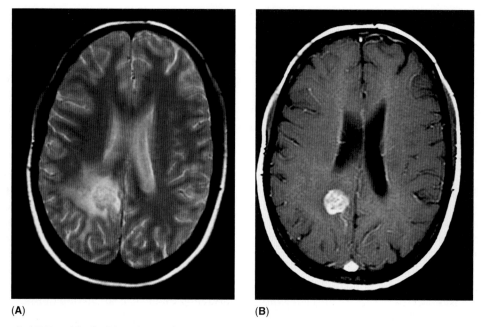

(A)   **(B)**

Figure 44.2 Cerebral metastasis. (**A**) T2-weighted axial MR image. The tumor mass is of higher signal intensity than surrounding brain. Surrounding edema returns high signal intensity. (**B**) T1-weighted MR image following Gd-DTPA shows an enhancing mass.

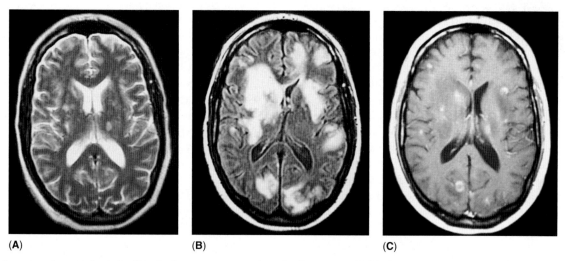

(A)   **(B)**   **(C)**

Figure 44.3 Patient presenting with headache following bone marrow transplantation for acute myeloid leukemia. (**A**) T2-weighted spin-echo MR sequence in axial plane shows vague areas of increased signal in white matter. These lesions did not enhance following injection of gadolinium. (**B**) Follow-up imaging performed three weeks later due to patient's increasing confusion. FLAIR image shows mass lesions with florid surrounding high signal intensity due to edema. (**C**) Following gadolinium administration, multiple enhancing lesions are seen. At biopsy, a diagnosis of cerebral toxoplasmosis was made.

Differential Diagnosis of Brain Metastases

In general, the diagnosis of brain metastasis in a patient known to have cancer presents few difficulties. The most difficult differential diagnosis is with primary tumors such as:

- Meningioma
- Pituitary adenoma
- Acoustic neuroma
- Glioma

Gliomas tend to be more diffuse in their growth pattern, but metastases in an appropriate anatomical situation may mimic meningioma and other primary tumors almost exactly. In one study, six of 54 patients with known cancer and solitary brain lesions did not have metastases on biopsy, and three of these had non-neoplastic lesions (30). However, if the clinical history and

appropriate imaging features, especially with multiple lesions, are present, the diagnosis of brain metastases can be established with reasonable certainty. Other clinical differential diagnoses include:

- Cerebral hemorrhage
- Cerebral embolus
- Abscess
- Viral infections
- Treatment related encephalopathy syndromes
- Radiation injury

Cerebral hemorrhage or embolus will have characteristic imaging features. Infections, particularly abscess formation, can cause problems of differential diagnosis, especially in patients with lymphoma and hematological malignancies (Fig. 44.3). Viral infections have a tendency to diffuse involvement of the brain without mass formation

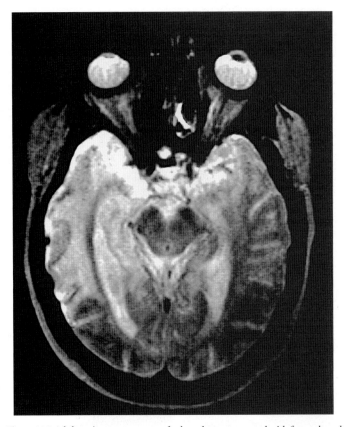

Figure 44.4 Adult patient on treatment for lymphoma presented with fever, altered mental state and seizures. T2-weighted axial MR image. There is diffuse high signal intensity in both temporal lobes. There is no discrete mass lesion, the abnormality affects grey and white matter, and is asymmetrical. The features are typical of herpes simplex encephalitis, and are unlikely to be confused with metastatic disease.

and often have a characteristic clinical syndrome. Examples are herpes simplex encephalitis (Fig. 44.4) and progressive multifocal leuco-encephalopathy (Fig. 44.5), which is thought to be a result of reactivation of papova virus infection during prolonged suppression of cellular immunity. Cytotoxic leuco-encephalopathy may be seen with drug regimens involving 5-fluorouracil and levamisole, or intrathecal methotrexate (Fig. 44.6) (31,32). Focal changes, detectable as reversible high signal lesions in the deep cerebral white matter on MR imaging, have also been demonstrated with a variety of high-dose IV chemotherapy regimens for common solid tumors (33). These lesions do not enhance with gadolinium-DTPA, and clinically present with non-specific problems such as headache and seizures.

A relatively frequent and often characteristic clinical entity which should be differentiated from relapse is the so-called posterior reversible encephalopathy syndrome. This is most often seen in patients who have undergone bone marrow transplantation (BMT) for hematological malignancies such as leukemia and lymphoma. The clinical presentation is with headache, decreased level of consciousness and seizures, with or without focal neurology such as cortical blindness or paralysis. CT may show some reduced attenuation in the posterior white and grey matter, but changes may be subtle. MR imaging is more sensitive and the observed changes reflect edema in certain areas of the brain, predominantly in the posterior cerebral hemispheres. However, the cerebellum, brain stem, basal ganglia, subcortical white matter, and frontal lobes may also be affected. Diffusion-weighted imaging may help to distinguish between areas of vasogenic edema, which show potentially reversible free diffusion, and areas of established infarction which will show cytotoxic edema and restricted diffusion. Neurological presentations following BMT are not uncommon,

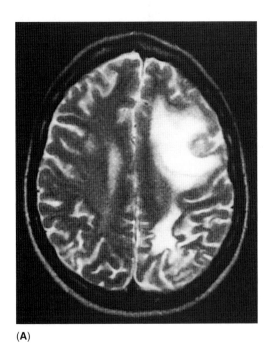

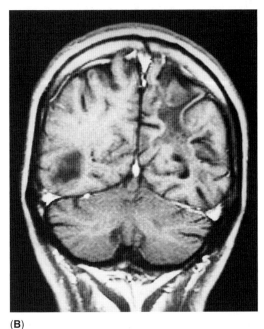

(A)   **(B)**

Figure 44.5 (A) T2-weighted axial MR image. Areas of diffuse grey and white matter abnormality are seen bilaterally. (B) T1-weighted MR coronal image. Rather than mass effect, there is a loss of substance within the grey and white matter. These appearances are typical of progressive multifocal leuco-encephalopathy.

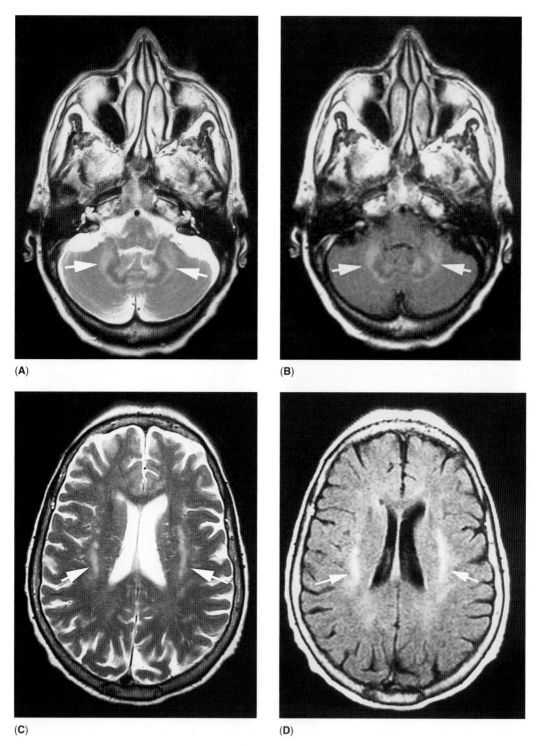

Figure 44.6 T2-weighted and FLAIR MR images through posterior fossa (A) and (B), and cerebral hemispheres (C) and (D), showing high signal intensity in cerebellar and cerebral white matter (arrows). Changes are seen on both pulse sequences and are slightly more pronounced on FLAIR images. The patient was receiving intrathecal methotrexate and had developed non-specific neurological symptoms, including headache and a mild confusional state. The appearance is consistent with white matter change seen in association with intrathecal chemotherapy. The observed abnormalities will frequently resolve on withdrawal or completion of treatment.

and cyclosporin A has increasingly been identified as a potential etiological factor. The mechanism of the neurotoxicity is not entirely clear, but the distribution of lesions suggests a vascular process. The imaging findings are very similar to those seen in hypertensive encephalopathy, and the clinical syndrome of posterior reversible encephalopathy syndrome is sometimes associated with a sustained increase in blood pressure which

resolves on withdrawal of cyclosporin. In most clinical circumstances, treatment-related encephalopathy syndrome should be distinguishable from metastatic disease (Fig. 44.7) (34–37).

Radiation necrosis may be difficult to differentiate from recurrent brain metastases as it tends to enhance and may form ring lesions. However, it is rarely a problem at initial diagnosis of brain metastases and is more often part of the differential diagnosis

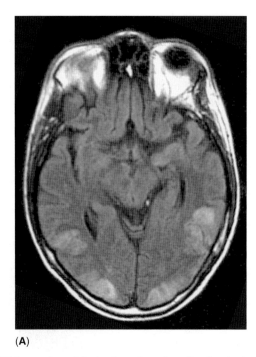

(A)

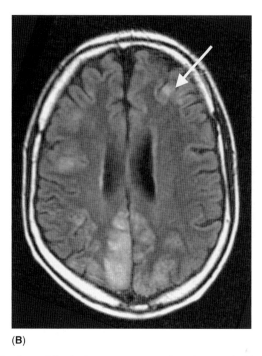

(B)

Figure 44.7 FLAIR MR images through brain of a patient who suffered tonic-clonic seizures following bone marrow transplantation, associated with non-specific neurological disturbance. (**A**) There are areas of high signal in grey and white matter in the occipital, parietal and posterior temporal regions. (**B**) Although the changes are predominantly posterior, some abnormality is detected in the frontal lobes (arrow). A diagnosis of posterior reversible encephalopathy syndrome (PRES) was made, and cyclosporine treatment was withdrawn. The clinical syndrome and imaging abnormalities resolved. Although the clinical entity is described as reversible, the imaging abnormality sometimes persists. *Source*: From Ref. 34.

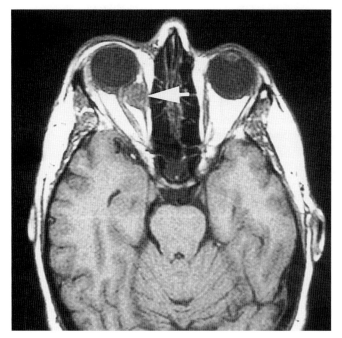

Figure 44.8 T1-weighted axial MR image in a patient with gaze paralysis interpreted as possible right 6th nerve palsy. A melanoma deposit is present in the right orbit (arrow), which was fixing the medial rectus and preventing normal eye movements.

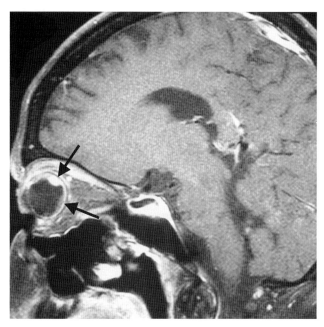

Figure 44.9 A patient with known metastatic breast cancer presented with visual disturbance and was referred for routine brain imaging. Supplementary gadolinium-enhanced T1-weighted sagittal MR sequences were obtained through the orbital regions and revealed diffuse enhancement of the retina and choroid, and an enhancing mass lesion lying superiorly in the globe, representing involvement by metastatic disease (arrows).

following treatment of primary brain tumors. Occasionally, intercurrent common diseases, such as multiple sclerosis, are seen in patients known to have cancer. In the absence of typical imaging features of metastatic disease, a review of the clinical features is of paramount importance and will frequently influence image interpretation. For example, patients presenting with disturbance of eye movements or other cranial nerve symptoms and signs may have disease around the skull base or in the orbit rather than brain metastases (Figs. 44.8 and 44.9).

Key Points: Brain Metastases

- Most brain metastases occur late in the natural history of malignant disease
- Gadolinium-enhance MR imaging is more sensitive than CT for detecting brain metastases
- [18]FDG PET is disadvantaged as a method for detection of brain metastases by high background glucose uptake in the grey matter
- Imaging for asymptomatic brain metastases is not routinely undertaken. Exceptions to this are patients with lung cancer being planned for thoracotomy with curative intent, and selected patients with non-seminomatous germ cell tumors of the testis
- The differential diagnosis of brain metastases includes primary brain tumors, cerebral hemorrhage, infection, treatment-related leuco-encephalopathy, and radiation injury

Imaging Features of Some Common Brain Metastases

Metastases from all primary tumors may look identical, but some of the common causes have "trademark" features, which if present, may increase confidence in diagnosis. Virtually all cancers are capable of metastasizing to the brain. Lung and breast are the commonest organs of origin, followed by malignant melanoma.

Bronchial tumors are the single commonest cause of metastatic deposits in the brain. Adenocarcinoma of the lung and squamous cell carcinoma typically metastasize to the grey/white junction, and both may produce ring-like enhancement on both CT and MR (Figs. 44.10 and 44.11). A small cell lung cancer may produce large masses, but frequently produces innumerable small metastases throughout the brain. These small lesions are best seen on enhanced T1-weighted MR imaging, emphasizing the increased sensitivity available with this technique (Figs. 44.12 and 44.13).

Carcinoma of the breast has a tendency to metastasize to the periphery of the brain. An association between breast cancer and

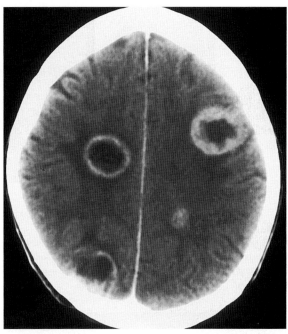

Figure 44.10 Contrast-enhanced CT showing multiple ring-enhancing lesions, a typical appearance in metastatic squamous cell carcinoma of the lung, but also seen with metastatic adenocarcinoma.

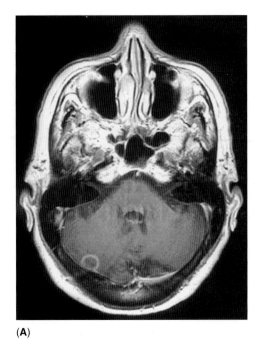

(A)

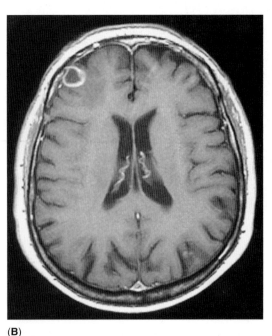

(B)

Figure 44.11 Gadolinium-enhanced T1-weighted MR image of brain demonstrating rim enhancing metastases from squamous carcinoma of the lung in (**A**) the cerebellum and (**B**) in the right frontal lobe.

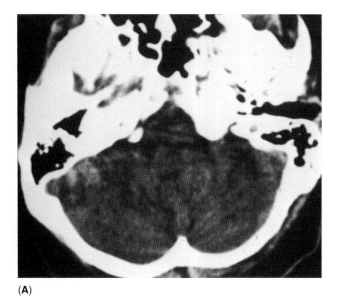

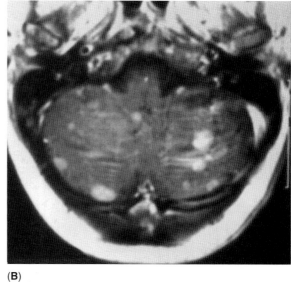

Figure 44.12 Small cell lung cancer. (**A**) Contrast-enhanced CT through posterior fossa is equivocal. Individual metastases cannot be reliably identified. (**B**) T1-weighted MR image following gadolinium administration performed two days later. Multiple small lesions were scattered throughout the posterior fossa.

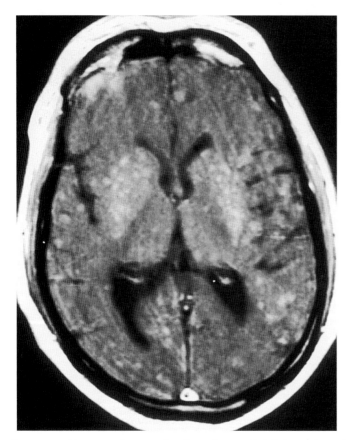

Figure 44.13 Metastases from small cell carcinoma. Gadolinium-enhanced T1-weighted spin-echo MR image shows multiple small enhancing lesions through the brain.

meningioma has created considerable interest among researchers. Some authors report a higher incidence of meningioma in women with breast cancer, although this has been disputed (38–40). Meningiomas have a relative lack of peritumoral edema, and show homogeneous contrast enhancement and attachment to

the dura. However, the practical problem is that metastases from breast carcinoma may mimic in every way the features of meningioma, and vice versa. Oncologists are naturally keen to establish the definitive diagnosis and consider surgery. An early follow-up scan is frequently helpful as it will establish the tempo of disease; a rapidly enlarging lesion, with or without new lesions, will confirm a diagnosis of metastatic disease and will avoid inappropriate craniotomy (Fig. 44.14). Breast carcinoma also has a tendency to metastasize to the pituitary gland where it can mimic an adenoma.

Metastases from malignant melanoma can exhibit some characteristic features. Like metastases from malignant testicular tumors and renal carcinoma, these tumors can be large and may have a prominent hemorrhagic component. The breakdown products of blood may have paramagnetic or superparamagnetic effects. In addition, melanin pigments have intrinsic paramagnetic properties as a result of their molecular structure (41). This can result in melanoma deposits having a high signal intensity on unenhanced T1-weighted images and a low signal intensity on T2-weighted images owing to the paramagnetic effect of pigments on proton relaxation (Fig. 44.15).

Colon cancer deposits may also exhibit paramagnetic effects, with a high signal intensity on T1-weighted images and a low signal intensity on T2 weighting. This is presumed to be caused by mucinous macromolecules (Fig. 44.16). Very occasionally, a similar appearance is seen in metastases from mucinous adenocarcinomas of ovary, breast, stomach, and pancreas.

Involvement of the brain by lymphoma is becoming more common, particularly in patients with human immunodeficiency virus (HIV) infection and other forms of immunosuppression. Lymphoma deposits are typically of higher attenuation than normal brain on unenhanced CT images and show only slight contrast enhancement (Fig. 44.17). There is relatively little edema, and the lesions are situated characteristically around the midline. On T2-weighted MR imaging, lesions may be of mixed signal

1057

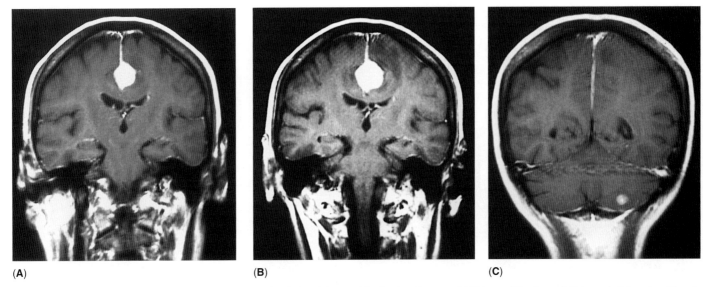

(A)   **(B)**   **(C)**

Figure 44.14 Patient with carcinoma of breast, presenting with headaches. (**A**) T1-weighted spin-echo coronal MR image following gadolinium administration. There is an enhancing mass apparently centered on the falx. The differential diagnosis lies between a deposit from carcinoma of the breast and a falx meningioma. (**B**) and (**C**) Rather than immediate craniotomy, a follow-up scan was obtained after a four week interval. This shows a clearly discernible enlargement of the falx lesion over a four week period, and further small lesions became detectable within the cerebellum during the interval. A diagnosis of cerebral metastatic disease was made.

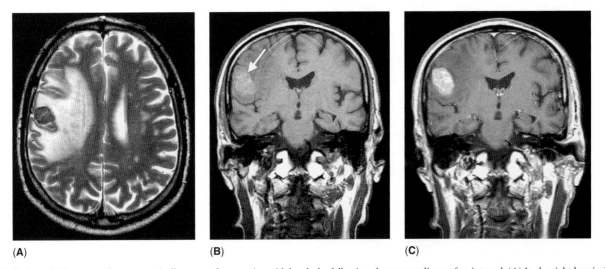

(A)   **(B)**   **(C)**

Figure 44.15 Patient with known melanoma surgically removed, presenting with headache following eleven-year disease-free interval. (**A**) In the right hemisphere there is a mass lesion returning low signal on a T2-weighted MR sequence with extensive surrounding white matter edema. The unenhanced T1-weighted coronal image (**B**) shows the mass lesion to return high signal (arrow). The mass enhances following gadolinium administration (**C**). The unusual signal characteristics, with reduced signal intensity on the T2-weighted image and increased signal intensity on unenhanced T1-weighted image, are a result of the paramagnetic effect of melanin pigment.

with some areas which are hypointense compared to normal brain (Fig. 44.18).

INTRACRANIAL MENINGEAL DISEASE

Cancer may reach the meninges by direct contact with tumor in brain or bone, or by hematogenous dissemination. Once contact is made with the CSF, tumor cells are likely to be shed and disseminate through CSF pathways to seed elsewhere in either a diffuse pattern or as multiple individual foci. Meningeal metastases are

increasingly recognized, and are common in the leukemias. They are sometimes seen in:

- Non-Hodgkin's lymphoma
- Breast carcinoma
- Lung carcinoma
- Malignant melanoma

Meningeal depotsits have also been described in a wide variety of other tumors. The clinical presentation can be obscure, with non-specific symptoms such as headache, mental change, nausea, and vertigo predominating. They can be difficult to diagnose with

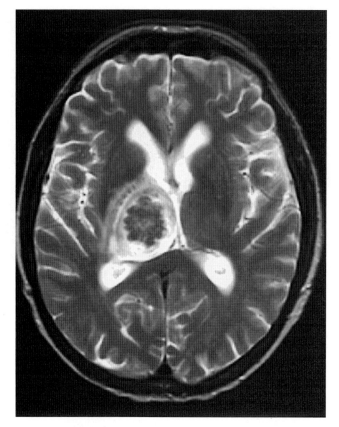

Figure 44.16 T2-weighted spin-echo axial MR image. Carcinoma of colon. Marked signal hypointensity is present in the central part of the deposit, which was not calcified on CT scanning. This appearance may be seen with mucinous adenocarcinoma deposits.

imaging studies, particularly if diffuse. Meningeal metastases enhance with contrast medium, but can be demonstrated on CT only if gross. Magnetic resonance (MR) imaging with gadolinium enhancement is more reliable but false negative examinations may occur (42–44). There are several causes of false positive results:

- Some meningeal enhancement can frequently be demonstrated in normal patients without meningeal disease
- Lumbar puncture with or without intrathecal chemotherapy can cause the meninges to enhance abnormally
- Previous surgery and radiation may also result in diffuse abnormality for months or years

However, despite these difficulties, MR is the most useful imaging technique, as its multiplanar imaging capability allows the demonstration of meningeal masses around the calvarium and skull base more readily than CT (Figs. 44.19 and 44.20). A meningeal mass lesion in the appropriate clinical setting is adequate confirmation of diagnosis of meningeal disease. Nodular enhancement of the leptomeninges deep in the cerebral sulci is the most convincing manifestation of intracranial meningeal metastasis. An important clinical circumstance in which meningeal deposits may arise is following surgery for primary brain tumors. The appearance of the meningeal disease is similar to metastases from distant common solid tumors, but often more florid (Figs. 44.21 and 44.22).

The majority of meningeal deposits affect the leptomeninges, and these are usually presumed to metastasize by the hematogenous route. A different pattern of imaging abnormality is seen in dural metastatic disease where asymmetrical or focal plaques of thickened enhancing dura are found, sometimes associated with adjacent bony disease, suggesting that metastatic disease may spread to the

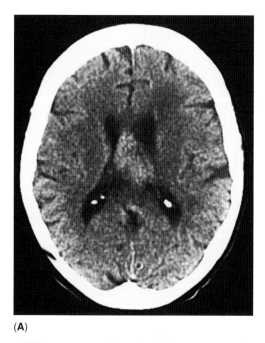

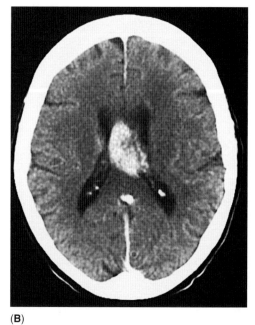

(A)　　　　　　　　　**(B)**

Figure 44.17 (**A**) Pre- and (**B**) post-contrast-enhanced CT. There is a mass involving the corpus callosum associated with a little edema and of attenuation slightly higher than normal brain. Modest enhancement is present after IV contrast. The distribution and appearance are characteristic of lymphoma. The patient had suffered several relapses of non-Hodgkin's lymphoma before presenting with headache.

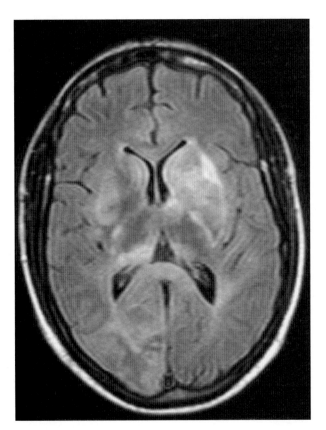

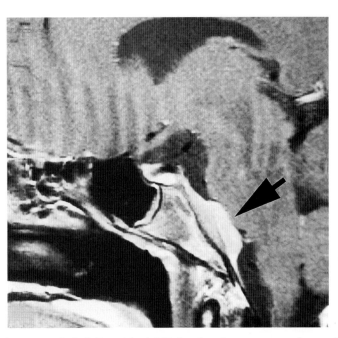

Figure 44.20 Sagittal T1-weighted MR imaging demonstrates a plaque of lymphoma (arrow) involving the basal meninges.

Figure 44.18 Adult patient presenting with previous history of lymphoma and clinical symptoms of headache. Axial FLAIR MR image demonstrates mixed signal intensity through thalamus and basal ganglia bilaterally. The midline site and relative lack of edema are characteristic of lymphoma. There was also little enhancement following contrast. Biopsy demonstrated diffuse large B-cell lymphoma.

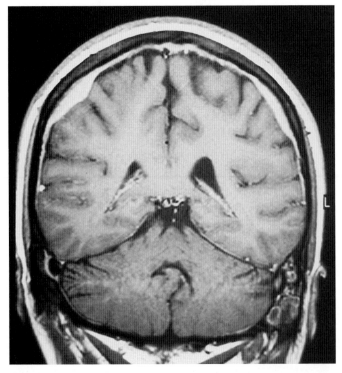

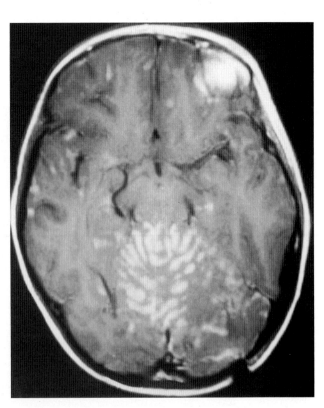

Figure 44.19 There is asymmetrical thickening and enhancement of the dura around the calvarium consistent with metastatic infiltration, demonstrated on gadolinium-enhanced T1-weighted coronal imaging.

Figure 44.21 T1-weighted spin-echo MR image with gadolinium enhancement shows extensive abnormal enhancement of the tentorium and further enhancing lesions in the leptomeninges, for example in the right sylvian fissure. The patient had been previously treated for medulloblastoma, and the appearance represents recurrent meningeal disease.

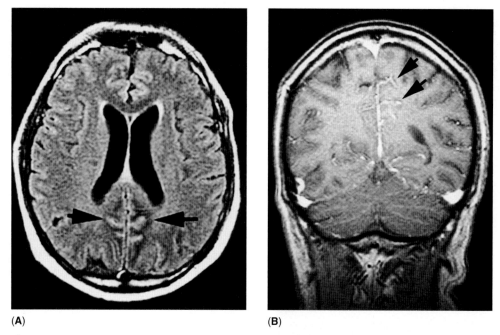

Figure 44.22 Subtle signs of meningeal metastatic disease. (**A**) Axial MR FLAIR sequence shows localized abnormality of signal in the para-falcine meninges and adjacent grey matter (arrows). (**B**) Gadolinium-enhanced T1-weighted coronal MR images show nodular asymmetrical enhancement in the leptomeninges of the medial parietal lobes. Some enhancement of the dura may be seen under normal circumstances, but nodular enhancement deep in the sulci (arrows), which was seen at several sites in this patient, is sufficient to make the diagnosis of meningeal metastatic disease in appropriate clinical circumstances. This patient had presented with headache and had known pulmonary metastases from melanoma.

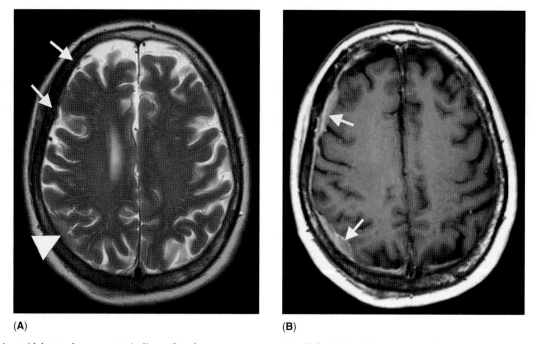

Figure 44.23 A patient with known bony metastatic disease from breast cancer presenting with headache. (**A**) T2-weighted MR image demonstrates low signal intensity in the bone marrow of the skull on the right (arrows). Abnormal signal intensity is also present on the surface of the brain in the right parietal region (arrowhead). (**B**) Gadolinium-enhanced T1-weighted imaging shows enhancement and focal thickening of the dura indicating the presence of metastatic disease (arrows). This pattern of disease suggests that metastatic spread to the meninges from adjacent tumor involved bone has occurred.

dura directly from adjacent bony metastases (Fig. 44.23). Dural metastatic disease is also seen in the absence of bony disease, indicating that hematogenous spread to the dura can occur (Fig. 44.19).

Cranial nerve abnormalities may be the presenting feature of meningeal disease, and when meningeal disease presents with non-specific symptoms, subtle cranial nerve signs may be detectable.

When cranial nerve symptoms and signs are present, a differential diagnosis must be made between involvement of the nerves at meningeal level or by tumor deposits in the bone around the skull base. Meningeal metastases affecting the cranial nerves are usually small, although occasionally they are large enough to mimic extrinsic tumors such as acoustic neuromas and meningiomas

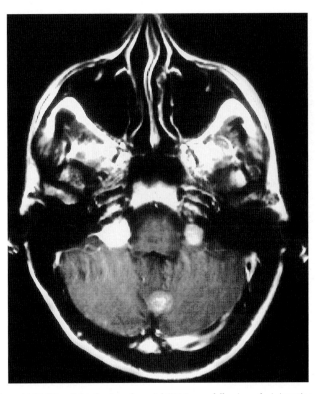

Figure 44.24 T1-weighted spin-echo axial MR image following administration of gadolinium. Bilateral enhancing masses are present in the cerebello-pontine angles mimicking acoustic neuromas. There is a further lesion between the cerebellar hemispheres. Postmortem examination confirmed meningeal metastases from melanoma.

(Fig. 44.24). As always, clinical correlation is useful in directing and informing the diagnostic search, for example, if a trigeminal neuropathy is clinically apparent, this will allow more confident diagnosis of lesions in an anatomically appropriate location (Fig. 44.25). In the absence of meningeal disease by imaging criteria, skull base deposits should initially be sought and sequences such as short tau inversion recovery (STIR) are frequently useful in highlighting bony pathology in the skull base. A deposit in the floor of the middle cranial fossa or clivus has the potential to cause multiple cranial nerve palsies and this pattern of disease is not uncommon in metastatic prostate and breast cancer. For example, an expansile deposit in the greater wing of the sphenoid might compress branches of the trigeminal nerve within the foramen ovale and rotundum.

The diagnosis of leptomeningeal metastatic disease is sometimes far from straightforward, and the combination of imaging and cerebrospinal fluid (CSF) cytology is necessary. Because the clinical presentation of meningeal disease may not be anatomically precise, it is useful to examine the part of the neuraxis which is symptomatic rather than imaging the whole of the brain and spine. There are fairly frequent false negative MR imaging examinations in patients who have positive CSF cytology, and this occurs more often in hematological malignancies such as leukemia and lymphoma than with solid tumors. Conversely, neuroimaging can be convincingly positive for meningeal disease where CSF remains negative, a phenomenon most frequently seen with solid tumors where presumably the malignant cells are adherent to a plaque of tumor and do not shed into the CSF. Because MR

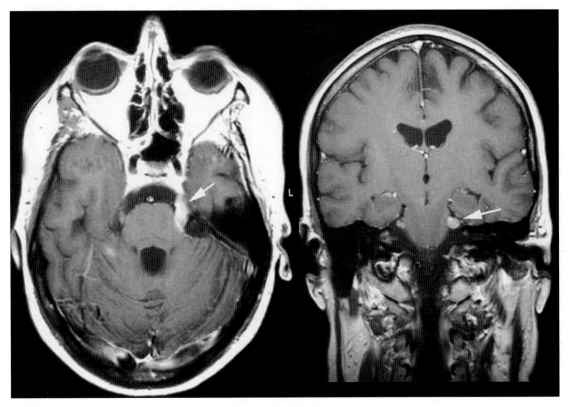

Figure 44.25 Gadolinium-enhanced T1-weighted axial and coronal MR images of a patient with breast carcinoma metastatic to lung and bone. Symptoms had developed of trigeminal neuropathy. Both trigeminal nerves are visible, but the left trigeminal nerve is thickened (arrows) in keeping with involvement by meningeal metastatic disease.

imaging with administration of IV contrast medium is less invasive, it is the investigation which is performed first but if clinical suspicion remains strong, CSF cytology should be obtained via lumbar puncture, which may need to be repeated to obtain positive cytology which has the advantage of 100% specificity (45,46).

The clinical background for meningeal metastatic disease is of paramount importance. Meningeal metastatic disease is very rarely identified as the first manifestation of distant metastatic disease. In the absence of established disease spread, the diagnosis should be made with great caution, as vascular events may lead to the development of hypertrophic vessels which give an imaging appearance which may mimic peripheral brain enhancement or meningeal enhancement (Fig. 44.26).

Key Points: Intracranial Meningeal Metastases

- Meningeal deposits are most frequently seen in the leukemias, non-Hodgkin's lymphoma, breast cancer, lung cancer, and malignant melanoma
- The clinical features are often non-specific
- Meningeal metastases enhance with contrast medium and are best demonstrated on MR imaging
- Some dural meningeal enhancement may be seen in normal patients

SPINAL CORD AND CAUDA EQUINA

Epidural Spinal Cord Compression

While most symptomatic intracranial metastases involve the brain parenchyma, in the spinal canal most symptomatic tumors compress the spinal cord or cauda equina from the epidural space, while intramedullary and meningeal disease is more unusual.

Most epidural compression is caused by a tumor that has metastasized to the vertebral body; the most frequent cancers are:

- Carcinoma of breast
- Carcinoma of lung
- Carcinoma of prostate
- Multiple myeloma

In patients with systemic cancer, incidences of symptomatic spinal cord compression reported in the literature vary from 1% to 5%, and at autopsy approximately 5% of patients dying from cancer exhibit spinal cord or cauda equina compression (47–50).

Clinical Presentation

Pain is the earliest and most frequent presenting symptom of spinal cord compression. It is usually mild at first but becomes progressively more severe. However, absence of pain does not mean absence of cord compression and very occasionally other clinical features of the clinical syndrome develop before pain is reported. The pain may be of several types:

- Local
- Radicular
- Funicular

In most patients the initial pain is local and perceived as a steady ache at the site of the involved vertebral body. Compression of nerve roots within the spinal canal or within the exit foramina generates radicular pain, which may precede local pain and is typically band-like if the lesion is in the thoracic region, and radiates to arms and legs in cervical and lumbar regions, respectively. Funicular pain is caused by compression of ascending (sensory) spinal cord tracts, causing symptoms that are apparently remote from the lesion and in a non-dermatomal distribution. For example, upper thoracic or cervical cord compression can cause funicular pain in the lower extremities, or band-like pain around the thorax and abdomen.

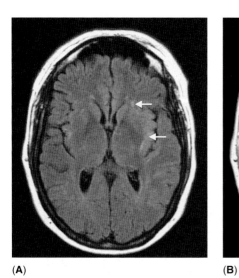 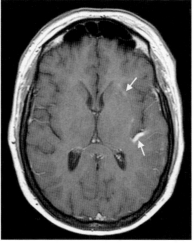 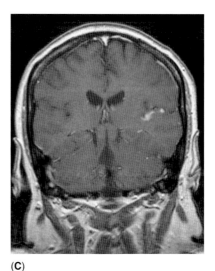

| (A) | (B) | (C) |

Figure 44.26 Patient with a history of carcinoma of cervix, presenting with loss of power in right leg. (A) FLAIR MR sequence shows barely detectable high signal in grey and white matter of left hemisphere (arrows). (B) and (C) Following injection of gadolinium, focal areas of enhancement are detected (arrows). These represent hypertrophic vessels in the aftermath of an episode of ischemia/infarction but could be interpreted as enhancing meningeal lesions. The key to diagnosis is correlation with the clinical history of a resolving hemiplegia. While a history of cervical cancer was known, no disease outside the pelvis had been reported.

Following the prodrome of pain which may be prolonged, other symptoms and signs develop rapidly, including:

- Weakness
- Sensory loss
- Autonomic dysfunction

Weakness is the second most common finding. It usually results from damage to the corticospinal tracts. The weakness begins in the legs, regardless of the level of compression and is more marked proximally early in the course of development of symptoms. The patient usually complains of difficulty in walking and climbing stairs, and this symptom should precipitate a sense of urgency in the investigative chain, as treatment at this stage may enable full recovery of power. In the early stages, typical signs of upper motor neuron weakness may be absent, with spasticity and hyper-reflexia developing later. If the onset of spinal cord compression is sudden and leads to complete paraplegia, most patients are flaccid with areflexia, as a result of distal spinal reflex inhibition.

Lower motor neuron weakness results from compression of the cauda equina, and is characterized by hypotonia, atrophy, and areflexia. Dysfunction of anterior horn cells in the spinal cord may also be seen, possibly as a result of vascular abnormality rather than true mechanical compression. The presence of lower motor neuron weakness will mask upper motor neuron signs at a higher level, so it should be remembered that in the presence of cauda equina compression, which explains lower motor neuron signs in the legs, an additional level of true cord compression may also be present.

Sensory loss follows shortly after the development of weakness, and the level will rise to arrive at the true level of compression given time. However, at the time of imaging, the sensory level may be several segments below the compressive lesion. Sensory loss is rarely as profound or disabling as weakness. Autonomic dysfunction causes bladder and bowel dysfunction, and impotence in men in more than 50% of patients by the time of diagnosis of spinal cord or cauda equina compression. Bladder dysfunction predominates, with urinary retention being associated with sudden onset of compression, while urgency with incontinence is a relatively frequent complaint if symptoms are evolving slowly.

Key Points: Spinal Cord Compression

- Most tumors that compress the spinal cord are situated in the epidural space
- Pain is the earliest presenting feature and may be local, radicular, or funicular
- In the early stages of spinal cord compression, upper motor neuron signs may initially be absent
- Lower motor neuron weakness will mask upper motor neuron signs from compression, at a higher level
- The sensory level may initially be several segments below the true compressive lesion
- Bladder dysfunction is the predominant autonomic disturbance

Pathophysiology

The neurological presentation of spinal cord compression can be variable and occasionally confusing, and this is partly explained by consideration of the site of the epidural compressive lesion and its relationship with the blood supply of the cord and the site of motor and sensory tracts within the cord.

The advent of MR has clearly demonstrated that the vertebral body is involved more often than the posterior elements in patients with spinal cord compression, but all parts of the vertebra are susceptible. Some tumors, notably lymphoma, can invade the epidural space without involving the vertebrae. The dura is up to a millimeter thick and relatively resistant to penetration by tumor. Epidural tumors rarely breach the dura to invade the cord, but may interfere with the delicate blood supply. The cord receives its blood supply predominantly from the anterior spinal artery which forms an anastomotic chain running the length of the cord and breaking into cauda equina arteries in the lumbar region (Fig. 44.27). The anterior spinal artery is supplied by radicular arteries which are branches of the vertebral artery in the cervical region. In the thoracic region the anterior spinal artery is supplied via the anterior radicular arteries, which come off the dorsal branch of the posterior intercostal arteries, which in turn emanate directly from the aorta. The anatomy is variable and some major anterior radicular arteries, such as the artery of Adamkiewicz, are well known to angiographers. The blood supply of the cord is vulnerable where the anterior radicular artery penetrates the neural foramen and where the anterior spinal artery runs immediately behind the vertebral body. The anterior spinal artery may be occluded by a deposit in the vertebral body, growing posteriorly on to the anterior aspect of the cord. At each segment the anterior spinal artery gives off branches supplying the anterior part of the cord that carries the anterior horn cells and major corticospinal pathways, and the damage resulting from ischemia and infarction is responsible for clinically catastrophic power loss. A small volume of epidural disease at these critical sites can cause vascular compromise.

Some deposits grow from the posterior elements, compressing the cord from a lateral or posterior direction. Because the sensory tracts occupy a peripheral position in the lateral and posterior cord, sensory symptoms may predominate in this instance. A limited part of the cord's blood supply comes from the posterior radicular artery, which branches from the anterior radicular artery in the neural foramen to form a posterior anastomotic chain. If the direction of compression is from the lateral or posterior aspect, the major part of the blood supply to the cord, from the anterior spinal artery, is likely to be preserved.

Technique of Examination with Imaging

Given the potential complexity of the neurological presentation, an imaging technique must take account of the fact that the clinically relevant lesion may be some distance away from the site suggested by the neurological signs. Abnormalities may be present within the vertebral bone marrow, epidural soft tissue, or both. As a result of its versatility in imaging the whole spine and surrounding soft tissues, MR imaging has replaced myelography (with or without CT myelography) as the investigation of choice in suspected spinal cord compression. Only when MR is contraindicated should other techniques be employed.

Plain radiographs remain a worthwhile investigation. If clinical signs point to a fairly definite level, many radiotherapists are prepared to commence steroids and plan an initial radiation field on a discrete bony abnormality if present. The sensitivity of plain radiographs in detecting lesions at other levels is low, and soft

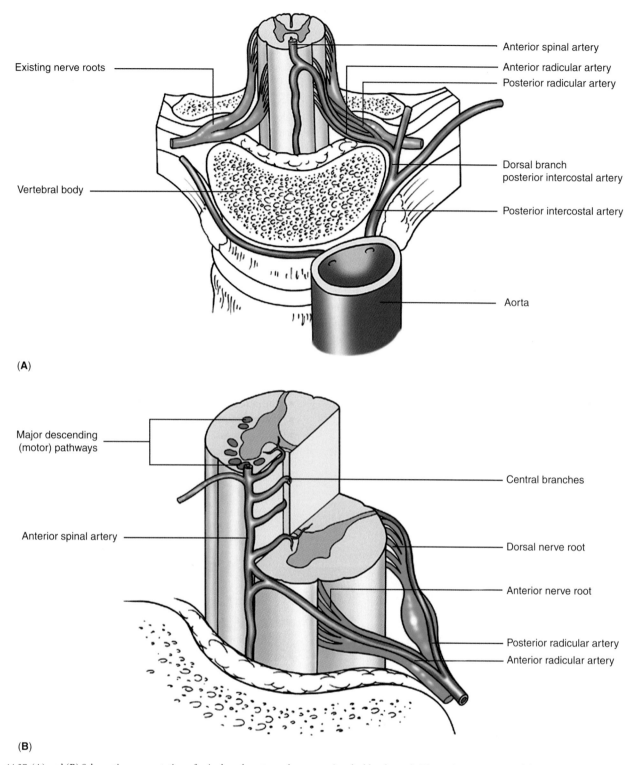

Figure 44.27 (**A**) and (**B**) Schematic representation of spinal cord anatomy demonstrating the blood supply. The major component of the cord's blood supply comes via the anterior radicular artery, which emanates from the dorsal branch of the posterior intercostal artery. The anterior radicular artery runs through the neural foramen where a small posterior radicular artery comes off. The anterior radicular artery feeds the spinal artery, which forms a single anastomotic chain running the length of the cord. From the anterior spinal artery, penetrating central branches supply the functionally crucial descending motor pathways. Some posterior and peripheral parts of the cord have some blood supply from a plexus of small pial vessels coming directly from the anterior and posterior radicular arteries. Interruption of the blood supply by compression of anterior radicular or anterior spinal arteries can cause infarction of the cord even in the absence of major mechanical compression.

tissue extension can rarely be evaluated accurately. However, little is lost by obtaining plain radiographs while MR is scheduled at the earliest opportunity. Isotope studies are sensitive in detecting bony deposits, but less so than MR (51). They are unlikely to be helpful in the acute management of spinal cord compression unless MR is unavailable.

If MR imaging is contraindicated, for example when a patient has a cardiac pacemaker, CT (without myelography) may demonstrate

vertebral bone and soft tissue disease extending into the spinal canal and the relationship of tumor to the spinal cord. Multidetector CT permits reconstruction of images in the sagittal and coronal planes with superb image quality; thus the full extent of disease can be shown in detail for radiotherapy planning (Fig. 44.28).

Myelography with water-soluble contrast agents should include the entire spine, with cervical as well as lumbar puncture if necessary. Subsequent CT scans (CT myelography) can identify paravertebral lesions growing into the spinal canal, and also bony lesions and herniated discs. For maximum information, CT myelography should be performed within a few hours, by the same radiologist or a radiologist with full access to the myelographic findings, so that all appropriate levels can be imaged.

The exact MR technique will depend on which sequences are available and how long the data acquisition takes but it is important to obtain a set of images of the entire spine. Levels of compression should be readily identifiable; most up-to-date scanners should be able to cover the spine from sacrum to foramen magnum in two sequences with a sufficient degree of overlap to identify levels confidently. If this is not possible, some form of skin marker will be necessary so that adequate overlap can be ensured and exact levels of compression accurately identified. A T1-weighted spin-echo sequence in the sagittal plane should be obtained initially. Contrast between normal marrow and metastatic deposits will normally allow detection of malignant infiltration of the vertebral bodies and posterior elements. If doubt exists, a high contrast sequence, for example STIR, a gradient-echo sequence with T2*-weighted or a T2-weighted spin-echo sequence may indicate the site of metastatic bony lesions. T2*-weighted gradient-echo or T2-weighted spin-echo sequences produce an excellent myelographic effect with high signal intensity CSF and a low signal intensity cord. Sagittal scans may be up to 4 to 5 mm thick, but the neural foramina must be covered, if necessary by widening slice thickness, inserting interslice gaps or obtaining two blocks. After review of sagittal images, the radiologist should maintain a low threshold for obtaining sequences in orthogonal planes, as important lesions in the paravertebral region and intervertebral foramina are easier to detect and interpret using the axial or occasionally the coronal plane. Gadolinium enhancement is not used routinely but, if the clinical presentation is suggestive of intramedullary or leptomeningeal disease, contrast-enhanced T1-weighted spin-echo sequences, initially in the sagittal plane, are mandatory (42–44).

Typical Imaging Features and Differential Diagnosis
The differential diagnosis of myelopathy includes:

- Epidural cord compression
- Meningeal metastases
- Intramedullary deposits
- Glioma of the spinal cord
- Meningioma
- Neurofibroma
- Radiation myelopathy
- Postinfection transverse myelitis
- Bone abscess, e.g., TB
- Osteoporotic vertebral collapse

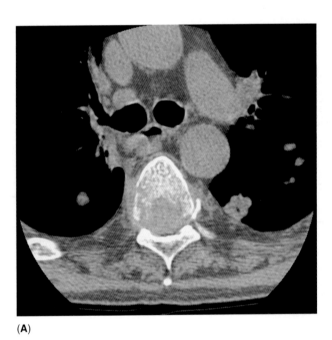

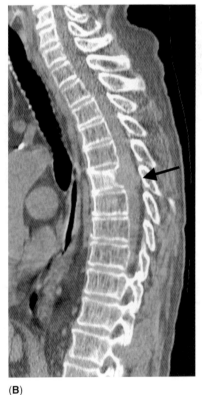

(A)   (B)

Figure 44.28 A patient with a history of renal cell carcinoma metastatic to the lungs, presenting with back pain and loss of power, but still ambulant. (A) During staging CT, a compressive lesion was identified in the midthoracic spine on axial imaging. (B) Sagittal reformats confirm a compressive lesion (arrow). If foramen magnum or sacrum can be identified, the level for treatment can be reliably identified. Although not the investigation of choice, multidetector CT is capable of depicting cord compression.

Most causes of myelopathy which may be confused clinically with epidural cord compression can be accurately diagnosed by MR imaging. In the patient with systemic cancer, meningeal metastases and intramedullary tumors are the principal differentials. Glioma of the cord, meningioma and neurofibroma are rare. Radiation myelopathy is unusual, and requires an appropriate history. Like postinfectious transverse myelitis, it will be seen as high signal intensity within the cord, which may enhance on T1-weighted sequence following IV gadolinium and shows little mass effect. Epidural hematoma usually has a precipitant such as recent lumbar puncture, while epidural abscess should be associated with clinical signs of sepsis, and both should have recognizable morphological features and signal intensity characteristics to enable differential diagnosis. However, an infection involving bone, for example a tuberculous abscess or fungal infiltration, may be difficult to differentiate from bone metastases. Infective processes destroy adjacent discs, whereas malignant involvement of bone, even in adjacent vertebrae, has a tendency to spare the disc, a feature which is useful in differential diagnosis. An osteoporotic acute vertebral collapse should be suspected if it is the solitary spinal lesion, particularly if the posterior elements of the vertebra are entirely normal and there is no evidence of a soft tissue mass. A herniated degenerative disc and malignant involvement of the spine may coexist, but imaging features of the two are rarely confused.

Tumor tissue in the epidural space typically returns low signal intensity on T1-weighted sequences, intermediate to high signal intensity on T2-weighted spin-echo sequences, and high signal intensity on T2* and STIR images. Bony lesions that are discrete and focal are easy to discern. It is more difficult to identify epidural spread of disease in very extensive diffuse bony metastatic disease. Where there is gross disease, several levels of compression may be present, underlining the necessity to cover the whole spine (Fig. 44.29). In the presence of diffuse disease, any subtle abnormality of cord morphology identified on the sagittal images should raise the index of suspicion, and orthogonal plane imaging should be performed, which may reveal lateral compression of the cord from expanded pedicles (Figs. 44.30 and 44.31). This type of compression is not infrequently seen in metastatic prostate and breast cancer.

Bony changes may be subtle or even absent. Soft tissue extension of tumor (in a "dumb-bell" fashion) may occur with a variety of tumors:

- Lymphoma
- Neurofibroma
- Neuroblastoma
- Malignant thymoma
- Mesothelioma
- Lung cancer

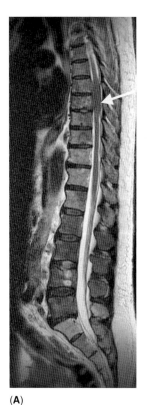
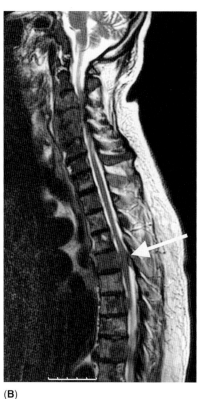
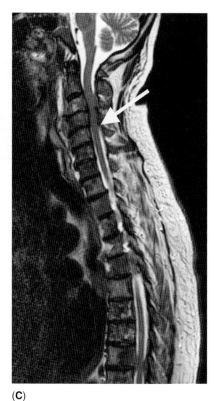

(A)   **(B)**   **(C)**

Figure 44.29 Patient with known carcinoma of the prostate metastatic to bone. The patient had a minor degree of scoliosis due to pain. Some power loss had been reported, and the sensory level was estimated at T10. T2-weighted sagittal MR imaging (**A**) shows a compressive lesion at T8 (arrow). Although this might explain the observed clinical syndrome, the thoracic and cervical spine must always be imaged. (**B**) A further compressive lesion is identified at T5 (arrow), and (**C**) an incipient compressive lesion, with loss of CSF signal around the cord, is observed in the upper cervical region (arrow).

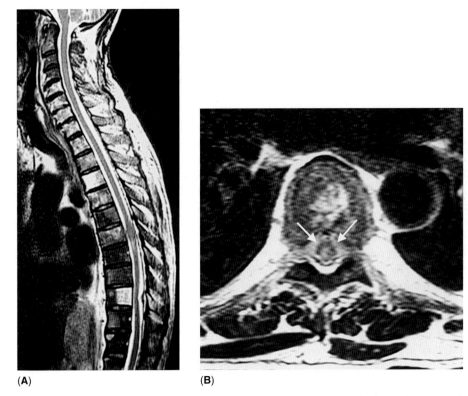

(A)   **(B)**

Figure 44.30 Spinal cord compression as a result of metastases to the spine from prostate carcinoma. (**A**) T2-weighted sagittal MR image shows anatomical distortion of the spinal cord at T7. Any abnormality such as this should precipitate orthogonal plane imaging. (**B**) T2-weighted axial imaging through T7 shows epidural soft tissue surrounding the spinal cord (arrows), and some high signal centrally within the cord. Although the imaging changes are not gross, the clinical syndrome of cord compression at mid-thoracic level was clear, and it is likely that ischemia or infarction of the cord was present.

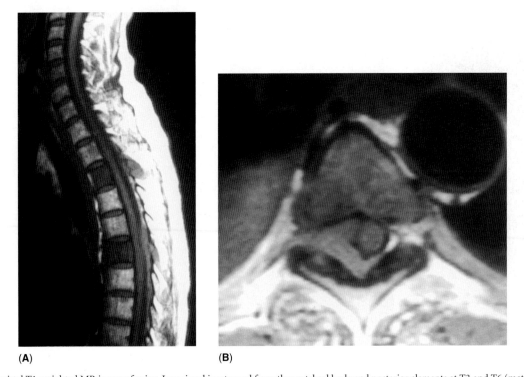

(A)   **(B)**

Figure 44.31 (**A**) Sagittal T1-weighted MR image of spine. Low signal is returned from the vertebral body and posterior elements at T3 and T6 (metastatic disease from breast carcinoma). There is a plaque of soft tissue apparently lying posteriorly to the cord at T6. (**B**) Orthogonal plane imaging (axial T1-weighted sequence) at T6 shows soft tissue epidural disease compressing the cord from the right. In this patient, pain was the major presenting clinical feature, and weakness was present but not profound. A good clinical response to steroids and radiation therapy was obtained.

Apart from the classical but uncommon neurofibroma and neuroblastoma, bronchial carcinoma can penetrate the intervertebral foramen while causing little bony destruction, particularly in superior sulcus tumors. Malignant thymoma and mesothelioma may also compress the cord by soft tissue extension (Fig. 44.32).

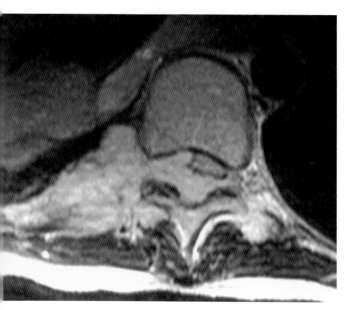

Figure 44.32 Malignant thymoma. Axial MR image in the thoracic region reveals a soft tissue mass involving the pleura and chest wall to the right of the midline. Tumor penetrates the neural foramen in a "dumb-bell" configuration and is displacing and compressing the spinal cord predominantly from a posterior and lateral direction. Pain was present, with relatively little power loss, indicating that the blood supply of the cord has not been significantly compromised by marked anatomical displacement.

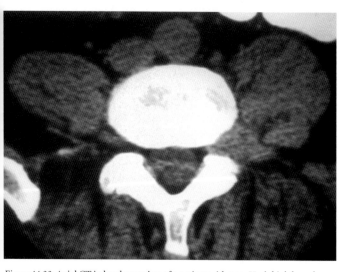

Figure 44.33 Axial CT in lumbar region of a patient with non-Hodgkin's lymphoma and back pain radiating to the left leg. A small soft tissue mass lies behind the left psoas, extending into the neural foramen. This is a characteristic site and appearance for epidural lymphoma. Patients may present with prolonged back pain, and if this is neglected, compression of the spinal cord or cauda equina may develop and lead to permanent neurological damage. However, if detected promptly, epidural lymphoma will respond to treatment and prognosis is no worse than for lymphoma at any other site. Note that the fat planes in and around the neural foramen are obliterated on the affected side but preserved on the normal side. The intervertebral foramina should be a "check area" on staging CT scans performed for lymphoma.

One of the most important dumb-bell tumors is lymphoma in the posterior mediastinum, retrocrural region, and retroperitoneum. The tendency of lymphoma to involve the epidural spaces has been recognized for many years (52). The reported incidence of spinal cord compression by lymphoma varies between 1% and 7%. Epidural masses may be small and subtle (Fig. 44.33) but any symptomatology should be vigorously investigated, as early treatment should result in a favorable response to treatment in keeping with the overall prognosis of the disease. If paraplegia is allowed to develop, it is unlikely to recover (53). In current practice it is most likely that a patient known to have lymphoma presenting with back pain and neurological symptoms will be referred for MR imaging. The same principles apply as for any tumor; the entire spine should be imaged, using orthogonal planes as necessary to elucidate soft tissue disease. In addition, when CT scans are performed as staging investigations for lymphoma, the epidural spaces should be an area subjected to special scrutiny as subtle signs, such as the obliteration of fat planes in the intervertebral foramina, may give early warning of epidural space invasion and incipient neurological dysfunction (Fig. 44.33).

Key Points: Magnetic Resonance Imaging Features of Spinal Cord Compression

- MR imaging is the investigation of choice in suspected spinal cord compression
- The entire spine should be evaluated as metastatic disease may produce multiple levels of compression
- T2-weighted sequences provide an excellent "myelographic" effect
- Most causes of myelopathy that mimic spinal cord compression can be accurately diagnosed with MR
- Lymphoma is a common malignant tumor which may invade the spinal canal through the intervertebral foramina without any bony destruction

Spinal Meningeal Disease

As is the case with leptomeningeal disease in the cranial cavity, disease may spread to the meninges by:

- The hematogenous route
- Cerebrospinal fluid pathways
- Direct extension along peripheral nerves

The clinical presentation may be somewhat obscure. Symptoms can be divided into two broad categories, namely those caused by invasion of spinal nerve roots (i.e., neural dysfunction) and those caused by invasion of the leptomeninges alone (i.e., meningeal irritation).

Neural dysfunction is likely to result in a constellation of symptoms and signs that are anatomically remote owing to the selective involvement of individual nerve roots. If an isolated lumbar nerve root is involved, radicular pain will result, mimicking a herniated lumbar disc. However, there are usually some vague symptoms attributable to meningeal irritation such as back pain, neck pain, or headache. When the referring clinician describes a neurological presentation which may be very vague or verging on the bizarre, it is important to consider the diagnosis of leptomeningeal disease,

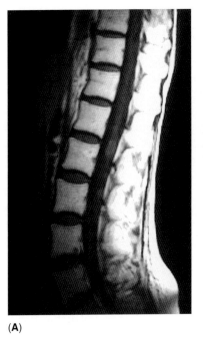
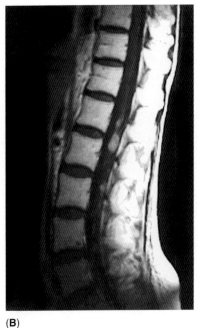

(A)   **(B)**

Figure 44.34 (**A**) and (**B**) T1-weighted spin-echo MR images before and after intravenous gadolinium administration. Meningeal deposits from carcinoma of the breast. Some thickening of the meninges is just discernible before contrast. After administration of gadolinium, enhancing masses on the meninges are clearly identifiable. This is the characteristic appearance of carcinoma metastatic to the meninges.

since the MR technique must involve T1-weighted sagittal sequences of the entire spine before and after IV Gd-DTPA administration. In contrast to the situation within the cranial cavity, any enhancement of the meninges in the spinal canal should be considered abnormal although faint enhancement is sometimes seen around the conus. Some tumors, notably carcinomas of lung and breast, produce enhancing masses within the meninges (Fig. 44.34). Leukemia and lymphoma tend to result in plaques or sheets of enhancing tissue (Fig. 44.35). Melanoma, which has a predilection to metastasize to the meninges, may do either (Fig. 44.36). When present, the appearance of enhancing plaques or masses of tumor is sufficiently characteristic to allow confident diagnosis. However, as in the cranial cavity, false negative MR imaging is not infrequent, particularly in leukemia and lymphoma. If MR imaging is negative, lumbar puncture can be used subsequently and may yield positive cytology (43–46).

Primary brain tumors that have a tendency to seed spinal meninges via CSF spread include:

- Ependymoma
- Medulloblastoma
- Pinealoblastoma
- Intracranial germ cell tumors
- Intracranial primitive neuro-ectodermal tumors (PNET)

MR imaging is frequently used as a staging technique, notwithstanding its relative lack of sensitivity. Changes may be subtle, and it is important to ensure coverage of the meninges in the neural foramina. An enhancing mass is diagnostic of drop metastases, which are more commonly found at the time of recurrence following treatment for primary brain tumors, particularly in children (Fig. 44.37). Myelography is capable of detecting meningeal nodules but is now rarely used.

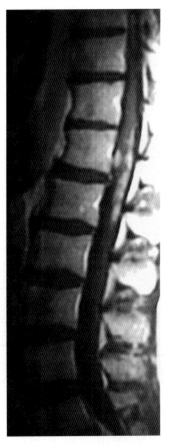

Figure 44.35 T1-weighted spin-echo MR image following gadolinium administration. Meningeal spread of lymphoma. The tumor appears as an enhancing sheet of tissue in the lumbar meninges. The patient had presented with backache and leg weakness as the initial clinical manifestation of non-Hodgkin's lymphoma. Biopsy at lumbar laminectomy confirmed the diagnosis. Staging CT revealed lymphadenopathy in mediastinum and retroperitoneum.

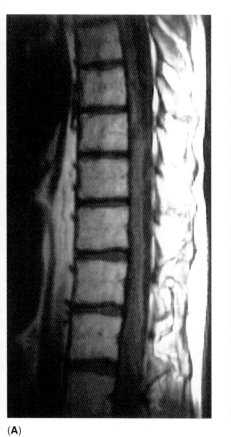

(A)

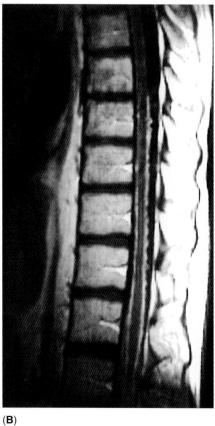

(B)

Figure 44.36 (A) and (B) T1-weighted spin-echo sagittal MR images before and after gadolinium injection. Diffuse nodular enhancement extends throughout the thoracic meninges. The appearance due to diffuse meningeal involvement by melanoma is seen better following intravenous contrast injection (**B**).

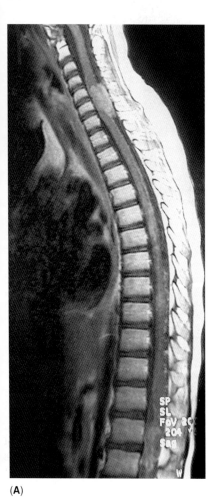

(A)

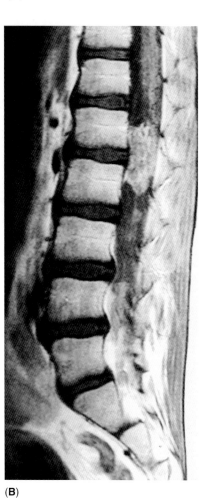

(B)

Figure 44.37 (**A**) and (**B**) Contrast-enhanced T1-weighted sagittal MR images through whole spine demonstrating gross drop metastases in cervical and lumbar regions in a child aged nine, with recurrent ependymoma following treatment for an intracranial primary tumor.

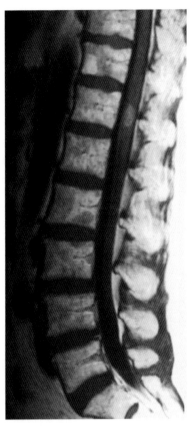

Figure 44.38 Gadolinium-enhanced T1-weighted spin-echo MR sequence demonstrating an enhancing nodule in the conus in a patient with disseminated metastatic disease from carcinoma of the breast.

Intramedullary Deposits

Tumor deposits are occasionally identified within the spinal cord. In these circumstances, clinical presentation is similar to meningeal disease, giving neurological symptoms and signs that may not correspond to a single anatomical site. Carcinoma of breast and lung and malignant melanoma are once again the most frequent culprits. Metastases to the spinal cord are seen as enhancing masses on MR imaging following Gd-DTPA injection, and appear to have a predilection for the conus (Fig. 44.38). Small cell lung cancer may give multiple small enhancing lesions throughout the cord, of similar appearance to small cell deposits, metastatic to the brain parenchyma (Fig. 44.39). The presence of a syrinx, which may be detected on T2-weighted imaging on patients being investigated for suspected cord compression, should raise the possibility of an associated small intramedullary deposit, and precipitate the use of a gadolinium-enhanced sequence (Fig. 44.40).

Key Points: Spinal Meningeal and Cord Involvement

- Spinal meningeal disease is caused by invasion of spinal nerve roots or by hematogenous spread to the leptomeninges
- Patients frequently present with neurological features that do not point to a single specific site
- T1-weighted sagittal sequences of the entire spine before and after IV contrast medium are mandatory
- MR imaging is a relatively insensitive technique and, if negative, lumbar puncture is indicated
- Primary brain tumors produce spinal seedlings
- Intramedullary metastases most frequently occur in breast and lung cancer and malignant melanoma

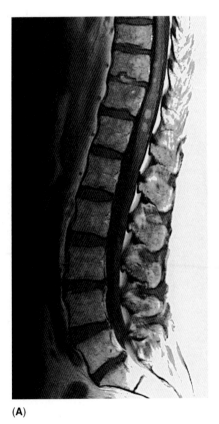

(A)

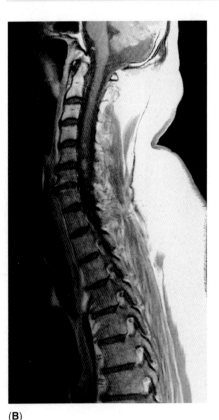

(B)

Figure 44.39 (A) and (B) T1-weighted sagittal MR images following gadolinium administration. Very small enhancing lesions are identified within the cord. The intramedullary lesions were scattered through the spinal cord and brain, and were due to metastases from small cell carcinoma.

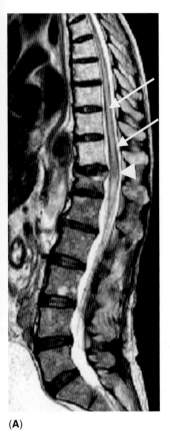
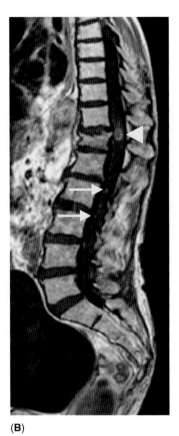

(A) **(B)**

Figure 44.40 MR imaging performed on a patient with power loss in legs. Pain was present but not severe. (**A**) T2-weighted sagittal MR sequence demonstrates high signal centrally within the cord throughout the lower thoracic region as a result of syrinx formation (arrows), extending down to an area of intermediate signal within the cord just above the conus (arrowhead). (**B**) Gadolinium-enhanced midline sagittal MR imaging demonstrates an enhancing deposit just above the conus (arrow head), which was responsible for the development of a syrinx which was not reliably identified on T1-weighted imaging. Note that there is also meningeal metastatic disease (arrows) in the lumbar region.

METASTATIC INVOLVEMENT OF PERIPHERAL NERVES AND MUSCLE

Major Nerve Plexuses

The two major areas of nerve plexus formation are the brachial plexus and the lumbosacral plexus. The brachial plexus is most commonly involved by superior sulcus tumors invading directly, or by lymph nodes metastatic from breast carcinoma (see chap. 26). Both of these pathologies usually invade the plexus from below, affecting those fibers that begin as C8 and T1 roots and end as the ulnar nerve. The primary symptom is pain, which may localize to the posterior aspect of the shoulder or around the elbow and may sometimes lead the physician to instigate fruitless investigations of the bony and soft tissue structures of the shoulder and elbow. Paresthesia and numbness are often present, particularly affecting the medial part of the hand. The differential diagnosis from radiation fibrosis of the brachial plexus can be difficult, and CT and MR can both be used to detect soft tissue masses in this region. MR, as a result of its multiplanar imaging capability and superior contrast resolution, has greater versatility but it may be impossible to discriminate between radiation fibrosis and infiltrative forms of tumor that do not present as a morphological mass (54–57). Brachial plexopathy in the context of recurrent breast cancer is further discussed in chapter 26.

Tumors that frequently affect the lumbosacral plexus include carcinomas of rectum, cervix, bladder, and prostate. The clinical presentation is dominated by pain, usually in a radicular distribution. Radiation damage to the lumbosacral plexus is less common than in the brachial plexus. Often, the crucial question is to establish whether the plexus is involved by a soft tissue mass or by bony involvement of the lumbosacral spine. CT is frequently adequate for detecting a soft tissue mass extending from the pelvic organs into the sacral plexus. However, in the absence of a soft tissue mass, MR is more sensitive for detecting malignant involvement of the sacrum (Figs. 44.41 and 44.42).

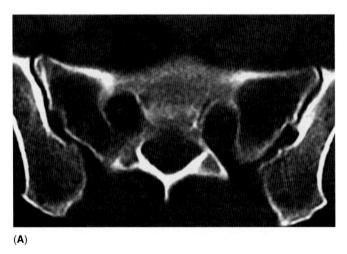
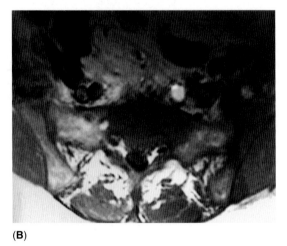

(A) **(B)**

Figure 44.41 This patient with a history of melanoma, presented with lower back pain radiating to the left leg. (**A**) CT with bony windows failed to reveal any explanation for the symptoms. (**B**) T1-weighted spin-echo axial MR image. Involvement of the sacral marrow cavity and impingement on the nerve root is clearly demonstrated, owing to the high sensitivity of MR in detecting bony lesions.

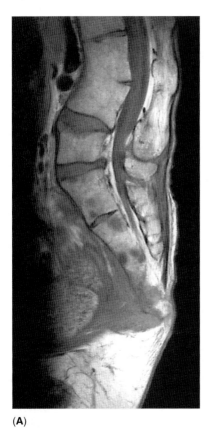

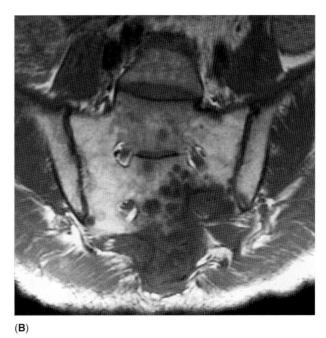

(A)   **(B)**

Figure 44.42 This patient had a history of transitional cell carcinoma of the bladder treated by cystectomy. He presented with radicular pain. (**A**) T1-weighted spin-echo sagittal MR image. There is a presacral soft tissue abnormality due to pelvic soft tissue recurrence. (**B**) T1-weighted spin-echo paracoronal MR image. Bony invasion affecting the sacrum and involving the nerve roots is clearly demonstrated.

Peripheral Nerves

Peripheral neuropathy in a patient with systemic cancer is usually due to chemotherapy. Diffuse or focal involvement of nerves by tumor, resulting in a sensorimotor neuropathy, is rare and usually associated with lymphoma, leukemia and other hematological malignancies (58,59). Isolated mononeuropathies may result from invasion by adjacent tumor, particularly if a nerve is located at a point where it passes directly over a bone, or through a bony canal. The radial and ulnar nerves may be affected by bony metastatic disease around the elbow or within the axilla. The sciatic nerve is also vulnerable to involvement by bony or soft tissue tumor at several sites in the pelvis, and the obturator nerve may be compressed or invaded as it passes through the obturator canal. Imaging studies are only likely to be useful if there is a strong clinical indication that an individual nerve has been affected by metastatic disease. In these circumstances, cross-sectional techniques including MR, CT, and US can give useful confirmation that there is a pathological mass in the vicinity of the affected nerve.

Key Points: Peripheral Nerves

■ The brachial plexus is most commonly involved in breast and lung cancer by direct soft tissue invasion
■ The lumbosacral plexus is usually involved by direct extension of bone metastases, e.g., carcinoma of the prostate

Muscle

Soft tissue metastases involving muscles are unusual, but may occasionally be seen in lymphoma and leukemia (chloroma).

Some solid tumors may also metastasize to the muscle:

- Malignant melanoma
- Lung cancer
- Rhabdomyosarcoma

Such lesions are usually obvious clinically, and cross-sectional imaging techniques can be used to determine the extent of the abnormality, but these lesions rarely have specific diagnostic features.

Summary

■ Neurological disorders are an increasingly common problem in the cancer patient
■ The radiologist should focus on the clinical findings so that the most appropriate investigation is performed
■ Many metastases arise from cancers of the lung, breast, and melanoma
■ Other primary sources of tumor include the kidneys and gastro-intestinal tract
■ In a significant number of patients the primary source of a brain metastasis remains unknown

- MR is the most sensitive imaging technique available for detecting brain metastases but screening is only undertaken in selected tumors (e.g., lung cancer preoperatively)
- Symptomatic spinal cord compression is seen in 1% to 5% of patients with disseminated malignancy
- Imaging of spinal cord compression should include the whole spine. MR is the preferred investigation
- Meningeal metastatic disease results in a wide range of neurological symptoms that cannot be unified to a single anatomical site, and for its detection gadolinium-enhanced MR imaging is the most sensitive imaging investigation
- The brachial plexus is most commonly involved in breast cancer and apical lung cancer by direct soft tissue invasion
- The lumbosacral plexus is usually involved as a result of direct extension of bone metastases
- Peripheral neuropathy is usually due to chemotherapy but, occasionally, a bone metastasis may involve an adjacent nerve

REFERENCES

1. Clouston PD, de Angelis LM, Posner JB. The spectrum of neurologic disease in patients with systemic cancer. Ann Neurol 1992; 31: 268–73.
2. Sculier JP, Feld R, Evans WK, et al. Neurological disorders in patients with small cell lung cancer. Cancer 1987; 60: 2275–83.
3. Gilbert MR, Grossman SA. Incidence and nature of neurological problems in patients with solid tumours. Am J Med 1986; 81: 951–4.
4. Eapen L, Vachet M, Catton G, et al. Brain metastases with an unknown primary: a clinical perspective. J Neurooncol 1988; 6: 31–5.
5. Nicholson GL. Organ specificity of tumour metastasis: role of preferential adhesion, invasion and growth of malignant cells at specific secondary sites. Cancer Metastasis Rev 1988; 7: 143–88.
6. Delattre J-Y, Kroll G, Thaler HT, et al. Distribution of brain metastases. Arch Neurol 1988; 45: 741–4.
7. Smith DB, Howell A, Harris M, et al. Carcinomatous meningitis associated with infiltrating lobular carcinoma of the breast. Eur J Surg Oncol 1985; 11: 33–6.
8. Nicholson GL, Kawaguchi T, Kawaguchi M, et al. Brain surface invasion and metastasis of murine malignant melanoma variants. J Neurooncol 1987; 4: 209–18.
9. Sze G, Milano E, Johnson C, et al. Detection of brain metastases: comparison of contrast-enhanced with unenhanced MR and enhanced CT. AJNR Am J Neuroradiol 1990; 11: 785–91.
10. Cherryman GR, Olliff JFC, Golfieri R, et al. A prospective comparison of Gadolinium-DTPA enhanced MRI and contrast-enhanced CT scanning in the detection of brain metastases arising from small cell lung cancer. Contrast media in MRI, International workshop, Berlin, Feb 1–3. The Netherlands: Medicom, 1990.
11. Sze G, Johnson C, Kawamura Y, et al. Comparison of single- and triple-dose contrast material in the MR screening of brain metastases. AJNR Am J Neuroradiol 1998; 19: 821–8.
12. Yuh WTC, Tall TE, Nguyen HD, et al. The effect of contrast dose, imaging time and lesion size in the MR detection of intracerebral metastases. Am J Neuroradiol 1995; 16: 73–80.
13. Black WC. High-dose MR in evaluation of brain metastases: will increased detection decrease costs? AJNR Am J Neuroradiol 1994; 15: 1062–4.
14. Boorstein JM, Wong KT, Grossman RI, et al. Metastatic lesions of the brain imaging with magnetisation transfer. Radiology 1994; 191: 799–803.
15. Okubo T, Hayashi N, Shirouzu I, et al. Detection of brain metastases: comparison of Turbo FLAIR imaging, T2-weighted imaging and double dose gadolinium-enhanced MR imaging. Radiat Med 1998; 16: 273–81.
16. Terae S, Yoshida D, Kudo K, et al. Contrast-enhanced FLAIR imaging in combination with pre- and postcontrast magnetization transfer T1-weighted imaging: usefulness in the evaluation of brain metastases. J Magn Reson Imaging 2007; 25: 479–87.
17. Kakeda S, Korogi Y, Hiai Y, et al. Detection of brain metastasis at 3T: comparison among SE, IR-FSE and 3D-GRE sequences. Eur Radiol 2007; 17: 2345–51.
18. Furutani K, Harada M, Mawlan M, Nishitani H. Difference in enhancement between spin echo and 3-dimensional fast spoiled gradient recalled acquisition in steady state magnetic resonance imaging of brain metastasis at 3-T magnetic resonance imaging. J Comput Assist Tomogr 2008; 32: 313–19.
19. Miller KD, Weathers T, Haney LG, et al. Occult central nervous system involvement in patients with metastatic breast cancer: prevalence, predictive factors and impact on overall survival. Ann Oncol 2003; 14: 1072–7.
20. Wong TZ, van der Westhuizen GJ, Coleman RE. Positron emission tomography imaging of brain tumors. Neuroimaging Clin N Am 2002; 12: 615–26.
21. Liu Y. Metastatic brain lesions may demonstrate photopenia on FDG PET. Clin Nucl Med 2008; 33: 255–7.
22. Konishi J, Yamazaki K, Tsukamoto E, et al. Mediastinal lymph node staging by FDG-PET in patients with non-small cell lung cancer: analysis of false-positive FDG-PET findings. Respiration 2003; 70: 500–6.
23. Yap KK, Yap KS, Byrne AJ, et al. Positron emission tomography with selected mediastinoscopy compared to routine mediastinoscopy offers cost and clinical outcome benefits for preoperative staging of non-small cell lung cancer. Eur J Nucl Med Mol Imaging 2005; 32: 1033–40.
24. Seute T, Leffers P, ten Velde GP, Twijnstra A. Detection of brain metastases from small cell lung cancer: consequences of changing imaging techniques (CT versus MRI). Cancer. 2008; 112: 1827–34.
25. Yokoi K, Kamiya N, Matsuguma H, et al. Detection of brain metastasis in potentially operable non-small cell lung cancer: a comparison of CT and MRI. Chest 1999; 115: 714–19.
26. Salbeck R, Grau HC, Artmann H. Cerebral tumour staging in patients with bronchial carcinoma by computed tomography. Cancer 1990; 66: 2007–11.
27. Rohren EM, Provenzale JM, Barboriak DP, et al. Screening for cerebral metastases with FDG-PET in patients undergoing whole body staging of non-central nervous system malignancy. Radiology 2003; 226: 181–7.

28. MacVicar D. Staging of testicular germ cell tumours. Clin Radiol 1993; 47: 149–58.

29. Recommendations for cross-sectional imaging in cancer management: CT, MRI, PET-CT. Royal College of Radiologists, London 2006; Issue 2.[Available from: www.rcr.ac.uk].

30. Patchell RA, Tibbs PA, Walsh JW, et al. A randomised trial of surgery in the treatment of single metastases to the brain. N Engl J Med 1993; 22: 495–500.

31. Hook CC, Kimmel DW, Kvols LK, et al. Multifocal inflammatory leuko-encephalopathy with 5-fluorouracil and levamisole. Ann Neurol 1992; 31: 262–7.

32. Asato R, Akiyama Y, Ito M, et al. Nuclear magnetic resonance abnormalities of the cerebral white matter in children with acute lymphoblastic leukaemia and malignant lymphoma during and after central nervous system prophylactic treatment with intrathecal methotrexate. Cancer 1992; 70: 1997–2004.

33. Stemmer SM, Stears JC, Burton BS, et al. White matter changes in patients with breast cancer treated with high-dose chemotherapy and autologous bone marrow support. Am J Neuroradiol 1994; 15: 1267–73.

34. Bratby M, MacVicar D. Seizures following bone marrow transplantation. Br J Radiol 2005; 78: 575–7.

35. Hinchey J, Chaves C, Appignani B, et al. A reversible posterior leukoencephalopathy syndrome. N Engl J Med 1996; 334: 494–500.

36. Casey SO, Sampaio RC, Michel E, Truwit CL. Posterior reversible encephalopathy syndrome: utility of fluid-attenuated inversion recovery MR imaging in the detection of cortical and subcortical lesions. AJNR Am J Neuroradiol 2000; 21: 1199–206.

37. Mukherjee P, McKinstry RC. Reversible posterior leukoencephalopathy syndrome: evaluation with diffusion-tensor MR imaging. Radiology 2001; 219: 756–65.

38. Rubinstein AB, Schein M, Reichenthal E. The association of carcinoma of the breast with meningioma. Surg Gynaecol Obstet 1989; 169: 334–6.

39. Smith FP, Slavik M, Macdonald JS. Association of breast cancer with meningioma: report of two cases and review of the literature. Cancer 1978; 42: 1992–4.

40. Jacobs DH, Holmes FF, McFarlane NJ. Meningiomas are not significantly associated with breast cancer. Arch Neurol 1992; 49: 753–6.

41. Enochs WS, Hyslop WB, Bennett HF, et al. Sources of the increased longitudinal relaxation rates observed in melanotic melanoma. An in vitro study of synthetic melanins. Invest Radiol 1989; 24: 794–804.

42. Yousem DM, Patrone PM, Grossman RI. Leptomeningeal metastases: MR evaluation. J Comput Assist Tomogr 1990; 14: 255–61.

43. Collie DA, Brush JP, Lammie GA, et al. Imaging features of leptomeningeal metastases. Clin Radiol 1999; 54: 765–71.

44. Singh SK, Leeds NE, Ginsberg LE. MR imaging of leptomeningeal metastases: comparison of three sequences. AJNR Am J Neuroradiol 2002; 23: 817–21.

45. Freilich RJ, Krol G, DeAngelis LM. Neuroimaging and cerebrospinal fluid cytology in the diagnosis of leptomeningeal metastasis. Ann Neurol 1995; 38: 51–7.

46. Zeiser R, Burger JA, Bley TA, et al. Clinical follow-up indicates differential accuracy of magnetic resonance imaging and immunocytology of the cerebral spinal fluid for the diagnosis of neoplastic meningitis–a single centre experience. Br J Haematol 2004; 124: 762–8.

47. Bansal S, Brady LW, Olsen A, et al. The treatment of metastatic spinal cord tumours. J Am Med Assoc 1967; 202: 686–8.

48. Hildebrand J. Lesions of the Nervous System in Cancer Patients. Monograph Series of the European Organisation for Research on Treatment of Cancer, Vol. 5. New York: Raven Press, 1978.

49. Klein SL, Sanford RA, Muhlbauer MS. Paediatric spinal epidural metastases. J Neurosurg 1991; 74: 70–5.

50. Barron KD, Hirano A, Araski S, et al. Experiences with metastatic neoplasms involving the spinal cord. Neurology 1959; 9: 91–106.

51. Jones AL, Williams MP, Powles TJ, et al. Magnetic resonance imaging in the detection of skeletal metastases in patients with breast cancer. Br J Cancer 1990; 62: 296–8.

52. Murphy WT, Bilge N. Compression of the spinal cord in patients with malignant lymphoma. Radiology 1964; 82: 495–501.

53. MacVicar D, Williams MP. CT scanning in epidural lymphoma. Clin Radiol 1991; 43: 95–102.

54. Moore NR, Dixon AK, Wheeler TK. Axillary fibrosis or recurrent tumour. An MRI study in breast cancer. Clin Radiol 1990; 42: 42–6.

55. Posniak HV, Olson MC, Dudiak CM. MR imaging of the brachial plexus. AJR Am J Roentgenol 1993; 161: 373–9.

56. Iyer RB, Fenstermacher MJ, Libshitz HI. MR Imaging of the treated brachial plexus. AJR Am J Roentgenol 1996; 167: 225–9.

57. Qayyum A, MacVicar D, Padhani AR, et al. Symptomatic brachial plexopathy following treatment for breast cancer: utility of MR imaging including surface coil techniques. Radiology 2000; 214: 837–42.

58. Sumi SM, Farrell DF, Knauss TA. Lymphoma and leukaemia manifested by steroid responsive polyneuropathy. Arch Neurol 1983; 40: 577–82.

59. McLeod JG. Peripheral neuropathy associated with lymphomas, leukaemias and polycythaemia vera. In: Dyck PJ, Thomas PK, eds. Peripheral Neuropathy, Vol. 2, 3rd edn. Philadelphia: W B Saunders, 1993: 1591–8.

45 Adrenal Metastases

Rodney H Reznek and Anju Sahdev

INTRODUCTION

The routine use of cross-sectional imaging in the staging of intra-abdominal and extra-abdominal malignancy has shown that the adrenal gland is a common site of unexpected metastatic disease. Although modern computed tomography (CT) and magnetic resonance (MR) imaging can be expected to detect nodules exceeding 5 to 10 mm, autopsy studies show that many adrenal metastases go undetected due to their small size.

Demonstration of adrenal metastases almost always alters the patient's management. Except for ipsilateral metastases in renal cancer, adrenal metastases indicate that the patient has Stage IV disease. However, a major problem exists in the radiological demonstration of metastases; benign cortical adenomas are common and always have to be distinguished from metastases before assuming that the patient has metastatic disease.

INCIDENCE

The adrenal glands are the fourth most common site of metastases after the lungs, liver, and bone. Common sites of origin of adrenal metastases are listed in Table 45.1. At autopsy, adrenal metastases are found in up to 27% of patients dying of cancer (1). Certain tumors show a higher incidence; around 30% to 40% of patients with breast and lung cancer have adrenal metastases (2,3). Fifty percent of melanomas spread to the adrenal glands (4). Adrenal metastases are found in gastro-intestinal and renal tumors in 10% to 20% of cases (5,6).

Infiltration is usually within the normal cortex and/or medulla but spread to adenomas has been reported (7,8). Metastases are asymptomatic as a rule but occasional cases of hypoadrenalism have been recorded (9).

Imaging by cross-sectional techniques will only detect metastases if there is a focal mass or distortion of the contour of the adrenal gland, but a normal-appearing gland does not exclude microscopic tumor infiltration (10). This is reflected in the low sensitivity of CT in the detection of metastases in patients with non-small-cell lung cancer (41%) but the specificity is high (91%) (10).

THE NORMAL ADRENAL GLAND

Normal adrenal glands are usually well visualized as an inverted 'Y' or 'V' shape against the surrounding retroperitoneal fat on both CT and MR. On ultrasound (US), identification of the normal adrenal gland is technically difficult; the gland is very small, and its echotexture is similar to that of the surrounding tissues. Bowel gas can often obscure the gland, particularly on the left.

To date, normal measurements have referred almost entirely to the body of the adrenal gland. However, in view of the predominance of cortical tissue within the limbs, measurement of their size

is important (11). Normal measurements of the body and limbs of the adrenal glands have been established for CT only and cannot be applied to MR. The maximum width of the body measured perpendicular to the long axis, at the junction of the adrenal body and limb, is 0.79 cm (SD 0.21) on the left and 0.6 cm (SD 0.2) on the right (11). The thickness of the limbs of the right adrenal are slightly less than the left, measuring 0.14 to 0.49 cm, compared with 0.13 to 0.52 cm on the left. In practice, the normal adrenal limb should not measure over 5 mm (11).

IMAGING APPEARANCES OF ADRENAL METASTASES

The radiological appearances of adrenal metastases are not specific. They can be large or small, unilateral or bilateral. Small adrenal metastases (<2 cm) are difficult to detect on US; however, large adrenal masses should be readily identifiable. Metastases are usually rounded or oval and hypoechoeic. US imaging will not differentiate between metastases and a benign adenoma.

On CT, metastases <3 cm in diameter are usually homogeneous. Larger lesions may show central necrosis or areas of hemorrhage (Fig. 45.1). They tend to be of inhomogeneous density and occasionally have a thick enhancing rim after intravenous (IV) contrast medium (Fig. 45.2) (12). Rarely, metastases may result in diffuse enlargement of the adrenal glands, retaining the normal adreniform contour with rim enhancement around the whole gland without a focal mass (Fig. 45.3).

On MR they are typically hypointense compared to the liver on T1-weighted images and relatively hyperintense on T2-weighted images (Fig. 45.4). Some adrenal metastases are atypical and either iso- or hypointense relative to liver on T2-weighted images (13,14).

In addition, some metastases have very long T2 relaxation times and can mimic pheochromocytomas, although pheochromocytomas can usually be differentiated on clinical grounds (Figs. 45.5 and 45.6). Thus, adrenal metastases often cannot be definitely distinguished from benign lesions such as an adenoma, hematoma, pseudocysts, or inflammatory masses on the basis of morphology (Fig. 45.7). As discussed below, CT attenuation and chemical-shift MR can be helpful in distinguishing between adenomas and metastases.

DIFFERENTIAL DIAGNOSIS OF AN ADRENAL MASS (TABLE 45.2)

The differential diagnosis of a non-hyperfunctioning adrenal mass includes a benign lipid-poor cortical adenoma, adrenal cyst, adrenal carcinoma, and a myelolipoma. Functioning adrenal masses such as pheochromocytomas should also be considered, especially if there is an underlying syndrome such as von Hippel–Lindau, or multiple endocrine neoplasia (Fig. 45.8). Some of these masses have specific imaging features that help in the diagnosis.

Table 45.1 Common Sites of Origin of Adrenal Metastases

Breast
Lung
Melanoma
Gastro-intestinal
Kidney

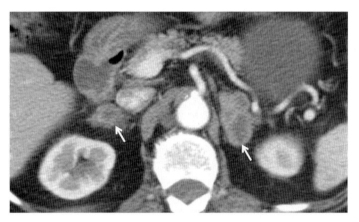

Figure 45.1 Bilateral adrenal metastases in a patient with malignant melanoma. Contrast enhanced CT image showing enhancing heterogenous masses (arrows) and areas of poor enhancement due to necrosis.

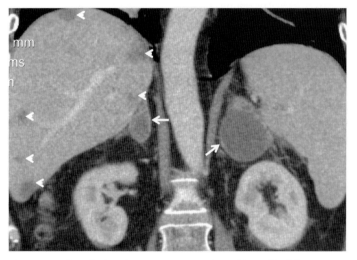

Figure 45.2 Bilateral adrenal metastases in a patient with small cell lung cancer. Contrast enhanced CT with coronal reformat showing the bilateral adrenal metastases with enhancement and central low attenuation (arrows). Multiple liver metastases are also present in the liver (arrow heads).

Adrenal cysts are rare and occur more commonly in women than men (15). They have a similar appearance on imaging to cysts elsewhere in the body, although the presence of proteinaceous fluid, infectious debris, or hemorrhage within a cyst will alter its appearance. *Primary adrenal carcinomas* are rare, highly malignant tumors. They are usually large (>6 cm) and are heterogeneous where there is necrosis and calcification (16). However, 16% of tumors are <6 cm and on imaging are homogeneous, morphologically resembling a non-hyperfunctioning adenoma (17) (Fig. 45.9).

Myelolipomas are composed of mature fat and hemopoietic tissue in varying proportions. The diagnosis is made by demonstrating the presence of fat within an adrenal mass. This can be accomplished with either CT or MR, although the presence of hemorrhage or

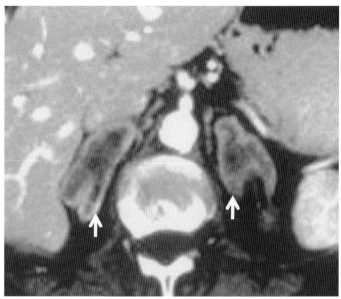

Figure 45.3 Bilateral adrenal metastases in a patient with non-small cell lung cancer. Contrast-enhanced CT showing bilateral enlarged adrenal glands retaining their adreniform contour and avid rim enhancement (arrows).

infection can complicate the diagnosis (18). Nevertheless, the use of narrow collimation on CT will usually allow demonstration of any fat that is present. On MR, the presence of fat is best demonstrated on T1-weighted images with and without fat suppression. The fat-containing area in a myelolipoma should be equal in signal intensity to that of subcutaneous and retroperitoneal fat on all pulse sequences (Fig. 45.10) (19).

Key Points

- The adrenal glands are a common site for metastases with lung and breast cancers being the commonest primary sources
- Adrenal metastases are asymptomatic and rarely cause adrenal insufficiency
- Adrenal metastases are homogenous when <3 cm, heterogenous when large but can also result in diffuse enlargement of the glands without focal mass lesions

EVALUATION OF THE ADRENAL MASS IN ONCOLOGICAL PATIENTS

Influence on Staging

Adrenal masses are frequently discovered during staging of patients with cancer. One autopsy study demonstrated the presence of microscopic and macroscopic adenomas in almost 54% of the population (20). In most cancers, the presence of adrenal metastases, even as the sole site of distant spread, will render the tumor Stage IV (i.e., distant metastases). The exception is in renal cell carcinoma when the demonstration of ipsilateral adrenal involvement does not increase the stage of the disease from Robson Stage II, but involvement of the contralateral gland upgrades the staging to IVB (Fig. 45.11).

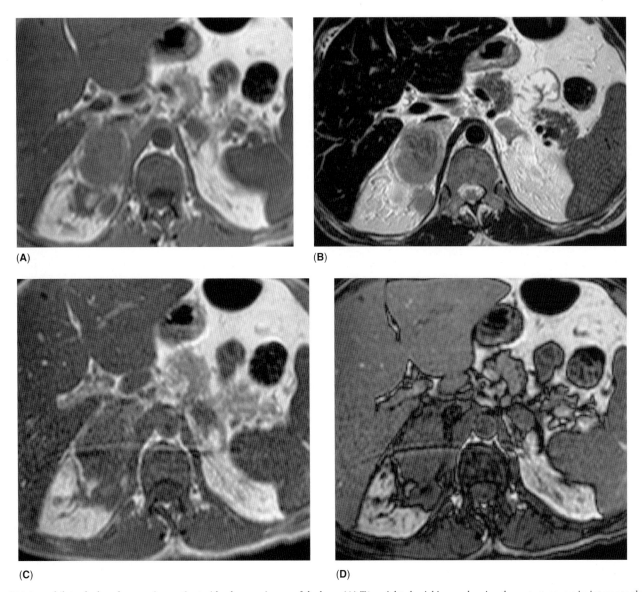

Figure 45.4 Large bilateral adrenal masses in a patient with adenocarcinoma of the lung. (A) T1-weighted axial image showing the metastases are isointense to the liver with a very irregular contour. (B) T2-weighted axial image demonstrating the metastases are hyperintense to the liver and spleen. (C) Axial T1-weighted in-phase image. (D) Axial T1-weighted opposed-phase image showing no loss of signal intensity within the adrenal masses compatible with metastases.

However, not all adrenal masses are metastases, even in patients with known malignancy (21). When an adrenal mass is the only finding suspicious of metastatic disease in an oncological patient, confirmation of its nature may be crucial in determining whether curative therapy of the primary tumor is warranted. This dilemma occurs most commonly in patients with carcinoma of the lung, because confirmation of an isolated adrenal metastasis will preclude a thoracotomy or curative radiotherapy. However, non-functioning macroscopic adrenal adenomas are very common, with a prevalence at autopsy in the general population of approximately 5% (20). Benign adrenal masses of at least 1 cm are found in up to 9% of the population during abdominal CT (22,23). The number and size of these nodules increase with age (0.2% in patients younger than 30 years and 6.9% in patients older than 70 years) (24), and they occur with increased frequency in obese, diabetic patients, and elderly women (25). Even in patients with lung cancer, an adrenal mass is more likely to be an adenoma than a metastasis (21).

When characterizing adrenal masses by non-invasive imaging the consequences of incorrectly characterizing a mass must be considered. In a patient with an extra-adrenal primary neoplasm it is unlikely that potentially curative treatment of the primary tumor would be withheld without biopsy confirmation of an adrenal lesion thought to be the sole site of metastatic spread. Non-invasive characterization of the adrenal mass as an adenoma, however, could result in a decrease in the number of percutaneous biopsies. Thus, the specificity for diagnosis of an adenoma needs to be very high, to ensure that a patient with an adrenal metastasis does not unnecessarily undergo curative resection of the primary tumor because of misdiagnosis of the adrenal lesion as an adenoma. The sensitivity for characterizing a mass as an adenoma is much less critical as the only consequence of a false negative diagnosis is that a percutaneous biopsy will be necessary to establish the diagnosis.

Adrenal masses >3 cm are malignant in 90% to 95% of cases, and 78% to 87% of lesions <3 cm are benign (26,27). However,

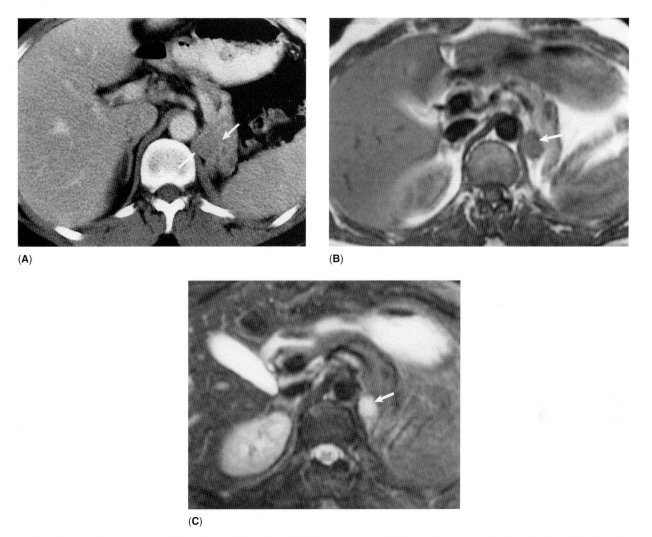

Figure 45.5 Adrenal metastasis in a patient with carcinoma of the kidney. (**A**) Contrast-enhanced CT scan showing normal right adrenal and left adrenal metastasis (arrows); (**B**) T1-weighted MR image showing the mass to be of intermediate signal intensity (arrow); (**C**) T2-weighted MR image of the same mass showing signal mimicking a pheochomocytoma (arrow).

several studies have shown that the size alone is poor at discriminating between adenomas and non-adenomas (28–30). Lee, using a threshold of 1.5 cm, found the specificity for the diagnosis of adenoma to be reasonably high (93%), but the sensitivity only 16% (29). In the same series, using 2.5 cm as the size cut-off, the specificity was 79% and the sensitivity 84%.

The presence of bilateral masses does not confirm a diagnosis of metastases. Katz and Shirkhoda showed that bilateral adrenal adenomas were almost as common as bilateral metastases even in patients with known malignant disease (31). Other causes of bilateral masses such as pheochromocytoma and tuberculosis also result in confusion (Figs. 45.7, 45.8, and 45.12).

The Role of Adrenal Metastectomy

Several small studies have reported a survival benefit following adrenelectomy for isolated adrenal metastases in non-small-cell lung cancer (NSCLC) and malignant melanoma (32–34). In NSCLC they have also shown that resection of the primary carcinoma (Stage 1) and adrenal metastases can be curative (32). The best results are obtained for adrenal metastases less than 4.5 cm

with a median survival of 30 months and an estimated five-year survival of 31% to 33%. In malignant melanoma, however, the median survival was only 6.4 months, but even this was still a statistically significant survival benefit when compared to the non-operative group (32,34,35). The adrenalectomy may be performed as an open or laproscopic procedure. Although the comparative studies are small, the initial results show laproscopic surgery performs as well as open surgery in terms of resection margins, complications, cost effectiveness, and survival and disease-free rates (35,36).

Computed Tomography

CT is extensively used for the characterization of adrenal masses. Many studies have now confirmed the usefulness of attenuation value measurements at non-enhanced, enhanced and delayed enhanced CT in differentiating benign from malignant masses (37–41). CT characterization uses two independent properties of adenomas: their intracellular lipid content, and the rapid enhancement and washout of contrast media after IV contrast enhancement. The majority of adrenal adenomas are

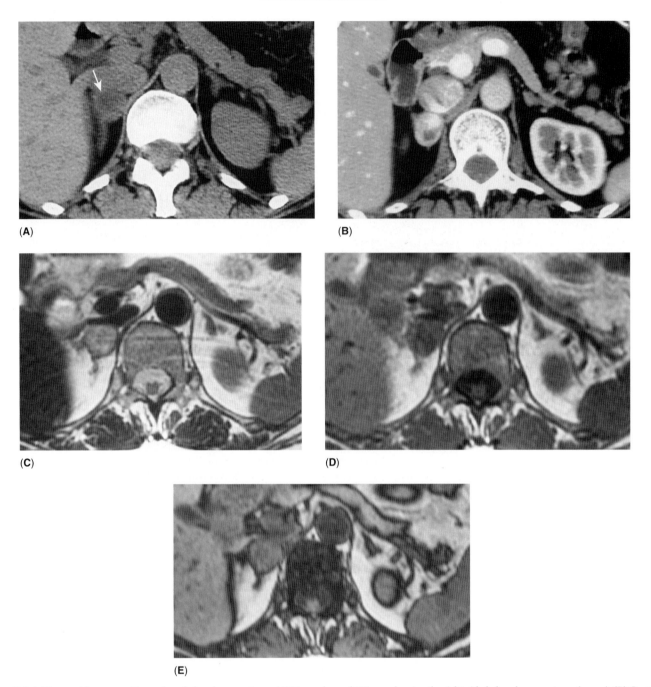

Figure 45.6 A 55-year-old woman with an adrenal pheochromocytoma. (A) Non-enhanced CT scan showing the right-sided pheochromocytoma (arrow). (B) Contrast-enhanced CT scan acquired 60 seconds after contrast administration with the pheochromocytoma demonstrating rim enhancement and central necrosis. (C) T2-weighted MR image showing the pheochromocytoma as an intermediate/ high signal intensity mass. (D) In-phase chemical shift image and (E) out-of-phase chemical shift image showing no loss of signal intensity within the mass.

lipid-rich, thus lowering their unenhanced attenuation values (Fig. 45.13). Analysis of the CT literature shows that the optimal sensitivity (74%) and specificity (96%) for the diagnosis of adrenal adenomas results from choosing a threshold attenuation value of 10 Hounsfield units on non-enhanced CT (29,37). Up to 30% of all adenomas are lipid-poor and cannot be characterized by non-enhanced CT alone (Fig. 45.14). Metastatic adrenal masses are also lipid-poor. This group of lesions therefore requires additional workup to establish the diagnosis.

Standard contrast medium-enhanced attenuation values obtained 60 seconds after contrast injection alone or dynamic enhanced scans show too much overlap between adenomas and malignant lesions (28). Enhanced attenuation values alone are therefore of limited value. Attenuation values of less than 30 Hounsfield units, one hour after contrast enhancement, are always adenomas (100% specificity and 95% sensitivity) (39). In addition to the one hour delayed CT attenuation value, the percentage of absolute contrast washout and the relative enhancement washout can be used to differentiate adenomas from malignant disease. These enhancement washout values are only applicable to relatively homogeneous masses without large areas of necrosis or hemorrhage. It has been demonstrated that washout of contrast

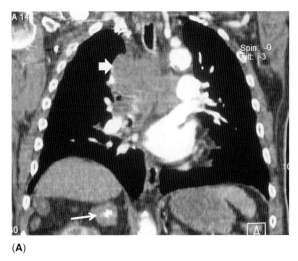
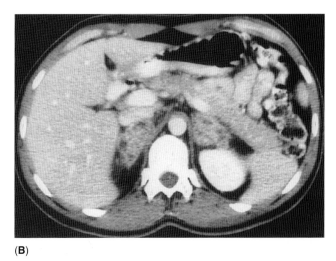

(A)　　　　　　　　　　　　　　　　　**(B)**

Figure 45.7 Adrenal masses in a patient with mediastinal tuberculosis. (**A**) Contrast-enhanced CT with coronal reformat showing extensive mediastinal nodal enlargement confirmed by biopsy as tuberculosis (block arrow). The right adrenal gland can be seen and shows enlargement with punctuate calcification (arrow). (**B**) The adrenal appearances following contrast enhancement showing typical non-enhancing areas within the gland corresponding to multiple small caseating granulomata.

Table 45.2 Differential Diagnosis of Adrenal Metastases

Unilateral	Bilateral
Adrenal adenoma	Bilateral adenoma
Adrenal cyst	Bilateral pheochromocytoma
Adrenal carcinoma	Tuberculosis
Myelolipoma	Lymphoma
Pheochromocytoma	

from adenomas occurs much faster than from a metastasis (41). Both lipid-rich and lipid-poor adenomas behave similarly as this property of adenomas is independent of their lipid content.

The percentage of absolute enhancement washout can be calculated thus:

$$\text{Absolute \% washout} = \frac{A^e - A^{d(15\,min)}}{A^e - A^u} \times 100$$

where A^e is the attenuation value of adrenal mass 60 seconds after IV contrast administration, $A^{d(15\,min)}$ is the attenuation value of the adrenal mass on 15-minute delayed images, and A^u is the attenuation value of the adrenal mass on non-enhanced CT.

At 15 minutes, if the percentage enhancement washout is 60% or higher, this has a sensitivity of 88% and a specificity of 96% for the diagnosis of an adenoma. However, the measurement of absolute contrast medium enhancement washout requires an unenhanced image. Frequently, in clinical practice, only post-contrast images are available. In these patients the percentage relative enhancement washout can be calculated:

$$\text{Relative \% washout} = \frac{A^e - A^{d(15\,min)}}{A^e} \times 100$$

where A^e is the attenuation value of adrenal mass 60 seconds after IV contrast administration and $A^{d(15min)}$ is the attenuation value of the adrenal mass on 15-minute delayed images.

At 15 minutes, if a relative enhancement washout of 40% or higher is achieved, this has a sensitivity of 96% to 100% and a specificity of 100% for the diagnosis of an adenoma (43).

More recently, absolute and relative contrast washout have been calculated using a shorter time delay (70 seconds for enhanced images and 10 minutes post-contrast enhanced delayed images) (44,45). Blake et al. assumed all lesions below 0 HU were benign and all lesions above 43 HU were malignant on unenhanced images. Using the shorter time delay they introduced different threshold criteria: absolute contrast washout criteria greater than 52% and relative contrast washout criteria of 38% for the diagnosis of an adenoma. The combined protocol had a sensitivity and specificity 100% and 98%, respectively for the diagnosis of an adenoma (45). Therefore, a combination of unenhanced CT and delayed enhanced CT with contrast washout correctly characterizes nearly all adrenal masses as adenomas or non-adenomas.

Histogram Analysis Method

This technique quantifies the number of pixels below 0 HU with an adrenal mass. These pixels are referred to as "negative pixels." Adenomas due to their lipid component will have negative pixels. Quantification of negative pixels in an adrenal mass can be performed from non-contrast enhanced and contrast-enhanced CT. A region of interest (ROI) cursor is drawn covering at least two-thirds of the adrenal mass. The individual attenuation values of all the pixels in the ROI are plotted against their frequency. This provides the range, mean, and number of pixels within the ROI. The number of negative pixels within a mass is proportional to the lipid component of the mass. Bae et al. demonstrated that all lipid rich adenomas (<10 HU) had negative pixels on unenhanced CT and 88% of lipid poor adenomas (>10 HU) demonstrated some negative pixels (46). On contrast-enhanced CT, only 53% of all adenomas had any negative pixels. No negative pixels were seen in adrenal metastases (Fig. 45.15). It remains unclear what threshold of negative pixels should be used to establish the diagnosis of an adenoma. The sensitivity and specificity for an adenoma is 92% and 100%, respectively if the mass contains more than 5% negative pixels (47).

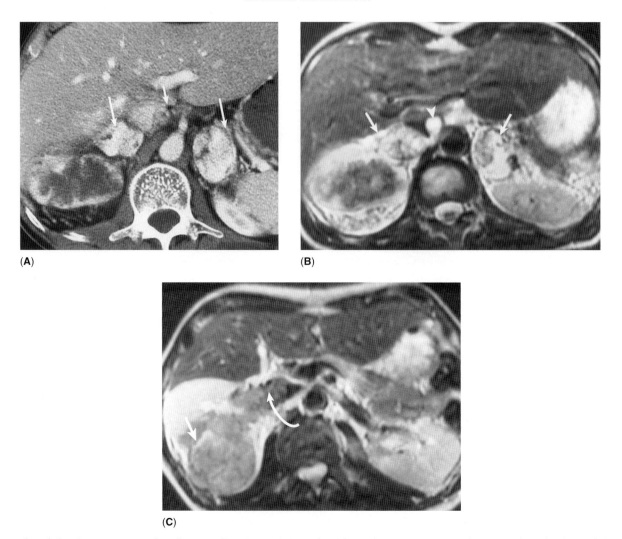

(A)

(B)

(C)

Figure 45.8 Bilateral pheochromocytomas and small paraganglioma in association with a right renal cancer in a patient with von Hippel–Lindau disease. (**A**) Computed tomography scan taken after injection of intravenous contrast medium showing large bilateral adrenal masses enhancing intensely (large arrows). A third smaller mass consistent with a paraganglioma can be seen lying just medial to the inferior vena cava (small arrow); (**B**) T2-weighted FSE MR sequence corresponding to CT scan showing the typical high signal intensity of the pheochromocytomas bilaterally (arrows) and the high signal intensity of the small paraganglioma (arrowhead); (**C**) T2-weighted MR image of the large right renal carcinoma (arrow) infiltrating the right renal vein (curved arrow).

Key Points: Computed Tomography

- On non-enhanced CT, a homogeneous adrenal mass measuring less than 10 HU will be an adenoma in 96% of cases
- On non-contrast-enhanced CT, an adrenal mass measuring >10 HU may be a lipid-poor adenoma or other pathology and contrast-enhanced 10-minute or 15-minutes delayed CT imaging is required
- If the absolute contrast medium enhancement washout is >60% or the relative enhancement washout is >40%, on 15-minute delayed images, the specificity of the mass representing an adenoma is 96%. If the absolute contrast medium enhancement washout is >50% or the relative enhancement washout is >38%, on 10 minute delayed images the specificity of the mass representing an adenoma is 98%
- If the absolute and relative contrast medium enhancement washout is less than specified above, the mass must still be considered indeterminate

Magnetic Resonance

A variety of MR protocols using different pulse sequences have been advocated in an attempt to distinguish between benign and metastatic lesions. Techniques include conventional spin-echo imaging, gadolinium (Gd)-enhanced imaging, chemical-shift and fat-saturation imaging.

Conventional Spin-Echo Imaging

Early reports were enthusiastic that MR would allow differentiation of benign from malignant adrenal masses on the basis of signal intensity differences on T2-weighted spin-echo images. Metastases frequently possess a longer T2 and are of higher signal intensity on T2-weighted images than the surrounding normal adrenal gland. Adenomas are homogeneously iso- or hypointense compared to the normal adrenal gland (13,48). Visual perception of signal intensity on T2-weighted images is problematic as most adrenal masses appear at least of moderately high signal intensity on fat-saturated T2-weighted images. This is because the suppression of fat leads to re-scaling of the signal intensities of abdominal organs. For similar reasons, most adrenal masses appear

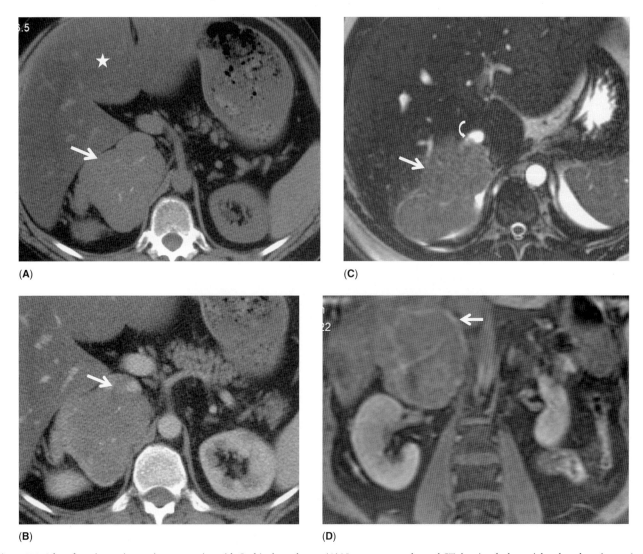

Figure 45.9 Adrenal carcinoma in a patient presenting with Cushing's syndrome. (A) Non-contrast-enhanced CT showing the large right adrenal carcinoma (arrow) with amorphous areas of calcification within it. There is marked fatty change in the liver commonly present in patients with Cushing's syndrome (star). (B) Contrast-enhanced CT demonstrating the heterogenous enhancement within the mass and direct invasion into the IVC (arrow). (C) Axial T2-weighted MR image showing the hyperintense signal intensity of the adrenal carcinoma compared to the liver (arrow). This appearance is similar to adrenal metastases. The curved arrow shows tumor invading the IVC. (D) Coronal T1-weighted post-gadolinium enhanced images with fat saturation. The adrenal carcinoma, similar to metastases, may demonstrate rim enhancement (arrow).

moderately low in signal intensity on spin-echo T2-weighted images because of the surrounding high fat signal intensity (49). Several studies performed on middle-field strength magnets reported that adrenal-to-liver and adrenal-to-fat signal intensity ratios could distinguish benign from malignant masses. However, considerable overlap was seen in most of these studies, with up to 31% of lesions being indeterminate, based on their signal intensity characteristics (13,50–53). The hepatic signal intensity may not be a reliable universal standard at high-field strengths; because of this some investigators have recommended the use of adrenal mass T2 calculations for differential diagnosis (14,43). However, even with this method there is still overlap between benign and malignant masses. In addition, T2 measurements are prone to numerous machine-related errors and may vary on different MR machines. Thus, neither of these techniques has proved useful clinically.

Gadolinium-Enhanced Magnetic Resonance

The accuracy of MR in differentiating benign from malignant masses can be improved by using IV gadolinium injection with gradient-echo imaging (54–56). On MR images obtained after administration of gadolinium, adenomas show mild enhancement with quick washout, whereas malignant tumors and pheochromocytomas show strong enhancement and slower washout. Uniform enhancement (capillary blush) on postgadolinium capillary phase images is common for adenomas, 70% in one series, but rare in other masses (57). Adenomas also commonly demonstrate a thin rim of enhancement in the late phase of Gd-enhanced images (58). Metastases frequently have heterogeneous enhancement. However, again there is considerable overlap in the characteristics of benign and malignant masses, limiting clinical applicability in distinguishing adenomatous from non-adenomatous masses.

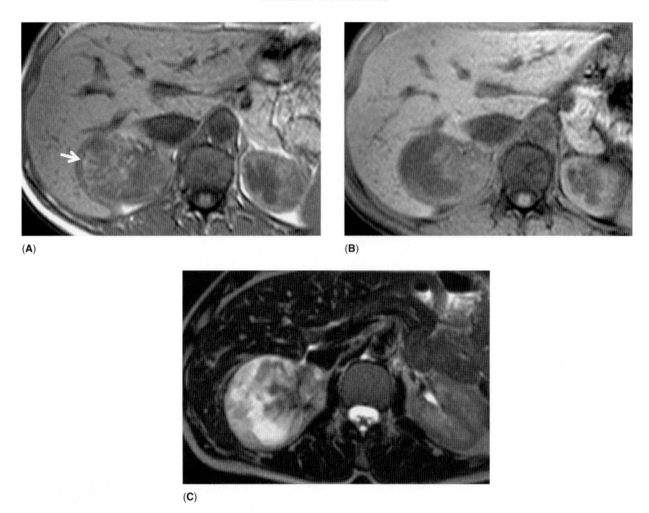

(A)

(B)

(C)

Figure 45.10 Adrenal myelolipoma. (A) Axial T1-weighted MR image showing a large right adrenal mass with multiple areas of high T1 signal intensity (arrow). (B) Axial T1-weighted MR image with fat saturation. The multiple areas of high T1 signal intensity lose signal after fat saturation indicating their fatty composition. (C) Axial T2-weighted MR image demonstrating the heterogenous and high signal intensity of the myelolipoma which may mimic adrenal metastases if viewed without the T1-weighted images.

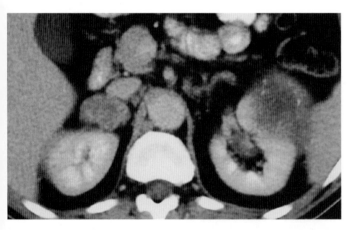

Figure 45.11 Contrast-enhanced CT scan of a patient with a left-sided renal cell carcinoma and a contralateral homogeneous adrenal metastasis. The contralateral metastasis upgrades the renal cell carcinoma to a stage IV-B.

Chemical-Shift Imaging

More recent attempts have been made to characterize adrenal masses with MR on the basis of fat content (59–65). Benign non-functioning adenomas generally contain large lipid-laden cells, in contrast to malignant lesions which contain little or none. Chemical-shift imaging (CSI) relies on the fact that protons in water molecules precess at a slightly different rate to the protons in lipid molecules in a magnetic field. As a result, water and fat protons cycle in- and out-of-phase with respect to one another. By selecting an appropriate TE, one can acquire an in-phase and an out-of-phase image. The signal intensity of a pixel on an in-phase image is derived from the signal of water plus fat protons. On out-of-phase images the signal intensity is derived from the difference of the signal of water and fat protons. Therefore, adenomas lose signal intensity on out-of-phase images compared with in-phase images, whereas metastases remain unchanged (Figs. 45.4 and 45.16). The most accurate method for demonstrating that a mass is an adenoma is to show loss of signal intensity on out-of-phase images.

There are several ways of assessing the degree of loss of signal intensity. Quantitative analysis can be made using a variety of ratios, essentially comparing the loss of signal in the adrenal with that of liver, paraspinal muscle, or spleen on in-phase and opposed-phase images. MR signal intensities are arbitrary units

1085

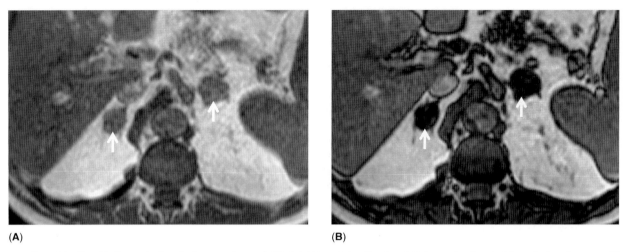

(A)   **(B)**

Figure 45.12 Bilateral incidentally detected adrenal adenomas (arrows). (**A**) Axial T1-weighted in-phase MR image showing the bilateral adrenal masses of isointense signal intensity to the liver. (**B**) Axial T1-weighted opposed-phase MR image showing marked loss of signal intensity within both adrenal masses in keeping with lipid-rich adenomas.

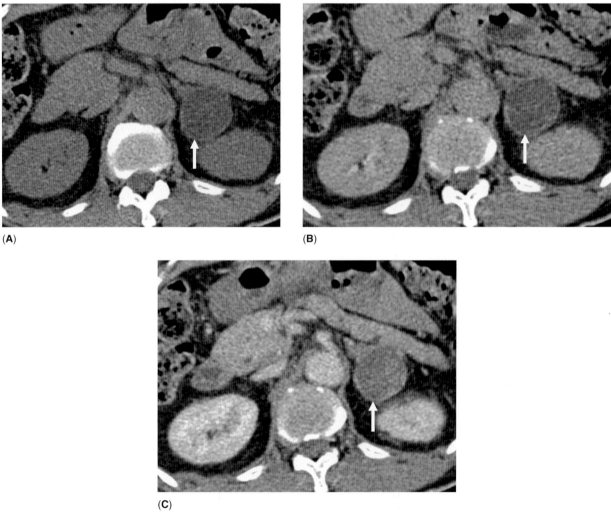

(A)   **(B)**

(C)

Figure 45.13 Lipid-rich adenoma (arrows). (**A**) Non-contrast-enhanced CT image showing a left adrenal mass with a CT attenuation of 6 HU. (**B**) Contrast-enhanced CT image acquired 60 seconds after intravenous contrast administration with enhancement of the adrenal mass. The attenuation value rises to 45 HU. (**C**) Delayed CT image acquired 15 minutes after intravenous contrast administration. There is contrast washout from the adrenal mass and the attenuation value is 15 HU. This provides an absolute % contrast washout of 71%, in keeping with a lipid-rich adenoma.

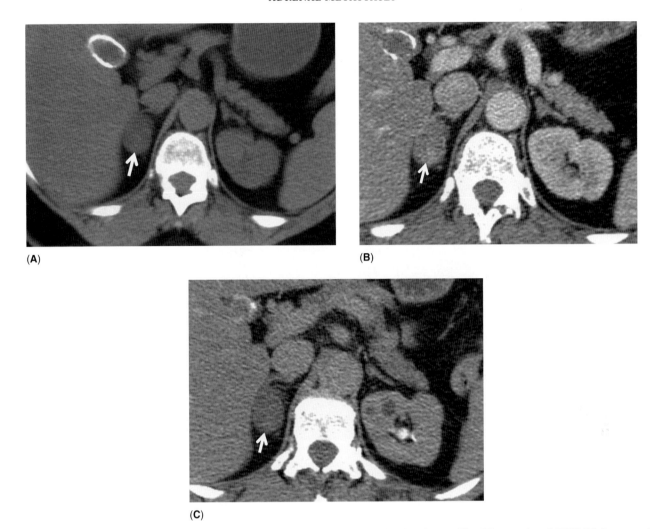

Figure 45.14 Lipid-poor adenoma (arrows). (A) Non-contrast-enhanced CT image showing a right adrenal mass with a CT attenuation of 15 HU. (B) Contrast enhanced CT image acquired 60 seconds after intravenous contrast administration with enhancement of the adrenal mass. The attenuation value rises to 76 HU. (C) Delayed CT image acquired 15 minutes after intravenous contrast administration. There is contrast washout from the adrenal mass and the attenuation value is 38 HU. This provides an absolute % contrast washout of 62%, in keeping with a lipid-poor adenoma.

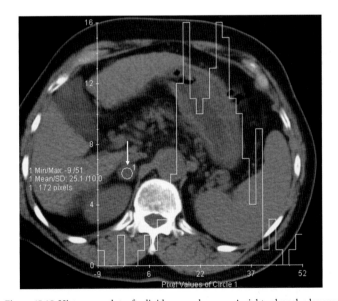

Figure 45.15 Histogram plot of a lipid poor adenoma. A right adrenal adenoma with a non-contrast CT attenuation value of 15 HU is demonstrated (arrow). A histogram obtained from the region of interest drawn within the adenoma is overlaid. The histogram shows 8% negative pixels with a minimum pixel value of −9 HU.

and, therefore, comparing the signal intensities of adrenal masses to an internal reference is necessary for accurate analyses. Fatty infiltration of the liver (particularly in oncology patients receiving chemotherapy) and iron overload make the liver an unreliable internal standard. Fatty infiltration may also affect skeletal muscle to a lesser extent. The spleen has been shown to be the most reliable internal standard, although this may also be affected by iron overload (62).

To calculate the adrenal lesion-to-spleen ratio (ASR) ROIs are used to acquire the signal intensity (SI) within the adrenal mass and the spleen from in-phase and opposed-phase images. The ASR reflects the percentage signal drop within the adrenal lesion compared to the spleen and it can be calculated as follows:

$$ASR = \frac{SI \text{ lesion (opposed - phase)/SI spleen (opposed - phase)}}{SI \text{ lesion (in - phase)/SI spleen (in - phase)}} \times 100$$

ASR ratio of 70 or less has been shown to be 100% specific for adenomas but only 78% sensitive. Crucially, this threshold does

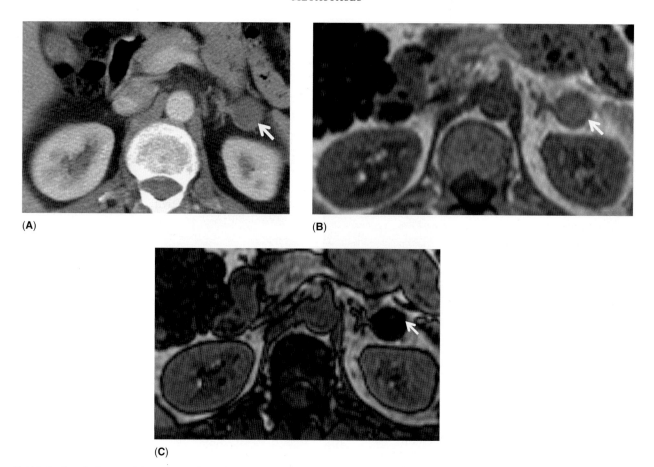

(A)

(B)

(C)

Figure 45.16 Left adrenal adenoma. (**A**) Contrast-enhanced CT acquired 60 seconds after intravenous contrast administration. A well defined left adrenal mass with an attenuation value of 60 HU is demonstrated (arrow). (**B**) Axial T1-weighted in-phase image. (**C**) Axial T1-weighted opposed-phase image showing a marked loss of signal intensity in keeping with a lipid-rich adenoma (arrows).

not label any metastases as adenomas but adenomas may have a higher ASR than 70 (66,67).

The second, better accepted quantitative method assesses the signal loss in adrenal masses as a ratio of signal intensities on the in-phase and opposed-phase images (signal intensity index) (67).

The signal intensity index (SII) is obtained as follows:

$$SII = \frac{SI\,in-phase - SI\,opposed-phase}{SI\,in-phase} \times 100$$

Adenomas characteristically have signal intensity indices greater than 5% whilst metastases have indices lower than 5%. Signal intensity indices have been shown to discriminate between adenomas and metastases with an accuracy of 100% (60). However, subsequent studies have used thresholds between 1% and 30% in identifying adenomas (61,62). This variability can in part be explained by increasing T1-weighting by increasing TR and increasing flip angles which overestimate the lipid content. Image noise, partial volume averaging, surrounding phase-cancellation at the fat-water interface and operator-selected regions of interest all affect the signal intensity measurements (63). The combination of spin-echo signal characteristics, gadolinium enhancement, and CSI is currently 85% to 90% accurate in distinguishing between adenomas and non-adenomas (64).

There are few direct comparisons between CT and MRI. Evidence from one histological study showed that because both non-contrast CT alone and chemical-shift imaging rely upon the same property of adenomas, namely their lipid content, the techniques correlate (61). Recent studies suggest that CSI may be more sensitive in the detection of intracellular lipid than CT (65–66). Whereas on non-contrast enhanced CT up to 30% of adenomas are lipid-poor, only 8% demonstrate no loss of signal intensity on CSI (61). In addition, more lipid-poor adenomas can be distinguished from non-adenomas using signal intensity indices. When CSI is applied to lipid-poor adenomas with non-contrast CT attenuation values between 10 and 30 HU, CSI detected adenomas with a sensitivity of 89%. Therefore, in this group of adrenal masses, CSI detects more adenomas than non-contrast enhanced CT.

Simple visual assessment of relative signal intensity loss, in comparison with the reference organ, is just as accurate as quantitative methods, but quantitative methods may be useful in equivocal cases (67,68). If only visual inspection is performed, it is necessary to ensure the same contrast window width and level on both the in-phase and opposed-phase images as image contrast may influence the perceived signal. Differences in image contrast do not influence the quantitative studies. A signal intensity loss of greater than 20% is diagnostic of adenomas (64). However, although specificities of 100% are reported, metastatic lesions from hepatocellular carcinomas, renal cell carcinomas, and liposarcomas can contain lipid, and two cases of adrenocortical carcinomas containing microscopic amounts of fat showing areas of loss of signal intensity on chemical-shift imaging have been

reported (69). However, in these cases, signal loss was heterogeneous and not uniform. Conversely, it is probable that some functioning adenomas may contain insufficient lipid to result in loss of signal on out-of-phase imaging (56,70). However, these would presumably be identified biochemically.

Key Points: Magnetic Resonance

- Conventional spin-echo techniques and Gad-enhanced MR demonstrate overlap in the appearances of adenomas and malignant lesions
- Chemical-shift imaging relies on the presence of intracellular lipid in adenomas and is the most accurate MR sequence for the diagnosis of an adenoma
- Qualitative assessment of loss of signal intensity on opposed-phase images is accurate in characterizing an adenoma. Quantitative analyses are useful in lesions with equivocal visual change

CT Vs. MRI in Characterizing Adrenal Masses

On unenhanced CT an adrenal mass with an attenuation value at or below 10 HU can be confidently diagnosed as an adenoma with a 96% specificity and require no further characterization (37). Thirty percent of adenomas are indeterminate on unenhanced CT (>10 HU). There is evidence that CSI is more sensitive than unenhanced CT in detecting lipid within adenomas with only 8% of adrenal adenomas characterized as indeterminate masses versus 30% on CT. Chemical shift imaging is therefore more sensitive for the detection of lipid in lipid-poor adenomas. CT contrast-washout dynamics and CSI have a comparable performance in the characterization of an adenoma with a sensitivity and specificity of 96% and 100%, respectively (42,44,45).

In patients with cancer, the first indication of an adrenal mass is usually at a staging post-contrast-enhanced CT. In these patients the unenhanced attenuation value of the adrenal mass is therefore unavailable. If the imaging is reviewed immediately, delayed imaging at 15 minutes should be obtained to allow calculation of relative contrast-washout of the mass. A relative washout of 40% or more indicates an adenoma with 100% specificity and no further imaging is required. The sensitivity of relative contrast-washout is 96% and, therefore, if the relative washout is less than 40%, the mass is indeterminate and requires further characterization. CSI may be contributory in detecting lipid within an adenoma as it is more sensitive than unenhanced CT.

When the imaging is not reviewed immediately and no unenhanced attenuation value is available, further characterization will be necessary and MRI has advantages over CT. CSI is preferred as it has a greater sensitivity to lipid and will perform as well as CT contrast-washout characteristics, thereby providing a greater chance of characterizing an adrenal adenoma than CT. The selection between CSI and CT contrast-washout dynamics will vary between institutions and is influenced by the local availability of expertise and equipment.

Nuclear Scintigraphy

Radiocholesterol agents [^{131}I-6-(beta)-iodomethyl-norcholesterol (NP-59) and 75-SE-selenomethyl-norcholesterol] are conveyed to the adrenal cortical tissue via low-density lipoprotein receptors. Their uptake is affected by adrenocorticotropic hormone (ACTH) and renin–angiotensin systems. Radiocholesterol scintigraphy can be used to identify functioning but not hypofunctioning adrenal masses in the adrenal cortex. This allows characterization of a mass as a benign functioning or a non-functioning lesion. Non-functioning lesions include malignant tumors and benign conditions such as hemorrhage and inflammatory lesions, resulting in an overlap between benign and malignant processes. In two studies the specificity of scintigraphy for the diagnosis of an adenoma was 100% even for masses as small as 1 to 2 cm in diameter (71,72). The sensitivity was comparable to CT density and chemical-shift MR.

Whole-body positron emission tomography with 2-[F-18] fluoro-2-deoxy-D-glucose (^{18}FDG PET) allows the recognition of malignant adrenal lesions. The contribution of ^{18}FDG PET has been well evaluated in large studies in relation to lung cancer and lymphoma (73–76). Using ^{18}FDG PET, these studies have shown a 100% sensitivity and specificity for the diagnosis of a malignant adrenal mass when CT or MR identify enlarged adrenal glands or a focal mass (72,77). For the diagnosis of a malignant adrenal tumor, the positive predictive value (PPV) of ^{18}FDG PET was 100%, and negative predictive value (NPV) to rule out malignancy was also 100% (Fig. 45.17). Within these study populations, ^{18}FDG PET also has the ability to detect metastatic lesions in non-enlarged adrenal glands but the accuracy of this has not

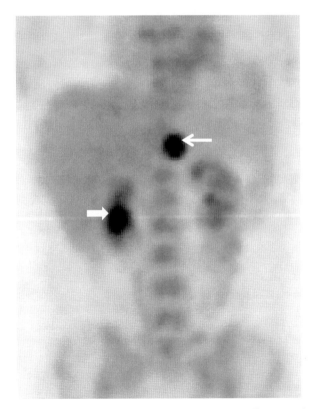

Figure 45.17 Adrenal metastases in a patient with renal cancer. ^{18}FDG-PET image showing the primary right-sided renal cancer (block arrow) as a focus of increased ^{18}FDG uptake. A further area of increased tracer, corresponding on CT to the left adrenal gland, is present (arrow), thereby indicating stage IV disease.

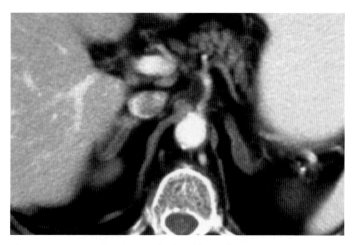

Figure 45.18 Non-metastatic smooth adrenal hyperplasia in patient with ovarian cancer. Contrast-enhanced CT showing mild bilateral enlargement of the adrenal glands in a patient with localized Stage I ovarian cancer.

been fully evaluated (73). ¹⁸FDG PET also has the advantage of simultaneously detecting metastasis at other sites. When evaluating all malignancies, a recent study comparing delayed contrast-enhanced CT with washout values and PET-CT has shown a better performance by CT (sensitivity and specificity of 100% vs. 88% and 75%, respectively) than PET-CT (78). False-positive findings are encountered in integrated PET-CT in approximately 5% of adrenal lesions which include adrenal adenomas, adrenal endothelial cysts, and inflammatory and infectious lesions. False negative findings may be seen in adrenal metastatic lesions with hemorrhage or necrosis, small-sized (<10 mm) metastatic nodules, and metastases from pulmonary bronchio-alveolar carcinoma or carcinoid tumors (79). The routine use of ¹⁸FDG PET is presently limited by availability and its high cost. Other PET radiopharmaceuticals such as 11-C-etiomidate and 11-C-metiomidate have been used to image the adrenals but require evaluation for routine clinical use (80–82).

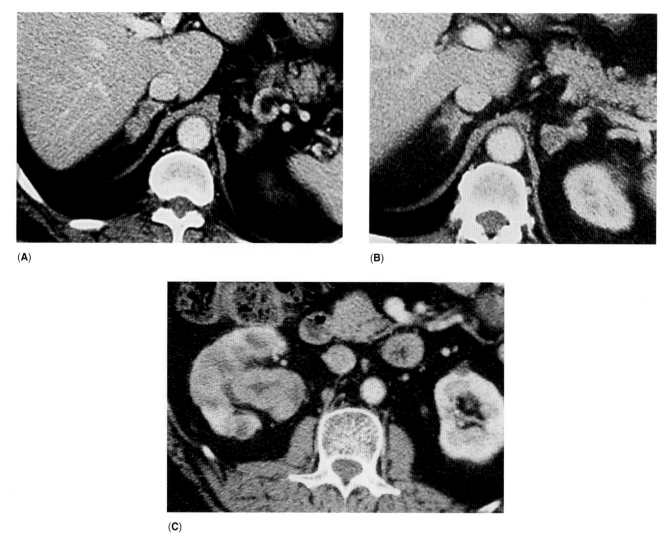

(A)

(B)

(C)

Figure 45.19 Bilateral adrenal hyperplasia in a patient with transitional cell carcinoma of the right renal pelvis. (A and B) Contrast-enhanced CT scans showing bilateral nodular enlargement of the adrenal glands. (C) Contrast-enhanced CT scan showing the primary tumor expanding the right renal pelvis and extending into the proximal ureter and the renal cortex.

Key Point: Radionuclide Imaging

■ Early studies indicate that ^{18}FDG PET has a 100% specificity and sensitivity for the diagnosis of a malignant adrenal mass. More recent and larger studies have reported false positive and more importantly false negative cases of adrenal metastases.

Percutaneous Adrenal Biopsy

With improved imaging and new techniques such as contrast medium washout measurement on CT and chemical-shift MR, only a small percentage of adrenal masses cannot be accurately characterized and require percutaneous biopsy for diagnosis. In a study of 33 patients with known malignancy, 48% were characterized as benign on CT and chemical-shift MR. Forty-six percent were thought to be malignant. Only 5% were considered indeterminate on MR and CT and required biopsy for diagnosis (64). Percutaneous CT-guided adrenal biopsy is a relatively safe procedure in patients with a known extra-adrenal malignancy. Silverman et al., in a study evaluating 101 percutaneous adrenal biopsies, showed the PPV for malignancy was 100% (83). In the study by Harisinghani et al., 225 adrenal biopsies were evaluated (84). For malignant disease, there were no false negative biopsies, giving an NPV of 100%. Adrenal biopsies can therefore safely exclude malignant disease. The reported accuracy ranges from 90% to 96%. One study showed accuracy was increased with the use of larger needles (85).

Minor complications of adrenal biopsy include abdominal pain, hematuria, nausea, and small pneumothoraces. Major complications, generally regarded as those requiring treatment, occur in 2.8% to 3.6% of cases and include pneumothoraces requiring intervention and hemorrhage, with isolated reports of adrenal abscesses, pancreatitis, and seeding of metastases along the needle track (83,85–87). The type of complication varies with the approach used but does not appear to be related to needle size (85,87).

Non-metastatic Adrenal Enlargement

Diffuse adrenal enlargement without metastatic adrenal involvement has been demonstrated in patients with malignant disease, including lymphoma, not known to produce ectopic ACTH (Figs. 45.18 and 45.19). The glands enlarge uniformly with preservation of the normal shape of the adrenal gland and without CT evidence of focal or multifocal masses. It is thought to be due to adrenal hyperplasia and is not related either to the site of primary disease or the stage of disease (88). These patients can be shown not to suppress serum cortisol levels on a low-dose dexamethasone-suppression test, indicating that they are biochemically cushingoid. Nevertheless, the ACTH levels are low, indicating that this phenomenon is not due to ectopic ACTH but is mediated through some other factor (89).

Summary

■ The adrenal glands are a relatively frequent site of metastatic disease
■ Demonstration of adrenal metastasis almost always indicates Stage IV disease

■ Adrenal metastases have to be distinguished from other adrenal masses, particularly adenomas, pheochromocytomas, and other inflammatory lesions
■ CT and MR have a high specificity for identifying benign adrenal adenomas
■ Whole-body ^{18}FDG PET has a high sensitivity and specificity for malignant adrenal masses
■ Occasionally, when an adrenal mass remains indeterminate on non-invasive imaging, percutaneous adrenal biopsy may be required

REFERENCES

1. Abrahams HL, Spiro R, Goldstein N. Metastases in carcinoma. Cancer 1950; 3: 74–85.
2. Cho SY, Choi HY. Causes of death and metastatic patterns in patients with mammary cancer. Am J Clin Pathol 1986; 73: 232–4.
3. Sahagian-Edwards A, Holland JF. Metastatic carcinoma of the adrenal glands with cortical hypofunction. Cancer 1954; 7: 1242–5.
4. Das Gupta T, Brasfield R. Metastatic melanoma. A clinico-pathological study. Cancer 1964; 17: 1323–39.
5. Cedermark BJ, Blumenson LE, Pickren JW, Holyoke DE, Elias EG. The significance of metastases to the adrenal glands in adenocarcinoma of the colon and rectum. Surg Gynaecol Obstet 1977; 144: 537–46.
6. Campbell CM, Middleton RG, Rigby OF. Adrenal metastases in renal cell carcinoma. Urology 1983; 21: 403–5.
7. Moriya T, Manabe T, Yamashita K, Arita S. Lung cancer metastases to adrenocortical adenomas. A chance occurrence or a predilected phenomenon? Arch Pathol Lab Med 1988; 112: 286–9.
8. McMahon RF. Tumor to tumor metastases: bladder carcinoma metastasising to an adrenocortical adenoma. Br J Urol 1991; 67: 216–17.
9. Travis WD, Oertel JE, Lack EE. Miscellaneous tumors and tumefaction lesions of the adrenal gland. In: Lack EE, ed. Pathology of the Adrenal Glands. Edinburgh: Churchill Livingstone, 1990: 351–78.
10. Allard P, Yankaskas BC, Fletcher RH, et al. Sensitivity and specificity of CT for the detection of adrenal metastatic lesions among 91 autopsied lung cancer patients. Cancer 1990; 66: 457–62.
11. Vincent JM, Morrison ID, Armstrong P, Reznek RH. The size of normal adrenal glands on computed tomography. Clin Radiol 1994; 49: 453–5.
12. Gillams A, Roberts CM, Shaw P, Spiro SG, Goldstraw P. The value of CT scanning and percutaneous fine needle aspiration of adrenal masses in biopsy-proven lung cancer. Clin Radiol 1992; 46: 18–22.
13. Reinig JW, Doppman JL, Dwyer AJ, Johnson AR, Knop RH. Adrenal masses differentiated by MR. Radiology 1986; 158: 81–4.
14. Kier R, McCarthy S. MR characterization of adrenal masses: field strength and pulse sequence considerations. Radiology 1989; 171: 671–4.
15. Ghandur-Mnaymneh L, Slim M, Muakassa K. Adrenal cysts: pathogenesis and histological identification with a report of six cases. J Urol 1979; 122: 87–91.

16. Dunnick NR, Heaston D, Halvorsen R, Moore AV, Korobkin M. CT appearance of adrenal cortical carcinoma. J Comput Assist Tomogr 1982; 6: 978–82.

17. Fishman EK, Deutch BM, Hartman DS, et al. Primary adrenocortical carcinoma. CT evaluation with clinical correlation. Am J Roentgenol 1987; 148: 531–5.

18. Cyran KM, Kenney PJ, Mernel DS, Yacoub I. Adrenal myelolipoma. Am J Roentgenol 1996; 166: 395–400.

19. Guo YK, Yang ZG, Li Y, et al. Uncommon adrenal masses: CT and MRI features with histopathologic correlation. Eur J Radiol 2007; 62: 359–70.

20. Reinhard C, Saeger W, Schubert B. Adrenocortical nodules in post-mortem series. Development, functional significance, and differentiation from adenomas. Gen Diagn Pathol 1996; 14: 203–8.

21. Oliver TW Jr, Bernardino ME, Miller JI, et al. Isolated adrenal masses in non-small-cell bronchogenic carcinoma. Radiology 1984; 153: 217–18.

22. Glazer HS, Weyman PJ, Sagel SS, Levitt RG, McClennan BL. Non-functioning adrenal masses: incidental discovery on computed tomography. Am J Roentgenol 1982; 139: 81–5.

23. Ambos MA, Bosniak MA, Lefleur RS, Mitty HA. Adrenal adenoma associated with renal cell carcinoma. Am J Roentgenol 1981; 136: 81–4.

24. Doppman JL, Travis WD, Nieman L, et al. Cushing syndrome due to primary pigmented nodular adreno cortical disease: findings at CT and MR imaging. Radiology 1989; 172: 415–20.

25. Gross MD, Wilton GP, Shapiro B, et al. Functional and scintigraphic evaluation of the silent adrenal mass. J Nucl Med 1987; 28: 1401–7.

26. Candel AG, Gattuso P, Reyes CV, Prinz RA, Castelli MJ. Fine needle aspiration of adrenal masses in patients with extra-adrenal malignancy. Surgery 1993; 114: 1132–7.

27. McGahan JP. Adrenal gland: MR imaging. Radiology 1988; 166: 284–5.

28. Korobkin M, Brodeur FJ, Yutzy GG, et al. Differentiation of adrenal adenomas from non-adenomas using CT attenuation values. Am J Roentgenol 1996; 166: 531–6.

29. Lee MJ, Hahn PF, Papanicolaou N, et al. Benign and malignant adrenal masses: CT distinction with attenuation coefficients, size, and observer analysis. Radiology 1991; 179: 415–18.

30. van Erkel AR, van Gils AP, Lequin M, et al. CT and MR distinction of adenomas and nonadenomas of the adrenal gland. J Comput Assist Tomogr 1994; 18: 432–8.

31. Katz RL, Shirkhoda A. Diagnostic approach to incidental adrenal nodules in the cancer patient. Cancer 1985; 55: 1995–2000.

32. Tanvetyanon T, Robinson LA, Schell MJ, et al. Outcomes of adrenalectomy for isolated synchronous versus metachronous adrenal metastases in non-small-cell lung cancer: a systematic review and pooled analysis. J Clin Oncol 2008; 26: 1142–7.

33. Kita M, Tamaki G, Okuyama M, Saga Y, Kakizaki H. Adrenalectomy for metastatic adrenal tumors. Hinyokika Kiyo 2007; 53: 761–6.

34. Mittendorf EA, Lim SJ, Schacherer CW, et al. Melanoma adrenal metastasis: natural history and surgical management. Am J Surg 2008; 195: 363–8.

35. Sebag F, Calzolari F, Harding J, et al. Isolated adrenal metastasis: the role of laparoscopic surgery. World J Surg 2006; 30: 888–92.

36. Strong VE, D'Angelica M, Tang L, et al. Laparoscopic adrenalectomy for isolated adrenal metastasis. Ann Surg Oncol 2007; 14: 3392–400.

37. Boland GW, Lee MJ, Gazelle GS, et al. Characterization of adrenal masses using unenhanced CT: an analysis of the CT literature. Am J Roentgenol 1998; 171: 201–4.

38. Boland GW, Hahn PF, Peña C, Mueller PR. Adrenal masses: characterization with delayed contrast-enhanced CT. Radiology 1997; 202: 693–6.

39. Korobkin M, Brodeur FJ, Francis IR, et al. Delayed enhanced CT for the differentiation of benign from malignant masses. Radiology 1996; 200: 737–42.

40. Szolar DH, Kammerhuber F. Quantitative CT evaluation of adrenal gland masses: a step forward in the differentiation between adenomas and nonadenomas? Radiology 1997; 202: 517–22.

41. Korobkin M, Brodeur FJ, Francis IR, et al. CT time-attenuation washout curves of adrenal adenomas and nonadenomas. Am J Roentgenol 1998; 170: 747–52.

42. Peña CS, Boland GW, Hahn PF, Lee MJ, Mueller PR. Characterization of indeterminate (lipid-poor) adrenal masses: use of washout characteristics at contrast-enhanced CT. Radiology 2000; 217: 798–802.

43. Dunnick NR, Korobkin M. Imaging of adrenal incidentalomas: current status. Am J Roentgenol 2002; 179: 559–68.

44. Szolar DH, Kammerhuber FH. Adrenal adenomas and nonadenomas: assessment of washout at delayed contrast-enhanced CT. Radiology 1998; 207: 369–75.

45. Blake MA, Kalra MK, Sweeney AT, et al. Distinguishing benign from malignant adrenal masses: multi-detector row CT protocol with 10-minute delay. Radiology 2006; 238: 578–85.

46. Bae KT, Fuangtharnthip P, Prasad SR, Joe BN, Heiken JP. Adrenal masses: CT characterization with histogram analysis method. Radiology 2003; 228: 735–42.

47. Jhaveri KS, Lad SV, Haider MA. CT histogram analysis in the diagnosis of lipid-poor adenomas: comparison to adrenal washout computed tomography. J Comput Assist Tomogr 2007; 31: 513–18.

48. Baker ME, Blinder R, Spritzer C, et al. MR evaluation of adrenal masses at 1.5 T. Am J Roentgenol 1989; 153: 307–12.

49. Semelka RC. Adrenal glands. Abdominal-Pelvic MRI. New York: Wiley-Liss, 2002: 695–740.

50. Chang A, Glazer HC, Lee JK, Heiken JP. Adrenal gland MR imaging. Radiology 1987; 163: 123–8.

51. Remer EM, Weinfeld RM, Glazer GM, et al. Hyperfunctioning and nonhyperfunctioning benign adrenal cortical lesions: characterization and comparison with MR imaging. Radiology 1989; 171: 681–5.

52. Glazer GM, Woolsey EJ, Borrello J, et al. Adrenal tissue characterization using MR imaging. Radiology 1986; 158: 73–9.

53. Baker ME, Spritzer C, Blinder R, et al. Benign adrenal lesions mimicking malignancy on MR imaging: report of two cases. Radiology 1987; 163: 669–71.

54. Krestin GP, Steinbrich W, Friedman G. Adrenal masses: evaluation with fast gradient-echo MR imaging and Gd DTPA enhanced dynamic studies. Radiology 1989; 171: 675–80.

55. Krestin GP, Friedmann G, Fishbach R, Neufang KF, Allolio B. Evaluation of adrenal masses in oncologic patients: dynamic contrast-enhanced MR vs CT. J Comput Assist Tomogr 1991; 15: 104–10.

56. Semelka RC, Shoenut JP, Lawrence PH, et al. Evaluation of adrenal masses with gadolinium enhancement and fat-suppressed MR imaging. J Magn Reson Imaging 1993; 3: 332–43.

57. Chung JJ, Semelka RC, Martin DR. Adrenal adenomas: characteristic postgadolinium capillary blush on dynamic MR imaging. J Magn Reson Imaging 2001; 13: 242–8.

58. Ichikawa T, Ohtomo K, Uchiyama G, et al. Adrenal adenomas: characteristic hyperintense rim sign on fat-saturated spin-echo MR images. Radiology 1994; 193: 247–50.

59. Mitchell DG, Crovello M, Matteucci T, Petersen RO, Miettinen MM. Benign adrenocortical masses: diagnosis with chemical shift MR imaging. Radiology 1992; 185: 345–51.

60. Tsushima Y, Ishizaka H, Matsumoto M. Adrenal masses: differentiation with chemical shift, fast low-angle shot MR imaging. Radiology 1993; 186: 705–9.

61. Korobkin M, Giordano T, Brodeur FJ, et al. Adrenal adenomas: relationship between histologic lipid and CT and MR findings. Radiology 1996; 200: 743–7.

62. Hussain HK, Korobkin M. MR imaging of the adrenal glands. Magn Reson Imaging Clin N Am 2004; 12: 515–44.

63. Al-Hawary MM, Francis IR, Korobkin M. Non-invasive evaluation of the incidentally detected indeterminate adrenal mass. Best Pract Res Clin Endocrinol Metab 2005; 19: 277–92.

64. McNicholas MM, Lee MJ, Mayo-Smith WW, et al. An imaging algorithm for the differential diagnosis of adrenal adenomas and metastases. Am J Roentgenol 1995; 165: 1453–9.

65. Inan N, Arslan A, Akansel G, et al. Dynamic contrast enhanced MRI in the differential diagnosis of adrenal adenomas and malignant adrenal masses. Eur J Radiol 2008; 65: 154–62.

66. Haider MA, Ghai S, Jhaveri K, Lockwood G. Chemical shift MR imaging of hyperattenuating (>10 HU) adrenal masses: does it still have a role? Radiology 2004; 231: 711–16.

67. Schwartz LH, Panicek DM, Koutcher JA, et al. Adrenal masses in patients with malignancy: prospective comparison of echo-planar, fast spin-echo, and chemical shift MR imaging. Radiology 1995; 197: 421–5.

68. Mayo-Smith WW, Lee MJ, McNicholas MM, et al. Characterization of adrenal masses (<5 cm) by use of chemical shift MR imaging: observer performance versus quantitative measures. Am J Roentgenol 1995; 165: 91–5.

69. Schlund JF, Kenney PJ, Brown ED, et al. Adrenocortical carcinoma: MR imaging appearance with current techniques. J MRI 1995; 5: 171–4.

70. Tsushima Y. Different lipid contents between aldosterone-producing and nonhyperfunctioning adreno cortical adenomas: in vivo measurement using chemical shift MRI. J Clin Endocrin Metab 1994; 79: 1759–62.

71. Kloos RT, Gross MD, Shapiro B, et al. The diagnostic dilemma of small incidentally discovered adrenal masses: a role for 131-I-6[beta]-iodomethyl-norcholesterol(NP-59) scintigraphy. World J Surg 1997; 21: 36–40.

72. Maurea S, Klain M, Mainolfi C, Zirielb M, Salvatore M. The diagnostic role of radionuclide imaging in evaluation of patients with nonhypersecreting adrenal masses. J Nucl Med 2001; 42: 884–92.

73. Lowe VJ, Naunheim KS. Current role of positron emission tomography in thoracic oncology. Thorax 1998; 53: 703–12.

74. Erasmus JJ, McAdams HP, Patz EF Jr. Non-small cell lung cancer: FDG-PET imaging. J Thorac Imag 1999; 14: 247–56.

75. Erasmus JJ, Patz EF Jr. Positron emission tomography imaging in the thorax. Clin Chest Med 1999; 20: 715–24.

76. Facey K, Bradbury I, Laking G, Payne E. Overview of the clinical effectiveness of positron emission tomography imaging in selected cancers. Health Technol Assess 2007; 11: iii–iv, xi–267.

77. Yun M, Kim W, Alnafisi N, et al. 18F-FDG PET in characterizing adrenal lesions detected on CT or MRI. J Nucl Med 2001; 42: 1797–9.

78. Park BK, Kim CK, Kim B, Choi JY. Comparison of delayed enhanced CT and 18F-FDG PET/CT in the evaluation of adrenal masses in oncology patients. J Comput Assist Tomogr 2007; 31: 550–6.

79. Chong S, Lee KS, Kim HY, et al. Integrated PET-CT for the characterization of adrenal gland lesions in cancer patients: diagnostic efficacy and interpretation pitfalls. Radiographics 2006; 26: 1811–24.

80. Bergström M, Bonasera TA, Lu L, et al. In vitro and in vivo primate evaluation of carbon-11-etomidate and carbon-11-metomidate as potential tracers for PET imaging of the adrenal cortex and its tumors. J Nucl Med 1998; 39: 982–9.

81. Bergström M, Juhlin C, Bonasera TA, et al. PET imaging of adrenal cortical tumors with the 11beta-hydroxylase tracer 11C-metomidate. J Nucl Med 2000; 41: 275–82.

82. Hennings J, Lindhe O, Bergström M, et al. [11C]metomidate positron emission tomography of adrenocortical tumors in correlation with histopathological findings. J Clin Endocrinol Metab 2006; 9: 1410–14.

83. Silverman SG, Mueller PR, Pinkney LP, Koenker RM, Seltzer SE. Predictive value of image-guided adrenal biopsy: analysis of results of 101 biopsies. Radiology 1993; 187: 715–18.

84. Harisinghani MG, Maher MM, Hahn PF, et al. Predictive value of benign percutaneous adrenal biopsies in oncology patients. Clin Radiol 2002; 57: 898–901.

85. Habscheid W, Pfeiffer M, Demmrich J, Muller HA. Metastases to the needle puncture track after ultrasound-guided fine needle adrenal biopsy. A rare complication? Dtsch Med Wochenschr 1990; 115: 212–15.

86. Welch TJ, Sheedy PF 2nd, Stephens DH, Johnson CM, Swensen SJ. Percutaneous adrenal biopsy: review of a 10-year experience. Radiology 1994; 193: 341–4.

87. Mody MK, Kazerooni EA, Korobkin M. Percutaneous CT-guided biopsy of adrenal masses: immediate and delayed complications. J Comput Assist Tomogr 1995; 19: 434–9.

88. Vincent JM, Morrison ID, Armstrong P, Reznek RH. Computed tomography of diffuse, non-metastatic enlargement of the adrenal glands in patients with malignant disease. Clin Radiol 1994; 49: 456–60.

89. Jenkins PJ, Sohaib SA, Trainer PJ, et al. Adrenal enlargement and failure of suppression of circulating cortisol by dexamethasone in patients with malignancy. Br J Cancer 1999; 80: 1815–19.

46 Peritoneal Metastases
Zahir Amin and Rodney H Reznek

INTRODUCTION

The detection of peritoneal metastases is essential in the staging of many tumors as their presence is often of major prognostic significance (1). Detection of peritoneal metastases allows decisions to be made regarding the need for surgery, response to treatment can be monitored and tumor recurrence identified. Although current imaging can depict peritoneal metastases as small as a few millimeters in size as well as very small volumes of ascites, sensitivities are variable and relatively low in detecting small deposits.

Causes of Peritoneal Metastases

Gynecological malignancy, mainly ovarian cancers, is the most common source of peritoneal metastases. Other primary sites are usually intra-abdominal and include gastric, colorectal, and pancreatic tumors. Approximately 71% of ovarian, 17% of gastric, and 10% of colorectal cancer cases have peritoneal metastases at the time of presentation (2).

Lymphoma can also give rise to peritoneal masses (see chap. 9). Less common causes include cholangiocarcinoma, gastrointestinal stromal tumor, carcinoid, hepatoma, renal cell cancer and bladder carcinoma. The main extra-abdominal primary cause is breast cancer and occasionally the primary site is not found.

Anatomy of the Peritoneal Spaces (Fig. 46.1)

The peritoneal cavity is a serous sac (or coelom) lying between the parietal and visceral peritoneum and consists of a series of communicating potential spaces not normally seen on imaging unless distended by fluid or air. The visceral peritoneum covers the abdominal organs and the parietal peritoneum lies against the abdominal wall and retroperitoneum, resulting in an extensive surface area as a potential site of tumor deposition. Ligaments are peritoneal folds connecting abdominal organs. The greater omentum consists of four layers of peritoneum, two from the greater curve of the stomach and two from the transverse mesocolon, which fuse and pass anterior to small bowel—this is often done by metastases. The lesser omentum (or gastrohepatic ligament) joins the lesser curve of the stomach to the liver. A mesentery is a peritoneal fold joining small bowel or parts of the colon to the posterior abdominal wall and containing vessels and nerves (3). Ligaments and mesenteries are suspended by the visceral peritoneum and so are not truly intraperitoneal (4).

The transverse mesocolon is the main dividing barrier, separating the supracolic and infracolic compartments. The left infracolic space is divided from the right by the small bowel mesentery and communicates inferiorly with the right pelvis.

The peritoneal cavity normally contains less than 100 ml of serous fluid which circulates and is preferentially drawn up to the right subphrenic space where it is absorbed (4).

MODES OF SPREAD

The development and spread of peritoneal metastases are related to the anatomical configuration of the peritoneal cavity, and its associated attachments to the abdominal/pelvic organs and bowel. The principle methods of spread are by direct invasion and intraperitoneal seeding, with many metastatic tumors likely to be using both (5).

Direct Invasion

Cancers of the stomach, colon, pancreas, liver, gallbladder, spleen, and ovary can invade directly into the adjacent ligaments and mesenteries and then into connecting organs as well as the GI tract and abdominal wall (5,6). Gastric cancer often spreads into the adjacent gastrohepatic ligament, and may then invade into the left lobe of the liver (7). Pancreatic cancer can extend from the retroperitoneum into the hepatoduodenal ligament (which contains the bile duct, hepatic artery, and portal vein) and then into the liver (8). Tumors of the colon, stomach, and pancreas often spread through the transverse mesocolon and greater omentum, and can invade the transverse colon. The right side of the transverse mesocolon forms the duodenocolic ligament providing a direct route for extension of colon cancer from the hepatic flexure to the duodenum (9). The phrenicocolic ligament, which extends from the splenic flexure to the diaphragm, prevents extension of metastases along the left side of the greater omentum. The gastrosplenic ligament extends from the greater curve of the stomach to the spleen and can be involved by extramural spread from gastric cancer. Direct involvement of the small bowel mesentery is commonly seen in carcinoid, pancreatic, breast, and colonic metastases. Lymphoma often spreads from the retroperitoneum through the root of the small bowel mesentery to the small bowel.

In the pelvis, ovarian carcinoma may spread through direct extension to surrounding tissues. The fallopian tubes, uterus, and contralateral adnexa are the most commonly involved tissues, but the rectum and bladder can also be directly invaded (10).

Intraperitoneal Seeding

This is the most common mode of tumor spread in ovarian cancer, with approximately 70% of patients having peritoneal metastases at staging laparotomy (10). Malignant cells are shed from the tumor surface into the peritoneal cavity, where they follow normal routes of peritoneal fluid circulation. The flow of peritoneal fluid is determined by gravity and pressure gradients related to respiration and bowel peristalsis, along pathways determined by the compartments of the peritoneal cavity (5,11). Metastases usually grow in sites where malignant ascites preferentially flows and pools, such as the pouch of Douglas, right lower quadrant, around the sigmoid colon, right paracolic gutter, right subhepatic, and subphrenic spaces, with flow to the left side limited by the phrenicocolic ligament (4,11). The oblique course of the small bowel mesentery and transverse course of the sigmoid mesocolon produce relative stasis of fluid (12). The omentum is bathed in peritoneal fluid and so is a common site of seeding. Eventually, dissemination of intraperitoneal

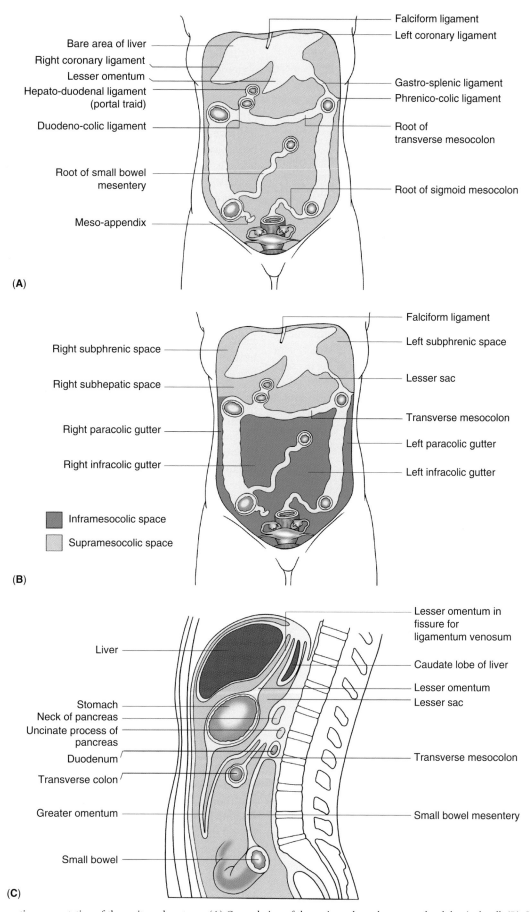

Figure 46.1 Diagrammatic representation of the peritoneal anatomy. (A) Coronal view of the peritoneal attachments to the abdominal wall. (B) Coronal view of the posterior peritoneal spaces. (C) Mid-sagittal section through the upper abdomen to show the peritoneal spaces and mesenteries.

tumor may involve all of the peritoneal surfaces, including the free peritoneal surfaces and bowel serosa. Other tumors that are spread in this way are cancers of the stomach, colon, pancreas, and endometrium, as well as cholangiocarcinoma, primary peritoneal cancer, and pseudomyxoma peritonei. Metastatic deposits to the ovaries are also due to transcoelomic spread (13) and probably result from seeding at sites of ovarian follicle rupture.

Lymphatic Invasion

This mainly relates to spread of lymphoma to mesenteric nodes, causing very large masses which surround the mesenteric vessels, and are separated from retroperitoneal lymphadenopathy by an intact anterior pararenal fat plane (14,15).

Since the lymphatics follow the course of the arteries, small bowel and colon cancers often extend via lymphatics to metastatic mesenteric or liver hilum nodes (12).

Hematogenous Spread

Peritoneal deposits from hematogenous spread are rare, usually from melanoma, breast cancer, lung cancer, and sarcoma, and deposits may occur in the bowel wall, peritoneal surface, mesentery, or omentum (5,16). Patients may present with bowel obstruction or GI bleeding, sometimes several years after treatment of the primary neoplasm. Hematogenous metastases to the stomach from breast cancer can produce marked gastric wall thickening with almost complete obliteration of its lumen (17). Breast cancer metastases are often plaque-like and difficult to clearly define on imaging, and the only abnormality may be slight stranding in the fat (6).

Key Points: Mode of Spread

- A good understanding of the anatomy of the peritoneal cavity and spaces aids CT and MRI interpretation
- Peritoneal metastases occur mainly by direct invasion into adjacent ligaments, mesenteries, and omentum, or by intraperitoneal seeding
- Intraperitoneal spread occurs mainly at sites where peritoneal fluid preferentially flows and pools—the pouch of Douglas/rectovesical pouch, around the sigmoid colon, right lower quadrant, right paracolic gutter, and around the liver.

IMAGING TECHNIQUES

Peritoneal imaging is difficult because of the extensive anatomical location of the peritoneal surface, and because peritoneal metastases may be just a few cells thick and disseminated but not visible on any imaging modality. Although there is no gold standard for imaging peritoneal metastases, they are identified most frequently on computed tomography (CT) as it is the principle technique for the staging of malignancy. Peritoneal metastases are also detected with ultrasound (US) and magnetic resonance (MR) imaging, but their role is secondary to CT. Positron emission tomography (PET) and in particular PET-CT is increasingly available. Barium studies are done less frequently and are only occasionally relevant in the current imaging of peritoneal metastases.

This section describes the different imaging modalities, with details of techniques and their role in imaging peritoneal metastases.

Computed Tomography

Multidetector computed tomography (MDCT) is now widely available, allowing very fast, thin-section scanning of the whole abdomen within a few seconds. Image artifact is reduced and multiplanar reformats easily viewed, resulting in improved assessment of subdiaphragmatic spaces, paracolic gutters, and pelvic deposits (18). Multiphasic enhancement is also possible, early scanning improving the sensitivity of detecting small peritoneal surface and bowel wall lesions, although in practice only one enhancement phase is usually performed. Although somewhat limited by poor contrast resolution, CT can still detect tiny peritoneal deposits without any special technique other than enhancement following intravenous (IV) contrast medium injection and thin slice multiplanar reconstructions (18). Many radiologists also use positive oral contrast to help differentiate extraluminal/serosal deposits from bowel lumen and its contents (10,12). However, with modern scanners and rapid interactive multiplanar display of images, positive oral contrast is less important. Using positive oral contrast separates bowel from cystic deposits, but may obscure calcified serosal deposits and reduces the advantage of mucosal/surface tumor enhancement with oral water/IV contrast (18). CT enteroclysis is a new technique which gives detailed views of the distended bowel lumen, bowel wall, and adjacent structures—it may be better for depicting serosal deposits, and be particularly useful in assessing patients with associated partial/intermittent small bowel obstruction (19).

Intraperitoneal positive contrast (20) and pneumoperitoneum (21) with CT, to try to improve detection of small peritoneal deposits, are techniques that are no longer used since there is no advantage over the improved image quality with multislice CT.

Magnetic Resonance Imaging

MR imaging can give comparable images to multislice CT and, in view of its excellent contrast resolution, has high sensitivity and accuracy for detecting tumors involving the peritoneum and can often show subtle peritoneal metastases (6,22). High-field strength magnet and phased-array surface coils should be used, and ideally an antiperistaltic agent should be administered. Standard T1 axial and T2 axial, coronal and sagittal sequences, with fat saturated T2 and, importantly, fat-suppressed T1-weighted sequences with contrast medium enhancement are recommended. Some authors advocate dynamic and 5 to 10 minute delayed post-contrast sequences, since enhancement improves on delayed images (6,23). Diffusion-weighted images can be useful since ascites and bowel content are suppressed, and peritoneal and serosal deposits seen as areas of high signal (6).

Distension and separation of bowel loops can be achieved with various agents: one of the simplest to use is dilute oral barium 30 minutes prior to the MR examination (6). The dilute barium acts as a positive oral contrast agent on the T2-weighted images and as a negative oral contrast agent on the T1-weighted images.

Although several studies have reported fat-suppressed T1-weighted post-contrast MR images to be superior to CT in detecting subtle peritoneal deposits, overall CT is generally the preferred imaging modality since it is much faster, has better spatial resolution, fewer artifacts, is more widely accessible, and is routinely used for the staging of most intra-abdominal malignancies. However, MR is routinely performed in assessing pelvic malignancies, and abdominal MR is useful in patients allergic to iodinated IV contrast, those with renal impairment, as well as for problem-solving.

Ultrasound

US image quality has improved significantly in recent years, and peritoneal/omental deposits are often seen well with graded compression and high frequency transducers (24). Tiny deposits of 2 to 3 mm can be seen, particularly in the presence of ascites which provides an acoustic window. Centrally located deposits may not be visualized because of overlying bowel gas, but this is also dependent on operator experience and whether the examination is specifically targeted towards searching for peritoneal/omental deposits (25,26). Therefore, although less objective than CT or MR, US may have a role for problem-solving if CT is inconclusive regarding peritoneal masses, and can also be used for guided biopsies (27). US may be the initial test to detect ascites and can then be used to assess the ovaries for a possible primary malignant source. Peritoneal deposits may also be detected during transvaginal US assessment of possible ovarian malignancy (28). In patients with gastric cancer, endoscopic US is more sensitive than conventional US or CT in detecting ascites and predicting the presence of peritoneal metastases (29,30).

PET and PET-CT

Positron emission tomography using 2-[F-18]fluoro-2-deoxy-D-glucose (^{18}FDG) is now being widely used in oncological practice, particularly in combination with CT (FDG PET-CT) and gives detailed anatomical as well as functional metabolic information (31–33). Fused PET-CT images allow precise anatomical location of abnormal FDG activity and help in correlating any equivocal CT findings with metabolic activity (34). Previous studies evaluating PET alone for the detection of peritoneal metastases have given variable results, reporting sensitivities and specificities of 83% to 86% and 54% to 86%, respectively (10). Sensitivity for small nodules and low volume disease is poor, and normal bowel and urinary activity give false positives, thus limiting specificity (35–37). PET has been reported to be poor in detecting mucinous neoplasms (e.g., from colon or ovary) as they have low cellularity and do not display a hypermetabolic state of glucose (38), although there is some conflicting data on this (39).

A few studies combining PET and unenhanced CT have involved small numbers, and mostly reported some advantage of PET-CT over PET or CT alone (34,40); these two studies reported low CT sensitivities of 22% (34) and 42% (40), increasing to 67% (34) and 78% (40) with PET-CT combination. However, a more recent study (39) reported that peritoneal tumours were correctly identified in only 16 patients out of 28 with PET-CT (sensitivity 57%), compared to 23 patients out of 28 on CT alone (sensitivity 82%), suggesting no advantage of PET over CT. Another recent study involving 31 patients (41) reported FDG PET-MDCT (IV contrast-enhanced MDCT) as showing peritoneal deposits in 30 patients compared to 26 patients for CT and 25 patients for PET, suggesting a significant benefit of PET-MDCT over CT or PET alone. Combining contrast-enhanced thin-collimation MDCT with FDG PET in this way is likely to be the most sensitive technique for imaging peritoneal metastases, but further evaluation is needed, since it may not be a practical or cost-effective approach.

PET may have a role in detecting tumor recurrence (42,43) and may also be useful in patients in whom CT/MR are negative but tumor markers rising (37,44). It may also have a role prior to surgery, since some peritoneal deposits picked up on PET may not be easily recognized on CT. Any inflammatory peritoneal process such as TB is likely to result in a false positive PET (45).

Oral Contrast Studies

Luminal contrast studies using barium or water soluble contrast (follow-through for small bowel or enema for colon) are not routinely used for assessing peritoneal metastases, but they may show indirect signs of serosal tumor deposits. With modern day CT scanners using positive or negative oral contrast and IV enhancement, luminal contrast studies no longer have any significant diagnostic role. Their main use is for evaluating patients with small bowel obstruction (water-soluble agents for acute small bowel obstruction), in order to assess the level of obstruction. However, CT is still the preferred modality in such patients and will usually more clearly show the site and possible cause of obstruction (46).

Image-Guided Biopsy

Imaging features of peritoneal metastases are often non-specific, and so tissue is needed to try to make a specific diagnosis. Image-guided biopsy usually provides enough tissue to identify the primary tumor site without needing to proceed to laparoscopy or laparotomy to make a tissue diagnosis.

The simplest and most effective modality for guided biopsy of peritoneal or omental masses is US, with CT scans being used for defining the position of the target and planning the approach, although direct CT guidance can also be used (27,47,48). For very small nodules, fine needle aspiration can be performed, but for the majority of lesions a core biopsy (usually 18G) should be feasible, and this allows immunohistochemical analysis. US can also be used for aspiration of ascites and cytological analysis. Endoscopic US has also been used for fine needle aspiration (FNA) of any nodules seen adjacent to the stomach, or to aspirate any fluid around the stomach (29).

Key Points: Imaging Techniques

- Although there is no gold standard imaging modality, multislice CT is the principle modality for detecting peritoneal metastases, using thin collimation and interactive multiplanar display

- Using negative oral contrast (water) maximizes the advantage of enhancement of bowel wall and peritoneal deposits, but positive oral contrast can help in differentiating cystic deposits from bowel lumen

- MR imaging gives comparable images to MDCT, but has a much longer examination time, is less widely available, and has more artifacts

- US can detect peritoneal metastases with good sensitivity, but overlying bowel gas may limit views; the acquired images are less objective than CT/MR, and it is more operator-dependent

- FDG PET and PET-CT can be used for problem-solving when CT/MR are inconclusive. Small deposits near bowel and mucinous metastases may be falsely negative. Contrast-enhanced MDCT combined with FDG PET and fused images is likely to be the best imaging combination, but further evaluation is needed to define its role

- Image-guided biopsy of most peritoneal metastases can be performed with US guidance and, in some cases, CT guidance might be needed

IMAGING APPEARANCES

Imaging identifies peritoneal tumors as small as a few millimeters, shows whether they are cystic or solid, and may demonstrate their site of origin. However, features on imaging are non-specific and often inadequate to demonstrate whether tumors are benign or malignant, primary or secondary. The various CT features are described in detail below, since this is the principle imaging modality, and an outline given of the appearances of peritoneal metastases on MRI, US and PET.

CT

Ascites is often seen in patients with peritoneal metastases, and the presence of loculated ascites is suggestive of carcinomatosis. The presence of ascites has a positive predictive value of up to 80% as a sign of peritoneal metastases in a patient with a known primary malignancy (2).

The anatomical "hot-spots" for tumor deposition based on ascites flow described earlier should be carefully evaluated—these are mainly the pouch of Douglas, sigmoid colon, terminal ileum, right paracolic gutter, posterior right subhepatic space, and the right subphrenic space.

The morphology and usual locations of peritoneal metastases are described below.

Tumor Morphology

Peritoneal metastases may be solitary or multiple nodules, typically of soft-tissue density (Fig. 46.2). Some deposits may be mucinous and are usually low density/cyst-like on CT, but may have the appearance of increased density fluid (Fig. 46.2). Small nodules can merge to form plaques—shown on CT as a thickened and/or nodular enhancing peritoneal surface (49) (Fig. 46.3). The nodules may be quite subtle, sometimes only a few millimeters in size, and the presence of ascites makes their detection easier (Fig. 46.3) (49). Peritoneal infiltration may initially be seen as increased density, stranding and enhancement of mesenteric, omental, or paracolic fat (Fig. 46.4). Progression occurs with nodules, plaques, or sheets of soft-tissue, and then discrete or diffuse masses (Fig. 46.4).

Peritoneal calcification may be seen, usually with mucin-producing cystadenocarcinoma of the ovary (especially after treatment), and also with carcinoid, and rarely gastric cancer (Fig. 46.5) (50–52).

After treatment with imatinib, many peritoneal metastases from GI stromal tumors become cystic in appearance, signifying a response to treatment even though some may increase in size (Fig. 46.6) (53).

Perihepatic Spaces and Fissures

The falciform ligament is a common site of tumor deposits, which may be plaque-like or nodular, and can extend into the liver parenchyma (Fig. 46.7). Similar deposits can occur in the fissures for the ligamentum teres and venosum (Fig. 46.7). Deposits also occur around the gallbladder (Fig. 46.8) and in the periportal region (Fig. 46.9), from where the tumor can extend into the liver by tracking along the portal vein branches. This is

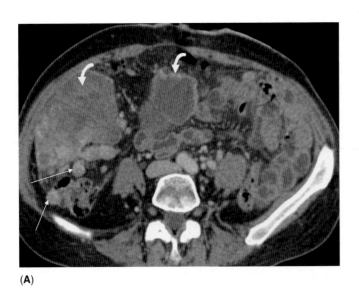

(A)

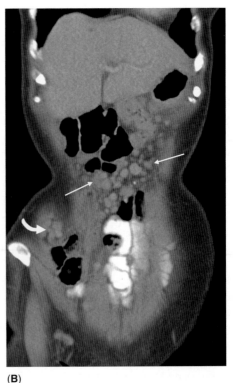

(B)

Figure 46.2 (A) CT density. Recurrent uterine leiomyosarcoma. Large subhepatic and mesenteric deposits (curved arrows), and small nodules around right colon, with one involving the lateral wall of the colon. The mesenteric deposit is very low density, but the smaller nodules are enhancing (white arrows). (B) Omental/abdominal wall nodules. Recurrent gastrointestinal stromal tumor with numerous small omental deposits (between arrows) as well as abdominal wall deposits (curved arrow).

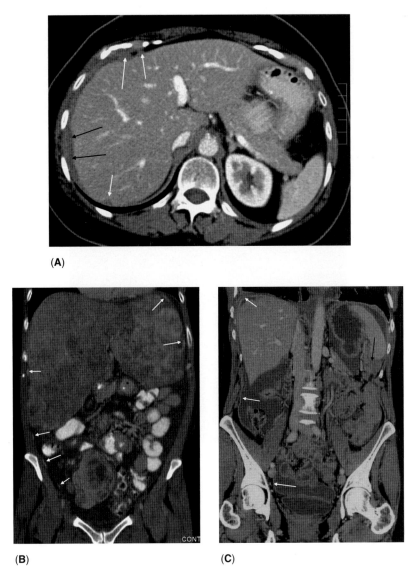

Figure 46.3 (**A**) Nodular peritoneal thickening. Patient with ovarian cancer and irregular thickening adjacent to the right lateral surface of the liver causing scalloping of the liver margin (black arrows). There are also small surface nodules anteriorly and a subcapsular deposit posteriorly (white arrows). (**B**) Focal peritoneal plaques. Patient with carcinoid, numerous liver metastases, and a large mesenteric mass. There is some ascites and several small enhancing peritoneal plaques (white arrows). (**C**) Diffuse peritoneal thickening. Recurrent ovarian cancer with ascites and diffuse peritoneal thickening, especially on the right (white arrows). There is also a peritoneal mass adjacent to the inferior tip of the spleen (black arrow).

shown on CT as thickening and enhancement around the portal veins within the liver.

Liver/Spleen Surface

Tumor deposits on the liver capsule must be differentiated from true parenchymal metastases since capsular lesions in ovarian cancer may still be resectable. Capsular masses are usually smooth and well defined, with an elliptic or biconvex appearance (Fig. 46.3A). The liver surface may show only slight irregularity (Figs. 46.8 and 46.10). Subcapsular extension may occur and so the deposits can appear intraparenchymal (Fig. 46.8). True parenchymal metastases are usually less well defined and surrounded by liver parenchyma (Fig. 46.11) (10). Scalloping of the liver surface may also be seen, indicating subcapsular involvement (Figs. 46.3A and 46.8). Similar deposits can occur around the spleen and splenic hilum (Fig. 46.3C). Deposits can also occur on the diaphragmatic

surfaces next to the liver/spleen causing diffuse thickening or nodularity (Fig. 46.12).

Gastrohepatic Ligament (Lesser Omentum)

Tumor deposits occur between the left lobe of liver and lesser curve of the stomach (Fig. 46.13). This also provides a pathway of direct organ invasion between tumors of the stomach and liver. Pancreatic cancer can invade into the gastrohepatic ligament and then into stomach and/or liver.

Hepatoduodenal Ligament

This lies along the free edge of the lesser omentum, extending from the porta hepatis to the duodenum, and contains portal vein, hepatic artery, and common bile duct. Pancreatic cancer commonly spreads along this ligament to the ligamentum venosum fissure, and then into liver and periportal space (Figs. 46.9 and 46.14).

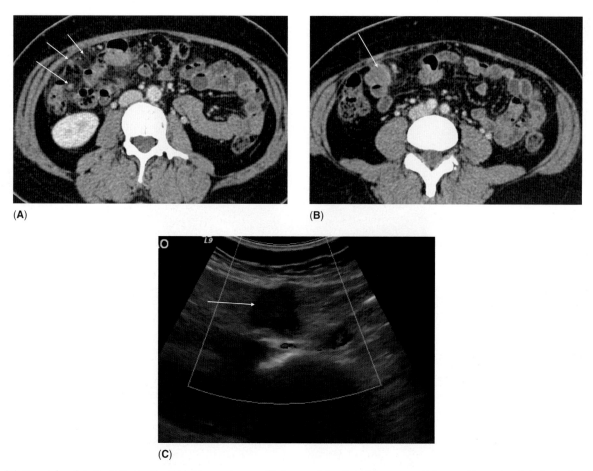

Figure 46.4 (**A**) Omental nodularity. Patient with gallbladder carcinoma with increased density/enhancement, slight stranding and nodularity in the right anterior omentum, in keeping with infiltration (arrows). Compare with normal left side. (**B**) Omental mass. Larger omental deposit in patient with gallbladder cancer also involving the serosal surface of an adjacent small bowel loop (arrow). (**C**) Same patient as in Figure 47.4B. Ultrasound also clearly shows the omental deposit as a hypoechoic solid mass (arrow).

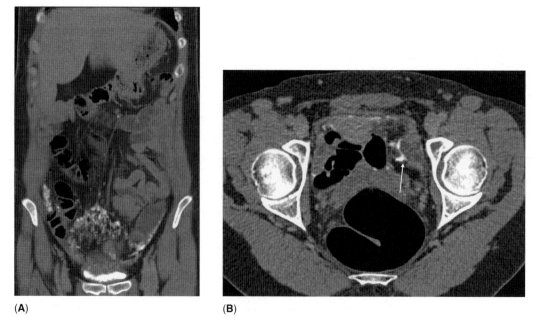

Figure 46.5 (**A**) Calcified peritoneal deposits. 33F, non-specific abdominal pain, coronal reformat CT showed nodular and plaque-like calcification in the omentum, right paracolic gutter, and serosal surface of sigmoid colon. Ultrasound-guided biopsy of the omentum showed serous papillary adenocarcinoma. (**B**) The axial CT in the same patient also shows calcification around the left ovary (arrow). There were no ovarian masses.

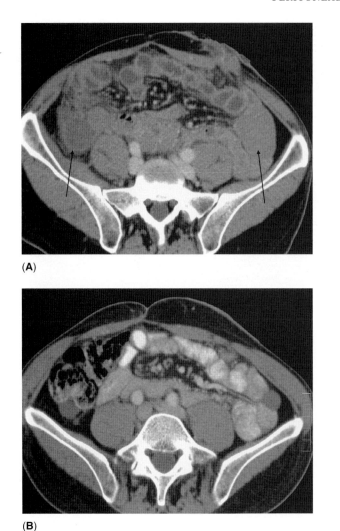

(A)

(B)

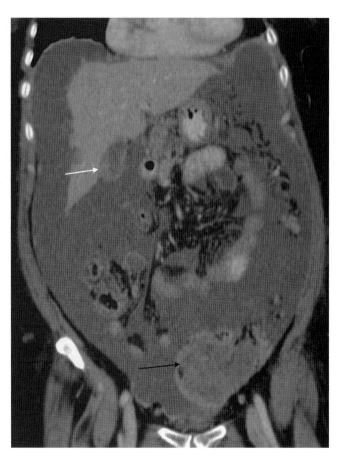

Figure 46.8 Gallbladder deposit. Coronal CT in patient with metastatic endometrial cancer. There is ascites, extensive nodular liver surface and thin peritoneal plaques. One of the surface nodules appears to extend into parenchyma. Subtle deposit adjacent to gallbladder fundus (white arrow). There is also an omental mass in the left iliac fossa (black arrow).

Figure 46.6 (**A**) Cystic change in peritoneal metastases. Recurrent peritoneal GI stromal tumor with masses in both flanks; relatively low density on the right (arrows). (**B**) Same patient after treatment with imatinib, the deposits have reduced in size and now appear cystic.

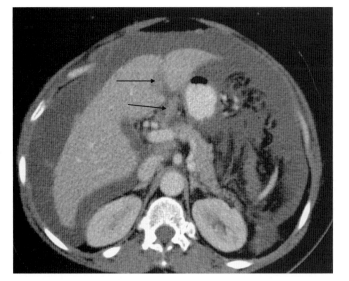

Figure 46.7 Hepatic ligament deposits. Axial CT shows stranding and nodularity adjacent to the liver surface, and soft-tissue deposits in the falciform ligament and gastrohepatic ligament (arrows).

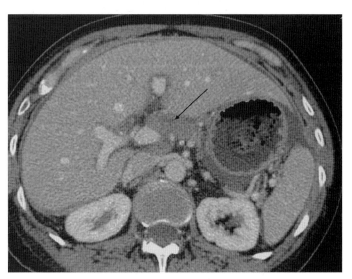

Figure 46.9 Periportal tumor. Recurrent ovarian cancer with periportal tumor deposit (arrow). There is also peritoneal thickening around the liver, particularly in Morrison's pouch.

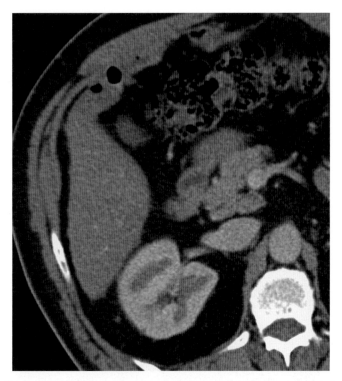

Figure 46.10 Subtle liver surface deposits. Patient with colorectal cancer and multiple peritoneal deposits. On this section there is only slight surface nodularity of lateral right lobe of liver, in keeping with tiny surface deposits.

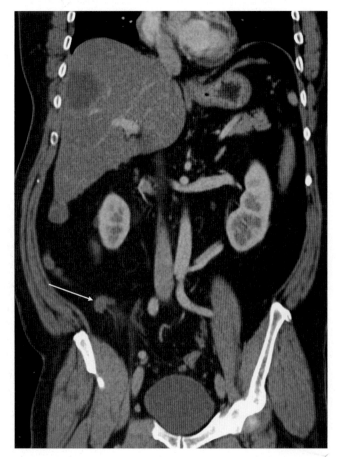

Figure 46.11 Subhepatic nodules on coronal scan. Metastatic colorectal cancer, with intraparenchymal liver metastasis, small subhepatic surface deposits (particularly well shown on this coronal reformat), and a deposit in the right iliac fossa (arrow).

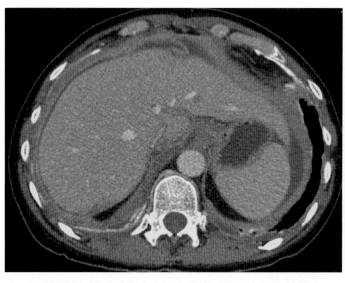

Figure 46.12 Diffuse bilateral diaphragmatic thickening. Recurrent ovarian cancer.

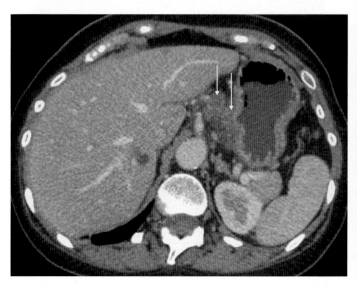

Figure 46.13 Patient with gastric cancer and tumor extension into gastrohepatic ligament (arrows).

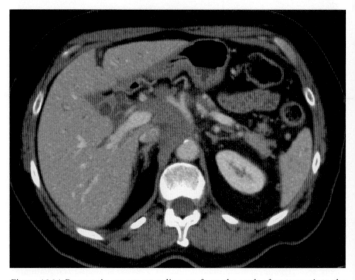

Figure 46.14 Pancreatic cancer extending up from the neck of pancreas into the hepatoduodenal ligament, encasing the portal vein and hepatic artery.

Transverse Mesocolon

This allows a pathway between pancreas and transverse colon (Fig. 46.15). The right side of the transverse mesocolon is thickened as the duodenocolic ligament and this provides a direct route for extension of colon cancer from hepatic flexure to duodenum (9).

Right Subhepatic Space

Also known as Morrison's pouch, this lies between the right lobe of liver and right kidney, and is contiguous with the gallbladder fossa. Tumor deposits may be seen as mild thickening and enhancement of the undersurface of the right lobe of liver, or as nodules and masses (Figs. 46.2A, 46.9, and 46.11). Gallbladder involvement may appear as wall thickening/enhancement mimicking cholecystitis.

Paracolic Gutters

These are the attachments of the ascending and descending colon to the posterior abdominal wall. There is preferential ascitic flow to the wider right side. Tumor here can extend into the colon (Figs. 46.2A, 46.3B and C, 46.5A, and 46.16).

Small Bowel Mesentery

This extends from the left upper quadrant to the right lower quadrant of the abdomen, and connects jejunum and ileum to the posterior abdominal wall. Ascites pools in the layers of folded small bowel mesentery and then collects in the right lower quadrant. Tumor deposits often occur around the terminal ileum, and this is an important area to evaluate carefully (Figs. 46.17 and 46.18). Tumor infiltration in the mesentery may be seen as stranding and enhancement in the fat or discrete masses. There may be separation and angulation of small bowel, tumor may extend into the bowel wall, and if encased and narrowed may lead to small bowel obstruction (Fig. 46.19). A stellate pattern of mesenteric infiltration is seen with pancreatic, colonic, breast, and ovarian cancer, resulting from diffuse infiltration (14,54) (Figs. 46.2A and 46.19).

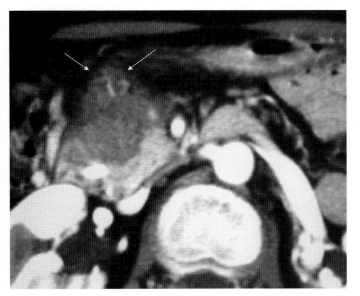

Figure 46.15 Pancreatic head cancer extending anteriorly into fat of transverse mesocolon (arrows).

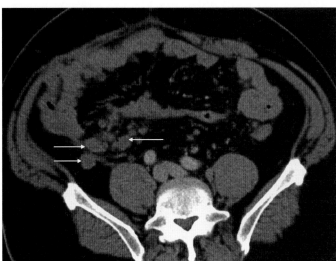

Figure 46.17 Multiple small deposits in the right iliac fossa (arrows), just superior to the terminal ileum (not shown).

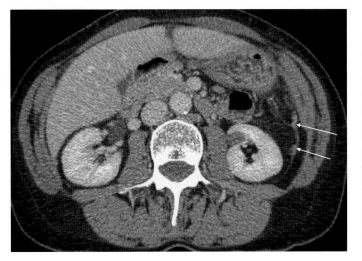

Figure 46.16 Recurrent ovarian cancer with nodular thickening in left paracolic gutter (arrows).

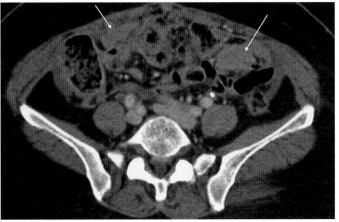

Figure 46.18 Recurrent endometrial cancer with deposits anterior to terminal ileum on the right and sigmoid on the left (arrows).

Nodal deposits may be present in the mesentery from lymphoma or sigmoid cancer.

Lymphoma can extend from the retroperitoneum, through the root of the small bowel mesentery, to the small bowel, producing soft tissue thickening within the mesenteric fat, perivascular encasement, and tethering of the bowel.

Greater Omentum

This consists of four layers of peritoneum, and is draped like an apron in the anterior abdominal cavity, over small bowel and colon. Peritoneal metastases are common here, may be seen as subtle infiltration with stranding and/or nodularity, larger discrete or irregular masses or an omental cake (55). Coronal images can be very useful for assessment (Figs. 46.2B, 46.4, 46.5, 46.8, and 46.20).

Small volume omental deposits may not be visible at surgery and up to 22% of omenta thought to be normal at laparotomy have tumor histologically (56).

Serosal Deposits

Gastrointestinal involvement usually affects the small bowel. Small nodules in the bowel wall are difficult to see on imaging. However, if small bowel is well distended with CT or MR enteroclysis, focal masses or enhancement are likely to be better seen. Tumor involvement can occur by serosal seeding or by direct bowel wall invasion from adjacent tumor (Figs. 46.2A, 46.19, 46.21, 46.22, and 46.23). Bowel obstruction may be from serosal metastases or associated

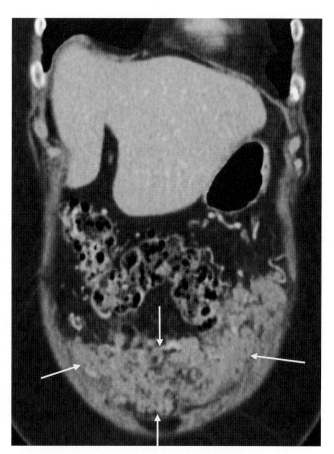

Figure 46.20 Ovarian cancer. Large omental "cake" (arrows) shown on coronal CT.

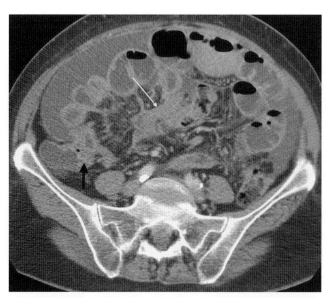

Figure 46.19 Mesenteric disease. Recurrent ovarian cancer with ascites, an irregular mesenteric mass (arrow), partial small bowel obstruction, and tumor thickening and narrowing bowel loops in the right iliac fossa (black arrow).

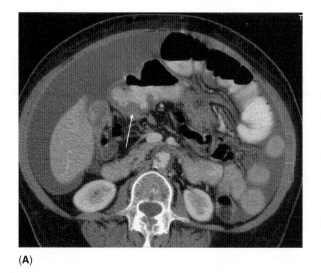

(A)

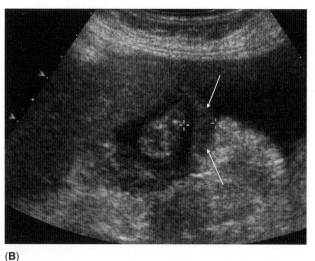

(B)

Figure 46.21 (A) Gastric wall deposit. Ovarian cancer with ascites, mesenteric mass, and serosal deposit in posterior gastric antrum (arrow). (B) The serosal deposit is shown clearly on ultrasound as hypoechoic focal thickening (arrows).

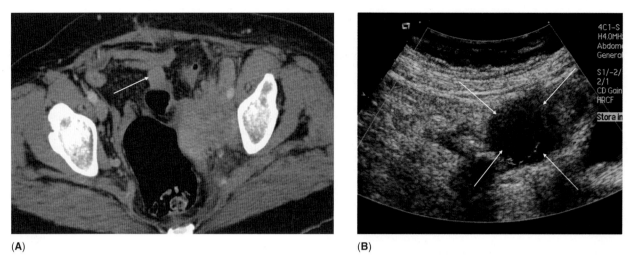

(A)　　　　　　　　　　　　　　　　**(B)**

Figure 46.22 (**A**) Small bowel deposit. Recurrent fallopian tube cancer with large left iliac fossa mass. CT-guided biopsy showed fibrosis only. A serosal deposit was not initially recognized on the CT (arrow). (**B**) Compression ultrasound clearly showed a hypoechoic mass with some blood flow in the midline pelvis (arrows), Ultrasound-guided biopsy of this confirmed recurrent adenocarcinoma consistent with the previously resected fallopian tube cancer.

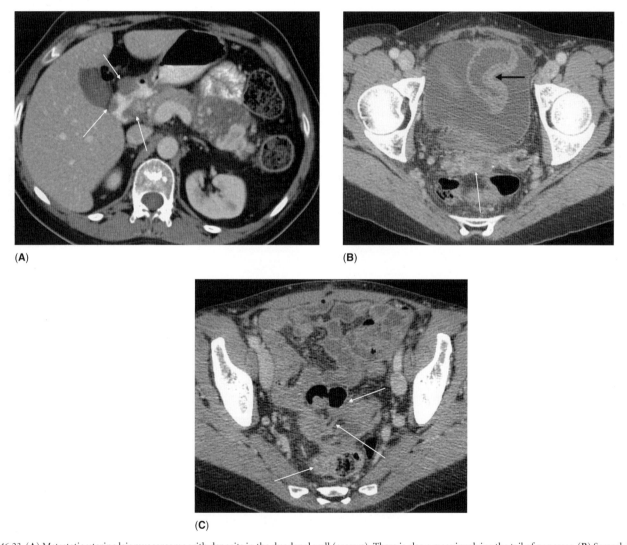

(A)　　　　　　　　　　　　　　　　**(B)**

(C)

Figure 46.23 (**A**) Metastatic uterine leiomyosarcoma with deposits in the duodenal wall (arrows). There is also a mass involving the tail of pancreas. (**B**) Serosal deposit. Recurrent ovarian cancer with ascites, tumor mass in the pouch of Douglas (arrow), and eccentric thickening of a dilated small bowel loop, in keeping with serosal tumor (black arrow). (**C**) Recurrent ovarian cancer with an irregular mass in the pelvis, and soft-tissue nodules and strands involving the serosal surface of adjacent bowel (arrows).

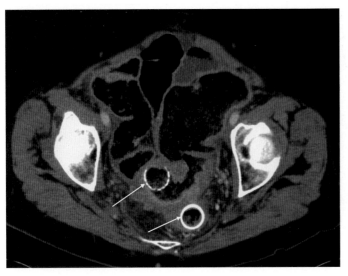

Figure 46.24 Recurrent ovarian cancer in the pelvis involving the distal sigmoid which was thickened and strictured, resulting in colonic obstruction. A metal stent has been inserted for palliation (arrows).

adhesions, but is most commonly seen when the intestinal wall is invaded (Fig. 46.24). Bowel obstruction has been reported in about 50% of cases at autopsy (57), CT findings suggesting bowel involvement include thickening and distorsion. Hematogenous metastases also occur to the bowel wall and may be seen as small submucosal nodules, cause bowel wall thickening, or larger discrete masses– —these may ulcerate or cavitate) (16). Breast cancer and lymphoma can cause diffuse gastric wall thickening, indistinguishable from primary scirrhous gastric carcinoma (17).

Abdominal Wall/Anterior Peritoneal Surface

The peritoneum may show thickening and enhancement, and this may be smooth, nodular, or irregular. Parietal peritoneal masses adjacent to the anterior abdominal wall may extend into the deeper abdominal wall (Figs. 46.2B and 46.25). Umbilical nodules can occur from seeding or lymphatic/hematogenous spread, usually from gastric, colon, pancreas, or ovary cancers (Fig. 46.26).

Pelvis

The rectovaginal pouch (pouch of Douglas) and the rectovesical pouch in males are common dependent sites for peritoneal

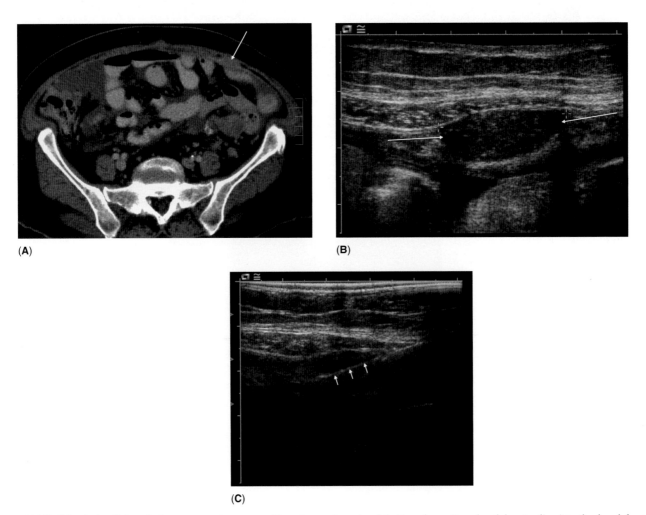

(A)   (B)

(C)

Figure 46.25 (A) Abdominal wall deposit. Recurrent ovarian cancer with ascites, peritoneal nodularity and a peritoneal nodule extending into the deep left anterior abdominal wall (arrow). (B) The peritoneal/abdominal wall mass is clearly shown on ultrasound (arrow). (C) Ultrasound-guided core biopsy with an 18G needle was quick and relatively safe, and histological confirmation obtained. Needle within mass shown with arrows.

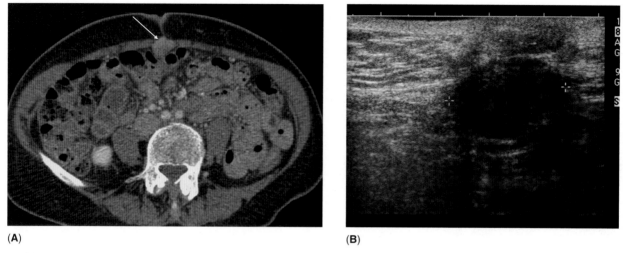

Figure 46.26 (A) Metastatic endometrial cancer with an abdominal wall/deep umbilical deposit (arrow). (B) Mass well shown on ultrasound (between cursors), and ultrasound-guided biopsy confirmed the diagnosis.

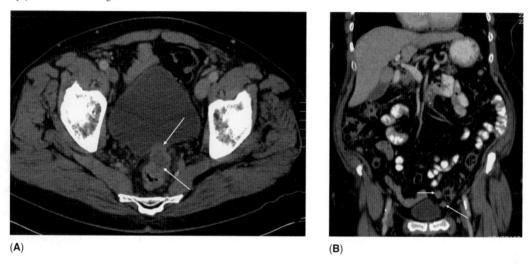

Figure 46.27 (A) Metastatic gallbladder cancer with a rectovesical mass invading into the anterior rectal wall and posterior bladder wall (arrows). (B) Recurrent ovarian cancer with small deposits around sigmoid colon (arrows).

metastases (Figs. 46.23B, 46.2C, and 46.27). The superior margin of the sigmoid colon is often involved, and this can progress to tumor encasement and bowel obstruction (Figs. 46.18, 46.24, and 46.27). Local extension of ovarian cancer is suggested by loss of tissue planes with the bladder or colon (10).

Pseudomyxoma Peritonei

Pseudomyxoma peritonei occurs if a mucinous cystadenoacarcinoma or cystadenoma of the ovary or appendix ruptures into the peritoneal cavity, and the gelatinous mucoid material surrounds mesenteric reflections, bowel and organs, and causes scalloping of the peritoneal surfaces, particularly adjacent to the liver (Fig. 46.28). Septations may be seen and bowel loops are displaced posteriorly. Scalloping, septations, locules, and variable fluid density distinguishes pseudomyxoma from ascites. In most cases of pseudomyxoma peritonei the primary tumor arises from the appendix (58).

MRI

MRI will show similar peritoneal tumor extent as on CT, but shows stronger enhancement of peritoneal thickening and nodules following IV injection of contrast medium (Figs. 46.29 and 46.30). Liver surface metastatic nodules which may appear intrahepatic on CT are well shown on MR, may appear partially cystic but tend to enhance strongly. Normal peritoneum enhances to a similar extent as the liver, but peritoneal enhancement greater than the liver suggests peritoneal metastases in patients with malignancy (6).

Omental and mesenteric masses are typically of low signal intensity on T1-weighted sequences and of slightly increased and heterogenous signal intensity on T2-weighted sequences compared to other soft-tissue (Figs. 46.29 and 46.31). The presence of adjacent ascites makes the metastases more conspicuous. In the absence of ascites, fat-suppressed T2-weighted sequences may show peritoneal deposits more clearly as bright signal lesions. Small peritoneal nodules and peritoneal thickening are best seen after contrast medium enhancement on fat-suppressed T1-weighted sequences (Figs. 46.29 and 46.30). Mesenteric involvement may be better shown on MR than CT (6). Direct invasion of ovarian cancer in the pelvis is often easier to identify with MR imaging than with CT because of its superior soft-tissue contrast (10).

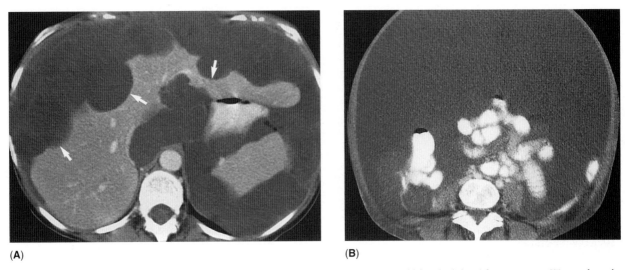

(A)   **(B)**

Figure 46.28   Pseudomyxoma peritonei in mucinous cystadenocarcinoma of the appendix in a 44-year-old female. (**A**) Axial postcontrast CT scan shows low density deposits producing scalloping of the liver margin (arrows). (**B**) The pressure of the gelatinous material prevents bowel loops floating up towards the anterior abdominal wall.

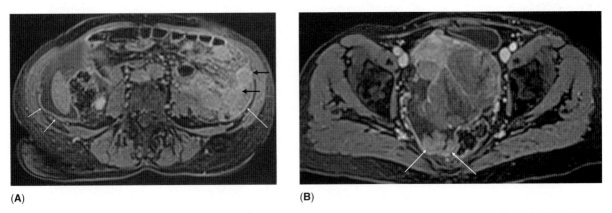

(A)   **(B)**

Figure 46.29   (**A**) MRI of metastatic ovarian cancer. Fat- saturated T-1 weighted MRI post-contrast. Ascites enhancing peritoneum (arrows) and enhancing nodules left flank (black arrows). (**B**) MRI of same patient. Large mass in the pelvis, and enhancing thickened peritoneum and soft-tissue deposits (arrows).

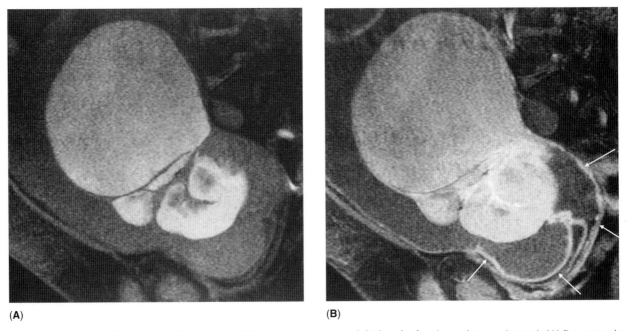

(A)   **(B)**

Figure 46.30   Sagittal fat-saturated T1-weighted MRI in patient with large ovarian cancer and thickened enhancing peritoneum (arrows). (**A**) Precontrast image. (**B**) Postcontrast.

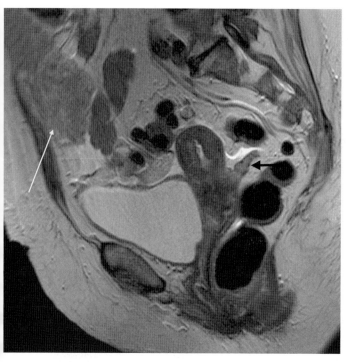

Figure 46.31 Sagittal T2- weighted MRI with a large omental cake (arrow) and tumor deposits in the pouch of Douglas (black arrow).

Mucinous tumors and pseudomyxoma may show increased signal intensity on T1-weighted MR images, and the complex nature of the fluid is better appreciated on MR (4,59).

Ultrasound

US can show many peritoneal nodules and masses, especially in the presence of ascites. Peritoneal metastases typically appear as hypoechoic masses, but their detection may be limited by operator experience, overlying bowel gas, and poor soft-tissue contrast (Figs. 46.4, 46.21, 46.22, 46.25, 46.26, and 46.32).

High-resolution US can show tiny nodules on the peritoneal surface of just a few millimeters in size.

Color Doppler US often shows the presence of blood vessels within peritoneal nodules.

Hypoechoic peritoneal nodules may also be visible on transvaginal US, particularly within the pouch of Douglas (28).

Mucinous tumors are likely to have low-level echoes on US.

Using compression US and correlating with CT appearances allows most omental/mesenteric masses to be well targeted for biopsy with US (Fig. 46.25).

FDG-PET

Peritoneal metastases cause abnormally intense FDG uptake near the abdominal wall on the peritoneal lining and on the surfaces of the solid organs. The uptake may be focal or uniform, corresponding to nodular or diffuse peritoneal involvement (Figs. 46.33, 46.34, 46.35, and 46.36) (40). Differentiating low-grade pathological uptake from normal physiological uptake can be difficult.

A standardized uptake value (SUVmax) of >5 has been reported to improve the diagnostic accuracy of FDG-PET (34), although an SUVmax > 3 with a corresponding nodule on CT is also consistent with a metastasis (37).

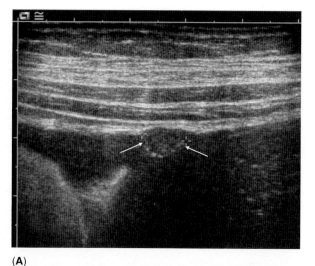

(A)

(B)

Figure 46.32 (A) Ultrasound showing a small peritoneal surface nodule arising from the parietal peritoneum layer (arrows). (B) Corresponding CT showing peritoneal surface nodule (arrow). Two tiny nodules also seen in the left flank.

Combination FDG PET-CT allows accurate anatomical localization of any suspicious FDG activity, and using enhanced MDCT significantly improves the detection of small peritoneal metastases; fused CT and PET images are particularly useful for assessing any equivocal lesions seen on the CT or PET images.

Oral Contrast Studies

Luminal contrast studies may show evidence of bowel obstruction, since peritoneal deposits on the bowel surface or adjacent mesentery can result in distortion, tethering, and stricturing. Often the level of obstruction and transition is not clearly defined on contrast studies, particularly if water-soluble contrast is used. Occasionally, bowel wall distortion and tethering is seen, suggesting an extra-luminal cause of the obstruction. Pancreatic cancer can cause tethering and pseudosacculation of the inferior margin of the transverse colon since the transverse mesocolon inserts here. However, gastric cancer spreading via the greater omentum causes similar change in the superior margin of the transverse colon (60).

Metastatic seeding in the pouch of Douglas produces a characteristic nodular mucosal impression on barium enema, with associated mucosal tethering on the ventral aspect of the rectosigmoid junction.

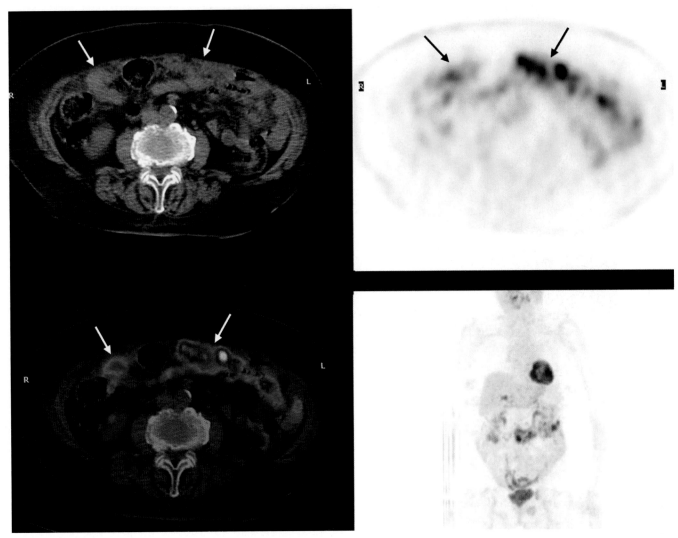

Figure 46.33 FDG PET-CT. Omental deposits (arrows) on unenhanced CT (*top left*) showing FDG uptake (*top right*) with fused PET-CT image bottom left.

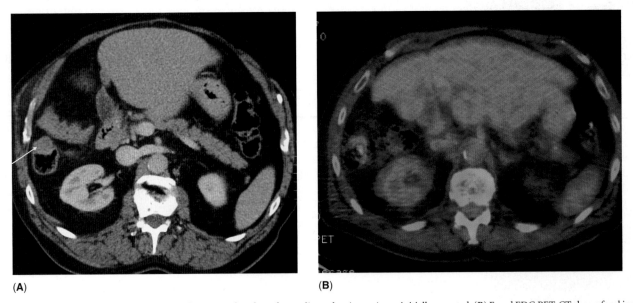

(A)   (B)

Figure 46.34 (**A**) Recurrent gallbladder cancer. Nodule on serosal surface of ascending colon (arrow), not initially reported. (**B**) Fused FDG PET-CT shows focal increased activity in colon wall nodule indicating likely deposit.

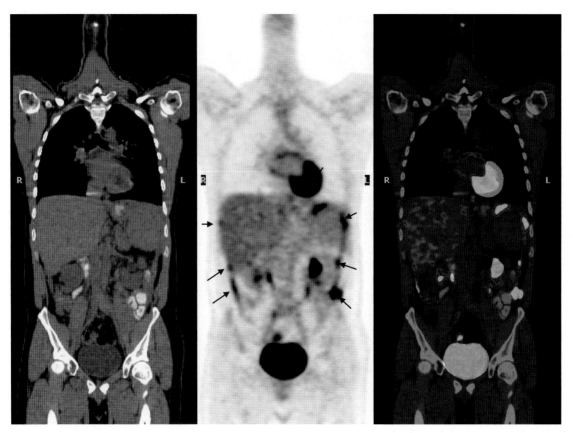

Figure 46.35 FDG PET-CT. Recurrent colorectal cancer with peritoneal deposits around the spleen and in the paracolic gutters (arrows). Unenhanced CT, PET, and fused PET-CT images.

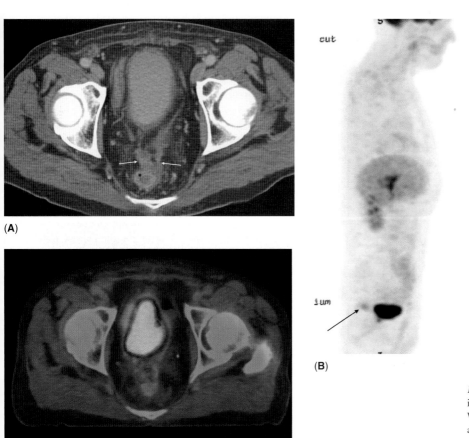

(A)

(B)

(C)

Figure 46.36 (**A**) Patient with cholangiocarcinoma and irregular mass in rectovesical pouch (arrows). (**B**) Whole body FDG-PET, sagittal view. Increased activity at liver hilum in keeping with the primary tumor and also increased focal activity behind bladder (arrow). Normal renal and bowel activity.

Metastatic seeding in the small bowel mesentery, especially in the right infracolic space, can produce separation of small bowel loops in a parallel configuration, known as "palisading", on barium follow-through studies. Marked bowel angulation and mucosal tethering of the ileal loops is also seen if the deposits stimulate a desmoplastic response, which can occur with pancreatic carcinoma and mucin-secreting gastric carcinoma. Metastases may also cause fold thickening or a nodular mass. Breast cancer metastases to the stomach can cause a "linitis plastica" type appearance.

Differential Diagnosis of Peritoneal Masses

Peritoneal nodules and stranding may be present in infectious peritonitis, particularly TB, mesenteric panniculitis, as well as primary peritoneal carcinoma (2,61). Mesothelioma should also be considered, and depending on the clinical setting, image-guided biopsy of the abnormal peritoneum considered for a definitive diagnosis.

Patients with portal hypertension and ascites can have omental varices and stranding/edema in the fat mimicking tumor infiltration (FIGs).

Key Points: Imaging Appearance

- Modern imaging can identify peritoneal metastases of just a few millimeters in size and this is made easier in the presence of ascites
- Peritoneal metastases may be solid or cystic, small nodules or plaques, larger discrete or diffuse masses
- The imaging appearance of peritoneal deposits is non-specific and causes other than malignancy should be considered in some cases. TB is the most likely pathology to mimic peritoneal carcinomatosis and a definitive diagnosis is usually made following biopsy
- Liver surface involvement is common and any irregularity or scalloping suggests deposits. Also, nodularity and thickening of the hepatic fissures, particularly the falciform ligament, indicate deposits
- Involvement of the mesentry or omentum can be subtle with slight nodular stranding, which can progress and coalesce to form an omental cake
- Bowel involvement may be by direct invasion and encasement, deposits in the serosa or submucosa, or diffuse wall thickening

Accuracy of CT and MRI in Identifying Peritoneal Metastases

As always with radiological research studies, reliable assessment and comparison of data is hampered by variations in patient groups and imaging techniques. This inevitably results in wide variations in the reported sensitivities and specificities. However, the detection of peritoneal metastases has improved greatly with spiral CT and in particular MDCT. Reported sensitivity for detecting peritoneal metastases using non-spiral CT was 63% to 79%, increasing to 85% to 93% with spiral scanning (2), although the main limitation remained in small deposits less than 1 cm with sensitivities of 25% to 50% (2). In one of the largest studies of 280 patients, the Radiology Diagnostic Oncology Group reported that spiral CT had a sensitivity of 92% and specificity of 82% in the detection of peritoneal metastases, similar to MR (95% and 80%), but the majority of the deposits were large (22). These studies used collimation of 5 to 10 mm, and a more recent study using MDCT for detecting peritoneal metastases showed improved sensitivity using 1 mm multiplanar reconstructions compared to 5 mm (62), the improvement likely to be due to interactive thin-section multiplanar display and absence of misregistration. Radiologist experience is also an important determinant of sensitivity of an imaging modality, and there is significant interobserver variation (40,62).

Laparoscopy can demonstrate deposits in as many as 75% of cases where CT has shown ascites but no peritoneal deposits (40,63). In the absence of ascites, MR may be more useful than CT in visualizing small or equivocal peritoneal deposits (10). Some older studies, not using MDCT, have reported that MR with oral and IV contrast is more sensitive in detecting small serosal and omental deposits (64,65). MR is probably more accurate in distinguishing between intrahepatic and peritoneal lesions on the liver surface.

Summary

- The detection of peritoneal metastases is essential in staging many tumors and allows assessment of resectability, monitoring of treatment response, and identification of recurrence. Image-guided biopsy (with US or CT) allows confirmation of diagnosis, and assists in determining the primary source
- Gynecological malignancy, in particular ovarian cancer, is the most common primary causing peritoneal metastases. Other primary sites include gastric, colorectal, pancreas, and cholangiocarcinoma. Lymphoma is also a cause and the main extra-abdominal primary is breast cancer
- A good understanding of peritoneal anatomy and the flow pathways of ascites helps in interpreting cross-sectional imaging and identifying peritoneal metastases
- Peritoneal metastases spread within the peritoneal cavity mainly by direct invasion into adjacent ligaments, mesenteries, and omentum, or by intraperitoneal seeding via the peritoneal fluid
- Intraperitoneal seeding occurs mainly at sites of preferential flow and stasis of peritoneal fluid. These include the pouch of Douglas or rectovesical pouch, around the sigmoid colon, right lower quadrant, right paracolic gutter, and around the liver
- Although there is no gold standard for imaging peritoneal metastases, multidetector CT is the key imaging modality; its ability to detect peritoneal deposits improved considerably with thin collimation scans, interactive multiplanar display, and excellent spatial resolution
- MRI has comparable sensitivity to CT for detecting peritoneal metastases and is better for evaluating tumor in the pelvis. However, it is less widely accessible, has a significantly longer examination time, has more artefacts, and needs greater expertise for image interpretation
- The role of FDG PET in detecting peritoneal metastases has not been defined, and it is best used combined with multislice CT and fused CT-PET images. It is currently mainly used for problem solving and may be useful in detecting tumor recurrence if CT/MR are inconclusive

REFERENCES

1. Harmon RL, Sugarbaker PH. Prognostic indicators in peritoneal carcinomatosis from gastrointestinal cancer. Int Semin Surg Oncol 2005; 2: 3.
2. Coakley FV, Choi PH, Gougoutos CA, et al. Peritoneal metastases: detection with spiral CT in patients with ovarian cancer. Radiology 2002; 223: 495–9.
3. Heiken JP, Aizenstein RI, Balfe DM, Gore RM. Peritoneal cavity and retroperitoneum: normal anatomy and examination techniques. In: Gore RM, Levine MS, eds. Textbook of Gastrointestinal Radiology, 2nd edn. Philadelphia: WB Saunders, 2000: 1930–47.
4. Coakley FV, Hricak H. Imaging of peritoneal and mesenteric disease: key concepts for the clinical radiologist. Clin Radiol 1999; 54: 563–74.
5. Meyers MA, Oliphant M, Berne AS, Feldberg MA. The peritoneal ligaments and mesenteries: pathways of intraabdominal spread of disease. Radiology 1987; 163: 593–604.
6. Low RN. MR imaging of the peritoneal spread of malignancy. Abdom Imaging 2007; 32: 267–83.
7. Dehn TC, Reznek RH, Nockler IB, White FE. The preoperative assessment of advanced gastric cancer by computed tomography. Br J Surg 1984; 71: 413–17.
8. Baker ME, Silverman PM, Halvorsen RA Jr, Cohan RH. Computed tomography of masses in periportal/hepatoduodenal ligament. J Comput Assist Tomogr 1987; 11: 258–63.
9. Diamond RT, Greenberg HM, Boult IF. Direct metastatic spread of right colonic adenocarcinoma to duodenum: barium and computed tomography findings. Gastrointest Radiol 1981; 6: 339–41.
10. Woodward PJ, Hosseinzadeh K, Saenger JS. Radiologic staging of ovarian carcinoma with pathologic correlation. Radiographics 2004; 24: 225–46.
11. Meyers MA. Distribution of intraabdominal malignant seeding: dependency on dynamics of flow of ascitic fluid. Am J Roentgenol 1973; 119: 198–206.
12. Raptopoulos V, Gourtsoyiannis N. Peritoneal carcinomatosis. Eur Radiol 2001; 11: 2195–206.
13. Cho KC, Gold BM. Computed tomography of Krukenberg tumours. Am J Roentgenol 1985; 145: 285–8.
14. Whitley NO, Bohlman ME, Baker LP. CT patterns of mesenteric disease. J Comput Assist Tomogr 1982; 6: 490–6.
15. Mueller PR, Ferrucci JT Jr, Harbin WP, et al. Appearance of lymphomatous involvement of the mesentery by ultrasonography and body computed tomography: the "sandwich sign". Radiology 1980; 134: 467–73.
16. Kawashima A, Fishman EK, Kuhlman JE, Schuchter LM. CT of malignant melanoma: patterns of small bowel and mesenteric involvement. J Comput Assist Tomogr 1991; 15: 570–4.
17. Caskey CI, Scatarige JC, Fishman EK. Distribution of metastases in breast carcinoma. CT evaluation of the abdomen. Clin Imaging 1991; 15: 166–71.
18. Pannu HK, Bristow RE, Montz FJ, Fishman EK. Multidetector CT of peritoneal carcinomatosis from ovarian cancer. Radiographics 2003; 23: 687–701.
19. Pilleul F, Penigaud M, Milot L, et al. Possible small-bowel neoplasms: contrast-enhanced and water-enhanced multidetector CT enteroclysis. Radiology 2006; 241: 796–801.
20. Nelson RC, Chezmar JL, Hoel MJ, Buck DR, Sugarbaker PH. Peritoneal carcinomatosis: preoperative CT with intraperitoneal contrast material. Radiology 1992; 182: 133–8.
21. Caseiro-Alves F, Goncalo M, Abraul E, et al. Induced pneumoperitoneum in CT evaluation of peritoneal carcinomatosis. Abdom Imaging 1995; 20: 52–7.
22. Tempany CM, Zou KH, Silverman SG, et al. Staging of advanced ovarian cancer: comparison of imaging modalities—Report from the Radiology Diagnostic Oncology Group. Radiology 2000; 215: 761–7.
23. Elsayes KM, Staveteig PT, Narra VR, et al. MRI of the peritoneum: spectrum of abnormalities. Am J Roentgenol 2006; 186: 1368–79.
24. Rioux M, Michaud C. Sonographic detection of peritoneal carcinomatosis: a prospective study of 37 cases. Abdom Imaging 1995; 20: 47–57.
25. Derchi LE, Solbiati L, Rizzatto G, De Pra L. Normal anatomy and pathologic changes of the small bowel mesentery: US appearance. Radiology 1987; 164: 649–52.
26. Goerg C, Schwerk WB. Malignant ascites: sonographic signs of peritoneal carcinomatosis. Eur J Cancer 1991; 27: 720–3.
27. Hewitt MJ, Anderson K, Hall GD, et al. Women with peritoneal carcinomatosis of unknown origin: efficacy of image-guided biopsy to determine site-specific diagnosis. BJOG 2007; 114: 46–50.
28. Savelli L, De Iaco P, Ceccaroni M, et al. Transvaginal sonographic features of peritoneal carcinomatosis. Ultrasound Obstet Gynecol 2005; 26: 552–7.
29. Lee YT, Ng EK, Hung LC, et al. Accuracy of endoscopic ultrasonography in diagnosing ascites and predicting peritoneal metastases in gastric cancer patients. Gut 2005; 54: 1541–5.
30. Schmulewitz N, Singh P, Safa M, Robinson-Smith T. Diagnosis of peritoneal carcinomatosis by EUS-guided FNA. Gastrointest Endosc 2007; 66: 825–6.
31. Hillner BE, Siegel BA, Liu D, et al. Impact of positron emission tomography/computed tomography and positron emission tomography (PET) alone on expected management of patients with cancer: initial results from the National Oncologic PET Registry. J Clin Oncol 2008; 26: 2155–61.
32. Cohade C, Wahl RL. Applications of positron emission tomography/computed tomography image fusion in clinical positron emission tomography—clinical use, interpretation methods, diagnostic improvements. Semin Nucl Med 2003; 33: 228–37.
33. Pfannenberg AC, Aschoff P, Brechtel K, et al. Value of contrast-enhanced multiphase CT in combined PET/CT protocols for oncological imaging. Br J Radiol 2007; 80: 437–45.
34. Suzuki A, Kawano T, Takahashi N, et al. Value of 18F-FDG PET in the detection of peritoneal carcinomatosis. Eur J Nucl Med Mol Imaging 2004; 31: 1413–20.
35. Fong Y, Saldinger PF, Akhurst T, et al. Utility of 18F-FDG positron emission tomography scanning on selection of patients for resection of hepatic colorectal metastases. Am J Surg 1999; 178: 282–7.
36. Rose PG, Faulhaber P, Miraldi F, Abdul-Karim FW. Positive emission tomography for evaluating a complete clinical response in patients with ovarian or peritoneal carcinoma: correlation with second-look laparotomy. Gynecol Oncol 2001; 82: 17–21.

37. Cho SM, Ha HK, Byun JY, et al. Usefulness of FDG PET for assessment of early recurrent epithelial ovarian cancer. Am J Roentgenol 2002; 179: 391–5.

38. Berger KL, Nicholson SA, Dehdashti F, Siegel BA. FDG PET evaluation of mucinous neoplasms: correlation of FDG uptake with histopathologic features. Am J Roentgenol 2000; 174: 1005–8.

39. Dromain C, Leboulleux S, Auperin A, et al. Staging of peritoneal carcinomatosis: enhanced CT vs PET/CT. Abdom Imaging 2008; 33: 87–93.

40. Turlakow A, Yeung HW, Salmon AS, Macapinlac HA, Larson SM. Peritoneal carcinomatosis: role of (18)F-FDG PET. J Nucl Med 2003; 44: 1407–12.

41. Dirisamer A, Schima W, Heinisch M, et al. Detection of histologically proven peritoneal carcinomatosis with fused 18F-FDG-PET/MDCT. Eur J Radiol 2008 (Epub ahead of print).

42. Makhija S, Howden N, Edwards R, et al. Positron emission tomography/computed tomography imaging for the detection of recurrent ovarian and fallopian tube carcinoma: a retrospective review. Gynecol Oncol 2002; 85: 53–8.

43. Chung HH, Kang WJ, Kim JW, et al. Role of [18F]FDG PET/CT in the assessment of suspected recurrent ovarian cancer: correlation with clinical or histological findings. Eur J Nucl Med Mol Imaging 2007; 34: 480–6.

44. Nakamoto Y, Saga T, Ishimori T, et al. Clinical value of positron emission tomography with FDG for recurrent ovarian cancer. Am J Roentgenol 2001; 176: 1449–54.

45. Takalkar AM, Bruno GL, Reddy M, Lilien DL. Intense FDG activity in peritoneal tuberculosis mimics peritoneal carcinomatosis. Clin Nucl Med 2007; 32: 244–6.

46. Nicolaou S, Kai B, Ho S, Su J, Ahamed K. Imaging of acute small-bowel obstruction. Am J Roentgenol 2005; 185: 1036–44.

47. Spencer JA, Swift SE, Wilkinson N, et al. Peritoneal carcinomatosis: image-guided peritoneal core biopsy for tumour type and patient care. Radiology 2001; 221: 173–7.

48. Yarram SG, Nghiem HV, Higgins E, et al. Evaluation of imaging-guided core biopsy of pelvic masses. Am J Roentgenol 2007; 188: 1208–11.

49. Walkey MM, Friedman AC, Sohotra P, Radecki PD. CT manifestations of peritoneal carcinomatosis. Am J Roentgenol 1988; 150: 1035–41.

50. Mitchell DG, Hill MC, Hill S, Zaloudek C. Serous carcinoma of the ovary: CT identification of metastatic calcified implants. Radiology 1986; 158: 649–52.

51. Matsuoka Y, Itai Y, Ohtomo K, Nishikawa J, Sasaki Y. Calcification of peritoneal carcinomatosis from gastric carcinoma: a CT demonstration. Eur J Radiol 1991; 13: 207–8.

52. Woodard PK, Feldman JM, Paine SS, Baker ME. Midgut carcinoid tumours: CT findings and biochemical profiles. J Comput Assist Tomogr 1995; 19: 400–5.

53. Vanel D, Albiter M, Shapeero L, et al. Role of computed tomography in the follow-up of hepatic and peritoneal metastases of GIST under imatinib mesylate treatment: a prospective study of 54 patients. Eur J Radiol 2005; 54: 118–23.

54. Kawamoto S, Urban BA, Fishman EK. CT of epithelial ovarian tumors. Radiographics 1999; 19: S85–S102.

55. Cooper C, Jeffrey RB, Silverman PM, Federle MP, Chun GH. Computed tomography of omental pathology. J Comput Assist Tomogr 1986; 10: 62–6.

56. Steinberg JJ, Demopoulos RI, Bigelow B. The evaluation of the omentum in ovarian cancer. Gynecol Oncol 1986; 24: 327–30

57. Dvoretsky PM, Richards KA, Angel C, et al. Distribution of disease at autopsy in 100 women with ovarian cancer. Hum Pathol 1988; 19: 57–63.

58. Ronnett BM, Zahn CM, Kurman RJ, et al. Disseminated peritoneal adenomucinosis and peritoneal mucinous carcinomatosis. A clinicopathologic analysis of 109 cases with emphasis on distinguishing pathologic features, site of origin, prognosis, and relationship to "pseudomyxoma peritonei". Am J Surg Pathol 1995; 19: 1390–408.

59. Jung SE, Lee JM, Rha SE, et al. CT and MR imaging of ovarian tumors with emphasis on differential diagnosis. Radiographics 2002; 22: 1305–25.

60. Meyers MA, Volberg F, Katzen B, Abbott G. Haustral anatomy and physiology: a new look. II. Roentgen interpretation of pathologic alterations. Radiology 1973; 108: 505–12.

61. Hamrick-Turner JE, Chiechi MV, Abbitt PL, Ros PR. Neoplastic and inflammatory processes of the peritoneum, omentum, and mesentery: diagnosis with CT. Radiographics 1992; 12: 1051–68.

62. Franiel T, Diederichs G, Engelken F, et al. Multi-detector CT in peritoneal carcinomatosis: diagnostic role of thin slices and multiplanar reconstructions. Abdom Imaging 2008 (Epub ahead of print).

63. De Rosa V, Mangoni di Stefano ML, Brunetti A, et al. Computed tomography and second-look surgery in ovarian cancer patients. Correlation, actual role and limitations of CT scan. Eur J Gynaecol Oncol 1995; 16: 123–9.

64. Low RN, Francis IR. MR imaging of the gastrointestinal tract with i.v., gadolinium and diluted barium oral contrast media compared with unenhanced MR imaging and CT. Am J Roentgenol 1997; 169: 1051–9.

65. Low RN, Barone RM, Lacey C, et al. Peritoneal tumor: MR imaging with dilute oral barium and intravenous gadolinium-containing contrast agents compared with unenhanced MR imaging and CT. Radiology 1997; 204: 513–20.

47 Spleen
S Aslam Sohaib and Rodney H Reznek

INTRODUCTION

The spleen is the largest collection of lymphoid tissue in the body and has important hematological and immunological functions. Metastatic disease in the spleen (i.e., secondary non-lymphoid tumors) is unusual and usually occurs late in the course of disseminated disease. This has to be distinguished from other splenic pathology as it has important prognostic implications.

IMAGING TECHNIQUES

Plain radiography is not routinely used in the evaluation of splenic pathology.

The spleen is readily visualized on ultrasound (US). The normal splenic parenchyma shows a homogeneous low-level echo pattern, which is generally of slightly lower reflectivity than hepatic parenchyma. US is useful for detecting and characterizing focal lesions within the spleen as cystic or solid.

On non-enhanced CT, the normal spleen is homogeneous and has an attenuation of 35 to 55 HU, which is 5 to 10 HU less than that of liver (1). Optimal visualization of the spleen includes the use of intravenous (IV) contrast material. The spleen normally demonstrates heterogeneous enhancement immediately after injection of a bolus of contrast material. Only after a minute or more does the splenic parenchyma achieve uniform homogeneous enhancement. This is thought to reflect the variable blood flow within different compartments of the spleen and should not be misinterpreted as pathology. Anatomical information from CT may be further supplemented with metabolic information with fused images from PET-CT using 18-fluro-2-deoxyglucose (FDG).

On MR imaging, the normal splenic parenchyma is of lower signal intensity than the liver and slightly greater signal than muscle on T1-weighted images. On T2-weighted images, the spleen shows higher signal intensity, appearing brighter than the liver. The signal intensities of normal splenic parenchyma and many pathologic processes are similar. Consequently, the use of contrast-enhanced MR is important for evaluating the spleen. Intravenous (IV) gadolinium-based contrast agents are most commonly used. Images are acquired using a dynamic breath-hold T1-weighted spoiled gradient-echo sequence after an IV bolus injection of gadolinium. As on CT, the spleen shows heterogeneous enhancement on dynamic contrast-enhanced MR (2). An alternative to gadolinium is to use superparamagnetic iron oxide particles taken up by the reticuloendothelial system. They lower the signal intensity of the normal spleen and therefore increase the conspicuity of focal abnormalities in the spleen (3).

NORMAL ANATOMY AND VARIANTS

The shape and position of the normal spleen can vary considerably. Prominent lobes may mimic a mass lesion. Ectopic splenic tissues of congenital origin give rise to an accessory spleen in 10% to 30% of the population (4). They usually occur near the splenic hilum (75%) but may sometimes be found in its suspensory ligaments or in the tail of the pancreas and rarely elsewhere in the abdomen (4). A single focus is found in 88% of cases (5). Accessory spleens vary in size from a few millimeters to several centimeters in diameter. After splenectomy, an accessory spleen can hypertrophy markedly, causing a recurrence of problems in patients who have undergone splenectomy for hypersplenism. The typical accessory spleen has a smooth round or ovoid shape. Its blood supply is usually derived from the splenic artery with drainage into the splenic vein. When there is doubt, ^{99m}Tc-sulphur colloid or heat-denatured red cell scintigraphy is useful, to diagnostically show functioning splenic tissue in areas of concern (6).

Spleen Size

The normal adult spleen measures approximately 12 to 15 cm in length, 4 to 8 cm in anteroposterior diameter, and 3 to 4 cm in thickness (7). However, the irregular shape and oblique orientation of the spleen means that these linear measurements are of limited use. Furthermore, splenic volume varies greatly from one individual to another. Normal *in vivo* adult splenic volume ranges from 100 to 310 cm³ (8). On US the long axis of the spleen is less than 12 cm in 95% of the population (9). Measurement of the length and width of the spleen has been shown to correlate extremely well with *in vivo* measurements of splenic volume (10). Determination of splenic volume on CT using summation of cross-sectional areas is very accurate, with errors in the range of 3% to 5% (10). However, this technique is cumbersome and, in practice, most observers judge splenic volume by subjective evaluation on CT or MR. Rounding of the normally crescentic shape, extension of the spleen anterior to the aorta or below the right hepatic lobe or rib cage are further clues to splenomegaly. On cross-sectional imaging a more accurate method for the assessment of the splenic volume is the splenic index, that is, the product of the length, width, and thickness (11). The normal splenic index is between 120 and 480 cm³ (11).

SPLENOMEGALY

There are many causes of splenomegaly (Table 47.1), which occasionally may be related to neoplastic disorders such as lymphoma, leukemia, primary benign or malignant tumors and metastases. A clue to the underlying cause can sometimes be identified on imaging, for example, abdominal lymph node enlargement may suggest lymphoma.

SPLENIC METASTASES

Metastases to the spleen are usually hematogenous. Transcelomic spread to the spleen within the abdominal cavity is less frequent.

Table 47.1 Causes of Splenomegaly

Neoplasms
Leukemia/lymphoma
Metastases

Congestive
Portal hypertension
Cirrhosis
Cystic fibrosis
Splenic vein obstruction

Storage disease
Gaucher's disease
Niemann–Pick disease
Amyloidosis
Histiocytosis

Collagen vascular disease
Systemic lupus erythematosus
Rheumatoid/Felty's syndrome

Hemolytic anemias
Hemoglobinopathies
Hereditary spherocytosis

Infections
Hepatitis
Malaria
Infectious mononucleosis
Tuberculosis
Typhoid

Extramedullary hematopoiesis
Myelofibrosis

Miscellaneous
Sarcoidosis
Porphyria

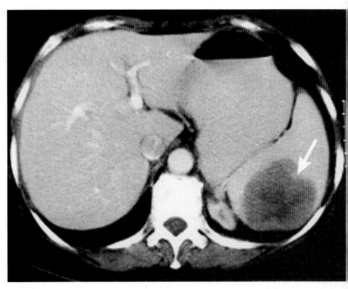

Figure 47.1 Isolated splenic metastasis in a patient with recurrent ovarian cancer. Contrast enhanced CT showing a large solitary deposit (arrow).

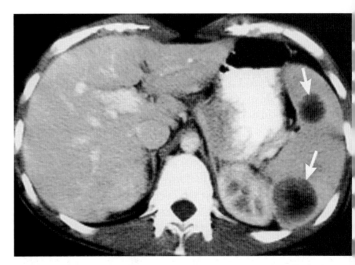

Figure 47.2 Splenic metastases. Contrast enhanced CT showing multiple deposits (arrows) from malignant melanoma.

Blood-borne spread usually results in parenchymal disease whilst peritoneal disease gives rise to surface disease. It has been postulated that the relative infrequency of splenic metastases may be due to the lack of afferent splenic lymphatics, filtering of the blood in the lung and the liver, or anti-tumor activity due to the high concentration of lymphoid tissue.

There are relatively few series reporting splenic metastases, the incidence ranging from 0.3% to 10.3% (12–21). In one large autopsy series of patients with metastatic disease, those with splenic metastasis were significantly younger (59 vs. 67 years) and had significantly more sites of metastastic disease (median: 6 vs. median: 1) (21). Prognosis of patients with splenic metastases may be worse than those without splenic metastases (21,22).

Adenocarcinomas are the most common source of splenic metastases, accounting for almost 95% of cases (12). Other tumors include melanoma and germ cell tumor. The primary carcinomas that most commonly spread to the spleen are (12,14,20):

- Breast
- Lung
- Colorectal
- Ovary
- Gastric

The majority of carcinomas are adenocarcinomas; others include squamous cell, undifferentiated and small cell cancer.

An *isolated splenic metastasis* in the absence of metastases to other organs is rare, found in only 5.3% of cases at autopsy (12), most frequently in ovarian carcinomas (Fig. 47.1). Other common primary sites that result in isolated splenic metastasis include colon and lung.

An even higher frequency of splenic metastasis from ovarian cancer has been reported by Spencer and Colleagues (13). In this study of 321 patients, 10.3% of patients had splenic metastases during the course of the disease with 5.3% at presentation. Splenic parenchymal metastases were present in 1.5% at presentation and in 3% during the course of disease. Disease on the splenic surface was more common, occurring in 5.3% at presentation and in 7.2% during the course of the disease. Parenchymal metastases were much less likely to respond to treatment than surface lesions. The splenic metastases behaved similarly to liver metastases in ovarian cancer (13). Ovarian cancer is the most common primary site in surgical series of patients undergoing splenectomies for metastases (23).

Melanoma has the highest frequency of splenic involvement (Fig. 47.2) as up to 34% of melanoma patients show splenic metastases on autopsy series (17). The risk of metastases increases with the depth of the melanoma lesions (24).

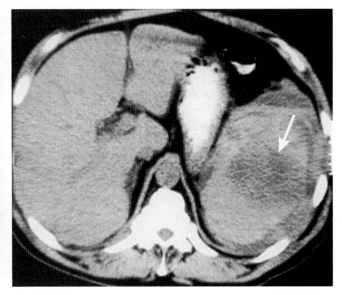

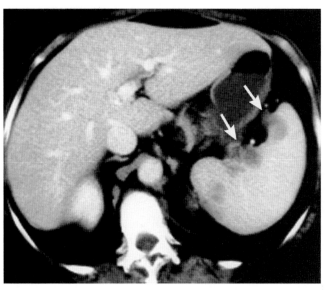

Figure 47.3 Spontaneous splenic rupture in a patient with a melanoma metastases to the spleen. Non-contrast enhanced CT shows a low density melanoma metastasis (arrow) within the spleen which is surrounded by a perisplenic hematoma.

Figure 47.4 Surface splenic metastases in a patient with ovarian cancer. Contrast enhanced CT showing multiple deposits (arrows) on the surface of the spleen.

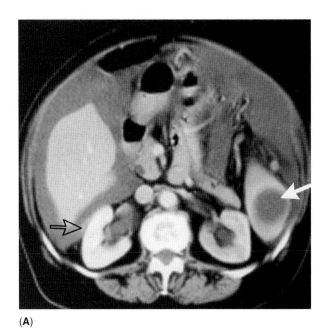

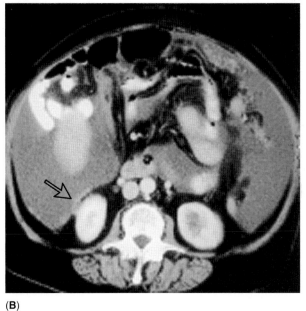

(A)

(B)

Figure 47.5 Cystic splenic metastasis. (A) Contrast enhanced CT shows a cystic splenic metastasis (arrow) in a patient with advanced ovarian cancer. (B) There are also peritoneal deposits (open arrow) and malignant ascites present.

Clinical Features

Splenic deposits are usually asymptomatic. Symptoms usually include abdominal pain or an enlarging mass. Spontaneous splenic rupture (Fig. 47.3) because of metastatic carcinoma is rare. The symptomatic splenic lesions are larger and more frequently found in women and younger patients (12).

Imaging Characteristics

Splenic metastases involve the splenic capsule/surface or parenchyma. Metastases to the splenic serosa are predominantly from the ovary, but may be from other tumors that spread via a peritoneal route. Serosal metastases result in scalloping or indentation of the splenic surface (Fig. 47.4). Surface implants are usually well defined, biconvex and peripheral, and indent rather than replace the splenic parenchyma. Parenchymal lesions are most frequently multiple but may be solitary. They are often circular and partially or completely surrounded by spleen tissue. Splenic metastases, parenchymal or serosal, are usually hypoechoic on US and hypodense on CT (Figs. 47.1 and 47.4).

Metastases may be cystic in character. Such metastases usually arise from primary tumors of the ovary (Fig. 47.5), breast, endometrium, and from melanoma.

Calcification is uncommon but occurs in patients with primary mucinous adenocarcinoma (Fig. 47.6).

Diagnosis

The diagnosis of splenic metastases is usually not difficult given the clinical setting. Rarely, where the diagnosis is uncertain, such as in an isolated splenic metastasis, patients usually undergo splenectomy. In other situations where a focal splenic abnormality is identified, and it is uncertain whether this is a metastasis or not, then the options are:

- Splenectomy or
- Image-guided biopsy or
- In the case of FDG–avid malignancy to image with FDG-enhanced PET-CT

Percutaneous biopsy may be performed for cytological or histological diagnosis. A diagnostic rate of 55% to 98% has been reported (25–28). The complication rate with fine-needle aspiration is low, but includes hemorrhage and pneumothorax.

An alternative to a percutaneous biopsy in patients with a FDG–avid malignancy is to image with FDG-PET. In this group of patients FDG-PET has been reported to be able to reliably (100%) discriminate between benign and malignant solid splenic masses (29). Furthermore, FDG PET has a high negative predictive value in patients with solid splenic masses, without known malignant disease (29). False positive FDG PET may arise in these patients without malignancy from other causes such as infection; hence patients without known malignancy with a FDG–avid splenic mass should be further evaluated with a percutaneous biopsy.

Key Points: Splenic Metastases

- Splenic metastases are uncommon and usually occur as a part of disseminated disease
- Splenic involvement may either be due to surface disease from peritoneal spread of cancer or parenchymal disease from hematogenous spread
- Isolated splenic metastases are rare but typically occur in recurrent ovarian cancer
- Splenic metastases are usually asymptomatic, and are usually found at autopsy or at imaging
- Melanoma has the highest frequency of splenic involvement
- In patients with known malignancy, FDG-PET will reliably identify or exclude splenic involvement

OTHER SPLEEN LESIONS IN ONCOLOGY PATIENTS

Malignant Lesions

Splenic lymphoma (see chap. 33) is the most common splenic malignancy. It is usually a manifestation of generalized lymphoma (Figs. 47.7 and 47.8) and therefore not regarded as metastatic disease to the spleen.

Other primary malignant tumors of the spleen are very rare. They include angiosarcoma, fibrosarcoma, leiomyosarcoma, malignant teratoma, and malignant fibrous histocytoma. Splenic angiosarcoma is the most common non-lymphoid primary malignant

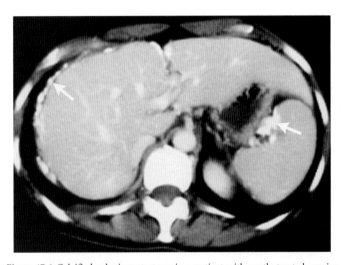

Figure 47.6 Calcified splenic metastases in a patient with partly treated ovarian cancer. Contrast enhanced CT showing multiple calcified peritoneal deposits (arrows).

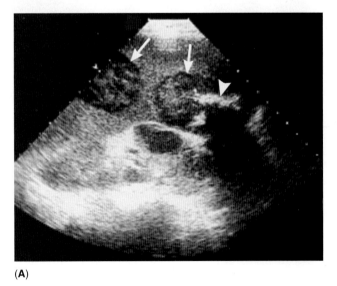

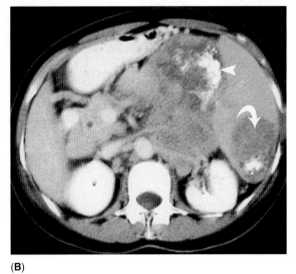

(A)

(B)

Figure 47.7 High-grade non-Hodgkin lymphoma involving the spleen. (**A**) Longitudinal ultrasound shows two large heterogeneous hypoechoic lesions (arrows). The inferior lesion contains a central area of hyperechoic area (arrowhead) casting an acoustic shadow in keeping with calcification. (**B**) Contrast-enhanced CT shows the partly calcified splenic lesion (curved arrow) as well as the bulky retroperitoneal calcified adenopathy (arrowhead).

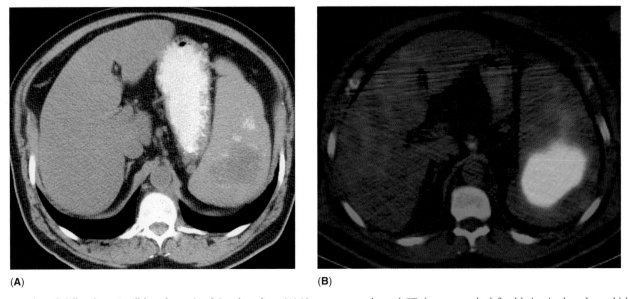

(A)　　　　　　　　　　　　　　　　**(B)**

Figure 47.8 Relapsed diffuse large B cell lymphoma involving the spleen. (A) Non-contrast-enhanced CT shows a poorly defined lesion in the spleen which shows markedly increased metabolic activity on (B) fused FDG-PET/CT images. *Source*: Images courtesy of Dr. Gary Cook, Royal Marsden Hospital, London.

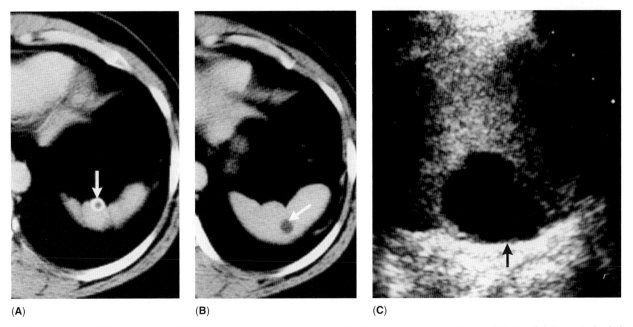

(A)　　　　　　　　　　**(B)**　　　　　　　　　　**(C)**

Figure 47.9 Simple cysts. (A, B) Contrast enhanced CT shows two simple cysts (arrows) within the spleen; one of which has a calcified wall. (C) Longitudinal ultrasound through the spleen in a different patient shows a subcapsular cyst (arrow).

tumor of the spleen (30). Prognosis is poor and almost all patients die within one year of diagnosis. Metastatic disease is common and typically involves the liver, lungs, bone, bone marrow, and lymphatic system, and approximately 30% undergo spontaneous rupture. Imaging reveals an enlarged spleen with a poorly defined mass, and there may be areas of hemorrhage within it (30).

Key Points: Splenic Malignancy

- Splenic lymphoma is the most common malignant disease to involve the spleen
- Other primary tumors of the spleen are extremely rare, the most common of which is an angiosarcoma

Benign Lesions

Splenic Cysts

Non-neoplastic splenic cysts may be true (primary) cysts which possess a cellular lining or false (secondary) cysts which have no cellular lining. True cysts are either parasitic (echinococcal) or non-parasitic (epithelial). True, non-parasitic, i.e., epithelial (also called epidermoid, mesothelial, or primary) cysts are congenital in origin. They are more common in females than males and are usually found in childhood or adolescence (31). In 80% of cases congenital splenic cysts are unilocular and solitary. A false cyst, i.e., pseudocyst, is post-traumatic in origin and is thought to represent the final stage in the evolution of a splenic hematoma.

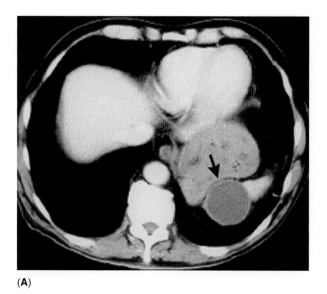
(A)

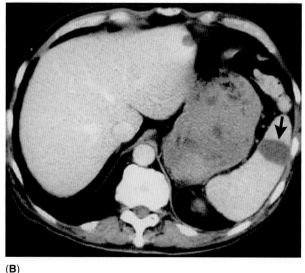
(B)

Figure 47.10 Multiple splenic abscesses. (A, B) Contrast-enhanced CT shows two well-defined low density lesions (arrows) from splenic abscesses.

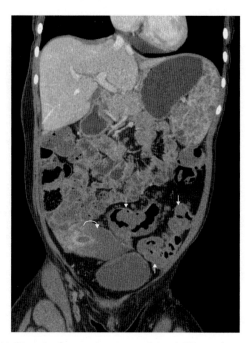

Figure 47.11 Coronal reformatted contrast-enhanced CT scan in a patient with Klippel-Trenaunay syndrome showing multiple splenic hemangiomas. As can be seen, the patient also has hemihypertrophy, multiple bowel wall (arrows) and uterine hemangiomas (curved arrow).

In general, the imaging characteristics of splenic cysts are similar to cysts elsewhere (Fig. 47.9). The differential diagnosis of a splenic cyst includes abscess (Fig. 47.10), acute hematoma, intrasplenic pancreatic pseudocyst, cystic neoplasm (lymphangioma or hemangioma), and cystic metastasis.

Hemangioma
Hemangioma is the most common primary benign neoplasm of the spleen occurring in 0.03% to 14% of cases at autopsy (1). Splenic hemangiomas can be multiple and form part of a generalized angiomatosis as in Klippel–Trenaunay–Weber syndrome (Fig. 47.11) (6). Most lesions are detected incidentally but in large hemangiomas, splenic rupture and anemia, thrombocytopenia, and coagulopathy (Kasabach–Merritt syndrome) have been reported (32).

The imaging characteristics of splenic hemangiomas range from solid to mixed to purely cystic lesions (33). The US appearance is non-specific and may show cystic areas (18). On CT, hemangioma may appear either solid or cystic, and may enhance in a similar pattern to hepatic hemangioma (34). Some lesions are relatively avascular or show slow filling of contrast material. The MR imaging appearance is also similar to hepatic hemangioma. The lesion with respect to the spleen is of low signal intensity or isointense on T1-weighted images with respect to the spleen and of high signal intensity on T2-weighted images. T2-weighted images may show heterogeneous signal intensity representing mixed solid and cystic components of the hemangioma (35). T1-weighted images may show areas of high signal due to subacute hemorrhage or proteinaceous fluid.

Lymphangioma
Lymphangiomas can occur as single or multiple lesions, are usually asymptomatic, and are categorized as capillary, cavernous, or cystic, depending on the size of the abnormal lymphatic channels (36). In the spleen, the cystic type is most common. On US, lymphangioma appears as a hypoechoic mass, occasionally containing septation and debris. CT shows multiple thin-walled, well-marginated cysts, often subcapsular in location. No enhancement is seen and the attenuation measurements vary from 15 to 35 HU (37). On MR, lymphangiomas (Fig. 47.12) may resemble cysts but usually show poor enhancement following IV injection of contrast medium (38).

Hamartoma
Splenic hamartomas (also called splenomas or nodular hyperplasia of the spleen) are rare benign lesions composed of an anomalous mixture of normal splenic elements with red pulp predominating. Hamartomas occur singly or less commonly as multiple nodules. On US, hamartomas are hyperechoic relative to the spleen and sometimes have a cystic component. On CT, they appear iso- or hypodense on the precontrast images with occasional lesions showing cystic components. On MR, they are isointense on T1-weighted images and hyperintense on T2-weighted images. On CT and MR, following injection of IV contrast material, they usually show gradual enhancement and filling (39).

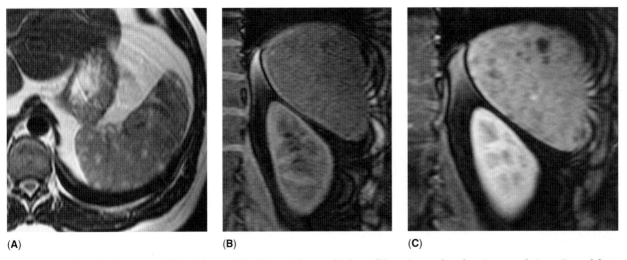

(A)   **(B)**   **(C)**

Figure 47.12 Multiple splenic lymphangiomas. (**A**) Axial T2-weighted images show multiple small hyperintense lymphangiomatous lesions. Coronal fat-suppressed T1-weighted images (**B**) before and (**C**) after intravenous gadolinium shows the poorly enhancing lesion.

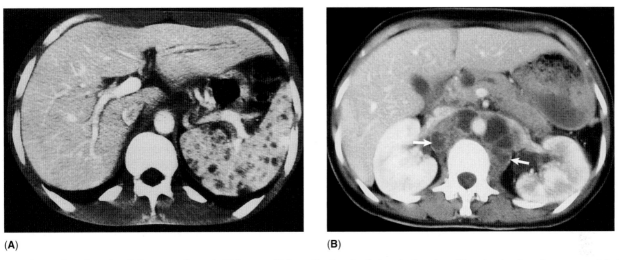

(A)   **(B)**

Figure 47.13 Splenic tuberculosis. (**A, B**) Contrast-enhanced CT shows multiple small enhancing lesions in the spleen. Note also the rim enhancement of the involved retroperitoneal nodes (arrows).

Infection

Splenic infection, especially fungal infection, may arise as a consequence of immunosuppression from chemotherapy. The most common pathogens are Candida, Aspergillus, and Cryptococcus. Fungal infection in the spleen is most likely to appear as a miliary or multifocal process. Hepatosplenic candidiasis may appear as multiple rounded areas of decreased attenuation, a so-called "bull's-eye" lesion (hypoattenuating foci with a central core of higher attenuation), or as tiny 2 to 5 mm lesions of increased attenuation due to calcification. Calcification is seen in treated Candida microabscesses and lesions caused by other fungi, especially Histoplasma, mycobacteria (Fig. 47.13) and *Pneumocystis carinii*. Fungal abscesses in neutropenic patients are often small and not always detectable with any imaging modality.

Infarcts

Splenic infarcts may occur from mass lesions compressing splenic vasculature, for example, pancreatic tumors (Fig. 47.14). Splenic infarction may be diffuse or focal. On CT, infarcts typically appear

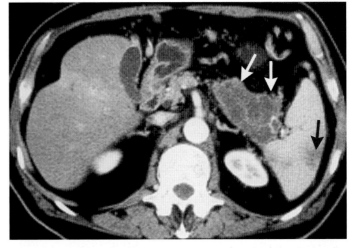

Figure 47.14 Splenic infarct. Contrast-enhanced CT shows a tumor mass (arrows) in the tail of the pancreas causing occlusion to the splenic vein and a splenic infarct (black arrow).

as sharply marginated, low-density wedge-shaped areas. Occasionally the infarct may be multiple, resulting in poorly defined hypodense lesions. When the entire spleen is infarcted only rim enhancement of the capsule occurs from capsular vessels. Splenic infarction can also be seen on MR: hemorrhagic infarcts have a high signal intensity on T1- and T2-weighted images.

Key Points: Benign Disease

- Non-neoplastic cysts of the spleen have the typical imaging appearances of cysts
- Hemangiomas are the most common benign primary tumor of the spleen and have similar imaging characteristics to hemangioma in the liver
- Focal splenic lesions in cancer patients may arise from other benign conditions such as infections and splenic infarcts

Summary

- Early heterogeneous enhancement in the spleen should not be misinterpreted as pathology
- The most common splenic malignancy is lymphoma. The spleen is involved as part of generalized lymphoma. An enlarged spleen is not a reliable indicator of lymphomatous involvement
- Metastases to the spleen are uncommon. The primary tumors most commonly metastasizing to the spleen include those of breast, lung, ovary, and colorectum, and melanoma
- Splenic metastases may be serosal from peritoneal spread of tumor or parenchymal from hematogenous metastases
- FDG-PET is of value in patients with malignancy in identifying or excluding splenic metastases

REFERENCES

1. Rabushka LS, Kawashima A, Fishman EK. Imaging of the spleen: CT with supplemental MR examination. Radiographics 1994; 14: 307–32.
2. Semelka RC, Shoenut JP, Lawrence PH, et al. Spleen: dynamic enhancement patterns on gradient-echo MR images enhanced with gadopentetate dimeglumine. Radiology 1992; 185: 479–82.
3. Weissleder R, Hahn PF, Stark DD, et al. Superparamagnetic iron oxide: enhanced detection of focal splenic tumors with MR imaging. Radiology 1988; 169: 399–403.
4. Wadham BM, Adams PB, Johnson MA. Incidence and location of accessory spleens [letter]. N Engl J Med 1981; 304: 1111.
5. Subramanyam BR, Balthazar EJ, Horii SC. Sonography of the accessory spleen. Am J Roentgenol 1984; 143: 47–9.
6. Freeman JL, Jafri SZ, Roberts JL, Mezwa DG, Shirkhoda A. CT of congenital and acquired abnormalities of the spleen. Radiographics 1993; 13: 597–610.
7. Warshauer DM, Koehler RE. Spleen. In: Lee JK, Sagel SS, Stanley RJ, Heiken JP, eds. CT with MRI Correlation. Philadelphia: Lippincott-Raven, 1998: 845–72.
8. Prassopoulos P, Daskalogiannaki M, Raissaki M, Hatjidakis A, Gourtsoyiannis N. Determination of normal splenic volume on computed tomography in relation to age, gender and body habitus. Eur Radiol 1997; 7: 246–8.
9. Dardenne AN. The Spleen. In: Cosgrove DO, Meire HB, Dewbury KCD, eds. Clinical Ultrasound. Edinburgh: Churchill Livingstone, 1993: 353–65.
10. Lamb PM, Lund A, Kanagasabay RR, et al. Spleen size: how well do linear ultrasound measurements correlate with three-dimensional CT volume assessments? Br J Radiol 2002; 75: 573–7.
11. Strijk SP, Wagener DJ, Bogman MJ, de Pauw BE, Wobbes T. The spleen in Hodgkin disease: diagnostic value of CT. Radiology 1985; 154: 753–7.
12. Lam KY, Tang V. Metastatic tumors to the spleen: a 25-year clinicopathologic study. Arch Pathol Lab Med 2000; 124: 526–30.
13. Spencer NJ, Spencer JA, Perren TJ, Lane G. CT appearances and prognostic significance of splenic metastasis in ovarian cancer. Clin Radiol 1998; 53: 417–21.
14. Warren S, Davis AH. Studies of tumor metastasis: the metastases of carcinoma to the spleen. Am J Cancer 1934; 21: 517–33.
15. Marymont JG, Gross S. Patterns of metastatic cancer in the spleen. Am J Clin Pathol 1963; 40: 58–66.
16. Nash DA Jr, Sampson CC. Secondary carcinoma of the spleen. Its incidence in 544 cases and a review of the literature. J Natl Med Assoc 1966; 58: 442–6.
17. Berge T. Splenic metastases. Frequencies and patterns. Acta Pathol Microbiol Scand [A] 1974; 82: 499–506.
18. Goerg C, Schwerk WB, Goerg K. Splenic lesions: sonographic patterns, follow-up, differential diagnosis. Eur J Radiol 1991; 13: 59–66.
19. Siniluoto T, Paivansalo M, Lahde S. Ultrasonography of splenic metastases. Acta Radiol 1989; 30: 463–6.
20. Abrams HL, Spiro R, Goldstein N. Metastases in carcinoma: analysis of 1000 autopsied cases. Cancer 1950; 3: 74–85.
21. Schon CA, Gorg C, Ramaswamy A, Barth PJ. Splenic metastases in a large unselected autopsy series. Pathol Res Pract 2006; 202: 351–6.
22. Sohaib SA, Houghton SL, Meroni R, et al. Recurrent endometrial cancer: patterns of recurrent disease and assessment of prognosis. Clin Radiol 2007; 62: 28–36.
23. Lee SS, Morgenstern L, Phillips EH, Hiatt JR, Margulies DR. Splenectomy for splenic metastases: a changing clinical spectrum. Am Surg 2000; 66: 837–40.
24. Shirkhoda A, Albin J. Malignant melanoma: correlating abdominal and pelvic CT with clinical staging. Radiology 1987; 165: 75–8.
25. Caraway NP, Fanning CV. Use of fine-needle aspiration biopsy in the evaluation of splenic lesions in a cancer center. Diagn Cytopathol 1997; 16: 312–16.
26. Silverman JF, Geisinger KR, Raab SS, Stanley MW. Fine needle aspiration biopsy of the spleen in the evaluation of neoplastic disorders. Acta Cytol 1993; 37: 158–62.
27. Kraus MD, Fleming MD, Vonderheide RH. The spleen as a diagnostic specimen: a review of 10 years' experience at two tertiary care institutions. Cancer 2001; 91: 2001–9.

28. Cavanna L, Lazzaro A, Vallisa D, Civardi G, Artioli F. Role of image-guided fine-needle aspiration biopsy in the management of patients with splenic metastasis. World J Surg Oncol 2007; 5: 13.

29. Metser U, Miller E, Kessler A, et al. Solid splenic masses: evaluation with 18F-FDG PET/CT. J Nucl Med 2005; 46: 52–9.

30. Abbott RM, Levy AD, Aguilera NS, Gorospe L, Thompson WM. From the archives of the AFIP: primary vascular neoplasms of the spleen: radiologic-pathologic correlation. Radiographics 2004; 24: 1137–63.

31. Dawes LG, Malangoni MA. Cystic masses of the spleen. Am Surg 1986; 52: 333–6.

32. Rolfes RJ, Ros PR. The spleen: an integrated imaging approach. Crit Rev Diagn Imaging 1990; 30: 41–83.

33. Duddy MJ, Calder CJ. Cystic haemangioma of the spleen: findings on ultrasound and computed tomography. Br J Radiol 1989; 62: 180–2.

34. Ros PR, Moser RP Jr, Dachman AH, Murari PJ, Olmsted WW. Hemangioma of the spleen: radiologic-pathologic correlation in ten cases. Radiology 1987; 162: 73–7.

35. Harris RD, Simpson W. MRI of splenic hemangioma associated with thrombocytopenia. Gastrointest Radiol 1989; 14: 308–10.

36. Ferrozzi F, Bova D, Draghi F, Garlaschi G. CT findings in primary vascular tumors of the spleen. Am J Roentgenol 1996; 166: 1097–101.

37. Pistoia F, Markowitz SK. Splenic lymphangiomatosis: CT diagnosis. Am J Roentgenol 1988; 150: 121–2.

38. Ito K, Murata T, Nakanishi T. Cystic lymphangioma of the spleen: MR findings with pathologic correlation. Abdom Imaging 1995; 20: 82–4.

39. Ohtomo K, Fukuda H, Mori K, et al. CT and MR appearances of splenic hamartoma. J Comput Assist Tomogr 1992; 16: 425–8.

48 Malignant Tumors of the Skin
Guy J Burkill and D Michael King

INTRODUCTION

Malignant tumors of the skin form a disparate group of cancers with a wide range of behaviors, but collectively they are the most frequently occurring human malignancy (1). Typically, these tumors are clinically obvious and radiology plays no role in their initial assessment. Increasingly, however, scintigraphy in the form of sentinel lymph node localization and biopsy (SLNB) is employed for staging certain skin cancers and for planning their treatment.

Computed tomography (CT) remains the mainstay for the assessment of metastatic disease supplemented by ultrasound (US), magnetic resonance (MR) imaging, and plain radiography. As with other malignancies, 2-[F-18]fluoro-2-deoxy-D-glucose positron emission tomography ([18]FDG PET) is increasingly replacing CT for the detection of distant spread.

Although the majority of cutaneous tumors are non-melanoma skin cancers (NMSC), this chapter is dominated by the imaging of melanoma, reflecting its increasing incidence, and the more established role of imaging in this malignancy.

PATHOLOGY

Cutaneous malignancies are categorized according to their cellular origin and have been summarized in Table 48.1 (2,3).

EPIDEMIOLOGY

Reliable epidemiological data, although sparse, are available for melanoma, basal cell carcinoma (BCC), and squamous cell carcinoma (SCC). Non-melanoma skin cancer (NMSC—BCC and SCC) is the most frequently occurring cancer in white populations. The reported ratio of BCC to SCC is 4:1 (4). Despite underreporting, over 72,000 new cases of NMSC were registered in the United Kingdom in 2004 (5).

The incidence ratio of NMSC to malignant melanoma is approximately 8:1 (5). Although melanoma remains a relatively rare cancer, the incidence is rising faster than any other tumor, doubling every 10 to 20 years (5). The United Kingdom has an above average incidence compared with other European Union countries with approximately 9000 new cases per annum (5). The United Kingdom incidence remains three times lower than that for Australia and New Zealand where the annual incidence is 30 to 40 per 100,000 population (5). In the United States it was estimated that there would be over 62,000 new cases of melanoma reported in 2008 (6).

Key Points: Epidemiology

- Skin cancer is the most common human malignancy
- BCC is the most common skin cancer
- The incidence of melanoma is rising faster than any other malignancy
- The United Kingdom has an above European Union average incidence for melanoma

RISK FACTORS

There are a number of risk factors for the development of both NMSC and melanoma. Common to both groups of cancers is exposure to ultraviolet (UV) radiation and burning of the skin before adolescence is of particular importance for fair- and freckled-skinned individuals (7–10). In addition, those with a history of previous skin cancer are at higher risk of developing new tumors (7). Overseas travel has undoubtedly been a factor in the rising incidence of malignant melanoma in the United Kingdom by over four-fold in men and three-fold in women over the last 25 years (5). This is also likely to explain a higher incidence in more affluent geographical areas in the United Kingdom (11). The use of sun beds was thought to result in a moderate increase in the risk of developing melanoma (5). However, following a meta-analysis the use of sunbeds has recently been re-classified by the International Agency for Research on Cancer (IARC) as carcinogenic to humans (12). The current advice from the International Commission on Non-Ionizing Radiation Protection (ICNIRP) and the World Health Organization (WHO) is that those with recognized risk factors for developing melanoma should not use sunbeds (13,14).

In SCC, additional risk factors include exposure to ionizing radiation and chemical carcinogens (e.g., soot, arsenic, and polycyclic aromatic hydrocarbons). Risk factors also include chronically injured or scarred skin following burning or ulceration. Viruses such as human papillomavirus Types 6, 11, and 16 have also been implicated. Precancerous conditions include Bowen's disease ("intraepidermal SCC") and epidermodysplasia verruciformis (9,10). Basal cell carcinomas may arise in the basal cell nevus syndrome (Gorlin's) and in organoid nevi (8). The presence of numerous or atypical moles increases the chance of developing melanoma. A two-fold risk of melanoma exists for individuals with a family history. Those families with three or more cases are likely to be carriers of a genetic mutation such as in the CDKN2A locus on chromosome 9p22 (5). However, routine genetic testing is not yet recommended (15).

Immunosuppression is an important risk factor for skin cancers, which form the most common malignancy in organ transplant recipients demonstrating an increased incidence compared with the normal population of 65-fold for SCC, 10-fold for BCC, 3.4-fold for melanoma, and 84-fold for Kaposi's sarcoma (KS) (16–18). Furthermore, skin tumors in transplant recipients appear to be more aggressive, resulting in a higher mortality (16,19–21).

Table 48.1 Classification of Malignant Tumors of the Skin According to Cellular Origin

Epidermal	Squamous cell carcinoma
	Keratoacanthoma Basal cell carcinoma
	Merkel cell carcinoma
	Paget's disease
Dermal	Dermatofibrosarcoma protuberans
	Malignant fibrous histiocytoma/atypical fibroxanthoma
Endothelial	Angiosarcoma
	Cutaneous Kaposi's sarcoma
Smooth muscle	Cutaneous leiomyosarcoma
Malignant appendageal tumors (cutaneous adnexal carcinomas)	Sweat gland carcinomas
	Malignant follicular tumors
	Sebaceous carcinoma
Melanocytes	Melanoma
Tumors of cellular immigrants to the skin	Primary cutaneous lymphomas
	Leukemia cutis
	Mastocytosis
	Primary cutaneous Langerhans' cell histiocytosis
Metastases	

Table 48.2 TNM Staging Classification of Skin Carcinomas, 2002 (22)

Primary tumor

TX	Primary tumor cannot be assessed
T0	No evidence of primary tumor
Tis	Carcinoma in situ
T1	Tumor 2 cm or less in greatest dimension
T2	Tumor >2 cm ≤5 cm in greatest dimension
T3	Tumor >5 cm in greatest dimension
T4	Tumor invades deep extradermal structures, i.e., cartilage, skeletal muscle, or bone

Regional lymph nodes

NX	Regional lymph nodes cannot be assessed
N0	No regional lymph node metastasis
N1	Regional lymph node metastasis

Distant metastasis

MX	Distant metastasis cannot be assessed
M0	No distant metastasis
M1	Distant metastasis

Key Points: Risk Factors

- For NMSC and melanoma, sun exposure is the most important factor
- Burning of the skin before adolescence is an important etiological factor
- Fair- and freckled-skin individuals are at greatest risk
- For SCC there are a number of predisposing chemical carcinogens and viruses
- There are premalignant lesions in both NMSC and melanoma
- Genetic mutations have been implicated in melanoma
- Immunosuppression is a risk factor for all skin malignancies

STAGING

Staging Classifications

TNM (tumor, node, metastases) staging for skin carcinomas is essentially pathological. T stage relates to tumor size up to T4, at which stage tumors invade deep extradermal structures (Table 48.2).

Table 48.3A AJCC Revised Version of the Melanoma TNM Classification (23)

T classification	Thickness	Ulceration status
T1	≤1.0 mm	a. Without ulceration and level II/III
		b. With ulceration or level IV/V
T2	1.01–2.0 mm	a. Without ulceration
		b. With ulceration
T3	2.01–4.0 mm	a. Without ulceration
		b. With ulceration
T4	>4.0 mm	a. Without ulceration
		b. With ulceration

N classification	No. of metastatic nodes	Nodal metastatic mass
N1	1 node	a. Micrometastasis[a]
		b. Macrometastasis[b]
N2	2–3 nodes	a. Micrometastasis[a]
		b. Macrometastasis[b]
		c. In transit met(s)/ satellite(s) without metastatic nodes
N3	Four or more metastatic nodes, or matted nodes, or in transit met(s)/satellites(s) with metastatic node(s)	

M classification	Site	Serum lactate dehydrogenase
M1a	Distant skin, subcutaneous, or nodal metastases	Normal
M1b	Lung metastases	Normal
M1c	All visceral metastases	Normal
	Any distant metastasis	Elevated

[a]Micrometastases are diagnosed after sentinel or elective lymphadenectomy.
[b]Macrometastases are defined as clinically detectable nodal metastases confirmed by therapeutic lymphadenectomy or when nodal metastasis exhibits gross extracapsular extension.

Staging of the regional lymph nodes for each skin site is also defined in the TNM classification, and staging as node-negative requires at least six tumor-free lymph nodes in the dissection specimen (22).

The staging system for malignant melanoma is also based on histopathological findings and in particular tumor thickness (23). The AJCC version of TNM for malignant melanoma has a number of refinements which are of prognostic importance such as ulceration within the T stage, inclusion of a number of metastatic lymph nodes and the distinction between micro- and macrometastases in the nodal staging. Site of distant metastases is also included and the serum lactate dehydrogenase level forms part of the M stage (Table 48.3A and B) (23).

A proposed staging system for Merkell Cell carcinoma (MCC) is based on 251 patients treated at one institution (Table 48.4) (24).

For the purposes of clinical trial participation and subsequent evaluation there is a staging system for KS devised by the AIDS Clinical Trials Group (ACTG) which may require modification due to the impact of highly active antiretroviral therapy (HAART) (25,26). The International Society for Cutaneous Lymphomas (ISCL) in collaboration with a sub-group of the European Organization for Research and Treatment of Cancer (EORTC) have proposed a staging system for primary cutaneous lymphoma and revisions to the staging system for mycosis fungoides and Sezary syndrome (27,28).

The staging of rarer cutaneous malignancies is dictated by their behavior as predicted by histological examination of biopsy material.

Table 48.3B Proposed Stage Groupings for Cutaneous
Melanoma (23)

	Clinical staging[a]			Pathological staging[b]		
	T	N	M	T	N	M
0	Tis	N0	M0	Tis	N0	M0
IA	T1a	N0	M0	T1a	N0	M0
IB	T1b	N0	M0	T1b	N0	M0
	T2a	N0	M0	T2a	N0	M0
IIA	T2b	N0	M0	T2b	N0	M0
	T3a	N0	M0	T3a	N0	M0
IIB	T3b	N0	M0	T3b	N0	M0
	T4a	N0	M0	T4a	N0	M0
IIC	T4b	N0	M0	T4b	N0	M0
III[c]	Any T	N1	M0			
		N2				
		N3				
IIIA				T1-4a	N1a	M0
				T1-4a	N2a	M0
IIIB				T1-4b	N1a	M0
				T1-4b	N2a	M0
				T1-4a	N1b	M0
				T1-4a	N2b	M0
				T1-4a/b	N2c	M0
IIIC				T1-4b	N1b	M0
				T1-4b	N2b	M0
				Any T	N3	M0
IV	Any T	Any N	Any M1	Any T	Any N	Any M1

[a]Clinical staging includes microstaging of the primary melanoma and clinical/
radiological evaluation for metastases. By convention, it should be used after
complete excision of the primary with clinical assessment for regional and
distant metastases.
[b]Pathological staging includes microstaging of the primary melanoma and
pathological information about the regional lymph nodes after partial or complete lymphadenectomy. Pathologic stage 0 or stage IA patients are the exception;
they do not require pathological evaluation of their lymph nodes.
[c]There are no stage III subgroups for clinical staging.

Table 48.4 Proposed Staging System for Merkel Cell
Carcinoma (24)

Stage	
I	Primary <2 cm T1, N0, M0
II	Primary ≥2 cm T2, N0, M0
III	Any T, N1, M1
IV	Any T, Any N, M1

Tumors that behave like BCCs require no further imaging. Those
with behavior similar to SCC require evaluation of the draining
lymph node basin while patients with soft tissue sarcoma-like tumors
exhibit a propensity for visceral spread and justify cross-sectional
imaging (29).

Local Staging

Using probe frequencies of up to 60 MHz, US has been used to
assess the thickness of primary cutaneous melanoma with good
correlation to histological thickness, but this technique has not
been further developed and cannot replace pathological staging (30–33).

Computed tomography may elegantly display local soft tissue
extension of some skin tumors (Fig. 48.1A and D), thus aiding
preoperative planning of surgery but it has no role in the routine
assessment of melanoma.

MR imaging has also been used to evaluate skin lesions
(Fig. 48.1B, C, and E) and, in melanoma, differences in the tumor-
to-fat contrast ratio (%T/F contrast) on T2-weighted imaging
allow the differentiation of primary malignant melanoma from
benign pigmented lesions. Benign lesions demonstrate a positive signal ratio whilst a negative value is obtained in primary
cutaneous melanoma. However, this technique is not sufficiently
accurate to avoid excision biopsy of clinically suspicious lesions
and application in clinical practice is seldom justified (34). Both
MR imaging and CT are able to detect perineural spread along
the V and VII cranial nerves by NMSCs of the face and scalp. The
features on imaging are enlargement or abnormal enhancement
of the nerve, loss of the surrounding fat plane, and enlargement
or destruction of the neural foramen. These imaging findings
can be used to plan radiotherapy and may help in predicting
prognosis (35).

Sentinel Node Localization
The technique of sentinel lymph node localization for biopsy was
initially based on the intradermal injection of the vital dyes patent blue-violet and isosulfan blue intraoperatively. However, the
blue dye technique fails to identify the sentinel node in approximately 20% of cases (36,37). Hence two further techniques have
been introduced to aid the identification of the sentinel node;
namely use of a gamma-detecting probe (GDP) and preoperative
dynamic lymphoscintigraphy. These two methods both utilize
intradermal injection of the same radiopharmaceutical but the
GDP method employs a handheld gamma probe during surgery
to identify the sentinel node. Both techniques are complementary
and, when used in combination, result in over 95% sentinel node
identification (37–40). Dynamic lymphoscintigraphy provides
the surgeon with a road map prior to surgery and is of particular
value in cases of unpredictable lymphatic drainage and in the
identification of in-transit lymph nodes lying between the primary tumor and the regional lymph node basin. [18]FDG PET can
detect in-transit disease and nodal basin metastases (Fig. 48.2)
but is not sufficiently sensitive to replace sentinel lymph node
biopsy (SLNB) (41,42).

Although melanoma, SCC, and MCC have a tendency towards
orderly lymph node spread, elective dissection of the draining
lymph node basin is not generally advocated (7,9,43,44). SLNB has
been shown to be of value as a prognostic tool and this has been
confirmed by recent data from the Multicenter Selective Lymphadenectomy Trial 1 (MSLT-1) (45–47). However, suggestions that
this procedure is also associated with a progression-free and overall
survival advantage have been severely criticized (48). At this time it
is reasonable to recommend the use of SLNB as a staging procedure, to stratify patients for clinical trials (48). In some centers
SLNB is being applied to stage other skin tumors (7,43,44,49).
However there is insufficient data to recommend adoption into
routine clinical practice.

Distant Staging
It is clear that the use of routine chest radiography for screening
patients with early-stage melanoma is not justified. A retrospective review of chest radiography in 876 asymptomatic patients
with localized cutaneous melanoma found a true positive rate of
just 0.1% for pulmonary metastases. Furthermore, 135 (15%) of

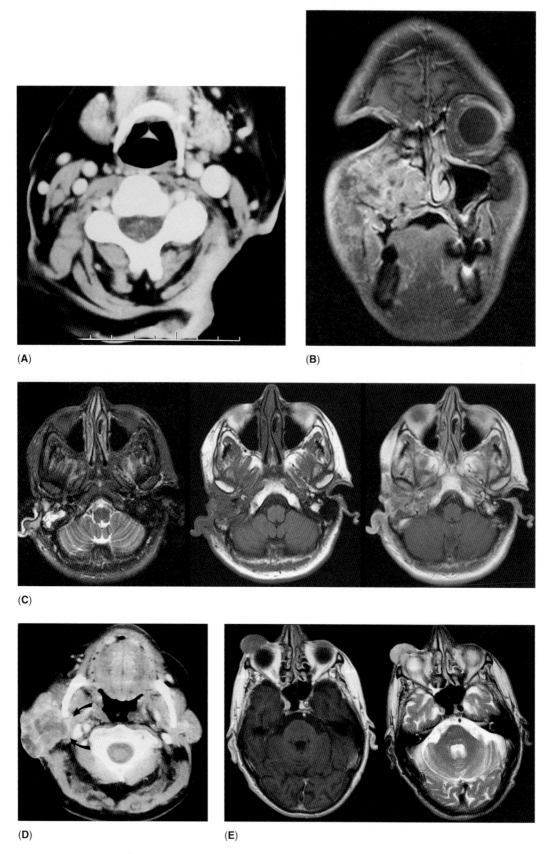

Figure 48.1 Skin involvement. (A) CT of a large, ulcerating, longstanding basal cell carcinoma involving left posterior neck. Note uniform enhancement of 1 cm thick tissue in the base of the ulcer and the characteristic "rolled edge." (B) Coronal T1-weighted post-gadolinium MR image of an advanced locally recurrent Basal cell carcinoma (BCC) in the right maxillary sinus and nasal airway following previous right eye enucleation. (C) STIR, T1 pre- and T1 post-gadolinium MR images of a locally advanced squamous cell carcinoma (SCC) arising in the skin of the right external auditory canal. (D) Contrast-enhanced CT showing a soft tissue mass centered on the right parotid gland involving the skin. Note heterogeneous enhancement and deep extension behind the mandible (arrows). (E) Axial T1- and T2-weighted MR images of a Merkel cell carcinoma (MCC) of the right eyelid.

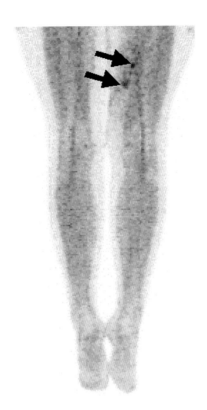

Figure 48.2 In-transit lower limb malignant melanoma metastases (arrows) demonstrated on coronal FDG PET.

patients had focal lesions unrelated to melanoma, necessitating further investigation (50). Thus patients with Stage I or IIA melanomas need no imaging investigation (7). The United Kingdom guidelines still recommend that those with Stage IIB disease and above undergo chest radiography and liver US or contrast-enhanced CT of the chest and abdomen with inclusion of the pelvis and groins when the primary site is a lower limb (7,51). There is a shift towards replacing body CT with PET-CT in high risk melanomas, that is, Stage IIB and above. The United Kingdom PET-CT Board have approved the use of PET-CT in disseminated melanoma to assess the extent of disease and for those with at least Stage II disease where a SLNB was not or cannot be performed (52). However the likelihood of detecting clinically occult distant disease remains very low and so its use has been called into question (53,54). Furthermore in the current context of limited treatment options for metastatic disease the need for imaging confirmation when metastases are clinically suspected should be discussed by a multidisciplinary team (MDT) on an individual patient basis.

The rarity of MCC militates against the establishment of imaging algorithms. Most experience lies with CT, with some authorities recommending coverage of the chest, abdomen, and pelvis to search for metastases after histological diagnosis (55,56). Given MCC's often high mitotic activity ^{18}F-FDG PET-CT is usually positive for metastases and so where available this latter technique can replace CT provided the assumed superior sensitivity is justified by an impact on management (57,58). Octreotide scanning has been successfully employed in the staging of MCC (56).

Key Points: Staging

- There are separate staging systems for NMSC, melanoma, MCC, and KS
- Local staging is pathological
- Elective lymph node dissection is not recommended
- Sentinel node biopsy for lymph node staging has been used in SCC and MCC but is most established for melanoma
- Patients with melanoma staged as IIB and above are currently recommended to undergo imaging investigation if SLNB cannot be performed, but imaging should be individually tailored through MDT discussion

CLINICAL FEATURES

Dermatological diagnosis is based on visual pattern recognition. Basal cell carcinoma is typically a smooth non-pigmented ulcerating nodule exhibiting a pearly appearance, telangiectasia, and a rolled edge.

Melanoma assumes several forms. The nodular type typically presents as a brown/black nodule whilst the superficial spreading form appears as a flat, irregular plaque. The trunk especially the back is the most frequent site in males whilst melanoma in females typically arises on the legs. The British Association of Dermatologists has published evidence-based guidelines for the prevention, surveillance, recognition, and referral of suspected melanoma (7). A typical MCC is less than 2 cm in diameter and is a red/violaceous dome-shaped nodule or indurated plaque on the head, neck, or limbs. Larger tumors may ulcerate (2).

Epidemiological descriptions of KS categorize the disease into four groups:

- Classical KS, a slowly progressive cutaneous tumor of the lower limbs
- Endemic African KS
- Epidemic (AIDS-related) KS
- Iatrogenic or transplant-related KS (25)

The clinical features and behavior of cutaneous KS vary according to the epidemiology of the disease. The lesions themselves are typically red, purple, or brown nodules, plaques, or patches (25).

PROGNOSIS

Prognosis in all skin cancers is markedly improved by early detection and this particularly applies to melanoma and MCC. Generally, local recurrence rates and metastatic potential for most cutaneous malignancies are highly variable and depend on the prognostic factors that have been determined for each tumor type. For SCC and BCC, prognostic factors include tumor site, size, depth (SCC), marginal definition (BCC), histological type/differentiation, local recurrence, and host immunocompetence (59). Most patients with SCC have an excellent prognosis but 10-year survival rate is dramatically reduced to 20% by the presence of regional nodal metastases and to 10% when there is disseminated disease (10).

Malignant melanoma confined to the epidermis is effectively curable. The five-year survival for patients in England and Wales diagnosed during the period 2000–2001 was 78% for men and

91% for women. Thin tumors without nodal spread have a five-year survival greater than 95% (5). Tumor thickness and ulceration are the most powerful predictors of survival in early-stage (I and II) disease. Sentinel lymph node status is overall the most powerful prognostic predictor in melanoma (53). Metastatic site determines the survival of Stage IV patients, with skin, subcutaneous, and distant nodes being more favorable than lung and other visceral organ involvement (59). Mean survival of patients with disseminated disease is seven to eight months (60).

MCC is potentially highly aggressive with doubling times measured in days (61). There is a tendency for local and nodal recurrence, which exceeds that of malignant melanoma (62,55). However there is variable behavior and like melanoma lymph node status is the most important prognostic predictor with long survival reported in pathologically node negative patients (61).

Other aggressive tumors which metastasize widely include:

- Sebaceous carcinoma—metastasizes to lacrimal system as well as hematogenous and lymph node sites (63)
- Malignant sweat gland tumors—five-year survival is less than 30% (64)
- Malignant fibrous histiocytoma with muscle invasion spreads to lung, liver, lymph nodes, and bone (2)
- Angiosarcomas metastasize widely, resulting in a five-year survival rate of only 10% (2)
- Cutaneous leiomyosarcoma rarely metastasizes, in contrast to leiomyosarcoma of the subcutis, which disseminates in 30% of patients, usually to the lungs (2)
- African KS and epidemic KS usually have a poor prognosis but newer therapies are having an impact. The prognosis in transplant-related KS is dependent on the degree of immunocompetence (25)

The survival of patients with primary cutaneous lymphoma is highly variable, being dependent on cell type and stage and has been detailed elsewhere (65).

The behavior of Langerhans' cell histiocytosis (LCH) is not uniform and there are reports of spontaneous regression in some cases, whereas highly aggressive forms may exhibit generalized cutaneous involvement, lymphadenopathy, and pulmonary metastases (66–68).

Key Points: Prognosis

- Prognosis is markedly improved by early detection
- NMSC prognosis is determined by site, size, depth, margin, and histological differentiation
- Melanoma prognosis is most dependent on thickness and ulceration in thin tumors
- SLN status is a powerful prognostic predictor in melanoma and MCC
- Survival in Stage IV melanoma is determined by site of metastasis

TREATMENT OPTIONS

Treatment of primary skin tumors is typically surgical and generally includes a wide excision margin (2,3,69). Surgical margins for various tumors have been studied and recommendations published (7–9,62,70,71). By way of example a 1 cm margin is adequate for melanomas smaller than 2 mm and a 2 cm margin is recommended for thicker melanomas (48).

A range of alternative surgical and non-surgical options are available for some cutaneous malignancies, for example, BCCs and SCCs, and include curettage, cryosurgery, carbon dioxide laser surgery, radiotherapy, topical 5-fluorouracil, and intralesional interferon. The choice of therapy depends on an assessment of tumor characteristics, patient performance status and preference, as well as local expertise (8,9).

Elective lymph node dissection is not routinely recommended in malignant melanoma and ideally, sentinel node biopsy for staging thicker tumors should be undertaken. When draining nodes are deemed suspicious clinically or radiologically, fine needle aspiration cytology (FNAC) should be performed and repeated if necessary. Open biopsy should be considered where there is continuing strong suspicion despite negative cytology. Node-positive patients should be fully staged by imaging and should undergo nodal dissection in limited disease (7).

Malignant melanoma is chemoresistent with decarbazine achieving a response rate of less than 10% (72). Hence the net has been cast wide to identify an effective novel therapy. However despite numerous trials the results have been uniformly disappointing. Most attention has focused on interferon-alpha which has gained the approval of international medicines agencies. However the survival benefits are marginal and its use in practice limited (48). A greater understanding of the behavior of individual melanomas and the host's response to it is more likely to yield positive results than treating the disease and patients as a homogenous group. Driven by the lack of effective therapies and the increasing health burden of the disease, research has now turned to gaining an understanding of angio- and lymphangiogenesis in melanoma and to identifying inhibitors to these tumor survival mechanisms (73).

Solitary local or regional recurrence is best treated surgically. When there is bulky or symptomatic locoregional/in-transit disease isolated limb perfusion with Melphalan and tumor necrosis factor alpha should be considered as it can be effective (74). Isolated or limited metastases might be considered for resection or aggressive radiotherapy (7,75).

For MCC, initial surgical excision forms the mainstay of treatment. Primary site radiotherapy is recommended for tumors greater than 2 cm or when a sufficient resection margin is not achievable. While as yet no clear conclusions can be drawn on the role or impact of SLNB, locoregional radiotherapy is recommended regardless of stage (61). Adjuvant chemotherapy is not supported by trial data (61). In metastatic disease there are a number of chemotherapy regimens which offer good response rates (61). Unfortunately, treatment responses are seldom sustained (76). Consistent with the neuroendocrine nature of MCC, responses to somatostatin have been reported (77).

HAART has significantly reduced the prevalence and improved survival in AIDS-related KS (78). Hence this forms the basis of treatment. There are several local therapeutic options. Palliative radiotherapy for selected symptomatic skin lesions is often effective. Photodynamic therapy, cryotherapy, laser, and intralesional chemotherapy can achieve local control (78). Systemic chemotherapy in the form of liposomal anthracyclines and taxanes are used in high burden disease or immune reconstitution flare when performance status and organ function allow (78). Novel therapies under investigation for AIDS-related KS include angiogenesis inhibitors, tyrosine kinase inhibitors such as imatinib, and matrix metalloproteinase inhibitors (78).

Key Points: Treatment

- Surgical resection is generally the treatment of choice
- There are recommended resection margins for the various skin tumors
- SLNB may be beneficial in selected melanoma patients
- Resection of limited malignant melanoma metastases should be considered
- Melanoma is a chemoresistant disease and novel therapies have been disappointing to date
- Limited stage MCC should be treated aggressively with surgery and radiotherapy

SURVEILLANCE

The merits of imaging in the follow-up of melanoma is dubious given that the majority (89–94%) of recurrences are detected by self-examination or by clinical assessment.

A 10-year review of Stage I malignant melanoma in a single practice found that just 10% of relapses were detected on chest radiography and abdominal US and CT conferred no benefit (79). Unsurprisingly, there is a lack of consensus as to the best method of postoperative surveillance but the cornerstone of follow-up appears to comprise clinic visits, chest radiography, full blood count, and liver function tests. More sophisticated radiological tests are rarely employed on a routine basis and should be reserved for clinically suspected relapse (80,81).

Follow-up US of the melanoma resection site, lymphatic track, and regional lymph node basin is more sensitive for the detection of recurrence (89.2%) than clinical examination (71.4%) (82). This US technique has not been widely adopted in United Kingdom practice. However the argument for its use may strengthen as there is a further movement away from a unified surgical approach towards more tailored treatment, provided biologically lower risk patients can be identified (48).

Key Points: Surveillance

- Self-examination and clinical examination detect most recurrences
- Recommendations for clinical surveillance are published
- Chest radiography detects few relapses
- US may prove useful in the early detection of lymph node metastases particularly as there is a move away from primary lymphadenectomy and SLNB

METASTATIC DISEASE

The known limitations of size as a marker of response assessment are compounded by the growing use of novel therapies where shrinkage may be delayed or minimal despite a good early response (see chap. 6). Metabolic imaging and blood flow changes using contrast-enhanced cross-sectional imaging and US microbubbles are being examined in such settings and are likely to become more attractive options are detecting and monitoring skin cancer metastases if anti-angiogenic therapies prove effective (83).

Melanoma

Initially, malignant melanoma has a predictable pattern of spread with involvement of the regional lymph node basin, and this is the rationale for sentinel lymph node sampling in staging and initial surgical management. Once the tumor escapes the regional draining nodes it becomes far less predictable and has the potential to involve virtually any site within the body. This wide and random dissemination potential has stimulated interest in [18]FDG PET in the identification of sites of metastatic melanoma but, to date, the use of CT remains predominant.

In descending order of frequency, the most common sites for metastases in malignant melanoma at autopsy are:

- Lymph nodes (74%)
- Lungs (71%)
- Soft tissues (68%)
- Liver (58%)
- Brain (55%)
- Bone (49%)
- Adrenal glands (47%)
- Gastrointestinal tract (44%) (84)

Lymph Nodes

On US, metastatic nodal disease is suspected when nodes have increased in size, show loss of their central echogenic hilum on grey scale US and loss of their hilar vessels on color Doppler, and tend to be round rather than oval shape (85). CT and MR imaging rely on established size criteria (see chap. 40) (Fig. 48.3). PET-CT is also able to detect in-transit and other lymph node metastases (Fig. 48.2) but is less accurate than SLNB. In our experience, splenic deposits are unusual in the absence of liver lesions. The size of splenic deposits and their characteristics on US and MR imaging are variable but typically they are hypodense on CT (Fig. 48.4) (86).

Lung

Pulmonary metastases in melanoma usually number at least five (Fig. 48.5), although a single lung nodule in a patient with melanoma is still more likely to be a metastasis than a primary bronchogenic carcinoma (87,88). When deposits are few in number, or preferably solitary, and there has been a long disease-free interval of at least 36 months, there is potential for prolonged remission following pulmonary metastasectomy (89,90).

Skin and Soft Tissues

Not surprisingly the skin and subcutaneous tissues are the most frequent soft tissue site for metastatic melanoma and the lesions are usually clinically evident. The distribution of muscle metastases reflects the relative muscle mass, hence the lower limb is most frequently affected (Fig. 48.6) (91). Sonographic appearances of melanoma metastases in the skin and subcutaneous tissues are typically those of a well-defined, smooth-bordered, heterogeneous mass, hypoechoic to muscle. One-third of deposits are isoechoic. Hyperechogenicity is a rare finding being seen in just 6% of patients. Over 70% of lesions demonstrate enhanced acoustics through transmission and internal arterial flow on color Doppler (92). On CT, skin, subcutaneous, and muscle deposits are often

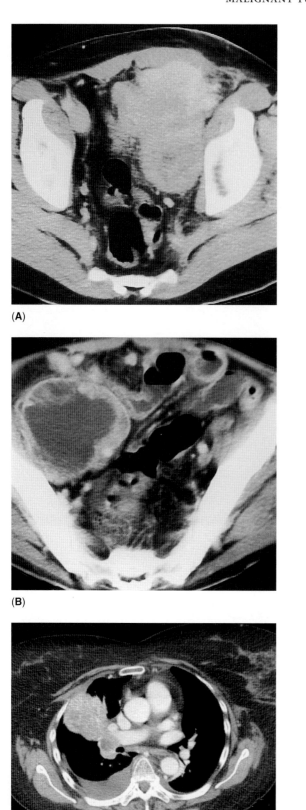

(A)

(B)

(C)

Figure 48.3 Nodal metastases. Large volume metastasis to pelvic lymph nodes from malignant melanoma. CT demonstrates the varying appearances ranging between (**A**) solid enhancing tumor and (**B**) cystic degeneration. Both masses remain relatively well-defined. (**C**) Contrast-enhanced CT showing large volume hilar nodal involvement from malignant melanoma with a large pulmonary metastasis and a pleural effusion.

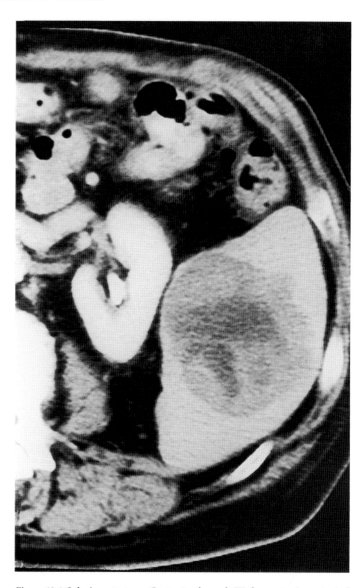

Figure 48.4 Splenic metastases. Contrast-enhanced CT demonstrating a typical well-defined, relatively non-enhancing malignant melanoma metastasis in the spleen.

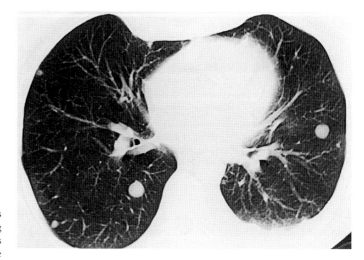

Figure 48.5 Pulmonary metastases. CT showing multiple well-defined pulmonary metastases from malignant melanoma.

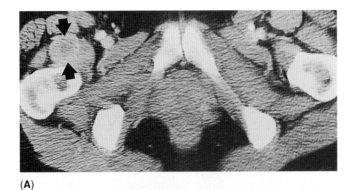

(A)

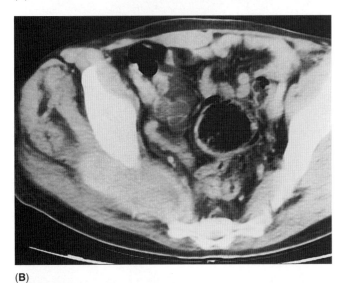

(B)

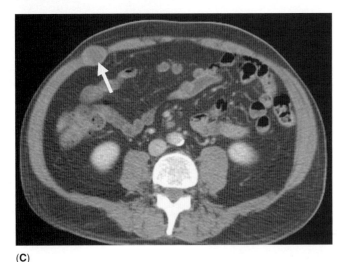

(C)

Figure 48.6 Muscle metastases. (**A**) A well-defined enhancing malignant melanoma metastasis in the right ileo-psoas on CT (arrows). (**B**) CT scan showing an enhancing metastasis replacing the right pyriformis and extending through the sciatic notch into overlying gluteal muscles. Note absence of bone erosion despite close application by soft tissue mass. (**C**) Muscle metastasis from malignant melanoma on staging CT (arrow).

well-defined and may show variable vascular enhancement (Figs. 48.6 and 48.7). Even small deposits can be avid enough for PET-CT detection (Fig. 48.8). On MR imaging, the majority of soft tissue melanoma metastases have non-specific signal intensity characteristics.

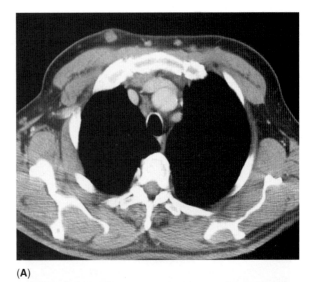

(A)

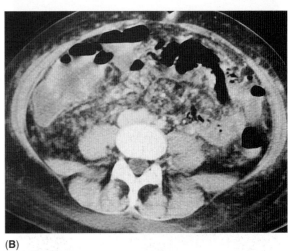

(B)

Figure 48.7 Subcutaneous metastases. (**A**) CT showing small volume mediastinal nodal enlargement and multiple subcutaneous deposits. (**B**) CT showing showers of metastases in the subcutaneous tissue, abdominal peritoneum, and mesentery.

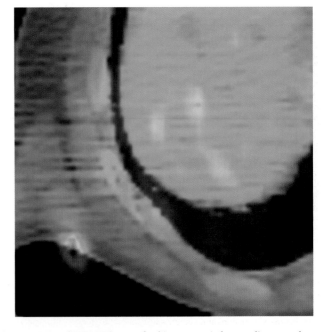

Figure 48.8 Fused PET-CT image of a skin metastasis from malignant melanoma.

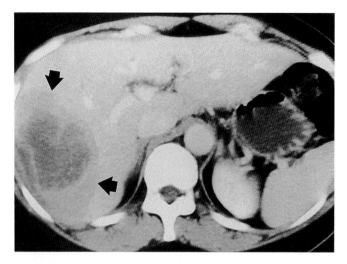

Figure 48.9 Liver metastases. Hepatic CT in the portal venous phase of contrast enhancement showing a large metastasis in the right lobe of the liver (arrows) from metastatic malignant melanoma.

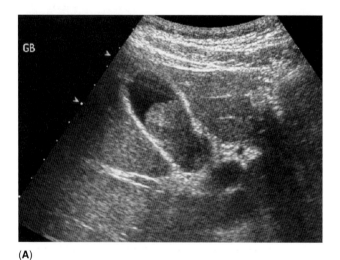

(A)

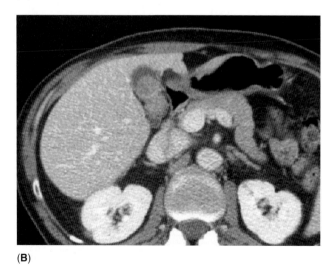

(B)

Figure 48.10 Gallbladder metastases. (A) Biliary ultrasound showing a large echogenic, non-shadowing polypoid metastasis in the gall bladder from malignant melanoma. (B) CT showing a soft tissue density mass in the gallbladder, subsequently shown to be malignant melanoma when the patient developed obstructive jaundice associated with occluding tumor in the biliary tree.

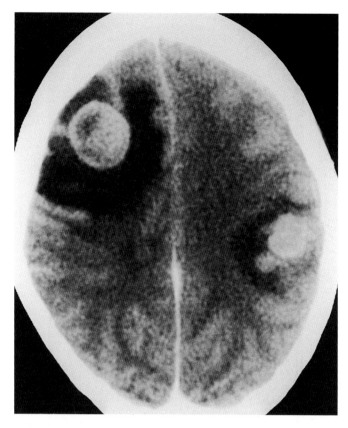

Figure 48.11 Brain metastases. Contrast-enhanced CT of the brain demonstrating typical avidly enhancing metastases from malignant melanoma with associated surrounding edema.

Liver and Biliary System

The majority of liver metastases from malignant melanoma are of low attenuation on CT when compared to the normal parenchyma (Fig. 48.9). Portal venous phase scanning alone fails to detect 14% of liver deposits but portal venous phase CT combined with either an unenhanced scan or an arterial phase scan shows improved conspicuity and both techniques have similar efficacy for the detection of liver metastases (93). On MR imaging, just 20% to 25% of liver deposits are hyperintense on T1-weighted images and hypo- or isointense on T2-weighted and short tau inversion recovery (STIR) images consistent with a paramagnetic effect of melanin. However, this signal pattern is not specific to melanin-containing deposits as it is also seen in other lesions such as focal fat deposits, intrahepatic hemorrhage or hematoma, and protein-containing lesions. Melanoma metastases are best demonstrated on fat-suppressed T1-weighted spin-echo or STIR images and there appears to be no advantage in using intravenous (IV) contrast medium (94,95). Diffusion-weighted imaging (DWI) may improve detection (96).

Melanoma accounts for more than half of all metastases to the gallbladder (97) (Fig. 48.10) and involvement of the gallbladder is seen in up to 20% of melanoma deaths at autopsy (84,98–100). Biliary involvement is usually clinically occult but, if symptomatic, is likely to mimic acute cholecystitis (99–101). Gallbladder deposits can be single or multiple and they are typically non-shadowing hyperechoic masses on US, with a diameter greater than 1 cm. They are attached to the gallbladder wall and project into the lumen (102,103).

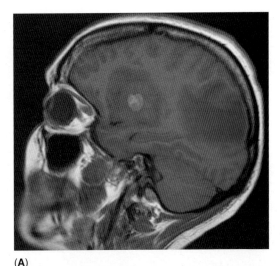

(A)

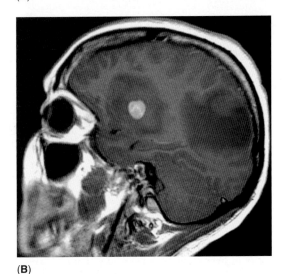

(B)

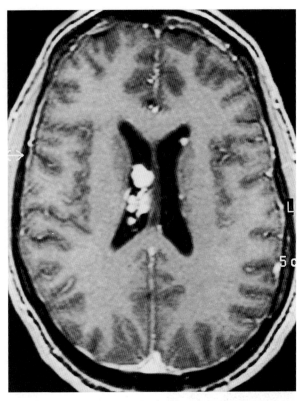

Figure 48.13 Unenhanced T1-weighted axial MR image showing high signal intensity choroidal metastases.

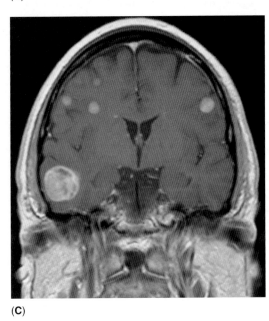

(C)

Figure 48.12 (**A**) T1-weighted pre- and (**B**) post-gadolinium MR images of the brain revealing an enhancing hyper-intense metastasis from malignant melanoma with surrounding vasogenic edema. (**C**) Unenhanced T1-weighted coronal MR images in another patient demonstrating typical well-defined high signal intensity cerebral metastases.

Central Nervous System

Historically the antemortem detection rate for cerebral metastases to the brain is 6% to 10%, but they carry a grave prognosis, with a median survival of four months (104,105). Survival can be prolonged with the use of combination treatment including aggressive targeted radiotherapy (75). Cerebral metastases are typically multiple and supratentorial, although any intracranial site can be involved (105). Peritumoral edema, a nodular contour, uniform enhancement following IV contrast medium and high attenuation on unenhanced CT are characteristic features (Fig. 48.11) (106,107). The MR imaging characteristics are highly variable, with only a quarter of lesions returning "typical" melanotic signal of hyperintensity on T1-weighted images and hypointensity on T2-weighted images relative to the cortex (Figs. 48.12 and 48.13). On histological examination, such metastases tend to have a higher proportion of melanin-containing cells (108). Due to the paramagnetic effect of intra-lesional hemorrhage and melanin, T2* imaging as an additional sequence improves detection (109). PET-CT is less sensitive than MR imaging for the detection of cerebral metastases due to relatively high physiological glucose uptake. However the brain should always be reviewed carefully on PET-CT as lesions can be detected (Fig. 48.14). Intramedullary spinal metastases have similar imaging features to intracerebral deposits (Fig. 48.15) (110).

Gastrointestinal Tract

Melanoma is the most frequently implicated tumor in bloodborne metastases to the gastrointestinal tract (111). In the upper

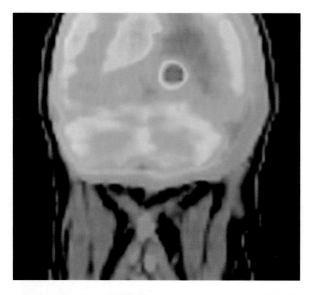

Figure 48.14 Solitary FDG avid brain metastasis on coronal PET-CT.

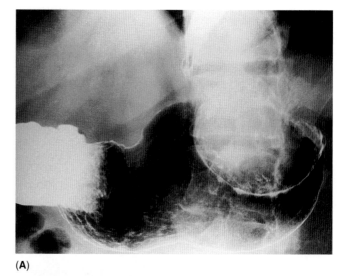

(A)

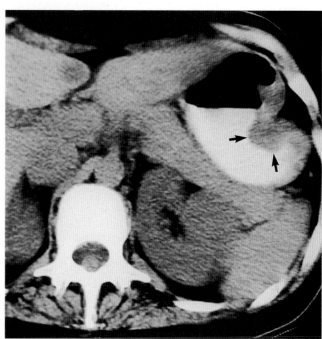

(B)

Figure 48.16 Gastric metastases. (**A**) A large rounded melanoma deposit in the fundus of the stomach is demonstrated on a double contrast barium meal. (**B**) CT showing a metastasis from malignant melanoma protruding into the stomach lumen (arrows).

- Colon
- Rectum
- Esophagus and anus (98)

Deposits within the small bowel often precipitate intussusception and small bowel obstruction. They are typically multiple and polypoid (113). Endoscopy and contrast studies are the investigations of choice as CT has a sensitivity of only 60% to 70% for small bowel metastases (Fig. 48.17). Peritoneal deposits have variable appearances ranging from extensive studding to scattered larger nodules leading to large volume confluent disease (Fig. 48.7B) (114).

Bone

Bone involvement is a late feature of melanoma, being detected in 0.8% to 6.9% of patients within clinical series, most of whom will

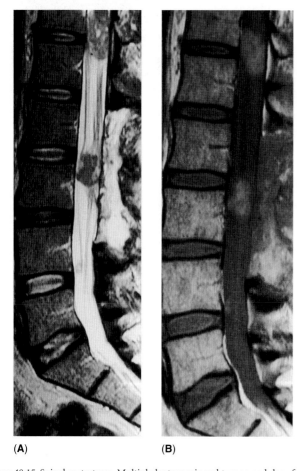

(A)   **(B)**

Figure 48.15 Spinal metastases. Multiple leptomeningeal tumor nodules of melanoma within the spinal canal. (**A**) T2-weighted sagittal MR image shows low signal intensity lesions, and (**B**) unenhanced T1-weighted image showing characteristic high signal intensity due to the paramagnetic features of melanin.

region, the tongue, and tonsil are the prime sites (112) but distal to the hypopharynx in descending order of frequency are:

- Small bowel
- Stomach (Fig. 48.16)

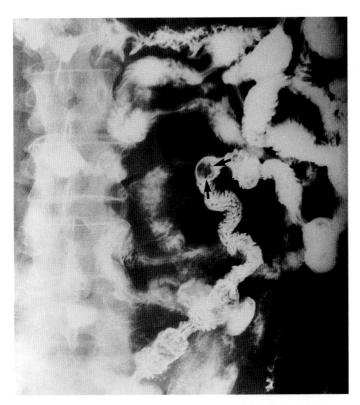

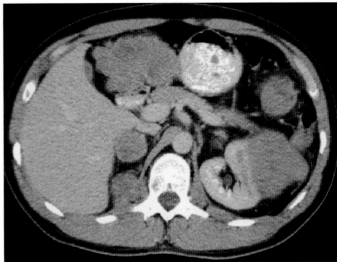

Figure 48.19 Abdominal metastases. Contrast-enhanced CT showing renal, adrenal, retroperitoneal, and peritoneal metastases.

Figure 48.17 A barium follow-through examination of a patient presenting with recurrent malignant melanoma. A polypoidal small bowel metastasis (arrows) was resected.

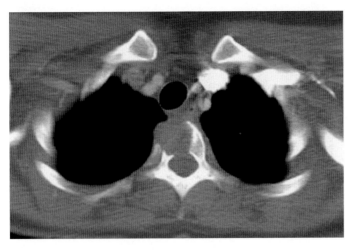

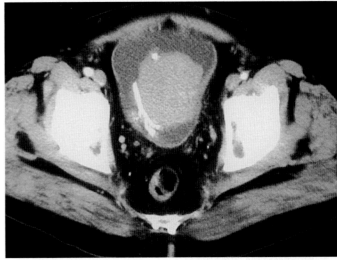

Figure 48.20 Bladder metastases. CT showing a large metastasis arising from the left wall of the bladder. Note urinary stent in situ.

Figure 48.18 Bone metastases. CT showing a metastasis in a thoracic vertebral body which subsequently collapsed despite radiotherapy.

have other sites of disease (115–117). They are indistinguishable from other osteolytic metastases on imaging and pathological fracture occurs in nearly a quarter of patients (Fig. 48.18), while soft tissue invasion (12.5%), marginal sclerosis (12.5%), and osteo-blastic deposits are atypical. Bone scintigraphy has a false negative rate of 15% in the spine, making MR imaging the investigation of choice in the search for metastatic disease (115,117).

Pancreas

The pancreas is an unusual site for metastases but up to 42% of patients with metastases will have multiple pancreatic deposits. The imaging features are broadly similar to primary adenocarcinoma

of the pancreas as compared with normal pancreatic parenchyma these lesions are hypoechoic on US and of relatively low attenua-tion on CT. However, peri-pancreatic fat infiltration, duct obstruc-tion, and vascular invasion are seldom featured in melanoma metastases (118).

Genito-Urinary Tract

The kidney is the most commonly involved site of metastatic disease in the urinary tract followed by the bladder and urinary collecting system (119). Melanoma metastasizing to the urethra has been described (120). Renal metastases are typically small, multiple, and cortical. Rarely, these lesions may manifest as a large parenchymal mass with similar appearances to those of renal cell carcinoma (Fig. 48.19) (119,121). Collecting system, ureteric, and bladder metastases (Fig. 48.20) are more likely to provoke symptom

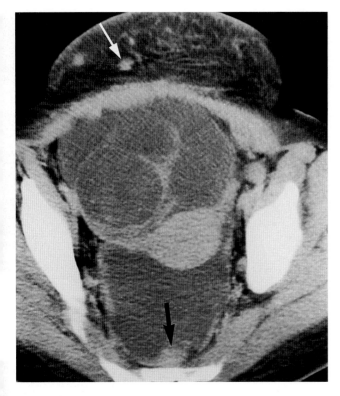

Figure 48.21 Ovarian metastases. CT showing a thick-walled multiloculate ovarian cyst in a patient with extensive metastatic malignant melanoma. Note fluid and peritoneal plaques (black arrow) in the Pouch of Douglas as well as subcutaneous deposits anteriorly (white arrow).

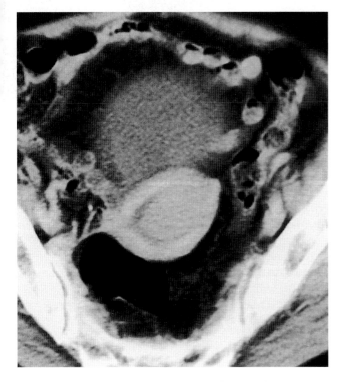

Figure 48.22 Uterine metastases. CT showing a malignant melanoma metasatsis as a poorly enhancing homogeneous density expanding the endometrial cavity. Diagnosis was confirmed when continuous bleeding required hysterectomy.

than renal disease and this will therefore trigger investigation. The urographic findings of single or multiple, smooth or irregular filling defects are clearly non-specific but, in the clinical context of malignant melanoma, the appearances should raise the suspicion of disseminated disease (119,121–123).

The female genital tract is more frequently and extensively involved than the male genital tract (124). The ovaries are the most commonly affected site presenting with uni- or bilateral involvement with large, smooth, lobulated solid or solid/cystic masses (Fig. 48.21). The imaging features tend to be non-specific on all modalities, including MR imaging, as only a minority contain significant quantities of melanin (125–127). Endometrial and placental metastases are rare (Fig. 48.22) (128).

The testis is more frequently involved than the penis and in itself is a rare antemortem diagnosis. The testicular mass is often suspected to be a primary testicular neoplasm and a history of primary melanoma may be crucial in aiding diagnosis (129,130). Melanoma metastasizing to the prostate has been reported (131).

Endocrine System

The adrenal gland is the most frequently involved endocrine organ. In clinical studies, adrenal metastases have a mean diameter of 4 cm although much smaller lesions can be resolved particularly on PET-CT (Fig. 48.23). They are usually unilateral but at autopsy they are typically found to be bilateral (84,94,132).

A new thyroid abnormality in a patient with disseminated malignancy has been reported as three times more likely to be due to a metastasis than a new primary tumor (133). Metastases to the thyroid from several primary sites, including malignant melanoma, exhibit diminished activity on scintigraphy and are typically solid, homogeneous, and hypoechoic on US, thus warranting FNAC. Thyroid function is almost invariably normal (133–135).

One-fifth of patients with cerebral metastases at autopsy also have disease involving the hypothalamus or pituitary gland (124).

Breast

Indistinguishable from a primary breast lesion, melanoma metastasizing to the breast often presents as a solitary, painless mass in the upper outer quadrant requiring tissue sampling for definitive diagnosis (Fig. 48.24) (136). In a case report of bilateral breast metastases, MR imaging showed that all five lesions had a high signal intensity on T1-weighted images and low signal intensity on T2-weighted images (137). It is recommended that, even in the presence of more widespread visceral disease, resection of melanoma metastases should be performed in order to achieve local control (137,138).

Cardiovascular System

Melanoma has a propensity for metastasizing to the heart, particularly the myocardium of the right-sided chambers (139,140). The discrepancy between ante- and postmortem detection rates of 1% and approximately 50% respectively, reflects the small size

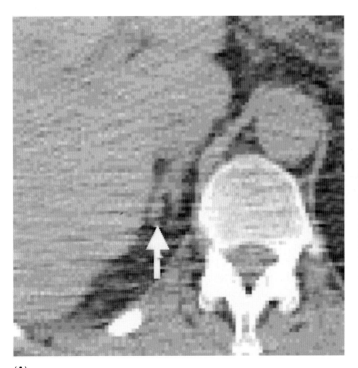

(A)

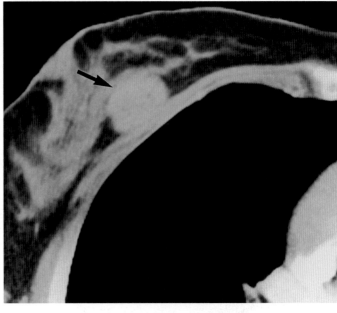

Figure 48.24 Breast metastases. Contrast-enhanced CT showing a well-defined ovoid enhancing malignant melanoma deposit (arrow) deep within the tissue of the right breast.

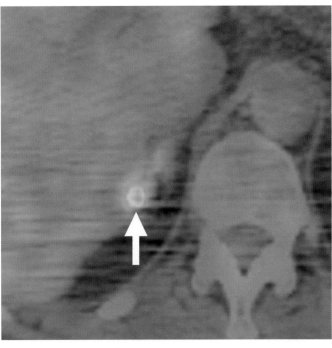

(B)

Figure 48.23 Adrenal metastases. (**A**) CT and (**B**) PET-CT of a small but intensely FDG-avid adrenal metastasis (arrows) from malignant melanoma.

Key Points: Malignant Melanoma Metastases

- Initial predictable route of spread is to locoregional lymph nodes
- On MR imaging the majority of melanoma metastases do not demonstrate high signal intensity on T1-weighted images
- Pulmonary metastasectomy may prolong survival in those with limited disease
- Lower limbs are the most frequent site of muscle deposits
- Twenty to twenty-five percent of liver metastases have high signal intensity on T1-weighting and low signal intensity on T2-weighting
- Melanoma accounts for more than 50% of all metastases to the gallbladder
- Brain metastases carry a poor prognosis
- Malignant melanoma is the most frequent cause of metastases to the gastrointestinal tract
- Bone involvement is a late feature of the disease
- Pancreatic deposits are uncommon and are multiple in 42% of cases
- Renal involvement may mimic primary renal cell carcinoma
- Ovarian metastases are the most common manifestation of involvement of the genital tract
- Most adrenal metastases identified on imaging are large (>4 cm) unilateral lesions
- Breast metastases are usually solitary and non-specific
- Cardiac metastases are seldom detected during life

of these deposits and lack of symptoms. Tachycardia, dyspnea, and features of right heart failure in a patient with malignant melanoma should prompt echocardiography (140,141). Cardiac MR imaging is complementary to echocardiography; CT can also demonstrate large melanoma metastases and pericardial disease (Fig. 48.25) (141,142).

Squamous Cell Carcinoma

Although considerably more common than melanoma, SCC demonstrates a comparatively low propensity to metastasize and

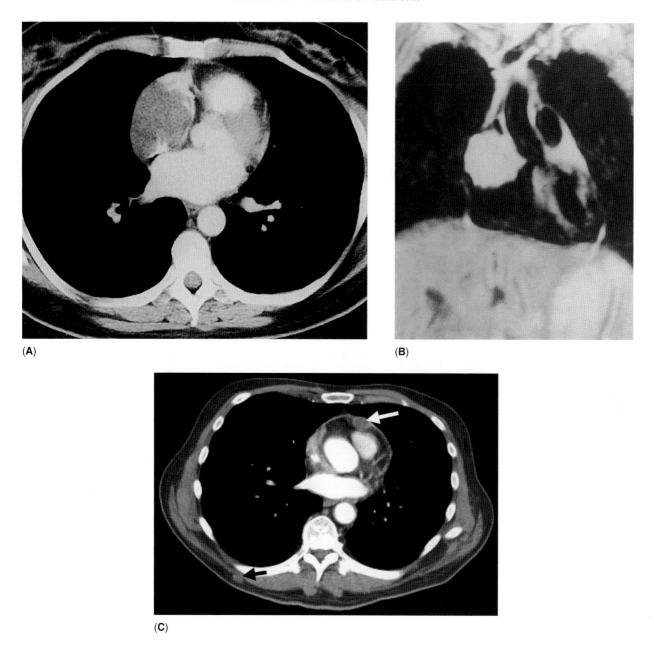

Figure 48.25 Cardiac metastases. (A) Contrast-enhanced CT and (B) coronal MR image demonstrating a large mass from malignant melanoma which almost fills the right atrium. (C) One of two pericardial metastases from malignant melanoma (white arrow). A subcutaneous metastasis is shown on the same image (black arrow).

deposits are seen in only 2% to 3% of cases (143–145). The majority of these will involve the locoregional lymph nodes and only 15% spread to more distant nodal sites (10). Lymph node metastases frequently exhibit central low density and avid rim enhancement on contrast-enhanced CT. Although rare, hematogenous spread to distant sites, including lungs, liver, brain, skin, and bone have been reported. Pulmonary metastases are typically multiple and may cavitate (146).

Basal Cell Carcinoma

Metastatic BCC is extremely rare, with a reported incidence of only 0.0028% to 0.55% (147). The median time interval from primary diagnosis to metastatic disease is nine years and the five-year survival thereafter is just 10% (148,149). The sites for metastatic disease in descending order of frequency are the lymph nodes, lungs, skin, liver, and pleura. Deposits in the kidney, spleen, heart, adrenal glands, brain, and bowel have also been reported (148).

Merkel Cell Carcinoma

Similar to malignant melanoma, once MCC has spread beyond the regional nodal basin it has a propensity for wide and unpredictable dissemination. There is a dearth of literature on the description of MCC metastases. Due to the propensity for head and neck involvement (>50% of cases), lymph node metastases in the neck, especially level 2, are a frequent finding (77). Beyond the draining nodal basin any nodal group may be involved. Lymph node metastases are hyper- or iso-attenuating to muscle on contrast-enhanced CT (56).

Subcutaneous and muscle deposits are described which once again show iso- or hyper-attenuation compared to muscle on contrast-enhanced CT (56). Chest involvement can present as nodal disease, intrapulmonary nodules, and masses or bone/chest

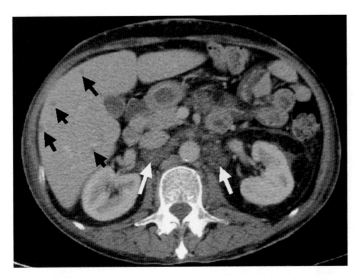

Figure 48.26 Kaposi sarcoma. Contrast-enhanced CT of a patient with Kaposi sarcoma showing retroperitoneal lymph node enlargement (white arrows) and small volume liver metastases (black arrows).

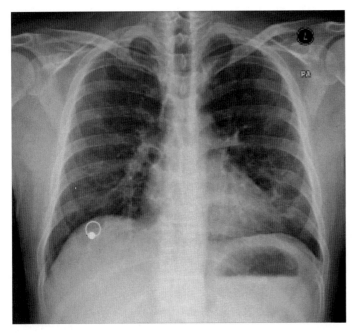

Figure 48.27 Pulmonary Kaposi sarcoma. Chest radiograph showing multiple irregular pulmonary nodules.

wall invasion. In common with melanoma, both solid-organ and hollow visceral disease can occur in the abdomen, and pelvis. The liver is a frequently targeted abdominal organ, with metastases typically demonstrating ring enhancement on contrast-enhanced CT (77,56).

The central nervous system (CNS) is not a frequent metastatic site but neurological symptoms/signs usually warrant MR examination. CNS metastases from MCC may show central necrosis (77,150).

Owing to the neuroendocrine origin of Merkel cells, assessment of recurrent and metastatic disease is amenable to somatostatin receptor scintigraphy (SRS) using indium-111-labelled octreotide. Although demonstrating good specificity in MCC, this technique lacks sensitivity, particularly in the skin and in organs that demonstrate physiological octreotide uptake, most notably the liver and spleen (77,151). 18FDG PET-CT has been successfully used in the assessment of response of MCC to isolated limb perfusion in a single case (152).

Kaposi's Sarcoma

Kaposi's sarcoma is a multifocal neoplasm with each new visceral lesion developing *de novo* from the endothelial cells lining the lymphatics or blood vessels rather than representing metastases from mucocutaneous neoplasms (153). In classical KS, skin lesions can regress whilst new lesions appear. The sites of involvement beyond the skin are numerous, including lymph nodes, bowel, liver, lungs, kidneys, and spleen (Fig. 48.26). Testicular and cerebral disease is rare. Visceral lesions are usually only seen in the presence of cutaneous disease (153). The lymphadenopathic form of endemic African KS is an aggressive form involving the lymph nodes, and occasionally visceral organs, of children (153).

Epidemic (AIDS-related) KS can affect the lymphatics and viscera, e.g., lungs, liver, gastrointestinal tract, spleen, and kidneys with mucocutaneous disease not being a prerequisite (153). Lymphedema can be marked and disproportionate to the degree of skin involvement (78). Chest radiographic findings in pulmonary KS include (Fig. 48.27):

- Peribronchovascular opacities (86%)
- Lung nodules (71%)
- Pleural effusion (41%)
- Interlobular septal thickening (29%)
- Lymphadenopathy (29%) (154)

CT may also reveal patchy ground glass attenuation surrounding or separate from nodules, and distortion and nodularity of the fissures (155). Iatrogenic or transplant-related KS is usually confined to the skin, with visceral involvement being atypical (153).

Key Points: Metastatic Disease

- SCC, melanoma, and MCC predictably metastasize to the draining nodal basin
- Melanoma and MCC have a tendency towards disseminated unpredictable spread beyond the regional lymph nodes
- SCC metastasizes in 2% to 3% of cases and BCC very rarely

Summary

- Malignant tumors of the skin form a disparate group of cancers with a wide range of behaviors
- Skin cancer is the most common human malignancy
- Skin tumors are categorized according to cellular origin and the common forms divided into non-melanoma skin cancer and melanoma
- Staging is pathological
- Elective lymph node dissection is not recommended
- Nodal staging with FNAC or sentinel node biopsy should be considered
- Surgical excision of the primary tumour is generally the treatment of choice

- Surveillance largely relies on self-examination and clinical follow-up
- Metastasis of SCC, melanoma, and MCC is usually initially to the regional lymph nodes
- Melanoma and MCC have a propensity to wide and unpredictable spread
- Increasingly, [18]FDG PET-CT forms the basis for investigation of metastatic disease
- Functional imaging techniques will need to evolve to deal with the shortcomings of established anatomical imaging techniques for both detection and response assessment

REFERENCES

1. Bruce AJ, Brodland DG. Overview of skin cancer detection and prevention for the primary care physician. Mayo Clin Proc 2000; 75: 491–500.

2. Brown MD. Recognition and management of unusual cutaneous tumors. Dermatol Clin 2000; 18: 543–52.

3. Skidmore RA Jr, Flowers FP. Non-melanoma skin cancer. Med Clin North Am 1998; 82: 1309–23.

4. Diepgen TL, Mahler V. The epidemiology of skin cancer. Br J Dermatol 2002; 146 (Suppl 61): 1–6.

5. Cancer Research UK CancerStats. [Available from: http://info.cancerresearchuk.org/cancerstats].

6. Cancer Facts and Figures 2008, American Cancer Society. [Available from: www.acs.org].

7. Roberts DL, Anstey AV, Barlow RJ, et al. The British Association of Dermatologists: The Melanoma Study Group. UK guidelines for the management of cutaneous melanoma. Br J Dermatol 2002; 146: 7–17.

8. Telfer NR, Colver GB, Bowers PW. Guidelines for the management of basal cell carcinoma. British Association of Dermatologists. Br J Dermatol 1999; 141: 415–23.

9. Motley R, Kersey P, Lawrence C. The British Association of Dermatologists: The British Association of Plastic Surgeons: The Royal College of Radiologists, Faculty of Clinical Oncology. Multiprofessional guidelines for the management of the patient with primary cutaneous squamous cell carcinoma. Br J Dermatol 2002; 146: 18–25.

10. Murad A, Ratner D. Primary care: cutaneous squamous cell carcinoma. N Engl J Med 2001; 344: 975–83.

11. Quinn M, Babb P, Brock A, Kirby L, Jones J. Cancer Trends in England & Wales 1950–1999, SMPS No. 66. Norwich: The Stationery Office, 2001.

12. El Ghissassi F, Baan R, Straif K, et al., on behalf of the WHO International Agency for Research on Cancer Monograph Working Group. A review of human carcinogens — Part D: radiation. Lancet Oncol 2009; 10: 751–2.

13. International Commission on Non-Ionizing Radiation Protection, Health Issues of Ultraviolet Tanning Appliances Used for Cosmetic Purposes. ICNIRP Statement, 2003.

14. World Health Organization. WHO guidance brochure: artificial tanning sunbeds—risks and guidance, 2003.

15. Kefford RF, Newton Bishop JA, Bergman W, Tucker MA. Counselling and DNA testing for individuals perceived to be genetically predisposed to melanoma: a consensus statement of the Melanoma Genetics Consortium. J Clin Oncol 1999; 17: 3245–51.

16. Berg D, Otley CC. Skin cancer in organ transplant recipients: epidemiology, pathogenesis, and management. J Am Acad Dermatol 2002; 47: 1–17.

17. Jensen P, Hansen S, Moller B, et al. Skin cancer in kidney and heart transplant recipients and different long-term immunosuppressive therapy regimens. J Am Acad Dermatol 1999; 40: 177–86.

18. Hartevelt MM, Bavinck JN, Kootte AM, et al. Incidence of skin cancer after renal transplantation in The Netherlands. Transplantation 1990; 49: 506–9.

19. Penn I, First MR. Merkel's cell carcinoma in organ recipients: report of 41 cases. Transplantation 1999; 68: 1717–21.

20. Veness MJ, Quinn DI, Ong CS, et al. Aggressive cutaneous malignancies following cardiothoracic transplantation: the Australian experience. Cancer 1999; 85: 1758–64.

21. Penn I. Malignant melanoma in organ allograft recipients. Transplantation 1996; 61: 274–8.

22. Sobin LH, Wittekind Ch, eds. TNM Classification of Malignant Tumours, 6th edn. San Francisco: Wiley-Liss, Inc., 2002.

23. Greene FL, Page DL, Fleming ID, et al., eds. American Joint Committee on Cancer (AJCC) Cancer Staging Handbook, 6th edn. Berlin: Springer, 2002.

24. Allen PJ, Bowne WB, Jaques DP, et al. Merkel cell carcinoma: prognosis and treatment of patients from a single institution. J Clin Oncol. 2005; 23: 2300–9.

25. Aboulafia DM. Kaposi's sarcoma. Clin Dermatol 2001; 19: 269–83.

26. Nasti G, Talamini R, Antinori A, et al. AIDS-related Kaposi's Sarcoma: evaluation of potential new prognostic factors and assessment of the AIDS Clinical Trial Group Staging System in the Haart Era—the Italian Cooperative Group on AIDS and Tumors and the Italian Cohort of Patients Naive From Antiretrovirals. J Clin Oncol 2003; 21: 2876–82.

27. Kim YH, Willemze R, Pimpinelli N, et al. ISCL and the EORTC. TNM classification system for primary cutaneous lymphomas other than mycosis fungoides and Sezary syndrome: a proposal of the International Society for Cutaneous Lymphomas (ISCL) and the Cutaneous Lymphoma Task Force of the European Organization of Research and Treatment of Cancer (EORTC). Blood. 2007; 110: 479–84.

28. Olsen E, Vonderheid E, Pimpinelli N, et al. Revisions to the staging and classification of mycosis fungoides and Sezary syndrome: a proposal of the International Society for Cutaneous Lymphomas (ISCL) and the cutaneous lymphoma task force of the European Organization of Research and Treatment of Cancer (EORTC). Blood 2007; 110: 1713–22.

29. Topping A, Wilson GR. Diagnosis and management of uncommon cutaneous cancers. Am J Clin Dermatol 2002; 3: 83–9.

30. Shafir R, Itzchak Y, Heyman Z, et al. Preoperative ultrasonic measurement of the thickness of cutaneous malignant melanoma. J Ultrasound Med 1984; 3: 205–8.

31. Hoffman K, Jung J, el Gammal S, Altemeyer P. Malignant melanoma in 20 MHz B scan sonography. Dermatology 1992; 185: 49–55.

32. Semple JL, Gupta AK, From L, et al. Does high frequency ultrasound imaging play a role in the clinical management of cutaneous melanoma? Ann Plast Surg 1995; 34: 599–606.

33. Shafir R. Re: Does high frequency ultrasound imaging play a role in the clinical management of cutaneous melanoma? Ann Plast Surg 1996; 36: 599–60.

34. Takahashi M, Kohda H. Diagnostic utility of magnetic resonance imaging in malignant melanoma. J Am Acad Dermatol 1992; 27: 51–4.

35. Williams LS, Mancuso AA, Mendenhall WM. Perineural spread of cutaneous squamous and basal cell carcinoma: CT and MR detection and its impact on patient management and prognosis. Int J Radiat Oncol Biol Phys 2001; 49: 1061–9.

36. Morton DL, Wen D-R, Wong JH, et al. Technical details of intraoperative lymphatic mapping for early-stage melanoma. Arch Surg 1992; 127: 392–9.

37. Gennari R, Bartolomei M, Testori A, et al. Sentinel node localisation in primary melanoma: preoperative dynamic lymphoscintigraphy, intraoperative gamma probe and vital dye guidance. Surgery 2000; 127: 19–25.

38. Alex JC, Weaver DL, Fairbank JT, et al. Gamma-probe-guided lymph node localization in malignant melanoma. Surg Oncol 1993; 2: 303–8.

39. Krag DN, Meijer SJ, Weaver DL, et al. Minimal access surgery for staging of malignant melanoma. Arch Surg 1995; 130: 654–8.

40. Yudd AP, Kempf JS, Goydos JS, et al. Use of sentinel node lymphoscintigraphy in malignant melanoma. Radiographics 1999; 19: 343–53.

41. Acland KM, Healy C, Calonje E, et al. Comparison of positron emission tomography scanning and sentinel node biopsy in the detection of micrometastases of primary cutaneous malignant melanoma. J Clin Oncol 2001; 19: 2674–8.

42. Schwimmer J, Essner R, Patel A, et al. A review of the literature for whole-body FDG PET in the management of patients with melanoma. Q J Nucl Med 2000; 44: 153–67.

43. Sian KU, Wagner JD, Sood R, et al. Lymphoscintigraphy with sentinel lymph node biopsy in cutaneous Merkel cell carcinoma. Ann Plast Surg 1999; 42: 679–82.

44. Hill AD, Brady MS, Coit DG. Intraoperative lymphatic mapping and sentinel lymph node biopsy for Merkel cell carcinoma. Br J Surg 1999; 86: 518–21.

45. Morton DL, Thompson JF, Cochran AJ, et al. MSLT Group. Sentinel-node biopsy or nodal observation in melanoma. N Engl J Med. 2006; 355: 1307–17.

46. Amersi F, Morton DL. The role of sentinel lymph node biopsy in the management of melanoma. Adv Surg. 2007; 41: 241–56.

47. Cochran AJ, Ohsie SJ, Binder SW. Pathobiology of the sentinel node. Curr Opin Oncol. 2008; 20: 190–5.

48. Eggermont AM, Gore M. Randomized adjuvant therapy trials in melanoma: surgical and systemic. Semin Oncol 2007; 34: 509–15.

49. Ross AS, Schmults CD. Sentinel lymph node biopsy in cutaneous squamous cell carcinoma: a systematic review of the English literature. Dermatol Surg. 2006; 32: 1309–21.

50. Terhune MH, Swanson N, Johnson TM. Use of chest radiography in the initial evaluation of patients with localized melanoma. Arch Dermtol 1998; 134: 569–72.

51. The Royal College of Radiologists. Recommendations for cross-sectional imaging in cancer management, 2006.

52. Clinical Indications for Positron Emission Tomography UK PET-CT Advisory Board Version 1.1 Approved 26 September 2006 [Available from: http://www.bnmsonline.co.uk, Last Updated: Wednesday, 23 January 2008].

53. Constantinidou A, Hofman M, O'doherty M, et al. Routine positron emission tomography and positron emission tomography/computed tomography in melanoma staging with positive sentinel node biopsy is of limited benefit. Melanoma Res 2008; 18: 56–60.

54. Yancovitz M, Finelt N, Warycha MA, et al. Role of radiologic imaging at the time of initial diagnosis of stage T1b-T3b melanoma. Cancer 2007; 110: 1107–14.

55. Medina-Franco H, Urist MM, Fiveash J, et al. Multimodality treatment of Merkel cell carcinoma: case series and literature review of 1024 cases. Ann Surg Oncol 2001; 8: 204–8.

56. Gollub MJ, Gruen DR, Dershaw DD. Merkel cell carcinoma: CT findings in 12 patients. Am J Roentgenol 1996; 167: 617–20.

57. Belhocine T, Pierard GE, Frühling J, et al. Clinical added-value of 18FDG PET in neuroendocrine-merkel cell carcinoma. Oncol Rep 2006; 16: 347–52.

58. Iagaru A, Quon A, McDougall IR, Gambhir SS. Merkel cell carcinoma: Is there a role for 2-deoxy-2-[f-18]fluoro-D-glucose-positron emission tomography/computed tomography? Mol Imaging Biol 2006; 8: 212–17.

59. Balch CM, Soong S-J, Gershenwald JE, et al. Prognostic factors analysis of 17,600 melanoma patients: validation of the American Joint Committee on Cancer melanoma staging system. J Clin Oncol 2001; 19: 3622–34.

60. Day CL Jr, Mihm MC Jr, Lew RA, et al. Cutaneous malignant melanoma: prognostic guidelines for physicians and patients. CA Cancer J Clin 1982; 32: 113–22.

61. Tai P. Merkel cell cancer: update on biology and treatment. Curr Opin Oncol 2008; 20: 196–200.

62. Goessling W, McKee PH, Mayer RJ. Merkel cell carcinoma. J Clin Oncol 2002; 20: 588–98.

63. Nelson BR, Hamlet KR, Gillard M, et al. Sebaceous carcinoma. J Am Acad Dermatol 1995; 33: 1–15.

64. Gortler I, Koppl H, Stark GB, Horch RE. Metastatic malignant acrospiroma of the hand. Eur J Surg Oncol 2001; 27: 431–5.

65. Gilliam AC, Wood GS. Primary cutaneous lymphomas other than mycosis fungoides. Semin Oncol 1999; 26: 290–306.

66. Itoh H, Miyaguni H, Kataoka H, et al. Primary cutaneous Langerhans' cell histiocytosis showing malignant phenotype in an elderly woman: report of a fatal case. J Cutan Pathol 2001; 28: 371–8.

67. Aoki M, Aoki R, Akimoto M, Hara K. Primary cutaneous Langerhans' cell histiocytosis in an adult. Am J Dermatopathol 1998; 20: 281–4.

68. Lichtenwald DJ, Jakubovic HR, Rosenthal D. Primary cutaneous Langerhans' cell histiocytosis in an adult. Arch Dermatol 1991; 127: 1545–8.

69. Balch CM, Urist MM, Karakousis CP, et al. Efficacy of 2-cm surgical margins for intermediate-thickness melanomas (1

to 4 mm). Results of a multi-institutional randomized surgical trial. Ann Surg 1993; 218: 262–7.

70. Veronesi U, Cascinelli N, Adamus J, et al. Thin Stage I primary cutaneous malignant melanoma. Comparison of excision with margins of 1 or 3 cm. N Engl J Med 1988; 318: 1159–62.

71. Heaton KM, Sussman JJ, Gershenwald JE, et al. Surgical margins and prognostic factors in patients with thick (>4 mm) primary melanoma. Ann Surg Oncol 1998; 5: 322–8.

72. Bedikian AY, Millward M, Pehamberger H, et al. Oblimersen Melanoma Study Group. Bcl-2 antisense (oblimersen sodium) plus dacarbazine in patients with advanced melanoma: the Oblimersen Melanoma Study Group. J Clin Oncol 2006; 24: 4738–45.

73. Facchetti F, Monzani E, La Porta CA. New perspectives in the treatment of melanoma: anti-angiogenic and anti-lymphangiogenic strategies. Recent Patents Anticancer Drug Discov 2007; 2: 73–8.

74. Grünhagen DJ, Brunstein F, Graveland WJ, et al. One hundred consecutive isolated limb perfusions with TNF-alpha and melphalan in melanoma patients with multiple in-transit metastases. Ann Surg. 2004; 240: 939–47.

75. Samlowski WE, Jensen RL, Shrieve DC. Multimodality management of brain metastases in metastatic melanoma patients. Expert Rev Anticancer Ther 2007; 12: 1699–705.

76. Smith DF, Messina JL, Perrott R, et al. Clinical approach to neuroendocrine carcinoma of the skin (Merkel cell carcinoma). Cancer Control 2000; 7: 72–83.

77. Nguyen BD, McCullough AE. Imaging of Merkel cell carcinoma. Radiographics 2002; 22: 367–76.

78. Di Lorenzo G, Konstantinopoulos PA, Pantanowitz L, et al. Management of AIDS-related Kaposi's sarcoma. Lancet Oncol 2007; 8: 167–76.

79. Basseres N, Grob JJ, Richard MA, et al. Cost-effectiveness of surveillance of Stage I melanoma. A retrospective appraisal based on a 10-year experience in a dermatology department in France. Dermatology 1995; 191: 199–203.

80. Provost N, Marghoob AA, Kopf AW, et al. Laboratory tests and imaging studies in patients with cutaneous malignant melanomas: a survey of experienced physicians. J Am Acad Dermatol 1997; 36: 711–20.

81. Virgo KS, Chan D, Handler BS, et al. Current practice of patient follow-up after potentially curative resection of cutaneous melanoma. Plast Reconstr Surg 2000; 106: 590–7.

82. Blum A, Schlagenhauff B, Stroebel W, et al. Ultrasound examination of regional lymph nodes significantly improves early detection of locoregional metastases during follow-up of patients with cutaneous melanoma. Cancer 2000; 88: 2534–9.

83. Lassau N, Chami L, Benatsou B, Peronneau P, Roche A. Dynamic contrast-enhanced ultrasonography (DCE-US) with quantification of tumor perfusion: a new diagnostic tool to evaluate the early effects of antiangiogenic treatment. Eur Radiol 2007; 17(Suppl 6): F89–F98.

84. Patel JK, Didolkar MS, Pickren JW, Moore RH. Metastatic pattern of malignant melanoma. A study of 216 autopsy cases. Am J Surg 1978; 135: 807–10.

85. Moehrle M, Blum A, Rassner G, Juenger MJ. Lymph node metastases of cutaneous melanoma: diagnosis by B-scan and colour Doppler sonography. J Am Acad Dermatol 1999; 41: 703–9.

86. Imada H, Nakata H, Horie A. Radiological significance of splenic metastases and its prevalence at autopsy. Nippon Igaku Hoshasen Gakkai Zasshi 1991; 51: 498–503.

87. Krug B, Dietlein M, Groth W, et al. Fluoro-18-fluorodeoxy-glucose positron emission tomography (FDG-PET) in malignant melanoma. Acta Radiol 2000; 41: 446–52.

88. Quint LE, Park CH, Iannettoni MD. Solitary pulmonary nodules in patients with extrapulmonary neoplasms. Radiology 2000; 217: 257–61.

89. Pastorino U, Buyse M, Friedel G, et al. Long-term results of lung metastasectomy: prognostic analysis based on 5206 cases. J Thorac Cardiovasc Surg 1997; 113: 37–49.

90. Leo F, Cagini L, Rocmans P, et al. Lung metastases from melanoma: when is surgical treatment warranted? Br J Cancer 2000; 83: 569–72.

91. Damron TA, Heiner J. Distant soft tissue metastases: a series of 30 new patients and 91 cases from the literature. Ann Surg Oncol 2000; 7: 526–34.

92. Nazarian LN, Alexander AA, Kurtz AB, et al. Superficial melanoma metastases: appearances on grey-scale and colour Doppler sonography. AJR Am J Roentgenol 1998; 170: 459–63.

93. Blake SP, Weisinger K, Atkins MB, Raptopoulos V. Liver metastases from melanoma: detection with multiphasic contrast-enhanced CT. Radiology 1999; 213: 92–6.

94. Premkumar A, Sanders L, Marincola F, et al. Visceral metastases from melanoma: findings on MR imaging. AJR Am J Roentgenol 1992; 158: 293–8.

95. Smirniotopoulos JG, Lonergan GJ, Abbott RM, et al. Image interpretation session 1998. Radiographics 1999; 19: 205–33.

96. Lichy MP, Aschoff P, Plathow C, et al. Tumor detection by diffusion-weighted MRI and ADC-mapping—initial clinical experiences in comparison to PET-CT. Invest Radiol 2007; 42: 605–13.

97. Backman H. Metastases of malignant melanoma in the gastrointestinal tract. Geriatrics 1969; 24: 112–20.

98. DasGupta TK, Brasfield R. Metastatic melanoma of the gastrointestinal tract. Arch Surg 1964; 88: 969–73.

99. Meyer JE. Radiographic evaluation of metastatic melanoma. Cancer 1978; 42: 127–32.

100. O'Connell JB, Whittemore DM, Russell JC, et al. Malignant melanoma metastatic to the cystic and common bile ducts. Cancer 1984; 53: 184–6.

101. McFadden PM, Krementz ET, McKinnon WMP, et al. Metastatic melanoma of the gallbladder. Cancer 1979; 44: 1802–8.

102. Daunt N, King DM. Metastatic melanoma in the biliary tree. Br J Radiol 1982; 55: 873–4.

103. Holloway BJ, King DM. Ultrasound diagnosis of metastatic melanoma of the gallbladder. Br J Radiol 1997; 70: 1122–5.

104. Moon D, Maafs E, Peterson-Schaefer K. A review of 567 cases of brain metastases from malignant melanoma. Melanoma Res 1993; 3: 40.

105. Sampson JH, Carter JH Jr, Friedman AH, Seigler HF. Demographics, prognosis, and therapy in 702 patients with brain metastases from malignant melanoma. J Neurosurg 1998; 88: 11–20.

106. McGann GM, Platts A. Computed tomography of cranial metastatic malignant melanoma: features, early detection and unusual cases. Br J Radiol 1991; 64: 310–13.

107. Reider-Groswasser I, Merimsky O, Karminsky N, Chaitchik S. Computed tomography features of cerebral spread of malignant melanoma. Am J Clin Oncol (CCT) 1996; 19: 49–53.

108. Isiklar I, Leeds NE, Fuller GN, Kumar AJ. Intracranial metastatic melanoma: correlation between MR imaging characteristics and melanin content. AJR Am J Roentgenol 1995; 165: 1503–12.

109. Gaviani P, Mullins ME, Braga TA, et al. Improved detection of metastatic melanoma by T2*-weighted imaging. AJNR Am J Neuroradiol 2006; 27: 605–8.

110. Crasto S, Duca S, Davini O, et al. MRI diagnosis of intramedullary metastases from extra-CNS tumours. Eur Radiol 1997; 7: 732–6.

111. Reintgen DS, Thompson W, Garbutt J, Siegler HF. Radiologic, endoscopic, and surgical considerations of melanoma metastatic to the gastrointestinal tract. Surgery 1984; 95: 635–9.

112. Sood S, Nair SB, Fenwick JD, Horgan K. Metastatic melanoma of the tonsil. J Laryngol Otol 1999; 113: 1036–8.

113. Schuchter LM, Green R, Fraker D. Primary and metastatic diseases in malignant melanoma of the gastrointestinal tract. Curr Opin Oncol 2000; 12: 181–5.

114. Kawashima A, Fishman EK, Kuhlman JE, Schuchter LM. CT of malignant melanoma: patterns of small bowel and mesenteric involvement. J Comput Assist Tomogr 1991; 15: 570–4.

115. Potepan P, Spagnoli I, Danesini GM, et al. The radiodiagnosis of bone metastases from melanoma. Radiol Med (Torino) 1994; 87: 741–6.

116. Stewart WR, Gelberman RH, Harrelson JM, Siegler HF. Skeletal metastases of melanoma. J Bone Joint Surg Am 1978; 60: 645–9.

117. Gokaslan ZL, Aladag MA, Ellerhorst JA. Melanoma metastatic to the spine: a review of 133 cases. Melanoma Res 2000; 10: 78–80.

118. Boudghene FP, Deslandes PM, LeBlanche AF, Bigot JMR. US and CT features of intrapancreatic metastases. J Comput Assist Tomogr 1994; 18: 905–10.

119. Goldstein HM, Kaminsky S, Wallace S, Johnson DE. Urographic manifestations of metastatic melanoma. AJR Am J Roentgenol 1974; 121: 801–5.

120. Das Gupta T, Grabstald H. Melanoma of genitourinary tract. J Urol 1965; 93: 607–14.

121. Spera JA, Pollack HM, Banner MP, et al. Metastatic malignant melanoma mimicking renal cell carcinoma. J Urol 1984; 131: 740–2.

122. Meyer J. Metastatic melanoma of the urinary bladder. Cancer 1974; 34: 1822–4.

123. Chin JL, Sales JL, Silver MM, Sweeney JP. Melanoma metastatic to the bladder and bowel: an unusual case. J Urol 1982; 127: 541–2.

124. de la Monte SM, Moore GW, Hutchins GM. Patterned distribution of metastases from malignant melanoma in humans. Cancer Res 1983; 43: 3427–33.

125. Fitzgibbons PL, Martin SE, Simmons TJ. Malignant melanoma metastatic to the ovary. Am J Surg Pathol 1987; 11: 959–64.

126. Young RH, Scully RE. Malignant melanoma metastatic to the ovary: a clinicopathological analysis of 20 cases. Am J Surg Pathol 1991; 15: 849–60.

127. Moselhi M, Spencer J, Lane G. Malignant melanoma metastatic to the ovary: presentation and radiological characteristics. Gynaecol Oncol 1998; 69: 165–8.

128. Bauer RD, McCoy CP, Roberts DK, Fritz G. Malignant melanoma metastatic to the endometrium. Obstet Gynecol 1984; 63: 264–8.

129. Richardson PGG, Millward MJ, Shrimankar JJ, Cantwell BMJ. Metastatic melanoma to the testis simulating primary seminoma. Br J Urol 1992; 69: 663–5.

130. Skarin A. Diagnostic dilemmas in oncology: melanoma metastatic to the testis. J Clin Oncol 2000; 18: 3187–92.

131. Zein TA, Huben R, Lane W, et al. Secondary tumours of the prostate. J Urol 1985; 133: 615–16.

132. Branum GD, Epstein RE, Leight GS, Seigler HF. The role of resection in the management of melanoma metastatic to the adrenal gland. Surgery 1991; 109: 127–31.

133. Ahuja AT, King W, Metreweli C. Role of ultrasound in thyroid metastases. Clin Radiol 1994; 49: 627–9.

134. Eftekhari F, Peuchot M. Thyroid metastases: combined role of ultrasonography and fine-needle aspiration biopsy. J Clin Ultrasound 1989; 17: 657–60.

135. Ferrozzi F, Campodonico F, De Chiara F, et al. Thyroid metastases: the echographic and computed tomographic aspects. Radiol Med (Torino) 1997; 94: 214–19.

136. Toombs BD, Kalisher L. Metastatic disease to the breast: clinical, pathological and radiographic features. AJR Am J Roentgenol 1977; 129: 673–6.

137. Ho LWC, Wong KP, Chan JHM, et al. MR appearance of metastatic melanotic melanoma in the breast. Clin Rad 2000, 55: 572–3.

138. Plesnicar A, Kovac V. Breast metastases from cutaneous melanoma: a report of three cases. Tumori 2000; 86: 170–3.

139. Klatt EC, Heitz DR. Cardiac metastases. Cancer 1990; 65: 1456–9.

140. Gibbs P, Cebon JS, Calafiore P, Robinson WA. Cardiac metastases from malignant melanoma. Cancer 1999; 85: 78–84.

141. Savoia P, Fierro MT, Zaccagna A, Bernengo MG. Metastatic melanoma of the heart. J Surg Oncol 2000; 75: 203–7.

142. Freedberg RS, Kronzon I, Rumancik WM, Liebskind D. The contribution of magnetic resonance imaging to the evaluation of intracardiac tumours diagnosed by echocardiography. Circulation 1988; 77: 96–103.

143. Epstein E, Epstein NN, Bragg K, Linden G. Metastases from squamous cell carcinomas of the skin. Arch Dermatol 1968; 97: 245–9.

144. Katz AD, Uraback F, Lilienfeld AM. The frequency and risk of metastases in squamous cell carcinoma of the skin. Cancer 1957; 10: 1162–6.

145. Moller R, Reymann F, Hou-Jensen K. Metastases in dermatological patients with squamous cell carcinoma. Arch Dermatol 1979; 115: 703–5.

146. Johnson TM, Rowe DE, Nelson BR, Swanson NA. Squamous cell carcinoma of the skin (excluding lip and oral mucosa). J Am Acad Dermatol 1992; 26: 467–84.

147. Lo JS, Snow SN, Reizner GT, et al. Metastatic basal cell carcinoma: report of 12 cases and a review of the literature. J Am Acad Dermatol 1991; 24: 715–19.

148. von Domarus H, Stevens PJ. Metastatic basal cell carcinoma. J Am Acad Dermatol 1984; 10: 1043–60.

149. Farmer ER, Helwig EB. Metastatic basal cell carcinoma: a clinicopathologic study of 17 cases. Cancer 1980; 46: 748–57.

150. Eggers SDZ, Salomao DR, Dinapoli RP, Vernino S. Paraneoplastic and metastatic neurological complications of Merkel cell carcinoma. Mayo Clin Proc 2001; 76: 327–30.

151. Guitera-Rovel P, Lumbroso J, Gautier-Gougis MS, et al. Indium-111 octreotide scintigraphy of Merkel cell carcinomas and their metastases. Ann Oncol 2001; 12: 807–11.

152. Lampreave JL, Benard F, Alavi A, et al. PET evaluation of therapeutic limb perfusion in Merkel's cell carcinoma. J Nucl Med 1998; 39: 2087–90.

153. Friedman-Kien AE, Saltzman BR. Clinical manifestations of classical, endemic African, and epidemic AIDS-associated Kaposi's sarcoma. J Am Acad Dermatol 1990; 22: 1237–50.

154. Haramati LB, Wong J. Intrathoracic Kaposi's sarcoma in women with AIDS. Chest 2000; 117: 410–14.

155. Traill ZC, Miller RF, Shaw PJ. CT appearances of intrathoracic Kaposi's sarcoma in patients with AIDS. Br J Radiol 1996; 69: 1104–7.

49 Radiological Investigation of Carcinoma of Unknown Primary Site
Christopher J Gallagher, Rodney H Reznek, and Janet E Husband

INTRODUCTION

Cancer of an unknown primary site is a commonly referred problem accounting for 3% to 9% of all patients seen in most tertiary treatment centers (1–3). In the United States, as estimated by the SEER statistics (Surveillance Epidemiology and End Results), 2% of cancers were registered as cancer of unknown primary site within the population as a whole. Of these cancers, adenocarcinoma comprised 55%, squamous carcinoma 14%, cancer undifferentiated 21% and 10% other specific diagnoses such as sarcoma, neuroendocrine cancer, and melanoma (4).

Patients present with the symptoms of their metastases without a clinically apparent primary site. The frequency of the site of presentation of the metastases varies in part due to differences in patient selection in the reported series. However, the most common sites of presentation (excluding head and neck) are shown in Table 49.1 (1,2).

The definition of a (metastatic) cancer of unknown primary site has shifted over the years largely due to changes in histological and radiological investigations. Thus, in the earlier clinical series, most patients simply had a careful clinical history, physical examination, and chest X-ray. However, in recent series, most patients have already undergone a computed tomography (CT) scan of chest, abdomen, and pelvis and, if appropriate, bilateral mammography before referral for investigation of the unknown primary site. Nevertheless, even after post mortem examination, the primary site will remain unknown in approximately 15% to 20% of patients diagnosed as having cancer of unknown primary site in historical series (5,6) and with improved clinical investigation in 49% (7,8).

Diagnostic pathology has improved remarkably over the past several years. Increased routine use of immunohistochemistry for panels of markers (9,10) and molecular genetics (11,12) are now contributing to a more precise diagnosis of neoplasms. In general, therefore, the term carcinoma of unknown origin is now a nonspecific light microscopical diagnosis, the most common cause of which is an inadequate or poorly handled biopsy specimen. If possible, fine-needle aspiration (FNA) should not be relied upon as a definitive diagnostic procedure because the histological pattern is not preserved and the ability to perform special studies is limited. Several instances have been documented in which FNA has suggested a specific diagnosis, which was proved later to be incorrect on tissue biopsy (13).

HISTOLOGY

The most critical step in the assessment of any patient with cancer of unknown primary site is a review of the histological findings, from which three main groups can be derived (14):

- Adenocarcinoma (50–60%)
- Squamous carcinoma (5%)
- Poorly differentiated tumors (35%)

Other malignancies include:

- Lymphoma (6%)
- Germ cell (1%)
- Melanoma, sarcoma, neuroendocrine (1%)

The most common histological type is that of adenocarcinoma, comprizing 50% to 60% of patients in all series. A panel of immunohistochemistry markers that includes thyroid transcriptor factor (TTF-1) for lung cancer (15), CK7 and CK20 cytokeratins, CdX, ER, PR, PSA and MUC1, can increasingly help identify likely primary sites. Squamous carcinomas are present in 5% of cases although perhaps underrepresented by the exclusion of head and neck cancers from some series. Poorly differentiated cancers comprise an important group because these patients may have the most highly treatable cancers. Careful histological and immunocytochemical review supplemented by molecular biology can identify chemotherapy-curable lymphoma in 6% and atypical germ cell tumors in 1% of cases (16).

Other specific histologies, such as melanoma, sarcoma, and poorly differentiated neuroendocrine tumors, are identified in a further 1% of cases.

Key Points: Histopathology

- The most critical step in the evaluation of any patient presenting with the diagnosis of cancer of unknown primary site is a review of the histology
- FNA should not be relied upon for a diagnosis and tissue should always be obtained

SQUAMOUS CARCINOMA OF UNKNOWN ORIGIN (SCUO)

Most patients with squamous carcinoma of unknown primary origin present with cervical lymphadenopathy although, rarely, inguinal lymphadenopathy may be the first sign of disease which originates in the vulva or the penis.

Squamous Carcinoma of Cervical or Supraclavicular Nodes

Most malignant lymph node masses in the neck are metastatic and the majority (85%) arise from primary head and neck tumors (17), especially when the upper or middle cervical lymph nodes are involved. When the lower cervical or supraclavicular lymph nodes are involved, a primary lung cancer should be suspected. The majority of primary sites are identified at routine clinical examination, with a further 16% being detected at panendoscopy and 4% by radiological investigation. This latter group usually comprises lung cancer presenting with enlarged nodes in the lower cervical region. However, between 3% and 9% have no identifiable primary site, even after such a program of investigation. FDG-PET

Table 49.1 Common Sites of Presentation of Metastases

Site	%
Lymph nodes	14–37
Thorax	28–30
Lung	28
Pleural	2–12
Liver	19–31
Adrenal	6
Abdomen pelvis (other)	15
Bone	16–28
CNS	8
Skin	2

can detect the primary source in 22% to 33% of patients, declared negative by all other investigations (18,19). When compared to CT and MRI, FDG-PET had the highest sensitivity at 69%, and negative predictive value of 87%, but a lower specificity than that of CT scan (87%), or MR (95%). However, FDG-PET cannot replace the need for a careful endoscopy which found lesions overlooked by PET in 16% of cases in one series (18).

The prognosis for patients identified as having head and neck primary tumors has improved from a 20% to 30% five-year survival rate, and a median survival of one year without a primary site (17), to a more recent series with modern chemoradiotherapy with a five-year survival of 40% to 68%, varying from 80% for N1 disease with surgery alone to 56% for N3 with surgery plus chemoradiotherapy. With such treatment there is no longer any difference in prognosis between those with or without an identified primary (20–22).

Radiological examination including PET-CT may be required for examination of:

- The paranasal sinuses
- Staging the extent of nodal enlargement
- Detection of mediastinal or lung disease prior to treatment

Patients without an identifiable primary tumor site and N1 disease (lymph nodes <3 cm on one side of the neck) have a better prognosis than those with N2 or N3 disease. Patients with low cervical and supraclavicular nodal involvement tend to have a worse prognosis because lung cancer is a frequent site of occult primary disease (23). Series reporting the results of surgical resection alone have found that up to 40% of patients subsequently develop a primary site in the head and neck region compared with 7% to 11% in series combining radiotherapy or chemoradiotherapy with surgery (19,20). Therefore, most authors would now recommend the inclusion of radiotherapy or chemoradiotherapy in the primary treatment to include the naso-, hypo-, and oropharynx as well as the contralateral neck nodes where there is a 15% likelihood of developing further deposits. This approach has led to a 62% to 67% five-year survival for these patients (19–25).

Squamous Carcinoma Involving Inguinal Lymph Nodes

In most cases of inguinal lymph node involvement, the primary tumor is genital or anorectal in origin; primary sites most commonly include the vulva, vagina, cervix, penis, or scrotum. In these cases imaging, notably MR imaging of the pelvis, is useful for planning surgical treatment particularly lymphadenectomy which may play a major part in treatment when the disease is limited to a resectable region.

Squamous Carcinoma Metastatic to Other Sites

Metastatic squamous carcinoma presenting in sites other than the cervical or inguinal nodes almost always represents spread from an occult primary lung cancer and, therefore, PET-CT of the chest should be considered under these circumstances. Very rarely, the primary site may lie in the head and neck, esophagus, or anus (13).

Key Points: Squamous Cell Carcinoma of Unknown Origin

- Most patients with squamous cell carcinoma of unknown origin (SCUO) present with cervical lymphadenopathy, and 85% of these cases represent head and neck tumors
- In SCUO in cervical lymph nodes, PET-CT may be required to identify base of tongue, tonsillar fossa, and paranasal sinus tumors, to detect lung cancer and to stage nodal disease
- Patients with unilateral cervical nodal disease have a better prognosis than those with bilateral disease or with supraclavicular nodal involvement

ADENOCARCINOMA OF UNKNOWN ORIGIN (ACUO)

Adenocarcinoma is the most frequent histology in cancers of unknown origin. In defining the plan of investigation, the likely incidence of the various primary diagnoses and the treatment options available following diagnosis need to be considered. The extent of investigation needs to be tailored to the patient's likely prognosis (qv). Exhaustive investigation of poor performance status patients with cancers of unknown primary site is often counterproductive because of the diminishing likelihood of identifying a primary site, the increasing expense of continuing investigation, and discomfort to the patient with limited life expectancy (2,3,6). Treatment options for this group of patients, though often limited except in certain special circumstances, have improved with new agents (see section "Treatment Opportunities and Radiological Strategy").

In early series, such as those reported by Le Chevalier and Nystrom, patients with adenocarcinoma of unknown primary site were subjected to post mortem examination and a primary site was identified in 82% to 84% (5,6), but more recently the yield has decreased as radiological investigation has improved (8). The most common sites were:

- Lung (17–28%)
- Pancreas (11–27%)
- Liver (3–6%)
- Colorectal (4–6%)
- Gastric (3–5%)
- Renal (3–7%)
- Ovary (2%)
- Prostate (2–3%)
- Thyroid (1–3%)
- Adrenal (1–3%)
- Breast (1%)
- Parotid (<1%)

Clinical series have revealed a similar distribution of primary sites of cancer (1,26).

Le Chevalier and Nystrom also compared post mortem findings with the investigations prior to death to define the investigational yield prior to the advent of CT and PET scanning (5,6). Their results revealed that primary tumor sites were identified prior to death by the following techniques:

- Chest radiography (12–24%)
- Intravenous urography (IVU) (6–9%)
- Barium enema (5–9%)
- Barium meal (4–6%)
- Thyroid scan (8%)

In other series, by contrast, with patients who did not undergo a post mortem, the primary site was identified in only 16% during life (1,2). There have been few attempts to define the diagnostic performance of these conventional studies and no such information is likely to become available for the more recent techniques of CT, MR imaging, and PET scanning. In one study summarized in Table 49.2 the authors showed that the radiological investigations had a low sensitivity, low positive predictive value, and variable specificity when correlated with post mortem findings (6).

Key Points: Adenocarcinoma—Clinical Presentation

- Three to nine percent of all referrals to an oncology unit are for investigation of a cancer of unknown primary site
- A careful histological examination of tissue biopsy by image-guided needle core or open biopsy with an appropriate panel of immunohistochemical markers can now identify the likely tissue of origin in the majority of cases
- Adenocarcinoma is the most common histological type in this group of patients
- Poorly differentiated cancers (35%) are an extremely important group as they frequently represent those patients with the most treatable cancers
- Most patients with SCUO present with cervical lymphadenopathy and 85% of these cases arise from head and neck tumors
- In patients presenting with adenocarcinoma of unknown origin, post mortem studies show that the primary tumor most commonly arises in the lung or pancreas

Computed Tomography and Magnetic Resonance

Overall, CT has proved to be the most successful technique for identifying the primary site in patients presenting with adenocarcinoma of unknown origin, showing up to 35% to 40% of all primary cancers discovered (2,26,27). In particular, CT of the chest can show over 70% of all primary tumors. Abdomino-pelvic CT is also successful and, in one series, CT revealed 86% of all pancreatic cancers, 67% of ovarian primaries, and 56% of renal primaries. At other sites the investigational yield of CT was considerably less: 36% of colorectal primary tumors, 33% of hepatobiliary tumors, and 20% of esophageal cancers. In addition to detecting the primary site of malignancy, CT may detect other clinically unsuspected sites of metastasis in two-thirds of patients examined (27). However, it is not possible to estimate the sensitivity and specificity of these findings in most studies.

MR has proved particularly advantageous in the pelvis (28) and in identifying occult breast cancers (29,30) in 50% to 86% of women with axillary lymph node metastases and facilitating breast conservation.

Positron Emission Tomography (Table 49.3)

The role of 2-[F-18]fluoro-2-deoxy-D-glucose positron emission tomography ([18]FDG PET) to detect occult primary carcinomas outside of the head and neck region has been reported in several small series of patients (31–35), and reviewed recently (36). In these studies, on average, a potential primary site was identified in 41% of patients (24–71%) but with confirmation from histology at biopsy or post mortem achieved in only half the cases; thus false positive and negative rates are unreliable. The lung was the detected primary site in 59% of cases, but there was a high false positive rate of detection of putative lower gastrointestinal tract primaries of 58%. Clinical management was changed as a result of PET scanning in 24% to 35%, mostly through the choice of chemotherapy agents for lung or pancreatic cancers, while in 12% treatment was directed to breast or prostatic primaries of a usually better prognosis. Further metastatses were found in 37%, but in 14% disease was confirmed as localized and suitable for potentially curative resection. Caution should be exercised in interpreting these combined

Table 49.2 Test Performance Compared with Postmortem Findings (13)

Test	Number performed	Sensitivity (%)	Specificity (%)	Positive predictive value (%)
Chest X-ray	302	69	63	38
Barium meal	150	75	92	30
Barium enema	105	71	96	55
Thyroid radio-iodine scan	45	57	76	31

Table 49.3 Role of [18]FDG PET to Detect Occult Primary Carcinomas

Author	Number patients	Primary site possible/confirmed	False positive/negative	Metastases	Treatment changed
Aasar	17	12/9	3/nd	0	2
Kole	29	7/nd	0/3	5	3
Jungelhulsing	27	7/nd	0/5	7	8
Bohulslavzki	53	27/20	6/0	nd	nd
Rades	42	27/20	nd	16	29
Lassen	20	13/9	nd	nd	4
Total	188	92/56 (49/30%)			46/133 (34%)

Abbreviation: nd, not done.

results as the number of patients in each of these series is small. However, three more recent studies, which have excluded cervical node presentations, have replicated these findings in single center studies (37–39). It is extremely difficult to evaluate the performance of ^{18}FDG PET in patients presenting with head and neck adenocarcinoma of unknown primary site. However, extracting data for this from three studies showed a 24% to 45% detection rate, especially for adenocarcinoma of the lung and primary sites in the head and neck, including the thyroid gland (33–35).

Poorly Differentiated Carcinoma of Unknown Primary Site (with or Without Features of Adenocarcinoma)

There is a distinctive subgroup of patients with poorly differentiated carcinoma or adenocarcinoma of unknown primary site in whom the clinical characteristics differ from patients with well differentiated adenocarcinomas (13). The median age group of this group is younger than those with well-differentiated disease. They have a history of rapid progression of symptoms (<30 days) with evidence of rapid tumor growth (40–42) and may express the germ cell tumor markers alpha-fetoprotein or beta-human chorionic gonadotrophin. Most importantly, from a radiological viewpoint, metastases occur more commonly in the lymph nodes, of the mediastinum, and retroperitoneum than in patients with well-differentiated adenocarcinoma (13). It is important to identify this subset of patients as they may have a high proportion of germ cell tumors that may be more responsive to chemotherapy and potentially curable (13). Indeed, Hainsworth and colleagues (43), using a multivariate analysis, showed that several features independently predicted a favorable treatment outcome. These included:

- A tumor location in the retroperitoneum, or
- Lymph nodes, limited to one or two metastatic sites, and
- A younger age (<35 years) (43)

It is recommended, therefore, that CT of the chest and abdomen should be performed as an initial investigation in this group of patients. However, further data are awaited before recommending the routine use of ^{18}FDG PET in this group.

Key Point: Poorly Differentiated Carcinoma or Adenocarcinoma of Unknown Origin

- Young patients presenting with poorly differentiated carcinoma with mediastinal or retroperitoneal disease at one or two sites may have potentially curable disease

NEUROENDOCRINE CARCINOMA OF UNKNOWN PRIMARY SITE

The majority of adult patients who present with features of a primary neuroendocrine tumor (NET) have a known primary site (see chap. 32). However, patients increasingly present with NETs of unknown primary site (4). These can be of three typical histological and clinical types:

- A well-differentiated or low-grade NET with an unknown primary site and indolent biological behavior

- A poorly differentiated tumor on light microscopy but with neuroendocrine features on imunohistochemistry with the same aggressive behavior as small cell carcinoma of the lung or other primary sites
- A group usually initially termed "poorly differentiated carcinoma" on light microscopy, but recognized as PNETs on immunoperoxidase staining. These too are aggressive tumors

The imaging investigation of these patients is considered in chapter 32. Paradoxically, poorly differentiated NETs are likely to achieve the greatest palliative benefit from chemotherapy (44).

METASTATIC MELANOMA OF UNKNOWN PRIMARY (MUP)

Radiological staging investigation by CT scan and PET scan of patients presenting with lymphadenopathy due to metastatic melanoma is necessary if the disease is apparently confined to a resectable nodal basin in order to exclude distant metastases. The prognosis following lymphadenectomy can be excellent with 55% to 58% five-year and 13.75-year median overall survival; significantly better than contemporaneous patients with a known primary site (45,46). The management of metastatic melanoma in other sites such as lung is also primarily surgical, and staging investigations can identify the few patients for whom resection may provide effective palliation such as those presenting with MUP only in the lung with a five-year survival of 42% and median survival of 2.7 years (47).

TREATMENT OPPORTUNITIES AND RADIOLOGICAL STRATEGY

Firstly, the investigational strategy for patients presenting with metastatic adenocarcinoma should aim to identify those primary tumors with the greatest treatment potential. The cancers that are likely to present as a cancer of unknown origin and for which treatment is most able to prolong life include:

- Breast
- Ovary
- Prostate

These cancers represent a small proportion (approximately 5–26%) (1–3) of the adenocarcinomas of unknown primary, but their treatment potential makes it important for them to be identified with a high degree of sensitivity. Before the use of newer cross-sectional imaging modalities and the greater choice of chemotherapy agents, only 11% to 14% of radiologically detectable primary adenocarcinomas were considered treatable (1,2,26). This proportion has increased, with a greater number being detected in the better prognostic groups in recent years and a greater number of specific chemotherapy treatment options now available.

Secondly, investigation should be directed to those sites most frequently presenting as ACUP though of lesser treatment potential. The most frequent primary diagnosis for ACUP is non-small

cell lung cancer (NSCLC). Chemotherapy treatment of metastatic NSCLC can improve survival by an average of six months. The second most common site of origin for ACUP is pancreatic cancer for which treatment benefits are even less certain. Thus the discovery of primary pancreatic cancer as the cause of ACUP, while not leading to significant gains in treatment outcomes in itself, can prevent inappropriate treatment for other cancers and aid the palliative management of the patient through the clearer identification of prognosis. Identification of other less common sites of origin of ACUP, such as metastatic upper or lower gastrointestinal cancers, can also lead to specific choices of chemotherapy and clinically useful benefits of up to a year on average in good prognosis patients.

PROGNOSIS

The overall median survival for all cancers of unknown primary site varies from 12 (26,48) to 22 weeks (26). In general, those patients with disease in limited nodal sites, or single-site of metastasis, a performance status of zero to two and weight loss of <10%, absence of liver metastases on CT scan, and in some series normal serum albumen and LDH, represent a better prognostic group, with a median survival up to 15 months compared to three months for those in the poor prognosis group (6,26,49–52). Those in whom a primary site is found at initial investigation may have a better prognosis than those in whom a primary tumor is not found. In some series, however, this is almost entirely due to the identification of patients with breast and ovarian primaries.

A selective policy of investigating and identifying the primary site of origin in patients with adenocarcinoma of unknown primary will avoid over investigation of patients with a poor prognosis while allowing the clinician to apply established tumor guidelines or experimental treatment protocols to palliate disease where appropriate. Finding the primary site often provides much psychological relief for patient and physician, although the practical benefit may be relatively small. The decision about how far to investigate should be linked to the likely prognosis and possibility of treatment and given the palliative nature of these treatments must involve the patient in the decision-making process throughout by careful communication of the relative risks and benefits. Bearing these points in mind, a radiological strategy should be agreed by clinician and radiologist to reflect locally available diagnostic facilities and treatment strategies. The cost of investigating such patients always needs to be considered. In one series the estimated cost of a limited assessment was United States $ 3350 per patient, 70% of which was accounted for by the cost of CT scanning.

There are special clinical situations in which well-defined guidelines for investigation can be recommended:

1. In women presenting with isolated axillary lymph node metastases, a primary breast cancer may be found in 40% to 70% of cases. In one series, only half of these were mammographically detectable, the remainder being found only on pathological examination of the mastectomy specimen (53). Recently, MR imaging has been found to be a valuable adjunct to mammography and US

in examination of these patients (29,30). The prognosis for the group as a whole with breast cancer type treatment and breast conservation (54) is similar to that of other women with Stage II breast cancer with a median survival of five years (53). On considering these statistics, it is clear that a thorough search for a primary breast cancer is justified. US, mammography and MR should be performed in this group of patients. If a primary tumor is found, then a thorough staging should be carried out as for patients presenting with a clinically diagnosed primary breast cancer.

2. Women presenting with peritoneal carcinomatosis, in particular those with papillary serous carcinoma on histological examination but no primary tumor within the ovary, are another group of potentially treatable patients with adenocarcinoma of unknown primary site. Image-guided biopsy can provide tissue to identify the likely site of origin in 93% of cases (55).

    These patients most often have either primary peritoneal carcinomatosis (56,57) or spread from an occult ovarian primary, and respond to platinum-based chemotherapy. The prognosis is similar to that in other women with Stage III ovarian carcinoma with a median survival of 17 to 23 months. Computed tomography (CT) is the initial investigation of choice, which should include the chest, abdomen, and pelvis. The information provided by CT gives an excellent baseline for monitoring response to platinum-based chemotherapy. Magnetic resonance (MR) should be reserved for those cases where the ovaries cannot be satisfactorily identified on CT or US.

3. For patients presenting with bone metastases, investigation with chest X-ray, radionuclide bone scan, abdominal US scan, and CT scan of chest and abdomen is likely to reveal a primary source in the lung in 24% of cases; prostate 17%; and breast or gynecological organs 16%; and with all other sites in less than 1% of patients, the majority are adenocarcinoma (54%), and squamous carcinoma (26%) (59). Men with adenocarcinoma of unknown primary and an elevated serum or tumor biopsy prostate-specific antigen (PSA) level and often bone metastases are usually found to have an unsuspected primary prostatic cancer and form another readily treatable group, with a clinical course similar to those presenting with prostatic cancer. Response to androgen-deprivation is approximately 70% and median survival is 18 to 24 months (58). In such patients, transrectal US or MR of the prostate gland should be performed in an attempt to identify the primary tumor. If a tumor is shown, then a biopsy may be helpful in patients with only minimal elevation of PSA in the serum.

    In patients suspected of harboring an occult prostatic tumor, full staging with a plain chest radiograph, CT of the abdomen, and pelvis to identify nodal disease, and a technetium bone scan is recommended.

4. Patients presenting with liver metastases, which are discovered incidentally or as a result of symptoms due to increasing abdominal discomfort and/or weight loss, are a common problem. In such patients the

immunohistochemical or radiological appearances of the liver metastases may occasionally point to the site of origin. For example, calcification within metastases is seen most commonly in gastrointestinal and ovarian tumors. Median survival in one series was seven months with chemotherapy directed at tumors of gastrointestinal origin depending upon performance status and serum lactate dehydrogenase levels (60). In patients with bowel symptoms suspected of harboring a gastrointestinal tumor, colonoscopy or imaging of the bowel are warranted, as the primary tumor may be excised to avoid obstruction either before or after chemotherapy with fluorouracil and oxaliplatin-based treatment.

5. Other treatable patients include those with multiple small-volume lung metastases due to thyroid carcinoma. This is a rare clinical situation, but response to treatment with radioiodine, if the tumor is shown to be metabolically active, can be achieved in a high proportion of patients.

6. Patients presenting with brain metastases or spinal cord compression from an unknown primary have a poor prognosis, irrespective of whether the primary is identified or not, with a median survival of five months, The good prognostic factors were age (<65), performance status, lack of symptoms, lack of other systemic metastases, and treatment with surgery and radiotherapy. Treatment with short course radiotherapy in five fractions is as effective as longer courses (61–63).

For the majority of other patients, investigation and treatment will be primarily determined by their performance status, and a realistic discussion of palliative options with the patient. Good prognosis patients may require fuller investigation with, for example, [18]FDG PET scans (qv) to identify localized squamous cell carcinoma or melanoma for resection, or primary sites in the lung, pancreas or colon, for which there are increasingly differentiated choices of multiagent chemotherapy. If, after all efforts, no primary site has been identified, palliative chemotherapy treatment with agents such as carboplatin and gemcitabine or etoposide can achieve median survival of 9 – 10 months in 20% to 40% of selected patientsand 5% to 10% surviving to five years (64–67).

Key Points: Imaging Investigation

- Currently, in patients presenting with cancer of unknown primary site, treatment will significantly prolong life in only 11% to 14% of radiologically identified primary tumors
- The majority of patients still present with poor prognosis disease with a short median survival of three months and do not warrant extensive investigation. However, imaging strategies should always take into account the likelihood of identifying those patients who are most suitable for treatment with surgery and radiotherapy for limited squamous carcinoma or melanoma, and chemotherapy for good prognosis patients with undifferentiated cancers and ACUOs

- In general, a good prognosis group can be identified by histology and by clinical presentation with limited nodal sites of disease, good performance status (0–2), weight loss <10%, absence of liver metastases, and normal serum albumen
- Special situations that warrant thorough imaging studies include a search for breast cancer in women with isolated axillary lymph node metastases, ovarian carcinoma in women with peritoneal carcinomatosis, and prostate cancer in men with elevated serum PSA and bone metastases

CONCLUSION

Patients presenting with cancers of unknown origin represent a heterogeneous group in which the detection of the primary site is becoming increasingly relevant to clinical oncological practice. There are now several tumors that present with metastatic disease and that are treatable with specific drugs, provided the organ of origin is known. Although the cost of investigation is high, there are certain situations in which a thorough search for the primary site is justified. In the future, it is likely that these special situations, in which the primary tumor is treatable, will be expanded to a much wider range of malignancies.

Summary

- The radiological investigation of patients with cancer of unknown primary site should be tailored to provide information that is relevant to prognosis and treatment
- All patients considered for treatment should have a chest radiograph, and CT scan of chest, abdomen, and pelvis.
- Women should also undergo bilateral mammography and examination of the pelvic organs by US
- Men should be screened for a prostatic primary by transrectal US if the PSA is elevated
- Further investigation, for example for thyroid carcinoma, by US or radioiodine scanning can be reserved for those cases with the appropriate histology and or metastatic pattern
- Further investigation may require MR scans for breast and ovarian masses, [18]FDG PET scans for head and neck, lung, melanoma, and possibly other primaries to guide the choice of surgery and radiotherapy, and radioisotope scans for thyroid and carcinoid tumors
- For good prognosis patients wishing to have palliative chemotherapy, endoscopy to identify lung, colon, or stomach primaries are indicated to guide the choice of chemotherapy agents
- The sophisticated information which can be obtained by increasingly sensitive imaging techniques is not yet matched by improvements in the prognosis for patients with the most commonly discovered primary tumor sites in the lung and pancreas

REFERENCES

1. Kirsten F, Chi CH, Leary JA, et al. Metastatic adeno- or undifferentiated carcinoma from an unknown primary site: natural history and guidelines for identification of treatable subsets. Q J Med 1987; 62: 143–61.
2. Abbruzzese JL, Abbruzzese MC, Lenzi R, Hess KR, Raber MN. Analysis of a diagnostic strategy for patients with

suspected tumors of unknown origin. J Clin Oncol 1995; 13: 2094–103.

3. Hamilton CS, Langlands AO. ACUPS (adenocarcinoma of unknown primary sites): a clinical and cost–benefit analysis. Int J Radiat Oncol Biol Phys 1987; 13: 1497–503.

4. Muir C. Cancer of unknown primary site. Cancer 1995; 75: 353–6.

5. Nystrom JS, Weiner JM, Wolf RM, Bateman JR, Viola MV. Identifying the primary site in metastatic cancer of unknown origin. JAMA 1979; 241: 381–3.

6. Le Chevalier T, Cvitkovic E, Caille P, et al. Early metastatic cancer of unknown primary origin at presentation. A clinical study of 302 consecutive autopsied patients. Arch Intern Med 1988; 148: 2035–9.

7. Al-Brahim N, Ross C, Carter B, Chorneyko K. The value of postmortem examination in cases of metastasis of unknown origin – 20-year retrospective data from a tertiary care center. Ann Diag Pathol 2005; 9: 77–80.

8. Pentheroudakis G, Golfinopoulos V, Pavlidis N. Switching benchmarks in cancer of unknown primary: from autopsy to microarray. Eur.J.Cancer 2007; 43: 2026–36.

9. Park SY, Kim BH, Kim JH, Lee S, Kang GH. Panels of immunohistochemical markers help determine primary sites of metastatic adenocarcinoma. Arch Pathol Lab Med 2007; 131: 1561–7.

10. Dennis JL, Hvidsten TR, Wit EC, et al. Markers of adenocarcinoma characteristic of the site of origin: development of a diagnostic algorithm. Clin Cancer Res 2005; 11: 3766–72.

11. Tothill RW, Kowalczyk A, Rischin D, et al. An expression-based site of origin diagnostic method designed for clinical application to cancer of unknown origin. Cancer Res 2005; 65: 4031–40.

12. Talantov D, Baden J, Jatkoe T, et al. A quantitative reverse transcriptase-polymerase chain reaction assay to identify metastatic carcinoma tissue of origin. J Mol Diagn 2006; 8: 320–9.

13. Greco FA, Hainsworth JD. Cancer of unknown primary site. In: de Vita VT, Hellman S, Rosenberg SA, eds. Cancer: Principles and Practice of Oncology, 6th edn. Philadelphia: Lippincott Williams and Wilkins, 2001: 2537–60.

14. Hainsworth JD, Greco FA. Treatment of patients with cancer of an unknown primary site. N Engl J Med 1993; 329: 257–63.

15. Srodon M, Westra WH. Immunohistochemical staining for thyroid transcription factor-1: a helpful aid in discerning primary site of tumor origin in patients with brain metastases. Hum Pathol 2002; 33: 642–5.

16. Summersgill B, Goker H, Osin P, et al. Establishing germ cell origin of undifferentiated tumors by identifying gain of 12p material using comparative genomic hybridization analysis of paraffin-embedded samples. Diagn Mol Pathol 1998; 7: 260–6.

17. Jones AS, Cook JA, Phillips DE, Roland NR. Squamous carcinoma presenting as an enlarged cervical lymph node. Cancer 1993; 72: 1752–61.

18. Miller FR, Hussey D, Beeram M, et al. Positron emission tomography in the management of unknown primary head and neck carcinoma. Arch Otolaryngol Head Neck Surg 2005; 131: 626–9.

19. Guntinas-Lichius O, Peter Klussmann J, Dinh S, et al. Diagnostic work-up and outcome of cervical metastases from an unknown primary. Acta Otolaryngol 2006; 126: 536–44.

20. Patel RS, Clark J, Wyten R, Gao K, O'Brien CJ. Squamous cell carcinoma from an unknown head and neck primary site: a "selective treatment" approach. Arch Otolaryngol Head Neck Surg 2007; 133: 1282–7.

21. Doty JM, Gossman D, Kudrimoti M, et al. Analysis of unknown primary carcinomas metastatic to the neck; diagnosis, treatment, and outcomes. J Ky Med Assoc 2006; 104: 57–64.

22. Aslani M, Sultanem K, Voung T, et al. Metastatic carcinoma to the cervical nodes from an unknown head and neck primary site: is there a need for neck dissection? Head Neck 2007; 29: 585–90.

23. Boscolo-Rizzo P, Gava A, Da Mosto MC. Carcinoma metastatic to cervical lymph nodes from an occult primary tumor: the outcome after combined-modality therapy. Ann Surg Oncol 2007; 14: 1575–82.

24. Colletier PJ, Garden AS, Morrison WH, et al. Postoperative radiation for squamous cell carcinoma metastatic to cervical lymph nodes from an unknown primary site: outcomes and patterns of failure. Head Neck 1998; 20: 674–81.

25. Iganej S, Kagan R, Anderson P, et al. Metastatic squamous cell carcinoma of the neck from an unknown primary: management options and patterns of relapse. Head Neck 2002; 24: 236–46.

26. Stewart JF, Tattersall MHN, Woods RL, Fox RM. Unknown primary adenocarcinoma: incidence of overinvestigation and natural history. Br Med J 1979; 1: 1530–3.

27. Abbruzzese JL, Abbruzzese MC, Hess KR, et al. Unknown primary carcinoma: natural history and prognostic factors in 657 consecutive patients. J Clin Oncol 1994; 12: 1272–80.

28. McMillan JH, Levine E, Stephens R. Computed tomography in the evaluation of metastatic adenocarcinoma from an unknown primary site. Radiology 1982; 143: 143–6.

29. Kurtz AB, Tsimikas JV, Tempany CM, et al. Diagnosis and staging of ovarian cancer, comparative values of doppler and conventional US, CT, and MRI imaging correlated with surgery and histopathologic analysis: report of the Radiologic Diagnostic Oncology Group. Radiology 1999; 212: 19–27.

30. Orel SG, Weinstein SP, Schnall MD, et al. Breast MR imaging in patients with axillary node metastases and unknown primary malignancy. Radiology 1999; 212: 543–9.

31. Olson JA, Jr, Morris EA, Van Zee KJ, Linehan DC, Borgen PI. Magnetic resonance imaging facilitates breast conservation for occult breast cancer. Ann Surg Oncol 2000; 7: 411–15.

32. Bohuslavizki KH, Klutmann S, Kroger S, et al. FDG PET detection of unknown primary tumors. J Nucl Med 2000; 41: 816–22.

33. Kole AC, Neiweg OE, Pruim J, et al. Detection of unknown occult primary tumors using positron emission tomography. Cancer 1998; 82: 1160–6.

34. Lassen U, Daugaard G, Eigtved A, Damgaard K, Friberg L. ^{18}F-FDG whole-body positron emission tomography (PET) in patients with unknown primary tumors (UPT). Eur J Cancer 1999; 35: 1076–82.

35. Rades D, Kühnel G, Wildfang I, et al. Localised disease in cancer of unknown primary (CUP): the value of positron emission tomography (PET) for individual therapeutic management. Annal Oncol 2001; 12: 1605–9.

36. Sève P, Billotey C, Broussolle C, Dumontet C, Mackey JR. The role of 2-deoxy-2-(F-18)fluoro-D-glucose positron emission tomography in disseminated carcinoma of unknown primary site. Cancer 2007; 109: 292–9.

37. Garin E, Prigent-Lejeune F, Lesimple T, et al. Impact of PET-FDG in the diagnosis and therapeutic care of patients presenting with metastases of unknown primary. Cancer Invest 2007; 25: 232–9.

38. Pelosi E, Pennone M, Deandreis D, et al. Role of whole body positron emission tomography/computed tomography scan with ^{18}F-fluorodeoxyglucose in patients with biopsy proven tumor metastases from unknown primary site. Q J Nucl Med Mol Imaging 2006; 50: 15–22.

39. Scott CL, Kudaba I, Stewart JM, Hicks RJ, Rischin D. The utility of 2-deoxy-2-(F-18)fluoro-D-glucose positron emission tomography in the investigation of patients with disseminated carcinoma of unknown primary origin. Mol Imaging Biol 2005; 7: 236–43.

40. Nystrom JS, Weiner JM, Heffelfinger-Juttner J, et al. Metastatic and histologic presentations in unknown primary cancer. Semin Oncol 1977; 4: 53–8.

41. van der Gaast A, Verweij J, Henzen-Logmans SC, Rodenburg CJ, Stoter G. Carcinoma of unknown primary: identification of a treatable subset? Ann Oncol 1990; 1: 119–22.

42. Greco FA, Vaughn WK, Hainsworth JD. Advanced poorly differentiated carcinoma of unknown primary site: recognition of a treatable syndrome. Ann Intern Med 1986; 104: 547–53.

43. Hainsworth JD, Johnson DH, Greco FA. Cisplatin-based combination chemotherapy in the treatment of poorly differentiated carcinoma and poorly differentiated adenocarcinoma of unknown primary site: results of a 12-year experience. J Clin Oncol 1992; 10: 912–22.

44. Lobins R, Floyd J. Small cell carcinoma of unknown primary. Semin Oncol 2007; 34: 39–42.

45. Cormier JN, Xing Y, Feng L, et al. Metastatic melanoma to lymph nodes in patients with unknown primary sites. Cancer 2006; 106: 2012–20.

46. Lee CC, Faries MB, Waneck LA, Morton DL. Improved survival after lymphadenectomy for nodal metastasis from an unknown primary melanoma. J Clin Oncol 2008; 26: 535–41.

47. de Wilt JH, Farmer SE, Scolyer RA, McCaughan BC, Thompson JF. Isolated melanoma in the lung where there is no known primary site: metastatic disease or primary lung tumor? Melanoma Res 2005; 15: 531–7.

48. Van de Wouw AJ, Janssen-Heijnen ML, Coebergh JW, Hillen HF. Epidemiology of unknown primary tumours: incidence and population-based survival of 1285 patients in Southeast Netherlands, 1984–1992. Eur J Cancer 2002; 38: 409–13.

49. Piga A, Gesuita R, Catalano V, et al. Identification of clinical prognostic factors in patients with unknown primary tumours treated with platinum based combination. Oncology 2005; 69: 135–44.

50. Seve P, Ray-Coquard I, Trillet-Lenoir V, et al. Low serum albumen levels and liver metastasis are powerful prognostic markers for survival in patients with carcinomas of unknown primary site. Cancer 2006; 107: 2698–705.

51. Seve P, Sawyer M, Hanson J, et al. The influence of comorbidities, age, and performance status on prognosis and treatment of patients with metastatic carcinomas of unknown primary site: a population-based study. Cancer 2006; 106: 2058–66.

52. Shaw PH, Adams R, Jordan C, Crosby TD. A clinical review of the investigation and management of carcinoma of unknown primary in a single cancer network. Clin Oncol 2007; 19: 87–95.

53. Rosen P. Axillary lymph node metastases in patients with occult noninvasive breast carcinoma. Cancer 1980; 46: 1298–306.

54. Varadarajan R, Edge SB, Yu J, Watroba N, Janarthanan BR. Prognosis of occult breast carcinoma presenting as isolated nodal metastasis. Oncology 2006; 71: 456–9.

55. Hewitt MJ, Anderson K, Hall GD, et al. Women with peritoneal carcinomatosis of unknown origin: efficacy of image guided biopsy to determine site specific diagnosis. Br J Obstet Gynaecol 2007; 114: 46–50.

56. Strand CM, Grosh WW, Baxter J, et al. Peritoneal carcinomatosis of unknown primary site in women. Ann Int Med 1989; 111: 213–17.

57. Ransom DT, Patel SR, Keeney GL, Malkasian GD, Edmonson JH. Papillary serous carcinoma of the peritoneum. Cancer 1990; 66: 1091–4.

58. CRC Cancer Fact Sheet. Prostate cancer. June 2002.

59. Destombe C, Botton E, Le Gal G, et al. Investigations for bone metastasis from an unknown primary. Joint Bone Spine 2008; 74: 85–9.

60. Pouessel D, Thezenas S, Culine S, et al. Hepatic metastases from carcinomas of unknown primary site. Gastroenterol Clin Biol 2005; 29: 1224–32.

61. Rades D, Bohlen G, Lohynska R, et al. Whole brain radiotherapy with 20 Gy in 5 fractions for brain metastases in patients with cancer of unknown primary. Strahlenther Onkol 2007; 183: 631–6.

62. Rades D, Fehlauer F, Veninger T, et al. Functional outcome and survival after radiotherapy of spinal cord compression in patients with cancer of unknown primary. Int J Radiat Oncol Biol Phys 2007; 67: 532–7.

63. D'Ambrosio AL, Agazzi S. Prognosis in patients presenting with brain metastasis from an undiagnosed primary tumour. Neurosurg Focus 2007; 22: E7.

64. Greco FA, Burris HA III, Litchy S, et al. Gemcitabine, carboplatin and paclitaxel for patients with carcinoma of unknown primary site: a Minnie Pearl cancer research network study. J Clin Oncol 2002; 20: 1651–6.

65. Schneider BJ, El-Rayes B, Muler JH, et al. Phase II trial of carboplatin, gemcitabine, and capecitabine in patients with carcinoma of unknown primary site. Cancer 2007; 110: 770–5.

66. Palmeri S, Lorusso V, Palmeri L, et al. Cisplatin and gemcitabine with either vinorelbine or paclitaxel in the treatment of carcinomas of unknown primary site: results of an Italian multicenter, randomised phase II study. Cancer 2006; 107: 2898–3905.

67. Pittman KB, Olver IN, Koczwara B, et al. Gemcitabine and carboplatin in carcinoma of unknown primary site: a phase 2 Adelaide Cancer Trials and Education collaborative study. Br J Cancer 2006; 95: 1309–13.

50 Interventional Imaging: General Applications
Tarun Sabharwal, Nicos Fotiadis, and Andreas Adam

INTRODUCTION

Over the past four decades, a variety of invasive diagnostic and therapeutic procedures have been developed by radiologists. Interventional Radiology (IR) uses all available imaging modalities [fluoroscopy, ultrasound (US), computed tomography (CT), magnetic resonance (MR), angiography] for guidance of interventional procedures for diagnostic or therapeutic purposes (1). The emergence of this specialty has been made possible by enormous technological advances in relation to catheter and instrument design and manufacture, imaging systems and radiological expertise. Interventional radiological procedures have virtually replaced several more invasive surgical and hazardous surgical alternatives. The need for open surgical biopsy or surgical insertion of tunneled central venous catheters has been significantly reduced since these procedures can be performed by radiologists under imaging guidance and local anesthetic as day-case procedures.

IR has a wide application in the diagnosis, active management, and palliation of malignant disease. However radiological interventions in cancer patients require a comprehensive assessment of the patient and careful consideration of the risks and benefits of the procedure. Factors unique to oncology patients must be evaluated, and decisions regarding therapeutic benefit must be made in light of the patient's prognosis and quality of life considerations. Effective communication of information about nature, benefits, and potential complications are an integral part of the treatment (2).

In this chapter emphasis is based on the indications, contraindications and likely outcomes rather than detailed technical considerations.

THORACIC INTERVENTION

Transthoracic Needle Biopsy

Percutaneous transthoracic biopsy is a rapid, safe, effective means of establishing a diagnosis in a patient with a pulmonary, pleural, or mediastinal lesion (3). In general percutaneous biopsy is performed when histological diagnosis will modify staging of the disease, influence therapeutic strategy, and when diagnosis cannot be established by bronchoscopic techniques (3).

Most central endobronchial lesions are biopsied bronchoscopically. The majority of the percutaneous biopsies are usually performed under CT guidance (Fig. 50.1) (3,4). It is easier to visualize small tumors with CT, to avoid vascular structures and also to biopsy from the viable part of the tumor rather than the necrotic areas.

Fluoroscopy could be used for large masses, which are clearly visible in posteroanterior and lateral projections. In these cases, transthoracic fluoroscopic-guided biopsy is unquestionably quicker and less expensive.

US guidance is useful for pleural biopsy, rib lesions, subcutaneous deposits, and peripheral lung lesions reaching a pleural surface.

CT-fluoroscopy has evolved in the last decade and can be extremely effective with lesions difficult to target but has the disadvantage of a significant amount of radiation for the operator (5).

Fine needle aspiration biopsy (FNAB) is usually sufficient for diagnosis especially with the new cytological techniques, for example, DNA cytofluorometry, immunocytochemistry, and tumor marker characterization (6). Diagnostic accuracy varies between 80% and 95% in different series (3,6). A cytologist should be in attendance whenever possible.

Cutting needle biopsy however provides larger cores of tissue for examinations, which can more reliably establish a benign diagnosis and are essential for diagnosis, subclassification, and immunotyping of lymphoreticular malignancies (7,8). There is no significant difference in rates of complications between FNAB and tru-cut biopsy of lung lesions (3). Pneumothorax (Fig. 50.2) is the commonest complication with an incidence that varies from 5% to 50%, with a mean of 20%. Less than 5% of patients have persistent clinical symptoms and require aspiration or drainage (3–7). Factors influencing pneumothorax are:

- Chronic obstructive pulmonary disease, especially emphysema
- Age
- Experience of the operator
- Number of transpleural needle passes (4,6,7)

If the use of a number of transpleural needle passes is anticipated then the use of coaxial needle technique is strongly recommended. In all cases, transgression of the needle through bullae should be avoided and needle passage through normal lung should be kept to a minimum (4,6,7). Hemorrhage, with or without hemoptysis, is encountered in less than 10% of cases, most of which are self-limited (4–7). If bleeding persists, bronchoscopic tamponade or bronchial artery embolization is indicated.

A relatively new technique for biopsying mediastinal masses is the application of endoscopic ultrasound (EUS) guidance with a multichannel scope introduced into the esophagus. With this technique, accessible mediastinal lesions can be biopsied using a fine needle, obviating invasive mediastinoscopy under general anesthesia (9).

Key Points: Transthoracic Needle Biopsy

- Percutaneous biopsy is performed when histological diagnosis will modify staging of the disease, influence the therapeutic strategy, and when diagnosis cannot be established by bronchoscopic techniques
- FNAB and cutting needle biopsy have the same diagnostic accuracy (80–95%) for lung malignancies and approximately the same low rate of complications
- Cutting needle biopsy may establish a benign diagnosis more reliably than FNAB and is essential for classification of primary lymphoreticular malignancies
- Coaxial needle technique and minimum needle passage through normal lung decrease the risk of pneumothorax
- CT-guided biopsy or EUS is recommended for lesions with poor accessibility

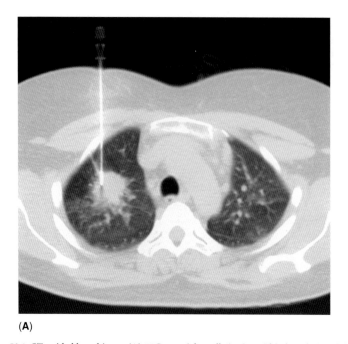 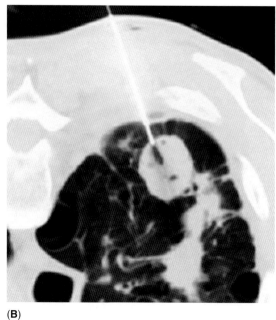

(A)   (B)

Figure 50.1 CT-guided lung biopsy. (A) 18G co-axial needle in situ within lung lesion. (B) Another example of co-axial guided biopsy. Note is made of the adjustment of needle to avoid multiple bulla. *Source*: Courtesy of Prof. A Gangi, France.

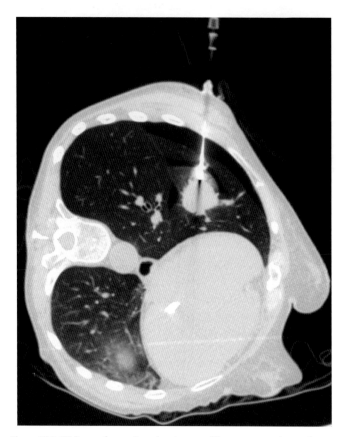

Figure 50.2 CT in another patient showing post biopsy pneumothorax that was subsequently aspirated via co-axial needle.

Thoracic Drainage Procedures

Malignant pleural effusions (MPEs) can produce significant respiratory symptoms and diminished quality of life in patients with cancer. A patient who presents with a MPE should have a diagnostic and therapeutic thoracocentesis, ideally under US guidance. It is important to assess for symptom improvement and the ability of the lung to re-expand. The fluid will re-accumulate in almost all patients, at which time local treatment should be needed. This typically consists of a small-bore tube (8–10 F) inserted under US guidance and installation of sclerosing agent (doxycycline, bleomycin, or talc) to chemically induce pleurodesis (10). A tunneled pleural catheter is also available for long-term out-patient palliation of malignant pleural effusions. The catheter is inserted under local anesthesia, with US and x-ray guidance in the interventional radiology suite (11). Infected thoracic collections are common in the immunocompromized oncologic patient; these include empyemas, parapneumonic and other pleural effusions, and pulmonary and mediastinal abscesses. Percutaneous drainage can be performed under US or CT guidance for the more complex cases and in general these need larger bore catheters 12 F to 20 F (12). Most organized collections do not adequately drain because of the presence of multiple loculi. In this situation intrapleural fibinolysis can be useful.

Key Points: Thoracic Drainage

■ US guidance is ideal for malignant pleural effusion drainage
■ CT guidance is indicated for complex multiloculated collections

Central Venous Obstruction

Superior vena cava obstruction (SVCO) syndrome often presents as a very distressing pre-terminal event in patients with thoracic malignancy. It is most commonly related to mediastinal neoplasia, particularly primary and secondary lung tumors and lymphoma. The obstruction, which can be partial or complete, can be caused by compression and/or invasion by tumor of the SVC; it is frequently complicated by venous thrombosis.

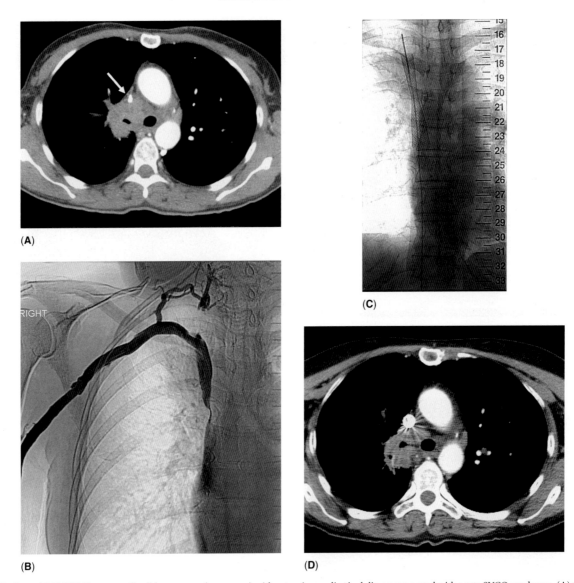

Figure 50.3 Patient with T4N3M1 non-small cell lung cancer (squamous) with extensive mediastinal disease presented with acute SVCO syndrome. (A) CT illustrating significant narrowing of SVC (arrow). (B) Right arm venogram confirming stenosis of SVC. The absence of collaterals is consistent with acute presentation. (C) SVC stent deployed via femoral route. (D) CT 14 months' post-procedure showing patent stent. The patient was now asymptomatic.

Superior venocavography delineates the site and extent of the obstruction. If extensive thrombosis is present, selective intravenous thrombolysis with a catheter placed within the thrombus is undertaken under local anesthesia. Percutaneous transfemoral or transjugular dilatation of the narrowed SVC is always followed by the insertion of a self-expandable metallic endoprosthesis (Fig. 50.3). Flow is restored immediately, providing excellent and immediate palliation of symptoms (13). This procedure of stenting can be performed prior to, in conjunction with, or after therapy, including radiotherapy or chemotherapy. It can also be performed in conjunction with airway stenting. In cases where there is obstruction of the central neck veins bilaterally, as well as the SVC, relief of obstruction on one side alone often provides adequate palliation (14).

Malignant involvement of the inferior vena cava can be managed in a similar fashion.

Tracheobronchial Stenting

Malignant airways obstruction can cause considerable distress to the patient. Tracheobronchial stenting is a useful, simple technique for the palliation of stridor caused by tumors within the upper mediastinum compromising the trachea and the main bronchus (15). Tracheobronchial stenting is best carried out under general anesthesia, as a combined effort between an interventional radiologist and a bronchoscopist. Bronchoscopic visualization is used to determine the position of the stricture, the limits of which are marked with a radio-opaque marker. The stricture is then dilated under fluoroscopic guidance. Following dilatation, a self-expandable metallic stent is released across the stricture, again under fluoroscopic guidance. This can result in significant symptomatic improvement and prevent collapse and/or infection and abscess formation beyond an obstructing lesion (Fig. 50.4) (16). Placement of covered metallic stents in the trachea is an effective method of managing tracheo-esophageal fistulae unsuitable for treatment with covered esophageal stents (17).

Techniques for Management of Hemoptysis

Massive hemoptysis is classically defined as an excess of 300 ml blood loss in 24 hours. Most frequent causes of major hemoptysis

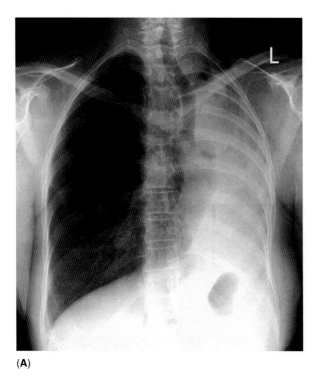

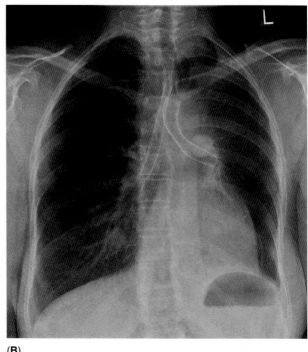

(A)   **(B)**

Figure 50.4 Chest radiographs in a patient suffering with severe respiratory distress. The patient was known to have metastatic lung cancer. (**A**) Left lung collapse due to complete occlusion of the left main bronchus. (**B**) Re-expansion left lung following insertion of bilateral bronchial stents.

in oncological patients include bronchogenic carcinoma, hypervascular metastasis, and post-transthoracic or transbronchial biopsy. Less frequently immunocompromised cancer patients present with hemoptysis due to tuberculosis or other infections, or radiation-induced pneumonitis. Bronchial artery embolization is a technically demanding but potential life-saving intervention for patients with massive hemoptysis. High quality angiographic images are pre-requisite to reveal a possible anastomosis with the artery of Adamkiewicz (anterior spinal artery supply) which if inadvertently embolized could cause tetraplegia. The application of microcatheters is extremely useful for super-selective embolization. Preferred embolic materials are polyvinyl alcohol particles (PVA), gelfoam, and tris-acryl gelatine microspheres.

Key Points: Thoracic Interventions

■ SVC stenting provides immediate and durable palliation for patients with malignant SVCO

■ Tracheobronchial stenting is a useful simple technique for the palliation of stridor secondary to airway compression by tumor

■ Bronchial artery embolization is a technically demanding but potential life-saving technique for massive hemoptysis

---

GASTROINTESTINAL INTERVENTIONS

Biopsy Techniques

Biopsy techniques have already been described in some detail in the previous section and the same general principles apply to the

gastrointestinal tract. In most cases percutaneous abdominal biopsy is performed under US or CT guidance (Fig. 50.5). Both these imaging techniques allow the radiologist to visualize not only the target lesion but also the intervening organs, thus increasing the accuracy and safety of the procedure. The choice between the two techniques depends on the experience and preference of the radiologist and on the precise location of the lesion to be biopsied. For example, retroperitoneal masses are usually easier to visualize with CT scans, whereas lesions in the dome of the liver immediately below the diaphragm are best biopsied under US guidance because this modality allows an oblique approach that avoids the lungs. US is usually quicker to perform, is cheaper, does not involve ionizing radiation and is available as a portable technique.

When lymphoreticular malignancy is suspected, larger 16 G to 18 G needles are used to supply large cores of tissue adequate for subclassification and immunotyping (8). For all other intra-abdominal lesions, a 18 G to 20 G cutting needle is usually sufficient.

Before a biopsy is performed every attempt should be made to correct any coagulopathy. In patients with uncorrectable coagulopathy and bleeding diathesis, percutaneous biopsy carries an increased risk of major, uncontrollable hemorrhage. In such patients embolization of the track can be performed. A co-axial biopsy needle is used. Under imaging guidance the coaxial introducer is inserted in the target lesion. The stylet of the introducer is removed and the biopsy needle is inserted in the lesion. Several samples should be obtained. The biopsy needle is withdrawn leaving the coaxial introducer in place. The biopsy tract is then embolized with gelfoam or steel coils as the co-axial introducer is withdrawn (18,19).

Remarkable developments have been made in endoluminal US technology allowing deep pelvic lesions to be accessed transrectally

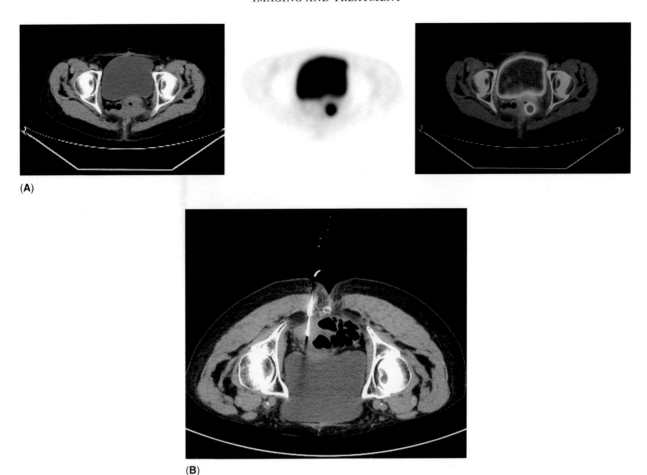

Figure 50.5 A 66-year-old female patient who had undergone AP resection and pelvic radiotherapy for rectal adenocarcinoma four years previously. She was being investigated for a suspicious lung nodule but CT and MR imaging showed no evidence of local recurrence. (A) PET-CT revealed a focus of increased metabolic activity in the left para-rectal space. (B) CT-guided biopsy needle in situ. This proved to be recurrent tumor.

(prostate biopsies) (20) or transvaginally (ovarian cysts aspiration). Endoscopic ultrasound (EUS) is particularly useful for biopsy and staging of locoregional lymph nodes in esophageal, gastric, and colonic cancer (21). Furthermore EUS is also often the safest way to biopsy small pancreatic tumors (22).

Key Points: Gastrointestinal Biopsy

- Co-axial plugged biopsy is indicated for vascular lesions and in patients with bleeding diathesis
- Transrectal and transvaginal US are commonly used for pelvic biopsy and drainage procedures
- EUS with biopsy is useful in staging esophageal, gastric, and colonic malignancy

Percutaneous Drainage Procedures

The accumulation of large volume ascites is a common occurrence in patients with intraperitoneal spread. Malignant ascites is distressing for the patient and frequently can be drained using a percutaneous technique without imaging guidance. In cases of difficulty or loculation of fluid, US guidance is extremely useful for achievement of complete drainage.

Abdominal and pelvic collections of fluid as well as abscesses may develop as a complication of medical or surgical treatment. These are easily drained using US or CT for guidance. Pelvic abscess drainage may be performed via transrectal or transvaginal approaches. These are safer and considerably less painful than the transgluteal approach.

Key Point: Percutaneous Drainage Procedures

- Transrectal and transvaginal approaches are safer and less painful than the transgluteal approach for pelvic abscess drainage

Management of Esophageal and Upper Gastrointestinal Strictures

Esophageal cancer is the commonest cause of a malignant stricture of the esophagus and leads to progressive dysphagia, malnutrition, and aspiration. The most rapid and durable relief of the dysphagia associated with esophageal cancer is provided by the insertion of a self-expandable metallic stent (23–26). Placement of the stent can be achieved under fluoroscopic or endoscopic guidance, or both. The procedure is relatively straightforward with negligible mortality and

low morbidity (24). Advantages of radiological placement of esophageal stents include:

- Accurate positioning under x-ray guidance
- Ability to traverse even tight stenoses or occlusions
- Ability to use small caliber catheters and wires which minimizes the risk of perforation and bleeding (24,25)

New advances in esophageal stent technology include smaller introductory devices, more flexible stents, retrievable stents which can be used as a bridge to surgery and devices with an anti-reflux valve which are used for stenting across the gastroesophageal junction (25,26).

Covered metallic esophageal stents are also integral to the management of malignant esophageal fistulas (Fig. 50.6). Unlike fistulas associated with benign diseases, which may heal with conservative therapy, malignant fistulas do not heal spontaneously. Without definitive treatment, most patients succumb to malnutrition and thoracic sepsis within weeks. Radiological insertion of a covered metallic stent can result in immediate sealing of the fistula and the patient can drink fluids within a few hours of the procedure, resuming a normal diet the following day (27).

Gastroduodenal obstruction is a preterminal event in many patients with advanced upper gastrointestinal malignant disease. Patients with gastric outlet and with duodenal obstruction often exhibit intractable nausea, vomiting, and inability to eat which leads to weight loss, dehydration and electrolyte disturbance, and a markedly impaired quality of life. Radiological insertion of a large-diameter, self-expanding stent (Fig. 50.7) can overcome gastroduodenal obstruction and re-establish oral feeding in such patients (28). The procedure of gastroduodenal stenting is performed via the peroral route. In a minority of

patients in whom there is failure to negotiate the stricture via the peroral approach, a shorter more direct route to the stricture via a gastrostomy may prove useful. The procedure can be guided under fluoroscopy alone or with fluoroscopy combined with endoscopy. However, fluoroscopy is essential for positioning of the stent.

Dilatation and Stenting of Lower Gastrointestinal Strictures

In the setting of acute malignant obstruction of the large bowel, the insertion of a self-expanding enteral stent can rapidly relieve the obstruction thereby providing immediate relief of symptoms (Fig. 50.8) (29,30). This may be a temporizing measure allowing stabilization of the patient prior to definitive surgery, or alternatively, for those who are not surgical candidates, the stent may provide adequate palliation (30). Rectosigmoid and descending colon lesions can be negotiated with fluoroscopic guidance alone whereas higher strictures may need a combined fluoroscopic-endoscopic approach (29,30). In cases of benign postoperative strictures following resection of a malignant lesion, balloon dilatation is usually sufficient to achieve alleviation of obstruction.

Percutaneous Gastrostomy–Gastrojejunostomy Feeding Tubes

In the management of patients with malignant disease, nutritional support is essential, particularly in those who are severely debilitated or unable to swallow. Parenteral nutrition can be provided using central venous catheters, but this is associated with significant morbidity and considerable expense. Enteral feeding

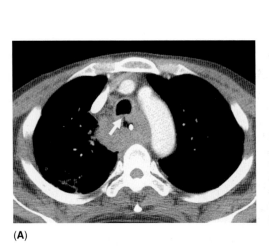

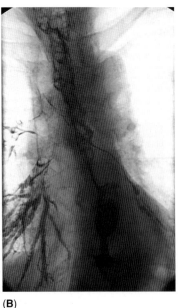

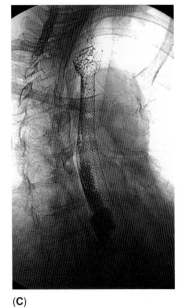

(A) **(B)** **(C)**

Figure 50.6 (A) CT demonstrating a tracheo-esophageal fistula (arrow) in a patient with known esophageal cancer. This was causing significant symptomatic distress. (B) Water-soluble contrast swallow image revealing the fistula and a considerable amount of contrast in the bronchial tree. (C) Water-soluble contrast swallow illustrating exclusion of the fistula following insertion of a covered esophageal stent.

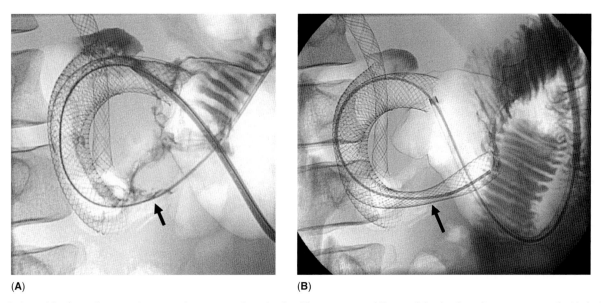

(A)   **(B)**

Figure 50.7 Patient with advanced pancreatic cancer who was treated previously with percutaneous biliary and duodenal stenting, now presented with further gastric outlet obstruction. (A) This was seen to be from tumor overgrowth in the third part of the duodenum (arrow). (B) This was treated with a longer duodenal stent inserted (arrow) over a wire and through a Mullins sheath.

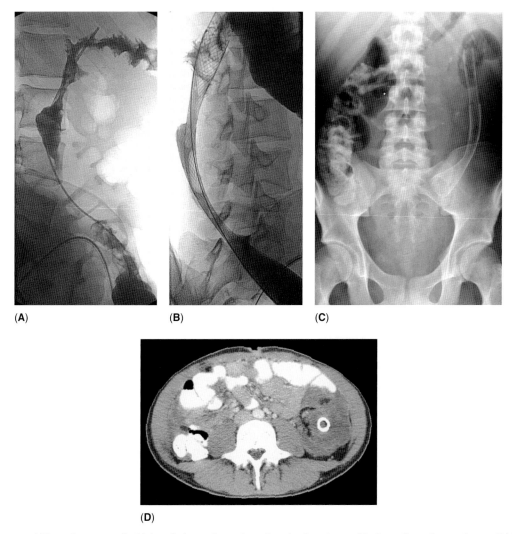

(A)   **(B)**   **(C)**

(D)

Figure 50.8 Seventeen-year-old boy who presented with bowel obstruction and was found to have inoperable descending colon carcinoma. (A) Radiological catheter study showing long colonic stricture. (B) Two colonic stents were deployed under fluoroscopic guidance. (C) An abdominal radiograph the next day showed satisfactory positioning and proximal bowel decompression. (D) CT demonstrating huge colonic tumor with patent stent in-situ.

is more desirable and can be provided by the insertion of gastrostomy tubes. Gastrojejunostomy tubes are preferable when there is gastric outlet obstruction or in cases of gastro-esophageal reflux (31). Several different techniques have been described for percutaneous gastrostomy insertion (32) with or without gastropexy under fluoroscopic guidance (Fig. 50.9).

If a stent in the pylorus fails to relieve obstruction, gastrostomy may also be useful for relieving symptoms in patients with gastric outlet obstruction due to retroperitoneal or mesenteric malignancy.

Key Points: Gastrointestinal Strictures

- Self-expandable metallic stents offer excellent palliation for obstructive (dysphagia) and locally invasive (fistulae and perforations) symptoms of esophageal carcinoma
- Enteral stents may provide palliation for malignant gastric outflow obstruction and acute large bowel obstruction
- The provision of enteral feeding through radiological placement of a gastrostomy–gastrojejunostomy tube is the preferable technique for palliation of patients who are unable to swallow or who have gastric outlet obstruction

MANAGEMENT OF MALIGNANT BILIARY STRICTURES

Recent advances in non-invasive imaging, in particular multidetector CT and MR cholangiography, have obviated the need for percutaneous transhepatic cholangiography (PTC) in the imaging investigation of the jaundiced patient. In many centers multi-detector CT and MR cholangiography, are increasingly used to determine the site and nature of biliary obstruction and to plan the approach for percutaneous or endoscopic drainage.

Patients with obstructive jaundice due to irresectable malignant biliary strictures can be palliated by the insertion of a stent. For surgical candidates, preoperative biliary drainage may be performed to correct metabolic disturbances and to stabilize the patient. Stents may be inserted endoscopically for lesions affecting the lower and mid common bile duct or percutaneously in patients with lesions at the hilum of the liver (Fig. 50.10) or when endoscopic retrograde cholangiopancreatography (ERCP) fails to relieve the obstruction (33). In most cases a unilateral approach is usually sufficient for relieving jaundice and pruritis. The procedure is usually carried out under fluoroscopic and US guidance. First a PTC is performed using a 22 G needle. It is important to visualize the entire biliary system prior to selecting the most suitable duct for insertion of a drainage catheter. Self-expanding metallic stents are widely available today and in general are preferable to conventional plastic endoprostheses (33). Such stents can be inserted using a small introducing catheter (5–7 French diameter) and yet they achieve a large internal diameter (10 mm) when released across the obstructing lesion. The large caliber of these devices ensures that the rate of occlusion is lower than that of plastic endoprostheses. In our experience, the incidence of hemorrhage and cholangitis is approximately three times lower with metallic endoprostheses than plastic stents. Most importantly the incidence of re-intervention to replace an occluded stent has also been found to be three times lower with metallic stents (34). A randomized trail comparing endoscopically inserted self-expanding metal stents with plastic stents has confirmed the longer patency of metallic endoprostheses and has shown that, although these stents are more expensive than the conventional plastic devices, the cost per patient is lower because of the lower rate of re-intervention (35).

Key Points: Management of Biliary Strictures

- Multidetector CT and MR cholangiography have cardinal roles in the initial non-invasive evaluation of biliary strictures
- ERCP is the procedure of choice for management of lower and mid-common bile duct strictures
- PTC has a higher success rate and lower complication rate for hilar strictures than ERCP
- Metal stents have higher rates of patency and lower rates of complications and re-interventions than plastic biliary stents

INTERVENTIONAL PROCEDURES IN THE MANAGEMENT OF LIVER TUMORS

Transarterial Chemoembolization of Liver Tumors

Image-guided catheter based therapies have revolutionized the non-surgical management of patients with primary and metastatic liver cancer. Currently various forms of catheter based therapies are used, including transcatheter arterial chemoembolization (TACE), transcatheter arterial embolization (TAE), and TAE with drug-eluting beads (DEB). TACE is conceptually appealing because

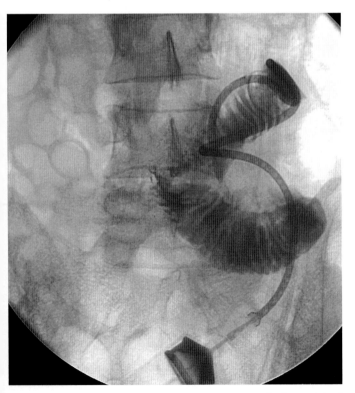

Figure 50.9 Percutaneous jejunostomy inserted fluoroscopically for nutritional support in a patient with gastric cancer.

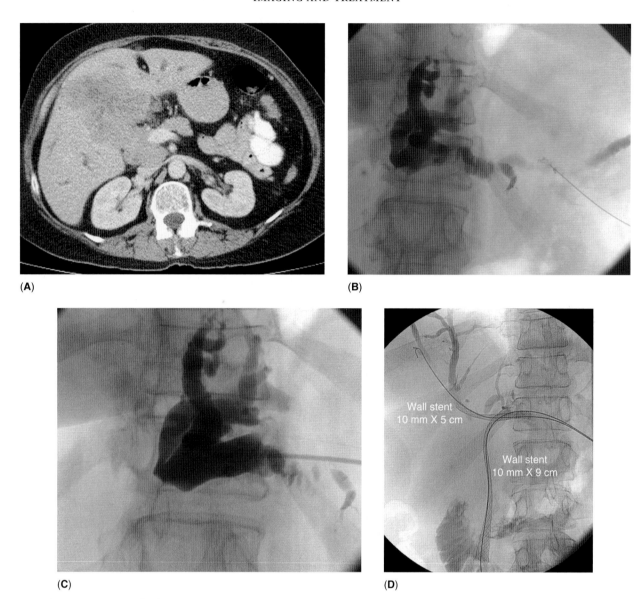

Figure 50.10 (A) CT in a patient with a large inoperable cholangiocarcinoma. (B) Peripheral segment III bile duct access under percutaneous fluoroscopy. (C) Cholangiogram showing central occlusion. (D) Successful decompression of both lobes via left access with biliary stents.

it causes some degree of ischemia within the tumor directly, which may increase death of tumor cells, and significantly extends tumor drug concentrations. The most widely used single chemotherapeutic agent is doxorubicin; in the United States a combination of drugs is the preferred option (cisplatin, doxorubicin, and mitomycin). Lipiodol almost always serves as a drug carrier and tumor seeking agent (Fig. 50.11). Some degree of embolization of the tumor-feeding arteries is also typically performed at the end of the procedure with a variety of embolic agents.

At present TACE is considered to be the mainstay of treatment for unresectable hepatocellular carcinoma (HCC). It provides significantly prolonged survival in selected patients with preserved liver function and adequate performance status (36). Prolonged survival can be achieved in selected patients with a combination of local ablative techniques (percutaneous ethanol injection, radiofrequency ablation) and TACE (37). TACE also has been used as a bridge for orthotopic liver transplantation (37).

In TAE with DEB, polyvinyl alcohol-based microspheres can be loaded with various types of chemotherapeutic agents and delivered intra-arterially in a manner similar to conventional TACE. Such a system loaded with doxorubicin has shown promising results in patients with unresectable HCC with an advantageous pharmacokinetic profile, reduced adverse effects, and improved tumor response as shown by imaging when compared with conventional TACE (38).

Radioembolization of Liver Tumors

Radioembolization is a local-regional liver-directed therapy that involves transcatheter delivery of particles embedded with the radioisotope yttrium-90 (^{90}Y). Particles are infused through a catheter into the hepatic artery from where they travel distally and lodge at the tumor arteriolar level. Once embedded within the arterioles, the ^{90}Y impregnated microspheres emit high energy and low penetrating radiation dose selectively to the tumor. Recently radioembolization

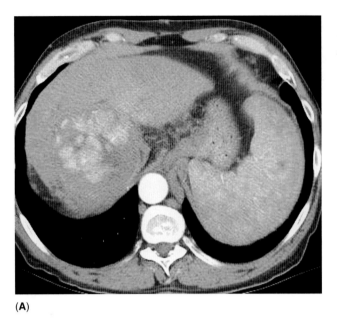

(A)

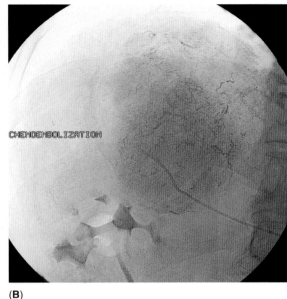

(B)

Figure 50.11 (**A**) CT demonstrating large arterial enhancing hepatocellular carcinoma in the right lobe of the liver. (**B**) TACE catheter directed embolization illustrating staining of tumor with lipiodol.

has shown promise for the treatment of uresectable hepatocellular carcinoma and metastatic liver disease (39,40).

Percutaneous Tumor Ablation

Ablation refers to local (rather than systemic) methods that destroy the tumor without removing it. The most frequent indication for percutaneous tumor ablation is for the treatment of liver tumors. This is largely due to the high incidence of liver metastases and the low number of patients who are deemed to have resectable disease. Other organs that are currently successfully treated with percutaneous ablation methods include the kidneys, lungs, adrenals, bone, breast, lymph nodes, and soft tissue tumors. Percutaneous techniques of local tumor ablation may be categorized into three major groups:

- Injection (ethanol, acetic acid, hot saline)
- Heating (radiofrequency, interstitial laser therapy, microwave coagulation therapy, high-intensity focused US)
- Freezing (cryotherapy)

Advantages of ablative therapies compared with surgical resection include reduced morbidity and mortality, low cost, and the ability to perform procedures on an out-patient basis (41). These techniques are described in detail in chapter 51.

Key Points: Embolization for Liver Tumors

- TACE is currently considered the mainstay of treatment for unresectable HCC providing a significantly prolonged survival in selected patients with preserved liver function and adequate performance status
- Combination of TACE with local-regional ablative techniques (ethanol injection-RFA) shows higher response rates than TACE alone
- HCC shows greater response to hepatic chemoembolization than metastases

PERCUTANEOUS NEUROLYSIS

Chronic abdominal pain can be associated with benign and malignant disease. Pain associated with pancreatic and gastric cancer can be severely debilitating with significant impairment in quality of life. Frequently, this chronic abdominal pain does not respond adequately to conventional analgesics including opioids. Celiac plexus neurolysis and celiac plexus block are aimed at either selectively destroying the celiac plexus or temporarily blocking visceral afferent nociceptors to alleviate chronic pain. Both techniques require injection of the chosen agent at the celiac axis. Agents most commonly used include alcohol for neurolysis and bupivacaine and triamcinolone for temporary block. The procedure may be performed percutaneously either under CT (Fig. 50.12) or fluoroscopic guidance or endoscopically under EUS guidance. Between 70% and 85% of patients experience pain relief lasting from one month up to one year post-procedure (42). Complications include transient diarrhea, orthostasis, and transient increase in pain but the incidence of these is low. Major complications occur in less than 1% of patients and include retroperitoneal bleeding, abscess formation, and transient or permanent paraplegia (42).

Key Point: Neurolytic Celiac Plexus Blockade

- Intractable pain from gastric or pancreatic malignancy may be alleviated with celiac ganglion neurolysis or blockade

VENOUS ACCESS

Central venous access is essential for most patients with malignant disease for the delivery of chemotherapy, parenteral nutrition and other fluids, blood and related products, as well as portal for

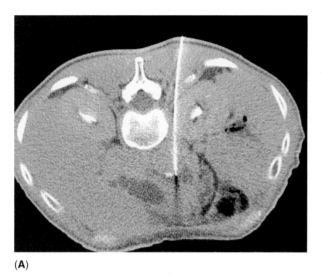
(A)

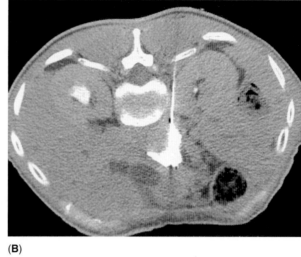
(B)

Figure 50.12 A patient who had extensive back pain from inoperable pancreatic cancer. (**A**) CT in the prone position. A 22G needle was inserted transaortically at position of the celiac plexus. (**B**) Post-insertion of lipiodol and alcohol for neurolysis blockade—note satisfactory distribution on both sides of the needle.

aspiration of blood samples. A variety of long-term venous access systems [e.g., tunneled central venous catheters, peripherally inserted central catheters (PICCs), and venous ports] have been developed for insertion under fluoroscopic and US guidance (43,44). The procedure is now usually performed in the radiology department under local anesthesia and strict asepsis (45). The procedure is rapid, well-tolerated by the patient, and associated with high success and low complication rates (46) (see chapter 53).

URINARY TRACT INTERVENTIONS

Percutaneous Nephrostomy and Antegrade Ureteric Stent Insertion

Percutaneous nephrostomy is one of the most frequently performed procedures in interventional oncology. The main indications include:

- Malignant obstruction of the urinary tract
- Patients with a recto-vesical or vesico-vaginal fistula secondary to pelvic malignancy
- Provision of urine-diversion in cases of chemotherapy related hemorrhagic cystitis

First the pelvicalyceal system is punctured under US guidance with a fine gauge needle through which radiographic contrast medium is instilled to demonstrate the anatomy and to determine the level of obstruction. Urine can be aspirated for microbiological and cytological examinations. Percutaneous nephrostomy entails the insertion into the collecting system of a pigtail configuration catheter with multiple, large side-holes. If drainage is to be of short duration, an external bag may be satisfactory. If long-term drainage is required and it is possible to cross the area of obstruction, an internal stent is preferred. This allows the patient to be free of "bags" (Fig. 50.13). It is noteworthy that, in most cases, it is possible to manipulate a catheter across an area of apparent complete obstruction. Although a contrast study may indicate total obstruction, a hydrophilic guide wire can usually be advanced

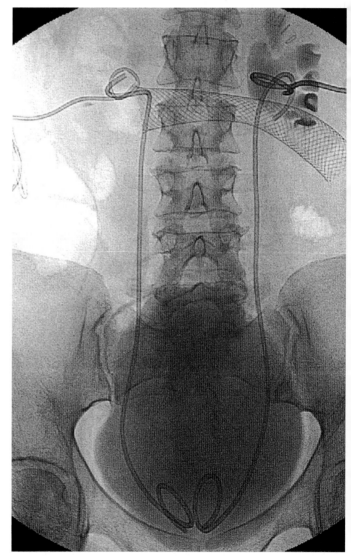

Figure 50.13 A 55-year-old female patient with metastatic esophageal cancer who presented with duodenal obstruction and bilateral hydronephrosis. Image following radiological insertion of a duodenal stent and bilateral ureteric stents. Nephrostomy tubes were subsequently removed leaving the patient with no external bags.

through the "obstruction" because the guide wire readily finds the very narrow lumen and follows it. The balloon catheter can then be advanced over the guide wire to dilate the stricture and restore patency before a stent is inserted.

In patients with pelvic malignancy complicated by fistulas to the perineum it may prove necessary to combine nephrostomy with ureteric embolization, using steel coils or segments of gelatine sponge, to prevent any urine reaching the skin of the perineum (47).

Renal Artery Embolization

Renal cell carcinoma (RCC) is a highly vascular tumor which presents frequently with local structural invasion. Although nephrectomy is the only curative form of treatment, surgical resection can present a daunting challenge to the surgeon due to intraoperative hemorrhage associated with excision of these highly vascularized and locally invasive tumors. Preoperative arterial embolization is a useful adjuvant therapy for the management of large hypervascular RCC. Preoperative embolization decreases intraoperative blood loss, facilitates excision of the tumor and there is evidence to indicate that improved survival can be achieved due to reduced dissemination of malignant cells during tumor mobilization (48).

Embolization is also a safe and minimally invasive management option for patients with inoperable RCC as a means of palliation of local symptoms (pain, hematuria) and of improving overall clinical status (49).

Key Points: Urinary Tract Interventions

- Percutaneous nephrostomy is used in the management of urinary obstruction, urinary leaks, and as a prelude for percutaneous ureteric stenting
- Renal artery embolization may be required as either a preoperative or a palliative measure

BREAST INTERVENTIONS

Mammography, especially when it is combined with US and MR imaging, can detect and accurately characterize the majority of palpable and non-palpable breast lesions. However, there is a significant percentage of breast lesions which require further characterization. Percutaneous biopsy is faster, less invasive, and less expensive than surgical biopsy and is therefore becoming the preferred alternative. It is recommended for lesions categorized as Breast Imaging Reporting and Data System (BI-RADS) 4 (suspicious abnormality) and 5 (highly suggestive of malignancy). Image guidance for percutaneous biopsy is provided by US, stereotaxis, and MR imaging (50).

Interventional US-guided techniques play an increasingly significant role in the management of breast disease. In general, US-guided interventions are patient friendly and avoid the discomfort of breast compression, waiting for films to be processed and repositioning of wires. Common indications are diverse and include biopsy of solid masses and microcalcifications, symptomatic cyst drainage, abscess drainage, tumor mapping with preoperative radiotracer injection or hookwires, and mapping with metallic markers in patients undergoing neoadjuvant chemotherapy.

Less frequent applications include ablation of benign lesions with vacuum biopsy devices, cryoablation of fibroadenomas, and radiofrequency ablation of small breast cancers. The radiologist should be aware of the limitations of the technique and should refer lesions which are not suitable for percutaneous procedures for surgical excision (radial scars, complex cysts) (50).

Stereotactic guidance is used for biopsy of lesions seen only by mammograms and not by US, particularly microcalcification clusters, small opacities in fatty breasts, and architectural distortion. Stereotactic equipment is designed to calculate the position of a designated site from the breast surface by localizing its position in the x, y, z axis. The same technique is extensively used for localization of breast lesions, to reduce the amount of tissue excised at surgery. A hookwire could be placed in a breast lesion, under stereotactic mammography guidance with a theoretical accuracy of 1 mm.

Key Points: Breast Intervention

- US guidance is the preferred method in most breast interventions since it is accurate, minimally invasive and more patient friendly
- Stereotactic biopsy and localization provide pin-point accuracy for mammographically visible lesions

MUSCULOSKELETAL INTERVENTIONS

Bone Biopsy

In the past, open biopsy was considered the gold standard for bone tumors; however many centers have now moved towards percutaneous needle biopsy because it offers advantages such as low cost and improved patient comfort. The procedure is usually performed under conscious sedation and has lower rates of complications than with open biopsy. Percutaneous needle biopsy includes both fine needle aspiration and core-needle biopsy. Depending on the location, type of the tumor and operator experience, CT, US, and fluoroscopy can be used for guidance. These targeted techniques allow a diagnosis to be made in 85% to 90% of cases (51). In order to optimize these methods there should be close co-operation between the surgeon, pathologist, and radiologist involved. The diagnosis of metastatic carcinoma and recurrent sarcoma are well suited to needle biopsy.

In a large review of 9500 percutaneous skeletal biopsies, Murphy et al. identified 22 complications (0.2%) (52). They reported nine pneumothoraces, three cases of meningitis, and five spinal cord injuries. Serious neurologic injury occurred in 0.08% of procedures. Death occurred in 0.02% of procedures.

In the future it is likely that MR directed biopsies will become increasingly used. The excellent tissue contrast resolution offered by MR imaging in conjunction with MR spectroscopy to help target viable tumor is likely to offer improved diagnostic rates as samples will be obtained from viable cancer tissue more readily than with conventional cross-sectional imaging techniques. Currently MR imaging can be used to place titanium marker coils. These coils are placed pre-operatively marking the periphery of the tumor. The coils are easily imaged with fluoroscopy intra-operatively allowing complete surgical resection of the tumor and equally important, reducing operating time.

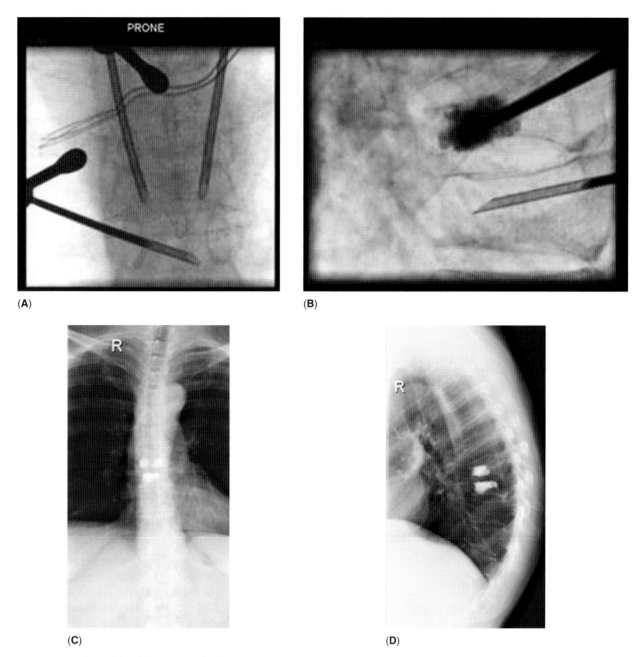

Figure 50.14 A patient with painful mid-thoracic vertebral body metastatic collapse. (A) Upper bilateral pedicular puncture and lower unilateral pedicular needle position as seen in the AP projection. (B) Lateral views demonstrating the injection of cement. Follow-up (C) AP and (D) lateral radiographs after cement injection. The patient was pain-free and suffered no further collapse in those vertebral bodies.

Bone Strengthening Techniques

Percutaneous Vertebroplasty, Kyphoplasty, and Osteoplasty

Percutaneous vertebroplasty (PVP) is a minimally invasive technique comprising injection of polymethylmethacrylate (bone cement) into a vertebral body (Fig. 50.14). The indication for its use is to relieve pain from vertebral disease (tumor infiltration or vertebral collapse). PVP was originally used to treat the painful aggressive variant of vertebral hemangioma, but its use has been extended to painful lesions caused by malignant disease, osteoporotic vertebral wedge fractures, and less common conditions such as Langerhans cell histiocytosis and osteogenesis imperfecta.

PVP can be performed using fluoroscopy alone or in tandem with CT (the latter being more useful in cervical and transthoracic procedures). The procedure is performed under sedation or general anesthesia, and vertebral body biopsy can be performed at the same time. A transpedicular route is most commonly used, though anterolateral (cervical), intercostovertebral (thoracic), posterolateral (lumbar), or even a trans-oral (C2) approach may be preferred. A single unipedicular approach is most frequently used although a bipedicular approach can be employed, the former reducing both trauma and procedural time. Patients are able to mobilize within their level of comfort immediately after the procedure.

Using this technique around 83% of patients with metastatic disease will obtain satisfactory pain relief (53). In cases of metastatic disease or myeloma, it should be noted that pain relief is not

directly related to the proportion of the lesion that is injected with cement. Complications are low:

- Asymptomatic epidural leak (6%)
- Neuralgic pain due to epidural leakage (1.6%)
- Asymptomatic pulmonary embolism (1%)(53)

Other rare complications include rib and pedicle fractures, post-procedure deep vein thrombosis, and spinal cord damage. The presence of bone cement does not preclude MR imaging which can be performed to assess disease progression.

Absolute contraindications to this technique include active infection and epidural extension of metastatic tumor with compression of neural structures. Relative contraindications include:

- Patients with more than five metastases or diffuse metastases
- The presence of radicular pain
- Fracture of the posterior column (increased risk of cement leak)
- Vertebral collapse >70% of body height (needle placement may be difficult)
- Spinal canal stenosis (asymptomatic retropulsion of a fracture fragment causing significant spinal canal compromise)

Kyphoplasty combines the techniques of vertebroplasty and angioplasty. The aim of kyphoplasty is pain-relief combined with restoration of vertebral body height and reduction in kyphosis. This is achieved by "expanding" the fractured vertebra with a balloon and then filling of the resultant cavity with bone cement. The indications for kyphoplasty are similar to those for vertebroplasty. However, currently there is no clear evidence that kyphoplasty is associated with better results than vertebroplasty, and the technique is much more expensive.

Percutaneous injection of methylmethacrylate (osteoplasty) (Fig. 50.15) allows pain reduction and bone strengthening in patients with malignant pelvic osteolysis who are unable to tolerate surgery. It is most commonly used to improve mobility in patients with osteolysis involving the weight-bearing part of the acetabulum (i.e., the acetabular roof). Excellent results can be obtained

with significant pain relief and improved mobility seen in up to 92% of patients in one series (54). Contraindications include local infection and uncorrected coagulopathy. The major complication encountered when treating acetabular lesions is intra-articular injection in acetabular lesions. The risk is minimized by monitoring the bone-filling procedure with fluoroscopic guidance.

Arterial Intervention
Arterial catheterization has two roles in orthopedic oncology:

1. To allow selective embolization of tumors to reduce their vascularity. This is performed preoperatively for pain relief or to reduce tumor size.
2. To allow regional infusion of a chemotherapeutic agent, that is, in osteosarcoma.

Arterial embolization has a role in devascularizing hypervascular tumors prior to resection (Fig. 50.16). This is particularly important for large tumors that are located in sites where tourniquet control is not possible. The procedure has the advantages of reducing tumor size, thereby decreasing intraoperative blood loss, and giving overall improved visualization of the tumor at surgery (55). In addition embolization can be a primary treatment for tumors that are refractory to other forms of treatment, for example, giant cell tumors and aneurysmal bone cysts. Embolization can be used to palliate patients who are poor candidates for surgery (55).

The goal of embolization is to occlude the blood supply to the tumor without impairing the circulation to surrounding normal tissue. Most experience of tumor embolization has involved metastatic renal cell carcinomas (70% of which are hypervascular) although potentially any hypervascular tumor supplied by large segmental arteries may benefit from embolization, for example, thyroid carcinoma, neuroendocrine tumors, leiomyosarcomas, and angiosarcomas. Myeloma and malignant melanoma are hypervascular due to a rich capillary network and respond poorly to embolization. Common bone metastases such as breast, colon, and lung carcinomas are relatively avascular and also respond poorly to embolization.

Complete embolization can be achieved in 50% to 86% of patients with tumors of the spine (56). Several studies have

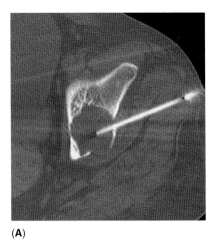
(A)

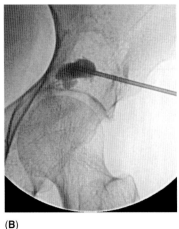
(B)

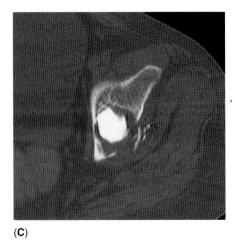
(C)

Figure 50.15 Symptomatic metastatic left acetabular deposit that was injected with cement for consolidation and pain relief. (**A**) Insertion of the needle under CT guidance into the lesion. (**B**) Injection of cement under fluoroscopic guidance. (**C**) CT confirming good fill with no leaks.

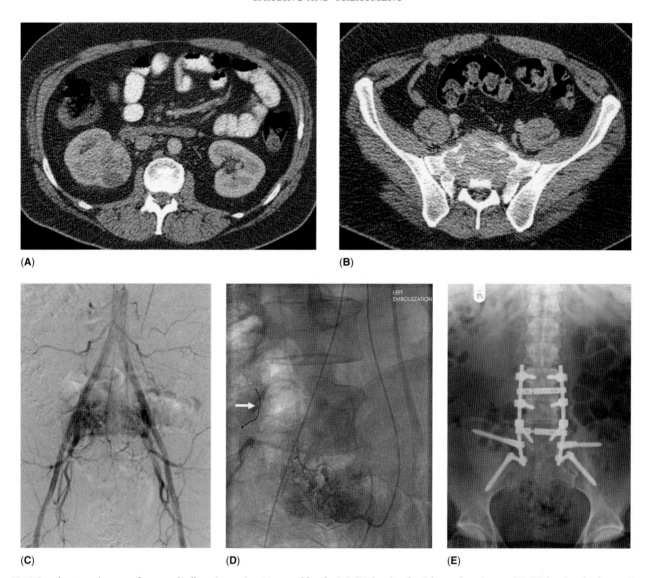

Figure 50.16 Sacral metastatic tumor from renal cell carcinoma in a 35-year-old male. (**A**) CT showing the right renal carcinoma. (**B**) CT showing the destructive tumor deposit within the sacrum. (**C**) Aortic flush angiogram illustrating large tumor blush. The tumor was supplied by multiple branches. (**D**) Selective embolization of the left internal posterior division trunk with particles. The right internal and lumbar branches were also selectively embolized. Note the arrow points to a microcoil within the lower right lumbar supply to the tumor. (**E**) Surgical stabilization was then successfully performed.

demonstrated a significant reduction in intraoperative blood loss following successful embolization (56). This has the potential to reduce operating time, allow a more extensive resection, and reduce complications due to the proximity to important anatomical structures, e.g., spinal cord.

Serious complication rates are low (1–2%) following embolization in most studies. Serious complications include paraplegia, quadraparesis, and aortic dissection. Following embolization procedures 43% of patients will experience post-embolization syndrome (local pain, low grade fever, and malaise) (57).

If a single vessel supplies an osteosarcoma, selective catheterization and infusion of chemotherapy is the optimal approach (58). The rationale for regional chemotherapy is two-fold: first it maximizes local delivery of the drug, thus theoretically increasing the local response rate while still allowing a sufficiently high concentration of the drug systemically to destroy micrometastases. The

procedure facilitates local resection and limb salvage and may obviate the need for amputation. The second indication is to identify the best chemotherapy agent for adjuvant therapy, a decision which is based on the degree of necrosis demonstrated in the resected specimen.

Key Points: Musculoskeletal Interventions

- Percutaneous image-guided musculoskeletal biopsies provide an accurate, rapid, and cost-effective method for histological diagnosis of musculoskeletal tumors
- Percutaneous vertebroplasty and kyphoplasty offer immediate pain relief in more than 80% of patients with painful spinal metastasis
- Therapeutic embolization for pelvic and musculoskeletal tumors may be preoperative or palliative measures

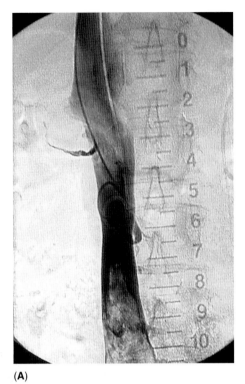
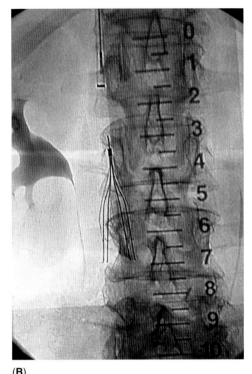

(A)   **(B)**

Figure 50.17 (A) Inferior venocavography showing extensive thrombus within the common iliac veins and distal IVC. (B) IVC filter was inserted via a jugular approach to prevent migration of thrombus.

OTHER INTERVENTIONS IN ONCOLOGY

Inferior Vena Cava Filtration

Inferior vena cava (IVC) filtration (Fig. 50.17) is indicated for selected patients as an adjunctive treatment for venous thromboembolism, or as an effective prophylactic measure in selected high-risk patients (59). While systemic anticoagulation remains the cornerstone of venous thromboembolism treatment, not all patients, especially oncology patients, are candidates for this therapy and in such patients IVC filtration offers an important alternative. Contraindications to anticoagulant therapy in the oncology setting include:

- Gastrointestinal bleeding
- Recent major surgery
- Malignancy of the central nervous system
- Widespread metastatic disease

Currently available devices may be classified as "optional" filters since they can function either as permanent or temporary filters. A retrievable IVC filter, that is optional either as a permanent or temporary filter, is an attractive alternative device for use in all oncology patients in whom the requirement for the device may be for a limited period.

Tumor Localization with Venous Sampling

Despite recent advances in cross-sectional and functional imaging, venous sampling remains a sensitive physiological investigation for localization of hormonal hypersecretion. The test requires technical expertise and reliable laboratory support and should be applied selectively to address individual clinical problems in

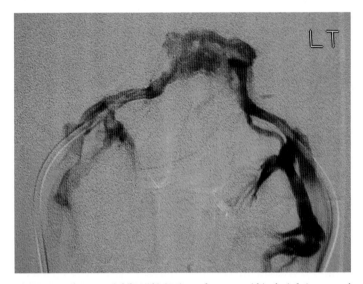

Figure 50.18 Fluoroscopic bilateral injections of contrast within the inferior petrosal sinuses prior to venous sampling. *Source:* Courtesy of Dr. Matthew Matson.

coordination with other imaging modalities (60). Depending on the venous anatomy, sampling may achieve either regional localization or lateralization of the endocrine tumor. Adrenal venous sampling serves to lateralize a functioning tumor and to differentiate tumor from hyperplasia. Inferior petrosal sinus sampling (Fig. 50.18) confirms pituitary Cushing's disease and lateralizes the adenoma. Systemic venous sampling identifies the site of ectopic hormonal secretion. In the localization of pancreatic islet cell tumors, the test is further enhanced by sampling after intra-arterial injection of hormonal secretagogue (60).

Percutaneous Retrieval Techniques

Percutaneous extraction of intravascular foreign bodies is becoming an increasingly common technique. It is an effective and minimally invasive way to avoid surgery. Multiple techniques have been developed by interventional radiologists and include:

- Wire loop snares
- Dormia baskets
- Fragment graspers
- Deflector wires

Retrieval techniques can be used safely to retrieve fragmented catheters, wires, misplaced coils, or stents. Such techniques are of particular relevance to the management of patients with malignancy who are often extremely ill and may have coagulopathy. In such patients, major surgery (e.g., thoracotomy) is particularly undesirable.

Gene Therapy

The most rapidly evolving area in medicine is gene therapy. The underlying principle is to identify and clone a gene, and then to insert it into a vector capable of directing expression in mammalian tissues (61). At present the main goal of gene therapy is to treat genetic deficiencies and malignant diseases which are refractory to conventional therapies. The delivery systems involved, include retroviral vectors (RNA viruses), adenoviral vectors (DNA viruses), and cationic liposomes, along with strategies that involve US-directed gene transfer, CT-guided gene transfer (62), and transcatheter gene delivery, in particular via the hepatic artery. Examples of genes being evaluated in clinical trials include oncogenes, tumor suppressor genes, suicide genes, and antiangiogenesis factors. The liver is an ideal therapeutic target for gene therapy. Hepatic lesions being considered for treatment include:

- Metastatic colorectal carcinoma
- Hepatoma
- Cholangiocarcinoma
- Lymphoma
- Metastatic melanoma
- Hemangioma

Gene therapy strategies for managing occluded biliary stents (resulting from tumor ingrowth) and vascular transjugular intrahepatic portosystemic stents (resulting from neoendothelialization) are also under consideration. In gene delivery, angiographic guidance will be of use for localizing tumor blood supply and directing the targeted intra-arterial delivery of genes of interest, so that vector–DNA complexes can be delivered with accuracy and specificity (63). Embolization techniques may also be of benefit, by prolonging vector contact with the target cells, thus delaying washout and further enhancing target cell uptake (64). Radiological monitoring will be of considerable importance during gene delivery, for example, the process of liposomal vector delivery can be monitored accurately with US because lipid vesicles are echogenic. Guided biopsy of transduced tissues for histopathological analysis after gene delivery should also improve the accuracy of tissue analysis in the evaluation of gene expression.

Key Points: Other Applications

- IVC filtration is indicated for patients with contraindication to anticoagulation therapy, failure of anticoagulation therapy, or complications from anticoagulation
- Venous sampling techniques may help to localize occult tumors that are biochemically active
- Percutaneous retrieval techniques may be used to retrieve fragmented or misplaced catheters and coils
- Interventional radiologists are an integral part of the multidisciplinary team working on gene therapy. Their role would be executing transmission of genetic material to the target cells

Summary

- Percutaneous transthoracic biopsy is a rapid, safe, effective means of establishing a diagnosis in a patient with a pulmonary, pleural, or mediastinal lesion
- SVC stenting provides immediate and durable palliation for patients with malignant SVCO
- Tracheobronchial stenting is a useful technique for the palliation of stridor secondary to airways compression by tumors
- In the gastrointestinal tract, EUS with biopsy is useful in the staging of esophageal gastric and colonic malignancy
- Co-axial plugged biopsy is indicated for vascular lesions and patients with bleeding diathesis
- Radiologically-placed self-expandable metallic stents offer excellent palliation for esophageal strictures and fistulas, gastric outflow obstruction, and acute large bowel obstruction
- In the management of obstructive jaundice, multidetector CT and MR cholangiography have cardinal roles in the initial non-invasive management of biliary strictures. ERCP is the procedure of choice for lower and mid-common bile duct strictures while PTC is indicated for hilar lesions and when ERCP fails
- TACE is currently considered the mainstay of treatment for unresectable HCC in selected patients with preserved liver function and adequate performance status
- Percutaneous vertebroplasty and kyphoplasty offer immediate pain relief in more than 80% of patients with painful spinal metastasis
- Therapeutic embolizations for pelvic and musculoskeletal tumors may be preoperative or palliative measures
- IVC filtration is indicated for patients with contraindications to anticoagulation, failure of anticoagulation therapy or complications from anticoagulation
- Percutaneous retrieval techniques may be used to retrieve fragmented or misplaced catheters and coils

REFERENCES

1. Adam A. Interventional radiology: there is no need for quotation marks. Eur Radiol 1997; 7: 944–5.
2. Bogda K. Radiological Interventions: special considerations in cancer patients. In: Ray CE, Hicks ME, Patel NH, eds. SIR syllabus: Interventions in oncology. Fairfax, VA: Society of Interventional Radiology, 2003: 1–7.

3. Ghaye B, Dondelinger RF. Imaging guided thoracic interventions. Eur Respir J 2001; 17: 507–28.

4. van Sonneberg E, Gasola G, Ho M, et al. Difficult thoracic lesions: CT guided biopsy experience in 150 cases. Radiology 1988; 167: 457–61.

5. Heck SL, Blom P, Berstad A. Accuracy and complications in computed tomography fluoroscopy guided needle biopsies of lung masses. Eur Radiol 2006; 16: 1387–92.

6. Wallace MJ, Krishnamurthy S, Broemeling LD, et al. CT-guided percutaneous fine-needle aspiration of small (<or=1cm) pulmonary lesions. Radiology 2002; 225: 823–8.

7. Yeow KM, Tsay PK, Cheung YC, et al. Factors affecting accuracy of CT-guided co-axial cutting needle lung biopsy: retrospective analysis of 631 procedures. J Vasc Interv Radiol 2003; 14: 581–8.

8. Husband JE, Golding SJ. The role of computed tomography-guided needle biopsy in an oncology service. Clin Radiol 1983; 34: 255–60.

9. Tournoy KG, Ryck FD, Vanwalleghem L, et al. The yield of endoscopic ultrasound in lung cancer staging: does lymph node size matter? J Thorac Oncol 2008; 3: 245–9.

10. Patz EF, McAdams HP, Erasmus JJ, et al. Sclerotherapy for malignant pleural effusions: a prospective randomized trial of bleomycin vs doxycycline with small-bore catheter drainage. Chest 1998; 113: 1305–11.

11. Musani AI, Haas AR, Seijo L, Wilby M, Sterman DH. Outpatient management of malignant pleural effusions with small-bore, tunneled pleural catheters. Respiration 2004; 71: 559–66.

12. Keeling AN, Leong S, Logan PM, Lee MJ. Empyema and effusion: outcome of image-guided small bore catheter drainage. Cardiovasc Intervent Radiol 2008; 31: 135–41.

13. Nicholson AA, Ettles DF, Arnold A, et al. Treatment of malignant superior vena cava obstruction: metal stents or radiation therapy. J Vasc Interv Radiol 1997; 8: 563–7.

14. Irving JD, Dondelinger RF, Reidy JF, et al. Gianturco self-expanding stents: clinical experience in the vena cava and large veins. Cardiovasc Intervent Radiol 1992; 15: 351–5.

15. Hatrick A, Sabharwal T, Adam A. Tracheobronchial stents. Semin Intervent Radiol 2001; 18: 243–50.

16. Tan BS, Watkinson AF, Dussek JE, Adam A. Metallic endoprosthesis for malignant tracheo-bronchial obstruction: initial experience. Cardiovasc Intervent Radiol 1996; 19: 91–6.

17. Morgan RA, Ellul JP, Denton ER, et al. Malignant esophageal fistulas and perforations: management with plastic-covered metallic endoprostheses. Radiology 1997; 204: 527–32.

18. Allison DJ, Adam A. Percutaneous liver biopsy and embolization of the track with steel coils. Radiology 1988; 169: 261–3.

19. Dawson P, Adam A, Edwards R. Technique for steel coil-embolization of liver biopsy track for use with the "Biopty" needle. Br J Radiol 1992; 65: 538–40.

20. Durkan GC, Sheikh N, Johnson P, et al. Improving prostate cancer detection with an extended-core transrectal ultrasonography-guided prostate biopsy protocol. BJU 2002; 89: 33–9.

21. Vazquez-Sequeiros E, Norton ID, Clain JE, et al. Impact of EUS-guided fine needle aspiration on lymph node staging in patients with esophageal carcinoma. Gastrointestinal Endosc 2001; 53: 751–7.

22. Horwhat JD, Paulson EK, McGrath K, et al. A randomized comparison of EUS-guided FNA versus CT guided FNA for the evaluation of pancreatic mass lesions. Gastrointest Endosc 2006; 63: 966–75.

23. Adam A, Ellul J, Watkinson AF, et al. Palliation of inoperable esophageal carcinoma: a prospective randomized trial of laser therapy and stent placement. Radiology 1997; 202: 344–8.

24. Sabharwal T, Morales JP, Irani FG, Adam A. Quality improvement guidelines for placement of oesophageal Stents. Cardiovascv Intervent Radiol 2005; 28: 284–8.

25. Sabharwal T, Morales JP, Salter R, Adam A. Esophageal cancer: self-expanding metallic stents. Abdom Imaging 2004; 29: 1–9.

26. Sabharwal T, Gulati MS, Fotiadis N, et al. Randomised comparison of the FerX Ella antireflux stent and the ultraflex stent-proton pump inhibitor combination for prevention of post-stent reflux in patients with esophageal carcinoma involving the esophago-gastric junction. J Gastroenterol Hepatol 2008; 23: 723–8.

27. Morgan RA, Ellul JPM, Denton ERE, et al. Malignant esophageal fistulas and perforations: Management with plastic covered metallic endoprostheses. Radiology 1997; 204: 527–32.

28. Sabharwal T, Irani FG, Adam A. Quality assurance guidelines for placement of gastroduodenal stents. Cardiovasc Intervent Radiol 2007; 30: 1–5.

29. Morgan R, Adam A. Use of metallic stents and balloons in the esophagus and the gastrointestinal tract. J Vasc Interv Radiol 2001; 12: 283–97.

30. Sebastian S, Johnston S, Geoghegan T, Torreggiani W, Buckley M. Pooled analysis of the efficacy and safety of self expanding metal stenting in malignant colorectal obstruction. Am J Gastroenterol 2004; 99: 2051–7.

31. Hicks ME, Surratt RS, Picus D, et al. Fluoroscopically guided percutaneous gastrostomy and gastroenterostomy: analysis of 158 consecutive cases. AJR Am J Roentgenol 1990; 154: 725–8.

32. Kuo YC, Shlansky-Goldberg RD, Mondschein JL, et al. Large or small bore, push or pull: a comparison of three classes of Percutaneous fluoroscopic gastrostomy catheters. J Vasc Interv Radiol 2008; 19: 557–63.

33. Adam A. Metallic biliary endoprostheses. Cardiovasc Intervent Radiol 1994; 17: 127–32.

34. Adam A, Chetty N, Roddie M, et al. Self-expandable stainless steel endoprostheses for treatment of malignant bile duct obstruction. AJR Am J Roentgenol 1991; 156: 321–5.

35. Davids PH, Groen AK, Rauws EA, et al. Randomized trial of self-expanding metal stents versus polyethelene stents for distal malignant biliary obstruction. Lancet 1992; 340: 1488–92.

36. Llovet JM, Bruix J. Systematic review of randomized trials for unresectable hepatocellular carcinoma: chemoembolization improves survival. Hepatology 2003; 37: 429–42.

37. Marelli L, Stigliano R, Triantos C, et al. Treatment outcomes for hepatocellular carcinoma using chemoembolization in combination with other therapies. Cancer Treat Rev 2006; 32: 594–606.

38. Varela M, Real MI, Burrel M, et al. Chemoembolization of hepatocellular carcinoma with drug eluting beads: efficacy and doxorubicin pharmacokinetics. J Hepatol 2007; 46: 474–81.

39. Salem R, Lewandowski RJ, Atassi B, et al. Treatment of unresectable hepatocellular carcinoma with the use of 90Y microspheres (TheraSphere): safety, tumour response, and survival. J Vasc Inter Radiol 2005; 16: 1627–39.

40. Sato KT, Lewandowski RJ, Mulcahy MF, et al. Unresectable chemorefractory liver metastases: Radioembolization with 90Y microspheres—Safety, Efficacy, and Survival. Radiology 2008; 247: 507–15.

41. Goldberg SN, Gazelle GS, Mueller PR. Thermal ablation therapy for focal malignancy: a unified approach to underlying principles, techniques, and diagnostic imaging guidance. AJR Am J Roentgenol 2000; 174: 323–31.

42. Eisenberg E, Carr DB, Chalmers TC. Neurolytic celiac plexus block for treatment of cancer pain: a meta-analysis. Anesth Analg 1995; 80: 290–5.

43. Robertson LJ, Mauro MA, Jaques PF. Radiologic placement of Hickman catheters. Radiology 1989; 170: 1007–9.

44. Parkinson R, Gandhi M, Harper J, Archibald C. Establishing an ultrasound guided peripherally inserted central catheter (PICC) insertion service. Clin Radiol 1998; 53: 33–6.

45. Adam A. Insertion of long term central venous catheters: time for a new look. BMJ 1995; 311: 341–2.

46. Page AC, et al. The insertion of chronic indwelling central venous catheters (Hickman lines) in interventional radiology suites. Clin Radiol 1990; 10: 105–9.

47. Farrell TA, Wallace M, Hicks ME. Long-term results of transrenal ureteral occlusion with the use of Gianturco coils and gelatin sponge pledgets. J Vasc Interv Radiol 1997; 8: 449–52.

48. Zielinski H, Szmigielski S, Petrovich Z. Comparison of preoperative embolization followed by radical nephrectomy with radical nephrectomy alone for renal cell carcinoma. Am J Clin Oncol 2000; 23: 6–12.

49. Maxwell NJ, Saleem Amer N, Rogers E, et al. Renal artery embolization in the palliative treatment of renal carcinoma. Br J Radiol 2007; 80: 96–102.

50. Pijnappel RM, van de Donk M, Holland R, et al. Diagnostic accuracy for different strategies of image-guided breast intervention in cases of nonpalpable breast lesions. Br J Cancer 2004; 90: 595–600.

51. Dupuy DE, Rosenberg AE, Punyaratabandhu T, Tan MH, Mankin HJ. Accuracy of CT-guided needle biopsy of musculoskeletal neoplasms. AJR Am J Roentgenol 1998; 171: 759–62.

52. Murphy WA, Destouet JM, Gilula LA. Percutaneous skeletal biopsy: a procedure for radiologists. Radiology 1981; 139: 545–9.

53. Gangi A, Dietemann JL, Guth S, et al. Computed tomography (CT) and fluoroscopy-guided vertebroplasty: results and complications in 187 patients. Semin Intervent Radiol 1999; 200: 525–30.

54. Kelekis A, Lovblad KO, Mehdizade A, et al. Pelvic osteoplasty in osteolytic metastases: technical approach under fluoroscopic guidance and early clinical results. J Vasc Interv Radiol 2005; 16: 81–8.

55. Sabharwal T, Salter R, Adam A, Gangi A. Image-guided therapies in orthopedic oncology. Orthop Clin North Am 2006; 37: 105–12.

56. Gottfried ON, Schloesser PE, Schmidt MH, Stevens EA. Embolization of metastatic spinal tumors. Neurosurg Clin N Am 2004; 15: 391–9.

57. Hemingway AP, Allison DJ. Complications of embolizations: analysis of 410 procedures. Radiology 1988; 166: 669–72.

58. Wallace MJ, Wallace S. Chemoembolization, Infusion and Embolization. In: Adam A, Dondelinger RF, Mueller PR, eds. Interventional Radiology in Cancer. Berlin: Springer-Verlag, 2004: 179–224.

59. Kinnet TB. Update on inferior vena cava filters. J Vasc Interv Radiol 2003; 14: 425–40.

60. Lau JH, Drake W, Matson M. The current role of venous sampling in the localization of endocrine disease. Cardiovasc Intervent Radiol 2007; 30: 555–70.

61. Voss SD, Kruskal JB. Gene therapy: a primer for radiologists. Radiographics 1998; 18: 1343–7.

62. Suh RD, Goldin JG, Wallace AB, et al. Metastatic renal cell carcinoma: CT-guided immunotherapy as a technically feasible and safe approach to delivery of gene therapy treatment. Radiology 2004; 231: 359–64.

63. Mahmood U. Can a clinically used chemoembolization vehicle improve transgene delivery? Radiology 2006; 240: 619–20.

64. Kim YI, Chung JW, et al. Intraarterial gene delivery in rabbit hepatic tumours: transfection with nonviral vector by using iodized oil emulsion. Radiology 2006; 240: 771–7.

51 Interventional Imaging: Tumor Ablation
Alice R Gillams

INTRODUCTION

Image-guided tumor ablation is a rapidly expanding field. Fifteen years ago there were a handful of pioneering centers; today hundreds of centers are practicing tumor ablation. Technical innovations and new applications are frequently reported with several hundred papers published annually. While it is accepted that ablation can be an effective therapy, there are still several unanswered questions and techniques are constantly being refined. It is still difficult to achieve large (>5 cm) areas of confluent necrosis and further modifications are needed. The optimal relationship between local ablation and systemic therapy is not known. Patient selection and the role of ablation relative to other therapies need to be studied.

TECHNICAL ASPECTS

Energy sources can be grouped into four major categories:

- Those employing thermal energy, either heating or cooling
- Direct injection therapies
- Photodynamic therapy (PDT)
- Ionizing radiation

Thermal Energy

With all heating techniques the aim is to raise the temperature of the tissue to be destroyed to between 60°C and 100°C. This is to produce coagulative necrosis yet avoid charring and vaporization of tissue. There are five thermal techniques: radio-frequency (RF), laser, microwave, cryotherapy, and high-intensity focused ultrasound (HIFU) (1). A summary of their characteristics is shown in Table 51.1.

Radio-Frequency

In the late 19th century, d'Arsonval, a physicist, reported the use of alternating RF to generate heat in biological tissue (2). RF current induces ionic agitation which, in turn, results in heating. RF has been used for many years to perform electrocautery in the operating room or to produce discrete, focal lesions that interrupt aberrant cardiac conduction pathways. Initial electrodes were unipolar of low power, <50 W, and were not internally cooled. Bipolar electrodes were effective in producing small, discrete lesions but had limited usefulness in the treatment of tumors. More recent RF technology has introduced arrays of electrodes that are activated either simultaneously or sequentially, internally water-cooled electrodes, high-power generators <200 W and simultaneous perfusion of the tissue with saline (3–8). Most experience has been gained with two multi-electrode designs, a water-cooled cluster of three parallel 17G electrodes (CoVidien, Colorado, United States) and an expanding electrode design (Fig. 51.1). The expanding

electrodes are introduced collapsed within a hollow (14–15G) needle. Once correctly positioned, multiple prongs or tines are deployed resulting in a final configuration that resembles a grappling hook or an umbrella (AngioDynamics, New York, United States, Boston Scientific, Massachusetts, United States) (9). An early comparison of water-cooled, triple cluster electrodes and the expandable, multi-tined electrodes showed that larger volumes of necrosis were produced using the water-cooled design (10). Since then, there have been modifications to the expandable electrode design, including an increase in the number of active tines, the use of higher power generators and combination with saline perfusion technology. Later technological developments include the development of MR-compatible electrodes, and new electrode designs, e.g., a multiprobe bipolar system which produces larger ablations than traditional bipolar electrodes, a two-tine expandable electrode for very small lesions and a bendable shaft expandable electrode to facilitate scanning within a gantry after electrode positioning.

Laser

Both neodymium yttrium aluminium garnet (Nd:YAG 1064 nm) and solid-state lasers (λ805 nm) have been used successfully in tumor ablation. Photon absorption and heat conduction produce hyperthermia and coagulative necrosis. Laser energy is delivered through flexible, thin fibers, 400 to 600 μm in diameter. Fiber morphology can be varied depending on the area to be treated. A point source from a bare-tip fiber will produce a sphere of necrosis, whereas a diffuser fiber will produce an elliptical ablation. Larger ablations can be achieved with increases in laser power <40 W and the addition of water-cooling. Although more expensive to set up and support than RF, laser ablations are more predictable. Laser energy is deposited around the fiber tip, whereas RF pathways and therefore energy deposition vary, are more complex and less predictable.

Microwave

Microwaves (915 MHz or 2450 MHz) cause rotation and vibration of water molecules thus producing heat. The equipment consists of a generator and a monopolar needle electrode which is introduced through a 14G access needle. Multiple percutaneous electrodes are generally required. Each microwave application produces a discrete focus of necrosis; for example, a single treatment for 120 seconds at 60 W provides approximately 1.6 cm of necrosis. For this reason, microwave ablation has most often been used for the treatment of small (<3 cm) hepatocellular carcinoma (HCC). New designs of microwave allow the delivery of more power <100 W. There is active research to develop specific applicators for specific tissues to improve the acoustic matching between the applicator and the tissue and increase the power deposited in the tumor. Theoretical advantages of microwave ablation

Table 51.1 Comparison of Thermal Ablation Techniques

Technique	Efficacy	Implementation	Cost
RF	+++	++	++
Laser	++	+	+++
Microwave	+	++	++
Cryotherapy	+++	+/–	+++
HIFU	+/–	+/–	+++

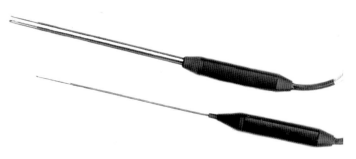

Figure 51.1 An example of a RF electrode. An internally cooled straight needle design—both a single and a cluster of three electrodes.

include a more predictable, linear dose response curve. The effect of microwave on adjacent blood vessels is under investigation but early reports suggest that it is less vulnerable to cooling from nearby vessels. Cooling can protect tumor and result in incomplete ablation.

Cryotherapy

Cryotherapy uses repetitive freezing and thawing of tissue to produce necrosis. Irreversible tissue destruction occurs at temperatures below –20°C to 30°C. Liquid nitrogen and argon gas are used as coolants. Traditional cryotherapy probes have been large, requiring laparotomy access for the treatment of liver tumors. Smaller cryotherapy probes <2.5 mm in diameter are available for percutaneous use. The development of the ice ball can be monitored using US, CT, or MR guidance. The edge of the ice ball represents 0°C and the anticipated –20°C isotherm is approximately 5 mm in from the edge of the ice-ball. One advantage is the clarity of real-time monitoring which is particularly valuable when treating near to vulnerable structures.

High-Intensity Focused Ultrasound

HIFU uses frequencies of 0.8 to 3.2 MHz and focal peak intensities of 5000 to 20,000 W/cm² (11). The basic mechanism is heat-induced coagulative necrosis. Pathological studies demonstrate particular damage to vessels, including tumor microvasculature (12). HIFU has the advantage of being a trackless technique, performed without anesthesia and with no risk of tumor seeding. A clear acoustic path from skin to the tissue to be ablated is required. The technique has been available since the 1940s but improvements in imaging and in HIFU technology, e.g., variable focusing and electronic beam steering, have renewed interest in the technique. The main problem is the limited amount of necrosis that can be achieved per unit time. Most work has been performed in the prostate using transrectal devices.

Key Points: Thermal Energy

- Five thermal techniques exist: RF, laser, microwave, cryotherapy, and HIFU
- RF ablation is currently the most widely used technique
- Laser tumor ablations are more predictable than RF
- Changing microwave technology is expected to increase efficacy
- Although HIFU is a trackless technique, without anesthesia and no risk of seeding, only a limited amount of necrosis can be achieved per unit time
- Cryotherapy provides the easiest real-time monitoring with US, CT, and MR. The iceball represents the 0°C isotherm and the zone of cell death is extrapolated from that

Direct Injection Therapies

Ethanol, acetic acid and gel-stabilized chemotherapeutic agents have all been used to ablate tumors with variable success. Gene therapy is hypothesized as the therapy of tomorrow.

Percutaneous Ethanol Injection

Percutaneous ethanol injection (PEI) was one of the first effective ablative techniques to be widely adopted for the treatment of small HCCs. Ethanol causes dehydration and, subsequently, necrosis (13). Under US guidance, a fine needle (21–22G) is introduced into the tumor and 95% to 100% ethanol injected. To achieve complete ablation, the ethanol must reach all parts of the tumor; however, ethanol spreads unevenly and the needle needs to be repositioned accordingly. Ethanol can reflux along the needle tract and cause pain; this limits the amount that can be injected at any one time in the conscious patient. PEI is, therefore, either performed as a multistage, outpatient technique under conscious sedation or as a single-stage procedure under general anesthesia. PEI is most effective in encapsulated HCC and of little benefit in infiltrating HCC or in metastases. The scirrhous nature of liver metastases restricts the amount of ethanol that can be injected, often leading to extravasation and thus incomplete necrosis. Thermal techniques are therefore preferred for the treatment of metastases. In HCC, thermal techniques provide more necrosis in less time and in fewer sessions. PEI still has a role in the treatment of HCC not amenable to RF, e.g., exophytic lesions, which can rupture with disastrous consequences during heating. It is also cheaper and therefore still commonly used in some parts of the world. A combination of PEI and thermal ablation shows a small incremental benefit.

Key Points: Direct Injection Therapy

- PEI is of value in encapsulated rather than infiltrating HCC, but its role lies in tumors not amenable to RF, which produces more necrosis in less time
- PEI is of little benefit in liver metastases as their scirrhous nature limits the quantity of injected ethanol

Photodynamic Therapy (PDT)

Principles

The combination of a photosensitizing agent and light of the appropriate wavelength in the presence of oxygen produces cell

death. This is the basis of PDT. The cytotoxic intermediaries are thought to be short-lived free oxygen radicals. The development of second-generation photosensitizing agents has rekindled interest in PDT (14–19). A literature search will reveal papers on multiple and diverse applications, e.g., photoangioplasty, treatment of dysplastic and early tumors, or palliation of advanced obstructing tumors in the lung and gastro-intestinal tract, treatment at surgery of the peritoneal surface in advanced ovarian carcinoma and open PDT for recurrent pituitary adenomas, to name just a few. Traditionally, PDT has been successfully applied to accessible tissue, e.g., skin, bladder, lung, and gastro-intestinal tract (20–24). Interstitial PDT is a more recent innovation requiring the introduction of a light source deep into the tissue to be treated. It was originally hoped that photosensitizing agents with selective tumor uptake could be developed. However, currently available agents exhibit only minimal selectivity. Therefore, image guidance is required to ensure exact delivery of light so that effective tumor ablation is achieved while minimizing collateral damage. Optimal tissue penetration is achieved with light of wavelengths 650 to 800 nm (25,26).

Photosensitizing Agents
There are a number of different porphyrin-based photosensitizing agents which vary in administration, tissue uptake, optimal wavelength, duration for which the patient remains photosensitized, and effectiveness. In the gastro-intestinal tract, oral 5-amino laevulinic acid (5-ALA) works well for superficial treatments with a short duration of photosensitivity. The optimal wavelength for 5-ALA is 635 nm, i.e., outside the range for optimal tissue penetration. Meso-tetra-hydro-phenylchlorin (mTHPC), which reacts to red light optimally of λ652 nm, is approved within the European Union for the palliation of head and neck cancer, and is available worldwide on a named-patient basis for the treatment of other tumors.

The Interstitial Technique
Using image guidance, 19G hollow needles are inserted into the tumor. Laser fibers are introduced through the needles such that the tip protrudes 5 to 10 mm beyond the needle and light of the appropriate wavelength can be delivered. Lasers are a good light source as they deliver monochromatic, coherent light. Optimal positioning depends on the photosensitizing agent, energy, and wavelength of light and tissue. For example, using mTHPC at a dose of 0.15 mg/kg administered intravenously three days prior to treatment and 20 J of red laser light (λ652 nm), a sphere of necrosis 9 mm (range 7–11) in diameter was produced in pancreatic tumors. To obtain large areas of confluent necrosis, multiple (up to eight) fibers are positioned, spaced appropriately. Diffuser fibers of 2 cm to 4 cm length can also be used in appropriate target tissues, e.g., central cholangiocarcinoma. Free oxygen radicals are short-lived and difficult to monitor with imaging. Maximal necrosis occurs some time after the treatment, e.g., using mTHPC, maximal necrosis is seen at 72 hours. Contrast-enhanced techniques, either computed tomography (CT) or MR, can be used to show the extent of necrosis produced. Treatments are usually performed under conscious sedation and local anesthesia. A drawback of mTHPC is that photosensitivity lasts 6 to 10 weeks and, therefore,

appropriate measures are required to avoid direct sunlight during this period.

Key Points: Photodynamic Therapy

- With interstitial PDT, a light source is introduced deep into the tumor under imaging guidance
- PDT requires administration of a photosensitizing agent, which is usually porphyrin-based and has only minimal tissue selectivity

Ionizing Radiation
Image-guided procedures include radioactive seed implantation in the prostate and transhepatic biliary access for cholangiocarcinoma. Although this concept is over 20 years old, improvements in seeds, three-dimensional US guidance and radiotherapy planning have increased its use as a treatment for T1 and T2 stage prostate cancer. Brachytherapy delivers conventional doses of radiotherapy over a period of months.

APPLICATIONS TO SPECIFIC ORGANS

Liver Tumors
Choice of Technique
More clinical experience has been gained in the treatment of liver tumors than in any other area. The liver is a relatively forgiving organ with substantial reserve and an ability to regenerate. Most techniques, including all the thermal techniques and PDT, have been tried in the liver. Today, PEI has been replaced by laser or RF ablation in most centers. Although both of these latter techniques are effective, currently RF is the preferred technique and the one most widely practiced. Laser has the advantage of being more MR-compatible, permitting direct MR monitoring (27). MR -compatible RF electrodes are available, but the application of RF current interferes with image acquisition so generator activation and image acquisition are alternated. Cryoablation, whilst effective, carries a higher complication rate. Animal work has shown that while cryoablation results in acute lung injury, RF does not (28). Comparisons of laparoscopic RF with cryoablation have shown a lower complication rate with RF (29,30). One study reported a 40.7% complication rate with cryotherapy as compared to 3.3% with RF (31). Comparisons of percutaneous cryotherapy and RF have shown a higher complete ablation rate with RF. Microwave has been used, particularly in China, and a few centers have performed PDT. HIFU is still experimental. RF is currently, therefore, the preferred technique for liver tumor ablation.

Pathological Validation of RF
The efficacy of RF has been validated in at least two cohorts of patients who subsequently underwent surgical resection (32,33). Pathological specimens resected immediately after ablation showed irreversible cell damage with an absence of enzymatic activity. Coagulative necrosis developed later and was consistently demonstrated on specimens resected three to seven days after thermal ablation.

Definitions of Success in Liver Tumor Ablation
The aim is complete tumor ablation with a margin of apparently normal tissue without collateral damage. Treatment efficacy is improved by intraprocedural imaging assessment. Treatment

efficacy can be assessed by dynamic contrast-enhanced US, CT, or MR (34). Complete ablation is defined as the absence of visible tumor on imaging so that there is an absence of enhancement following intravenous (IV) injection of contrast medium. Despite the appearance of complete ablation, recurrence adjacent to the ablated area can occur, particularly where blood flowing in adjacent vessels results in tissue cooling and protects microscopic quantities of tumor. Wide variations in early reported recurrence rates reflect different definitions and assessment techniques. The accepted definition is the development on follow-up of hypo- or hypervascular tumor adjacent to or within the ablation zone, with or without an increase in the size of the lesion. In patients with colorectal metastases, new tumors develop in the liver at a distance to the ablated site in 57% of cases (35). For HCC, the five-year recurrence rate in the liver following successful resection varies from 67.6% to 100% (36–40). Therefore, an important aspect of ablation is careful, structured imaging follow-up with dynamic contrast-enhanced US, CT, or MR to detect new lesions and recurrence, such that further ablation can be offered as appropriate.

Key Points: Liver Tumor Ablation—Choice of Technique and Assessing Efficacy

- RF ablation is currently the preferred technique for liver tumor ablation and its effect has been histologically validated
- Recurrence is defined as evidence of hypo- or hypervascular tumor adjacent to or within the ablation zone with or without an increase in the size of the lesion

Liver Metastases
Colorectal

Limited colorectal liver metastases are the most commonly treated metastatic lesion. The liver is often the first and only site for metastases. There is good evidence that most patients will succumb from their liver metastases and therefore, local control can improve life expectancy. This has been the reasoning behind hepatic resection. Surgical resection is the accepted first-line treatment for patients with resectable disease. Five-year survival figures range from 25% to 39% (41). Traditionally, most patients (80–90%) are not candidates for surgical resection due to the extent or distribution of disease, or co-morbidity (42). Although historical chemotherapy results have been disappointing, there are now several chemotherapy regimes that impact survival. Irinotecan was the first agent reported to significantly improve survival to a median 17.4 months and one-year survival of 69% (43). Oxaliplatin and the newer biological agents (Cetuximab and Avastin) also significantly increase survival (44). The sequential use of multiple chemotherapy regimes, if tolerated, can allow survival <24 months. Neoadjuvant chemotherapy can be used to downsize inoperable/unablatable disease to the point where ablation or resection can be performed (45,46).

Between 1993 and 1995 we performed laser thermal ablation and reported a median survival of 27 months (47). We have previously published our results in 167 patients treated with RFA and recently analyzed survival in a cohort of 309 patients with inoperable colorectal liver metastases treated with RFA (48). These patients were not candidates for resection because the location and distribution of tumors meant that resection would have resulted in inadequate liver reserve or because of concomitant medical morbidity. Of the 309 patients, we identified a subgroup of 123 patients with ≤5 metastases, ≤5 cm with no extrahepatic disease whose median survival was 46 months from diagnosis and 36 months from ablation (Fig. 51.2). Three and five-year survival rates were 63%, 34% and 49%, 24%, respectively. The most important factors in survival were the absence of extrahepatic disease and liver tumor volume. Sixty-nine of the 123 patients had three tumors or less with a maximum diameter <3.5 cm and their five-year survival was better at 40%. Finally, for those patients who only have small solitary tumors <4 cm, the survival is even better at >80% at three years (49). These figures compare reasonably well with surgical resection data (50,51). Other thermal ablation groups have reported similar survival results (52–55).

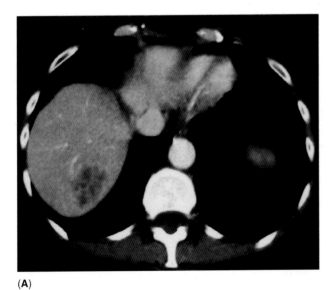

(A)

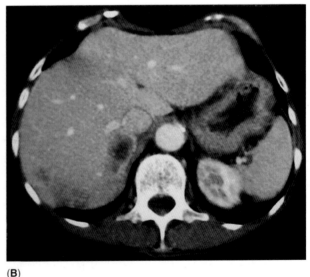

(B)

Figure 51.2 A 61-year-old woman presenting with multiple colorectal liver metastases. *(Continued)*

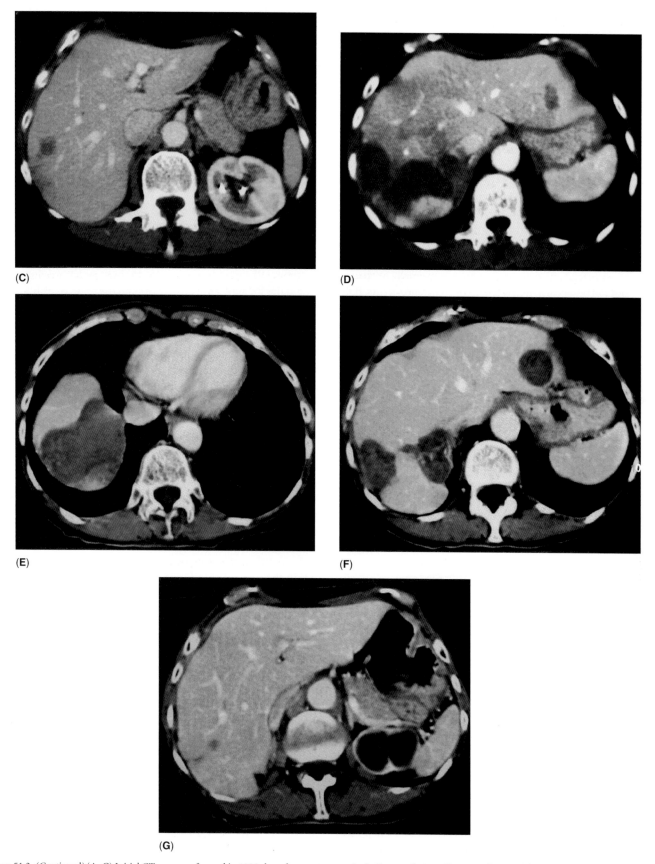

Figure 51.2 (Continued) (**A–C**) Initial CT scans performed in 1999 show four metastases, including one lesion adjacent to the cava. These were treated with RF ablation. (**D**) On follow-up in 2000, a fifth metastasis developed in the left lobe. There is also some recurrence adjacent to the cava. Further RF ablation was performed and followed by systemic chemotherapy. (**E–G**) CT scans performed in October 2002 showing areas of ablation without evidence of tumor recurrence. This patient is tumor-free three years after presentation with inoperable liver metastases.

Patient Selection

Our current recommendation is to accept patients with five metastases or less, each with a maximum diameter not exceeding 5 cm, more numerous tumors as long as the largest is <4 cm, and larger tumors <7 cm if they are solitary.

Where the distribution of disease is not amenable to surgery, the use of a combination of RF and resection can be considered. For those with co-morbidity, RF ablation is a much less invasive alternative than surgery and has lower complication rates. Other applications of RF ablation include use in patients with limited liver disease who have insufficient residual liver to allow resection, usually post-hemihepatectomy patients with new metastases in the residual lobe.

RFA, like surgery, is most effective in small tumors. Retrospective comparisons of RF and repeat hepatic resection show similar survival benefits (53). At our institution, a retrospective comparison of RF and surgery in solitary metastases showed a similar survival rate (56). RF can be performed either concurrently or sequentially to chemotherapy, and can be repeated if new lesions or recurrence occurs. If the patient develops more extensive disease, such that RF can no longer be performed, then chemotherapy should be considered.

Key Points: Colorectal Liver Metastases

- Surgical resection remains the first-line treatment for patients with resectable disease but this may change in certain circumstances
- In disease not amenable to surgery, or in patients who have undergone surgery, RF ablation is used to good effect
- Three and five-year survival following RF ablation in inoperable patients compares well with survival following resection

---

Neuroendocrine

The treatment options for these patients are limited. Few patients are eligible for surgery and the alternatives produce symptomatic improvement but have less impact on tumor load (57). Aggressive cytoreduction followed by octreotide analogues can be the best way to achieve prolonged symptom control (58). RF can be used to reduce hormone secretion and/or to reduce tumor load. Siperstein et al. initially reported on laparoscopic RF ablation in 15 patients (59). Our experience with 17 patients showed benefits in 11, local control of tumor volume in seven, and relief or reduction in hormone-related symptoms in four of six with secreting tumors (60). Control of liver tumor load should translate into improved survival but this is harder to prove. Median survival of 5.5 years from the diagnosis of liver metastases and 3.9 years from ablation has been reported in a series of 63 patients with various neuroendocrine primaries treated with laparoscopic RFA (61).

Non-colorectal, Non-neuroendocrine Including Breast

Isolated liver metastases are an uncommon occurrence in breast cancer. Breast cancer patients with liver metastases are a heterogeneous population and the tumor biology is unpredictable. Some surgeons will perform hepatic resection for limited liver metastases, others are more reluctant. Nevertheless, a 22% five-year survival post-resection has been reported (62). RF has also been used in small cohorts of patients. Livraghi reported on 24 patients of whom 10 were free of disease at a mean follow-up of 10 months (63).

A more common clinical scenario is liver metastasis in the presence of extrahepatic disease. Current chemotherapeutic regimes are less effective in controlling liver disease than extrahepatic disease. We achieved a 30-month survival of 41.6% in 19 patients, 11 of whom had extrahepatic disease (64). Sofocleous et al. performed ablation in 12 patients, 10 of whom had extrahepatic disease and achieved a median progression-free survival of 13 months (65). The largest group treated to date included 232 patients, 72 (31%) of whom had bone metastases, who underwent laser ablation in conjunction with chemotherapy (66). The mean survival was 4.8 years for patients with no extrahepatic disease and 4.3 years for those with bone metastases; this difference was not significant. There is limited experience of RF in other non-colorectal, non-neuroendocrine metastases, but good surgical results have been reported when there has been an interval of more than two years between the primary tumor and the development of detectable metastatic disease (67). Therefore, RF could be considered in these patients if they are not candidates for surgery.

Hepatocellular Carcinoma

Unlike liver metastases, local ablative therapy is well established in HCC. Historically, ablation was performed using pure ethanol. Trials of PEI and liver resection suggest comparable survival. In one trial, Childs Pugh Class A patients had a three-year survival of 71% following PEI compared to 79% following surgery, and Childs Pugh Class B patients had a three-year survival of 41% and 40%, respectively (68). Several randomized, prospective comparisons of PEI and RFA in patients with small tumors have shown that RFA is superior to PEI as it has lower local recurrence rates, less operator variability, longer disease-free survival, and a better overall increase in survival (69,70). There are still some indications for PEI (e.g., in patients with exophytic tumors) and PEI is very cost competitive. Microwave therapy has been shown to be effective in small HCC (71). Encapsulated HCC is generally easier to destroy than metastases as the heat is contained and amplified within the lesion. Several centers use laser effectively in the treatment of HCC and, to date, there has been no comparison of laser and RF in HCC (72). Current recommendations for RF in HCC are Childs Pugh Class A or B cirrhosis and no more than three lesions no larger than 3 cm, or a single tumor <5 cm in diameter (Fig. 51.3) (73). Long-term results for patients treated with RFA from several groups in Europe and Asia confirm the efficacy of RFA. Three-year survival rates for Childs A patients treated with RFA vary between 71% and 87%. These data compare well with three-year survival rates of 76% to 86% for resection. Five-year survival following RFA is 48% to 64%, which is not dissimilar to the 44% to 59% achieved following resection (74–76).

Screening programs for the detection of early HCC in patients with hepatitis C or B are not widespread and, therefore, many patients present with large tumors. Although the survival advantage of transarterial chemoembolization (TACE) remains controversial (77), the combination of selective TACE and thermal ablation has been explored with some success in this cohort (78,79). Different techniques have been used, e.g., laser followed weeks later by TACE, or balloon occlusion of the hepatic artery during RF followed by selective catheterization of the tumor-feeding vessels and chemoembolization immediately afterwards. The optimal sequence and timing of the two therapies is not yet known.

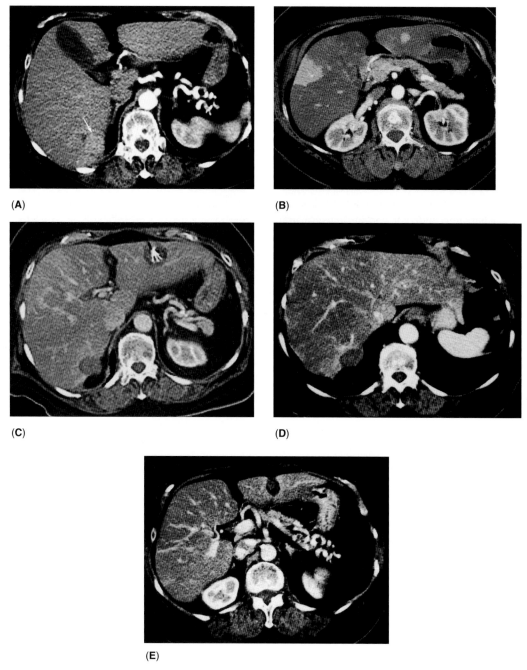

Figure 51.3 HCC treated with RF. A 78-year-old woman with a previous colorectal primary. (**A**) Initial scans performed in November 1999 showing a solitary hypervascular tumor in the postero-medial aspect of the right lobe (arrow). The AFP was normal and therefore this lesion was biopsied. Histology showed HCC. This was treated with RF. (**B**) During follow-up a new hypervascular lesion develops in the left lobe. There is also a wedge-shaped perfusion anomaly in the right lobe. (**C**) CT scan performed immediately after RF ablation showing an expandable electrode with surrounding low attenuation necrosis. (**D, E**) CT scans performed in October 2002 showing complete ablation with no active tumor. This patient is tumor-free three years after her original ablation.

Key Point: Hepatocellular Carcinoma Ablation

■ Current recommendations for RF ablation in HCC are Childs Pugh Class A or B cirrhosis and no more than three lesions no larger than 3 cm, or a single lesion <5 cm.

Complications

The complication rate following ablation varies from 2% to 10% and the mortality is less than 0.8% (80,81). Needle puncture or thermal injury can result in:

- Subcapsular hematoma
- Occlusion or thrombosis of hepatic veins or portal vein branches
- Bile duct strictures
- Injury to adjacent viscera such as stomach, duodenum, gall bladder, colon (manifested as perforation or fistula formation), or the lung or pleura (pneumothorax or pleural effusions). This complication has largely been prevented by infusing 5% dextrose into the periablation zone and displacing any vulnerable structures away

Complication rates will increase with increasing numbers of punctures, larger volumes of necrosis, more advanced Child Pugh class, and treatment of lesions close to the diaphragm, into the liver hilum, close to vessels or viscera. The worst morbidity is associated with infection of necrotic-ablated metastases, and the major etiological factor for this is the presence of a biliary endo-prosthesis or a previous bilio-enteric anastomosis.

Approach—Percutaneous, Laparoscopic, or Open?

RFA can be performed using image guidance and a percutaneous approach (82–84), laparoscopic guidance (59,85–87), or at open laparotomy (88,89). At open laparotomy, RF ablation can be combined with liver resection, i.e., resection of one area of the liver and ablation of another. If a patient is undergoing laparotomy for some other surgical procedure then it is reasonable to perform RF at the same time. With this exception it is difficult to justify the added morbidity, invasiveness, and expense of a laparotomy compared to a percutaneous procedure. The laparoscopic approach has been used when tumor is adherent to structures that would be damaged by thermal ablation, e.g., tumor adherent to stomach, colon, or duodenum. Some centers prefer the laparoscopic approach where there is poor tumor visualization transcutaneously and also for large HCCs requiring multiple punctures (90,91). RFA will most commonly be performed in the radiology department, but there is a subgroup of patients who will benefit from open or laparoscopic RF.

Thermal Ablation and Blood Flow Manipulation

Normal liver responds to thermal injury with an increase in perfusion. Using CT we have quantified this effect in a group of 32 patients (92). There was a mean 3.3-fold increase in hepatic arterial flow adjacent to the ablated area. Tissue perfusion has a direct impact on the volume of necrosis that can be produced. This has been confirmed using pharmacological manipulation where, for example, a halothane-induced reduction in blood flow of 46% resulted in a 50% increase in the diameter of the ablation (93). Several groups have explored vascular occlusion as a method for increasing the volume of necrosis (94,95). Vascular occlusion, either portal venous, hepatic arterial, or both, has been shown to be beneficial in animal models with increases in measured temperature at the treatment site and increases in the size of ablation (96,97). Surgeons have the option of clamping the vascular pedicle during RF ablation, and percutaneous balloon occlusion is also effective. Although vascular occlusion increases the volume of ablation, it also removes the protective effect of blood flow and, as a result, there is an associated increase in bile duct injury. An alternative approach, favored by our group, is the use of hypotensive general anesthesia, similar to that used at hepatic resection, i.e., maintenance of a systolic pressure of approximately 80 mmHg (98).

Key Points: Ablation Techniques

- Ablation techniques have been successfully applied to both primary and secondary tumors
- The number and size of tumors that can be ablated varies with the technique and primary pathology
- Percutaneous techniques have a lower morbidity and complication rate than intraoperative techniques

- Retrospective analysis suggests that ablation improves patient survival in both colorectal liver metastases and HCC
- Ablation can be used in conjunction with other therapies to good effect

Pancreas

The median survival for a patient with pancreatic adenocarcinoma is five months, and for those with operable disease the median is 18 to 20 months. However, most patients present with inoperable disease (99,100). The most common cause for inoperability is vascular invasion, which occurs early in the disease process, despite a relatively small tumor load. Alternatives to surgery include chemotherapy and/or radiotherapy. Currently, Gemcitabine is the best chemotherapeutic option, offering symptomatic relief and a small increase in survival (101). External beam radiotherapy in combination with chemotherapy also produces a modest improvement in survival. Given the lack of good alternative therapies, we evaluated photodynamic therapy in a pilot study (102).

We studied the use of interstitial PDT in the treatment of 16 patients with localized but inoperable pancreatic adenocarcinoma. Biliary stents were always positioned prior to PDT. Three to five days after administration of IV mTHPC, up to eight percutaneous hollow needles were positioned within the tumor (Fig. 51.4). Then, 20 J of red light were delivered at each treatment station. Treatment was performed at multiple stations to produce confluent necrosis. Median total light energy delivered was 240 J (range 40–480 J).

The median volume of necrosis as measured on contrast-enhanced CT was 36 cc (range 9–60 cc). Endoscopic evaluation of the duodenum showed hemorrhagic necrosis, which healed rapidly over four to six weeks. The median survival was 12.5 months (range 6–34 months). There were six complications: hemorrhage in two patients, needle track seeding in one, and the subsequent development of fibrous duodenal strictures in three. The results of this pilot study suggest that necrosis can be produced in pancreatic cancer; further studies are required to see if this will impact survival.

RFA has also been performed as a palliative debulking procedure in inoperable pancreatic carcinoma. The proximity of a number of vulnerable structures has limited this to an intraoperative approach. One non-randomized study suggests an improvement in survival (103). Novel approaches such as using endoscopic US guidance are also under investigation.

Head and Neck

Therapeutic options for recurrent head and neck cancer are limited, and in most instances PDT is palliative. Surface illumination for mucosal PDT has been applied to dysplasia and localized carcinoma in the oropharynx, as well as for recurrent head and neck cancer when other therapeutic options have been exhausted. One group treated 51 patients with a range of different head and neck primaries, and reported both symptomatic benefit and improvements in tumor control. Laser has also been applied with some success to recurrent head and neck tumors (104,105).

The Breast

The aim of surgery to the breast in breast cancer is to obtain local control of a systemic disease. Extent or type of surgery performed does not affect the ultimate outcome. This is determined by the

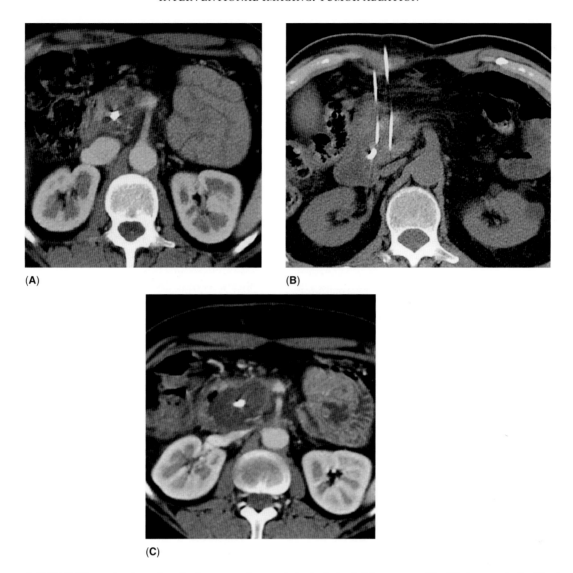

Figure 51.4 Pancreatic PDT. (A) CT scan showing an irregular, low attenuation mass lesion in the head of the pancreas with a bile duct stent in situ. Biopsies showed adeno-carcinoma. (B) Axial CT scan performed during treatment showing multiple needles positioned through the anterior abdominal wall into the pancreatic tumor. (C) Axial contrast enhanced CT scan performed three days after PDT. There is a large confluent area of absent enhancement consistent with necrosis in the head of the pancreas.

systemic spread of the disease. However, the extent of local surgery is determined by the spread of tumor within the breast. Most screen-detected cancers are small and show little evidence of spread. A major goal in the management of breast cancer is to reduce the psychological and physical trauma of biopsy and surgery, and, in particular, to compress the duration of the process from suspicion, screening, and diagnosis to therapy as much as possible. RF, laser, and cryotherapy techniques have all been applied to the breast (106–111). In our experience in over 100 tumors in a phase 1 study, with no attempt to destroy the whole tumor, complete response was achieved in 40% (106). A series of studies in which RFA was performed prior to resection achieved complete tumor kill in 96/108 (88%) tumors. Challenges arise due to the multifocality of breast cancer, the difficulty of image-guided detection and exact targeting. Skin burns have been reported and the cosmetic results are not always excellent. Photodynamic therapy has been used for the treatment of superficial, locally recurrent breast cancer (112–114).

An alternative technique, radiosurgery was developed by the Photoelectron Corporation in Boston. They have manufactured a battery-powered electron gun, which fires low kilovoltage electrons down an evacuated needle to a tungsten target to generate soft X-rays. The delivery system is only 3 mm in diameter and is small enough to be combined with stereotactic mammography, US, or MR.

The advantages of radiosurgery are:

- Energy deposition is precisely known and its distribution within tissue can be calculated using radiotherapy planning methods
- Biological effects of ionizing radiation are well understood
- Effects of X-irradiation are reproducible and have some selectivity between tissue types. Radiotherapy in the breast is used for two reasons: first, to sterilize the margins of a resected tumor to avoid a local recurrence; second, to suppress multifocal disease elsewhere in the breast. Radiosurgery not only destroys residual tumor tissue *in situ* but can also act as a local boost to external beam radiotherapy. The radiosurgery needle is sufficiently small to be guided into position by US. There is no immediate treatment effect that can be recognized by imaging techniques

Key Points: Breast Cancer Ablative Therapy

- RF, laser and cryotherapy techniques have all been applied in the treatment of breast cancer
- PDT has been used for the treatment of superficial, locally recurrent, breast cancer

The Prostate

The introduction of PSA screening has resulted in the earlier detection of small tumors, yet the best treatment for localized prostate cancer remains controversial. Reported long-term cure rates are 19% to 46% for radiotherapy and 40% to 75% for radical prostatectomy. These results are achieved at the expense of significant complications. Urinary incontinence occurs in <40% and impotence in <60% of patients following radical prostatectomy, and <7% and <66%, respectively, after radiotherapy (115–117).

The 20-year old technique of radioactive seed implantation is increasingly popular. This has been revived through persistent development of better ultrasound control, three-dimensional planning of the irradiation, and new isotopes. Despite this, both brachytherapy and external beam radiotherapy have a significant local failure rate (10–15% within 18 months for DXR) and there is a great need for a method to treat these recurrences. Salvage radical prostatectomy carries a much higher complication rate than *de novo* radical prostatectomy.

Thermal Ablation

Prostate cancer is an example of field change and is frequently multifocal at presentation. Multiple mapping biopsies using a grid system can provide more accurate detection of small foci of cancer than any imaging technique. Successful ablation may require treatment of the whole gland.

All the thermal techniques have been used in the prostate. There are no controlled trials and the length of follow-up in many studies is still very short. Enthusiasm for cryotherapy has varied over time and reports of high complications have led many centers to abandon this technique (118). Yet other centers have reported five-year results that are competitive to established treatments while emphasizing the need for substantial training and meticulous technique (119). Third generation cryotherapy machines, available since 2000, carry a lower complication rate. The other main contender is HIFU; complications have been reduced by using HIFU in combination with transurethral resection. HIFU has projected progression-free survival rates of 63% to 87%, and cryosurgery of between 36% and 92%. Research continues into these techniques which are currently offered to patients who are unfit for conventional therapy (120). We have studied the feasibility of using PDT in the treatment of recurrent prostate cancer following radiotherapy in 11 patients who have declined salvage prostatectomy (Fig. 51.5) (121).

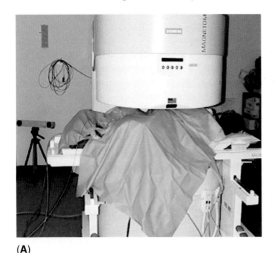

(A)

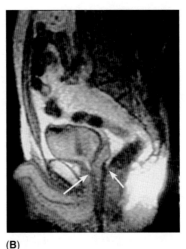

(B)

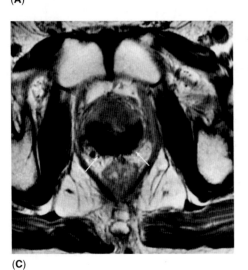

(C)

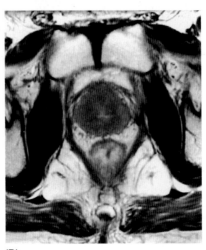

(D)

Figure 51.5 Prostate photodynamic therapy. (A) Patient set-up during MR-guided transperineal photodynamic therapy in an open (0.2 T) MR. (B) Intraprocedural sagittal image showing the needle positions (arrows). (C) Post-procedural contrast enhanced T1-weighted axial image performed at 1.5 T showing absent enhancement in the peripheral zone posteriorly (arrows). Compare to (D), the pretreatment contrast-enhanced axial T1-weighted image.

Lung Tumors

This is predicted to be the single largest growth area in ablation over the next few years. Laser, radiofrequency, cryotherapy, and microwave have all been used (122–125). Currently, the most widely used technique is RF. Good results can be achieved in small peripheral tumors. Both inoperable primary and limited numbers of metastatic tumors have been treated. CT fluoroscopy facilitates electrode placement as small scirrhous lung lesions can be difficult to penetrate with a large calibre needle. The complication profile is well described. Pneumothorax occurs in about 40% of cases, a similar incidence to that seen with trucut biopsy, but only a small percentage (10–15%) require drainage. The likelihood of a pneumothorax increases with the length of aerated lung that is traversed by the electrode and is more common when treating multiple tumors (126). The second most common complication is pleural effusion. Other complications include infection, hemorrhage and bronchopleural fistulae.

During treatment a penumbra of ground glass opacification develops around the tumor representing the ablation zone and a surrounding inflammatory reaction (Fig. 51.6). Histological studies have shown that the zone of cell death lies 2 to 4 mm inside the outer margin of the ground glass shadowing. Over time the ablation zone becomes increasingly dense and then reduces in size. At 12 months, up to 33% of successfully treated small lesions will have shrunk to a linear scar. Recurrence is identified by enlargement of the ablation zone, or a change in the shape of the zone indicating enlargement in one area or the development of focal nodular enhancement. Tumors <3.0 cm can usually be ablated at a single session, larger tumors (3–5 cm) may require more than one ablation or other additional therapy (127–129). Multivariate analysis has shown size to be the dominant feature determining complete ablation, but contact with >3 mm blood vessels or bronchi also increases the chance of recurrence (130,131). Current indications include patients with small volume but inoperable metastases and early primary lung cancer in patients inoperable for medical reasons. Early clinical studies report three- and five-year survival of between 46% and 57% in patients with colorectal metastases (128,129,132). Combinations of

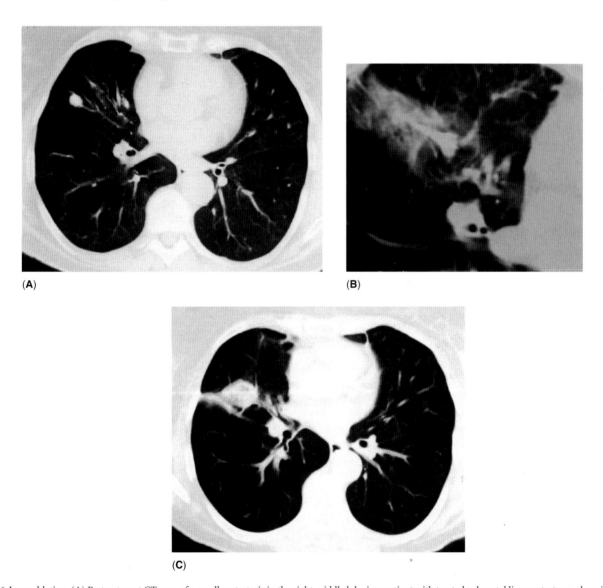

(A) **(B)**

(C)

Figure 51.6 Lung ablation. (**A**) Pretreatment CT scan of a small metastasis in the right middle lobe in a patient with treated colorectal liver metastases, chronic bronchitis, and emphysema. (**B**) Magnified view of the right middle lobe. CT scan during treatment showing the expandable electrode around the metastasis. There is some associated pulmonary contusion which was not clinically significant. (**C**) Follow-up CT scan at one month showing a large area of ablation with some associated pleural thickening.

radiotherapy and RFA have been used to good effect in primary lung cancer in inoperable patients (133). Photodynamic therapy has been extensively explored in lung malignancy both via the endoscopic and percutaneous route (134–137).

Key Points: Lung Cancer Ablative Therapy

- RF, microwave, laser, and cryotherapy have all been shown to be effective in small volume primary and secondary lung tumors
- Ablation has a much lower morbidity than conventional therapies and is anticipated to have a significant role in the management of primary and secondary lung cancer

Tumors of the Kidney

Nephron-sparing surgery presents a challenge to the surgeon. Yet there is increasing evidence that even moderate degrees of renal failure can significantly impact on survival following cardiovascular events. This will increase the focus of all physicians on the need to preserve renal function wherever and whenever possible (138). Local ablative techniques are the optimal nephron-sparing treatment for small renal tumors. One study found that 95.2% of patients had a GFR >60 ml/min/1.73m^2 at three years post-RFA as compared with 70.7% of patients post-partial nephrectomy and only 39.9% of patients post-radical nephrectomy (139). Therefore, patients with a solitary kidney and others with borderline renal function will increasingly be treated with ablation. Both tumor size and location are important predictors of outcome following ablation. Renal tumors up to 3.5 cm in diameter can be destroyed *in situ* by laser, RF, or cryotherapy with virtually no damage to the surrounding normal renal tissue (140–143). Some authors advocate cryotherapy for larger renal tumors <5 cm in diameter (144). Exophytic tumors are more readily ablated than central tumors (145). Multiple renal tumors are not rare and can be difficult to resect without complications, which are rare after ablation, particularly if a percutaneous approach is used (146). Hemorrhage is the most common; bowel injury can be prevented by dextrose isolation but it remains necessary to maintain a distance of >1 cm from the proximal ureter as ablation can result in ureteral stricturing.

Several series have now been published (140–142,147,148) including one retrospective comparison with partial nephrectomy which showed comparable oncologic efficacy, albeit with a shorter mean follow-up in the RF group (30 vs. 47 months) (149). Unfortunately, the urological literature has been muddied by the use of basic histopathological stains to assess ablation efficacy. As stated earlier, only enzyme stains provide the necessary information to assess the efficacy of the heating techniques. The question as to whether cryotherapy or RF is better has yet to be resolved.

Key Points: Renal Cancer Ablative Therapy

- Ablation is the ultimate nephron-sparing intervention for renal cell cancer
- Currently accepted for patients who cannot undergo resection, or for whom nephron sparing is critical, the role of ablation is likely to expand to include most small, particularly exophytic, renal tumors

Adrenal

There are a few reports of adrenal ablation. Adrenal adenomas are relatively easy to destroy either with chemical injection or thermal methods. Adrenal metastases have been treated successfully. Very careful patient selection is required as adrenal metastasis is often a marker of more systemic disease; however, in selected cases, where PET has shown no other site of disease, adrenal ablation may be of value (150). Ablation of normal functioning adrenal tissue can result in marked hypertension. We advocate intra-arterial monitoring of blood pressure during adrenal ablation and that IV alpha- and beta-blockers are at hand in the event of severe blood pressure rises.

Abdominal and Pelvic Nodes or Local Recurrence

Where nodal recurrence has occurred despite maximal radiotherapy treatment, local ablative techniques can be effective (150,151). The main problem is the potential for collateral neural injury. For most thermal techniques, a distance of 1 cm is required between the area to be ablated and any important local structure. A thermocouple placed at the interface with the structure to be protected is advocated so that treatment can be discontinued if temperatures rise unacceptably. For cryotherapy, many operators discontinue treatment when the ice-ball, the 0°C isotherm, approaches the potentially vulnerable structure.

Gynecological Malignancy

In the majority of cases the first-line approach to pelvic tumors is either surgery or chemoradiation. Many patients with recurrent pelvic tumors will experience multiple surgical procedures and will have reached their maximum tolerance of radiotherapy. Effective therapeutic options do not remain. Both RF and laser techniques can be very effective in this circumstance. Collateral damage is the main problem; the tumor destruction is relatively easy.

Bone Tumors

One of the first accepted indications for ablation was the minimally invasive treatment of benign osteoid osteomas (152). Malignant primary bone tumors will be treated by chemotherapy, radiotherapy, and surgery. However, if aggressive therapy is delivered at an early stage, recurrence can be very difficult to treat. Treatment by RF ablation may be curative, but is more likely to form part of a palliative treatment regimen. Either CT or MR are the usual guidance methods (Fig. 51.7).

RFA has been advocated in the symptomatic palliation of bone metastases following radiotherapy (153). Initial results suggest that ablation can produce significant reductions in pain levels and analgesic requirements. Only limited numbers of metastases can be treated. It is important to select patients with a clearly defined and understood dominant site of bone pain. Some authors promote the combination of ablation and cementoplasty, others argue that cementoplasty alone would be adequate. A trial to establish the relative merits of the two techniques has been suggested.

COMBINATION THERAPY AND CHEMOPREVENTION

Selected patients with small volume disease in more than one organ can also be treated with ablation. Where two major surgical procedures would be difficult to tolerate, two minimally invasive

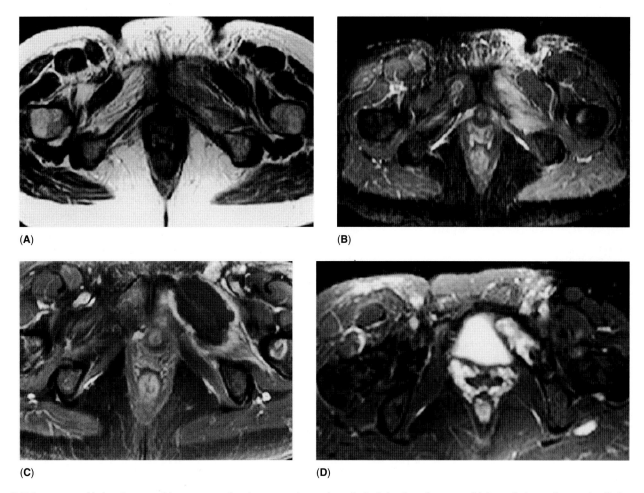

Figure 51.7 Bone tumor ablation. Recurrent biopsy-proven chondrosarcoma in a patient who had already undergone multiple surgical procedures and radiotherapy such that further radiotherapy or surgery were not feasible. This was treated with ultrasound and MR-guided RF ablation. (**A**) Gadolinium-enhanced axial T1-weighted image showing a mildly enhancing mass next to the left inferior pubic ramus. (**B**) Axial inversion recovery sequence showing the tumor as indistinct high signal intensity. (**C**) Immediate postablation: gadolinium-enhanced fat-suppressed, T1-weighted image showing an area of absent enhancement that embraces the original tumor. There is a surrounding inflammatory reaction seen as enhancement at the periphery. (**D**) Axial inversion recovery image at follow-up showing the area of necrosis has reduced in size and become well defined. This patient has had no further recurrence in three years.

treatments or even treatment of two organs at the same session is quite feasible with ablation. Examples of combined treatments include patients with both liver and lung metastases from colorectal cancer or synchronous primary lung cancers (154). The great promise of ablation, namely its focality and minimal invasiveness, is also its limitation. Local ablative techniques need to be used carefully, preferably within the context of multidisciplinary meeting and consensus. It is important to recognize the need for more extensive treatment in those cancers that arise within field change (e.g., the prostate), and also to combine ablation with systemic therapies for those cancers that are part of a systemic process. There is also a role for chemoprevention in conjunction with local ablation, for example, in HCC.

Summary

- There are multiple different technologies available for tumor ablation and each technology continues to improve
- The preferred technique and guidance will vary with the area treated
- The current preferred technique for liver tumors is RF ablation

- There are multiple applications for ablation ranging from symptomatic palliation in bone metastases to complete ablation of liver tumors
- Initial experience has been gained in inoperable tumors but retrospective evidence suggests ablation may supplant resection for small liver tumors
- Ablation will form one part of the oncologic therapeutic armamentarium. Local therapy is often combined with systemic therapy. The role of ablation within oncologic therapy needs to be established. This will be an area of active study in the next few years

REFERENCES

1. Dodd G, Soulen M, Kane R, et al. Minimally invasive treatment of malignant hepatic tumors: at the threshold of a major breakthrough. Radiographics 2000; 20: 9–27.
2. d'Arsonval MA. Action physiologique des courants alternatifs. CR Soc Biol 1891; 43: 283–93.
3. Lorentzen T. A cooled-needle electrode for radiofrequency tissue ablation: thermodynamic aspects of improved performance

compared with conventional needle design. Acad Radiol 1996; 3: 556–63.

4. Goldberg SN, Gazelle GS, Dawson SL, et al. Tissue ablation with radiofrequency using multiprobe arrays. Acad Radiol 1995; 2: 670–4.

5. Miao Y, Ni Y, Yu J, Marchal G. A comparative study on validation of a novel cooled-wet electrode for radiofrequency liver ablation. Invest Radiol 2000; 35: 438–44.

6. Miao Y, Ni Y, Mulier S, et al. Ex vivo experiment on radiofrequency liver ablation with saline infusion through a screw-tip cannulated electrode. J Surg Res 1997; 71: 19–24.

7. Livraghi T, Goldberg SN, Monti F, et al. Saline-enhanced radio-frequency tissue ablation in the treatment of liver metastases. Radiology 1997; 202: 205–10.

8. Goldberg SN, Ahmed M, Gazelle GS, et al. Radio-frequency thermal ablation with NaCl solution injection: effect of electrical conductivity on tissue heating and coagulation – phantom and porcine liver study. Radiology 2001; 219: 157–65.

9. McGahan JP, Dodd GD. Radiofrequency ablation of the liver. Current status. Am J Roentgenol 2001; 176: 3–16.

10. de Baere T, Denys A, Johns Wood BJ, et al. Radiofrequency liver ablation: experimental comparative study of water-cooled versus expandable systems. Am J Roentgenol 2001; 176: 187–92.

11. ter Haar G. High intensity ultrasound. Semin Laparosc Surg 2001; 8: 77–89.

12. Wu F, Chen W, Bai J, et al. Pathological changes in human malignant carcinoma treated with high-intensity focused ultrasound. Ultrasound Med Biol 2001; 27: 1099–106.

13. Livraghi T. Percutaneous ethanol injection in the treatment of hepatocellular carcinoma in cirrhosis. Hepatogastroenterology 2001; 48: 20–4.

14. Moore JV, West CM, Whitehurst C. The biology of photodynamic therapy. Phys Med Biol 1997; 42: 913–35.

15. Dougherty TJ. Photodynamic therapy (PDT) of malignant tumors. Crit Rev Oncol Hematol 1984; 2: 83–116.

16. Keller SM. Photodynamic therapy. Biology and clinical application. Chest Surg Clin N Am 1995; 5: 121–37.

17. Li JH, Guo ZH, Jin ML, et al. Photodynamic therapy in the treatment of malignant tumors: an analysis of 540 cases. J Photochem Photobiol B 1990; 6: 149–55.

18. McCaughan JS Jr. Photodynamic therapy: a review. Drugs Aging 1999; 15: 49–68.

19. Koren H, Alth G, Schenk GM, Jindra RH. Photodynamic therapy: an alternative pathway in the treatment of recurrent breast cancer. Int J Radiat Oncol Biol Phys 1994; 28: 463–6.

20. Patelli M, Lazzari Agli L, Poletti V, Falcone F. Photodynamic laser therapy for the treatment of early-stage bronchogenic carcinoma. Monaldi Arch Chest Dis 1999; 4: 315–18.

21. Furuse K, Fukuoka M, Kato H, et al. A prospective phase II study on photodynamic therapy with photofrin II for centrally located early-stage lung cancer. The Japan Lung Cancer Photodynamic Therapy Study Group. J Clin Oncol 1993; 11: 1852–7.

22. Karanov S, Kostadinov D, Shopova M, Kurtev P. Photodynamic therapy in lung and gastrointestinal cancers. J Photochem Photobiol B 1990; 6: 175–81.

23. Chang SC, Bown SG. Photodynamic therapy: applications in bladder cancer and other malignancies. J Formos Med Assoc 1997; 96: 853–63.

24. Puolakkainen P, Schroder T. Photodynamic therapy of gastrointestinal tumors: a review. Dig Dis 1992; 10: 53–60.

25. Fielding DI, Buonaccorsi GA, MacRobert AJ, et al. Fine-needle interstitial photodynamic therapy of the lung parenchyma: photosensitizer distribution and morphologic effects of treatment. Chest 1999; 115: 502–10.

26. Hornung R, Jentsch B, Crompton NE, Haller U, Walt H. In vitro effects and localization of the photosensitizers m-THPC and m-THPC MD on carcinoma cells of the human breast (MCF-7) and Chinese hamster fibroblasts (V-79). Lasers Surg Med 1997; 20: 443–50.

27. Vogl T, Müller P, Hammerstingl R, et al. Malignant liver tumors treated with MR imaging-guided laser-induced thermotherapy: technique and prospective results. Radiology 1995; 196: 257–65.

28. Chapman WC, Debelak JP, Wright Pinson C, et al. Hepatic cryoblation, but not radiofrequency ablation, results in lung inflammation. Ann Surg 2000; 231: 752–61.

29. Bilchik AJ, Wood TF, Allegra D, et al. Cryosurgical ablation and radiofrequency ablation for unresectable hepatic malignant neoplasms: a proposed algorithm. Arch Surg 2000; 135: 657–64.

30. Pearson AS, Izzo F, Fleming RY, et al. Intraoperative radiofrequency ablation or cryoablation for hepatic malignancies. Am J Surg 1999; 178: 592–9.

31. Adam R, Hagopian E, Linhares M, et al. A comparison of percutaneous cryosurgery and percutaneous radiofrequency for unresectable hepatic malignancies. Arch Surg 2002; 137: 1332–40.

32. Scudamore CH, Lee SI, Patterson EJ, et al. Radiofrequency ablation followed by resection of malignant liver tumors. Am J Surg 1999; 177: 411–17.

33. Goldberg SN, Gazelle GS, Compton CC, Mueller PR, Tanabe KK. Treatment of intrahepatic malignancy with radiofrequency ablation: radiologic–pathologic correlation. Cancer 2000; 88: 2452–63.

34. Cioni D, Lencioni R, Rossi S, et al. Radiofrequency thermal ablation of hepatocellular carcinoma: using contrast-enhanced harmonic power doppler sonography to assess treatment outcome. Am J Roentgenol 2001; 177: 783–8.

35. Solbiati L, Livraghi T, Goldberg SN, et al. Percutaneous radiofrequency ablation of hepatic metastases from colorectal cancer: long-term results in 117 patients. Radiology 2001; 221: 159–66.

36. Izumi N, Asahina Y, Noguchi O, et al. Risk factors for distant recurrence of hepatocellular carcinoma in the liver after complete coagulation by microwave or radiofrequency ablation. Cancer 2001; 91: 949–56.

37. Ikeda K, Saitoh S, Tsubota A, et al. Risk factors for tumor recurrence and prognosis after curative resection. Cancer 1993; 71: 19–25.

38. Adachi E, Maeda T, Matsumata T, et al. Risk factors for intrahepatic recurrence in human small hepatocellular carcinoma. Gastroenterology 1995; 108: 768–75.

39. Nagashima I, Hamada C, Naruse K, et al. Surgical resection for small hepatocellular carcinoma. Surgery 1996; 199: 40–5.

40. Belghiti J, Panis Y, Farges O, Benhamou JP, Fekete F. Intrahepatic recurrence after resection of hepatocellular carcinoma complicating cirrhosis. Ann Surg 1991; 214: 114–17.

41. Fong Y, Cohen AM, Fortner JG, et al. Liver resection for colorectal metastases. J Clin Oncol 1997; 15: 938–46.

42. Steele G, Ravikumar T. Resection of hepatic metastases from colorectal cancer. Ann Surg 1989; 210: 127–38.

43. Douillard JY. V303 Study Group. Irintoecan and high-dose fluorouracil/leucovorin for metastatic colorectal cancer. Oncology 2000; 14: 51–5.

44. Giacchetti S, Perpoint B, Zidani R, et al. Phase III multicenter randomized trial of oxaliplatin added to chronomodulated fluorouracil–leucovorin as first-line treatment of metastatic colorectal cancer. J Clin Oncol 2000; 18: 136–47.

45. Bismuth H, Adam R, Levi F, et al. Resection of nonresectable liver metastases from colorectal cancer after neoadjuvant chemotherapy. Ann Surg 1996; 224: 509–22.

46. Shankar A, Leonard P, Renaut AJ, et al. Neo-adjuvant therapy improves respectability rates for colorectal liver metastases. Ann R Coll Surg Engl 2001; 83: 85–8.

47. Gillams A, Lees WR. Survival after percutaneous, image-guided thermal ablation of hepatic metastases from colorectal cancer. Dis Colon Rectum 2000; 43: 656–61.

48. Gillams AR, Lees WR. Radio-frequency ablation of colorectal liver metastases in 167 patients. Eur Radiol 2004; 14: 2261–7.

49. Gillams AR, Lees WR. Five-year survival following radiofrequency ablation of small, solitary, hepatic colorectal metastases. J Vasc Interv Radiol 2008; 19: 712–17.

50. Jenkins LT, Millikan KW, Bines SD, Staren ED, Doolas A. Hepatic resection for metastatic colorectal cancer. Am Surg 1997; 63: 605–10.

51. Nordlinger B, Guiguet M, Vaillant JC, et al. Surgical resection of colorectal carcinoma metastases to the liver. A prognostic scoring system to improve cse selection based on 1568 patients. Assocation Française de Chirugie. Cancer 1996; 77: 1254–62.

52. Vogl TJ, Müller PK, Mack MG, et al. Liver metastases: interventional therapeutic techniques and results, state of the art. Eur Radiol 1999; 9: 675–84.

53. Elias D, de Baere T, Smayra T, et al. Percutaneous radiofrequency thermoablation as an alternative to surgery for treatment of liver tumor recurrence after hepatectomy. Br J Surg 2002; 89: 752–6.

54. Sørensen SM, Mortensen FV, Nielsen DT. Radiofrequency ablation of colorectal liver metastases: long-term survival. Acta Radiol 2007; 48: 253–8.

55. Jakobs TF, Hoffmann RT, Trumm C, Reiser MF, Helmberger TK. Radiofrequency ablation of colorectal liver metastases: mid-term results in 68 patients. Anticancer Res 2006; 26: 671–80.

56. Oshowo A, Gillams A, Harrison E, Lees WR, Taylor I. Comparison of resection and radiofrequency ablation for treatment of solitary colorectal liver metastases. Br J Surg 2003; 90: 1240–3.

57. Clouse ME, Perry L, Stuart K, Tokes KR. Hepatic arterial chemoembolization for metastatic neuroendocrine tumors. Digestion 1994; 55: 92–7.

58. Chung MH, Pisegna J, Spirt M, et al. Hepatic cytoreduction followed by a novel long-acting somatostatin analogue: a paradigm for intractable neuroendocrine tumors metastatic to the liver. Surgery 2001; 130: 954–62.

59. Siperstein A, Rogers S, Hansen P, Gitomirsky A. Laparoscopic thermal ablation of hepatic neuroendocrine tumor metastases. Surgery 1997; 122: 1147–55.

60. Gillams AR, Lees WR. Thermal ablation of neuroendocrine liver metastases Eur Radiol 2001; 11: 340.

61. Mazzaglia PJ, Berber E, Milas M, Siperstein AE. Laparoscopic radiofrequency ablation of neuroendocrine liver metastases: a 10-year experience evaluating predictors of survival. Surgery 2007; 142: 10–19.

62. Selzner M, Morse MA, Vredenburgh JJ, Meyers WC, Clavien PA. Liver metastases from breast cancer: long-term survival after curative resection. Surgery 2000; 127: 383–9.

63. Livraghi T, Goldberg SN, Solbiati L, et al. Percutaneous radiofrequency ablation of liver metastases from breast cancer: initial experience in 24 patients. Radiology 2001; 220: 145–9.

64. Lawes D, Chopada A, Gillams A, Lees W, Taylor I. Radiofrequency ablation (RFA) as a cytoreductive strategy for hepatic metastasis from breast cancer.Ann R Coll Surg Engl 2006; 88: 639–42.

65. Sofocleous CT, Nascimento RG, Gonen M, et al. Radiofrequency ablation in the management of liver metastases from breast cancer. Am J Roentgenol 2007; 189: 883–9.

66. Mack MG, Straub R, Eichler K, et al. Breast cancer metastases in liver: laser-induced interstitial thermotherapy—local tumor control rate and survival data. Radiology 2004; 233: 400–9.

67. Laurent C, Rullier E, Feyler A, Masson B, Saric J. Resection of noncolorectal and nonneuroendocrine liver metastases: late metastases are the only chance of cure. World J Surg 2001; 25: 1532–6.

68. Livraghi T, Bolondi L, Buscarini L, et al. No treatment, resection and ethanol injection in hepatocellular carcinoma: a retrospective analysis of survival in 391 patients with cirrhosis. Italian Cooperative HCC Study Group. J Hepatol 1995; 22: 522–6.

69. Livraghi T, Goldberg SN, Lazzaroni S, et al. Small heptocellular carcinoma: treatment with radiofrequency ablation versus ethanol injection. Radiology 1999; 210: 655–61.

70. Lencioni RA, Allgaier HP, Cioni D, et al. Small hepatocellular carcinoma in cirrhosis: randomized comparison of radiofrequency thermal ablation versus percutaneous ethanol injection. Radiology 2003; 228: 235–40.

71. Shibata T, Iimuro Y, Yamamoto Y, et al. Small hepatocellular carcinoma: comparison of radio-frequency ablation and percutaneous microwave coagulation therapy. Radiology 2002; 223: 331–7.

72. Pacella CM, Bizzarri G, Magnolfi F, et al. Laser thermal ablation in the treatment of small hepatocellular carcinoma: results in 74 patients. Radiology 2001; 221: 712–20.

73. Livraghi T, Goldberg SN, Lazzaroni S, et al. Hepatocellular carcinoma: radio-frequency ablation of medium and large lesions. Radiology 2000; 214: 761–8.

74. Choi D, Lim HK, Rhim N, et al. Percutaneous radiofrequency ablation for early-stage hepatocellular carcinoma as a first-line treatment: long-term results and prognostic factors in a large single-institution series. Eur Radiol 2007; 17: 684–92.

75. Lencioni R, Cioni R, Crocetti L, et al. Early-stage hepatocellular carcinoma in patients with cirrhosis: long-term results of percutaneous image-guided radiofrequency ablation. Radiology 2005; 234: 961–7.

76. Tateishi R, Shiina S, Teratani T, et al. Percutaneous radiofrequency ablation for hepatocellular carcinoma. An analysis of 1000 cases. Cancer 2005; 103: 1201–9.

77. Llovet JM, Bruix J. Systematic review of randomized trials for unresectable hepatocellular carcinoma: chemoembolization improves survival. Hepatology 2003; 37: 429–42.

78. Pacella CM, Bizzarri G, Cecconi O, et al. Hepatocellular carcinoma: long-term results of combined treatment with laser thermal ablation and transcatheter arterial chemoembolization. Radiology 2001; 219: 669–78.

79. Lencioni R, Cioni D, Donati F, Bartolozzi C. Combination of interventional therapies in hepatocellular carcinoma. Hepatogastroenterology 2001; 48: 8–14.

80. Mulier S, Mulier P, Ni Y, et al. Complications of radiofrequency coagulation of liver tumors. Br J Surg 2002; 89: 1206–22.

81. Rhim H, Dodd G D. Radiofrequency thermal ablation of liver tumors. J Clin Ultrasound 1999; 27: 221–9.

82. Solbiati L, Goldberg SN, Ierace T, et al. Hepatic metastases: percutaneous radio-frequency ablation with cooled-tip electrodes. Radiology 1997; 205: 367–73.

83. Rossi S, DiStasi M, Buscarini E, et al. Percutaneous RF interstitial thermal ablation in the treatment of hepatic cancer. Am J Roentgenol 1996; 167: 759–68.

84. Lencioni R, Goletti O, Armillotta N, et al. Radio-frequency thermal ablation of liver metastases with cooled tip electrode needle: results of a pilot clinical trial. Eur Radiol 1998; 8: 1205–11.

85. Cuschieri A, Bracken J, Boni L. Initial experience with laparoscopic ultrasound-guided radiofrequency thermal ablation of hepatic tumours. Endoscopy 1999; 31: 318–21.

86. Siperstein A, Garland A, Engle K, et al. Local recurrence after laparoscopic radiofrequency thermal ablation of hepatic tumours. Ann Surg Oncol 2000; 7: 106–13.

87. Curley SA, Izzo F, Delrio P, et al. Radiofrequency ablation of unresectable primary and metastatic hepatic malignancies: results in 123 patients. Ann Surg 1999; 230: 1–8.

88. Jiao L, Hansen P, Havlik R, et al. Clinical short-term results of radiofrequency ablation in primary or secondary liver tumors. Am J Surg 1999; 177: 303–6.

89. Wood TF, Rose DM, Chung M, et al. Radiofrequency ablation of 231 unresectable hepatic tumors: indications, limitations, and complications. Ann Surg Oncol 2000; 7: 593–600.

90. Montorsi M, Santambrogio R, Bianchi P, et al. Radiofrequency interstitial thermal ablation of hepatocellular carcinoma in liver cirrhosis. Role of the laparoscopic approach. Surg Endosc 2001; 15: 141–5.

91. Podnos YD, Henry G, Ortiz JA, et al. Laparoscopic ultrasound with radiofrequency ablation in cirrhotic patients with hepatocellular carcinoma: technique and technical considerations. Am Surg 2001; 67: 1181–4.

92. Gillams AR, Lees WR. Thermal ablation-induced changes in hepatic arterial perfusion. Radiology 1999; 213P: 382.

93. Goldberg S, Hahn P, Halpern E, Fogle RM, Gazelle GS. Radiofrequency tissue ablation: effect of pharmacological modulation of blood flow on coagulation diameter. Radiology 1998; 209: 761–7.

94. Patterson EJ, Scudamore CH, Owen DA, Nagy AG, Buczkowski AK. Radiofrequency ablation of porcine liver in vivo: effects of blood flow and treatment time on lesion size. Ann Surg 1998; 227: 559–65.

95. Goldberg SN, Hahn PF, Tanabe KK, et al. Percutaneous radiofrequency tissue ablation: does perfusion-mediated tissue cooling limit coagulation necrosis? J Vasc Interv Radiol 1998; 9: 101–11.

96. de Baere T, Bessoud B, Dromain C, et al. Percutaneous radiofrequency ablation of hepatic tumors during temporary venous occlusion. Am J Roentgenol 2002; 178: 53–9.

97. Denys A, Portier F, Lamarre A, Wicky S. Hepatic vascular occlusions and radiofrequency liver ablation: from animal experiment to clinical observation? Am J Roentgenol 2001; 177: 1215–16.

98. Lees WR, Gillams AR, Schumillian C. Hypotensive anaesthesia improves the effectiveness of radiofrequency ablation in the liver. Radiology 2000; 217: 228.

99. Livingston EH, Welton ML, Reber HA. Surgical treatment of pancreatic cancer. The United States Experience. Int J Pancreatol 1991; 9: 153–7.

100. Warshaw AL, Fernandez-del Castillo C. Pancreatic carcinoma. N Engl J Med 1992; 326: 455–65.

101. Burris HA 3rd, Moore MJ, Andersen J, et al. Improvements in survival and clinical benefit with gemcitabine as first-line therapy for patients with advanced pancreas cancer: a randomized trial. J Clin Oncol 1997; 15: 2403–13.

102. Bown SG, Rogowska AZ, Whitelaw DE, et al. Photodynamic therapy for cancer of the pancreas. Gut 2002; 50: 549–57.

103. Spiliotis JD, Datsis AC, Michalopoulos NV, et al. Radiofrequency ablation combined with palliative surgery may prolong survival of patients with advanced cancer of the pancreas. Langenbecks Arch Surg 2007; 392: 55–60.

104. Bockmuhl U, Knobber D, Vogl T, Mack M. Use of MR-controlled laser-induced thermotherapy in recurrent squamous epithelial carcinoma of the head-neck area. Laryngorhinootologie 1996; 75: 597–601.

105. Vogl T, Mack MG, Muller P, et al. Recurrent nasopharyngeal tumors: preliminary clinical results with interventional MR imaging-controlled laser-induced thermotherapy. Radiology 1995; 196: 725–33.

106. Harries SA, Amin Z, Smith ME, et al. Interstitial laser photocoagulation as a treatment for breast cancer. Br J Surg 1994; 81: 1617–19.

107. Robinson DS, Parel JM, Denham DB, et al. Interstitial laser hyperthermia model development for minimally invasive therapy of breast carcinoma. J Am Coll Surg 1998; 186: 284–92.

108. Jeffrey SS, Birdwell RL, Ikeda DM, et al. Radiofrequency ablation of breast cancer: first report of an emerging technology. Arch Surg 1999; 134: 1064–8.

109. Böhm T, Hilger I, Müller W, et al. Saline-enhanced radiofrequency ablation of breast tissue: an in vitro feasibility study. Invest Radiol 2000; 35: 149–57.

110. Pfleiderer SO, Freesmeyer MG, Marx C, et al. Cryotherapy of breast cancer under ultrasound guidance: initial results and limitations. Eur Radiol 2002; 12: 3009–14.

111. Dowlatshahi K, Francescatti D, Bloom K. Laser therapy for small breast cancers. Am J Surg 2002; 184: 359–63.

112. Allison R, Mang T, Hewson G, Snider W, Dougherty T. Photodynamic therapy for chest wall progression from breast carcinoma is an underutilized treatment modality. Cancer 2001; 91: 1–8.

113. Schuh M, Nseyo UO, Potter WR, Dao TL, Dougherty TJ. Photodynamic therapy for palliation of locally recurrent breast carcinoma. J Clin Oncol 1987; 5: 1766–70.

114. Taber SW, Fingar VH, Wieman TJ. Photodynamic therapy for palliation of chest wall recurrence in patients with breast cancer. J Surg Oncol 1998; 68: 209–14.

115. Carlson K, Nitti V. Prevention and management of incontinence following radical prostatectomy. Urol Clin North Am 2001; 28: 595–612.

116. McCullough A. Prevention and management of erectile dysfunction following radical prostatectomy. Urol Clin North Am 2001; 28: 613–27.

117. D-Amico D, Coleman C. Role of interstitial radiotherapy in the management of clinically organ-confined prostate cancer: the jury is still out. J Clin Oncol 1996; 14: 304–15.

118. Aus G, Pileblad E, Hugosson J. Cryosurgical ablation of the prostate: 5-year follow-up of a prospective study. Eur Urol 2002; 42: 133–8.

119. Donnelly BJ, Saliken JC, Ernst DS, et al. Prospective trial of cryosurgical ablation of the prostate: five-year results. Urology 2002; 60: 645–9.

120. Aus G. Current status of HIFU and cryotherapy in prostate cancer—a review. Eur Urol 2006; 50: 927–34.

121. Nathan TR, Whitelaw DE, Chang SC, et al. Photodynamic therapy for prostate cancer recurrence after radiotherapy: a Phase I study. J Urol 2002; 168: 1427–32.

122. Dupuy DE, Zagoria RJ, Akerly W, et al. Percutaneous radiofrequency ablation of malignancies in the lung. Am J Roentgenol 2000; 174: 57–9.

123. Brookes JA, Lees WR, Bown SG. Interstitial laser photocoagulation for the treatment of lung cancer. Am J Roentgenol 1997; 168: 357–8.

124. Brenner M, Shankel T, Waite TA, et al. Animal model for thoracoscopic laser ablation of emphysematous pulmonary bullae. Lasers Surg Med 1996; 18: 191–6.

125. Wolf FJ, Grand DJ, Machan JT, et al. Microwave ablation of lung malignancies: effectiveness, CT findings, and safety in 50 patients. Radiology 2008; 247: 871–9.

126. Gillams AR, Lees WR. Analysis of the factors associated with radiofrequency ablation-induced pneumothorax. Clin Radiol 2007; 62: 639–44.

127. de Baère T, Palussière J, Aupérin A, et al. Midterm local efficacy and survival after radiofrequency ablation of lung tumors with minimum follow-up of 1 year: prospective evaluation. Radiology 2006; 240: 587–96.

128. Yamakado K, Hase S, Matsuoka T, et al. Radiofrequency ablation for the treatment of unresectable lung metastases in patients with colorectal cancer: a multicenter study in Japan. J Vasc Interv Radiol 2007; 18: 393–8.

129. Simon CJ, Dupuy DE, DiPetrillo TA, et al. Pulmonary radiofrequency ablation: long-term safety and efficacy in 153 patients. Radiology 2007; 243: 268–75.

130. Gillams AR, Lees WR. Radiofrequency ablation of lung metastases: factors influencing success. Eur Radiol 2008; 18: 672–7.

131. Hiraki T, Mimura H, Gobara H, et al. Repeat radiofrequency ablation for local progression of lung tumors: does it have a role in local tumor control? J Vasc Interv Radiol 2008; 19: 706–11.

132. Yan TD, King J, Sjarif A, et al. Percutaneous radiofrequency ablation of pulmonary metastases from colorectal carcinoma: prognostic determinants for survival. Ann Surg Oncol 2006; 13: 1529–37.

133. Dupuy DE, DiPetrillo T, Gandhi S, et al. Radiofrequency ablation followed by conventional radiotherapy for medically inoperable stage I non-small cell lung cancer. Chest 2006; 129: 738–45.

134. Lam S. Photodynamic therapy of lung cancer. Semin Oncol 1994; 21: 15–19.

135. McCaughan JS Jr. Survival after photodynamic therapy to non-pulmonary metastatic endobronchial tumors. Lasers Surg Med 1999; 24: 194–201.

136. Ost D. Photodynamic therapy in lung cancer. Oncology (Huntingt) 2000; 14: 379–86, 391–2.

137. Pass HI, Pogrebniak H. Photodynamic therapy for thoracic malignancies. Semin Surg Oncol 1992; 8: 217–25.

138. Anavekar NS, McMurray JJ, Velazquez EJ, et al. Relation between renal dysfunction and cardiovascular outcomes after myocardial infarction. N Engl J Med 2004; 351: 1285–95.

139. Lucas SM, Stern JM, Adibi M, et al. Renal function outcomes in patients treated for renal masses smaller than 4 cm by ablative and extirpative techniques. J Urol 2008; 179: 75–9, discussion 79–80.

140. Zagoria RJ, Traver MA, Werle DM, et al. Oncologic efficacy of CT-guided percutaneous radiofrequency ablation of renal cell carcinomas. Am J Roentgenol 2007; 189: 429–36.

141. Park S, Anderson JK, Matsumoto ED, et al. Radiofrequency ablation of renal tumors: intermediate-term results. J Endourol 2006; 20: 569–73.

142. Breen DJ, Rutherford EE, Stedman B, et al. Management of renal tumors by image-guided radiofrequency ablation: experience in 105 tumors. Cardiovasc Intervent Radiol 2007; 30: 936–42.

143. Littrup PJ, Ahmed A, Aoun HD, et al. CT-guided percutaneous cryotherapy of renal masses. J Vasc Interv Radiol 2007; 18: 383–92.

144. Atwell TD, Farrell MA, Callstrom MR, et al. Percutaneous cryoablation of large renal masses: technical feasibility and short-term outcome. Am J Roentgenol 2007; 188: 1195–200.

145. Gervais DA, Arellano RS, McGovern FJ, McDougal WS, Mueller PR. Radiofrequency ablation of renal cell carcinoma: part 2, Lessons learned with ablation of 100 tumors. Am J Roentgenol 2005; 185: 72–80.

146. Bandi G, Wen CC, Hedican SP, et al. Cryoablation of small renal masses: assessment of the outcome at one institution. BJU Int 2007; 100: 798–801.

147. Ogan K, Jacomides L, Dolmatch B, et al. Percutaneous radio-frequency ablation of renal tumors: technique, limitations and morbidity. Urology 2002; 60: 954–8.

148. Pavlovich C, Walther MM, Choyke PL, et al. Percutaneous radio frequency ablation of small renal tumors: initial results. J Urol 2002; 167: 10–15.

149. Stern JM, Svatek R, Park S, et al. Intermediate comparison of partial nephrectomy and radiofrequency ablation for clinical T1a renal tumours. BJU Int 2007; 100: 287–90.

150. Lees WR, Gillams A. Radiofrequency ablation: other abdominal organs. Abdom Imaging 2005; 30: 451–5.

151. Mack MG, Straub R, Eichler K, et al. MR-guided laser-induced thermotherapy in recurrent extrahepatic abdominal tumours. Eur Radiol 2001; 11: 2041–6.

152. Rosenthal DI, Hornicek FJ, Wolfe MW, et al. Ercutaneous radiofrequency coagulation of osteoid osteoma compared with operative treatment. J Bone Joint Surg Am 1998; 80: 815–21.

153. Callstrom MR, Charboneau JW, Goetz MP, et al. Painful metastases involving bone: feasibility of percutaneous CT- and US-guided radio-frequency ablation. Radiology 2002; 224: 87–97.

154. Gillams A. Minimally invasive treatment for liver and lung metastases in colorectal cancer. Br Med J 2007; 334: 1056–7.

52 Imaging for Radiotherapy Treatment Planning
Vincent Khoo

INTRODUCTION

Imaging has always been central to radiotherapy practice. Apart from the use of radioisotopes that are administered systemically, the methodology for external beam radiotherapy and brachytherapy (interstitial or intra-cavitary therapy) remains a localized treatment where the radiation source needs to be aimed or placed at the tumor or target volume. Thus appropriate imaging is crucial for radiotherapy practice in order to identify the target volume(s) in question and to accurately direct the radiation beams to the nominated target(s). Radiation has been utilized for medical treatments since the discovery of ionizing radiation by WC Röntgen in 1895. In the early days of radiation use, visual identification or physical palpation of abnormal masses was used to guide radiotherapy. Subsequently radiological imaging using plain X-rays and anatomical landmarks directed the clinician in the placement of radiotherapy fields. The advent of cross-sectional imaging and advances in medical equipment technology has consequently led to a revolution in the practice of radiotherapy and will be described in the next section.

The rationale and application of imaging for radiotherapy is briefly summarized in Table 52.1 for the various steps that comprise the radiotherapeutic treatment chain. It is clear that imaging has a role in each step of the entire radiotherapy process. It is appropriate to define what is meant by radiotherapy treatment planning (RTP) as this process can include the initial step of cancer staging to designing the radiotherapy plan, which is outside the scope of this chapter. In the context of this chapter, it is intended that a more specific definition for RTP is used, namely the application of imaging for target volume delineation in the RTP process. This chapter intends to review and summarize the use and impact of imaging for modern radiotherapy methods to provide a background for its role, the utility of multimodality imaging in RTP, the rationale and use of functional/biological imaging for RTP, innovations in technological imaging for image guided radiotherapy and future directions.

IMPACT OF IMAGING DEVELOPMENTS FOR RADIOTHERAPY

The practice of radiotherapy has undergone substantial and significant changes largely as a result of innovations in cross-sectional and multimodality imaging, advances in medical and radiotherapy equipment, developments in medical computer technology as well as better understanding of the biological basis of tumors and normal tissue responses to irradiation. The ability to visualize and define internal anatomy by cross-sectional imaging means that tumor or target volumes can be shaped to a three-dimensional volume (3D) with several advantages for the patient (see section "Conformal Radiotherapy"). In addition, the introduction of telecobalt units and subsequently linear accelerators (LINACS) to produce high energy photons have allowed deeper seated tumors to receive

tumoricidal radiation doses without exceeding skin tolerance and thereby avoiding severe late skin fibrosis. At the same time, developments in radiotherapy hardware such as automated radiotherapy beam-shaping using multileaf collimators (MLC), advances in computer engineering and visual graphics such as 3D planning, computer-derived planning algorithms, and automated computer-controlled delivery processes together with electronic portal imaging devices (EPID) for field verification have enabled the introduction of modern high precision 3D radiation treatments. More recently the availability of on-line and cross-sectional imaging in the radiotherapy treatment room and/or linear accelerator has refined the radiotherapy process for image-guided strategies.

As outlined previously, traditional or "conventional" RTP was based mainly on palpation of tumor masses or the use of plain radiographs to identify visible masses seen on X-rays and/or anatomical and bony landmarks to design relevant radiotherapy fields (Figs. 52.1A and 52.2A). Computed tomography (CT) can be used to define a 3D volume that includes the tumor with its relevant nodal regions in spatial relationship to its surrounding anatomy rather than a cube or rectangular volume of tissue for treatment. A study undertaken during the early days of the introduction of CT for RTP in the late 1970s prospectively assessed the contribution of CT to conventional methods of RTP (1). These conventional imaging methods included regular radiographic examinations, xerograms, lymphangiograms, arteriograms, air contrast studies, isotopic studies, and ultrasound (US). This study revealed that 52% (44/77 of the cases) had their conventional treatment changed as a result of using CT. Inadequate coverage of the target volume was noted in 42% (32/77) of the treatment plans and up to 31% (24/77) of cases had some portion of the target outside of the 50% isodose region, which is a substantial geographical miss. It is clear that the target volumes clinically estimated from plain radiographs cannot accurately define the entire tumor extent compared to CT information. Using this information with an empirical mathematical model to estimate the probability of local tumor control, it was suggested that the improved tumor delineation and target coverage using CT could result in an increase in local tumor control probability by an average of 6% with the chance of five-year survival increasing by an average of 3.5% (2).

Key Points: Impact of Imaging Developments for Radiotherapy

- Traditional or conventional radiotherapy techniques rely on palpation or visualization of masses using plain X-rays to define treatment fields. It cannot reliably define the tumor extent
- Conventional radiotherapy fields are usually square or rectangular shapes and may include unnecessary volumes of normal tissue during irradiation
- CT provides 3D spatial volumes for better tumor definition and reduces geographical miss of the tumor

Table 52.1 The Process Pathway in Radiotherapy

Radiotherapy step	Imaging needs and rationale
Cancer staging	To determine the extent of disease
	To determine the intent of radiotherapy (curative, high dose local control, or palliative intent)
Target volume determination	To define the treatment volumes of the tumour for treatment planning
	To identify the relevant organs-at-risk for treatment planning
Treatment planning	To evaluate the defined 3D target volumes and organs-at-risk for selection of the number of beams, the orientation of the beams, design of the treatment plan, selection of the plan technique, use of intensity modulation or image-guided strategy, and computing plan distributions
	To review plan dosimetry in 3D and permit creation of dose–volume histograms
	To provide opportunity for plan optimization
Simulation	To determine patient positioning and set-up in 3D
	To assess position and use of radiotherapy immobilisation aids or anatomical markers
Radiotherapy delivery	To provide accuracy and reliability of treatment delivery
	To offer opportunity for image guided radiotherapy such as adaptive or predictive treatments
	To permit options of target tracking and target gating
Radiotherapy verification	To confirm placement of treatment fields or delivery of radiotherapy.
	To evaluate in vivo treatment dosimetry
Patient monitoring	To assess uncertainties in patient tolerance to treatment
Patient follow-up	To determine tumor response
	To assess treatment related side effects
	To evaluate disease recurrence

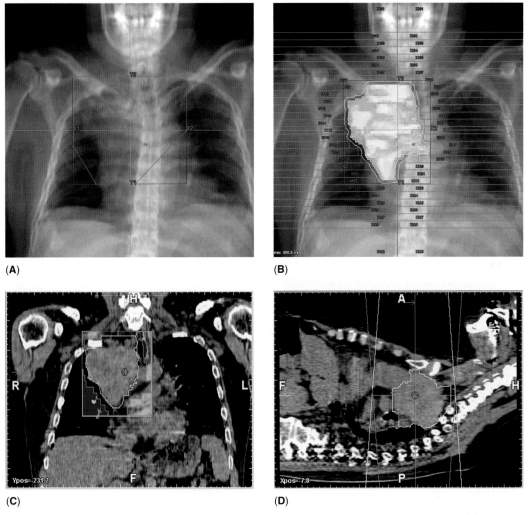

(A) (B) (C) (D)

Figure 52.1 (**A**) An example of a lung radiotherapy case where the anterior treatment field was planned using conventional radiotherapy planning methods with a simple chest radiograph image and (**B–D**) the same lung case planned using CT simulation planning where the anterior treatment field in shown in **B** and the corresponding coronal and sagittal views are shown in **C** and **D**, respectively. Note that shaping of the treatment field for **A** is crude and does not provide estimation of the tumor shape. By using CT scanning, the 3D shape of the tumor can be determined. The treatment fields can then be shaped to the profile of the tumor using multileaf collimation and taking into account the surrounding organs-at-risk such as the heart, esophagus, and lung tissue as demonstrated in **B**.

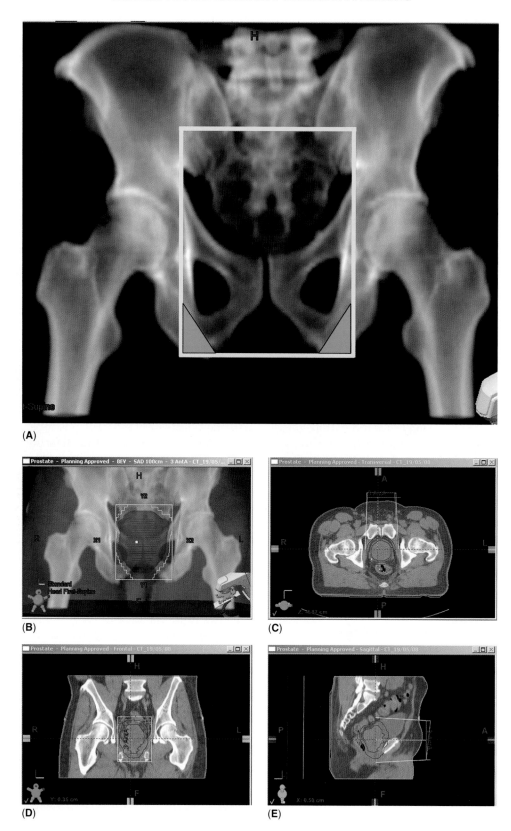

Figure 52.2 (**A**) An example of a prostate radiotherapy field where the anterior treatment field was planned using conventional radiotherapy planning methods with a simple pelvic radiograph and (**B–E**) the same case planned using CT scanning. **B** is the anterior treatment field whilst **C**, **D**, and **E** are the corresponding axial, coronal, and sagittal CT views, respectively. Note that the shaping of the treatment field in **A** remains crude and is usually based on clinical experience. The use of CT planning allows the prostate gland to be defined in 3D together with its surrounding organs-at-risk such as the rectum and bladder. **B** provides a comparison where the anterior treatment field is now shaped to the profile of the prostate gland or CTV (represented by the red horizontal lines). The PTV is represented by the blue cloud. The treatment field is defined by the outer yellow border and the multileaf collimation is denoted by the inner yellow lines.

CONFORMAL RADIOTHERAPY (CFRT)

The development of CT for visualization of internal anatomy was a significant advance that enabled the introduction of conformal radiotherapy (CFRT). This term was first coined by Shinji Takahashi in the 1960s (3). The goal of CFRT is based on a principle that attempts to maintain or improve the intended therapeutic ratio of radiotherapy. The therapeutic ratio in radiotherapy relates dose to local control and expected treatment-related complications. The aim is to achieve the highest level of local tumor control with the lowest possible level of clinically relevant side-effects or complications. The intent of the therapeutic ratio concept is to provide the clinician with a framework to better understand the issues of delivering tumoricidal doses relative to the radiation tolerance of surrounding normal tissues. The slopes of the local control and complication curves will vary for different tumor types and organs-at-risk (OAR). For example, lymphomas and germ cell tumors are considered more radiosensitive with steeper dose curve gradients than melanomas or renal cell tumors with shallow dose curve gradients. If these tumors are located very close to OAR or dose-sensitive structures then high local control rates are not possible without incurring substantial normal tissue damage. This concept is schematically illustrated in Figure 52.3. It is possible to improve the therapeutic ratio in Figure 52.3 by separating the curves of local tumor control and treatment-related complication further apart. This may be achieved by methods that better define tumor extent or better target the treatment volume so as not to unnecessarily irradiate normal tissue. Such methods include the use of multimodality imaging for improved target volume definition, better

radiation delivery through dose-shaping and/or dose modulation, image-guided radiation, and combined modality therapies.

CFRT attempts to separate these two curves and consequently improve the therapeutic ratio in two ways. CFRT techniques can tailor radiotherapy fields to the shape of the tumor. In this manner, the high dose region can be made to conform more closely to the tumor volume and reduce the quantity of adjacent normal tissue within the irradiated volume. This is likely to translate into decreased normal tissue complication rates. Radiotherapy planning studies have outlined that the volume of irradiated tissue can be reduced by 30% to 50% using CFRT compared to conventional planning techniques (4,5). By accurate shaping of the delivered beams and sparing of the normal tissues, especially critical structures, CFRT has the potential benefit to allow escalation of the prescribed dose for reduced or equivalent clinically acceptable normal tissue complication rates. It has been postulated that if the dose can be safely escalated by 20%, this may result in demonstrable improvements in local tumor control rates and therefore increase the probability of cancer-specific survival for some cancer types (6,7).

The general availability of CT dramatically changed the RTP environment by allowing the tumor not only to be accurately defined in 3D but also in relation to its anatomical surroundings. This is the foundation for CFRT and is a prerequisite for 3D beam-shaping. The intended target volume can now be fully appreciated in the individual patient and "conformal avoidance" of dose-limiting normal organs may be attempted. The standard method of incorporating CT for RTP has been to obtain a series of axial images of the patient in the treatment position. After appropriate volumes-of-interest (VOI) are outlined, these corresponding segmented axial outlines can then be stacked to create a reconstructed 3D volume for RTP (Figs. 52.1B–D and 52.2B–E). The radiotherapy treatment portals are usually designed using beams-eye-view (BEV) imaging facilities in the treatment planning systems. The BEV is the view of a virtual observer as seen along the projection of the treatment field from the source of radiation within the treatment machine. This visual perspective allows a projection of the treated anatomy in relation to the treatment field edges (Fig. 52.4). Using the BEV facilities, the proposed CFRT treatment portals can be assessed to determine accurate shaping of the tumor but also to permit maximal sparing or avoidance of the OAR.

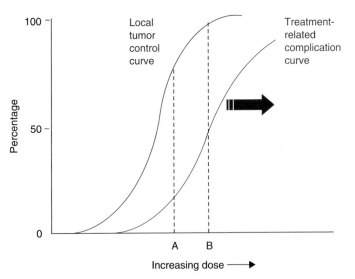

Figure 52.3 The therapeutic ratio in radiotherapy can be demonstrated by the sigmoid shaped dose-response curves for local tumor control (left blue curve) and treatment-related complications (right red curve). Different clinical outcomes may be produced by different clinical dose prescriptions. For example, prescribing the dose at B may be expected to produce a higher level of local tumor control than using a dose at A, but this also results in a potentially higher level of complications. If the two curves can be separated further apart, for example by pushing the complication curve to the right (solid arrow), then the therapeutic ratio of B would be improved. This may be achieved by a variety of means such as combined modality therapy or improvements in radiotherapy planning and delivery techniques (CFRT, IMRT, IGRT).

Key Points: Conformal Radiotherapy (CFRT)

- CFRT uses CT to define 3D spatial volumes for individualized patient treatment planning
- CFRT uses beams-eye-view imaging facilities to tailor the shape of the treatment fields to the profile of the tumor volume
- CFRT provides the opportunity to spare or avoid organs at risk and potentially reduce treatment-related side-effects

The Benefits of CFRT

The value of CFRT has been addressed in randomized trials. A good example is in external beam prostate radiotherapy where both acute and late toxicity has been significantly reduced by the use of CFRT compared to conventional radiotherapy techniques when the prescribed dose was kept constant in the randomized treatment arms (8,9). Based on these results, the National Institute

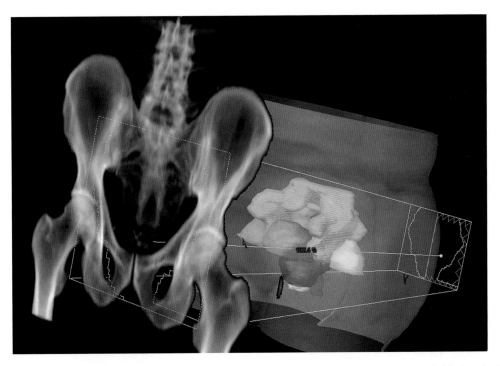

Figure 52.4 Beams-eye-view (BEV) of a single radiotherapy field for a pelvic plan treating the prostate (blue), seminal vesicles (hidden), and pelvic lymph nodes (light blue). This view is that of a virtual observer as seen along the projection of the treatment field from the source of radiation within the treatment machine. This visual perspective allows a projection of the treated pelvic anatomy in relation to the treatment field edges. The bladder (light orange) is located anteriorly, the rectum (brown) is posterior and the femoral heads are light pink and light green.

of Clinical Excellence (NICE) in the United Kingdom in its "Guidance on Cancer Services in Improving Outcomes for Urological Cancers" recommended CFRT as the new technique standard for prostate external beam radiotherapy (10). It would be reasonable to extrapolate this recommendation for all other cancer subsites needing radical radiotherapy treatment.

The other potential benefit of CFRT is the opportunity for dose escalation with less or similar levels of side-effects. In prostate cancer, the benefit for dose escalation is suggested by a review of 1465 men from four randomized controlled Radiation Therapy Oncology Group (RTOG) trials that reported improved 10-year disease-specific survival and overall survival rates when treated with doses ≥66 Gy, particularly for those with poor prognostic features such as Gleason score 8 to 10 and pretreatment prostate specific antigen (PSA) levels >10 ng/mL (11). This is now supported by randomized trials of CFRT dose escalation for localized prostate cancer (Table 52.2). These clinical trials have escalated the dose from 64–70 Gy to 74–79.2 Gy and reported improvements in biochemical (b) PSA control rates of between 6% and 19% with the escalated dose arms (12–16). However, the magnitude of dose escalation is limited as CFRT can only spare the rectum if it lies outside of the concavity of the target volume. Often the rectum lies within the prostate/seminal vesicle target concavity and despite optimization of CFRT techniques, will thus receive the full prescription dose (17,18). This physical limitation has restrained the extent of dose escalation possible with CFRT. Data from these randomized dose escalation trials report that the incidence of late GI toxicity (RTOG grade ≥2) is also approximately doubled by the dose escalation. This limitation can be overcome by using intensity-modulated radiotherapy (IMRT).

Key Points: Benefits of CFRT

- CFRT improves the therapeutic ratio by reducing radiotherapy related side-effects compared to conventional radiotherapy in randomized trials
- CFRT can permit dose escalation for improved local control rates in randomized trials but treatment related side-effects can also be increased
- CFRT has recognized limitations in its technique that will restrict the level of safe dose escalation. This limitation may be overcome by intensity-modulated radiotherapy

INTENSITY MODULATED RADIOTHERAPY (IMRT)

IMRT can address the limitations of CFRT by providing the opportunity to manipulate the dose distribution to treat concave-shaped targets and avoid structures lying in the concavity of the targets. Conceptually, in IMRT, the radiation dose or "beam fluence" of each radiotherapy field can be extensively varied by producing a series of many smaller beamlets within that individual field (Fig. 52.5A). This is in stark contrast to the uniform dose fluence afforded by CFRT techniques (Fig. 52.5B). By using several of these IMRT fields to vary the 3D intensity of the dose distribution across the target volume, the high dose region may be better shaped to cover irregular or concave volumes. This technique can offer improved dose homogeneity, sharper dose gradients between target and normal tissues, and better avoidance of dose to important surrounding OAR to minimize side-effects (19). This method of "dose painting" using IMRT can also permit boosting of the

Table 52.2 Randomized Trials of Dose Escalation in Prostate Cancer

Site (reference)	No. Pats	5-Yr bPSA control		Late GI toxicity (%) (RTOG ≥ 2)	
		Standard (dose)	Escalated (dose)	Standard	Escalated
MDACC (12)[a]	301	64% (70 Gy)	70% (78 Gy)	8	17
MGH (13)	394	61% (70.2 GyE)	80% (79.2 GyE)	12	26
RMH (14)	126	59% (64 Gy)	71% (74 Gy)	11	23
Dutch (15)	664	54% (68 Gy)	64% (78 Gy)	16	21
MRC (16)	843	60% (64 Gy)	71% (74 Gy)	24	33
GETUG	306	TBA (70 Gy)	TBA (80 Gy)	TBA	TBA

[a]6-yr bpSA rates.

Abbreviations: No.Pats, number of patients; bPSA, biochemical prostate specific antigen; GyE, Gray equivalent; TBA, results to be announced.

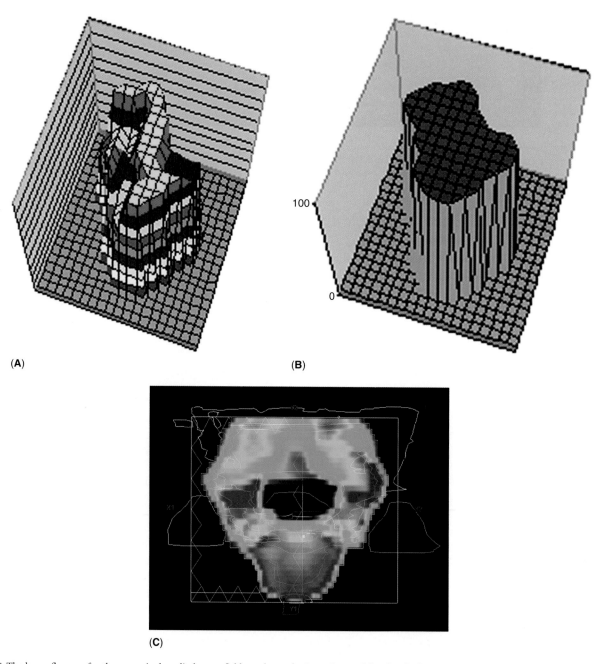

(A)

(B)

(C)

Figure 52.5 The beam fluences for the same single radiotherapy field are shown for intensity-modulated radiotherapy (IMRT) methods and conformal radiotherapy (CFRT) in 3D where in **A** the IMRT field has varying beam intensities across its field with each color representing a different dose intensity compared to **B** where the CFRT field has a constant beam intensity across its entire field. In **C**, the varying beam intensities within an IMRT field treating the prostate and pelvic nodes are illustrated in 2D. *Source*: From Ref. 20.

target by using different dose fractions to different volumes at the same time; an alternative method of dose escalation termed "simultaneous integrated boost".

The design of these beamlets and their dose is achieved by inverse planning algorithms. The use of MLCs for automated shaping of the treatment fields has increased the efficiency for both CFRT and IMRT. These MLC leaves can be manipulated to provide a "step and shoot," dynamic window or tomotherapy-type methods of IMRT dose-delivery (20). Specific descriptions for these different types of IMRT are outside the scope of this chapter but can be found in most radiotherapy oncology or physics books (20).

Key Points: Intensity-Modulated Radiotherapy (IMRT)

- IMRT is a refinement of the CFRT process whereby the beam fluence of each radiotherapy field can be substantially varied across its field
- IMRT can overcome some of the limitations with CFRT techniques
- The combination of several IMRT fields can permit volumetric "dose painting" for improved dose coverage, or dose homogeneity of the target volume and dose minimization, or dose avoidance of OARs

The Benefits of IMRT

The clinical use of IMRT is rapidly increasing and is based on the numerous planning studies outlining its dosimetric benefits for improved dose coverage and 3D avoidance of dose-limiting OAR. In the brain, some planning studies have reported IMRT improves conformality by 10% and dose coverage by 36% compared to CFRT (21), while other studies do not (22). A factor in the discrepancies from these studies may lie in the 3D shape of the target. Tumor volumes with complex irregular and concave 3D shapes are more likely to benefit from IMRT planning than spherical shapes which can just as easily be treated using CFRT. Early clinical feasibility studies for complex shaped base-of-skull meningiomas suggest that IMRT offers the opportunity to adequately treat these complex base-of-skull meningiomas safely with improved sparing of critical OAR compared to CFRT (23). The major thrust of current developments in CNS treatment planning is to integrate the use of functional data for target volume determination (24). This will be discussed later in this chapter.

IMRT has been employed in head and neck radiotherapy to reduce the morbid side-effect of treatment-induced xerostomia. Several prospective studies have reported good and acceptable recovery of xerostomia using IMRT to partially spare dose to the parotid glands, resulting in improvements in swallowing, speech and quality of life for patients (25,26). Randomized trials are now going on to formally assess the value of parotid-sparing IMRT (27).

Breast radiotherapy is one of the few clinical sites where randomized data for IMRT is now available. In a randomized study of 306 women, those who were treated using IMRT experienced less unwanted late skin side-effects and better breast cosmesis compared to those treated using conventional radiotherapy (28). However, this reduction in treatment-related side-effects did not translate into significant improvements in quality of life scores, suggesting that a more complex set of endpoints than cosmesis is required for breast cancer patients.

In prostate cancer, one large single institution study of 1571 men reported that safe dose escalation is possible using IMRT with reduced rates of rectal toxicity (29). With a median follow-up of 10-year, bowel/rectal toxicities were reduced from 13% using CFRT to 5% using IMRT, even with doses up to 81 Gy (29). There is emerging evidence that intermediate to high risk prostate cancer subsets may benefit from pelvic nodal irradiation and IMRT can be used to reduce the bowel dose from 18% to 5% during pelvic radiotherapy (30) as well as permit safe dose escalation to the nodal regions.

IMRT can also permit the use of simultaneous integrated boosting of disease where larger doses per fraction are delivered to sub-volumes within the main target volume. These sub-volumes may represent a dominant, rapidly proliferating tumor nodule or perhaps a hypoxic tumor region. The simultaneous delivery of a larger dose per fraction to these sub-volumes may overcome potential radioresistance. The use of biological imaging may be helpful in defining these sub-volumes and will be discussed subsequently in this chapter.

Key Points: Benefits of IMRT

- Planning studies have outlined potential dosimetric benefits for using IMRT in almost all radiotherapy treatment sites
- IMRT has permitted safe dose escalation and clinical IMRT studies have confirmed a reduction in treatment-related side-effects
- IMRT may be used for biological treatment planning

IMAGE-GUIDED RADIOTHERAPY (IGRT)

One of the main limitations in the reliability of any precision radiotherapy technique is the accuracy of defining the exact spatial location for the target volume on a daily basis during each treatment fraction. Treatment delivery uncertainties may result from a variety of causes such as internal physiological activity that can displace or deform the target, to errors in patient set-up and delivery. These uncertainties are as important as defining appropriate target volumes for treatment because temporal spatial variations for either the target or patient set-up/delivery can lead to geographical misses and a loss of the therapeutic ratio, particularly when using IMRT where the margins and high-dose regions are greatly refined. Treatment strategies to overcome or minimize both systematic and random errors associated with tumor and organ temporal spatial variations or patient set-up and delivery uncertainties have been collectively termed image-guided radiotherapy (IGRT). A variety of terminologies has also been applied to this concept and includes 4D-radiotherapy where the 4th dimension being evaluated is time. Conceptually, the term IGRT can have a broader meaning and may relate not only to strategies of reliable beam targeting but also to improved means of identifying the extent of the tumor, and OAR or functional and molecular aspects of the tumor that may be targeted differently with radiation. This will be addressed below.

Usually a safety margin accounting for these uncertainties (see Radiotherapy Nomenclature) is used to ensure that the target

volume is not missed during treatment. However, having a large safety margin also increases the irradiation of normal tissue and limits the therapeutic ratio of radiotherapy. A good example of this is a tumor within the lung parenchyma that can move and deform with respiration. The safety margin for treatment delivery may be large if one takes into account the magnitude of the peak and trough of respiration to avoid missing the tumor but, in doing so, the potential for treatment-related side-effects will also increase. IGRT methods aim to increase the reliability of targeting such that treatment margins may be reliably reduced. These methods include strategies such as adaptive IGRT whereby the range of target motion during the first week of radiotherapy is used to define a composite planning margin; predictive IGRT whereby individual patient's pattern of motion or deformity is modeled and treatment plans are based on this modeling; breath-hold treatment delivery; gated respiration-based IGRT, where treatment delivery is pulsed to the section of the breathing cycle, to real-time tracking of the target position during treatment delivery using on-line, in-room imaging and verification systems. A full description of IGRT and its methods are outside the scope of this chapter and can be found in most radiotherapy books (20).

Key Points: Image-Guided Radiotherapy (IGRT)

- Temporal spatial variation for the target and OAR exist due to physiological activity and uncertainties in patient setup and treatment delivery
- If these temporal spatial uncertainties are not accounted for then there is the potential for geographical miss of the target
- Radiotherapy strategies that aim to reduce or minimize systematic and random errors for target and organ temporal spatial variations or set-up and delivery uncertainties are collectively termed image guided radiotherapy (IGRT)

RADIOTHERAPY NOMENCLATURE

The fundamental step for both CFRT and IMRT techniques is the use of cross-sectional imaging to accurately define the spatial volumetric relationship of the target with its surrounding normal tissues for maximum coverage of the target and sparing of OAR. This step remains the most crucial and often the most difficult aspect of the radiotherapy planning process as inappropriate definition of the tumor volume can either lead to a geographical miss of the tumor or a systematic error that will be perpetuated throughout therapy. Target volumes in radiotherapy require a definition of treatment volumes that is distinct from a simple description of the visualized gross tumor. Treatment volumes need to be defined in order to account for both macroscopic and microscopic disease that may be treated to different prescribed total doses and dose fraction sizes during a fractionated (up to 40 fractions) course of radiotherapy over a six- to eight-week period.

The International Commission for Radiation Units (ICRU) Report 50 published in 1993 defines a series of volumes which takes into consideration factors such as the subclinical extent of disease, internal organ motion due to physiological activity, patient movement, treatment set-up variability and penumbral effects of the treating beam (31). These definitions are outlined in Table 52.3 and illustrated in Figure 52.6. These planning terms have been modified and refined in the ICRU Report 62 in 1999 (32). The additional concepts introduced in ICRU Report 62 were to more accurately define some of the limitations of the ICRU Report 50. In addition to subdividing the planning target volume (PTV) into two further volumes, that is, the internal and set-up margins, OAR were further defined. The planning organ-at-risk volume (PRV) is defined as that volume that is needed to account for movements or changes in the shape and/or size of the OAR as well as set-up uncertainties. Therefore, the PRV for the OAR provides the same concept as the PTV for the CTV. These new definitions provide areas of further refinement and assessment for RTP. A further update for this nomenclature was expected in late 2008 and this was expected to take into account recent developments in image-guided strategies for radiotherapy. The use of this nomenclature allows for uniformity in designing treatment volumes for RTP and delivery as well as in consistency in reporting. This standardization is important to enable comparisons of radiotherapy reports from different centers and in published literature.

One of the most difficult areas in RTP is in defining the extent of microscopic or subclinical nodal disease spread, termed the clinical target volume (CTV). These microscopic extensions cannot be visualized with standard morphological cross-sectional imaging methods but have to be estimated using the clinician's

Table 52.3 The Nomenclature Use in Radiotherapy Treatment Planning: ICRU 50 and 62 Treatment Planning Volume Definitions

Nomenclature	Definition	
Gross target volume (GTV)	This is the radiologically visible or clinically palpable extent of tumor and represents macroscopic disease	
Clinical target volume (CTV)	This is the GTV with a margin that includes the presumed microscopic extent of disease or subclinical nodal involvement. These microscopic extension of disease cannot be seen on cross-sectional imaging	
Planning target volume (PTV)	This is the CTV with a margin added to account for patient movement, internal organ and target motion, uncertainties in patient set-up, and treatment beam penumbra. This margin may be further subdivided into the internal margin and the set-up margin	
	Internal margin	This is the volume needed to account for variation in size, shape, and position of the CTV in relation to anatomical reference set-up points
	Set-up margin	This is the volume needed to account for uncertainties in patient-beam positioning
Treated volume (TV)	This is the volume of tissue actually treated to the prescribed dose as specified by the clinician (e.g., 95% isodose volume)	
Irradiated Volume (IV)	This is the volume of tissue irradiated to a clinically significant dose in relation to normal tissue tolerance (e.g., 50% isodose volume)	

Source: Adapted from Ref. 31, 32.

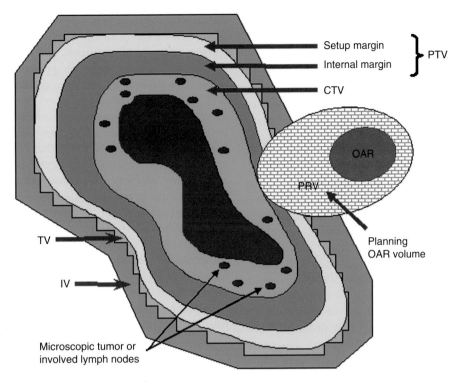

Figure 52.6 Planning target volumes for radiotherapy treatment planning. *Abbreviations*: CTV, clinical target volume; GTV, gross target volume; IV, irradiated volume; OAR, organs-at-risk; PTV, planning target volume; TV, treated volume.

experience and examination of the disease site, knowledge of the cancer's usual patterns of spread, and interpretation of the prognostic clinical and histological features of the cancer such as tumor subtype, tumor grade, lymphovascular involvement, and any post-operative histopathology. More recently, data from functional and biological imaging studies are being used to aid in the definition of target volumes and normal tissue function in RTP.

Key Points: Radiotherapy Nomenclature

- ICRU Reports 50 and 62 provide standard nomenclature for RTP
- This RTP nomenclature creates standardization for delineating target volumes, allows uniformity in designing radiotherapy treatment plans, provides consistency in reporting and permits comparison of data between different centers

Clinical Issues for Target Volume Delineation

In RTP, the clinician has to define a target boundary during the delineation process on which lies either the gross tumor for the GTV or the microscopic edge of the tumor for the CTV. Defining the GTV, and especially the CTV, is often the most difficult aspect of the RTP process as the patterns of spread and local failures differ substantially, not only for different tumor types but also within subcategories of the same tumor type. No current imaging modality to-date can define the presence of every single clonagenic tumor cell. Furthermore, data on which boundary is likely to exist is lacking from many tumor sites. This perceived boundary or margin will have to be inferred based on the clinician's experience and expertise for the tumor subtype and its clinical behavior as well as from an interpretation of the patient's imaging, biopsy results or operation.

Tumor factors which may have to be taken into account include the following: histological subtype; tumor grade which may correlate with degree of invasion; the presence or absence of lymphovascular permeation; and natural history of patterns of disease spread.

In some tumor sites such as the brain, the surrounding edema around a malignant tumor may also contain tumor cells or infiltrate along fascial planes such as with meningiomas. Target volumes can also change dramatically following chemotherapy when tumor shrinkage has been substantial but where in some cases, there may be islands of residual cancer cells left behind in a fibrotic matrix such as in soft tissue sarcomas. Another well known treatment scenario is following radical surgery in the primary or recurrent disease situation, where the original tumor has been removed and the normal anatomy is also altered. In the recurrent disease scenario, the nodal drainage may also be different. Here the challenge will be to determine the post-operative CTV for the primary disease and, where appropriate, a separate CTV for the nodal regions. This process may require image correlation or co-registration between preoperative and post-operative scans. In addition, there are the temporal spatial uncertainties previously mentioned above that will need to be taken into account.

Key Points: Clinical Issues for Target Volume Delineation

- Defining the subclinical extent of disease or the CTV remains the most difficult task faced by clinicians as standard morphological anatomical imaging cannot define microscopic disease involvement
- CTV definition will be based on clinical expertise and knowledge as well as taking into account tumor and therapy factors

The Multidisciplinary Team for Target Volume Delineation

It is obvious that one of the first steps in cancer management is staging the patient to determine the extent of disease (Table 52.1). Most tumors are classified according to staging systems such as the TNM system but these systems do not advise on the optimal imaging method to define the tumor extent. There are many reports of substantial inter- and intraobserver variability in defining target volumes for RTP in a variety of cancer subsites such as CNS (33), lung (34,35), esophagus (36), breast (37,38), and prostate (39). This marked extent of observer variability has implications for any radiotherapy trials, especially multicenter national or international studies, and can limit the outcome of the study. It is important to have thorough protocols describing the process of target volume delineation in any radiotherapy trial, and this process will also need careful audit and quality assurance. Much of this uncertainty in target volume delineation can be reduced by optimizing the imaging, such as selection of the appropriate imaging modality and use of multimodality imaging, as well as incorporating the expertise of trained radiologists familiar with oncology. This latter aspect cannot be underestimated and has been highlighted by the Working Party for The Royal College of Radiologists in their publication on "Recommendations for Cross-Sectional Imaging in Cancer Management" (40).

It is important that the specialist radiologist understands the imaging rationale for RTP and the radiotherapy nomenclature used, namely the GTV and CTV. The imaging information needed by the radiation oncologist is listed in Table 52.4. Often there may not be a clear distinction between the GTV and its surrounding tissues, such that the extent of adjacent microscopic spread becomes a dilemma. Good examples of this includes microscopic tumor spread into surrounding edema in brain tumors, the distinction between tumor and atelectasis or collapsed lung in lung cancers, and extracapsular extension or seminal vesicle involvement in prostate cancer. In these situations, it is difficult to outline a confident boundary between GTV and CTV, let alone the extent of the CTV particularly in the post-operative situation, as outlined above. Often determination for the GTV and CTV may be arbitrary and based on knowledge of the clinical tumor behavior, intent of radiotherapy, and other treatment considerations such as the dose tolerance of any adjacent critical normal structures, for example, optic chiasma, brain stem, spinal cord, salivary glands, heart, bowel, and kidneys.

It is imperative that there is close dialogue between the clinician and radiologists and issues of uncertainty are discussed in the context of the individual clinical case. In some cases, particularly following an operative procedure, it can be very helpful to canvass the viewpoint of the surgeon and histopathologist. This collaborative effort is more likely to provide an improved assessment of treatment volumes than working in isolation.

Key Points: The Multidisciplinary Team for Target Volume Delineation

- There can be substantial inter- and intraobserver variability in target volume delineation for a wide variety of treatment sites
- Interobserver variability can limit outcomes in radiotherapy trials
- Interobserver variability may be reduced by dedicated target volume delineation protocols by using the appropriate imaging modality, discussing cases with your radiologists, and obtaining help from them in determining target volumes

Table 52.4 Imaging Information Needed by the Radiation Oncologist for Target Volume Delineation

The patient	• The position of the patient when imaged for target volume delineation should reproduce the patient's setup position for radiotherapy treatment • Any devices used for treatment set-up such as patient positioning or immobilization devices should also be used during the radiotherapy planning scan. Examples include the stereotactic head frames for brain radiotherapy, thermoplastic casts for head and neck radiotherapy, chest/arm setup for breast and thoracic radiotherapy (Fig. 52.7), vacuum bags and/or knee and ankle stocks in pelvic radiotherapy (Fig. 52.8) • Specific conditions needed for treatment should also be reproduced such as breath-hold in lung and abdominal radiotherapy or a full bladder and empty rectum in pelvic radiotherapy
The tumor	• The spatial location of the tumor • Its 3D size and shape • Details of the edge of the tumor where it forms a clear boundary with adjacent normal tissue • Details of adjacent anatomy where no clear boundary exists • Details of any potential microscopic disease extension • Information regarding functional tumor activity and its relationship to the morphological and anatomical status of the tumor • Details of the temporal spatial variation that may exist for the tumor
The nodal regions	• Details of the relevant nodal drainage regions • Details of any abnormal size or suspicious nodes
The organs-at-risk	• Details of the relevant critical organs-at-risk for the region under treatment • Details of the adjacent normal tissues and its potential functional activity • Information on the potential temporal spatial variation that may exist for relevant normal structures or tissues • Knowledge of any unusual anatomy such as a horse-shoe or solitary kidney

Source: Modified from Dobbs and Barrett [Dobbs, 2004 #274].

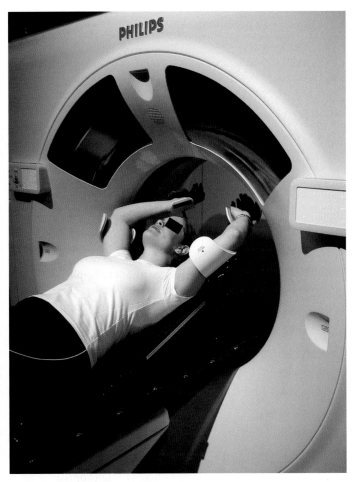

Figure 52.7 An example of an immobilization device for chest wall and arms setup for breast radiotherapy.

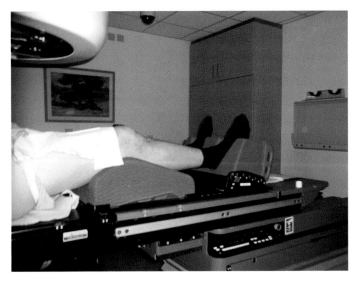

Figure 52.8 An example of immobilization devices for the knee and ankles in pelvic radiotherapy.

MULTIMODALITY IMAGING

CT is the current standard imaging modality used in RTP. It is widely available and the imaging data is easily handled by all commercial treatment planning systems. There are two main reasons for its utilization. Firstly, it provides geometrically accurate and reliable cross-sectional images with 3D external contours of the patient; secondly, the tissue or electron density information available from the Hounsfield units on the CT slices can be directly used, after applying correction factors, to calculate radiation absorbed doses for planning dosimetry. However, CT has certain limitations in determining the extent of cancer disease for a number of anatomical regions due to its restrictive ability to discriminate between the tumor and tissues of similar electron density or if the tumor is close to thick bone, which can absorb X-rays from CT and reduce soft tissue image quality. Other imaging modalities can confer better morphological visualization of the tumor extent such as magnetic resonance imaging (MRI) for regions in the brain, pelvis, and limbs, while positron emission tomography (PET) may provide functional and biological information on the nature of the cancer activity. Multimodality imaging combines information from the different imaging modalities to take advantage of the complementary information available from them to aid the determination of treatment volumes for RTP.

Key Points: Multimodality Imaging

- CT is the standard imaging modality used in radiotherapy planning but has known limitations for target volume delineation in some clinical sites
- Multimodality imaging aims to combine the benefits from different imaging modalities, often providing complementary information to aid target volume delineation

Rationale for the Use of MRI for RTP

MRI is being increasingly used in oncology for staging, assessing tumor response, and evaluating disease recurrence. Indeed, MRI has replaced CT as the diagnostic imaging modality of choice for many regions in the body and its applications for RTP will be discussed below. The advantage of MRI compared to CT is in the enhanced ability of MRI to better characterize soft tissues, even when these structures possess very similar X-ray attenuation properties or electron densities. By using different MRI sequences, better tissue discrimination can be obtained between the extent of tumor with its boundaries of infiltration and the adjacent normal structures. Therefore, MRI can provide better visualization of the tumor extent and improved reliability for target volume delineation in RTP (41). It can also provide better delineation of OARs for dose avoidance in RTP. An obvious benefit for increasing the reliability and consistency of target definition with MRI is that it will reduce both interobserver and intraobserver variability for outlining (42). This is valuable for institutional and multicenter trials in radiotherapy where it is important to maintain consistent and accurate target and OAR volumes. MRI may also be useful in assessing the need for re-treatments by offering the opportunity to differentiate between changes due to recurrent cancer and those secondary to post-treatment fibrosis. Further advantages and disadvantages of MRI for RTP are outlined in Table 52.5. It is vital that if MRI is used for RTP, oncology clinicians should have the necessary training to comprehend the MR images and understand how to use them appropriately for target volume delineation. Thus it is important to undertake suitable supervised training (43) and, even if there is relevant clinician experience, it is still

Table 52. 5 Advantages and Disadvantages of MRI for RTP

Features	Advantages	Disadvantages
Patient	Non- or minimally invasive procedure. Few patient risks No radiation associated with imaging. This may be advantageous to pediatric patients and pregnant women. This may be useful for follow-up scanning	Claustrophobia due to the smaller patient bore Contraindicated in patients with loose metal foreign bodies within the body, particularly the orbits or pacemakers
Imaging	Increased imaging parameters for more imaging flexibility Superior soft tissue imaging with excellent spatial resolution to provide better visualization for the following: • Determining the tumor/GTV extent and degree of tumour infiltration/CTV extent • Understanding the surgical bed or altered anatomy secondary to surgery • Distinguishing between post-treatment fibrosis or tumour recurrence • Improved definition of normal soft tissue structures and tissue planes • Avoidance of image artefact from metal prosthesis and large bony regions • True multiplanar capability to image in any oblique plane and reduction of the partial volume imaging effect • Increased accuracy, reliability and consistency of target definition to reduce both inter- and intra-observer variability • Providing functional and biological information for functional avoidance or biological targeting Ultrafast volumetric and cine mode acquisitions to assess temporal-spatial variations in target positioning or deformation Can be registered with CT information for use in RTP systems	MR image distortion • Systems • Object-induced distortions Lack of electron density information for dosimetry and needs additional steps to permit dose calculations Lack of cortical bone information to create DRR in radiotherapy May have longer scan times than CT with more potential for motion artfact Need for specific training to comprehend and understand MR images for RTP use RTP systems can only import transverse MR images and cannot take full advantage of sagittal and coronal in-plane MR images Most immobilization devices used in radiotherapy may not be MR compatible The smaller imaging bore may not allow larger body immobilization devices such as breast boards
Contrast agents	New contrast agents (USPIO) to define nodal status Less incidence of allergic reactions to gadolinium than iodine-based contrast agents	
Machine	New bore flange openings to lessen patient claustrophobia Open MR systems for easier patient access, tolerance and positioning for radiotherapy	Not as readily available and accessible Smaller bore than CT (52 cm vs. 82–85 cm). Curved table top

Source: Modified from Ref. 66.

Abbreviations: CT, computed tomography, CTV, clinical, target volume; DRR, digitally reconstructed radiographs; GTV, gross target volume; MR, magnetic resonance; RTP, radiotherapy treatment planning; USP10, ultrasmall superparamagnetic particles of iron oride.

beneficial to liaise closely with subsite specialized radiologists who have necessary MR expertise.

Key Points: MRI Rationale for Radiotherapy Planning

■ MRI has replaced CT as the imaging modality of choice for several cancer sub-types, such as CNS cancers, pelvic cancers, and musculo-skeletal tumors
■ MRI can offer imaging advantages in identifying tumor extent for RTP
■ MRI can reduce inter- and intraobserver variability in assessing target volumes for RTP

Applications for MRI for RTP

In the CNS, MRI is used extensively for staging and planning for radiotherapy. Quantitative RTP improvements of up to 80% in target coverage have been reported by several investigators when MRI has been utilized to aid CT-based treatment planning (44–46). There are also situations where the use of both CT and MRI data is complementary and can provide for improved target volume delineation when compared to either MRI or CT alone (47). For base of skull meningiomas, where CT artifact from these large skull bones may obscure soft tissue detail, the use of MRI was reported to provide better visualization of tumor extent, especially for disease that crept along the skull bones (48). However, CT provided detail on tumor-related bony erosion that was not available on MRI demonstrating that the information from CT and MRI was complementary and useful in optimizing target volume delineation. In many radiotherapy centers, the use of CT-MRI co-registration for RTP may now be considered as standard practice. To aid the planning process, the use of both automated and atlas-based segmentation algorithms for the CNS region are being actively studied with promising results (49,50).

Determining the extent of tumor infiltration in the head and neck region can be difficult because of the complex anatomy at this site. In studies of nasopharyngeal tumors, multimodality imaging with CT-MRI changed disease staging and RTP in approximately 50% of cases (51,52). In another study of over 250 patients, CT imaging missed up to 40% of intracranial infiltration detected by MRI (53). MRI can further aid RTP in this region by defining the extent of tumor infiltration at the following sites:

- The extent of perineural infiltration and intracranial extension, for example, nasopharyngeal tumors
- Tumor infiltration of soft tissue structures and tissue planes such as the pterygoids and tongue
- Longitudinal tumor infiltration along the upper aerodigestive tract and adjacent fascial planes, for example, prevertebral fascia

Specific MRI segmentation algorithms based on the contrast enhancement ratio of T1-weighted images and signal intensity of T2-weighted images are being developed to aid the delineation process and this methodology may further assist the reliability of using MRI for RTP (54).

In rectal carcinoma, CT planning has improved RTP by providing 3D visualization of the rectum, rectal tumor and wall abnormalities, the mesorectum boundaries, and drainage nodal regions compared to traditional planning using plain X-rays and rectal contrast (55). Some limitations in CT definition of the extent of rectal cancers, especially the superior-inferior tumor boundaries, may occur due to no contrast between feces and tumor, partial volume effects due to the curves/valves of Houston in the rectum, and imaging of the horizontal sigmoid. It may also be difficult to assess anal canal/sphincter infiltration in low rectal cancers unless there is an obvious mass effect. MRI can reduce these visualization problems by better defining the depth of rectal wall invasion similar to endorectal US, the spread into the mesorectum and the extent of the longitudinal tumor spread along the rectum (56,57). It also avoids the limitations in importing and correlating US data in treatment planning systems. MRI can also improve evaluation of invasion into adjacent local organs such the bladder, prostate or seminal vesicles in men, and vagina and uterus in women (58–60). By improving the accuracy and reliability of the tumor extent, strategies of anal sphincter sparing, tumor boosting, and dose escalation with or without concurrent chemotherapy may be initiated.

Similar improvements for target volume delineation are achieved using MRI which provides better assessment of the prostate and seminal vesicle than CT for disease extent, extracapsular extension, and seminal vesicle involvement (61–63). MRI can improve determinations of the prostatic apex and between the prostate boundaries with the recto-vesicle fascia of Denonvillier, and adjacent rectal or bladder walls. It also provides better delineation of other pelvic structures such as the urogenital diaphragm, penile bulb, periprostatic venous plexus, neurovascular bundle, levator ani, and anal sphincters (64–66). Radiotherapy planning studies have compared co-registered CT-MRI scans and have reported that CT-defined prostate volumes are approximately 27% to 33% larger than those defined by MRI, suggesting that there is an overestimation with CT and that this is due to the uncertainty in defining pelvic soft tissues using CT (67–70). In prostate radiotherapy, better delineation of erectile tissues by MRI can permit dose-sparing of these structures by IMRT (71) and may lead to improved patient outcomes.

MRI can also be useful where the internal pelvic anatomy has been substantially altered due to previous extensive surgery such as abdomino-perineal resections (72). This improved ability to delineate prostate and seminal vesicles can also reduce interobserver and intraobserver variation with advantages for minimizing planning variance within departments and clinical trials. The main advantage is that MR-based prostate planning volumes can result in more appropriate treatment volumes leading to better shaping of the treatment fields and thereby reduce the risk of treatment-related complications to important normal structures such as the rectum and penile bulb (73).

Multimodality CT-MRI imaging has also been used in brachytherapy. In both low dose-rate and high dose-rate prostate brachytherapy, investigators have reported improved definition of target volumes, reduced observer variability, and increased confidence in guiding needle placement compared to either US or CT imaging (74,75). This is particularly useful for postimplant dosimetry as delineating the prostate gland using CT is considerably more difficult following seed implantation due to seed-induced artefact and the intrinsic poor tissue contrast of CT (76,77). Co-registered MR-CT images have also been reported to be useful in other sites where brachytherapy has been used for head and neck cancers, sarcomas, and gynecology (78). The use of MRI for cervical cancer brachytherapy has been endorsed by the Gynecological GEC-ESTRO Working Group (79).

Key Points: Applications for MRI for Radiotherapy Planning

- MRI can provide better visualization of the tumor extent as well as improved reliability for target volume delineation for a number of cancers
- MRI can complement CT planning information
- MRI for RTP can be used in both external beam radiotherapy and brachytherapy procedures

MRI Issues for RTP

In order to use MRI information for RTP, there are several issues that need to be addressed. These include:

- Defining and correcting MR image-related distortions
- Overcoming the lack of electron density information in MR images which are needed for assessing tissue in homogeneities
- Calculating dose distributions
- Ensuring any immobilization devices to be used are MRI compatible and can be fitted into the imaging bore

MR image distortion is of concern as inaccuracies resulting from this will limit the value of precision radiotherapy, that is, 3D-CFRT or IMRT, and reduce the therapeutic ratio. MR image distortions can be grouped into two main categories: system-related and object-induced. An illustration of these distortion effects is shown in Figure 52.9.

System-related distortions are due to the imperfections of the magnet, its operating system and imaging procedures. The effects of magnet field inhomogeneity, gradient field non-linearities, and

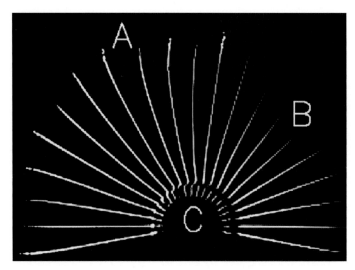

Figure 52.9 An illustration of the various forms of image distortion that may exist in MRI using a phantom consisting of a co-planar array of water-filled tubes embedded within a circular solid plastic block. System-related distortion effects are seen in the apparent curvature of the tubes at **A** and their disappearance at **B**, which was due to warping distortion of the imaging plane. Magnetic susceptibility differences due to the presence of the plastic block at **C** give rise to the object-induced distortion in the form of discontinuities at the point where each tube enters the support plastic block. *Source*: From Ref. 80.

eddy currents can contribute to system-related image distortion. In general, the effect of system-related distortion is least at the center of the magnet and worsens with increasing distance from the magnet center. The distortion magnitude is largest at the periphery of the field-of-view (FOV). This may provide spatially incorrect volumes of interest if they lie at the periphery of the image and can limit co-registration if the body outline or external fiducials are being used for image registration.

Object-induced distortion arises when any object, that is, the patient, is placed within a magnetic field. This type of distortion can result from magnetic susceptibility and chemical-shift effects. Different body tissues have different magnetic susceptibilities and this effect can be pronounced at different tissue boundaries such as between air cavities and soft tissues. Chemical shift effects result from the different behavior of protons in fat and tissue. Fat protons "precess" at a slower rate than water protons and this can result in a chemical-shift effect where the positions of fat/water protons are shifted from their true spatial locations. While chemical-shift effects are manipulated for diagnostic sequences or for any spatial discrepancies arising, MR images with substantial distortion will incorporate a systematic error in the treatment plan from inaccurate delineation and be propagated throughout the course of radiotherapy.

In order to utilize MR images for RTP, these image distortions must be evaluated, quantified, minimized, and/or corrected. Several investigators have reported methods for evaluation and correction of both system-related and object-induced distortions as well as the procedures for quality assurance programs (81–84). System-related distortion can be quantified and mapped using a phantom (linearity test object) that has a predetermined 3D set of markers which can provide spatial assessments of the whole imaging volume to be used for RTP. An inverted U-shaped reference frame with another predetermined 3D set of markers is used to cover the periphery of the imaging volume. The linearity test object or the patient is then housed within this reference frame. A separate set of markers is placed on the patient's body surface to provide assessment of object-induced effects. The spatial positions of all these arrays of markers within the imaging volume are subsequently mapped using a dedicated automated algorithm and can then be post-processed to provide correction for any image distortion. The use of read-out gradient reversal imaging and post-processing image corrections can account for object-induced effects. Distortional shifts of up to 5 mm can be corrected (81–84). Other correction methods have also been developed and can reduce distortions by a factor of two (85). Site-specific phantoms have also been created with air cavities to assess the use of MRI for lung RTP (86). It is important to ensure that the same MR scanner and imaging sequence used for mapping is also used to image the patients. Once the magnitude of any MR image distortions has been quantified and corrected, appropriate image co-registration can be undertaken. By combining the two imaging modalities, the improved imaging information from MRI can be transposed over the CT images and subsequently be used for treatment planning and dosimetry.

Key Points: MRI Issues for Radiotherapy Planning

- Some of the major limitations of using MRI for RTP include MR image-related distortions and the lack of electron density information needed to account for tissue inhomogeneities and to calculate radiotherapy dose distributions
- MR-related image distortion can introduce incorrect target volumes for RTP causing propagation of a systematic error in the course of a patient's radiotherapy
- MR image distortion can be grouped into two main categories: system-related and object-induced
- In order to utilize MR images for RTP, MR-related image distortions must be evaluated, quantified, minimized, and/or corrected. Methods are available to assess and correct MR-related image distortion
- MR image co-registration with CT can overcome the lack of electron density data and permit the improved target volume delineation from MRI to be incorporated for RTP

Recent and Future Developments of MRI for RTP

There are many current developments in MR sequences that can also aid RTP. Cine MR imaging or ultrafast MR sequences such as echoplanar imaging can model in 4D the effects of internal organ motion or the spatial position of targets that are affected by physiological activity such as bowel motion, organ filling or emptying, and respiration. Examples of this include the modeling of motion and deformation for the liver (87,88), the bladder (89), and the prostate (90,91). Knowledge of intrathoracic tumor displacement can allow individualized treatment planning margins for lung radiotherapy (92) and permit the assessment of free-breathing gating techniques for lung radiotherapy (93). These 4D studies can provide assessment of the temporal-spatial uncertainties that can occur during a fractionated course of radiotherapy and data for the estimation of site-specific planning margins and IGRT strategies.

Ultrasmall superparamagnetic iron oxide (USPIO) particles are discussed in chap. 40. It has been reported to have high sensitivity and specificity of up to 90% for discriminating microscopic tumor

involvement in nodal tissue (94,95). Nodal volumes are often included in the CTV for radiotherapy. Inadequate nodal coverage can either compromise local control or unnecessarily irradiate normal structures (96,97). This new MR contrast agent may provide a new method to map lymph nodes and optimize selection of nodal regions for radiotherapy as well as permit boosting of involved nodes. USPIO can aid the selection and delineation of CT-defined nodal regions in head and neck radiotherapy (98) and has also been used in the pelvis to define pelvic fields for prostate radiotherapy (99). However, the use of USPIO remains a structural imaging modality with size limitations but it may be combined with PET to provide disease correlation.

Open MR scanners can be used as radiotherapy simulators to provide a planning environment similar to CT simulation for RTP. These scanners will have some of the imaging advantages of MR over CT imaging but may also have some advantages over conventional MR scanners such as lower purchase cost, greater T1 image contrast, reduced vessel flow/ghosting artefacts, and the capability of using standard radiotherapy patient immobilization devices without size restriction. However, MR material compatibility of these devices is still needed. Open MR systems may have less object-induced distortions due to the lower magnetic field strength but larger systems related distortions which can be corrected (78,100). A potential limitation of MRI for radiotherapy simulation is lack of bony structure information to create the digitally reconstructed radiographs needed for radiotherapy field verification, but this can be overcome by post-processing software or image fusion (101). In a study of 243 patients, open low-field MR simulation provided adequate imaging for 95% of treatment planning cases and led to planning improvements in up to 33% and 40% of lung and prostate cases, respectively (78). It has also been used in glioma radiotherapy for both target delineation and to derive dose calculations with acceptable results (102).

Another very interesting concept is the integration of an MRI scanner with a megavoltage LINAC. While this concept and prototype was first initiated at the University of Utrecht in the Netherlands (103), there are now several other systems being developed (104). Given the known advantages of MRI for target volume delineation, MRI-LINAC can offer further opportunities to refine target volumes during radiotherapy and implement IGRT strategies for improved patient outcomes. However, there are still many technical issues that need to be reviewed and dealt with before it becomes a practical reality (105,106). This development is similar to the integration of a CT scanner with a megavoltage LINAC that is already a commercial product produced by Tomotherapy Inc (Wisconsin, United States).

Key Points: Recent and Future Developments of MRI for Radiotherapy Planning

- Ultrafast and cine MRI studies can provide non-invasive methods to obtain 4D information useful for implementing IGRT
- USPIO may aid identification of microscopic nodal disease to optimize and individualize the intended nodal CTV for RTP
- Open MRI scanners can function similarly to standard radiotherapy CT simulators with the added benefits of MR imaging functionality
- Developments in progress include the opportunity for integrated MR LINACS similar to CT LINACS

FUNCTIONAL IMAGING FOR RTP

There has been increasing interest by clinicians in the use of functional imaging in radiotherapy in the past couple of years. Much of this interest lies in the awareness that simple morphological imaging does not fully represent the extent of the tumor or its biological characteristics. It is assumed that better knowledge of the tumor's characteristics will enable improved radiotherapy strategies to be designed to enhance the therapeutic ratio for patient outcomes. A thought provoking radiotherapy review in 2000 by Ling et al. (107) highlighted the potential of using functional and molecular imaging modalities to define a new radiotherapy target concept, namely the "biological target volume," moving away from the simplistic model of morphologically-based target volumes that is discussed earlier in this chapter. Integrating molecular imaging with advances in radiotherapy such as IMRT now confers the opportunity to improve the therapeutic ratio of radiotherapy by permitting IMRT-based dose escalation via the technique of simultaneous integrated boosts or "dose painting" to regions of increased biological activity or radioresistance. This section will review the applications of both MRI and positron emission tomography (PET) for target volume delineation in RTP. The use of MRI or PET for tumor response assessment or to evaluate normal organ function following irradiation will not be discussed here.

Functional MR Imaging for RTP

The principles and methodology of functional MRI in oncology is reviewed in chapters 63 and 65. MRI techniques such as dynamic contrast-enhanced MR, diffusion-weighted MR; blood oxygen level dependent (BOLD) MRI; diffusion tensor MRI; and MR spectroscopy (MRS) may provide further characterization of tissue that can aid identification of tumor regions for irradiation boosts using methods such as IMRT or IGRT (108–111). In addition, functional MRI may also be used to delineate regions of the brain that would result in significant patient morbidity if excessively irradiated. These regions may be considered as functional OAR and avoided in stereotactic radiosurgery to improve patient outcomes (112).

Tumor features of vascular angiogenesis and increased cellular growth are exploited by MR techniques such as dynamic contrast-enhanced MRI (dcMRI) and MR diffusion. The use of fast MR sequences to capture the sequential vascular perfusion changes in tissue provides characterization for normal, tumor, and irradiated tissues (108). T2-based dcMRI methods have been used to evaluate brain tumors, particularly gliomas (113), whereas T1-based dcMRI methods have been used more widely in breast, musculoskeletal, gynecological, and urological cancers (114–117). Tumor recurrence in previously irradiated breast (114) and prostate cancer sites (115,118) can also be detected using dcMRI. Nodal regions may also be assessed as involved nodes may possess tumor enhancement patterns on their signal intensity time curves, but a limitation of this technique is that it can assess only one specific region at a time and not all nodal sites. Tumor-related regions may be delineated and preferentially selected for radiotherapy targeting or tumor boosting.

Diffusion-weighted MRI (dwMRI) relies on the tumor regions having increased cellular density due to tumor proliferation with a corresponding reduction of water diffusion in this region (109).

This is quantified through apparent diffusion coefficient (ADC) maps with a lower ADC being more likely to contain tumor. Most of the published literature has explored its use in assessing response to therapy for a variety of the different tumors or normal tissues (119–122). A recent histopathological-dwMRI study in head and neck cancers following chemoradiation suggests reasonable correlation in identifying active disease (123); thus there is an opportunity to manipulate this finding to either select regions of poor response during radiotherapy for additional boosts or to initiate alternative therapies.

Similar histopathological work has been undertaken to correlate the ability of BOLD MRI to map regions of hypoxia in tumors, with reports suggesting high sensitivity but low specificity in identifying regions of intraprostatic tumor hypoxia (111). This offers a non-invasive method to delineate specific regions for biologically planned, image-guided IMRT or to implement other strategies such as high-dose rate brachytherapy.

Diffusion tensor MRI (DTI) can demonstrate white matter abnormalities based on cerebral tissue anisotropy and provide information on white matter infiltration by occult tumor that was not identified by other imaging methods (124). This information provided by DTI may be used to optimize and individualize target volumes to reduce normal tissue irradiation and for dose escalation to involved tumor regions (125). If the extent of invasion is a determinant of disease outcome, then this prognostic information may also be used to select patients for more aggressive treatments (126). Magnetoencephalography can be combined with DTI to identify relevant neuro-functional regions for specific-dose reduction to lower the probability of late neurological dysfunction in individual patients (127).

MR spectroscopy (MRS) is another useful method under investigation capable of detecting low molecular weight metabolites that reflect cellular processes. Its basis and methodology is described in several chapters previously (mainly those dedicated to prostate cancer and the CNS: chaps. 19 and 31, respectively). MRS, together with other functional imaging methods, may also indicate the presence of tumor and degree of infiltration that may not be noted by standard MRI sequences, such as that reported in studies of brain gliomas (Fig. 52.10) (128,129). Detection of increased spectra profiles of lipids/creatine and lactate/creatine has been noted in the peritumoral region of high-grade tumors, suggesting this region remains at high risk for recurrence (130) and would need to be included in the CTV for radiotherapy. Other investigators have reported that an elevated spectra profile for choline and the neuronal marker, NAA, may indicate regions of higher cellular activity and potential radiosensitivity, while regions with higher lactate spectra profiles may indicate hypoxia and hence radioresistance. The opportunity to define these regions would be beneficial in optimizing RTP. Similarly, in prostate cancer, an elevated spectra profile of choline with substantially reduced citrate is found (131). Correlation between MRS findings for prostate cancer and histopathological biopsies has supported the match and may even allude to tumor grade (132,133). Using MRS data, investigators have delineated apparent dominant intraprostatic lesions for dose-boosting using either IMRT or high-dose rate brachytherapy (134,135).

Key Points: Functional Imaging

- Functional MRI methods remain active areas of research and are currently being investigated for their applications in RTP
- Functional MR methods such as dcMRI, dwMR; BOLD MRI; DTI; and MRS can provide characterization of tissue for identification of active tumor; radiosensitive or radioresistant tumor regions for biological targeting using boost methods such as IMRT; and brachytherapy with or without IGRT
- Functional MR methods may also provide delineation of normal tissue regions as clinically relevant OAR where irradiation should be minimized or avoided in order to maintain acceptable clinical function

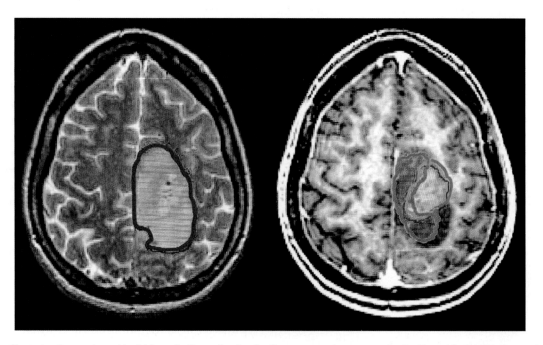

Figure 52.10 A case illustration for a patient with a high-grade glioma showing the disease extent when measured using T2-weighted MRI sequence (red), T1-weighted post-contrast medium (green), and MRS measuring high choline/NAA spectra (orange). *Source*: From Ref. 172.

PET for RTP

The rationale for using PET in oncology is reviewed in chapter 61. A similar rationale exists for its use for target volume delineation in RTP. PET scanning can improve staging of cancers by defining localized versus more extensive locoregional or metastatic disease and thereby ensure patients are selected appropriately for radical radiotherapy. There is also an opportunity to use PET for assessing XRT response both during and post-irradiation. For target-volume delineation, PET can be used to locate disease not readily identified by morphological imaging, differentiate tumor from necrosis or benign processes such as atelectasis, and potentially reduce the extent of observer variability.

PET can provide physiological and biological data for both the tumor and any important adjacent normal organs. The most commonly used PET tracer is 2-[F-18]fluoro-2-deoxy-D-glucose (^{18}F-FDG) and relates glucose metabolism via a combination of mechanisms to the increased metabolic activity usually seen in cancers. More PET tracers are now available to assess different aspects of tumor metabolism such as hypoxia and proliferation. By quantifying different aspects of tissue metabolism with different PET tracers, details of hypoxia and perfusion may be used to aid target volume delineation. In addition, molecular imaging may be used to identify different tumor-related phenotypes and genotypes that may also be useful in determining subclinical target volumes or CTV for RTP (136,137). The following sections will address the current rationale and subsite cancer applications of PET for target volume delineation.

The use of FDG-PET in determining target volumes for CNS tumors is limited due to the normally high glucose uptake in the brain, so there is less of a differential between tumor and normal brain tissue for target-volume delineation (138). More specific PET tracers are being used, such as radiolabeled amino acids; methionine (MET), alanine, and tyrosine, on the basis that cellular turnover in much greater in tumors than in cerebral tissues (137). The use of Met-PET has been reported to have a sensitivity of 87% and specificity of 89% for the detection of tumor tissue relative to normal brain tissue using stereotactically-guided biopsies (139). There are only a few reports outlining the use of MET-PET for target volume delineation. One study of 13 patients with low-grade gliomas reported that MET-PET aided tumor delineation in 36% of cases and was complimentary in 46%. Investigators from Munich reported the application of MET-PET for RTP in high-grade gliomas and meningiomas (140,141). For their study on-high grade gliomas, there was substantial difference between MRI and MET-PET (140). The use of MET-PET improved localization of tumor compared to MRI as MRI was unable to reliably distinguish post-operative changes from the residual tumor. MET-PET also aided identification of menigioma disease, particularly in the base of the skull, and increased interobserver concordance for target delineation (141).

Although the intent of this chapter is not to discuss the staging of cancers using PET, it is clear that PET can substantially alter the staging status of patients by confirming nodal or metastatic involvement and by visualizing disease in radiologically normal sized nodes. This will change the treatment intention and radiotherapy plans for these patients. This is particularly true for lung cancer. An in-depth tabulation of all the published PET trials (mainly using ^{18}F-FDG) up to 2001 with over 4000 patients illustrates that PET can change patient management in over one-third of cases (142). This will also impact on radiotherapy plans. In lung radiotherapy, the use of FDG-PET resulted in a substantial change in treatment plans between 22% and 62% of cases (143–147) and in two smaller studies the change was 100% (148,149). The two main contributions of PET for RTP were in the identification of involved mediastinal nodes and the improved ability to better distinguish between tumor and atelectasis. Using CT, clinicians tend to overestimate the potential CTV for lung irradiation due to the uncertainty in determining the boundaries between tumor and atelectasis. This can limit the prescribed dose, if dose escalation was being contemplated, or lead to increased lung side-effects, if larger than necessary lung tissue was irradiated. One important feature of using integrated PET-CT information for RTP is that interobserver variability is also substantially reduced for lung RTP (147,150) and this benefit is most pronounced for the regions in the mediastinum and presence of atelectasis (151). The added value of using PET-CT for RTP was highlighted by the American Radiation Therapy Oncology Group (RTOG) with recommendations that it should be utilized for all dose escalation trials in lung cancer (152).

There is a similar impact on RTP for head and neck radiotherapy, where it is estimated that treatment plans were changed in 10% to 100% (149,153–155). A landmark study was reported by Daisne et al. where surgical pathological data was correlated with imaging using CT, MRI, and FDG-PET (154). This small but robust study examined 9/29 cases that had surgical pathological correlation. It was shown that both CT and MRI substantially overestimated the tumor volume. There was a smaller discrepancy between FDG-PET and the resected specimens but the key feature is that none of the three imaging modalities was able to accurately depict the extent of microscopic disease. It was reported that false positive results were seen for cartilage, extralaryngeal, and pre-epiglottic extensions. This study demonstrates the value of correlating imaging findings with histopathology in order to establish the reliability of any imaging modality in defining target volumes for RTP. This research is needed for more subsites. FEG-PET has also reduced interobserver variability for head and neck planning target volumes (156) and, based on the reduced target volumes using PET-CT, planning studies have outlined a dosimetric benefit with more normal tissues sparing (157).

For gastrointestinal tumors, the use of PET is mainly focused on staging, assessing response, and recurrence. The impact of PET for colorectal staging changed management in about one-third of cases. In colorectal cancers, the mainstay of therapy is surgery and systemic chemotherapy; thus the few reports of PET use for RTP. In esophageal cancers, upstaging of disease can occur in up to 38% of cases (158). One study examined 30 cases with reported discrepancies of up to 47% between CT with transesophageal US and FDG-PET for abnormal adenopathy that could change the CTV (159). The investigators also noted the potential for false-negatives and suggested that planning volumes should not be reduced in regions where there are suspected nodes on other imaging. However, the investigators also suggested, due to the high specificity of FDG-PET, that planning volumes should be enlarged for PET-avid nodal sites when other

imaging for this region is negative. In a smaller study of 16 patients planned for radical chemoradiation, the CT-based CTV excluded PET-defined disease in 69% of cases (158). The investigators outlined that the main disparity was in defining the longitudinal extent of the CTV with discrepancies of 75% at the cranial extent and 81% at the caudal extent. Moreover, the investigators reported that without the aid of FDG-PET for RTP a geographical miss of gross tumor would have occurred in 31% of cases. In rectal cancers the use of FDG-PET altered GTV delineation in 15% to 67% cases (149,150). For anal radiotherapy these groups reported that FDG-PET altered target volumes in 33% to 57% of cases (149,160), while another larger study reported an impact on RTP in 19% (9/48) of cases (161). In all these studies, the target volumes defined by PET may either be larger or smaller than their respective VCT-defined volumes. Further work is needed to define the utility of PET for RTP here.

In prostate cancer the use of FDG-PET for RTP has been minimal, largely due to the urinary excretion of FDG. Efforts are being directed to the use of choline-PET which is a promising marker of cellular membrane synthesis with encouraging results of high uptake in prostate cancer (162–164), but caution is still needed as prostatic disorders other than cancer can also cause uptake (165). Working is on-going to assess if choline-PET may adequately identify significant intraprostatic proliferative regions for image-guided functional radiotherapy boosts (166).

Similarly, functional imaging has been applied in gynecological cancer radiotherapy. In RTP for cervix cancer, target volumes were altered in 20% (2/8) of cases (149). The principle of radiation boosts to FDG-PET-avid nodal regions was explored in a small feasibility study of four cases in cervix cancer (167) and subsequently assessed in an on-going clinical trial that treated the PET-avid para-aortic nodes to doses as high as 60 Gy (168). This prospective report of 10 patients confirmed that it is possible to dose escalate para-aortic nodes whilst respecting the dose tolerances of the adjacent normal tissues, but longer follow-up and more rigorous studies are needed to determine the late side-effect profile and efficacy of this strategy. PET has also been used to guide treatment volumes in gynecological brachytherapy. In cervix brachytherapy, it was reported that PET can guide applicator positioning for brachytherapy (169) and its use enable better dose coverage of the tumor without increasing dose to the rectum or bladder (170).

Although PET is used extensively for lymphomas, there are only a few reports of PET being used for RTP in lymphomas. This is not surprising as the mainstay of treatment is with systemic agents. The role of PET in the selection of patients for radiotherapy remains unclear as it has been reported that a negative PET scan following therapy does not exclude residual microscopic disease (171). In a study of 17 cases of thoracic lymphomas undergoing radiotherapy, mixed results were obtained where 6/17 cases noted CT-defined masses of up to 367 cc whilst no masses were declared using PET; and in the 10 CT/PET-positive cases, 6/10 PET-defined GTV were smaller than the CT-defined GTV with differences as large as 12 cm in inferior extent. Although the investigators suggested that FDG-PET could reduce the subjectivity of RTP in thoracic lymphomas, much more work is needed here.

Key Points: PET for Radiotherapy Planning

- PET can identify abnormal activity in primary tumor and nodal regions that can alter management of the disease by clarifying the intent of treatment and impact on radiotherapy treatment planning by clarifying the target volume
- There is no consistency with regard to the change of target volumes when using PET for treatment planning in the individual cancer subtypes as PET-based target volumes can be either larger or smaller than its respective CT-based target volumes
- Both MRI and PET can reduce interobserver variability in target volume delineation. Examples include the use of PET to distinguish between tumor and atelectasis in lung cancer

Issues Using Functional Imaging for RTP

In MRI functional studies, the accuracy with which the tumor extent and its biology are depicted by the MR method remains uncertain and, therefore, it is difficult to pinpoint with confidence the line between active or resistant tumor regions and normal tissue. In most studies using PET for RTP, the identification of active tumor in lymph nodes has aided clinicians in determining the CTV and intent of treatment, but it is unable to detect every clonogenic tumor cell. For lung radiotherapy, PET can help in differentiating regions of atelectasis from tumor but it cannot provide accurate identification of exactly where this boundary between atelectasis and tumor exists. The greatest issue comes to a pinnacle when the clinician has to draw "the line" that denotes the boundary or "edges" of the GTV and/or the CTV. There is much controversy in how to determine where this line should lie, particularly when using PET scans, as the numerical values of the PET intensity levels selected for use, such as standardized uptake value (SUV), are quite arbitrary. Furthermore, many different parameters can affect PET intensity levels, such as patient characteristics, scanner and scanning technique, organ motion, and deformation. For improved clarification of this issue, more clinico-pathological-imaging studies, similar to that reported by Daisne et al. for head and neck cancers, are needed to verify the "true" meaning and depiction of the disease identified by the different imaging modalities.

Key Points: Issues Using Functional Imaging for Radiotherapy Planning

- There are limitations in using functional imaging for RTP and recognition of these limitations is useful when considering the added value of using functional imaging for RTP
- Where possible, it is important to undertake careful histopathological correlation with multimodality imaging in order to verify the "true" value of the imaging modality in question when defining the microscopic extent or biological parameters of the disease

Summary

- Imaging is central to radiotherapy and is needed for each and every step in the RTP process
- CT for RTP provides 3D spatial volumes for identification of tumor volumes and the surrounding normal tissues

- CFRT provides for 3D shaping of the radiation fields, reduces geographical miss of the tumor, and minimizes unnecessary dose to OAR
- Level 1 evidence from randomized trials demonstrates that CFRT can significantly reduce treatment-related side-effects
- IMRT refines the CFRT concept by improving the shaping of the high-dose regions through dose modulation, allows "dose painting," and permits safer dose escalation with better avoidance of adjacent critical OAR
- Treatment uncertainties can exist due to temporal spatial variation for the target and OAR resulting from physiological activity as well as uncertainties in patient set-up and treatment delivery
- RT strategies that aim to reduce or minimize systematic and random errors for target and organ temporal spatial variations or set-up and delivery uncertainties are collectively termed image-guided radiotherapy (IGRT)
- IGRT can also be used in the broader sense to encompass the need for more accurate and reliable means of target volume delineation for RTP
- There is an international standard nomenclature to define target volumes for RTP and this nomenclature provides uniformity in creating treatment volumes for RTP, consistency in reporting, and comparison of data between different centers
- One of the most difficult tasks in RTP is in the delineation of target volumes
- Definition of target volumes will need clinical expertise to take into account tumor and therapy factors, and the method of imaging the known disease
- There can be substantial inter- and intraobserver variability in target volume delineation for a wide variety of treatment sites
- It is important to have specific training for oncologists to understand how to utilize specific imaging modalities such as MRI or PET for RTP
- Close collaboration between diagnostic and therapeutic clinicians are needed to optimize the process of target volume delineation
- Multimodality imaging aims to combine the benefits from different imaging modalities, often providing complementary information to aid target volume delineation
- MRI can offer improved imaging functionality for more reliable identification of the extent of tumor compared to CT for a number of clinical sites and reduce observer variability
- There are many advances in MRI that can be used to aid target volume delineation and IGRT strategies such as ultrafast and cine MRI, contrast agents such as USPIO, MR simulators, and potentially MR LINACS
- Functional and molecular imaging may improve the therapeutic ratio of radiotherapy by offering the opportunity for biological target volumes, IGRT and treatment individualization for patients
- The added information from functional imaging on active or radioresistant tumor regions may be exploited for radiotherapy boost volumes, dose escalation, combined therapy with chemotherapy or radiosensitisers, or to select prospective non-responders during a course of radiotherapy for more aggressive therapies
- Functional imaging may also permit functional avoidance of normal tissue function to maintain patient outcomes and reduce observer variability in target volume delineation. One example involves the use of PET to distinguish between tumor and atelectasis in lung radiotherapy
- Many functional MRI and PET methods remain active areas of research and are currently being investigated for their applications in RTP
- It is important to undertake careful histopathological correlation with multimodality imaging in order to verify the "true" value of the imaging modality in question in defining the microscopic extent or biological parameters of the disease

REFERENCES

1. Goitein M, Wittenberg J, Mendiondo M, et al. The value of CT scanning in radiation therapy treatment planning: a prospective study. Int J Radiat Oncol Biol Phys 1979; 5: 1787–98.
2. Goitein M. The utility of computed tomography in radiation therapy; an estimate of outcome. Int J Radiat Oncol Biol Phys 1979; 5: 1799–807.
3. Takahashi S. Conformation radiotherapy: rotation techniques as applied to radiography and radiotherapy of cancer. Acta Radiol 1965; (Suppl): 242.
4. Robinson MH, Bidmead AM, Harmer CL. Value of conformal planning in the radiotherapy of soft tissue sarcoma. Clin Oncol (R Coll Radiol) 1992; 4: 290–3.
5. Crosby TD, Melcher AA, Wetherall S, Brockway S, Burnet NG. A comparison of two planning techniques for radiotherapy of high grade astrocytomas. Clin Oncol (R Coll Radiol) 1998; 10: 392–8.
6. Williams MV, Denekamp J, Fowler JF. Dose response relationships for human tumours: implications for clinical trials of dose modifying agents. Int J Radiat Oncol Biol Phys 1984; 10: 1703–7.
7. Thames HD, Schultheiss TE, Hendry JH, et al. Can modest escalations of dose be detected as increased tumor control? Int J Radiat Oncol Biol Phys 1992; 22: 241–6.
8. Koper PC, Stroom JC, van Putten WL, et al. Acute morbidity reduction using 3DCRT for prostate carcinoma: a randomized study. Int J Radiat Oncol Biol Phys 1999; 43: 727–34.
9. Dearnaley DP, Khoo VS, Norman AR, et al. Comparison of radiation side-effects of conformal and conventional radiotherapy in prostate cancer: a randomised trial. Lancet 1999; 353: 267–72.
10. NICE. (National Institute of Clinical Excellence). Improving outcomes in urological cancers. The Manual (NICE: London, September 2002) 67.
11. Valicenti R, Lu J, Pilepich M, Asbell S, Grignon D. Survival advantage from higher-dose radiation therapy for clinically localized prostate cancer treated on the Radiation Therapy Oncology Group trials. J Clin Oncol 2000; 18: 2740–6.
12. Pollack A, Zagars GK, Starkschall G, et al. Prostate cancer radiation dose response: results of the M. D. Anderson phase III randomized trial. Int J Radiat Oncol Biol Phys 2002; 53: 1097–105.

13. Zietman AL, DeSilvio ML, Slater JD, et al. Comparison of conventional-dose vs high-dose conformal radiation therapy in clinically localized adenocarcinoma of the prostate: a randomized controlled trial. JAMA 2005; 294: 1233–9.

14. Dearnaley DP, Hall E, Lawrence D, et al. Phase III pilot study of dose escalation using conformal radiotherapy in prostate cancer: PSA control and side effects. Br J Cancer 2005; 92: 488–98.

15. Peeters ST, Heemsbergen WD, Koper PC, et al. Dose-response in radiotherapy for localized prostate cancer: results of the Dutch multicenter randomized phase III trial comparing 68 Gy of radiotherapy with 78 Gy. J Clin Oncol 2006; 24: 1990–6.

16. Dearnaley DP, Sydes MR, Graham JD, et al. Escalated-dose versus standard-dose conformal radiotherapy in prostate cancer: first results from the MRC RT01 randomised controlled trial. Lancet Oncol 2007; 8: 475–87.

17. Rowbottom CG, Khoo VS, Webb S. Simultaneous optimization of beam orientations and beam weights in conformal radiotherapy. Med Phys 2001; 28: 1696–702.

18. Khoo VS, Bedford JL, Webb S, Dearnaley DP. Class solutions for conformal external beam prostate radiotherapy. Int J Radiat Oncol Biol Phys 2003; 55: 1109–20.

19. Khoo VS. Radiotherapeutic techniques for prostate cancer, dose escalation and brachytherapy. Clin Oncol 2005; 17: 560–71.

20. Khoo V. Conformal radiotherapy, intensity-modulated radiotherapy and image-guided radiotherapy. In: Price P, Sikora K, Illidge T, eds. Treatment of Cancer, 5th edn. London: Hodder Arnold Health Sciences, 2008: Chapter 53.

21. Pirzkall A, Carol M, Lohr F, et al. Comparison of intensity-modulated radiotherapy with conventional conformal radiotherapy for complex-shaped tumors. Int J Radiat Oncol Biol Phys 2000; 48: 1371–80.

22. Khoo VS, Oldham M, Adams EJ, et al. Comparison of intensity-modulated tomotherapy with stereotactically guided conformal radiotherapy for brain tumors. Int J Radiat Oncol Biol Phys 1999; 45: 415–25.

23. Pirzkall A, Debus J, Haering P, et al. Intensity modulated radiotherapy (IMRT) for recurrent, residual, or untreated skull-base meningiomas: preliminary clinical experience. Int J Radiat Oncol Biol Phys 2003; 55: 362–72.

24. Levivier M, Massager N, Wikler D, Goldman S. Modern multimodal neuroimaging for radiosurgery: the example of PET scan integration. Acta Neurochir Suppl 2004; 91: 1–7.

25. Lee N, Xia P, Quivey JM, et al. Intensity-modulated radiotherapy in the treatment of nasopharyngeal carcinoma: an update of the UCSF experience. Int J Radiat Oncol Biol Phys 2002; 53: 12–22.

26. Lin A, Kim HM, Terrell JE, et al. Quality of life after parotid-sparing IMRT for head-and-neck cancer: a prospective longitudinal study. Int J Radiat Oncol Biol Phys 2003; 57: 61–70.

27. Guerrero Urbano MT, Clark CH, Kong C, et al. Target volume definition for head and neck intensity modulated radiotherapy: pre-clinical evaluation of PARSPORT trial guidelines. Clin Oncol 2007; 19: 604–13.

28. Donovan E, Bleakley N, Denholm E, et al. Randomised trial of standard 2D radiotherapy (RT) versus intensity modulated radiotherapy (IMRT) in patients prescribed breast radiotherapy. Radiother Oncol 2007; 82: 254–64.

29. Zelefsky MJ, Levin EJ, Hunt M, et al. Incidence of late rectal and urinary toxicities after three-dimensional conformal radiotherapy and intensity-modulated radiotherapy for localized prostate cancer. Int J Radiat Oncol Biol Phys 2008; 70: 1124–9.

30. Nutting CM, Convery DJ, Cosgrove VP, et al. Reduction of small and large bowel irradiation using an optimized intensity-modulated pelvic radiotherapy technique in patients with prostate cancer. Int J Radiat Oncol Biol Phys 2000; 48: 649–56.

31. ICRU-50. ICRU Report 50: Prescribing, recording, and reporting photon beam therapy. Bethesda, MD: International Commission on Radiation Units and Measurement, 1993: 3–16.

32. ICRU-62. ICRU Report 62: Prescribing, recording, and reporting photon beam therapy. Besthesda, MD: International Commission on Radiation Units and Measurement, 1999: 3–20.

33. Cattaneo GM, Reni M, Rizzo G, et al. Target delineation in post-operative radiotherapy of brain gliomas: interobserver variability and impact of image registration of MR (pre-operative) images on treatment planning CT scans. Radiother Oncol 2005; 75: 217–23.

34. Van de Steene J, Linthout N, de Mey J, et al. Definition of gross tumor volume in lung cancer: inter-observer variability. Radiother Oncol 2002; 62: 37–49.

35. Giraud P, Elles S, Helfre S, et al. Conformal radiotherapy for lung cancer: different delineation of the gross tumor volume (GTV) by radiologists and radiation oncologists. Radiother Oncol 2002; 62: 27–36.

36. Tai P, Van Dyk J, Yu E, et al. Variability of target volume delineation in cervical esophageal cancer. Int J Radiat Oncol Biol Phys 1998; 42: 277–88.

37. Hurkmans CW, Borger JH, Pieters BR, et al. Variability in target volume delineation on CT scans of the breast. Int J Radiat Oncol Biol Phys 2001; 50: 1366–72.

38. Landis DM, Luo W, Song J, et al. Variability among breast radiation oncologists in delineation of the postsurgical lumpectomy cavity. Int J Radiat Oncol Biol Phys 2007; 67: 1299–308.

39. Seddon B, Bidmead M, Wilson J, Khoo V, Dearnaley D. Target volume definition in conformal radiotherapy for prostate cancer: quality assurance in the MRC RT-01 trial. Radiother Oncol 2000; 56: 73–83.

40. The Royal College of Radiologists. Recommendations for Cross-Sectional Imaging in Cancer Management: Computed Tomography (CT), Magnetic Resonance Imaging (MRI), Positron Emission Tomography (PET), 2nd edn. London: The Royal College of Radiologists, 2006.

41. Khoo VS. MRI—"magic radiotherapy imaging" for treatment planning? Br J Radiol 2000; 73: 229–33.

42. Debois M, Oyen R, Maes F, et al. The contribution of magnetic resonance imaging to the three-dimensional treatment planning of localized prostate cancer. Int J Radiat Oncol Biol Phys 1999; 45: 857–65.

43. Sundar S, Symonds RP. Diagnostic radiology for radiotherapist: the case for structured training in cross-sectional imaging (CT and MRI). Clin Oncol 2002; 14: 413–14.

44. Thornton AF, Sandler HM, Ten Haken RK, et al. The clinical utility of magnetic resonance imaging in the 3-dimensional

treatment planning of brain tumors. Int J Radiat Oncol Biol Phys 1992; 24: 767–75.

45. Heester MA, Wijrdeman HK, Strukmans H, Witkamp T, Moerland MA. Brain tumor delineation based on CT and MR imaging. Strahlenther Onkol 1993; 169: 729–33.

46. Sultanem K, Patrocinio H, Lambert C, et al. The use of hypo-fractionated intensity-modulated irradiation in the treatment of glioblastoma multiforme: preliminary results of a prospective trial. Int J Radiat Oncol Biol Phys 2004; 58: 247–52.

47. Ten Haken RK, Thornton AF, Sandler HM, et al. A quantitative assessment of the addition of MRI to CT-based, 3-D treatment planning of brain tumors. Radiother Oncol 1992; 25: 121–33.

48. Khoo VS, Adams EJ, Saran F, et al. A comparison of clinical target volumes determined by CT and MRI for the radiotherapy planning of base of skull meningiomas. Int J Radiat Oncol Biol Phys 2000; 46: 1309–17.

49. Mazzara GP, Velthuizen RP, Pearlman JL, Greenberg HM, Wagner H. Brain tumor target volume determination for radiation treatment planning through automated MRI segmentation. Int J Radiat Oncol Biol Phys 2004; 59: 300–12.

50. Bondiau PY, Malandain G, Chanalet S, et al. Atlas-based automatic segmentation of MR images: validation study on the brainstem in radiotherapy context. Int J Radiat Oncol Biol Phys 2005; 61: 289–98.

51. Manavis J, Sivridis L, Koukourakis MI. Nasopharyngeal carcinoma: the impact of CT-scan and of MRI on staging, radiotherapy treatment planning, and outcome of the disease. Clin Imaging 2005; 29: 128–33.

52. Emami B, Sethi A, Petruzzelli GJ. Influence of MRI on target volume delineation and IMRT planning in nasopharyngeal carcinoma. Int J Radiat Oncol Biol Phys 2003; 57: 481–8.

53. Chung NN, Ting LL, Hsu WC, Lui LT, Wang PM. Impact of magnetic resonance imaging versus CT on nasopharyngeal carcinoma: primary tumor target delineation for radiotherapy. Head Neck 2004; 26: 241–6.

54. Lee FK, Yeung DK, King AD, Leung SF, Ahuja A. Segmentation of nasopharyngeal carcinoma (NPC) lesions in MR images. Int J Radiat Oncol Biol Phys 2005; 61: 608–20.

55. Joon D, Butcher M, Marr M, et al. Evaluation of the use of CT planning vs. orthogonal films in the treatment of rectal carcinoma. In: Proceedings of the 12th International Congress of Radiation Research (ICRR). Brisbane, Australia, 2003: 258.

56. Khoo V, Joon D, Tan J, et al. The utility of multimodality imaging with MRI to determine treatment volumes for chemoradiation in rectal cancer. Eur J Cancer 2005; 3: 408.

57. Ferri M, Laghi A, Mingazzini P, et al. Pre-operative assessment of extramural invasion and sphincteral involvement in rectal cancer by magnetic resonance imaging with phased-array coil. Colorectal Dis 2005; 7: 387–93.

58. Urban M, Rosen HR, Holbling N, et al. MR imaging for the preoperative planning of sphincter-saving surgery for tumors of the lower third of the rectum: use of intravenous and endorectal contrast materials. Radiology 2000; 214: 503–8.

59. Blomqvist L, Holm T, Nyren S, et al. MR imaging and computed tomography in patients with rectal tumours clinically judged as locally advanced. Clin Radiol 2002; 57: 211–18.

60. Beets-Tan RG, Lettinga T, Beets GL. Pre-operative imaging of rectal cancer and its impact on surgical performance and treatment outcome. Eur J Surg Oncol 2005; 31: 681–8.

61. Huch Boni RA, Boner JA, Debatin JF, et al. Optimization of prostate carcinoma staging: comparison of imaging and clinical methods. Clin Radiol 1995; 50: 593–600.

62. Barentsz JO, Engelbrecht MR, Witjes JA, de la Rosette JJ, van der Graaf M. MR imaging of the male pelvis. Eur Radiol 1999; 9: 1722–36.

63. Heenan SD. Magnetic resonance imaging in prostate cancer. Prostate Cancer Prostatic Dis 2004; 7: 282–8.

64. Khoo VS, Padhani AR, Tanner SF, et al. Comparison of MRI with CT for the radiotherapy planning of prostate cancer: a feasibility study. Br J Radiol 1999; 72: 590–7.

65. Wachter S, Wachter-Gerstner N, Bock T, et al. Interobserver comparison of CT and MRI-based prostate apex definition. Clinical relevance for conformal radiotherapy treatment planning. Strahlenther Onkol 2002; 178: 263–8.

66. Khoo VS, Joon DL. New developments in MRI for target volume delineation in radiotherapy. Br J Radiol 2006; 79 Spec No 1: S2–S15.

67. Roach M, Faillace-Akazawa P, Malfatti C, Holland J, Hricak H. Prostate volumes defined by magnetic resonance imaging and computerized tomographic scans for 3-dimensional conformal radiotherapy. Int J Radiat Oncol Biol Phys 1996; 35: 1011–18.

68. Kagawa K, Lee WR, Schultheiss TE, et al. Initial clinical assessment of CT-MRI image fusion software in localization of the prostate for 3D conformal radiation therapy. Int J Radiat Oncol Biol Phys 1997; 38: 319–25.

69. Rasch C, Barillot I, Remeijer P, et al. Definition of the prostate in CT and MRI: a multi-observer study. Int J Radiat Oncol Biol Phys 1999; 43: 57–66.

70. Sannazzari GL, Ragona R, Ruo Redda MG, et al. CT-MRI image fusion for delineation of volumes in three-dimensional conformal radiation therapy in the treatment of localized prostate cancer. Br J Radiol 2002; 75: 603–7.

71. Buyyounouski MK, Horwitz EM, Price RA, et al. Intensity-modulated radiotherapy with MRI simulation to reduce doses received by erectile tissue during prostate cancer treatment. Int J Radiat Oncol Biol Phys 2004; 58: 743–9.

72. Lau HY, Kagawa K, Lee WR, et al. Short communication: CT-MRI image fusion for 3D conformal prostate radiotherapy: use in patients with altered pelvic anatomy. Br J Radiol 1996; 69: 1165–70.

73. Steenbakkers RJ, Deurloo KE, Nowak PJ, et al. Reduction of dose delivered to the rectum and bulb of the penis using MRI delineation for radiotherapy of the prostate. Int J Radiat Oncol Biol Phys 2003; 57: 1269–79.

74. Menard C, Susil RC, Choyke P, et al. MRI-guided HDR prostate brachytherapy in standard 1.5T scanner. Int J Radiat Oncol Biol Phys 2004; 59: 1414–23.

75. Citrin D, Ning H, Guion P, et al. Inverse treatment planning based on MRI for HDR prostate brachytherapy. Int J Radiat Oncol Biol Phys 2005; 61: 1267–75.

76. Polo A, Cattani F, Vavassori A, et al. MR and CT image fusion for postimplant analysis in permanent prostate seed implants. Int J Radiat Oncol Biol Phys 2004; 60: 1572–9.

77. Crook J, McLean M, Yeung I, Williams T, Lockwood G. MRI-CT fusion to assess postbrachytherapy prostate volume and the effects of prolonged edema on dosimetry following transperineal interstitial permanent prostate brachytherapy. Brachytherapy 2004; 3: 55–60.

78. Krempien RC, Daeuber S, Hensley FW, Wannenmacher M, Harms W. Image fusion of CT and MRI data enables improved target volume definition in 3D-brachytherapy treatment planning. Brachytherapy 2003; 2: 164–71.

79. Haie-Meder C, Potter R, Van Limbergen E, et al. Recommendations from Gynaecological (GYN) GEC-ESTRO Working Group (I): concepts and terms in 3D image based 3D treatment planning in cervix cancer brachytherapy with emphasis on MRI assessment of GTV and CTV. Radiother Oncol 2005; 74: 235–45.

80. Khoo VS, Dearnaley DP, Finnigan DJ, et al. Magnetic resonance imaging (MRI): considerations and applications in radiotherapy treatment planning. Radiother Oncol 1997; 42: 1–15.

81. Finnigan DJ, Tanner SF, Dearnaley DP, et al. Distortion-corrected magnetic resonance images for pelvic radiotherapy treatment planning. In: Faulkner K, Carey B, Crellin A, Harrison RM, eds. Quantitative Imaging in Oncology. London: British Institute of Radiology, 1997: 72–6.

82. Tanner SF, Finnigan DJ, Khoo VS, et al. Radiotherapy planning of the pelvis using distortion corrected MR images: the removal of system distortions. Phys Med Biol 2000; 45: 2117–32.

83. Doran SJ, Charles-Edwards L, Reinsberg SA, Leach MO. A complete distortion correction for MR images: I. Gradient warp correction. Phys Med Biol 2005; 50: 1343–61.

84. Reinsberg SA, Doran SJ, Charles-Edwards EM, Leach MO. A complete distortion correction for MR images: II. Rectification of static-field inhomogeneities by similarity-based profile mapping. Phys Med Biol 2005; 50: 2651–61.

85. Petersch B, Bogner J, Fransson A, Lorang T, Potter R. Effects of geometric distortion in 0.2T MRI on radiotherapy treatment planning of prostate cancer. Radiother Oncol 2004; 71: 55–64.

86. Koch N, Liu HH, Olsson LE, Jackson EF. Assessment of geometrical accuracy of magnetic resonance images for radiation therapy of lung cancers. J Appl Clin Med Phys 2003; 4: 352–64.

87. Rohlfing T, Maurer CR Jr, O'Dell WG, Zhong J. Modeling liver motion and deformation during the respiratory cycle using intensity-based nonrigid registration of gated MR images. Med Phys 2004; 31: 427–32.

88. Kirilova A, Lockwood G, Choi P, et al. Three-dimensional motion of liver tumors using cine-magnetic resonance imaging. Int J Radiat Oncol Biol Phys 2008; 71: 1189–95.

89. Mangar SA, Scurr E, Huddart RA, et al. Assessing intra-fractional bladder motion using cine-MRI as initial methodology for Predictive Organ Localization (POLO) in radiotherapy for bladder cancer. Radiother Oncol 2007; 85: 207–14.

90. Padhani AR, Khoo VS, Suckling J, et al. Evaluating the effect of rectal distension and rectal movement on prostate gland position using cine MRI. Int J Radiat Oncol Biol Phys 1999; 44: 525–33.

91. Ghilezan MJ, Jaffray DA, Siewerdsen JH, et al. Prostate gland motion assessed with cine-magnetic resonance imaging (cine-MRI). Int J Radiat Oncol Biol Phys 2005; 62: 406–17.

92. Plathow C, Ley S, Fink C, et al. Analysis of intrathoracic tumor mobility during whole breathing cycle by dynamic MRI. Int J Radiat Oncol Biol Phys 2004; 59: 952–9.

93. Liu HH, Koch N, Starkschall G, et al. Evaluation of internal lung motion for respiratory-gated radiotherapy using MRI: Part II-margin reduction of internal target volume. Int J Radiat Oncol Biol Phys 2004; 60: 1473–83.

94. Harisinghani MG, Saini S, Weissleder R, et al. MR lymphangiography using ultrasmall superparamagnetic iron oxide in patients with primary abdominal and pelvic malignancies: radiographic-pathologic correlation. Am J Roentgenol 1999; 172: 1347–51.

95. Mack MG, Balzer JO, Straub R, Eichler K, Vogl TJ. Superparamagnetic iron oxide-enhanced MR imaging of head and neck lymph nodes. Radiology 2002; 222: 239–44.

96. Portaluri M, Bambace S, Perez C, et al. Clinical and anatomical guidelines in pelvic cancer contouring for radiotherapy treatment planning. Cancer Radiother 2004; 8: 222–9.

97. Martin J, Joon DL, Ng N, et al. Towards individualised radiotherapy for Stage I seminoma. Radiother Oncol 2005; 76: 251–6.

98. Gregoire V, Coche E, Cosnard G, Hamoir M, Reychler H. Selection and delineation of lymph node target volumes in head and neck conformal radiotherapy. Proposal for standardizing terminology and procedure based on the surgical experience. Radiother Oncol 2000; 56: 135–50.

99. Shih HA, Harisinghani M, Zietman AL, et al. Mapping of nodal disease in locally advanced prostate cancer: rethinking the clinical target volume for pelvic nodal irradiation based on vascular rather than bony anatomy. Int J Radiat Oncol Biol Phys 2005; 63: 1262–9.

100. Mizowaki T, Nagata Y, Okajima K, et al. Development of an MR simulator: experimental verification of geometric distortion and clinical application. Radiology 1996; 199: 855–60.

101. Ramsey CR, Arwood D, Scaperoth D, Oliver AL. Clinical application of digitally-reconstructed radiographs generated from magnetic resonance imaging for intracranial lesions. Int J Radiat Oncol Biol Phys 1999; 45: 797–802.

102. Weber DC, Wang H, Albrecht S, et al. Open low-field magnetic resonance imaging for target definition, dose calculations and set-up verification during three-dimensional CRT for glioblastoma multiforme. Clin Oncol 2008; 20: 157–67.

103. Lagendijk JJ, Raaymakers BW, Raaijmakers AJ, et al. MRI/linac integration. Radiother Oncol 2008; 86: 25–9.

104. Raaijmakers AJ, Raaymakers BW, Lagendijk JJ. Magnetic-field-induced dose effects in MR-guided radiotherapy systems: dependence on the magnetic field strength. Phys Med Biol 2008; 53: 909–23.

105. Raaymakers BW, Raaijmakers AJ, Kotte AN, Jette D, Lagendijk JJ. Integrating a MRI scanner with a 6 MV radiotherapy

accelerator: dose deposition in a transverse magnetic field. Phys Med Biol 2004; 49: 4109–18.

106. Raaijmakers AJ, Hardemark B, Raaymakers BW, Raaijmakers CP, Lagendijk JJ. Dose optimization for the MRI-accelerator: IMRT in the presence of a magnetic field. Phys Med Biol 2007; 52: 7045–54.

107. Ling CC, Humm J, Larson S, et al. Towards multidimensional radiotherapy (MD-CRT): biological imaging and biological conformality. Int J Radiat Oncol Biol Phys 2000; 47: 551–60.

108. Padhani AR, Husband JE. Dynamic contrast-enhanced MRI studies in oncology with an emphasis on quantification, validation and human studies. Clin Radiol 2001; 56: 607–20.

109. Koh DM, Padhani AR. Diffusion-weighted MRI: a new functional clinical technique for tumour imaging. Br J Radiol 2006; 79: 633–5.

110. Payne GS, Leach MO. Applications of magnetic resonance spectroscopy in radiotherapy treatment planning. Br J Radiol 2006; 79 Spec No 1: S16–S26.

111. Hoskin PJ, Carnell DM, Taylor NJ, et al. Hypoxia in prostate cancer: correlation of BOLD-MRI with pimonidazole immunohistochemistry-initial observations. Int J Radiat Oncol Biol Phys 2007; 68: 1065–71.

112. Stancanello J, Cavedon C, Francescon P, et al. BOLD fMRI integration into radiosurgery treatment planning of cerebral vascular malformations. Med Phys 2007; 34: 1176–84.

113. Sugahara T, Korogi Y, Kochi M, et al. Correlation of MR imaging-determined cerebral blood volume maps with histologic and angiographic determination of vascularity of gliomas. Am J Roentgenol 1998; 171: 1479–86.

114. Dao TH, Rahmouni A, Campana F, et al. Tumor recurrence versus fibrosis in the irradiated breast: differentiation with dynamic gadolinium-enhanced MR imaging. Radiology 1993; 187: 751–5.

115. Hawnaur JM, Zhu XP, Hutchinson CE. Quantitative dynamic contrast enhanced MRI of recurrent pelvic masses in patients treated for cancer. Br J Radiol 1998; 71: 1136–42.

116. De Vries A, Griebel J, Kremser C, et al. Monitoring of tumor microcirculation during fractionated radiation therapy in patients with rectal carcinoma: preliminary results and implications for therapy. Radiology 2000; 217: 385–91.

117. Mayr NA, Yuh WT, Arnholt JC, et al. Pixel analysis of MR perfusion imaging in predicting radiation therapy outcome in cervical cancer. J Magn Reson Imaging 2000; 12: 1027–33.

118. Rouviere O, Valette O, Grivolat S, et al. Recurrent prostate cancer after external beam radiotherapy: value of contrast-enhanced dynamic MRI in localizing intraprostatic tumor – correlation with biopsy findings. Urology 2004; 63: 922–7.

119. Dzik-Jurasz A, Domenig C, George M, et al. Diffusion MRI for prediction of response of rectal cancer to chemoradiation. Lancet 2002; 360: 307–8.

120. Kremser C, Judmaier W, Hein P, et al. Preliminary results on the influence of chemoradiation on apparent diffusion coefficients of primary rectal carcinoma measured by magnetic resonance imaging. Strahlenther Onkol 2003; 179: 641–9.

121. Mardor Y, Roth Y, Ochershvilli A, et al. Pretreatment prediction of brain tumors' response to radiation therapy using high b-value diffusion-weighted MRI. Neoplasia 2004; 6: 136–42.

122. Dirix P, De Keyzer F, Vandecaveye V, et al. Diffusion-weighted magnetic resonance imaging to evaluate major salivary gland function before and after radiotherapy. Int J Radiat Oncol Biol Phys 2008; 71: 1365–71.

123. Vandecaveye V, De Keyzer F, Nuyts S, et al. Detection of head and neck squamous cell carcinoma with diffusion weighted MRI after (chemo)radiotherapy: correlation between radiologic and histopathologic findings. Int J Radiat Oncol Biol Phys 2007; 67: 960–71.

124. Price SJ, Burnet NG, Donovan T, et al. Diffusion tensor imaging of brain tumours at 3T: a potential tool for assessing white matter tract invasion? Clin Radiol 2003; 58: 455–62.

125. Jena R, Price SJ, Baker C et al. Diffusion tensor imaging: possible implications for radiotherapy treatment planning of patients with high-grade glioma. Clin Oncol 2005; 17: 581–90.

126. Price SJ, Jena R, Burnet NG, et al. Predicting patterns of glioma recurrence using diffusion tensor imaging. Eur Radiol 2007; 17: 1675–84.

127. Aoyama H, Kamada K, Shirato H, et al. Integration of functional brain information into stereotactic irradiation treatment planning using magnetoencephalography and magnetic resonance axonography. Int J Radiat Oncol Biol Phys 2004; 58: 1177–83.

128. Nelson SJ, Graves E, Pirzkall A, et al. In vivo molecular imaging for planning radiation therapy of gliomas: an application of 1H MRSI. J Magn Reson Imaging 2002; 16: 464–76.

129. Catalaa I, Henry R, Dillon WP, et al. Perfusion, diffusion and spectroscopy values in newly diagnosed cerebral gliomas. NMR Biomed 2006; 19: 463–75.

130. Walecki J, Tarasow E, Kubas B, et al. Hydrogen-1 MR spectroscopy of the peritumoral zone in patients with cerebral glioma: assessment of the value of the method. Acad Radiol 2003; 10: 145–53.

131. Kurhanewicz J, Swanson MG, Nelson SJ, Vigneron DB. Combined magnetic resonance imaging and spectroscopic imaging approach to molecular imaging of prostate cancer. J Magn Reson Imaging 2002; 16: 451–63.

132. Burns MA, He W, Wu CL, Cheng LL. Quantitative pathology in tissue MR spectroscopy based human prostate metabolomics. Technol Cancer Res Treat 2004; 3: 591–8.

133. Cheng LL, Burns MA, Taylor JL, et al. Metabolic characterization of human prostate cancer with tissue magnetic resonance spectroscopy. Cancer Res 2005; 65: 3030–4.

134. Xia P, Pickett B, Vigneault E, Verhey LJ, Roach M 3rd. Forward or inversely planned segmental multileaf collimator IMRT and sequential tomotherapy to treat multiple dominant intraprostatic lesions of prostate cancer to 90 Gy. Int J Radiat Oncol Biol Phys 2001; 51: 244–54.

135. Kim Y, Hsu IC, Lessard E, et al. Class solution in inverse planned HDR prostate brachytherapy for dose escalation of DIL defined by combined MRI/MRSI. Radiother Oncol 2008; 88: 148–55.

136. Hustinx R, Pourdehnad M, Kaschten B, Alavi A. PET imaging for differentiating recurrent brain tumor from radiation necrosis. Radiol Clin North Am 2005; 43: 35–47.

137. Chen W, Silverman DH, Delaloye S, et al. 18F-FDOPA PET imaging of brain tumors: comparison study with 18F-FDG

PET and evaluation of diagnostic accuracy. J Nucl Med 2006; 47: 904–11.

138. Gross MW, Weber WA, Feldmann HJ, et al. The value of F-18-fluorodeoxyglucose PET for the 3-D radiation treatment planning of malignant gliomas. Int J Radiat Oncol Biol Phys 1998; 41: 989–95.

139. Kracht LW, Miletic H, Busch S, et al. Delineation of brain tumor extent with [11C]L-methionine positron emission tomography: local comparison with stereotactic histopathology. Clin Cancer Res 2004; 10: 7163–70.

140. Grosu AL, Weber WA, Riedel E, et al. L-(methyl-11C) methionine positron emission tomography for target delineation in resected high-grade gliomas before radiotherapy. Int J Radiat Oncol Biol Phys 2005; 63: 64–74.

141. Grosu AL, Weber WA, Astner ST, et al. 11C-methionine PET improves the target volume delineation of meningiomas treated with stereotactic fractionated radiotherapy. Int J Radiat Oncol Biol Phys 2006; 66: 339–44.

142. Gambhir SS, Czernin J, Schwimmer J, et al. A tabulated summary of the FDG PET literature. J Nucl Med 2001; 42(Suppl 5): 1S–93S.

143. Vanuytsel LJ, Vansteenkiste JF, Stroobants SG, et al. The impact of (18)F-fluoro-2-deoxy-D-glucose positron emission tomography (FDG-PET) lymph node staging on the radiation treatment volumes in patients with non-small cell lung cancer. Radiother Oncol 2000; 55: 317–24.

144. Macmanus M, D'Costa I, Everitt S, et al. Comparison of CT and positron emission tomography/CT coregistered images in planning radical radiotherapy in patients with non-small-cell lung cancer. Australas Radiol 2007; 51: 386–93.

145. Mah K, Caldwell CB, Ung YC, et al. The impact of (18)FDG-PET on target and critical organs in CT-based treatment planning of patients with poorly defined non-small-cell lung carcinoma: a prospective study. Int J Radiat Oncol Biol Phys 2002; 52: 339–50.

146. van Der Wel A, Nijsten S, Hochstenbag M, et al. Increased therapeutic ratio by 18FDG-PET CT planning in patients with clinical CT stage N2-N3M0 non-small-cell lung cancer: a modeling study. Int J Radiat Oncol Biol Phys 2005; 61: 649–55.

147. Ashamalla H, Rafla S, Parikh K, et al. The contribution of integrated PET/CT to the evolving definition of treatment volumes in radiation treatment planning in lung cancer. Int J Radiat Oncol Biol Phys 2005; 63: 1016–23.

148. Erdi YE, Rosenzweig K, Erdi AK, et al. Radiotherapy treatment planning for patients with non-small cell lung cancer using positron emission tomography (PET). Radiother Oncol 2002; 62: 51–60.

149. Ciernik IF, Dizendorf E, Baumert BG, et al. Radiation treatment planning with an integrated positron emission and computer tomography (PET/CT): a feasibility study. Int J Radiat Oncol Biol Phys 2003; 57: 853–63.

150. Steenbakkers RJ, Duppen JC, Fitton I, et al. Reduction of observer variation using matched CT-PET for lung cancer delineation: a three-dimensional analysis. Int J Radiat Oncol Biol Phys 2006; 64: 435–48.

151. Fitton I, Steenbakkers RJ, Gilhuijs K, et al. Impact of Anatomical Location on Value of CT-PET Co-Registration for Delineation of Lung Tumors. Int J Radiat Oncol Biol Phys 2008; 70: 1403–7.

152. Chapman JD, Bradley JD, Eary JF, et al. Molecular (functional) imaging for radiotherapy applications: an RTOG symposium. Int J Radiat Oncol Biol Phys 2003; 55: 294–301.

153. Nishioka T, Shiga T, Shirato H, et al. Image fusion between 18FDG-PET and MRI/CT for radiotherapy planning of oropharyngeal and nasopharyngeal carcinomas. Int J Radiat Oncol Biol Phys 2002; 53: 1051–7.

154. Daisne JF, Duprez T, Weynand B, et al. Tumor volume in pharyngolaryngeal squamous cell carcinoma: comparison at CT, MR imaging, and FDG PET and validation with surgical specimen. Radiology 2004; 233: 93–100.

155. Paulino AC, Koshy M, Howell R, Schuster D, Davis LW. Comparison of CT- and FDG-PET-defined gross tumor volume in intensity-modulated radiotherapy for head-and-neck cancer. Int J Radiat Oncol Biol Phys 2005; 61: 1385–92.

156. Geets X, Daisne JF, Arcangeli S, et al. Inter-observer variability in the delineation of pharyngo-laryngeal tumor, parotid glands and cervical spinal cord: comparison between CT-scan and MRI. Radiother Oncol 2005; 77: 25–31.

157. Geets X, Daisne JF, Tomsej M, et al. Impact of the type of imaging modality on target volumes delineation and dose distribution in pharyngo-laryngeal squamous cell carcinoma: comparison between pre- and per-treatment studies. Radiother Oncol 2006; 78: 291–7.

158. Leong T, Everitt C, Yuen K, et al. A prospective study to evaluate the impact of FDG-PET on CT-based radiotherapy treatment planning for oesophageal cancer. Radiother Oncol 2006; 78: 254–61.

159. Vrieze O, Haustermans K, De Wever W, et al. Is there a role for FGD-PET in radiotherapy planning in esophageal carcinoma? Radiother Oncol 2004; 73: 269–75.

160. Anderson C, Koshy M, Staley C, et al. PET-CT fusion in radiation management of patients with anorectal tumors. Int J Radiat Oncol Biol Phys 2007; 69: 155–62.

161. Nguyen BT, Joon DL, Khoo V, et al. Assessing the impact of FDG-PET in the management of anal cancer. Radiother Oncol 2008; 87: 376–82.

162. de Jong IJ, Pruim J, Elsinga PH, Vaalburg W, Mensink HJ. Visualization of prostate cancer with 11C-choline positron emission tomography. Eur Urol 2002; 42: 18–23.

163. de Jong IJ, Pruim J, Elsinga PH, Vaalburg W, Mensink HJ. Preoperative staging of pelvic lymph nodes in prostate cancer by 11C-choline PET. J Nucl Med 2003; 44: 331–5.

164. Scattoni V, Picchio M, Suardi N, et al. Detection of lymph-node metastases with integrated [11C]choline PET/CT in patients with PSA failure after radical retropubic prostatectomy: results confirmed by open pelvic-retroperitoneal lymphadenectomy. Eur Urol 2007; 52: 423–9.

165. Farsad M, Schiavina R, Castellucci P, et al. Detection and localization of prostate cancer: correlation of (11)C-choline PET/CT with histopathologic step-section analysis. J Nucl Med 2005; 46: 1642–9.

166. Ciernik IF, Brown DW, Schmid D, et al. 3D-segmentation of the 18F-choline PET signal for target volume definition in radiation therapy of the prostate. Technol Cancer Res Treat 2007; 6: 23–30.

167. Mutic S, Malyapa RS, Grigsby PW, et al. PET-guided IMRT for cervical carcinoma with positive para-aortic lymph nodes-a dose-escalation treatment planning study. Int J Radiat Oncol Biol Phys 2003; 55: 28–35.

168. Esthappan J, Chaudhari S, Santanam L, et al. Prospective clinical trial of positron emission tomography/computed tomography image-guided intensity-modulated radiation therapy for cervical carcinoma with positive para-aortic lymph nodes. Int J Radiat Oncol Biol Phys 2008; 72: 1134–9.

169. Wahab SH, Malyapa RS, Mutic S, et al. A treatment planning study comparing HDR and AGIMRT for cervical cancer. Med Phys 2004; 31: 734–43.

170. Lin LL, Mutic S, Low DA, et al. Adaptive brachytherapy treatment planning for cervical cancer using FDG-PET. Int J Radiat Oncol Biol Phys 2007; 67: 91–6.

171. Lavely WC, Delbeke D, Greer JP, et al. FDG PET in the follow-up management of patients with newly diagnosed Hodgkin and non-Hodgkin lymphoma after first-line chemotherapy. Int J Radiat Oncol Biol Phys 2003; 57: 307–15.

172. Laprie A, Pirzkall A, Haas-Kogan DA, et al. Longitudinal multivoxel MR spectroscopy study of pediatric diffuse brain-stem gliomas treated with radiotherapy. Int J Radiat Oncol Biol Phys 2005; 62: 20–31.

INTRODUCTION

Acute complications of treatment in the cancer patient typically occur within days or weeks of initiation of therapy. Acute complications are defined as those encountered up to three months; sub-acute complications between 3 and 12 months; and delayed or late complications after 12 months. However, there is variation in susceptibility among individuals and there may be overlap of the acute, sub-acute, and early delayed effects in the first few weeks to months following treatment. Radiological manifestations are often non-specific and thus the clinical context and temporal relationship to induction of therapy are important considerations. Good communication between the radiologist and the oncologist is vital for the early recognition and accurate diagnosis of complications related to treatment.

The role of the radiologist is to help clinical colleagues to make a distinction between the effects of the cancer and the effects of its treatment so that ineffective or toxic therapies can be discontinued. Cancer patients with treatment complications usually present with common and non-specific symptoms such as headache, confusion, vomiting, breathlessness, and abdominal pain. The differential diagnosis includes:

- Acute complications of treatment
- Complications or progression of the primary tumor
- Metastatic spread of tumor
- Problems related to co-morbid conditions

In this chapter, acute and early delayed complications, mainly related to chemotherapy, will be discussed concentrating on those processes that are likely to be encountered by the radiologist. Emphasis is placed upon complications whose recognition may spare the patient unnecessary harm or require specific changes in management. Complications of therapy which may mimic malignant disease are highlighted. Historically, these complications have been seen most commonly with treatment of hematological malignancies, but with more intensive chemotherapy for solid tumors these are increasingly seen in general oncology. For convenience, complications are discussed by anatomic site: the chest, the abdomen and pelvis, and the brain and spine.

While the majority of complications relate to direct organ toxicity and to the effects of myelosuppression there are a variety of complications related to newer agents which target tumor vascularity including perforation of bowel and the tracheobronchial tree. There have also been devastating multiorgan complications of novel agents using monoclonal antibodies which have proved fatal. A section on novel agents covers some of these aspects.

The complications associated with radiotherapy have been covered in detail elsewhere (see chaps. 54, 55, and 56). Late delayed complications related to chemotherapy are considered in other chapters as appropriate.

THE CHEST

A variety of complications of treatment are seen. These relate to:

- Drug-related toxicity
- Infectious complications of therapy
- Intravenous (IV) lines and catheters

A particular constellation of pulmonary problems, both infective and non-infective, are associated with bone marrow transplantation (BMT).

Drug-Related Toxicity

Identifying the etiology of pulmonary disorders in the treated cancer patient is a challenging problem requiring good communication between the oncologist and radiologist to arrive at the correct diagnosis. Drug-related toxicity is a diagnosis of exclusion having investigated treatable infections and by recognizing patterns in patient groups.

Cytotoxic drugs have a relatively high incidence of pulmonary complications due to a combination of direct cytotoxicity and immune mediated effects (1). Drug toxicity is a potentially reversible cause of respiratory disease which, if not recognized, may progress to fatal respiratory failure. However, identifying drug toxicity as the cause of respiratory disease is complicated by the wide range of pulmonary manifestations, and the many potential alternative causes for respiratory symptoms in patients undergoing treatment for cancer. These include:

- Drug toxicity
- Infections secondary to immunosuppression
- Manifestations of malignancy, primary and metastatic
- Post-radiotherapy complications
- Venous thrombo-embolic disease
- Pulmonary hemorrhage

Due to the sporadic reporting of cases and the concomitant use of radiotherapy, the incidence of pulmonary toxicity related to chemotherapy is uncertain. A review of the long-term effects of treatment of germ cell tumors with a combination of bleomycin, etoposide, and cisplatin reported an incidence of clinically apparent acute pulmonary toxicity of 0% to 4% and of late pulmonary toxicity of 8%. However, up to 20% of patients had sub-clinical evidence of deterioration in pulmonary function tests (2). Increased rates are reported in high risk subgroups treated with bleomycin and depend upon the criteria used for diagnosis (3).

A wide range of manifestations of pulmonary drug toxicity are described. Many drugs cause several patterns of pulmonary toxicity and more than one pattern of disease may be seen in a single patient. Furthermore, pulmonary toxicity is more likely when cytotoxic drugs are used in combination. Agents associated with

Table 53.1 Pulmonary Complications of Chemotherapy

Complication	Drugs associated
Bronchospasm	Etoposide, interleukin-2, mitomycin C, monoclonal anti-bodies, taxanes
Pleural effusion	ATRA, filgrastim (G-CSF), gemcitabine, interleukin-2, taxanes
Non-cardiogenic pulmonary edema	ATRA, cytarabine, cytosine, arabinoside, filgrastim (G- CSF), gemcitabine, imatinib, interleukin-2, mitomycin C, monoclonal anti-bodies
Pulmonary hemorrhage	Bevacizumab, cyclophosphamide, mitomycin C
Diffuse alveolar damage and acute respiratory distress syndrome	Bleomycin, busulfan, carmustine, cyclophosphamide, etoposide, gefitinib, gemcitabine, mitomycin C, mephalan, monoclonal antibodies, taxanes, tyrosine kinase inhibitors
Hypersensitivity pneumonitis/Eosinophilic pneumonia	Bleomycin, carmustine, cyclophosphamide, methotrexate, oxaliplatin, procabazine, rituximab, taxanes, tyrosine kinase inhibitors
Organizing pneumonia	Bleomycin, cyclophosphamide, cytarabine, doxorubicin, methotrexate, mitomycin-C
Pneumonitis and pulmonary fibrosis	Bleomycin, busulfan, carmustine, chlorambucil, cyclophosphamide, mitomycin C
Pneumothorax	Bleomycin, carmustine
Veno-occlusive disease	Nitrosoureas
Alveolar proteinosis	Busulfan
Granulomatous disease	Methotrexate

these various manifestations are included in Table 53.1, although the list is not comprehensive and continues to grow.

Fortunately, the radiological manifestations frequently fall into one of four groups (4–6):

- Interstitial pneumonitis and fibrosis
- Hypersensitivity pneumonitis
- Organizing pneumonia
- Acute onset non-cardiogenic pulmonary edema or diffuse alveolar damage

The lung has a limited range of responses to injury and the radiological appearances are often indistinguishable from idiopathic forms of interstitial lung disease.

Clinical Manifestations

The clinical manifestations clearly depend on the underlying mechanism of injury. In pneumonitis and pulmonary fibrosis, clinical features typically consist of slowly progressive dyspnea and non-productive cough associated with a low-grade fever and hypoxemia. Bibasal crackles and, occasionally, finger clubbing may develop. Hypersensitivity pneumonitis and organizing pneumonia follow a more sub-acute course. There is often an associated pulmonary or peripheral blood eosinophilia. Non-cardiogenic pulmonary edema and diffuse alveolar damage may develop over a few hours with a rapid onset of respiratory distress and hypoxemia. The onset of symptoms frequently has a clear temporal relationship with the drug and occurs with the initial onset of treatment. However, symptoms may occur idiosyncratically during a subsequent course of treatment, or many months to years after the initiation of therapy when a causal relationship may be less easy to identify (4,7).

Imaging

The chest radiograph (CXR) is usually the initial method of radiological evaluation of symptomatic respiratory disease and is also usually the first diagnostic test to demonstrate sub-clinical disease. Chest radiography is useful for documenting the time frame and evolution of pulmonary abnormalities and can identify the pattern of radiographic abnormalities.

Computed tomography (CT) is more sensitive than chest radiography in the detection of pulmonary abnormalities and should be considered in the presence of persisting respiratory symptoms when the CXR is normal (8,9). High resolution CT (HRCT) is particularly useful in identifying both the presence and morphology of lung parenchymal abnormalities and may allow differentiation from other causes of diffuse lung disease, such as lymphangitic spread of tumor. When no definitive diagnosis can be made, HRCT provides an accurate baseline for assessment of progression of disease and a guide to the optimal site for invasive tests such as broncho-alveolar lavage and surgical biopsy.

Interstitial Pneumonitis and Pulmonary Fibrosis

This is the most frequent presentation associated with drug induced pulmonary disease and is seen in almost all categories of chemotherapeutic agents, and is particularly associated with bleomycin (1). The clinical and radiological findings are insidious in onset and slowly progressive. Early features consist of subpleural irregular linear opacities. This may be associated with groundglass opacification which may progress into areas of peripheral consolidation. The findings are typically bilateral and most marked within the dependent portion of the lung bases (4,8,9). A variable amount of pulmonary fibrosis may develop, indicated by the presence of consolidation associated with architectural distortion, traction bronchiectasis, and honeycomb fibrosis (Fig. 53.1). The extent of abnormalities correlates with both respiratory function tests and the likelihood of resolution of changes.

Hypersensitivity Pneumonitis

Hypersensitivity pneumonitis typically has a sub-acute onset ranging from hours to days and once present may persist for several months. As in other hypersensitivity reactions, the development of pulmonary complications is often unrelated to the duration or cumulative dose of the drug. This pattern of disease is well described with the use of methotrexate. Radiological findings are most clearly identified on HRCT and predominantly consist of widespread or occasionally patchy ground-glass opacities. Typically these have a diffuse distribution or appear as ill-defined centrilobular nodules (Fig. 53.2). In general, hypersensitivity pneumonitis has a favorable prognosis. It is likely to resolve following the withdrawal of the drug and administration of corticosteroids.

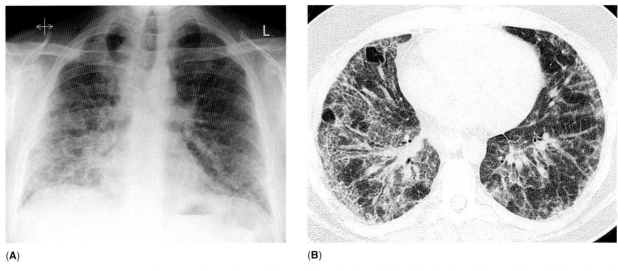

(A)   **(B)**

Figure 53.1 Bleomycin induced pulmonary fibrosis. (**A**) Chest radiograph shows a bilateral and mainly basal distribution of abnormal interstitial markings. (**B**) HRCT demonstrates a pattern of ground-glass opacities with septal thickening and early traction bronchiectasis. The changes are most marked in the sub-pleural lung.

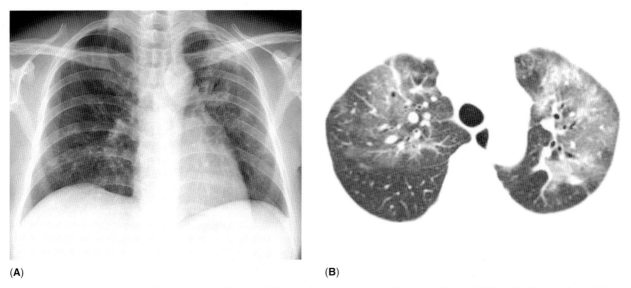

(A)   **(B)**

Figure 53.2 Hypersensitivity pneumonitis which developed sub-acutely following the administration of a tyrosine kinase inhibitor. (**A**) Chest radiograph demonstrates subtle opacification which appears localized to the left upper lobe. (**B**) HRCT reveals more diffuse ground-glass opacification throughout both lungs. The abnormalities resolved following administration of steroids.

Organizing Pneumonia

Organizing pneumonia has a sub-acute onset. Radiological features consist of bilateral asymmetric patchy or nodular consolidation with a peribronchial or subpleural distribution. This consolidation occurs without evidence of fibrosis. Occasionally the consolidation is solitary and has a nodular appearance, measuring up to several centimeters in diameter. Organizing pneumonia is usually very responsive to treatment with corticosteroids. The findings may be mistaken for persisting multifocal consolidation, due to infection or when more nodular, pulmonary metastases (1,4,10,11)

Non-cardiogenic Pulmonary Edema/Diffuse Alveolar Damage

Several drug reactions have a similar clinical and radiological onset and can be conveniently grouped together, although the underlying pathophysiology and prognosis vary. These conditions present with rapid onset of dyspnea and cough accompanied by radiographic findings of rapidly developing bilateral, predominantly bibasal heterogeneous opacities often progressing to complete pulmonary opacification. Non-cardiogenic pulmonary edema is thought to be due to increased permeability of basement membranes and is a well-described complication of treatment with interleukin 2. Diffuse alveolar damage consists of an acute phase of alveolar proteinaceous exudates and interstitial edema followed by a late proliferative phase of healing with fibrosis, and is the underlying pathological mechanism of adult respiratory distress syndrome (ARDS). It has a correspondingly poorer outcome. The CT features initially consist of bilateral, typically bibasal, ground-glass change, septal thickening, and consolidation. The subsequent proliferative phase demonstrates radiological evidence of healing

with progressive fibrosis and features traction bronchiectasis and honeycomb fibrosis. The main radiological differentials often include acute pulmonary edema or hemorrhage, aspiration pneumonitis, and other causes of ARDS including sepsis (1,4,5,12–14).

A rare but unique complication of chemotherapeutic drugs is "radiation recall" pneumonitis. This presents following the administration of chemotherapy with the development of ground-glass change and consolidation within a radiotherapy field previously deemed to be normal. This condition can occur many months after the completion of radiotherapy but often presents within several hours of administration of the drugs. The mechanism is thought to be due to the additive effect of the pulmonary toxicity of a chemotherapy agent on an area of sub-clinical injury within the lung. Agents associated with this syndrome include adriamycin carmustine, gemcitabine, gefitinib, and paclitaxel (15–19). A related clinical syndrome, also termed "radiation recall," is the rapid development of dermatitis within a previously irradiated area of skin following the administration of chemotherapy.

Specific Drugs
Although a wide range of cytotoxic drugs have been reported to cause pulmonary toxicity, several agents deserve particular attention due to their wide use and well-documented association with pulmonary toxicity.

Bleomycin
Bleomycin has been used since the 1970s in the treatment of testicular germ cell tumors (GCT) and lymphoma. The young age of these patients and high likelihood of curative therapy makes long-term drug toxicity an important consideration in the choice of treatment. Long-term follow-up of 835 patients with GCT demonstrated an incidence of pulmonary toxicity of 6.8%, with a median time of onset of 4.2 months. A mortality of 14% occurred within patients affected by bleomycin pulmonary toxicity (20). Pulmonary toxicity is predominantly due to pulmonary fibrosis due to the generation of oxygen radicals within the lungs. The risk of fibrosis is strongly related to cumulative dose with a sporadic incidence in doses of 100,000 to 450,000 IU rising to a reported mortality of up to 10% with doses in excess of 550,000 IU. Important related risk factors include:

- Renal impairment
- Supplemental oxygen therapy
- Radiotherapy

Weaker associations are with older age, prior lung disease, advanced stage disease, and bolus drug delivery. CT identifies disease at an earlier stage than the CXR and the degree of CT abnormalities correlates with impairment of pulmonary function tests and the likelihood of recovery (9). Increased uptake may be identified on [18]FDG PET which may have the potential to distinguish active pneumonitis from residual pulmonary fibrosis (Fig. 53.3) (21).

Bleomycin has also been reported to cause a hypersensitivity pneumonitis which is not dose dependent and can occur within hours of administration.

Busulfan
Busulfan is an alkylating agent used in the treatment of myeloproliferative disorders and has the dubious distinction of being the first cytotoxic agent with which pulmonary toxicity was reported. An incidence of 6% is reported and is related to cumulative dose and is unlikely to occur in total doses of less than 500 mg (1). Onset of complications is insidious and significantly later than other agents with an average delay of 3.5 years post-treatment (range 6 months to 10 years). The radiological pattern is of pneumonitis and progressive fibrosis with rare reports of alveolar proteinosis.

Nitrosoureas
Nitrosoureas, including carmustine, are alkylating agents with a key property of being able to cross the blood brain barrier. They are used in the treatment of high-grade gliomas, multiple myeloma, lymphoma, and in the preparatory phase of bone marrow transplantation. They carry a high risk of early pneumonitis and late onset fibrosis if used at an early age. In a study of children (median age 12 years) treated with carmustine, cisplatin, and vincristine 9.6% developed pneumonitis within 12 months, with an 86% mortality (22). Fatal pulmonary fibrosis occurs many years after treatment. A further study of carmustine use in the treatment of childhood gliomas demonstrated a 53% mortality at 25 years with progressive radiological and physiological evidence of fibrosis amongst all of the survivors (23,24). Unusually, carmustine related fibrosis tends to occur predominantly within the periphery of the upper zones rather than the lung bases.

Methotrexate
Methotrexate is a folic acid analogue used in the treatment of hematological malignancies. Pulmonary complications occur in 2% to 8% of patients and usually within a month of the onset of treatment (7). Pulmonary complications occur with small doses and even after non-systemic routes of treatment such as intrathecal therapy. The imaging findings are of a hypersensitivity pneumonitis occasionally associated with pleural effusions. The prognosis is good with the use of corticosteroids or discontinuation of therapy. Unusually, the pulmonary complications do not always recur if treatment is re-initiated.

Mitomycin C
Mitomycin C inhibits DNA synthesis and is used in the treatment of lung, breast, and upper gastrointestinal malignancies. Recognized complications are pneumonitis with pulmonary fibrosis and an increase in complications associated with pulmonary radiotherapy (25–27). The risk of pneumonitis is approximately 5% and occurs with a cumulative dose greater than 30 mg. A rare but frequently fatal complication is hemolytic-uremic syndrome, a combination of renal failure, hemolytic anemia, and thrombocytopenia, associated with non-cardiogenic pulmonary edema (28).

Vinca alkaloids are a class of drugs which cause few pulmonary complications. However, when combined with Mitomycin C there is a reported 4% incidence of acute respiratory insufficiency (29).

Cyclophosphamide
Cyclophosphamide is an alkylating agent widely used in the treatment of hematological and solid tumors. The incidence of pulmonary toxicity is low. Most cases present as late onset pneumonitis and progressive fibrosis up to five years post therapy (30). Rarely an acute pneumonitis occurs within a week of onset of therapy (31).

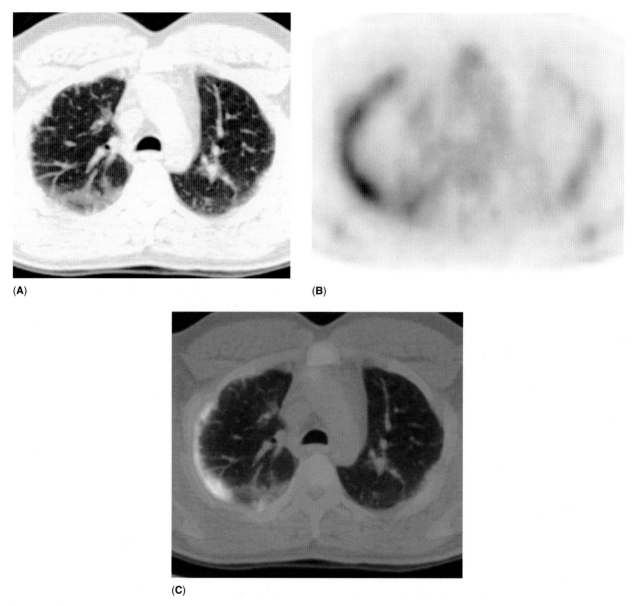

(A)

(B)

(C)

Figure 53.3 Interstitial pneumonitis in early bleomycin induced pulmonary fibrosis identified with ¹⁸F-FDG PET-CT. During combined chemotherapy including bleomycin for Hodgkin's lymphoma low-dose CT images (**A**) obtained during ¹⁸F-FDG PET-CT showed new areas of sub-pleural ground-glass opacification. (**B**) PET and (**C**) fused PET-CT images demonstrate more extensive avid uptake of ¹⁸F-FDG on PET and fused images within the sub-pleural lung. The findings probably indicate active pneumonitis in the early stages of bleomycin lung toxicity. *Source*: Courtesy of Dr. P. Manorahan, Christie Hospital, Manchester, U.K.

This may respond to withdrawal of therapy and administration of steroids or can progress to fatal ARDS (32).

Taxanes

Taxanes prevent cell mitosis by interfering with microtubule function. Both Paclitaxel and Docetaxel are used to treat a wide range of tumors including breast, lung, and ovarian carcinomas. Due to a castor oil carrier medium, Paclitaxel is associated with an infusion related acute hypersensitivity reaction similar to that of radiological contrast agents (33). The incidence of this reaction is reduced from 30% to 3% by the use of prophylactic anti-histamines and steroids. Docetaxel has an ethanol and water carrier medium and a much lower incidence of immediate reactions.

Both agents are associated with a delayed hypersensitivity pneumonitis which typically occurs during or soon after the completion of therapy. This has radiographic features of upper zone reticular-nodular opacities which correlate to patchy upper-zone ground-glass opacities on CT (34,35). These may resolve spontaneously, with withdrawal of the drug, or following the administration of steroids. Rarely, there is progression to diffuse alveolar damage and ARDS with the development of widespread septal thickening, patchy consolidation, and evidence of fibrosis (35–37).

Novel Molecular Targeted Therapies

Advances in molecular biology have resulted in the development of a range of novel therapies which inhibit cellular function. These include monoclonal antibodies and small molecules which inhibit specific aspects of tumor growth or progression which are different or over-expressed in malignant cells. Despite being highly selective in their mechanism of action they may still interfere with

normal cell metabolism and result in a wide range of toxic side effects (38,39).

Monoclonal Antibodies

A wide range of monoclonal antibodies have been recently developed which inhibit specific cell functions, particularly receptors associated with growth factors and angiogenesis. Almost all are associated with immediate hypersensitivity reactions including fever, skin rashes, dyspnea, hypotension, and vomiting. This reaction may be associated with the development of pulmonary opacities and small effusions on the chest radiograph (40).

Interstitial lung disease is an unusual but serious complication which has been described with Trastuzumab and Rituximab (41,42). Rituximab binds to CD20 and is used in the treatment of hematological malignancies (42). Rapid onset dyspnea, cough, and fever are accompanied by the development of widespread radiographic and CT opacities consistent with a pneumonitis. The mortality reported in a series of 16 cases was 38% (42).

Bevacizumab acts against vascular endothelial growth factors (VEGF) and is used in the treatment of non-small cell lung cancer (NSCLC), colorectal, and renal tumors and has been associated with major bleeding and thrombotic complications. In a study of the treatment of NSCLC with Bevacizumab plus Carboplatin, 6% developed life-threatening hemoptysis. The risk was associated with squamous cell carcinoma and cavitation in response to treatment (43). In a separate study of the benefit of adding Bevacizumab in the treatment of colorectal carcinoma, venous thrombo-embolic disease occurred in 26% of the treatment group compared with 9% of the control group (44).

Small Molecules

One group of small molecules bind to and inhibit tyrosine kinase and thereby interfere with the function of specific cell receptors.

Gefitinib (Iressa) impairs the function of epidermal growth factor receptors and is used in the treatment of a wide range of malignancies particularly metastatic NSCLC. A significant degree of pulmonary toxicity has been reported since its widespread use with an incidence of 3.5% to 5.4% and specific mortality of 1.6% to 3.6% (45,46). The risk of pulmonary toxicity is greatest in men, heavy smokers, and in the presence of underlying interstitial lung disease with symptoms developing a median of 31 days following the start of therapy (interquartile range 18–50 days). A review of the CT features of 70 cases of Gefitinib associated pulmonary toxicity indicates that the two commonest patterns of disease are patchy ground-glass opacities in 44%, and evidence of diffuse alveolar damage with a combination of ground-glass opacities, septal thickening, and consolidation with fibrosis, in 29% (47). Imaging features predict prognosis with a mortality of 31% and 75% respectively for the two patterns of disease. Erlotinib (Tarceva) has a similar mechanism of action to Gefitinib and is used in the treatment of NSCLC and pancreatic carcinomas. It has a lower incidence of pulmonary toxicity of less than 1% although cases of fatal interstitial lung disease similar to Gefitinib have been reported (48–50).

Imatinib (Glivec/Gleevec) also inhibits tyrosine kinase and interferes with the bcr-abl protein identified in chronic myelogenous leukemias (CML) and c-KIT protein in gastrointestinal stromal tumors (GIST). As with Gefitinib, Imatinib has a low incidence of serious pulmonary toxicity. A review of 5500 cases of CML or GIST treated with Imatinib identified only 27 cases (51). The commonest pattern of disease is a hypersensitivity pneumonitis which usually resolves spontaneously or with administration of steroids. Life-threatening pleural and pericardial effusions have been occasionally reported (52).

All-Trans-Retinoic Acid

All-trans-retinoic acid (ATRA) is a derivative of vitamin A used in the treatment of acute promyelocytic leukemia (APL), a specific form of acute myeloid leukemia. It allows the differentiation of leukemic promyelocytes into normal mature cells. ATRA syndrome is a unique cardio-pulmonary complication which occurs in 15% to 25% of cases. It is thought to be due to an inflammatory response and organ infiltration by APL cells. Respiratory distress, fever, cardiac, and renal failure occur usually on days 7 to 12 of treatment (53). The chest radiograph and HRCT are invariably abnormal. A review of radiographic and HRCT features indicated that 87% develop cardiac enlargement, 73% pleural effusions, and 60% ground-glass opacities, consolidation or septal lines (54). Nineteen percent develop a pericardial effusion (53). The radiological features are similar to cardiogenic interstitial pulmonary edema (Fig. 53.4). Features of pulmonary hemorrhage with centrilobular ill-defined ground-glass opacities occur in 20% of cases. Mortality is estimated to be 14%.

Cardiac Complications of Treatment

Cardiac failure and its radiological manifestations should be recognized as a potential complication of cytotoxic therapy itself and not only as a result of the fluid load which may be administered with the agents. Treatment regimes may include monitoring of cardiac function with echocardiography, MR imaging, or radionucleotide ventriculography to identify and monitor sub-clinical cardiomyopathy.

Anthracyclines (doxorubicin, daunorubicin, and epirubicin) are widely used in the treatment of lymphomas, leukemias, sarcomas, small cell, breast, and gastric carcinomas. The risk of cardiomyopathy is related to cumulative dose. A retrospective study demonstrated a 7.5% incidence of clinical cardiac failure following a dose of 550 mg/m^2 with a linear increase in risk above this dose and a mortality rate of 40% (55). The majority of cases develop within one year of completion of treatment, although there may be a delay of several years. There is an increasing recognition of sub-clinical disease. In children treated for leukemia and sarcomas, cardiac failure may occur up to 20 years following completion of treatment with a cumulative risk of between 5% and 10% at 15 years post-treatment. Factors that increase the risk of cardiac failure with anthracyclines include:

- Young age
- Mediastinal radiotherapy
- Combined use with other cardiotoxic agents, particularly taxanes

Trastuzumab (Herceptin) is a monoclonal antibody used in the treatment of breast carcinoma. Used alone, it has risk of sub-clinical cardiac impairment of 3% to 7% and a non-dose dependent risk of clinical cardiac failure of 1% to 4%. This is increased if used with other cardiotoxic agents such as anthracyclines (2,38).

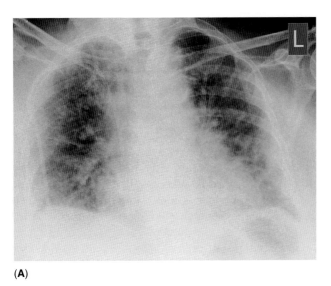

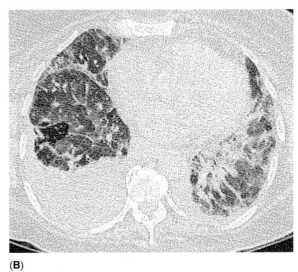

(A)   **(B)**

Figure 53.4 All-Trans-Retinoic Acid (ATRA) syndrome in acute promyelocytic leukemia. The development of acute dyspnea on day 7 of treatment was accompanied by new rapidly developing diffuse interstitial opacities on (A) the chest radiograph. (B) HRCT showing widespread septal thickening and ground-glass opacities accompanied by large bilateral pleural effusions.

Pericarditis and pericardial effusions are a rare side-effect of chemotherapy and have been described with the use of anthracyclines and cyclophosphamide (55,56).

Key points: Drug-Related Pulmonary Toxicity

- Identifying drug-induced lung disease relies on recognizing the temporal relationship between the drug and onset of respiratory disease
- Four key patterns of disease frequently occur: interstitial pneumonitis and fibrosis; hypersensitivity pneumonitis; organizing pneumonia; acute onset pulmonary edema and diffuse alveolar damage
- HRCT is the most sensitive and specific diagnostic imaging test but a conclusive diagnosis is frequently impossible
- The clinical and radiological features of drug toxicity can be non-specific. If these do not conform to a well-recognized pattern of disease, invasive tests for histopathological confirmation should be considered

---

Infectious Complications of Therapy

Infection is a major life-threatening complication of the treatment of malignancy with chemotherapy, with the lower respiratory tract being the most likely site of disease (57). Rates of pulmonary infection depend on the combination of drugs used but have been described in up to 13% of patients overall (58). Cytotoxic drugs, particularly alkylating agents such as cyclophosphamide are potent immunosuppressants, inducing neutropenia and impairing neutrophil function.

The risk of infection and the likelihood of complications are primarily related to the intensity of chemotherapy and depth and duration of neutropenia (58,59). Impaired skin and mucosal barriers as a result of pulmonary radiotherapy, chemotherapy, vascular access, and surgery, predispose to bacteremia and increase the likelihood of sepsis. Hematological malignancies and cases of advanced stage disease are particularly prone to pulmonary infections due to defects in underlying immunity. In high risk patients with leukemia being treated with cytotoxic drugs the incidence of pneumonia is as high as 24% with a mortality rate in those affected of up to 39% (60). Furthermore bone marrow transplantation (BMT), used in the treatment of many leukemias and lymphomas, is associated with infectious and non-infectious pulmonary complications due to a combination of neutropenia, toxic anti-rejection therapies, and graft versus host disease (GVHD).

HRCT is superior to CXR in the early identification of pulmonary infection and in its differentiation from non-infective causes. HRCT should be used in the investigation of persisting pyrexia when the CXR is normal or non-specifically abnormal. In 188 neutropenic patients with pyrexia persisting more than 48 hours who had a normal CXR, HRCT identified abnormalities suggestive of pneumonia in 60% of cases (61). Furthermore these appeared on HRCT a median of five days before the CXR abnormalities (61,62). Conversely, only 4% to 6% of those with a normal HRCT were subsequently found to have pneumonia (61,63). In a separate study of febrile BMT patients with non-specific CXR abnormalities, HRCT altered clinical decision making in 17 of 22 cases (64). Early diagnosis and the initiation of specific therapies reduce mortality (62). Specific radiological findings can occasionally indicate a likely organism or direct invasive tests such as broncho-alveolar lavage (BAL).

Radiological Features of Specific Organisms
Bacterial Pneumonias
Bacteria are the most likely cause of infection in both the general oncology population and post-BMT (60,65,66). The organisms most frequently cultured following BAL include Staphylococcus, *Streptococcus pneumoniae*, *Hemophilus influenzae*, Moraxella, Pseudomonas, *Klebsiella pneumoniae*, and *Escherichia coli* (65,67). There may be more than one organism involved. The CXR and HRCT appearances are not specific enough to differentiate between

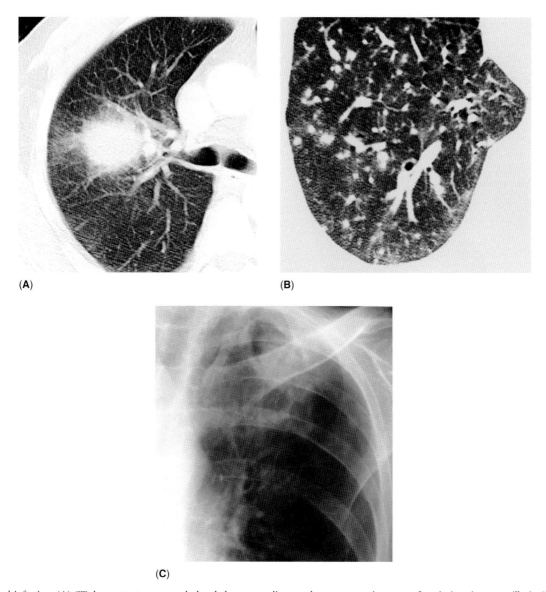

(A) (B)

(C)

Figure 53.5 Fungal infection. (A) CT demonstrates a ground-glass halo surrounding a pulmonary mass in a case of angio-invasive aspergillosis. (B) Multiple small (<1 cm) nodules with ground-glass halos are present in a case of infection with candida. This is a less frequent and less specific radiological pattern of fungal infections. (C) Chest radiograph demonstrates a cavity with a filling defect and an "air-crescent" sign in an aspergillus infection.

different pathogens or from non-bacterial causes of pneumonia (63). The main CXR findings are of consolidation, most frequently with a unilateral lobar pattern, but often with a segmental, multi-focal, and bilateral distribution (67,68). HRCT studies reflect this pattern of disease with additional features of diffuse or focal ground-glass opacities, small (<1 cm) and larger nodules and bronchial wall thickening with tree-in-bud opacities (63). Only 10% have an associated pleural effusion and, importantly in the presence of malignancy, lymph node enlargement is an unusual finding (63,67).

Fungal Pneumonias

The most frequent CXR features of invasive aspergillosis are ill-defined nodules or masses without evidence of cavitation and less frequently multi-focal areas of peripheral consolidation (68). Occasionally there are small pleural effusions. As with the CXR, the most frequent HRCT sign is the presence of large nodules measuring greater than 10 mm in diameter present in 62% of

cases (63,69). Small nodules are less frequent and are associated with tree-in-bud opacities. A ground-glass halo due to localized vascular invasion and infarction surrounds nodules early in the course of infection in 25% to 50% of cases (62,63,69). Although occasionally seen in bacterial or viral infections and hemorrhagic metastases, this is the most specific sign of invasive aspergillosis (Fig. 53.5A) (69). Less frequent findings of peripheral wedge shaped areas of consolidation thought to be due to vascular invasion and infarction, and multifocal consolidation, do not accurately differentiate bacterial from fungal infections. Cavitation, mycetoma formation, and the development of the "air crescent" sign are features of hematological reconstitution and are not generally seen during the neutropenic phase of bone marrow transplantation.

Less frequently occurring fungal agents include *Candida albicans* which shares some radiological features of aspergillosis (Fig. 53.5B) (63). Infection can occur via the airways and appear as consolidation and nodules, or occur via a hematogenous route particularly

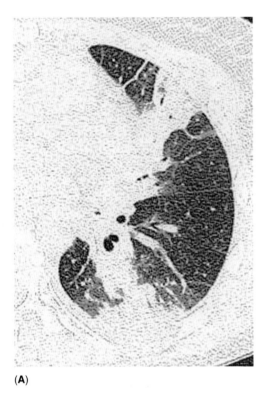 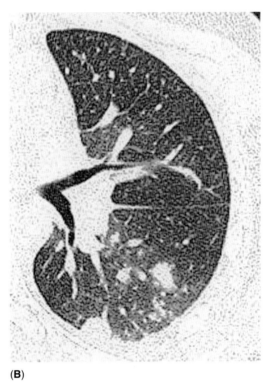

(A) (B)

Figure 53.6 HRCT in a patient with RSV pneumonitis post-BMT. (A) The most specific features on HRCT are of multiple small nodules measuring <10 mm in diameter associated with ground-glass opacification. (B) Larger areas of consolidation with ground-glass halos can develop.

from central lines with hemorrhagic and necrotic nodules. Ground-glass halos may be present. In summary, HRCT appearances of fungal infection include:

- Nodules >1 cm
- Smaller nodules with "tree-in-bud" appearance
- Ground-glass halo
- Peripheral wedge shaped consolidation
- Cavitation
- Mycetoma formation
- "Air crescent" sign (Fig. 53.5C)

Viral Pneumonias

Viral infections are characteristic of the early (post-engraftment) phase of BMT occurring typically within 6 to 12 weeks of transplant and usually do not occur after one year (68,70). The most common pathogen is cytomegalovirus (CMV) which involves 10% to 40% of recipients particularly with allogenic transplants (68,70). The infection is thought to derive from re-activation of latent host CMV or transmission of the virus in the transplant or blood products. If treatment with anti-viral therapies is delayed until pneumonitis develops the mortality reaches 85%(70). The early diagnosis is facilitated by routine blood assays for CMV titers and immuno-fluorescence with monoclonal antibodies to CMV antigens in BAL samples (70,71).

Radiographic features are of bilateral small nodules measuring less than 5 mm in diameter associated with more diffuse parenchymal opacification. The abnormalities do not occur in the upper zones without concomitant mid and lower zone abnormalities. Small effusions occasionally occur (68). The most specific HRCT features are of small nodules (<10 mm) with no evidence of necrosis or cavitation associated with ground-glass halos or a background ground-glass opacification (71–73). This makes differentiation from fungal infections difficult. Larger nodules and consolidation may occur (Fig. 53.6).

Less common viral pneumonias include Respiratory Syncytial Virus (RSV), Adenovirus, Influenza A and B, and Varicella Zoster. These all share similar radiological features to CMV.

In summary, the HRCT appearances of viral infections include:

- Widespread bilateral abnormalities
- Nodules measuring <1cm
- Ground-glass opacification

Pneumocystis Pneumonias

Pneumocystis jirovecii (formerly *Pneumocystis carinii*) pneumonia has significantly reduced in incidence due to routine anti-microbial prophylaxis. Onset occurs with a median of two months following transplantation and an increased long-term risk persists in the presence of GVHD (70). The radiographic findings are relatively non-specific and vary from focal to widespread parenchymal opacification and are occasionally associated with small nodules. Typical early HRCT features are peri-hilar or diffuse ground-glass opacities progressing to widespread consolidation (Fig. 53.7). Lymph node enlargement and effusions are atypical findings (68,74).

Bone Marrow Transplantation (BMT)—Infectious Complications
Pulmonary complications are the most common cause of death following BMT (66). In an autopsy series, pulmonary complications

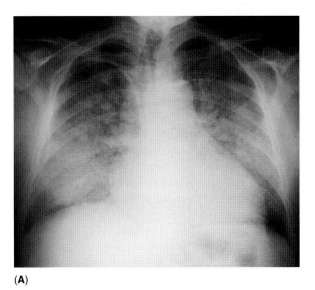
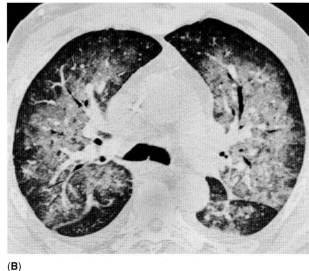

(A)   **(B)**

Figure 53.7 Pneumocystis pneumonia. (A) Chest radiograph demonstrates non-specific widespread parenchymal consolidation. (B) HRCT reveals this to be ground-glass opacification with a peri-hilar distribution typical of Pneumocystis pneumonia.

were the direct cause of death in 52% of patients and were identified in a total of 89% of cases. However, 72% of complications were not identified ante-mortem (66). Because of the reduced use of immunosuppressants and absence of graft versus host disease (GVHD), complications are less frequent in autologous compared to allogenic grafts. An important feature of BMT is the typically temporal pattern of the degree of immunosuppression and graft function which then influences the likeliest cause of infectious and non-infectious pulmonary complications (70). This temporal pattern is usually divided into three phases: neutropenic, early (post-engraftment), and late.

Neutropenic Phase
Various combinations of high dose chemotherapy and radio-therapy are used to suppress the recipient's marrow in preparation for bone marrow transplantation (75). The resulting profound neutropenia lasts for up to 30 days post-transplantation. The infections that characterize this period are bacterial and fungal, particularly invasive aspergillosis and occasionally *Candida albicans* (70). The prognosis for fungal infections is poor, in part due to delays in obtaining an accurate diagnosis and instituting specific therapies (66). Non-infective complications seen during the neutropenic phase include pulmonary edema, diffuse alveolar hemorrhage, and pulmonary drug toxicity (70,71,73,76).

Early (Post-Engraftment) Phase
Typically from days 30 to 100 neutrophil function has returned but there are persisting defects in humoral and cell-mediated immunity (70,71,73). The predominant infectious risk is from viral infections, most notably cytomegalovirus. *P. jirovecii* infections are less common due to the routine use of prophylactic therapies. The main non-infective complication is the development of idiopathic pulmonary syndrome.

Late Phase
After 100 days the immune system has reconstituted and infections are less common. Long-term infective complications are

associated with allogenic bone marrow transplantation due to the presence of chronic graft versus host disease and the use of immunosuppresive drugs. The most common pulmonary pathogens are bacterial sino-pulmonary and fungal infections and occasionally CMV or Pneumocystis infections. The main non-infective complications are obliterative bronchiolitis and organizing pneumonia associated with GVHD, and rarely alveolar proteinosis or the development of lymphoproliferative malignancies.

Non-infective Complications of BMT
The non-infective pulmonary complications of BMT are a significant cause of morbidity post-BMT. They are identified in 72% of autopsy studies but are less likely than pulmonary infection to be diagnosed ante-mortem (66). As with infective complications, they have a typical temporal pattern related to the time of transplantation.

Neutropenic Phase Complications
These include:

- Pulmonary edema
- Diffuse alveolar hemorrhage
- Acute drug toxicity

Pulmonary edema is a frequent finding due to the use of intravenous fluids, sepsis, and drug-induced pulmonary and cardiac toxicity often augmented by radiotherapy (70,71,73). The radiological features of bilateral consolidation with septal thickening and pleural effusions are similar to those seen in the general population.

Diffuse alveolar hemorrhage (DAH) occurs in 2% to 14% of recipients typically between days 7 to 19 post transplantation (77). The cause is unknown but thought to be an inflammatory process perhaps related to multiple factors including the preparatory chemotherapy and radiotherapy and perhaps sub-clinical infection. It is not related to thrombocytopenia or clotting abnormalities. Clinical features are of rapid onset respiratory distress associated with fever but without hemoptysis. In a study of 39 cases, the

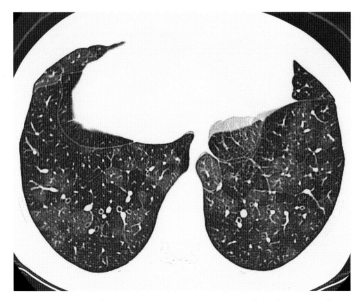

Figure 53.8 HRCT demonstrates mosaic attenuation of the lung parenchyma which is accentuated on expiratory images and indicates air-trapping in early obliterative bronchiolitis.

radiographic abnormalities preceded the clinical diagnosis by four days and consisted of rapidly progressive reticular or small nodular opacities in 73%, with consolidation in the remainder. Abnormalities are typically bilateral and peri-hilar, but unilateral in 26%, and associated with effusion in 15% (78). HRCT features are of ground-glass opacities with septal thickening progressing to consolidation. The diagnosis is confirmed with BAL. Untreated the condition has a high mortality but is very responsive to high dose steroid therapy.

Early (Post-Engraftment) Phase Complications
The main non-infective complication during this period is the idiopathic pneumonia syndrome (IPS) (70,79) which is defined as a diffuse lung injury in which an infective component is not found. The incidence is between 7.3% and 12% and as with DAH the etiology of this inflammatory process is unknown. It differs from DAH in its time of onset, has an increased incidence in allogenic grafts, and a poor prognosis which is not influenced by steroids (70,77,79). The syndrome presents between days 21 to 87 (median 42 days) with cough and dyspnea and a rash associated with hypoxemia and pulmonary opacities. The radiographic features reflect the underlying histological process of diffuse alveolar damage with bilateral patchy ground-glass opacities progressing to consolidation (73). IPS may resolve spontaneously, but in those that fail to recover, CT demonstrates the onset of fibrosis and features of ARDS. The diagnosis is one of exclusion with the main differentials being that of infection (excluded by BAL), drug reactions, and other causes of ARDS.

Late Phase Complications
The late non-infective complications are almost exclusively seen in allogenic (as opposed to autologous) transplants due to the presence of chronic GVHD and the continued use of immunosuppressive drugs (70). This systemic disorder manifests itself in the lungs as obliterative bronchiolitis (OB) and cryptogenic

organizing pneumonias (COP) (formerly known as bronchiolitis obliterans with organizing pneumonia, BOOP). In OB an allogenic peribronchiolar inflammation leads to the constriction and obliteration of the airways. COP is characterized by extension of the inflammatory process into the alveoli. The incidence is 10% and with a poor clinical outcome due to progressive respiratory failure (80). Clinical features are of dyspnea and cough with evidence of airways obstruction on pulmonary function tests. Radiographic features of OB are minimal and consist of hyperinflation of the lungs. There is an association with spontaneous pneumothoraces and pneumomediastinum (81). HRCT is a sensitive test with specific findings of mosaic attenuation of the lung parenchyma due to air-trapping in the early stages, and bronchiectasis as the condition progresses (Fig. 53.8) (82).

COP is characterized by bilateral patchy asymmetrically distributed areas of consolidation. CT may reveal a characteristic peribronchovascular or subpleural distribution of ground-glass opacities and consolidation. In the immunocompromised single or multiple nodules and masses may be seen (83,84). The condition is very responsive to steroids. The initial differential diagnosis of COP usually includes infection and possibly malignancy.

Rare non-infective complications reported include alveolar proteinosis, pulmonary veno-occlusive disease, granulomatous disease, and post-transplant lymphoproliferative disease (79).

Key Points: Pulmonary Infectious Complications of Therapy

- Pulmonary infections are a major complication in oncology patients and the leading cause of post-treatment death in some groups
- Patients with hematological malignancies and BMT recipients are in the highest risk group for infective and non-infective complications
- The likely organism can often be predicted from the clinical history
- Infectious organisms may give rise to specific radiological features
- HRCT is a sensitive method for detecting pulmonary complications, is useful in excluding the chest as a source of sepsis and can direct specific tests such as BAL

Intravenous Lines and Catheters

Long-term central venous catheters are frequently used in oncology patients for the infusion of cytotoxic agents and blood products. These are increasingly sited under imaging guidance in radiological departments. Complications related to catheter placement may be identified at the time of placement or on the post-procedural "check" CXR. More specialized investigations may include contrast venography or cross-sectional imaging, including Doppler US and contrast-enhanced CT. Typical sites of placement are the internal jugular, subclavian, and brachial or basilic veins. Subclavian catheters have a higher rate of acute complications and an increased risk of long-term line fracture (85,86). Brachial/cephalic/basilic vein catheters have the advantages of ease of access and low risk of immediate complications such as pneumothorax, but due to their smaller

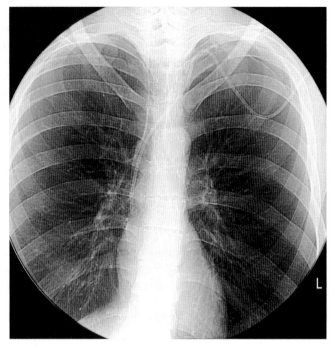

Figure 53.9 Immediate complications. A post-procedural film following insertion of a left sub-clavian line demonstrates a left apical pneumothorax, the commonest immediate complication of central line placement.

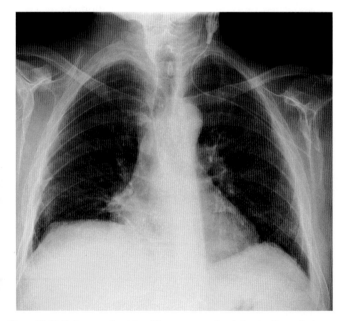

Figure 53.10 Catheter malposition. The post-procedural chest radiograph demonstrates that the tip of the left internal jugular catheter lies within the left axillary vein.

caliber have a higher rate of occlusion and thrombogenic complications (85,87).

The method and type of central venous catheter placed varies with local practice and the needs of the patient. For example, the side of line placement may be determined by the need to avoid the

site of previous breast surgery. Long-term catheters are tunneled subcutaneously to reduce the risk of infection. Immediate complications occur at the time of line placement due to malposition or trauma. Important late complications relate to the development of line thrombus and fibrin sheaths and the associated complication of line sepsis.

Immediate Complications
The most frequent complications at the time of line placement are: (85)

- Pneumothorax
- Traumatic injury to the great vessels
- Catheter malposition
- Air embolism

The risk of acute complications is increased with a subclavian approach and if the practitioner is inexperienced. US guidance significantly reduces the number of attempts required, the duration of the procedure, and rate of acute complications.

Both pneumothorax and traumatic injury occur more frequently with subclavian punctures. Pneumothorax is the most frequent complication with rates of 0% to 12%, the rate depending on the experience of the practitioner. Hemothorax, mediastinal hematoma, and cardiac tamponade are less common but potentially fatal. The post-procedural CXR is performed to identify these potentially fatal complications (Figs. 53.9 and 53.10). This and subsequent films should be evaluated for an unusual course of the catheter, pleural effusion, widening or loss of the normal mediastinal contour, or enlargement of the cardiac silhouette. A raised hemi-diaphragm may indicate phrenic nerve injury.

Sub-optimal positioning occurs in 40% of procedures performed without image guidance but it is unlikely to occur if fluoroscopic guidance has been used. The optimal position for the tip of the catheter is within the superior vena cava (SVC) 3 cm to 5 cm above the right atrium. Intracardiac positioning is associated with dysrhythmias, thrombus formation, infection, and cardiac tamponade. Positioning in the upper third of the SVC also has an increased risk of thrombus formation. Occasionally the catheter tip may be within the contralateral brachiocephalic or azygous veins. Although the catheter may appear to be positioned correctly on a single view CXR it should be remembered that it could potentially lie outside the vessel anterior or posterior to the SVC.

Air embolism is a rare but potentially serious complication avoided by measures used to increase intrathoracic pressure such as the Trendellenberg position and Valsalva maneuvers.

Late Complications
The three main late complications are:

- Formation of a fibrin sheath around the catheter
- Catheter related thrombus
- Line infections

Fibrin sheaths may cause catheter dysfunction by preventing aspiration from the catheter and predispose to infection and thrombus formation but are otherwise benign (Fig. 53.11). Catheter

related thrombus occurs in 1.5% to 34% and approximately two-thirds of cases are clinically silent (88). Catheter dysfunction, similar to that with fibrin sheaths, with swelling of the upper limbs and/or head and neck, erythema and pain are the main clinical features (Fig. 53.12). The complications are of pulmonary embolism (15–25%) and predisposition to catheter related infections. Compression and Doppler US is a highly specific diagnostic test

and has a sensitivity of 56% to 100%. If the clinical suspicion of thrombus remains high and US examinations are negative the gold standard test is considered to be contrast venography. There is currently no consensus as to whether the presence of thrombus should be treated with anti-coagulation or warrants catheter removal.

Catheter related infections occur in up to 21% of oncology patients with long-term central venous lines but with the neutropenic and post-BMT patients at greatest risk. It is important to differentiate colonization of the catheter and local port related infections from true catheter infections which lead to bacteremia and sepsis (87). True catheter infections are typically due to Staphyloccocal and Candida organisms and may be complicated by septic emboli, endocarditis, osteomyelitis, shock, and multi-organ failure. Identifying the site of sepsis without the surgical removal of the tunneled catheter is a difficult problem requiring simultaneous catheter and peripheral blood samples for culture and, rarely, endoluminal brushings may also be required. Infections may occasionally be successfully treated with antibiotics but catheter removal is usually warranted.

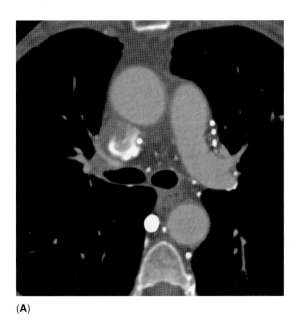

Figure 53.11 Late complications. Lineogram demonstrates contrast pooling along the outer aspect of the distal catheter within the SVC, indicating the presence of a fibrin sheath.

Key Points: Intravenous Lines and Catheters

- Subclavian catheters have the highest rate of immediate complications
- Peripheral catheters have the lowest rate of immediate complications but more long-term complications
- The post-procedural chest radiograph may identify a range of immediate complications
- US is useful in the diagnosis of late complication of catheter thrombosis
- Central venous catheters are a frequent source of sepsis

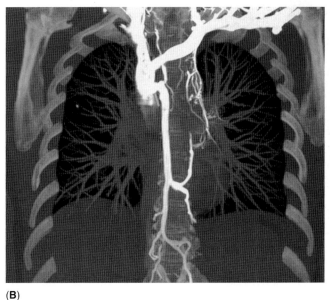

(A) **(B)**

Figure 53.12 Late complications: CT in a patient with a malfunctioning Hickman line which was removed but who developed acute swelling of the head and neck. (A) CT demonstrates a filling defect within the distal SVC indicating the presence of thrombus and a maximum intensity projection. (B) Demonstrates the presence of multiple mediastinal collateral vessels and retrograde flow within the azygos vein.

THE ABDOMEN AND PELVIS

A variety of drug-related complications affect the gastrointestinal (GI) and genitourinary (GU) systems. Most are predictable and self-limiting and result from bowel irritation with nausea, vomiting, and diarrhea or bladder irritability. Opiates and other drugs result in disordered gut motility in the cancer patient ranging from diarrhea to fecal impaction. More serious complications may result from direct toxicity to selected organs or are secondary to myelosuppression with its attendant risks of bleeding and infection. There is considerable overlap with early symptoms of more serious surgical conditions. Patients may, understandably, attribute their symptoms to the chemotherapy and delay their presentation until the situation becomes serious and life threatening. It is important to recognize that cancer patients are still at risk from general surgical conditions and, in the setting of a patient presenting with an acute abdomen, the radiologist should consider these conditions as well as treatment-related complications. For convenience acute complications are divided into:

- Surgical emergencies
- Severe infections
- Drug toxicity in specific organs

Acute complications of radiotherapy and post-surgical complications are discussed in chapter 56.

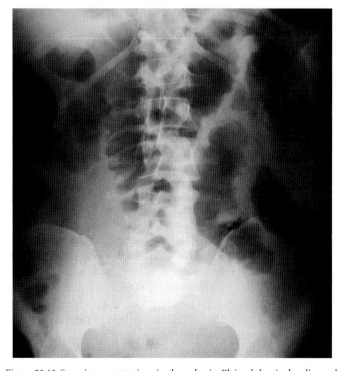

Figure 53.13 Superior mesenteric vein thrombosis. Plain abdominal radiograph showing small bowel wall and fold thickening with thumbprinting, suggesting either intestinal ischemia or hemorrhage. Venous ischemia and intramural bleeding was found at surgery in this leukemic patient and was fatal.

Surgical Emergencies

The aim of imaging assessment is to:

- Provide a specific surgical diagnosis
- Determine if cancer therapy is responsible
- Determine if tumor is responsible for the clinical features
- Define the prevailing extent of tumor
- Consider image-guided options for treatment or palliation of symptoms

Some therapies increase the likelihood of an acute abdomen. Treatment with both corticosteroids and non-steroidal anti-inflammatory drugs may result in intestinal perforation. Disordered coagulation may result in either bleeding into the bowel, the peritoneum, the body wall, or into a tumoral cavity. Conversely thrombosis of a vascular pedicle may also be seen.

Some therapies increase the production of urinary tract calculi.

Marrow suppression also results in acute intestinal inflammation with both infectious and non-infectious colitis, notably neutropenic colitis (typhlitis), other severe infections, and GVHD. A common pattern to these conditions is "mucosal barrier injury" or "mucositis" (89) which consists of four phases:

- Inflammatory
- Epithelial
- Ulcerative
- Healing

There is a considerable overlap in the clinical and imaging features of these conditions. Symptoms such as diarrhea and vomiting may be expected side effects of treatment as well as early symptoms of more serious complications. The severity of pain and tenderness may be reduced by analgesia and corticosteroid medication thereby masking clinical features. Some patients do not have specific gastrointestinal symptoms, merely generalized constitutional symptoms and fever and thus investigation begins as for pyrexia of unknown origin (PUO). Given the paucity of specific clinical pointers the radiologist has a key role in the diagnosis and management of the sick undiagnosed cancer patient.

Plain abdominal radiographs are useful to identify common conditions such as bowel obstruction/pseudo-obstruction and to exclude pneumoperitoneum. It may be difficult to obtain satisfactory horizontal beam films of the chest and abdomen in the sick patient who cannot travel to the radiology department and decubitus films may be required. Plain radiographic signs of gastrointestinal complications of therapy include:

- Dilatation of loops, which may be segmental particularly affecting the cecum
- Wall thickening, irregularity, and mucosal islands (Fig. 53.13)
- Pneumatosis intestinalis (Fig. 53.14)
- Pneumoperitoneum, localized (sealed) or generalized

Pneumatosis intestinalis is an uncommon condition that is not well understood. Whilst its radiographic findings are striking, its clinical significance is variable, particularly when only shown by CT. In some cases it is merely a reversible radiological fascination

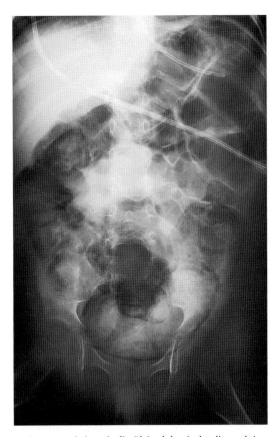

Figure 53.14 Pneumatosis intestinalis. Plain abdominal radiograph in a two-year old leukemic boy who settled on conservative management and whose follow-up CT was normal. *Source*: Courtesy of Dr. William Ramsden, St. James's University Hospital, Leeds, U.K.

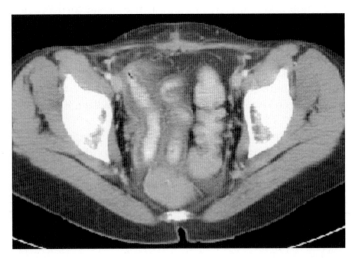

Figure 53.15 Taxane related enteritis. CT showing wall edema in several loops of pelvic small bowel in a patient with lower abdominal pain and diarrhea which resolved with conservative measures.

of no clinical significance (Fig. 53.14) (90). However, a number of complications which affect the cancer patient are associated with pneumatosis and it may therefore herald severe complications (91). Pneumatosis is predominantly right-sided and has a poor prognosis in the context of systemic infection and/or shock (92).

CT is used at an early stage in assessment of cancer patients with an acute abdomen. There are usually prior CT examinations with which to compare. Additionally, CT offers the therapeutic intervention of aspiration or drainage of fluid collections. CT demonstrates the layers of the bowel wall as well as its surrounding fat, the peritoneal cavity, mesenteric vascular pedicle, and solid organs. Further it allows distinction of whether tumor is the cause of the problem and a re-assessment of tumor burden which may influence whether treatment options are radical or palliative. IV contrast is valuable to show bowel wall vascularity. The bowel may be better shown in contrast to intestinal fluid contents rather than with administration of oral contrast. Iodinated oral contrast agents routinely used in cancer CT of the abdomen, such as dilute gastrografin, may be poorly tolerated and should be avoided when preliminary abdominal radiographs show dilated small bowel with suspected obstruction, ischemia, or ileus. When there is genuine concern for body wall or intestinal hemorrhage, preliminary unenhanced CT should be performed looking for a high density of fresh hemorrhage within the bowel wall or other affected areas (93).

With inflammatory complications, CT findings in both the small and large bowel are (94):

- Mucosal hyperemia
- Wall thickening and edema between the enhancing mucosa and serosa (the "halo" sign)
- Dilatation or luminal narrowing
- Mucosal irregularity and nodularity
- Pneumatosis intestinalis
- Perienteric stranding and mesenteric edema
- Localized or free intraperitoneal fluid
- Mesenteric lymphadenopathy
- Para-enteric abscess
- Localized (sealed) or free (generalized) pneumoperitoneum

These signs do not lead to specific diagnoses but indicate to some degree an increasing severity, and the need for surgical or image-guided intervention, moving down the list. The CT signs may be seen with a whole range of inflammatory and infectious conditions and following vascular insults to the bowel. Not all the signs are seen with the same condition in different patients and many of the complications resolve on conservative management (Fig. 53.15).

Neutropenic Colitis/Typhlitis

This is a necrotizing inflammatory process originally described after chemotherapy for leukemia (95) and childhood tumors but is increasingly recognized in treatment of lymphoma, AIDS (91), and solid tumors as regimens become more intensive. A wide variety of chemotherapeutic agents have been implicated. Neutropenia is defined as <1000 cells/mm³. It is believed that mucosal injury from the chemotherapy initiates the process which may be limited to mucosal inflammation or progress through transmural inflammation to perforation with overgrowth by a variety of organisms. Gram-negative bowel organisms are common pathogens but Gram-positive organisms, viruses, and fungi are recognized pathogens.

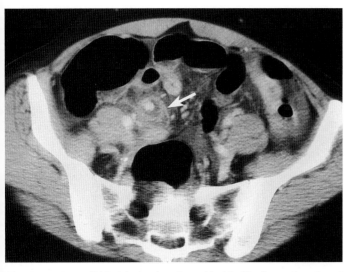

Figure 53.16 Appendicitis. A leukemic patient with right iliac fossa pain and cecal distension. CT shows an appendicolith (arrow), not seen on the abdominal radiograph, with surrounding appendix wall thickening and hyperemia.

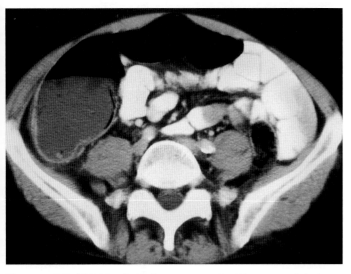

Figure 53.17 Typhlitis. The diagnosis was presumed in this neutropenic leukemic man. CT shows a distended cecum with pneumatosis in its medial wall. Although the wall is hyperemic it is only minimally thickened.

There are three forms of neutropenic colitis but the right colon is predominantly involved. In the commonest form of neutropenic colitis, typhlitis, the cecum is involved and dilates (in Greek a typhlon is a blind-ended sac). Another form also involves the terminal ileum, and in a third there is more generalized bowel ulceration. Patients present with right iliac fossa pain suggestive of appendicitis and, if untreated, may progress rapidly to perforation. CT is performed to assess common alternative surgical diagnoses such as appendicitis (Fig. 53.16) and to look for perforation and abscess formation. In typhlitis, CT usually shows cecal distension, circumferential wall thickening with a halo sign of wall edema. Surgeons are wary of operating. CT may facilitate aspiration and drainage of any collection. Imaging findings overlap with other right iliac fossa inflammatory conditions but the finding of pneumatosis intestinalis with gas in the bowel wall is suggestive of typhlitis (Fig. 53.17). There is a great reluctance to operate on sick

neutropenic patients and if CT excludes a free perforation, generalized peritonitis or an abscess, patients are often treated supportively with the diagnosis presumed to represent a manifestation of neutropenic colitis (Fig. 53.17).

Pseudomembranous Colitis

Pseudomembranous colitis (PMC) is classically associated with prior broad-spectrum antibiotic use and is due to toxin production by *Clostridium difficile*, the growth of which is promoted by changes in the intestinal flora. It is increasingly seen in cancer patients where the association with antibiotic use is more speculative. Rather than the distal colitis or pancolitis seen in earlier reports it is now recognized to be predominantly right sided in 30% to 40% of cases. Stool culture, toxin analysis, and proctosigmoidoscopy are usually diagnostic. Plain films show mucosal edema and irregularity with thumbprinting (Fig. 53.18). There may be progressive dilatation leading to mucosal destruction and perforation. It is now uncommon to perform contrast studies of the bowel but these show a non-specific colitis. If complications are suspected or the diagnosis remains uncertain, CT may be useful. With more proximal colonic involvement there may be fewer symptoms and occasionally the diagnosis only comes to light on the staging CT study of a patient who has attributed symptoms to the chemotherapy (Fig. 53.19). CT shows bowel wall thickening and mucosal hyperemia which may spare the rectum. In more severe cases there is marked thickening of the haustra, usually exceeding a centimeter but up to 3 cm, a helpful discriminator as this degree of thickening is rare in other colitides (96–98).

Graft Vs. Host Disease

GVHD occurs in patients following bone marrow transplant and represents an immunological response by donor lymphocytes against host tissues. Acute GVHD occurs within the first 100 days after transplant, causing a skin rash, severe mucosal inflammation, and diarrhea. Chronic GVHD may occur as early as 45 to 50 days after transplantation, with a skin rash resembling scleroderma. Severe mucosal inflammation is followed by fibrosis and stricture formation. The esophagus is principally affected, less commonly the small and large bowel (90,98). Plain radiographic findings are non-specific and include air–fluid levels, bowel wall and mucosal fold thickening, dilatation of bowel loops but occasionally a gasless abdomen (99). Barium studies are uncommonly performed nowadays but confirm the mucosal thickening and flattening with a "ribbon bowel" appearance, and a rapid transit time. In severe cases, prolonged coating of the bowel wall is seen as barium fills ulcers in the wall and may even be incorporated (100). Both the colon and small bowel may be simultaneously involved although the ileo-colic region is most prone to attack. CT findings are non-specific and show a spectrum of inflammatory changes (101). With small bowel disease, a long length of involvement acts as a clue to the diagnosis but the clinical context is the key indicator (Fig. 53.20) (102).

In one large series neutropenic patients with gastrointestinal complications who underwent CT the commonest causes in order were pseudomembranous colitis, neutropenic colitis, and then GVHD (103). Bowel wall thickening was greatest in pseudomembranous

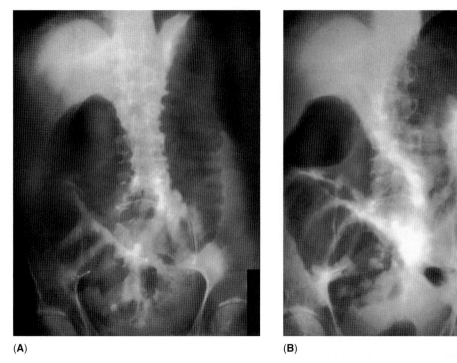

(A)   **(B)**

Figure 53.18 Severe and progressive pseudomembranous colitis. (A) and (B) Serial plain radiographs showing disease progression to mucosal sloughing. Colectomy was required.

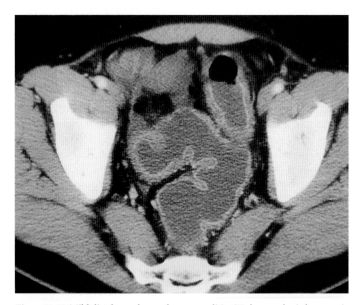

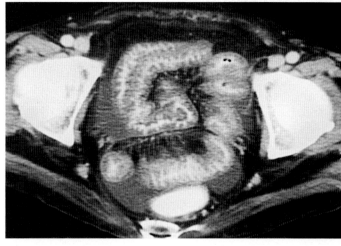

Figure 53.20 Graft versus host disease. CT showing a long length of abnormal small bowel with nodular wall thickening and a small amount of free fluid. This bone marrow transplant patient also had skin signs of GVHD.

Figure 53.19 Mild distal pseudomembranous colitis. CT shows colonic hyperemia and wall thickening in an out-patient who had attributed symptoms to a side-effect of chemotherapy.

colitis (12 mm) and least in GVHD (5 mm). Pneumatosis was limited to neutropenic enterocolitis and bowel ischemia and wall nodularity was significantly more common in pseudomembranous colitis. Findings in neutropenic enterocolitis and GVHD could involve any bowel segment. With high grade GVHD, involvement is particularly of the ileum and cecum but with a tendency to involve multiple small bowel loops which help to distinguish GVHD from neutropenic and pseudomembranous colitis (103). A number of solid malignancies as well as leukemias are now managed by high

dose chemotherapy followed by stem cell rescue or transplantation. As well as the above conditions these profoundly neutropenic patients may be subject to infection with a wide range of viruses and fungi (104).

Other Complications Resulting in an Acute Abdomen

Hemorrhage may occur at a variety of sites in thrombocytopenic patients, including the body wall musculature, notably the iliopsoas and rectus compartments (Fig. 53.21), the bowel, the peritoneal cavity and within pre-existing lesions, especially those undergoing rapid necrosis. Bleeding at any of these sites may result in acute abdominal symptoms; rectus sheath hematoma

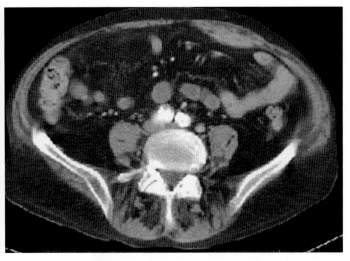

Figure 53.21 Rectus sheath hematoma. This patient, with chemotherapy related thrombocytopenia, developed severe left sided abdominal pain and guarding but CT shows only body wall hemorrhage.

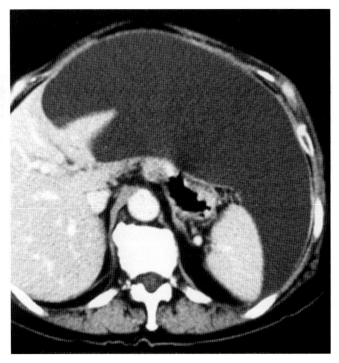

Figure 53.22 Encysted fluid. CT showing a huge encysted fluid collection around the tip of the left lobe of the liver which developed from a surface tumor deposit after experimental therapy for advanced ovarian cancer.

gives a worrying combination of a mass and severe tenderness mimicking peritonism. Plain film findings are typically normal unless mural hemorrhage results in intestinal obstruction but there may be wall thickening (Fig. 53.13). The distinction from intestinal ischemia is difficult with enhanced CT. A short segment with greater than one centimeter of wall thickening favors hemorrhage (105).

Response to some chemotherapies may lead to bowel complications. As well as bleeding into lesions there may be cystic enlargement

or loculation of ascites leading to compression or obstruction (Fig. 53.22) (106). Tumor lysis within bowel may lead directly to perforation or fistulation into adjacent involved solid organs (107). This is seen with lymphoma (especially high-grade) and other chemosensitive tumors such as gastro-intestinal stromal tumors (Fig. 53.23). Another phenomenon seen with tumor deposits, notably lymphoma and melanoma, affecting the bowel is intussusception (Fig. 53.24). This may be seen in patients receiving treatment but whether this is a true complication of therapy induced by changes in the deposits or happenstance is unclear (108).

Severe Infections
Candida albicans
Disseminated candidiasis may be seen in the severely immunocompromised patient and can affect almost any site but with few specific radiological features. In the gut it may cause mucosal erosion and ulceration. A highly suggestive appearance in the esophagus is multiple pseudodiverticula. Abscess formation is common and there may be multiple microabscesses in the liver, spleen, and kidneys (Fig. 53.25). US and CT have been used traditionally to demonstrate visceral lesions that are typically less than 1 cm in size. The frequency of involvement is liver, spleen, and then kidneys, and most patients have hematological malignancy (109). Many conditions affecting the cancer patient can cause multiple liver and spleen lesions but some pattern recognition is possible (110). Larger lesions cause a typical bull's eye appearance. In suspected cases, MR imaging may show more lesions but their appearances are not unique and other infections such as tuberculosis and GVHD may mimic these findings (111).

Other fungal infections which affect the neutropenic patient include *Aspergillus* and Mucorales. Aspergillus can affect the bowel by thrombosis of small vessels leading to both hemorrhage and infarction (104).

Cytomegalovirus (CMV)
Abdominal radiographs in patients with CMV infection reveal bowel wall thickening, dilated bowel, and fluid levels. Pneumatosis intestinalis may occur (112). Patients who have undergone whole-body irradiation, and stem cell transplantation with whole-body irradiation, are at risk for CMV infection and thus it can be difficult to distinguish CMV enteritis from neutropenic colitis and GVHD in these patients. CMV enteritis usually has more perienteric stranding and fluid than neutropenic colitis. Small bowel involvement may be a clue but similar findings also arise with adenovirus and herpes simplex virus infection (104). A feature of adenovirus infection is mural hemorrhage (104).

Clostridial Infection
As well as the toxin-induced colitis which may result from intestinal Clostridial infection, there are other severe and often fatal forms of invasive Clostridial infection including gas gangrene. Patients undergoing chemotherapy, particularly with leukemia, are susceptible and again it is thought that mucosal injury allows invasion by normal gut pathogens. Recognition of gas formation within serosal cavities and tissue planes is crucial in suggesting the diagnosis and CT may be diagnostic well before clinical or radiographic signs are apparent. Here the radiologist has

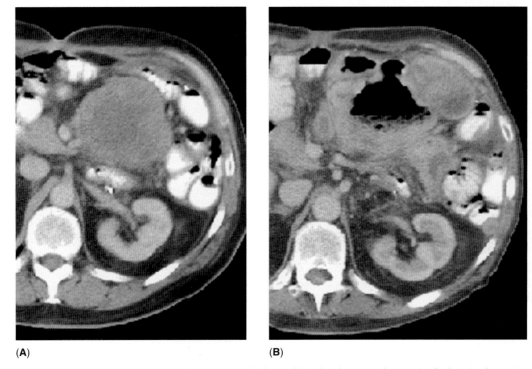

(A)

(B)

Figure 53.23 Perforation of tumor into bowel following chemotherapy. CT (**A**) before and (**B**) after therapy with necrosis of a deposit of gastrointestinal stromal tumor and perforation into an adjacent small bowel loop.

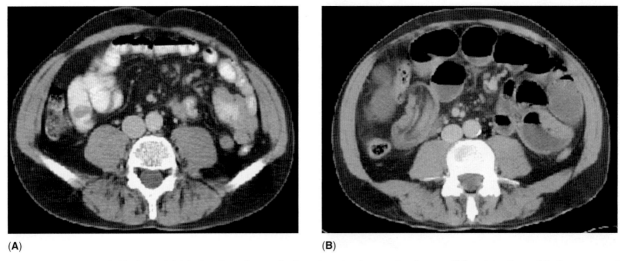

(A)

(B)

Figure 53.24 Intussusception. CT (**A**) before and (**B**) during chemotherapy for disseminated melanoma showing a small deposit in a loop of the ileum next to the cecum and subsequent acute presentation with an ileo-ileal intussusception.

a key role in suggesting the diagnosis in the peritonitic or septic cancer patient (Fig. 53.26) (113). Soft tissue abscesses in neutropenic patients also result from *S. aureus* and gram-negative bacteria but gas formation suggests Clostridial infection (Fig. 53.27).

Drug Toxicity in Specific Organs

Gastrointestinal Tract

Although many cancer patients have gastrointestinal symptoms, there are few radiological manifestations. Complications are due to disordered motility, malabsorption, inflammation, and ischemia. 5-Fluorouracil (5-FU) causes gut toxicity and a clinical picture which mimics inflammatory bowel disease. Ischemic colitis has been described with cisplatin and 5-FU (114). Recently, docetaxel-based chemotherapy for metastatic breast cancer has been associated with a severe colitis, with some suggestion of exacerbation when in combination with vinorelbine (115). Vincristine causes a neuropathy that may result in a chronic ileus with dilated, air-filled small bowel loops on the plain film.

Liver

Fatty infiltration, with increased echogenicity seen using US and decreased attenuation on CT, is the most common manifestation and may be due to a variety of chemotherapies and corticosteroids (116).

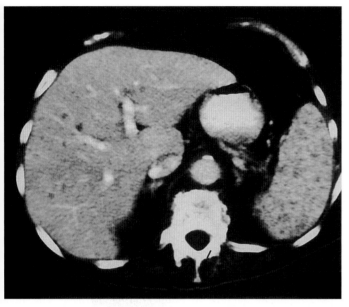

Figure 53.25 Candidiasis. CT showing microabscesses within the liver and spleen.

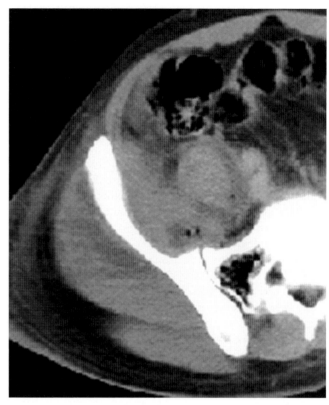

Figure 53.27 Gas gangrene in the right pelvis. CT was performed because of suspected appendicitis or typhlitis in this leukemic man but showed gas forming infection in the right side of the sacrum and muscles around the right iliac bone.

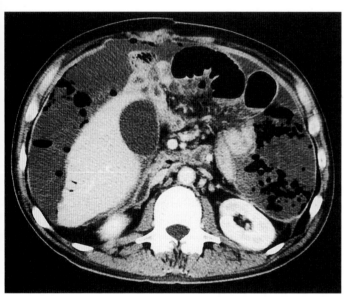

Figure 53.26 Clostridial infection of the peritoneal cavity. CT shows multiple tiny gas bubbles and peripheral portal venous gas.

Several drugs cause hepatic veno-occlusive disease, resulting in a clinical Budd–Chiari syndrome characterized by hepatomegaly and ascites (116). Characteristic findings are a mosaic pattern within the liver which is well demonstrated by contrast-enhanced CT or MR. The latter has the advantage of direct imaging along the plane of the hepatic veins (117).

Pancreas

Acute pancreatitis may occur secondary to high-dose steroid therapy but it has also been described in patients receiving chemotherapy,

notably L-asparaginase (118). Pancreatitis is usually diagnosed on clinical and biochemical features, but in more severe cases US and contrast-enhanced CT may be useful to assess the extent of the condition, including the degree of necrosis and complications such as pseudocyst and abscess formation. Both allow aspiration and drainage of complicated fluid collections. About 2% of children with acute lymphoblastic leukemia develop pancreatitis that is hemorrhagic. US is the key imaging study in children (118).

Genitourinary Tract

Patients may present with acute renal failure due to nephrotoxic chemotherapy agents but urinary tract obstruction must be excluded. In any patient with deteriorating renal function, US is the investigation of choice to distinguish parenchymal disease from vascular disease and obstruction. Cytotoxic agents may cause radiographically non-opaque renal calculi, and treatment of myeloproliferative disorders can result in a uric acid neph-ropathy. These stones are, however, visible on unenhanced CT. Treatment of AIDS patients with protease inhibitors such as indivar also results in radiolucent stones, which may result in severe renal colic (119). These matrix stones may be non-opaque even on CT but this may still be valuable in confirming second-ary signs of ureteric obstruction and excluding other causes of obstruction (120).

- Gastrointestinal complications of chemotherapy include disordered motility, inflammation, and ischemia
- Bleeding diatheses may result in intramural or body wall hemorrhage
- Neutropenic colitis (typhlitis) is a transmural inflammatory process causing thickening of the bowel wall particularly around the cecum and terminal ileum
- Immunocompromised patients are susceptible to gut infection with Candida, CMV, and other viruses and Clostridium including toxin related pseudomembranous colitis
- GVHD may affect the whole gastrointestinal tract and is typically associated with skin changes
- Plain radiological signs of GVHD are usually non-specific but pneumatosis intestinalis may indicate serious complications
- CT of GVHD shows the bowel wall changes, perienteric inflammation, and local or free perforation
- The liver may show fatty infiltration as a response to many agents
- Tumor lysis within bowel tumors, notably high-grade lymphoma, may result in perforation or fistulation
- Urinary tract complications of drug treatment include acute renal failure, renal calculi (which can be radiolucent in AIDS patients receiving protease inhibitors), and hemorrhagic cystitis

THE CENTRAL NERVOUS SYSTEM

In assessment of patients with possible acute complications of therapy the radiologist is required to consider whether the patient has a potentially remediable problem:

- An acute complication of therapy requiring cessation or alteration of therapy
- An infection requiring a specific therapy
- A surgically remediable condition such as hydrocephalus or an extra-axial collection
- Metastatic disease requiring treatment with curative or palliative intent

Clinical presentations, whether with a localized symptom or with generalized confusion or coma, may all result from any of the above. More than one therapy may have been instituted as with leukemia where both intrathecal chemotherapy and craniospinal radiation therapy are administered to this sanctuary site of disease.

Not surprisingly, for some categories of patient with leukemia, complications of treatment are more common than manifestations of the primary disease (121).

Simple and predictable complications resulting from corticosteroid therapy, craniospinal radiotherapy, and chemotherapy, such as white matter change and atrophy may be reversible. When atrophy is persistent after combination therapy it is usually the result of radiation damage.

Myelosuppressive therapies lead to increased risks of infection and bleeding within the CNS. The profound and prolonged neutropenia experienced during treatment for leukemia and some high dose therapies for solid tumors place these individuals at particular risk. Complications to be discussed are:

- Thrombosis and hemorrhage
- Stroke like syndromes, e.g., posterior reversible encephalopathy syndrome
- Drug-related toxicity
- Infectious complications

In a cancer patient with new intracranial symptoms, the main concern is to exclude metastatic disease and brain CT should be the first investigation. With new spinal symptoms, MR imaging is valuable in distinguishing between an intrinsic cord abnormality caused by tumor or myelitis (Fig. 53.28) and the various causes of spinal cord or cauda equina compression, including post-treatment complications such as epidural infection or hemorrhage.

Thrombosis and Hemorrhage

Patients with thrombocytopenia and other bleeding diatheses may develop intracranial or intraspinal hemorrhage. This may be intra-axial or affect any of the dural layers. Hemorrhage may complicate pre-existing primary tumors and metastases, leading to sudden deterioration. A particular concern is for bleeding complications in patients undergoing lumbar puncture or other spinal interventions including intrathecal therapies, epidural anesthesia, and other spinal interventions for pain palliation.

Patients with cancer may also have a generalized "pro-coagulant" tendency to thrombosis and this also predisposes to cerebral venous thrombosis. This diagnosis remains elusive especially as the hemorrhage and/or infarction resulting from this may give a ready explanation for symptoms. Contrast-enhanced CT is valuable in investigation of this entity by showing the "delta" sign as a triangular filling defect in the superior sagittal sinus but MR venography is the investigation of choice where available in the emergent setting (Fig. 53.29). Unenhanced CT is often the initial study and findings of venous thrombosis may be subtle, including a non-arterial territory distribution of infarcts, especially if bilateral and hemorrhagic. The presence of hyperdensity along the line of venous sinuses should alert to the diagnosis (Fig. 53.29). CT features suggesting cerebral venous thrombosis include:

- Hyperdensity along the line of venous sinuses, the "cord" sign, on unenhanced CT
- A non-arterial territory distribution of infarction, especially if bilateral and hemorrhagic
- The "delta" sign with contrast-enhanced CT

Some chemotherapeutic agents such as L-asparaginase used in treatment of leukemia may result in a disseminated intravascular coagulopathy with either bleeding or thrombotic sequelae including cerebral venous thrombosis (122). Intra-axial bleeding is more common than extra-axial. Up to 2% of leukemic patients treated with L-asparaginase develop hemorrhagic or non-hemorrhagic infarcts (123).

Posterior Reversible Encephalopathy Syndrome

Stroke-like syndromes can also result from vasospasm and small vessel ischemia. A syndrome similar to the eclamptic encephalopathy of late pregnancy has been recognized in cancer patients receiving acute therapy. As in eclampsia there are a variety of manifestations, but dominant features are seizure and cortical

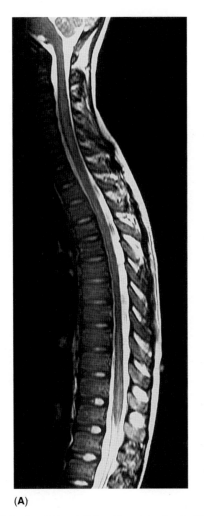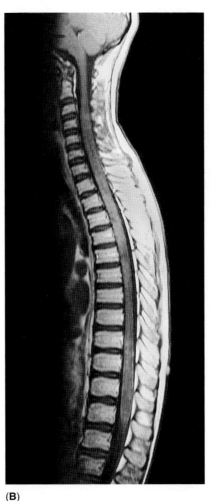

(A)   **(B)**

Figure 53.28 Myelitis. (**A**) T2-weighted and (**B**) gadolinium T1-weighted sagittal MR imaging in a leukemic boy with paraparesis. There is patchy non-enhancing abnormality with slight cord expansion. CSF examination showed no leukemic cells.

visual loss. The syndrome has been given a variety of names: posterior reversible encephalopathy syndrome (PRES); posterior leucoencephalopathy syndrome (PLES); posterior ischemic encephalopathy (PIE) and is also discussed in chapter 58. MR imaging typically shows posterior T2 signal increase with parieto-occipital edema involving the visual areas but the findings may be more widespread affecting the posterior frontal lobes, temporal lobes, thalamus, brainstem, and cerebellum (Fig. 53.30) (124). In some cases hemorrhage occurs leading to some irreversible changes (125). With non-hemorrhagic PRES, diffusion-weighted imaging (DWI) may be useful to show areas of high DWI signal or pseudonormalized apparent diffusion coefficient (ADC) which herald progression to cerebral infarction (126).

Drug-Related Toxicity

A variety of drugs may be directly neurotoxic but the majority of these do not cause changes that can be identified radiologically (Table 53.2). The most common imaging abnormality that can be identified is craniospinal white matter change (leuco-encephalopathy) (127). The neurotoxic effects of chemotherapy may be potentiated by radiotherapy (128). Drugs that cause leucoencephalopathy include methotrexate, 5-FU, cytarabine, and cyclosporin A (129). The probable mechanism of chemotherapeutic toxicity is vascular injury, causing endothelial leakage with fluid accumulation or endothelial thickening and eventual infarction and necrosis (128). As with the lung and the bowel, the brain and spinal cord have limited and overlapping responses to a variety of insults. The other mechanism in leucoencephalopathy is (re)activation of viral particles as seen with progressive multifocal leucoencephalopathy (PML). These complications are discussed in chapter 58.

With severe and established cases, focal or diffuse white matter low attenuation is seen with CT (130). With MR imaging there is high signal intensity on T2-weighted images (127). MR usually reveals a greater burden of white matter lesions, especially with sequences using fluid-attenuated inversion recovery (FLAIR). There may be marginal enhancement with contrast media on either modality. A more aggressive focal or diffuse necrotizing leucoencephalopathy with associated demyelination and necrosis is described as a later complication occurring

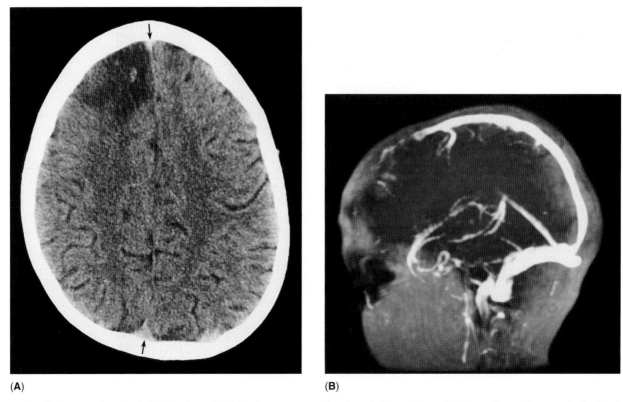

(A) **(B)**

Figure 53.29 Cerebral venous thrombosis. (**A**) Unenhanced CT showing a non-arterial territory infarct with petechial hemorrhage with arrows indicating the sagittal sinus which is abnormally dense anteriorly. (**B**) MR venography confirming thrombosis.

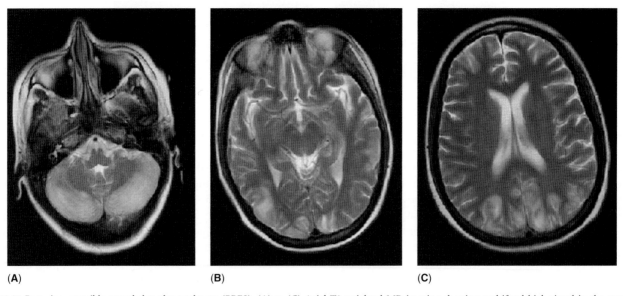

(A) **(B)** **(C)**

Figure 53.30 Posterior reversible encephalopathy syndrome (PRES). (**A**) to (**C**) Axial T2-weighted MR imaging showing multifocal high signal in the cerebellum, occipital, and parietal lobes. This leukemic woman developed seizures and cortical blindness during induction therapy but recovered fully.

Table 53.2 Drugs Causing Neurotoxicity

Drug	Toxicity
Vincristine	Peripheral neuropathy
Cisplatin	Peripheral neuropathy, encephalopathy
Cytarabine	Cerebellar dysfunction
Ifosfamide	Personality change, cerebellar dysfunction, cranial nerve lesions
5-Fluorouracil	Cerebellar dysfunction
Methotrexate	Focal neurological defects

after weeks or months of treatment. This is typically seen in treatment of leukemia and is more common with combinations of IV and intrathecal methotrexate and radiotherapy. It may be reversed if intrathecal infusion of methotrexate is discontinued (131). MR imaging reveals patchy involvement of the periventricular white matter and centrum semiovale, which becomes confluent. The subcortical U-fibres, corpus callosum, brain stem, and cerebellum are usually spared. Enhancement

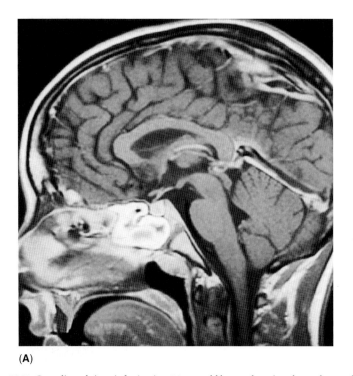

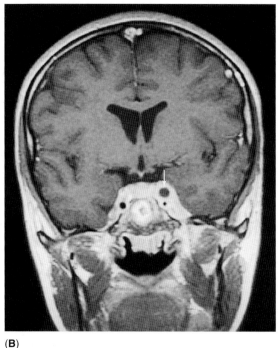

(A)　　　　　　　　　　　　　　　　　　　　　　　(B)

Figure 53.31 Complicated sinus infection in a 14-year-old boy undergoing chemotherapy for soft tissue sarcoma who developed left ophthalmoplegia. MR imaging with (A) sagittal and (B) coronal post-gadolinium images showing (A) an infected sphenoid sinus and (B) a left sided cavernous sinus thrombosis (arrow) compressing the carotid artery below.

and mass effect are only seen in the most severe cases mimicking tumor infiltration. Treatment of colonic cancer with 5-FU and levamisole may cause acute demyelination, with multifocal enhancing white matter lesions on MR imaging (132). It may preferentially affect the cerebellum causing ataxia.

DWI may show abnormality earlier than FLAIR which relies upon T2 contrast to identify potentially reversible areas of abnormality in the acute phase of toxicity. In leukemic patients with clinical features of methotrexate toxicity DWI showed abnormalities which correlated well with clinical deficits when there was little or no T2 abnormality (129).

Investigation of patients with suspected acute cerebral complications of treatment should:

- Begin with pre-and post-contrast CT in the emergency setting
- Utilize MR imaging wherever possible with younger and potentially curable patients
- Use FLAIR sequences to maximize detection of peri-ventricular lesions
- Use gadolinium-enhanced images to exclude underlying mass lesions
- Consider the use of DWI with unexplained acute presentations

There are also spinal effects of intrathecal therapies, resulting in a myelitis (Fig. 53.28) or radiculopathy. An anterior lumbosacral radiculopathy has been described with intrathecal methotrexate therapy. This entity is not well understood but may reflect gravitational dose-dependent toxicity on the nerve roots (133). If the diagnosis is considered, IV injection of contrast medium is needed as root enhancement on MR imaging may be the only abnormal finding in an examination which is usually performed to exclude an epidural collection.

Infectious Complications

Neutropenic patients are predisposed to many infections of the CNS, including fungal and yeast infections, particularly Aspergillosis, Cryptococcus, and Candida. The risk is related to the degree of neutropenia and patients with neutrophil counts of less than 100 cell/mm³ sustained for more than two weeks are at particular risk of fungal infection (134). Broad-spectrum antibiotic therapy also compounds this risk. Bacterial meningitis with *H. influenzae* and *S. pneumoniae* may occur in splenectomized patients (135).

Infection of the meninges and brain may result from direct spread of aggressive infection in the paranasal sinuses and middle ear and these should always be carefully inspected on CT and MR imaging sections of the face and skull base, looking for bony changes on appropriate window settings (Fig. 53.31) (136). Complex sinus disease may also encroach into the orbit and there may be secondary involvement and thrombosis of venous sinuses. In such cases the role of the radiologist is to be alert to such complications, to look for abscess formation and, importantly, to consider the safety of lumbar puncture for microbiological assessment. In immunocompromised patients there may not be the immune response to infection seen in competent hosts and thus contrast enhancement may be reduced making distinction of masses and abscesses from infarcts more difficult.

It is not possible to provide a microbiological diagnosis on the basis of imaging features but a few key signs may be valuable in guiding antibiotic, antifungal, or antiviral therapies.

Aspergillosis (136) invades vascular structures with hemorrhagic infarction as well as abscess formation. Pulmonary or sinus infection is usually coincident. Cryptococcus (137) results in a meningitis with extension into basal perforating substances with enhancing lesions in the midbrain and basal ganglia. Other organisms to consider in a patient with basal meningitis are listeria and tuberculosis which may show marked meningeal enhancement and lead to a secondary communicating hydrocephalus. Cytomegalovirus infection affects the periventricular region with a nodular rim of subependymal enhancement. Many agents may result in encephalitis but herpes simplex virus preferentially attacks the temporal lobes. Imaging findings are often asymmetric.

Complications of Novel Agents in the Abdomen and CNS

The new agents which attack tumor vascularity such as bevacizumab have been associated with a variety of abdominal complications. It is believed that they interfere with vascular growth factors in healing or result in necrosis of tissues due to other vascular effects. Acute complications described have included perforation of bowel, anastomotic breakdown, and delayed wound healing with dehiscence (138,139).

As yet, we are not aware of any major recognized CNS complications of these agents.

Key Points: CNS Complications

- MR imaging is the most sensitive imaging modality for identifying the neurotoxic effects of cancer treatment
- MR venography is the preferred examination to show cerebral venous sinus thrombosis, a recognized complication of L-asparaginase therapy for leukemia
- Posterior reversible encephalopathy syndrome is increasingly recognized as a complication of toxic induction therapies, especially for leukemia
- Necrotizing leucoencephalopathy is usually seen in combination therapy with IV or intrathecal methotrexate and radiotherapy for the treatment of leukemia
- Immunocompromised patients are susceptible to CNS infection producing meningitis and encephalitis and this may spread from the paranasal sinuses
- Patients with neutrophil counts of less than 100 cells/mm^3 sustained for more than two weeks are at particular risk of fungal infection

Summary

- Complications of treatment in the chest are the result of drug toxicity, infection, and those related to IV lines and catheters
- Drug-induced lung disease relies on recognizing the temporal relationship between the drug and the onset of respiratory disease, and the exclusion of other potentially treatable causes

- Patients with hematological malignancies and BMT recipients are in the highest risk groups for developing infective and non-infective complications
- Chest radiography is usually the first diagnostic test to demonstrate subclinical disease and is useful for documenting the evolution of parenchymal abnormalities
- HRCT is the most sensitive and specific radiological test but frequently a definitive diagnosis cannot be made
- Neutropenic colitis (typhlitis) is a transmural inflammatory process causing thickening of the bowel wall particularly around the cecum and terminal ileum. It is most commonly seen in patients treated for leukemia, lymphoma, and AIDS
- Immunocompromised patients are susceptible to gut infection with Candida, CMV, and other viruses, and Clostridium, including toxin-related pseudomembranous colitis
- GVHD occurs following BMT and may be acute or chronic. Acute GVHD may affect the whole gastrointestinal tract and is typically associated with skin changes
- Hemorrhage, tumor lysis within bowel leading to perforation and intussusception may present as an acute complication of treatment
- MR imaging is the most sensitive imaging modality for identifying the neurotoxic effects of cancer treatment
- MR venography is the preferred examination to show cerebral venous sinus thrombosis, a recognized complication of L-asparaginase therapy for leukemia
- PRES is increasingly recognized as a complication of toxic induction therapies, especially in leukemia
- Spinal MR imaging helps to distinguish between tumor, myelitis, epidural infection or hematoma, which may particularly complicate intrathecal and epidural therapies

REFERENCES

1. Cooper JA Jr, White DA, Matthay RA. Drug-induced pulmonary disease: part 1: cytotoxic drugs. Am Rev Respir Dis 1986; 133: 321–40.
2. Carver JR, Shapiro CL, Ng A, et al. American Society of Clinical Oncology clinical evidence review of the ongoing care of adult cancer survivors: cardiac and pulmonary late effects. J Clin Oncol 2007; 25: 3991–4008.
3. Sleijfer S. Bleomycin induced pneumonitis. Chest 2001; 120: 617–24.
4. Cleverley JR, Screaton NJ, Hiorns MP, Flint JD, Müller NL. Drug-induced lung disease: high-resolution CT and histological findings. Clin Rad 2002; 57: 292–99.
5. Rossi SE, Erasmus JJ, McAdams HP, Sporn TA. Goodman PC. Pulmonary drug toxicity: radiologic and pathologic manifestations. Radiographics 2000; 20: 1245–59.
6. Ellis SJ, Cleverley JR, Müller NL. Drug-induced lung disease: high-resolution CT findings. AJR Am J Roentgenol. 2000; 175: 1019–24.
7. Meadors M, Floyd J, Perry MC. Pulmonary toxicity of chemotherapy. Semin Oncol, 2006; 33: 98–105.

8. Padley SP, Adler B, Hansell DM, Müller NL. High-resolution computed tomography of drug-induced lung disease. Clin Radiol 1992; 46: 232–6.

9. Bellamy EA, Husband JE, Blaquiere RM, Law MR. Bleomycin-related lung damage: CT evidence. Radiology 1985; 156: 155–8.

10. Rosenow EC 3rd. Drug-induced pulmonary disease. Dis Mon 1994; 40: 253–310.

11. Rosenow EC, Myers JL, Pisani RJ. Drug-induced pulmonary disease. An update. Chest 1992; 102: 239–50.

12. Cooper JAD, White DA, Matthay RA. Drug-induced pulmonary disease. Part 2: Noncytotoxic drugs. Am Rev Respir Dis 1986; 133: 488–505.

13. Saxon RR, Klein JS, Bar MH, et al. Pathogenesis of pulmonary edema during interleukin-2 therapy: correlation of chest radiographic and clinical findings in 54 patients. AJR Am J Roentgenol 1991; 156: 281–5.

14. Conant EF, Fox KR, Miller WT. Pulmonary edema as a complication of interleukin-2 therapy. AJR Am J Roentgenol 1989; 152: 749–52.

15. Ma LD, Taylor GA, Wharam MD, Wiley JM. "Recall" pneumonitis: adriamycin potentiation of radiation pneumonitis in two children. Radiology 1993; 187: 465–7.

16. Schwarte S, Wagner K, Karstens JH, Bremer M. Radiation recall pneumonitis induced by gemcitabine. Strahlenther Onkol 2007; 183: 215–17.

17. Miya T, Ono Y, Tanaka H, Koshiishi Y, Goya T. [Radiation recall pneumonitis induced by Gefitinib (Iressa): a case report] Nihon Kokyuki Gakkai Zasshi. 2003; 41; 565–8.

18. Thomas PS, Agrawal S, Gore M, Geddes DM. Recall lung pneumonitis due to carmustine after radiotherapy. Thorax 1995; 50: 1116–18.

19. Schweitzer VG, Juillard GJ, Bajada CL, Parker RG. Radiation recall dermatitis and pneumonitis in a patient treated with paclitaxel. Cancer 1995; 76: 1069–72.

20. O'sullivan JM, Huddart RA, Norman AR, et al. Predicting the risk of bleomycin lung toxicity in patients with germ-cell tumors. Ann Oncol 2003; 14: 91–6.

21. Buchler T, Bomanji J, Lee SM. FDG-PET in bleomycin-induced pneumonitis following ABVD chemotherapy for Hodgkin's disease—a useful tool for monitoring pulmonary toxicity and disease activity. Haematologica, 2007; 92: e120–1.

22. Chastagner P, Kalifa C, Doz F, et al. Outcome of children treated with preradiation chemotherapy for a high-grade glioma: results of a French Society of Pediatric Oncology (SFOP) Pilot Study. Pediatr Blood Cancer 2007; 49: 803–7.

23. O'Driscoll BR, Kalra S, Gattamaneni HR, Woodcock AA. Late carmustine lung fibrosis. Age at treatment may influence severity and survival. Chest 1995; 107: 1355–7.

24. Lohani S, O'Driscoll BR, Woodcock AA. 25-year study of lung fibrosis following carmustine therapy for brain tumor in childhood. Chest 2004; 126: 1007.

25. Castro M, Veeder MH, Mailliard JA, Tazelaar HD, Jett JR. A prospective study of pulmonary function in patients receiving mitomycin. Chest 1996; 109: 939–44.

26. Verweij J, van Zanten T, Souren T, Golding R, Pinedo HM. Prospective study on the dose relationship of mitomycin C-induced interstitial pneumonitis. Cancer 1987; 60: 756–61.

27. Rancati T, Ceresoli GL, Gagliardi G, Schipani S, Cattaneo GM. Factors predicting radiation pneumonitis in lung cancer patients: a retrospective study. Radiother Oncol 2003; 67: 275–83.

28. Lesesne JB, Rothschild N, Erickson B, et al. Cancer-associated hemolytic-uremic syndrome: analysis of 85 cases from a national registry. J Clin Oncol 1989; 7: 781–9.

29. Rivera MP, Kris MG, Gralla RJ, White DA. Syndrome of acute dyspnea related to combined mitomycin plus vinca alkaloid chemotherapy. Am J Clin Oncol 1995; 18: 245–50.

30. Hamada K, Nagai S, Kitaichi M, et al. Cyclophosphamide-induced late-onset lung disease. Intern Med 2003; 42: 82–7.

31. Segura A, Yuste A, Cercos A, et al. Pulmonary fibrosis induced by cyclophosphamide. Ann Pharmacother 2001; 35: 894–7.

32. Brieva J. Cyclophosphamide-induced acute respiratory distress syndrome. Respirology 2007; 12: 769–73.

33. Rowinsky EK, Donehower RC. Paclitaxel (taxol) N Engl J Med 1995; 332: 1004–14.

34. Wong P, Leung AN, Berry GJ, et al. Paclitaxel-induced hypersensitivity pneumonitis: radiographic and CT findings. AJR Am J Roentgenol 2001; 176: 718–20.

35. Read WL, Mortimer JE, Picus J. Severe interstitial pneumonitis associated with docetaxel administration. Cancer 2002; 94: 847–53.

36. Suzaki N, Hiraki A, Takigawa N, et al. Severe interstitial pneumonia induced by paclitaxel in a patient with adenocarcinoma of the lung. Acta Med Okayama 2006; 60: 295–8.

37. Ostoros G, Pretz A, Fillinger J, Soltesz I, Dome B. Fatal pulmonary fibrosis induced by paclitaxel: a case report and review of the literature. Int J Gynecol Cancer 2006; 16(Suppl 1): 391–3.

38. Widakowich C, de Castro G Jr, de Azambuja E, Dinh P, Awada A. Review: side effects of approved molecular targeted therapies in solid cancers. Oncologist 2007; 12: 1443–55.

39. de Castro G Jr, Awada A. Side effects of anti-cancer molecular-targeted therapies (not monoclonal antibodies). Curr Opin Oncol 2006; 18: 307–15.

40. Byrd JC, Waselenko JK, Maneatis TJ, et al. Rituximab therapy in hematologic malignancy patients with circulating blood tumor cells: association with increased infusion-related side effects and rapid blood tumor clearance. J Clin Oncol 1999; 17: 791–5.

41. Vahid B, Mehrotra A. Trastuzumab (Herceptin)-associated lung injury. Respirology 2006; 11: 655–8.

42. Wagner SA, Mehta AC, Laber DA. Rituximab-induced interstitial lung disease. Am J Hematol 2007; 82: 916–19.

43. Johnson DH, Fehrenbacher L, Novotny WF, et al. Randomized phase II trial comparing bevacizumab plus carboplatin and paclitaxel with carboplatin and paclitaxel alone in previously untreated locally advanced or metastatic non-small-cell lung cancer. J Clin Oncol 2004; 22: 2184–91.

44. Kabbinavar F, Hurwitz HI, Fehrenbacher L, et al. Phase II, randomized trial comparing bevacizumab plus fluorouracil (FU)/leucovorin (LV) with FU/LV alone in patients with metastatic colorectal cancer. J Clin Oncol 2003; 21: 60–5.

45. Ando M, Okamoto I, Yamamoto N, et al. Predictive factors for interstitial lung disease, antitumor response, and survival

in non-small-cell lung cancer patients treated with gefitinib. J Clin Oncol 2006; 24: 2549–56.

46. Takano T, Ohe Y, Kusumoto M, et al. Risk factors for interstitial lung disease and predictive factors for tumor response in patients with advanced non-small cell lung cancer treated with gefitinib. Lung Cancer 2004; 45: 93–104.

47. Endo M, Johkoh T, Kimura K, Yamamoto N. Imaging of gefitinib-related interstitial lung disease: multi-institutional analysis by the West Japan Thoracic Oncology Group. Lung Cancer 2006; 52: 135–40.

48. Shepherd FA, Rodrigues Pereira J, Ciuleanu T, et al. Erlotinib in previously treated non-small-cell lung cancer. N Engl J Med 2005; 353: 123–32.

49. Liu V, White DA, Zakowski MF, et al. Pulmonary toxicity associated with erlotinib. Chest 2007; 132: 1042–4.

50. Makris D, Scherpereel A, Copin MC, et al. Fatal interstitial lung disease associated with oral erlotinib therapy for lung cancer. BMC Cancer 2007; 7: 150.

51. Ohnishi K, Sakai F, Kudoh S, Ohno R. Twenty-seven cases of drug-induced interstitial lung disease associated with imatinib mesylate. Leukemia 2006; 20: 1162–4.

52. Breccia M, D'Elia GM, D'Andrea M, Latagliata R, Alimena G. Pleural-pericardic effusion as uncommon complication in CML patients treated with Imatinib. Eur J Haematol 2005; 74: 89–90.

53. De Botton S, Dombret H, Sanz M, et al. Incidence, clinical features, and outcome of all trans-retinoic acid syndrome in 413 cases of newly diagnosed acute promyelocytic leukemia. The European APL Group. Blood 1998; 92: 2712–18.

54. Jung JI, Choi JE, Hahn ST, et al. Radiologic features of all-trans-retinoic acid syndrome. AJR Am J Roentgenol 2002; 178: 475–80.

55. Ng R, Better N, Green MD. Anticancer agents and cardiotoxicity. Semin Oncol 2006; 33: 2–14.

56. Bock J, Doenitz A, Andreesen R, Reichle A, Hennemann B. Pericarditis after high-dose chemotherapy: more frequent than expected? Onkologie 2006; 29: 321–4.

57. Gençer S, Salepçi T, Ozer S. Evaluation of infectious etiology and prognostic risk factors of febrile episodes in neutropenic cancer patients. J Infect 2003; 47: 65–72.

58. Ozer H, Armitage JO, Bennett CL, et al. 2000 update of recommendations for the use of hematopoietic colony-stimulating factors: evidence-based, clinical practice guidelines. American Society of Clinical Oncology Growth Factors Expert Panel. J Clin Oncol 2000; 18; 3558–85.

59. Joos L, Tamm M. Breakdown of pulmonary host defense in the immunocompromised host: cancer chemotherapy. Proc Am Thorac Soc 2005; 2: 445–8.

60. Rossini F, Verga M, Pioltelli P, et al. Incidence and outcome of pneumonia in patients with acute leukemia receiving first induction therapy with anthracycline-containing regimens. Haematologica 2000; 85; 1255–60.

61. Heussel CP, Kauczor HU, Heussel GE, et al. Pneumonia in febrile neutropenic patients and in bone marrow and blood stem-cell transplant recipients: use of high-resolution computed tomography. J Clin Oncol 1999; 17; 796–805.

62. Caillot D, Casasnovas O, Bernard A, et al. Improved management of invasive pulmonary aspergillosis in neutropenic

patients using early thoracic computed tomographic scan and surgery. J Clin Oncol 1997; 15; 139–47.

63. Escuissato DL, Gasparetto EL, Marchiori E, et al. Pulmonary infections after bone marrow transplantation: high-resolution CT findings in 111 patients. AJR Am J Roentgenol 2005; 185; 608–15.

64. Barloon TJ, Galvin JR, Mori M, Stanford W, Gingrich RD. High-resolution ultrafast chest CT in the clinical management of febrile bone marrow transplant patients with normal or nonspecific chest roentgenograms. Chest 1991; 99; 928–33.

65. Joos L, Chhajed PN, Wallner J, et al. Pulmonary infections diagnosed by BAL: a 12-year experience in 1066 immunocompromised patients. Respir Med 2007; 101: 93–7.

66. Sharma S, Nadrous HF, Peters SG, et al. Pulmonary complications in adult blood and marrow transplant recipients: autopsy findings. Chest 2005; 128: 1385–92.

67. Carratalà J, Rosón B, Fernández-Sevilla A, Alcaide F, Gudiol F. Bacteremic pneumonia in neutropenic patients with cancer: causes, empirical antibiotic therapy, and outcome. Arch Intern Med 1998; 158: 868–72.

68. Leung AN, Gosselin MV, Napper CH, et al. Pulmonary infections after bone marrow transplantation: clinical and radiographic findings. Radiology 1999; 210; 699–710.

69. Bruno C, Minniti S, Vassanelli A, Pozzi-Mucelli R. Comparison of CT features of Aspergillus and bacterial pneumonia in severely neutropenic patients. J Thorac Imaging. 2007; 22: 160–5.

70. Soubani AO, Miller KB, Hassoun PM. Pulmonary complications of bone marrow transplantation. Chest 1996; 109: 1066–77.

71. Wah TM, Moss HA, Robertson RJ, Barnard DL. Pulmonary complications following bone marrow transplantation. Br J Radiol 2003; 76: 373–9.

72. Franquet T, Lee KS, Müller NL. Thin-section CT findings in 32 immunocompromised patients with cytomegalovirus pneumonia who do not have AIDS. AJR Am J Roentgenol 2003; 181: 1059–63.

73. Gosselin MV, Adams RH. Pulmonary complications in bone marrow transplantation. J Thorac Imaging. 2002; 17: 132–44.

74. Bergin CJ, Wirth RL, Berry GJ, Castellino RA. Pneumocystis carinii pneumonia: CT and HRCT observations. J Comput Assist Tomogr 1990; 14: 756–9.

75. Socié G, Clift RA, Blaise D, et al. Busulfan plus cyclophosphamide compared with total-body irradiation plus cyclophosphamide before marrow transplantation for myeloid leukemia: long-term follow-up of 4 randomized studies. Blood 2001; 98; 3569–74.

76. Worthy SA, Flint JD, Müller NL. Pulmonary complications after bone marrow transplantation: high-resolution CT and pathologic findings. Radiographics 1997; 17: 1359–71.

77. Afessa B, Tefferi A, Litzow MR, et al. Diffuse alveolar hemorrhage in hematopoietic stem cell transplant recipients. Am J Respir Crit Care Med 2002; 166: 641–5.

78. Witte RJ, Gurney JW, Robbins RA, et al. Diffuse pulmonary alveolar hemorrhage after bone marrow transplantation: radiographic findings in 39 patients. AJR Am J Roentgenol 1991; 157: 461–4.

79. Afessa B, Peters SG. Noninfectious pneumonitis after blood and marrow transplant. Curr Opin Oncol 2008; 20: 227–33.

80. Krowka MJ, Rosenow EC 3rd, Hoagland HC. Pulmonary complications of bone marrow transplantation. Chest 1985; 87: 237–46.

81. Kumar S, Tefferi A. Spontaneous pneumomediastinum and subcutaneous emphysema complicating bronchiolitis obliterans after allogeneic bone marrow transplantation—case report and review of literature. Ann Hematol 2001; 80: 430–5.

82. Sargent MA, Cairns RA, Murdoch MJ, et al. Obstructive lung disease in children after allogeneic bone marrow transplantation: evaluation with high-resolution CT. AJR Am J Roentgenol 1995; 164: 693–6.

83. Dodd JD, Müller NL. Bronchiolitis obliterans organizing pneumonia after bone marrow transplantation: high-resolution computed tomography findings in 4 patients. J Comput Assist Tomogr 2005; 29: 540–3.

84. Lee KS, Kullnig P, Hartman TE, Müller NL. Cryptogenic organizing pneumonia: CT findings in 43 patients. AJR Am J Roentgenol 1994; 162: 543–6.

85. Ganeshan A, Warakaulle DR, Uberoi R. Central venous access. Cardiovasc Intervent Radiol 2007; 30: 26–33.

86. Jensen MO. Anatomical basis of central venous catheter fracture. Clin Anat 2008; 21: 106–10.

87. Vescia S, Baumgärtner AK, Jacobs VR, et al. Management of venous port systems in oncology: a review of current evidence. Ann Oncol 2008; 19: 9–15.

88. Boersma RS, Jie KS, Verbon A, van Pampus EC, Schouten HC. Thrombotic and infectious complications of central venous catheters in patients with hematological malignancies. Ann Oncol 2008; 19: 433–42.

89. Niscola P, Romani C, Cupelli L, et al. Mucositis in patients with hematologic malignancies: an overview. Haematologica 2007; 92: 222–31.

90. Ho LM, Paulson EK, Thompson WM. Pneumatosis intestinalis in the adult: benign to life-threatening causes. AJR Am J Roentgenol 2007; 188: 1604–13.

91. Jones B, Wall SD. Gastrointestinal disease in the immunocompromised host. Radiologic Clin North Am 1992; 30: 555–77.

92. Day DL, Ramsey NKC, Letourneau JG. Pneumatosis intestinalis after bone marrow transplantation. AJR Am J Roentgenol 1988; 151: 85–7.

93. Lane MJ, Katz DS, Mindelzun RE, et al. Spontaneous intramural small bowel haemorrhage: importance of non-contrast CT. Clin Radiol 1997; 52: 378–80.

94. Macari M, Balthazar EJ. CT of bowel wall thickening: significance and pitfalls of interpretation. AJR Am J Roentgenol 2001; 176: 1105–16.

95. Wagner ML, Rosenberg HS, Fernbach DJ, et al. Typhlitis: a complication of leukemia in childhood. AJR Am J Roentgenol 1970; 109: 341–50.

96. Fishman EK, Kavuru M, Jones B, et al. Pseudomembranous colitis: CT evaluation of 26 cases. Radiology 1991; 180: 57–60.

97. Kawamoto S, Horton KM, Fishman EK. Pseudomembranous colitis: spectrum of imaging findings with clinical and pathologic correlation. Radiographics 1999; 19: 887–97.

98. Horton KM, Corl FM, Fishman EK. CT evaluation of the colon: inflammatory disease. Radiographics 2000; 20: 399–418.

99. Jones B, Cramer SS, Saral R, et al. Gastrointestinal inflammation after bone marrow transplantation: graft-versus-host disease or opportunistic infection? AJR Am J Roentgenol 1988; 150: 277–81.

100. Belli AM, Williams MP. Graft versus host disease: findings on plain abdominal radiography. Clin Radiol 1988; 39: 262–4.

101. Kalantari BN, Mortelé KJ, Cantisani V, et al. CT features with pathologic correlation of acute gastrointestinal graft-versus-host disease after bone marrow transplantation in adults. AJR Am J Roentgenol 2003; 181: 1621–5.

102. Horton KM, Corl FM, Fishman EK. CT of non-neoplastic diseases of the small bowel: spectrum of disease. J Comput Assist Tomogr 1999; 23: 417–28.

103. Kirkpatrick ID, Greenberg HM. Gastrointestinal complications in the neutropenic patient: characterization and differentiation with abdominal CT. Radiology 2003; 226: 668–74.

104. Schmit M, Bethge W, Beck R, et al. CT of gastrointestinal complications associated with hematopoietic stem cell transplantation. AJR Am J Roentgenol 2008; 190: 712–19.

105. Macari M, Chandarana H, Balthazar E, et al. Intestinal ischemia versus intramural haemorrhage: CT evaluation. AJR Am J Roentgenol 2003; 180: 177–84.

106. Spencer JA, Crosse BA, Mannion RA, et al. Gastroduodenal obstruction from ovarian cancer: imaging features and clinical outcome. Clin Radiol 2000; 55: 264–72.

107. Scott J, Spencer JA, MacLennan KA. Choledochoduodenal fistula complicating non-Hodgkin's lymphoma of the duodenum during chemotherapy. Clin Radiol 2001; 56: 508–10.

108. Bender GN, Maglinte DD, McLarney JH, Rex D, Kelvin FM. Malignant melanoma: patterns of metastasis to the small bowel, reliability of imaging studies, and clinical relevance. Am J Gastroenterol 2001; 96: 2392–400.

109. Shirkhoda A. CT findings in hepatosplenic and renal candidiasis. J Comput Assist Tomogr 1987; 11: 795–8.

110. Bean MJ, Horton KM, Fishman EK. Concurrent focal hepatic and splenic lesions: a pictorial guide to differential diagnosis. J Comput Assist Tomogr 2004; 28: 605–12.

111. Semelka RC, Kelekis NL, Sallah S, et al. Hepatosplenic fungal disease: diagnostic accuracy and spectrum of appearances on MR imaging. AJR Am J Roentgenol 1997; 169: 1311–16.

112. Olliff JFC, Williams MP. Radiological appearances of cytomegalovirus infections. Clin Radiol 1989; 40: 463–7.

113. Spencer JA, Elliot L. Clostridial infection of the abdomen: CT findings in two successfully treated patients. AJR Am J Roentgenol 1996; 166: 1094–6.

114. Zilling TL, Ahren B. Ischaemic pancolitis. A serious complication of chemotherapy in a previously irradiated patient. Acta Chirurgica Scand 1989; 155: 77–9.

115. Ibrahim NK, Sahin AA, Dubrow RA, et al. Colitis associated with docetaxel-based chemotherapy in patients with metastatic breast cancer. Lancet 2000; 355: 281–3.

116. Gatenby RA. The radiology of drug-induced disorders in the gastrointestinal tract. Semin Roentgenol 1995; 30: 62–76.

117. Ward J, Spencer JA, Guthrie JA, et al. Liver transplantation: dynamic contrast-enhanced magnetic resonance imaging of the hepatic vasculature. Clin Radiol 1996; 51: 191–7.

118. Sahu S, Saika S, Pai SK, Advani SH. L-Asparaginase (Leunase) induced pancreatitis in childhood acute lymphoblastic leukemia. Pediatr Hematol Oncol 1998; 15: 533–8.

119. Kohan AD, Armenkas NA, Fracchia JA. Indivar urolithiasis: an emerging cause of renal colic in patients with human immunodeficiency virus. J Urol 1999; 161: 1765–8.

120. Schwartz BF, Schenkman N, Armenakas NA, Stoller ML. Imaging characteristics of indinavir calculi. J Urol 1999; 161: 1085–7.

121. Vazquez E, Lucaya J, Castellote A, et al. Neuroimaging in pediatric leukaemia and lymphoma: differential diagnosis. Radiographics 2002; 22: 1411–28.

122. Kieslich M, Porto L, Lanfermann H, et al. Cerebrovascular complications of L-asparaginase in the therapy of acute lymphoblastic leukemia. J Pediatr Hematol Oncol 2003; 25: 484–7.

123. Ho CL, Chen CY, Chen YC, et al. Cerebral dural sinus thrombosis in acute lymphoblastic leukaemia with early diagnosis by fast fluid-attenuated inversion recovery (FLAIR) image: a case report and a review of the literature. Ann Hematol 2000; 79: 90–4.

124. McKinney AM, Short J, Truwit CL, et al. Posterior reversible encephalopathy syndrome: incidence of atypical regions of involvement and imaging findings. AJR Am J Roentgenol 2007; 189: 904–12.

125. Morris EB, Laningham FH, Sandlund JT, Khan RB. Posterior reversible encephalopathy syndrome in children with cancer. Pediatr Blood Cancer. 2007; 48: 152–9.

126. Covarrubias DJ, Luetmer PH, Campeau NG. Posterior reversible encephalopathy syndrome: prognostic utility of quantitative diffusion-weighted MR images. AJNR Am J Neuroradiol 2002; 23: 1038–48.

127. Packer RJ, Zimmerman RA, Bilaniuc LT. Magnetic resonance imaging in the evaluation of treatment-related central nervous system damage. Cancer 1988; 61: 928–30.

128. Paakko E, Vainionpaa L, Lanning M, et al. White matter changes in children treated for acute lymphoblastic leukaemia. Cancer 1992; 70: 2728–33.

129. Inaba H, Khan RB, Laningham FH, et al. Clinical and radiological characteristics of methotrexate-induced acute encephalopathy in pediatric patients with cancer. Ann Oncol 2008; 19: 178–84.

130. Pagani JJ, Libshitz HI, Wallace S, et al. Central nervous system leukaemia and lymphoma: computed tomographic manifestations. AJR Am J Roentgenol 1981; 137: 1195–201.

131. Asato R, Akiyama Y, Ito M, et al. Nuclear magnetic resonance abnormalities of the cerebral white matter in children with acute lymphoblastic leukaemia and malignant lymphoma during and after central nervous system prophylactic treatment with intrathecal methotrexate. Cancer 1992; 70: 1997–2004.

132. Hook CC, Kimmel DW, Kvols LK, et al. Multifocal inflammatory leukoencephalopathy with 5-fluorouracil and levamisole. Ann Neurol 1992; 31: 262–7.

133. Koh S, Nelson M, Kovanlikaya A, et al. Anterior lumbosacral radiculopathy after intrathecal methotrexate treatment. Pediatr Neurol 1999; 21: 576–8.

134. Parisi MT, Fahmy JL, Kaminsky CK, et al. Complications of cancer therapy in children: a radiologists guide. Radiographics 1999; 19: 283–97.

135. Davenport C, Dillon WP, Sze G. Neuroradiology of the immunosuppressed state. Radiol Clin North Am 1992; 30: 611–37.

136. Ashdown BC, Tien RD, Felsberg GJ. Aspergillosis of the brain and paranasal sinuses in immunocompromised patients: CT and MR imaging findings. AJR Am J Roentgenol 1994; 162: 155–9.

137. Mathews VP, Alo PL, Glass JD, et al. AIDS-related CNS cryptococcus: radiologic–pathologic correlation. AJNR Am J Neuroradiol 1992; 13: 1477–86.

138. Scappaticci FA, Fehrenbacher L, Cartwright T, et al. Surgical wound healing complications in metastatic colorectal cancer patients treated with bevacizumab. J Surg Oncol 2005; 91: 173–80.

139. Saif MW, Elfiky A, Salem RR. Gastrointestinal perforation due to bevacizumab in colorectal cancer. Ann Surg Oncol 2007; 14: 1860–9.

54 Effects of Treatment on Normal Tissue: Thorax
Revathy B Iyer, Harmeet Kaur, Reginald F Munden, and Herman I Libshitz

INTRODUCTION

Radiotherapy and/or chemotherapy affect all tissues of the thorax. The evidence of these effects and the timing of their appearance vary from organ to organ. Radiation change is almost always seen in the lungs within weeks of completion of therapy. It is usually far less obvious in bone and takes years to be seen on conventional radiographs.

The details of the radiotherapy, including the volume and shape of the area treated, dose, time from completion of therapy, possible effects of other treatment, including chemotherapy, and the variability of human response are all factors that influence the appearance of radiotherapy change. The changes secondary to chemotherapy are usually dose-related. The radiotherapy changes described are for radiotherapy given with linear accelerators or Co-60 at 180 to 200 cGy/day with treatment given five days a week. The advent of three-dimensional conformal radiotherapy allows target volumes that minimize dose to normal structures and findings of radiation injury to the lung after such therapy will also be described.

LUNG

Radiation injury of the lung manifests as an acute phase radiation pneumonitis and a chronic phase radiation fibrosis. The radiological appearances of these phases have been well described and follow relatively predictable patterns. Radiologists define radiation pneumonitis as evidence of acute radiotherapy changes in the lungs regardless of the clinical findings. Clinicians require that cough, fever and/or shortness of breath accompany the radiographic changes (1). It has long been recognized that the radiographic changes of radiation pneumonitis are not necessarily accompanied by symptoms (2).

Radiation injury of the lung is generally not apparent below 3000 cGy, variably seen between 3000 and 3500 cGy, and almost always evident at doses over 4000 cGy. Radiation pneumonitis is usually evident six to eight weeks following radiotherapy; for each 1000 cGy over 4000 cGy, it presents a week earlier following completion of therapy.

Radiation pneumonitis is most extensive about three to four months following completion of radiotherapy. From this point, the changes gradually organize, contract and evolve into radiation fibrosis. There are no pathognomonic histological findings of radiation pneumonitis (3). The histological appearance of radiation pneumonitis is that of diffuse alveolar damage (4). Diffuse alveolar damage is seen in other entities such as immunologic insult, chemotherapeutic injury and infections, so the histologic and radiographic findings are not pathognomic for radiation injury. The histological appearance of radiation fibrosis is that of

organizing alveolar disease with fibroblast proliferation and fibrosis. The radiologic hallmark of radiation fibrosis is consolidation, volume loss, and bronchiectasis.

Key Points: radiation injury to the Lung

- Radiographic changes of radiation pneumonitis are not necessarily accompanied by symptoms
- Radiation pneumonitis is usually evident six to eight weeks following completion of at least 3000 to 4000 cGy
- Radiation pneumonitis is most extensive about three to four months following completion of therapy
- Conventional and CT findings of radiation pneumonitis gradually evolves into radiation fibrosis
- Radiation fibrosis is characterized by consolidation, volume loss, and bronchiectasis
- On conventional radiographs, the radiation fibrosis is usually stable 9 to 12 months following completion of therapy

Conventional Radiographic Findings

Radiation pneumonitis, when extensive, has sharp, well-defined areas of consolidation that conform to the radiation portals, not anatomic boundaries (5–7). Less extensive radiation pneumonitis may present as patchy consolidation in the irradiated fields (Fig. 54.1), or when early or minimal in extent, indistinctness of vessels. Familiarity with standard portals and the availability of prior radiographs facilitates identification of minimal changes. Reports of radiation change outside the radiation field are usually the result of oblique, rotational, or misplaced fields (8). A possible humoral cause has also been postulated (9).

Our experience indicates that radiation fibrosis or evidence of contraction secondary to fibrosis is seen in virtually all patients who received therapeutic doses of radiotherapy. Fibrosis usually presents as strand-like opacities with volume loss.

When extensive, there is significant volume loss with associated bronchiectatic changes. While the fibrosis is usually obvious, it can be subtle (Fig. 54.2). Less obvious findings include minimal pleural thickening, slight elevation of one or both hila or the minor fissure, slight medial retraction of upper lobe pulmonary vessels, minimal tenting or elevation of a hemidiaphragm, and minor blunting of cardiophrenic angles. The fibrotic changes usually become stable 9 to 12 months following completion of therapy (Fig. 54.1). Any alteration in stable radiation fibrosis suggests either superinfection or recurrent disease.

The combined effect of radiotherapy and chemotherapy on normal lung is difficult to evaluate. Combined therapy regimens are quite variable and chemotherapy has been given before, during

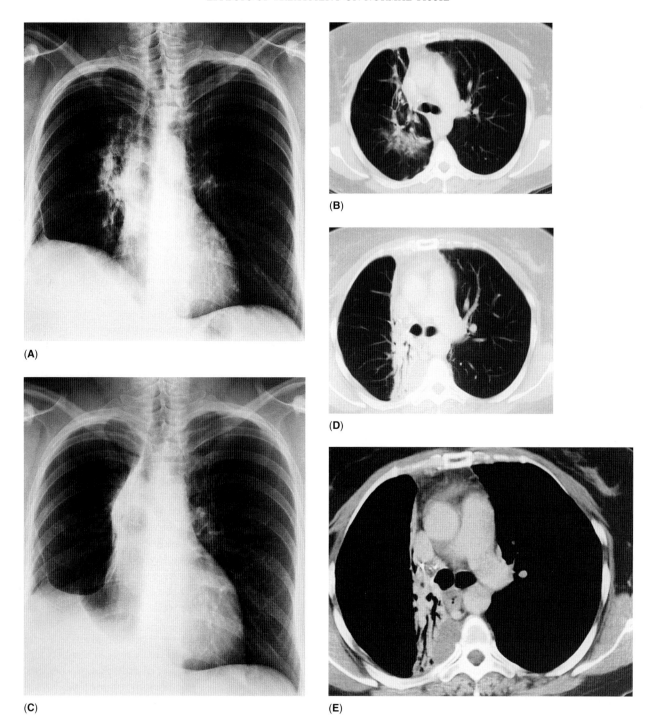

Figure 54.1 Radiation pneumonitis and fibrosis. (A) Radiation pneumonitis is seen in the right lung six weeks following 6000 cGy. A right upper lobectomy had also been performed for bronchogenic carcinoma. (B) CT scan at the same time as (A) showing patchy consolidation in the right lung. (C) Radiation fibrosis is present in the right lung eight months following; (D) CT scan at the same time as (C) showing solid consolidation on lung windows. The sharp margin of the radiation changes is evident. (E) Same CT scan as (D) on soft tissue windows showing the bronchiectatic changes to better advantage. A small loculated pleural effusion is present medially.

and after radiotherapy. Empiric observation and small animal experimentation (10) have shown that the use of drugs that enhance the effects of radiation cause greater radiation damage and a shorter time to the onset of radiation pneumonitis. The radiation-enhancing drugs include:

- Actinomycin D
- Adriamycin
- Bleomycin
- Cyclophosphamide
- Mitomycin C
- Vincristine (10)

There is disagreement regarding the effect of methotrexate (10,11).

Bleomycin, busulfan, and methotrexate are recognized to cause pulmonary parenchymal injury independent of associated radiotherapy (12). Bleomycin is used in the treatment of squamous cell carcinoma, lymphoma and testicular carcinoma.

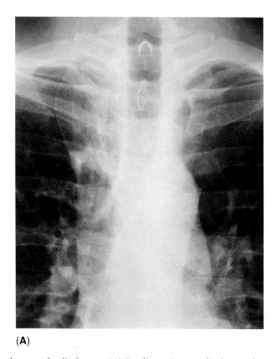 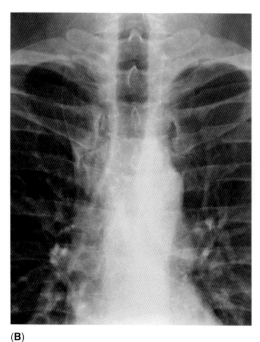

(A)   **(B)**

Figure 54.2 Subtle changes of radiotherapy. (A) Baseline prior to radiotherapy for Hodgkin's disease. (B) Twelve months following radiotherapy there is slight retraction of the azygous fissure medially and slight medial contracture of the upper lobe vessels bilaterally as well as minimal elevation of the left hilum.

The toxicity is related to accumulation of drugs in the lung and is directly related to the cumulative dose administered (12). The use of concomitant radiation, other chemotherapy, or oxygen therapy compounds the pulmonary toxicity. The early changes on chest radiography include a reticulonodular interstitial pattern, which is initially seen in the basal segments. Lung injury may be progressive, resulting in alveolar damage and eventual pulmonary fibrosis (13). Gallium-67 is known to accumulate in damaged lungs and is helpful in identifying bleomycin toxicity (14). Busulfan used to treat leukemia may also cause interstitial lung damage, resulting in a reticular pattern on conventional radiographs (13). Methotrexate is also used in the treatment of leukemia and other malignancies. A hypersensitivity reaction may occur resulting in alveolar infiltrates. Mediastinal adenopathy may also occur. The diffuse alveolar damage may result in fibrosis (13).

Computed Tomography and Magnetic Resonance Findings

Computed tomography (CT), with its greater sensitivity to minimal differences in radiographic density, can identify radiation pneumonitis earlier than conventional radiographs (15,16). It is also presumed that CT demonstrates radiation pneumonitis at lower radiotherapeutic doses than conventional radiographs. A dose-related effect with greater changes at higher doses has been described with CT (17).

There have been four patterns of radiation change described at CT after conventional radiotherapy (15):

- Homogeneous consolidation
- Patchy consolidation
- Discrete consolidation
- Solid consolidation

Homogeneous consolidation is a diffuse, minimal, or early radiation pneumonitis that uniformly involves the irradiated lung. The appearance is of ground glass opacities, whereby the pulmonary vessels are present within the generalized areas of increased lung attenuation and uniformly affects the treated portions of the lungs. It may be seen within two to three weeks of completion of therapy. Patchy consolidation (Fig. 54.1) is thought to be the CT analogue of radiation pneumonitis on plain films. The consolidation is contained within the irradiated lung, is not uniform in distribution and does not exhibit significant fibrosis. Discrete consolidation is defined by the irradiated field with well-demarcated borders but does not involve it uniformly (Fig. 54.3). Traction changes may be seen at the boundary of the treated lung. It is felt to represent fibrotic changes in treated lung with areas of relative sparing. It is usually seen in the 3500 to 4000 cGy range as used in the therapy of Hodgkin's disease rather than in the higher doses used in treating lung cancer. Solid consolidation, which is generally seen at doses of 5000 cGy and higher, more uniformly involves the treated lung causing consolidation and volume loss (Fig. 54.1). Bronchiectatic changes are seen within the area of volume loss in this pattern. It is the CT analogue of a dense radiation fibrosis seen on conventional radiographs.

Conventional radiotherapy results in the delivery of higher doses of radiation to surrounding tissues than to the primary tumor because of attenuation of the radiation. As more normal lung is included in the treatment, there is an increased risk of side-effects (18). Three-dimensional conformal radiation therapy is used by radiation therapists to limit the amount of radiation injury to the lung and surrounding tissues. This technique uses multiple smaller beams of radiation aimed at the tumor so that large areas of surrounding tissues are not irradiated. This ensures that the entire target volume is adequately treated, while minimizing dose to normal structures.

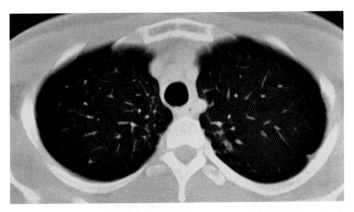

Figure 54.3 Discrete consolidation is seen in the paramediastinal portions of both lungs eight years following radiotherapy to the mediastinum for Hodgkin's disease (4000 cGy). The irradiated volume is well defined with traction changes at the periphery of the field.

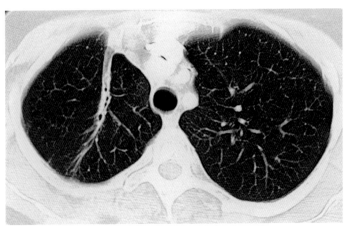

Figure 54.4 Scar like pattern of three-dimensional conformal radiation therapy. CT of a patient treated for squamous cell carcinoma shows a linear band of radiation fibrosis at the site of original tumor.

Treatment planning for three-dimensional conformal radiation is accomplished using CT data to generate three-dimensional images of the patient. Computer software determines the best orientations of the radiation beams that will deliver therapeutic dosages to the tumor while at the same time limiting the dosage of radiation to the surrounding tissues. Each beam will have a portion of the total amount of radiation delivered. The radiation from these multiple ports is additive at the tumor and ensures that the entire tumor volume is adequately treated, allowing higher dosages of radiation to be delivered to the tumor without increasing injury to the surrounding tissues. This technique also potentially improves local tumor control and decreases toxicity from injury to normal structures (19,20).

Three-dimensional radiation therapy is well suited to patients who are not surgical candidates because of pre-existing cardiac disease or who do not have adequate pulmonary reserve to tolerate lobectomy or standard radiation therapy. It is particularly useful in those patients with Stage I disease who cannot tolerate standard treatment; the radiation therapist can offer these patients treatment with curative intent.

However, this complex distribution of radiation dose to the tumor and surrounding lung tissue manifests as patterns of lung injury that are different than those reported after conventional radiotherapy. With less radiation of the surrounding tissue, the majority of radiation-induced injury is at the tumor site. Three patterns have been described as a result of three-dimensional conformal radiation therapy: mass-like, modified conventional, and scar-like (21). Mass-like opacities occur when the radiation fibrosis forms a mass appearance immediately surrounding the tumor. Modified conventional patterns occur when the radiation fibrosis looks like conventional radiation fibrosis, but the extent is limited to the lobe involved with tumor. The lung in the same plane as the tumor that is located peripherally, is not involved as compared to conventional therapy. Scar-like patterns occur when only a thin band of 1 cm or less of fibrosis remains after treatment (Fig. 54.4). This thin band forms a scar-like appearance and without prior studies one may not know a tumor existed.

The edema and inflammatory change of radiation pneumonitis are seen on MR imaging as increased signal intensity on T2-weighted images and low signal intensity on T1-weighted images (22). Radiation fibrosis would be expected to demonstrate low signal intensity at both T1- and T2-weighted images. Unfortunately, increased signal intensity on T2-weighted images (23) and contrast enhancement (24) may be seen in irradiated lung at a time when fibrosis would be expected. These non-specific signal intensity changes have made MR evaluation of recurrent disease in irradiated patients problematic.

Other Imaging Findings

Other less common complications include:

- Hyperlucency of lung adjacent to irradiated lung (25)
- Spontaneous pneumothorax (26)
- Pleural effusions secondary to radiotherapy (27)
- Calcification in lymph nodes (28)

Effusions are usually small and more frequently seen with CT (Fig. 54.5). They are indistinguishable from malignant pleural effusions. They usually develop within six months of therapy and may resolve spontaneously (27). Rapid increase or reaccumulation after thoracocentesis speaks for a malignant origin. If cytological examination is negative, prolonged follow-up may be necessary.

Calcification may occur in lymph nodes following therapy for lymphoma (28). This is more frequent in Hodgkin's disease and far more common following radiotherapy than in patients treated only with chemotherapy. The calcification begins about a year after therapy and gradually gets denser over years. Cystic changes that may calcify have been described in the thymus in patients irradiated for Hodgkin's disease (Fig. 54.6) (29). Very rarely, malignant pleural mesotheliomas may develop after radiotherapy (30).

Key Points: Imaging Findings of Radiation Injury

- Ground glass opacities of pneumonitis can be seen on CT within two to three weeks after completion of therapy
- Bronchiectatic changes of radiation fibrosis occur within the areas of volume loss
- Three-dimensional conformal radiotherapy results in radiation-induced injury that is usually localized to the tumor site and are different in distribution than conventional therapy patterns

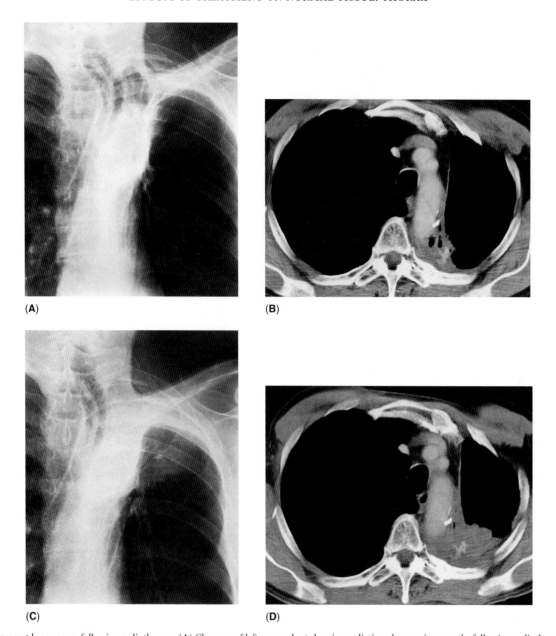

Figure 54.5 Recurrent lung cancer following radiotherapy. (A) Close-up of left upper chest showing radiation change nine months following radiotherapy. (B) CT scan at the same time as (A) showing solid consolidation. (C) Mass is now seen three months following (A) in the left upper chest and the air-containing lung above the aortic knuckle has been obliterated. (D) CT scan at the same time as (C) showing mass and filling in of bronchiectatic changes.

Evaluation of Treated Areas

Identification of residual or recurrent malignancy in the thorax may be made more difficult by the superimposition of radiation changes in the areas of concern. In these cases, CT most often provides adequate visualization of pulmonary parenchymal masses and/or the mediastinum following radiotherapy (see also chap. 8, Lung Cancer). In irradiated lymphoma, a residual mediastinal mass need not represent viable disease and, in patients who have been appropriately treated, further therapy is not warranted (31,32). Enlarging nodes or mass does speak for recurrence. By comparison, a residual mass in bronchogenic carcinoma often represents residual disease.

Awareness of the timing of radiation change is most helpful in identifying recurrent disease. Routine follow-up studies at two to three monthly intervals following completion of radiotherapy aids in making these observations. Features that should suggest recurrent disease include:

- Alteration in stable contours of radiation fibrosis (Fig. 54.5)
- Failure of contracture of an area of radiation pneumonitis when expected four months or more after completion of therapy
- Absence of air-containing ectatic bronchi in an area of solid consolidation at CT, especially if ectatic bronchi were present previously (33). The filling in of radiation therapy-induced ectatic bronchi may be the first sign of recurrence, or may be seen along with other signs of recurrence, and is a reliable CT sign of locally recurrent lung cancer (34)

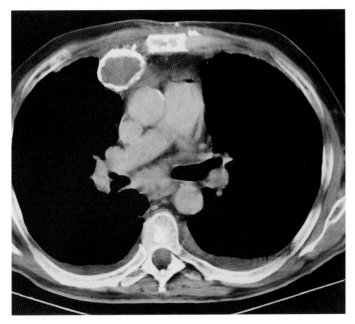

Figure 54.6 Calcified thymic cyst 30 years following radiation therapy in a patient treated for Hodgkin's disease. The subcarinal adenopathy and small bilateral pleural effusions are related to a current non-small cell lung cancer.

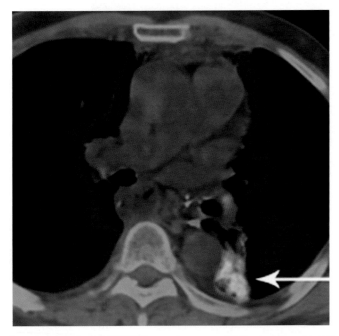

Figure 54.7 Fused axial PET/CT image shows consolidation and bronchiectatic changes that is FDG-avid and has a straight linear border (arrow) in the left lung after radiotherapy. The sharply defined border is more suggestive of radiation injury than tumor recurrence.

Infection can usually be distinguished from radiation pneumonitis both by knowledge of the field size and shape, and the date of completion of therapy. However, it is virtually impossible to exclude superimposed infection in an area of radiation pneumonitis with imaging. However, PET/CT can be valuable in distinguishing recurrent tumor from progressive fibrosis and infections (Fig. 54.7) (35). Further bronchial ectasia or tissue destruction in a treated area suggests superinfection. Recurrent malignancy causing distal pneumonia may be confusing.

Key Point: Evaluation of Treated Areas

■ Awareness of the timing of radiation change, knowledge of the field size and shape, and the date of completion of therapy, are essential for radiological identification of superinfection or of residual or recurrent malignant disease

HEART

The spectrum of radiation-induced heart disease includes:

- Acute and chronic pericarditis
- Coronary artery disease
- Valvular dysfunction
- Cardiomyopathy
- Conduction abnormalities

Radiation-induced heart disease, particularly ischemic disease, is more frequent and of greater clinical significance than had been previously thought (36,37). Evaluation of myocardial perfusion of asymptomatic long-term survivors, primarily patients treated for Hodgkin's disease, has shown a high incidence of subclinical myocardial lesions (38). Radiation injury to the heart is related to total dose, fractionated dose, volume of heart exposed, age at exposure, and lapse of time since radiation. An increased risk of radiation-induced heart disease is seen at cardiac doses exceeding 35 to 40 Gy and fractionated doses exceeding 2 Gy/day (39,40). A radiated left ventricular volume of >5% is associated with development of perfusion defects in 57% of patients (41). Younger patients are at a higher risk for cardiotoxic effects. A study evaluating patients treated at <21 years of age with 42 Gy for mediastinal Hodgkin's disease found a relative risk of fatal myocardial infarction of 41.5 over the age-matched population (42).

The pathogenesis of radiation changes in both the pericardium and myocardium is related to diffuse interstitial fibrosis. The common pathophysiologic pathway appears to be microcirculatory damage. Acute damage is marked by inflammation of the small and medium sized vessels, and subsequently endothelial cells demonstrate damage, occluding the vessel lumen, leading to ischemia, myocardial cell damage, and finally fibrosis. The coronary arteries, particularly the left anterior descending, show accelerated atherosclerosis (43).

Pericardial Disease

Fajardo and Berthrong have described thickening of the pericardium with fibrosis, fibrin deposition, and protein-rich pericardial effusions. Myocardial fibrosis also occurs but, unlike the focal fibrosis seen after infarction, it has a patchy involvement that follows the collagen framework of the myocardium (44).

The incidence of pericarditis is related to the dose, fraction size, volume irradiated, and technique. Below 4000 cGy the incidence is quite low. At 4000 cGy it ranges from 2% to 6% (45–48) and has been reported to be as high as 20% at 4500 cGy (48). Cosset et al. reported an incidence of 4.1% at 3500 to 3700 cGy that rose to 10.4% at 4100 to 4300 cGy (47). Moderate-sized mediastinal fields have a 1% incidence of pericardial disease that rises to 17% when the fields are larger with treatment of extensive disease (46). Techniques previously used with only anterior fields gave a 50% greater

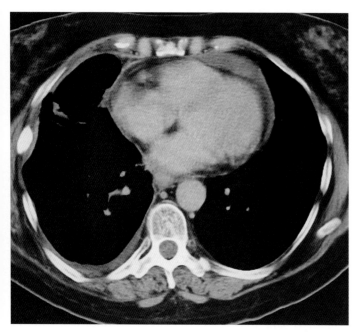

Figure 54.8 Small right pleural effusion and eccentric small pericardial effusion eight months following radiotherapy to a non-small cell bronchogenic carcinoma centrally in the right lung.

dose to the pericardium than the dose delivered to the midplane (49). The dose relationship of coronary artery disease has not yet been demonstrated (47).

Radiation pericarditis generally presents six to nine months after therapy and the majority of cases will occur within 12 to 18 months of therapy, but it may appear many years after radiotherapy. Acute and chronic pericarditis is seen with equal frequency. Both are indistinguishable clinically from other causes of pericarditis (50).

Symmetrical increase in the size of the cardiac silhouette is the typical appearance of radiation-induced pericardial effusion. Eccentric effusions may occur, presumably because of adhesions in the treated area of the pericardium, that prevent uniform distribution of the fluid (Fig. 54.8) (51). Small pericardial effusions or pericardial thickening are more easily identified with cross-sectional imaging techniques, ultrasound (US), CT, or MR. Far higher incidences of pericardial effusion will be found with these techniques. In a series of breast cancer patients treated with radiotherapy, Ikäheimo et al. found that 33% had pericardial effusions on US examination (52).

Evidence of radiation change in the lungs, either pneumonitis or fibrosis depending on the timing following therapy, is almost always present and can raise the possibility of radiation as the cause of pericardial disease. The major differential consideration is malignant pericardial effusion, which may be suggested by nodularity of the pericardium or mediastinal adenopathy. Cytological evaluation of pericardial fluid is necessary for a definitive diagnosis and is not always positive even in malignant disease. Exclusion of a pericardial effusion as the cause of cardiac enlargement in a patient whose heart has been irradiated raises the question of cardiomyopathy or ischemic heart disease.

Key Points: Pericardial Disease

- The incidence of pericardial disease is related to the dose, fraction size, volume irradiated, and technique—below 4000 cGy the incidence is low
- Radiation pericarditis generally presents six to nine months after therapy and the majority occur within 12 to 18 months after therapy
- Evidence of radiation change in the lungs is almost always present in association with pericardial disease

Myocardial Disease

Myocardial abnormalities, particularly ischemic in etiology, can result from radiation. Acute changes seen during the course of radiotherapy include repolarization abnormalities, transient decrease in ejection fraction and perfusion defects (41,53). Cardiac effects become more significant with the passage of time, with increased mortality from ischemic heart disease seen 10 to 15 years after therapy. Valvular abnormalities, most commonly mitral and aortic regurgitation, and conduction defects, such as prolongation of the QT interval, are also long-term consequences of radiation therapy (54).

In the myocardium, radiation affects both systolic and diastolic function, a study of Hodgkin's disease treated with modern techniques showed 4% had abnormal left ventricular filling and 16% had abnormal peak filling rate (55). While dilated, restrictive, and hypertrophic cardiomyopathy result from radiotherapy, ischemic heart disease remains the most common clinical presentation. Risk factors such as smoking, hypertension, and diabetes accentuate the risk of ischemic disease from radiation.

The use of newer techniques such as three-dimensional treatment planning, CT, decreased fraction size, total dose electron beam radiotherapy, and cardiac shielding have decreased cardiac exposure. Intensity modulated radiation can further reduce cardiac dose.

A study evaluating treatment with older radiation protocols revealed an increased relative risk of 1.98 for patients with left-sided breast cancer compared to right-sided cancers (56). The modification of regimens with incorporation of planning with CT particularly in breast cancer has lead to a decrease in cardiotoxicity. However, the clinical consequence of this still remains controversial. A recent study showed a comparable rate of ischemic heart disease in right and left-sided breast cancers (57). However, a report in Hodgkin's disease, shows that with modern radiotherapy techniques cardiac morbidity has declined, but the incidence of myocardial infarction remains unchanged (58). A recent prospective study using the latest techniques irradiating less then 7% of the left ventricle evaluated myocardial perfusion, wall motion, and ejection fractions with gated SPECT and echocardiography. It showed perfusion defects in 50% to 63% of women 6 to 24 months after therapy. These defects are of uncertain clinical significance, they persisted on a six-year follow-up, but were not associated with changes in ejection fraction or wall motion abnormalities. A longer term follow-up for evaluating the cardiac effects of new radiation techniques is required (41).

The development of cardiomyopathy may also result from the use of chemotherapeutic agents. Anthracyclines such as doxorubicin and HER2 antibodies like trastuzumab may lead to dilated

1251

cardiomyopathy. At a total cumulative dose of 550 mg/m² of doxorubicin, 1% to 2% of patients have overt congestive heart failure (59). The cardiotoxic effects of radiation are also compounded by chemotherapy. Studies on long term survivors of Hodgkin's disease demonstrated an increased mortality in those treated with doxorubicin and radiation over patients receiving radiation alone (60). A three- to four-fold increased risk of cardiac events was reported in breast cancer patients receiving a total cumulative dose 450 mg/m² and radiation compared to non-irradiated patients (61). When the total dose of doxorubicin was <225 mg/m² there was no increase in the incidence of cardiac events. Non-invasive diagnostic modalities, such as echocardiography and radionuclide cine-angiogram, as well as invasive tests such as endomyocardial biopsy, aid to assess risk-status of individuals receiving doxorubicin chemotherapy.

Using these techniques some degree of cardiac injury is demonstrated in more than 50% of asymptomatic patients treated with doxorubicin (59). While the total dose is the most significant factor contributing to the development of cardiomyopathy, other factors associated with an increased cardiotoxicity are:

- Age
- Pre-existing cardiac disease
- Mediastinal irradiation
- Concomitant administration of cyclophosphamide, actinomycin D, and mitomycin C (58)

Stenosis, thrombosis, and aneurysms in vessels such as the aorta, carotid, and subclavian arteries have been associated with radiation (62).

Key Points: Myocardial Disease

■ Ischemic heart disease is a common and long-term consequence of radiotherapy, the effect is compounded by chemotherapy with anthracyclines and trastuzumab, and other risk factors such as smoking

■ The use of modern radiation techniques has reduced cardiac dose and with a decrease in cardiac morbidity, a definitive assessment of clinical consequences requires longer term follow-up

ESOPHAGUS

Radiation-induced injury to the esophagus may be a limiting factor in therapy of thoracic neoplasms. Doses that result in radiation injury are of the order of 4500 cGy and higher (63). Chemotherapeutic agents such as adriamycin exacerbate these effects. More recent approaches for lung cancer favor treatment intensification in order to improve patient survival through the use of dose-intense chemotherapy regimens and/or higher doses of radiation therapy. Concurrent treatment is often used in patients for non-operative management and this can increase the incidence of severe esophagitis by 14% to 49% as compared to 1.3% with radiotherapy alone (64).

The abnormalities seen on esophograms following radiotherapy include:

- Abnormal peristalsis
- Mucosal edema
- Stricture (Fig. 54.9)
- Ulceration and fistula formation
- Esophageal dysmotility which is the earliest and most common change

These, generally, occur within 4 to 12 weeks after completion of therapy. Focal segments with either decreased peristalsis or aperistalsis are seen and correspond to the portals used (62). A serrated appearance of the esophageal mucosa is seen when mucosal edema is present (65). Marked esophagitis is usually seen endoscopically. In patients with breast cancer treated with radiotherapy, esophageal transit time as measured by esophageal scintigraphy has been shown to increase (66). The development of swallowing dysfunction over time may also occur.

Cross-sectional imaging may demonstrate thickening of the esophagus and mucosal enhancement corresponding to the inflammatory changes (Fig. 54.10). The differential diagnosis includes other causes of esophagitis in the absence of an appropriate history.

Esophageal strictures corresponding to the portals used are not infrequent and in general develop four to eight months following therapy (63). Barium swallow shows narrowing, usually with smoothly tapered margins, although ulceration may also

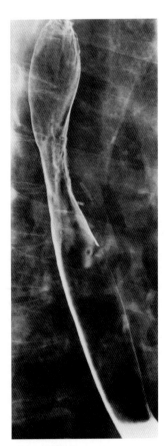

Figure 54.9 Barium swallow shows slight narrowing of the mid-esophagus with mucosal irregularity in a patient irradiated three months earlier for lung carcinoma. Endoscopy demonstrated esophagitis.

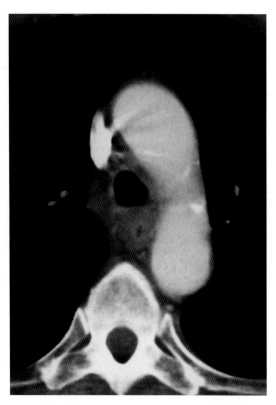

Figure 54.10 CT scan of the chest demonstrates thickened esophageal wall and mucosal enhancement (arrow) in a patient who received radiotherapy four months earlier for small cell carcinoma of the lung. The patient developed progressive dysphagia and odynophagia.

occur. Development of fistulae between the esophagus and tracheobronchial tree is uncommon and is likely to be related to extrinsic tumor involvement of the esophageal wall, with resultant erosion and fistula formation following therapy (63). Radiation-induced strictures may be indistinguishable radiographically from those caused by other injury such as ingestion of caustic material or prolonged nasogastric intubation. Esophageal cancers that respond to radiotherapy also frequently result in stricture formation.

A rare but well-described complication of therapeutic irradiation is carcinoma of the esophagus. Squamous cell carcinoma is most common. The mean latency period is 14 years (67).

Patients with malignancies may also develop infectious esophagitis as a result of immune compromise due to cytotoxic and/or immunosuppressive drugs, or the malignancy itself. The most common pathogen in such patients is *Candida albicans*, normal flora in the pharynx that grows in the esophagus as a result of the altered immunity. Clinical signs include odynophagia and dysphagia. The appearance on double-contrast esophagrams is usually characteristic (68). Mucosal plaques are seen which are generally diffuse and, in severe cases, a shaggy irregular contour of the esophagus results. Candida esophagitis can result in stricture and tracheo-esophageal fistula formation (69). Herpes simplex virus also may cause esophagitis in cancer patients. Discrete superficial ulcers can be seen with esophagrams (54).

Key Points: Esophageal Disease

- Abnormalities within the esophagus generally occur within 4 to 12 weeks after completion of radiotherapy with dysmotility and development of swallowing dysfunction over time
- Esophageal strictures generally develop four to eight months following radiotherapy and are radiographically indistinguishable from those caused by other injury
- Carcinoma of the esophagus is a rare but well-described complication of radiotherapy, occurring usually about 14 years after radiation
- Compromised immunity due to cytotoxic or immunosuppressive drugs can result in infectious esophagitis most commonly due to *C. albicans*

BONE

A detailed account of changes to the bone marrow following radiotherapy is given in chapter 55. The radiographic changes in adult bone following radiotherapy follow a temporal pattern. There is a latent period of 12 months or more during which no change is evident on conventional radiographs (70). Following this, some degree of demineralization may be seen. With progression, small lytic areas are seen through the cortex with thickening of the remaining trabeculae. This pattern usually develops two to three years or more following radiotherapy. These changes can be likened to multiple small foci of aseptic necrosis that are slowly progressive (71).

Should the radiotherapy changes continue to progress, the lytic areas can reach 1 to 2 cm in size and may be similar to metastatic disease. It generally takes at least five years for the more pronounced changes to occur and in most patients metastatic disease will have developed earlier in the course of disease. The extent of the changes is generally much less with current megavoltage therapy than is seen with orthovoltage irradiation (70). The presence of similar changes affecting adjacent bones in the irradiated field point to the correct diagnosis (72). Absence of recurrent mass in the soft tissues with CT or MR speaks against local recurrence or soft tissue sarcoma.

Spontaneous fractures and aseptic necrosis can occur. Radiation-induced fractures may heal quite slowly, taking months to years to heal (Fig. 54.11). Non-union is not uncommon. Abnormal callus formation may be seen. Resorption of fracture fragments may occur. Despite the decreased incidence with current therapy techniques, the changes still occur and long-term survivors from the orthovoltage era remain at risk. Bones subjected to muscular pull or constant weight-bearing tend to fracture more frequently. Radiation-induced fractures may be asymptomatic in non-weight-bearing bones (73).

Rib fractures are far less common following megavoltage than orthovoltage irradiation (55) and more frequent when higher doses per fraction are used (74). The current incidence of rib fractures is slightly less than 2% (75). The fractures may be quite subtle and generally involve the anterior aspects of the ribs included in tangential fields of the chest wall. The abnormal callus at the fractures may simulate a radiation-induced sarcoma. Radiation brachial plexopathy may accentuate demineralization of a treated

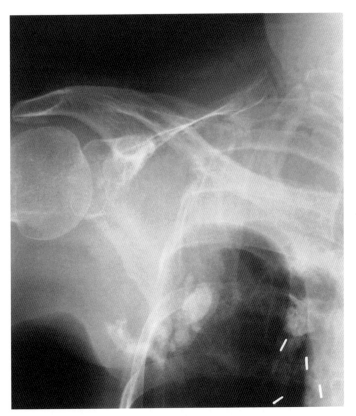

Figure 54.11 Extensive chest wall changes, following postoperative radiation therapy for breast cancer 20 years earlier, are present. Multiple rib fractures with resorption, abnormal callus formation, and dystrophic calcifications are present. The metallic clips are from coronary artery surgery. Radiation fibrosis is present in the upper right lung.

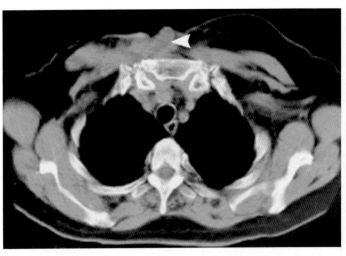

Figure 54.13 Chest wall ulcer and radiation-induced soft tissue sarcoma. Twenty years earlier, this woman underwent subcutaneous mastectomies and radiotherapy for a right breast cancer. The soft tissue fullness beneath the skin ulcer (arrowhead) proved to be a malignant fibrous histiocytoma rather than inflammation related to the ulcer.

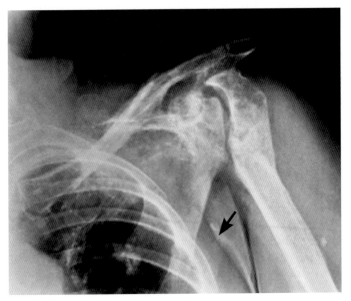

Figure 54.12 Marked destruction of the left shoulder joint due in part to a radiation-induced brachial plexopathy 16 years following postoperative radiotherapy for breast cancer. Vascular calcification is seen (arrow). Rib and lung changes are also present.

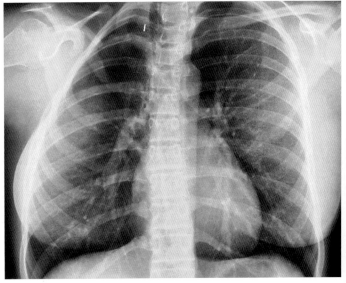

Figure 54.14 Marked asymmetry is seen in the upper right thorax of this 17-year-old female who received postoperative radiotherapy at aged three years for a rhabdomyosarcoma. The clavicle spontaneously fractured and resorbed nearly completely several years before.

shoulder joint and may also result in the appearance of a neuropathic-like shoulder joint superimposed on the radiation change (Fig. 54.12). Radiation-induced ulcers of the chest wall may also develop (Fig. 54.13).

Radiation change in the adult spine is not generally obvious on conventional radiographs. However, therapeutic levels of radiotherapy cause conversion of hematopoietic bone marrow to fatty marrow. This is seen at MR as increased signal intensity on T1-weighted images (76). The transformation begins as early as two weeks into a course of radiotherapy at a dose of approximately 1600 cGy (77).

The effects of therapeutic irradiation on growing bone are far more dramatic than those seen in adult bone because of associated

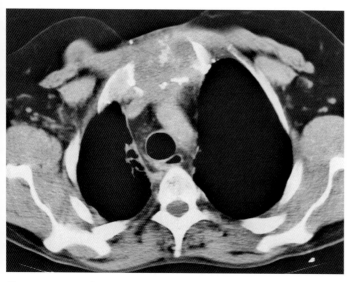

Figure 54.15 Postradiation osteosarcoma of the sternum showing mass and bony destruction. The sarcoma developed 12 years after mediastinal irradiation at 3600 cGy for metastases of a testicular seminoma.

growth impairment (Fig. 54.14). In the spine these changes in progressive order of severity include:

- Growth arrest lines
- End-plate irregularity
- Anterior beaking
- Asymmetry of vertebral development (78)

Significant scoliosis or kyphosis following radiotherapy is rare using modern techniques, but minor scoliotic changes are commonly seen (79).

Postradiation Sarcomas

Postradiation sarcomas are an infrequent but well-recognized complication of radiotherapy. They are estimated to occur in approximately 0.1% or fewer patients who receive radiotherapy and survive five years (80,81). Postradiation sarcomas may occur in either bone or soft tissue. Osteosarcoma is more frequent in bone (Fig. 54.15) and malignant fibrous histiocytoma (Fig. 54.13) more common in soft tissue (82–85). Review of Finnish data indicates soft tissue sarcomas are more common than osseous sarcomas (82). In a review by Sheppard and Libshitz, 83% of postradiation sarcomas probably arose in bone, with 63% representing osteosarcoma (83).

Postradiation sarcomas more commonly occur around the shoulder girdle and pelvis because of the more frequent use of radiotherapy in malignancies in these regions and better survival of patients with those malignancies. A higher incidence in women reflects the malignancies treated more often with radiotherapy (84). Most postradiation sarcomas are now related to radiation for soft tissue neoplasms, particularly breast cancer, lymphoma, and genito-urinary cancer (83).

A long latent period, averaging 10 to 15 years, is usually present between irradiation and the development of the sarcoma. However, postradiation sarcomas have developed as soon as two to three years following therapy, and as long as 45 to 55 years after treatment (82–87).

The appearance of soft tissue sarcomas caused by radiotherapy is not different from the spontaneously developing sarcomas

except that evidence of radiotherapy may be seen in adjacent bone or other tissues. They may get quite large if clinically silent.

With conventional radiographs postradiation sarcomas, arising in bone, most frequently present as an area of bony destruction (71). A soft tissue mass may be evident but is better appreciated with CT or MR. Tumor matrix may be seen. An expansile area in a previously irradiated bone suggests the development of sarcoma. Similarly, an area of lucency that is larger than the background pattern of radiation change is suspect.

At CT, a soft tissue mass and bony destruction are the most common findings (86). A soft tissue density, rather than fat, in the marrow cavity of irradiated bones may be the earliest indicator that a sarcoma has developed.

The occasional late metastatic lesion may mimic a postradiation sarcoma. Infection that has developed in a treated bone may also mimic postradiation sarcoma. Biopsy may be necessary to make the distinction. The absence of a soft tissue mass is helpful in distinguishing between extensive benign radiation change and a postradiation sarcoma.

Radiation-induced osteochondromas (cartilaginous exostoses) may occur in children until growth stops. The incidence is about 12% (88). Most are small and asymptomatic. Occasionally, the size and/or location cause symptoms. The appearance is that of the spontaneous osteochondromas and the same concerns apply.

Key Points: Radiation-Induced Bone Disease

- Bone demineralization results only after 12 months following radiotherapy
- Small lytic areas are seen only two to three years following radiotherapy and larger lytic areas 1 to 2 cm in size occur only after five years
- Radiation-induced fractures may take months or years to heal
- Radiation-induced sarcomas occur in about 0.1% of patients who receive radiotherapy
- A latent period of 10 to 15 years usually exists between radiotherapy and the development of a sarcoma, but some have developed within two to three years or as late as 45 to 55 years after treatment
- Radiation-induced osteochondromas may occur in children until growth stops

Summary

- Radiation pneumonitis is evident six to eight weeks following completion of radiotherapy, and is most extensive three to four months after radiotherapy
- Radiation pulmonary fibrosis usually becomes stable 9 to 12 months after completion of therapy; any alteration thereafter suggests infection or recurrence
- Drugs that enhance radiation effect cause greater radiation damage and result in a shorter time for onset of radiation pneumonitis
- Bleomycin, busulfan, and methotrexate cause pulmonary parenchymal damage independent of radiotherapy

- Identification of recurrent or residual malignant disease is made difficult by the presence of radiation change, usually requires CT and an awareness of the timing of radiation change and follow-up at two- to three-monthly intervals
- Radiation-induced heart disease includes pericarditis, coronary artery disease, valvular dysfunction, cardiomyopathy, and conduction abnormalities
- Chemotherapeutic agents, particularly doxorubicin, can result in cardiomyopathy
- Radiation injury to the esophagus can result in edema, dysmotility, stricture, ulceration, and fistula formation or carcinoma
- Postradiation sarcomas occur after a long latent period, many more commonly in soft tissue than in bone

REFERENCES

1. Maasilta P. Radiation-induced lung injury. From the chest physician's point of view. Lung Cancer 1991; 7: 367–84.

2. Chu FC, Phillips R, Nickson JJ, McPhee JG. Pneumonitis following radiation therapy of the breast by tangential technique. Radiology 1955; 64: 642–53.

3. Fajardo LF. Respiratory system. In: Pathology of Radiation Injury. New York: Masson Publishing, 1982: 34–46.

4. Katzenstein AA, Astin FB. Surgical Pathology of Non-Neoplastic Lung Disease, 2nd edn. Philadelphia: W B Saunders, 1990: 9–57.

5. Libshitz HI, Brosof AB, Southard ME. Radiographic appearance of the chest following extended field radiation therapy for Hodgkin's disease. A consideration of time-dose relationship. Cancer 1973; 32: 206–15.

6. Libshitz HI, North LB. Lung. In: Libshitz HI, ed. Diagnostic Roentgenology of Radiotherapy Change. Baltimore: Williams & Wilkins, 1979: 33–46.

7. Libshitz HI. Radiation changes in the lung. Semin Roentgenol 1993; 28: 303–20.

8. Wechsler RJ, Ayyangar K, Steiner RM, Yelovich R, Moylan DM. The development of distant pulmonary infiltrates following thoracic irradiation: the role of computed tomography with dosimetric reconstruction in diagnosis. Comput Med Imaging Graph 1990; 14: 43–51.

9. Morgan GW, Breit SN. Radiation and the lung: a re-evaluation of the mechanisms mediating pulmonary injury. Int J Radiat Oncol Biol Phys 1995; 31: 361–8.

10. Von der Maase H. Experimental drug-radiation interactions in critical normal tissues. In: Hill BT, Bellamy SA, eds. Antitumor Drug–Radiation Interactions. Boca Raton, FL: CRC Press, Inc, 1990: 191–205.

11. Phillips TL. Effects of chemotherapy and irradiation on normal tissues. In: Meyer JL, Vaeth JM, eds. Radiotherapy/Chemotherapy Interactions in Cancer Therapy. Series: Frontiers in Radiation Therapy in Oncology. Basel: Karger, 1992: 26, 45–54.

12. Cooper JA, Jr, White DA, Matthay RA. Drug-induced pulmonary disease. Part 1: Cytotoxic drugs. Am Rev Respir Dis 1986; 133: 321–40.

13. Morrison DA, Goldman AL. Radiographic patterns of drug-induced lung disease. Radiology 1979; 131: 299–4.

14. Richman SD, Levenson SM, Bunn PA, et al. [67]Ga accumulation in pulmonary lesions associated with bleomycin toxicity. Cancer 1975; 36: 1966–72.

15. Libshitz HI, Shuman LS. Radiation-induced pulmonary change: CT findings. J Comput Assist Tomogr 1984; 8: 15–19.

16. Ikezoe J, Takashima S, Morimoto S, et al. CT appearance of acute radiation-induced injury in the lung. Am J Roentgenol 1988; 150: 765–70.

17. Mah K, Poon PY, van Dyk J, et al. Assessment of acute radiation-induced pulmonary changes using computed topography. J Comput Assist Tomogr 1986; 10: 736–43.

18. Graham MV, Purdy JA, Emami B, et al. Clinical dose-volume histogram analysis for pneumonitis after 3D treatment for non-small cell lung cancer (NSCLC). Int J Radiat Oncol Biol Phys 1999; 45: 323–9.

19. Armstrong JG. Three-dimensional conformal radiotherapy. Precision treatment of lung cancer. Chest Surg Clin North Am 1994; 4: 29–43.

20. Graham MV, Matthews JW, Harms WB, Sr, et al. Three-dimensional radiation treatment planning study for patients with carcinoma of the lung. Int J Radiat Oncol Biol Phys 1994; 29: 1105–7.

21. Koenig TR, Munden RF, Erasmus JJ, et al. Radiation injury of the lung after three-dimensional conformal radiation therapy. Am J Roentgenol 2002; 178: 1383–8.

22. Davis SD, Yankelevitz DF, Henschke CI. Radiation effects on the lung: clinical features, pathology and imaging findings. Am J Roentgenol 1992; 159: 1157–64.

23. Glazer HS, Lee JK, Levitt RG, et al. Radiation fibrosis: differentiation from recurrent tumor by MR imaging. Radiology 1985; 156: 721–6.

24. Werthmuller WC, Schiebler ML, Whaley RA, Mauro MA, McCartney WH. Gadolinium-DTPA enhancement of lung radiation fibrosis. J Comput Assist Tomogr 1989; 13: 946–8.

25. Wencel ML, Sitrin RG. Unilateral lung hyperlucency after mediastinal irradiation. Am Rev Respir Dis 1988; 137: 955–7.

26. Twiford TW, Zornoza J, Libshitz HI. Recurrent spontaneous pneumothorax after radiation therapy to the thorax. Chest 1978; 73: 387–8.

27. Bachman AL, Macken K. Pleural effusions following supervoltage radiation for breast carcinoma. Radiology 1959; 72: 699–709.

28. Brereton HD, Johnson RE. Calcification in mediastinal lymph nodes after radiation therapy of Hodgkin's disease. Radiology 1974; 112: 705–7.

29. Kim HC, Nosher J, Haas A, Sweeney W, Lewis R. Cystic degeneration of thymic Hodgkin disease following radiation therapy. Cancer 1985; 55: 354–6.

30. Shannon VR, Nesbitt JC, Libshitz HI. Malignant pleural mesothelioma after radiation therapy for breast cancer. A report of two additional patients. Cancer 1995; 76: 437–41.

31. Jochelson M, Mauch P, Balikian J, Rosenthal D, Canellos G. The significance of the residual mediastinal mass in treated Hodgkin's disease. J Clin Oncol 1985; 3: 637–40.

32. Radford JA, Cowan RA, Flanagan M, et al. The significance of residual mediastinal abnormality on the chest radiograph

following treatment for Hodgkin's disease. J Clin Oncol 1988; 6: 940–6.

33. Bourgouin P, Cousineau G, Lemire P, Delvecchio P, Hébert G. Differentiation of radiation-induced fibrosis from recurrent pulmonary neoplasm by CT. Can Assoc Radiol J 1987; 38: 23–6.

34. Libshitz HI, Sheppard DG. Filling in of radiation therapy-induced bronchiectatic change: a reliable sign of locally recurrent lung cancer. Radiology 1999; 210: 25–7.

35. Choi YW, Munden RF, Erasmus JJ, et al. Effects of radiation therapy on the lung: radiological appearances and differential diagnosis. Radiographics 2004; 24: 985-98.

36. Cosset JM, Henry-Amar M, Meerwaldt JH. Long-term toxicity of early stages of Hodgkin's disease therapy: the EORTC experience. EORTC Lymphoma Cooperative Group. Ann Oncol 1991; 2: 77–82.

37. Boivin J, Hutchison GB, Lubin JH, et al. Coronary artery disease mortality in patients treated for Hodgkin's disease. Cancer 1992; 69: 1241–7.

38. Pierga JY, Maunoury C, Valette H, et al. Follow-up thallium-201 scintigraphy after mantle field radiotherapy for Hodgkin's disease. Int J Radiat Oncol Biol Phys 1993; 25: 871–6.

39. Glanzmann C, Kaufmann P, Jenni R, Hess OM, Huguenin P. Cardiac risk after mediastinal irradiation for Hodgkin's disease. Radiother Oncol 1998; 46; 51–62.

40. Stewart JR, Fajardo LF. Radiation–induced heart disease. Clinical and experimental aspects. Radiol Clin North Am 1971; 9: 511–31.

41. Prosnitz RG, Hubbs JL, Evans ES, et al. Prospective assessment of radiotherapy-associated cardiac toxicity in breast cancer patients analysis of data 3 to 6 years after treatment. Cancer 2007; 110: 1840–50.

42. Hancock SL, Donaldson SS, Hoppe RT. Cardiac disease following treatment of Hodgkin's disease in children and adolescents. J Clin Oncol 1993; 11: 1208–15.

43. Adams MJ, Hardenbergh PH, Constine LS, Lipshultz SE. Radiation-associated cardiovascular disease. Crit Rev Oncol/Hematol 2003; 45: 55–75.

44. Fajardo LF, Berthrong M. Radiation injury in surgical pathology. Part I. Am J Surg Pathol 1978; 2: 159–99.

45. Tarbell NJ, Thompson L, Mauch P. Thoracic irradiation in Hodgkin's disease: disease control and long-term complications. Int J Radiat Oncol Biol Phys 1990; 18: 275–81.

46. Cosset JM, Henry-Amar M, Ozanne F, et al. Les péricardites radiques: études des cas observés dans une série de 160 maladies de Hodgkin irradiées en mantelet a l'Institut Gustave-Roussy, de 1976 à 1980. J Eur Radiother 1984; 5: 297–308.

47. Cosset JM, Henry-Amar M, Pellae-Cosset B, et al. Pericarditis and myocardial infarctions after Hodgkin's disease therapy. Int J Radiat Oncol Biol Phys 1991; 21: 447–9.

48. Dana M, Colombel P, Bayle-Weisgerber C, et al. Periarditis after widefield irradiation for Hodgkin's disease study of dosimetry in relation to therapeutic concentrations.[French] J Radiol Electrol Med Nucl 1978; 59: 335–41.

49. Kinsella TJ, Fraass BA, Glatstein E. Late effects of radiation therapy in the treatment of Hodgkin's disease. Cancer Treat Rep 1982; 66: 991–1001.

50. Loyer EM, Delpassand ES. Radiation-induced heart disease: imaging features. Semin Roentgenol 1993; 28: 321–32.

51. Green B, Zornoza J, Ricks JP. Eccentric pericardial effusion after radiation therapy of left breast carcinoma. Am J Roentgenol 1977; 128: 27–30.

52. Ikäheimo MJ, Niemelä KO, Linnaluoto MM, et al. Early cardiac changes related to radiation therapy. Am J Cardiol 1985; 56: 943–6.

53. Larsen RL, Jakacki RI, Vetter VL, et al. Electrocardiographic changes and arrhythmias after cancer therapy in children and young adults. Am J Cardiol 1992; 70: 73–7.

54. Carlson RG, Mayfield WR, Normann S, Alexander JA. Radiation-associated valvular disease. Chest 1991; 9: 538–45.

55. Constine LS, Schwartz RG, Savage D, King V, Muhs A. Cardiac function, perfusion, and morbidity in irradiated long-term survivors of Hodgkin's disease. Int J Radiat Oncol Biol Phys1997; 39: 897–906.

56. Paszat LF, Mackillop WJ, Groome PA, et al. Mortality from myocardial infarction after adjuvant radiotherapy for breast cancer in the surveillance, epidemiology, and end-results cancer registries. J Clin Oncol 1998; 16: 2625–31.

57. Hojris I, Overgaard M, Christensen JJ, Overgaard J. Morbidity and mortality of ischemic heart disease in high-risk breast cancer patients after adjuvant postmastectomy systemic treatment with or without radiotherapy: analysis of DBCG 82b and 82c randomized trials. Radiotherapy Committee of the Danish Breast Cancer Cooperative Group. Lancet 1999; 354: 1425–30.

58. Hancock SL, Hoppe RT. Long term complication of treatment and causes of mortality after Hodgkin's disease. Semin Radiat Oncol 1996; 6: 225–42.

59. Gerling B, Gottdiener J, Borer JS. Cardiovascular complications of the treatment of Hodgkin's disease. In: Lacher MJ, Redman JR, eds. Hodgkin's Disease: The Consequences of Survival. Philadelphia: Lea & Febiger, 1990: 267–95.

60. Leonard GT, Green DM, Spangenthel EL, et al. Cardiac mortality and morbidity after treatment for Hodgkin disease during child hood and adolescence (Abstract). Pediatr Res 2000; 47: 46A.

61. Shapiro CL, Hardenbergh PH, Gelman R, et al. Cardiac effects of adjuvant doxorubicin and radiation therapy in breast cancer patients. J Clin Oncol 1998; 16: 3493–501.

62. Benson EP. Radiation injury to large arteries: 3. Further examples with prolonged asymptomatic intervals. Radiology 1973; 106: 195–7.

63. Lepke RA, Libshitz HI. Radiation-induced injury of the esophagus. Radiology 1983; 148: 375–8.

64. Werner-Wasik M. Treatment-related esophagitis. Semin Oncol 2005; 32(Suppl 3): S60–S66.

65. DuBrow RA. Radiation changes in the hollow viscera. Semin Roentgenol 1994; 29: 38–52.

66. Türkölmez S, Atasever T, Akmansu M. Effects of radiation therapy on esophageal transit in patients with inner quadrant breast tumour. Nucl Med Commun 2005; 26: 721–6.

67. Ogino T, Kato H, Tsukiyama I, et al. Radiation-induced carcinoma of the esophagus. Acta Oncol 1992; 31: 475–7.

68. Levine MS, Macones AJ, Jr, Laufer I. Candida esophagitis: accuracy of radiographic diagnosis. Radiology 1985; 154: 581–7.

69. Yee J, Wall SD. Infectious esophagitis. Radiol Clin North Am 1994; 32: 1135–45.

70. Howland WJ, Loeffler RK, Starchman DE, Johnson RG. Post-irradiation atrophic changes of bone and related complications. Radiology 1975; 117: 677–85.

71. Libshitz HI. Radiation changes in bone. Semin Roentgenol 1994; 29: 15–37.

72. de Santos LA, Libshitz HI. Adult bone. In: Libshitz HI, ed. Diagnostic Roentgenology of Radiotherapy Change. Baltimore: Williams and Wilkins, 1979: 137–50.

73. Dalinka MK, Neustafler LM. Radiation changes. In: Resnick D, Niwayama G, eds. Diagnosis of Bone and Joint Disorders. Philadelphia: WB Saunders, 1988: 3024–56.

74. Overgaard M. Spontaneous radiation-induced rib fractures in breast cancer patients treated with postmastectomy irradiation. A clinical radiobiological analysis of the influence of fraction size and dose–response relationships on late bone damage. Acta Oncol 1988; 27: 117–22.

75. Pierce SM, Recht A, Lingos TI, et al. Long-term radiation complications following conservative surgery (CS) and radiation therapy (RT) in patients with early stage breast cancer. Int J Radiat Oncol Biol Phys 1992; 23: 915–23.

76. Ramsey RG, Zacharias CE. MR imaging of the spine after radiation therapy: easily recognizable effects. Am J Roentgenol 1985; 144: 1131–5.

77. Yankelevitz DF, Henschke CI, Knapp PH, et al. Effect of radiation therapy on thoracic and lumbar bone marrow: evaluation with MR imaging. Am J Roentgenol 1991; 157: 87–92.

78. Neuhauser EB, Wittenborg MH, Berman CZ, Cohen J. Irradiation effects of roentgen therapy on the growing spine. Radiology 1952; 59: 637–50.

79. Heaston DK, Libshitz HI, Chan RC. Skeletal effects of megavoltage irradiation in survivors of Wilms' tumor. Am J Roentgenol 1979; 133: 389–95.

80. Taghian A, de Vathaire F, Terrier P, et al. Long-term risk of sarcoma following radiation treatment for breast cancer. Int J Radiat Oncol Biol Phys 1991; 21: 361–7.

81. Tountas AS, Fornasier VL, Harwood AR, Leung PM. Postirradiation sarcoma of bone: a perspective. Cancer 1979; 43: 182–7.

82. Wiklund TA, Blomqvist CP, Räty J, et al. Post irradiation sarcoma. Analysis of a nationwide cancer registry material. Cancer 1991; 68: 524–31.

83. Sheppard DG, Libshitz HI. Post-radiation sarcomas: a review of the clinical and imaging features in 63 cases. Clin Radiol 2001; 56: 22–9.

84. Huvos AG, Woodard HQ, Cahan WG, et al. Postradiation osteogenic sarcoma of bone and soft tissues. A clinicopathologic study of 66 patients. Cancer 1985; 55: 1244–55.

85. Laskin WB, Silberman TA, Enzinger FM. Postradiation soft tissue sarcomas. An analysis of 53 cases. Cancer 1988; 62: 2330–40.

86. Lorigan JG, Libshitz HI, Peuchot M. Radiation-induced sarcoma of bone: CT findings in 19 cases. Am J Roentgenol 1989; 153: 791–4.

87. Weatherby RP, Dahlin DC, Ivins JC. Postradiation sarcoma of bone: review of 78 Mayo Clinic cases. Mayo Clin Proc 1981; 56: 294–306.

88. Libshitz HI, Cohen MA. Radiation-induced osteochondromas. Radiology 1982; 142: 643–7.

55 Effects of Treatment on Normal Tissue: Bone and Bone Marrow
Lia Moulopoulos

INTRODUCTION

Osseous changes believed to be related to radiation-induced vascular damage were reported as early as 1926 (1). Ewing introduced the term "radiation osteitis" to describe these radiation-induced abnormalities. Since then, many other investigators have described changes related to the effect of radiation on bone and have introduced many terms, such as osteonecrosis and radionecrosis.

Howland and his colleagues suggested that, because atrophy is the main event that takes place in the irradiated bone, the term "atrophic changes" more accurately defines the expected, uncomplicated postradiation bony changes (2). All other superimposed conditions, such as fractures, infection, and aseptic necrosis can be considered complications of radiation therapy. The number of complications of radiation therapy that affect the osseous skeleton has been reduced, but not eliminated, since the advent of megavoltage therapy.

PATHOPHYSIOLOGY OF TREATMENT-RELATED OSSEOUS CHANGES

The effect of radiation therapy on bone has been documented by pathological studies (3–5). The changes that occur in irradiated bone are due to destruction of the cellular bony matrix and the fine vasculature that supplies the bone. Radiation therapy induces an immediate inflammatory reaction in the bone marrow. All cellular elements die early in the postradiation period and, as early as the first week of therapy, the marrow becomes hypocellular accompanied by edema and hemorrhage. Endarteritis occurs later in the postradiation period and is responsible for the late postradiation manifestations observed on radiographic examinations. Destruction of the microvasculature of the bone prevents the migration of hematopoietic elements from contiguous healthy bone marrow. Vascular compromise leads to bone necrosis. Necrotic bone is gradually removed by "creeping substitution" and new bone is deposited over a period of years.

The development and the severity of postradiation changes of bone depend on:

- Dose
- Fractionation
- Field size
- Type of radiation treatment

Regeneration of the bone marrow is possible if the microvasculature of the affected bone has not been completely obliterated. However, histological studies have not shown recovery of hematopoietic marrow with doses greater than 30 to 40 Gy (5,6). Magnetic resonance (MR) imaging and radionuclide studies have shown similar results (7–11).

The changes that occur in the bone marrow after chemotherapy have been studied on serial bone marrow specimens from patients with acute myeloid leukemia (12). Immediately after initiation of chemotherapy, depletion of the cellular elements takes place and the bone marrow becomes edematous. The vascular sinuses dilate and large, unilocular adipocytes (structured fat), which are produced by multilocular precursor fat cells, appear in the irradiated marrow. It is only within these areas of structured fat that foci of regenerating hematopoietic marrow appear after the first week of treatment, suggesting the potential role of structured fat in the proliferation of stem cells (Fig. 55.1).

POSTRADIATION ATROPHIC CHANGES

Local demineralization and osteopenia is the earliest and, most often, the only postradiation change on conventional bone radiographs, together with coarsening of the bony trabecula and thickening of the cortex of the long bones, changes that have been likened to Pagetoid bone (2). Such changes occur a year after radiation therapy and may become more pronounced with time. Later, both sclerotic and lytic foci representing dead and resorbed bone, respectively, may appear (Fig. 55.2). Postradiation atrophic changes are more obvious on computed tomography (CT). Occasionally, lytic foci grow and simulate primary or secondary malignant bone tumors. Appearances that support the diagnosis of postradiation lytic change rather than neoplasm include:

- Localization to the radiation portals
- Absence of an extra-osseous mass
- Absence of a periosteal reaction
- A sharp transition zone to the uninvolved bone
- Slow growth of the lesion (13–15)

CT should be obtained if review of conventional bone radiographs poses the question of malignancy. If findings are equivocal on CT, MR imaging may help in the detection of extra-osseous or bone marrow involvement.

POSTRADIATION COMPLICATIONS

Fractures
The irradiated, atrophic bone is brittle and may fracture, even under physiological stress such as muscular contractions, particularly in weight-bearing bones. The first radiation-induced fracture was described in the femoral neck, in 1927 (16). Since the introduction of megavoltage therapy, radiation-induced fractures are seen less often. They are infrequently observed earlier than two or three years after therapy (15). They may be discovered incidentally on routine imaging studies or the patient may present with pain, particularly when weight-bearing bones are involved. Radiation-induced

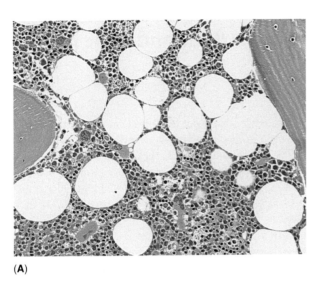

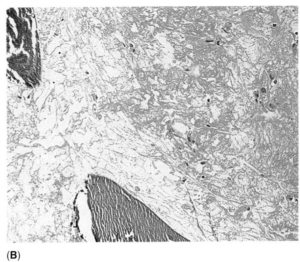

(A) **(B)**

Figure 55.1 (**A**) Bone marrow showing fatty change and fibrosis following chemotherapy. (**B**) Normal cellular bone marrow for comparison.

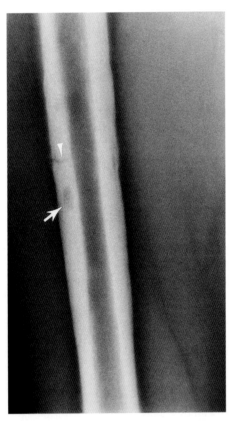

Figure 55.2 Cortical lucency (arrow) and insufficiency fracture (arrow head). Anteroposterior radiograph of the femur of a patient with soft tissue sarcoma who received 70 Gy five years ago. *Source*: Courtesy of H I Libshitz.

fractures heal more slowly than fractures of healthy bone. Formation of abnormal, exuberant callus, non-union of the osseous fragments or bony resorption may occur.

Radiation-induced insufficiency fractures of the pelvis occur earlier than fractures in other parts of the skeleton, at a median interval of six months from completion of radiation therapy (Figs. 55.3 and 55.4) (15,17–19). After treatment with pelvic radiation, the sacrum loses its elasticity and may fracture under

the stress of normal activity. Fractures of the pubic rami and subcapital fractures of the femoral head may also occur in such patients. A 13% to 20% five-year cumulative index for pelvic insufficiency fractures has been reported in patients treated with radiotherapy for gynecological malignancies (17,20). In patients who developed pelvic insufficiency fractures after radiotherapy for cervical cancer, important predisposing factors included patient age over 55 years and radiation dose over 50 Gy (20). In postmenopausal women, osteoporosis increases the probability of insufficiency fractures of irradiated bones. On conventional radiographs, findings may be absent or very subtle (21). An H-shaped appearance of increased uptake on radionuclide studies is characteristic of sacral insufficiency fractures, which course vertically in the sacral alae (22,23). The horizontal bar of the "H" corresponds to a third transverse fracture of the sacrum that may not be identified on radiographs. In patients with known malignancies, it may be difficult to differentiate sacral insufficiency fractures, especially unilateral ones, from metastatic disease with conventional radiographs and radionuclide scans alone. CT or MR imaging can provide a definitive diagnosis in most cases. On T1-weighted MR images of sacral insufficiency fractures, the expected bright signal intensity of irradiated marrow is replaced by decreased signal intensity produced by the presence of free water in the edematous marrow (24). The water, and consequently the decreased signal intensity, extends well beyond the margins of the fracture (Fig. 55.5). A fracture line may be visible and it usually parallels the sacroiliac joint. Symmetric alteration of sacral signal intensity is more often observed and must be distinguished from bone metastases which are usually patchier in distribution and more sharply defined. MR imaging studies may demonstrate sacral insufficiency fractures well before any changes appear on CT images because of the higher contrast resolution, capability for multiplanar image acquisition and depiction of bone marrow edema.

In patients who receive radiation therapy for breast cancer, rib fractures may occur. The incidence of this complication is about 1.8% but may be even higher when radiation doses exceed 50 Gy and if chemotherapy is administered as well (25,26).

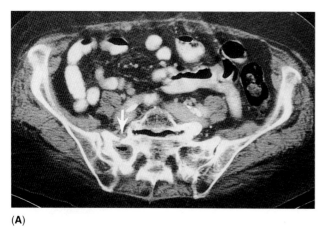

(A)

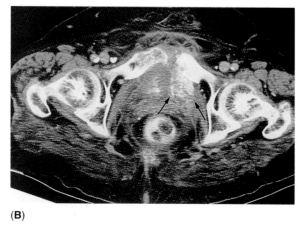

(B)

Figure 55.3 Insufficiency fractures of the pelvis. CT scan of the pelvis of a 66-year-old woman who was treated with radiotherapy for vaginal cancer two years previously. In (A) the arrow points to a fracture of the right sacral wing. (B) Note healed insufficiency fracture of the left pubic bone and extra-osseous calcification (arrows).

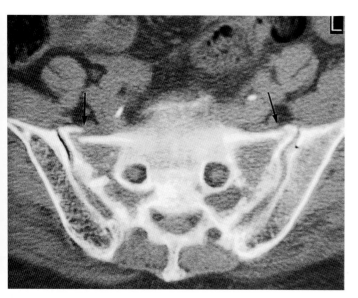

Figure 55.4 Bilateral insufficiency fractures (arrows) on CT scan of the pelvis of a 60-year-old woman who underwent radiotherapy of the pelvis for colon cancer one year previously. The patient presented with severe back pain and a positive bone scan (not shown).

AVASCULAR NECROSIS

Radiation therapy and steroids are known causes of avascular necrosis. Avascular necrosis develops several years after radiation treatment (Fig. 55.6) and has been reported to occur in 19% of bone marrow transplant recipients (27). Cumulative prednisolone-equivalent doses over 3 g have been associated with a 13% risk of osteonecrosis (28). In such cases, necrosis occurs as a result of decreased local blood flow caused by fatty marrow hypertrophy or lipid emboli (28). Before the introduction of MR imaging, radionuclide examination was the procedure of choice for the diagnosis of avascular necrosis. With this modality, however, false negative radionuclide scans of 18% have been reported (29). In another study, radionuclide studies failed to detect 10% of cases of avascular necrosis which were positive on MR studies (30).

Early in its clinical course, avascular necrosis presents as bone marrow edema and is indistinguishable from other causes of bone marrow edema, such as transient osteoporosis, occult fracture, etc. The presence of the double-line sign on T2-weighted MR images is characteristic of avascular necrosis (Fig. 55.7). This consists of an outer dark line, which is produced by reactive sclerosis at the interface of the lesion with the healthy marrow, and a bright inner line, which corresponds to areas of hyperemia and inflammation at the periphery of the ischemic marrow (30). Changes of early avascular necrosis may be accompanied by bone marrow edema and joint effusion, both of which have been associated with transient bone pain even in the absence of collapse (31). At the early stages of avascular necrosis, articular cartilage is not involved because it is not supplied by vessels. Recognition of the presence of avascular necrosis before the occurrence of a subchondral fracture is important for the success of conservative treatment. MR studies can detect avascular necrosis within days of the vascular insult. MR imaging has also been shown to identify those patients at particular risk for developing avascular necrosis when exposed to known predisposing factors. In a study of patients treated with chemotherapy for testicular tumors, asymptomatic avascular necrosis was detected on MR images of 9% of patients (32). The presence of a sealed-off epiphyseal scar in the femoral head has been associated with an increased risk for avascular necrosis (33). MR imaging can also reliably assess the location and the extent of the necrotic bone relative to the weight-bearing area, factors that influence the course of avascular necrosis and affect the management of the patient (34).

Avascular necrosis should be distinguished from bone marrow necrosis, a rare entity which has been reported to occur after chemotherapy, before the diagnosis of malignancy or at recurrence. In bone marrow necrosis myeloid tissue is destroyed but spicular architecture is preserved (35). Changes on MR images are similar in avascular and bone marrow necrosis but in the latter they are more extensive and affect predominantly the spine and pelvis (36).

Key Points: Fractures and Aseptic Necrosis

- Radiation-induced fractures occur earlier in the pelvis than in other parts of the skeleton
- Sacral insufficiency fractures may be difficult to distinguish from metastases on conventional radiographs and radionuclide scans
- MR is the most sensitive and most specific technique in the detection of avascular necrosis
- Bone marrow necrosis is a rare entity which may mimic avascular necrosis

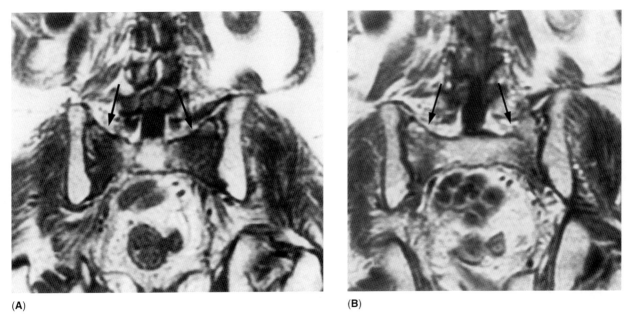

Figure 55.5 Bilateral insufficiency fractures of the sacrum. T1-weighted (**A**) and contrast-enhanced T1-weighted (**B**) coronal MR images of the sacrum in a 70-year-old woman who was treated with radiotherapy for cervical cancer one year previously. Note edematous marrow (arrows) with faint enhancement in (**B**).

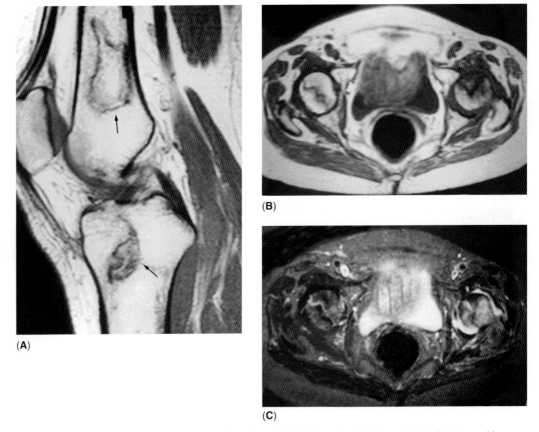

Figure 55.6 T1-weighted sagittal (**A**) MR image of the knee shows bone infarcts (arrows) of the femoral and tibial metaphysis of a 26-year-old woman treated for Hodgkin's lymphoma 10 years previously. In another patient who received chemotherapy for multiple myeloma, T1-weighted fast spin echo (**B**) and STIR (**C**) axial MR images of the proximal femurs show early avascular necrosis of the right and more advanced avascular necrosis of the left femoral head.

EFFECTS OF RADIATION ON THE GROWING SKELETON

The effect of radiation on the osseous skeleton depends on the type of bone involved, the dosage and, in particular, the patient's age at the time of therapy. The younger the child at the time of radiation therapy, the more pronounced the radiation-induced osseous changes become due to impairment of bone growth. The epiphysis, which is radiosensitive, may show signs of radiation-induced changes with doses as low as 400 cGy. Widening of the epiphyseal plate, and irregularity and sclerosis of the metaphysis are common findings in

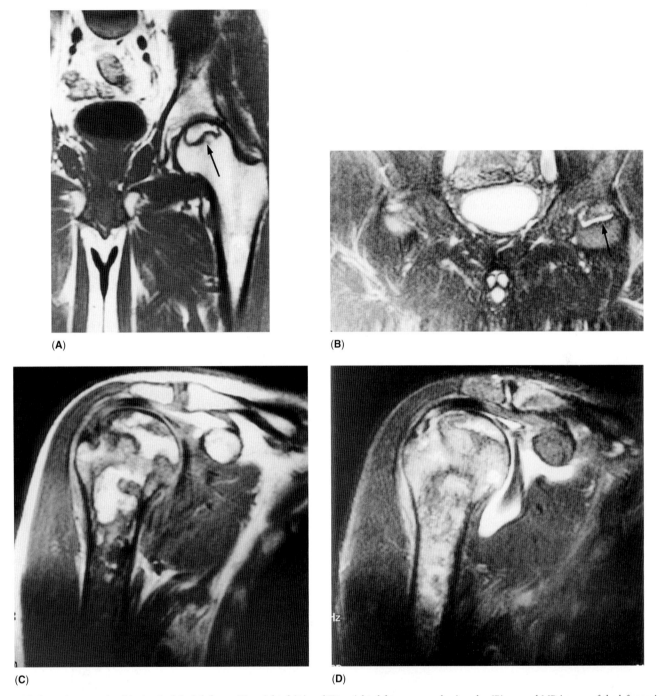

(A)   (B)

(C)   (D)

Figure 55.7 Avascular necrosis of the head of the left femur. T1-weighted (**A**) and T2-weighted fat-suppressed spin-echo (**B**) coronal MR images of the left proximal femur of a 51-year-old man with a history of lymphoma and radiation treatment to the pelvis, show changes of avascular necrosis (arrows). In another male patient with aplastic anemia who was treated with bone marrow transplantation, T1-weighted (**C**) and fast spin-echo T2-weighted fat-suppressed (**D**) coronal MR images of the right shoulder show advanced avascular necrosis of the humeral head.

the growing skeleton which is exposed to radiation (15). These findings may appear early after therapy and may resemble the osseous changes observed in rickets. In the diaphyses, changes are minimal and include narrowing of the shaft and some degree of osteopenia.

Slipped capital femoral epiphysis and, less frequently, slipped capital humeral epiphysis represent serious complications which occur one to seven years after treatment and at an earlier age than their idiopathic counterparts (15,37,38). Administration of chemotherapy increases the possibility of epiphyseal slippage. Slipped epiphysis may be accompanied by avascular necrosis of the femoral

or humeral head (39). Because of the late manifestation of post-radiation epiphyseal injuries, it is obvious that long-term follow-up is warranted for patients with a history of radiation therapy.

Radiation-induced changes of the growing spine are more pronounced in patients treated before the age of six years or at puberty, both being periods of increased skeletal growth (39). Growth arrest lines, which are dense lines parallel to the vertebral end-plates, are a common manifestation of growth arrest related to prior radiotherapy. They appear within a year from therapy

with doses greater than 10 Gy and may cause a "bone within bone" appearance. Doses greater than 20 Gy are associated with more pronounced changes of growth disturbance that become apparent within five years of completion of therapy (40). Such changes include loss of height of vertebral bodies, irregularity of the end-plates and, less frequently, contour abnormalities, which may resemble changes observed in mucopolysaccharidoses (Fig. 55.8) (41). Mild scoliosis, concave to the irradiated side, is a common complication when the spine is included in the radiation field. With megavoltage therapy, it is unusual for scolioses greater than 5° to occur, because of more even distribution of the radiation beam to the vertebrae (39,40). Kyphosis may accompany scoliosis but it is extremely rare for it to occur alone.

Osteochondroma is the only benign tumor associated with a history of radiotherapy. While the incidence of spontaneous osteochondromas is less than 1%, the incidence of osteochondromas developing within a previously irradiated field has been reported to be as high as 12% (42). An incidence of over 20% has been reported in patients who were treated with total body irradiation before the age of five (43,44). Osteochondromas appear at an average of eight years after radiotherapy (42). Histologically, these tumors do not differ from those that occur spontaneously and should be treated accordingly (41).

Radiation-induced sarcomas of the bone are extremely rare with reported relative increased risks at doses greater than 60 Gy (45). They occur 14 to 17 years after radiotherapy and with aggressive treatment survival rates approach those of primary bone sarcomas (45–48).

Key Points: Effects of Radiotherapy on the Growing Skeleton

- In children, epiphyseal changes can occur with doses as low as 400 cGy
- Slipped epiphyses occur one to seven years after radiation and warrant long-term follow-up
- Spinal changes are more pronounced in patients treated before age six or at puberty, both periods of increased skeletal growth
- Osteochondromas occur in the irradiated field in up to 12% of patients
- Osteochondromas develop approximately eight years after radiotherapy
- Radiation-induced bone sarcomas are extremely rare

EFFECTS OF CHEMOTHERAPY ON THE GROWING SKELETON

Pediatric oncology patients may suffer from complications related to the effect of certain chemotherapeutic agents on the growing skeleton (49). Prolonged administration of steroids may cause diffuse osteopenia and fractures, particularly in the spine. Avascular necrosis is a well-known complication of long-term steroid treatment. Methotrexate osteopathy is a rare syndrome, which was first described as a complication of maintenance treatment for children with acute lymphoblastic leukemia (50). It is also known to occur in 9% of children with osteosarcoma who receive high doses of methotrexate and the condition has been reported also in children under three years of age who were treated for brain tumors (51,52). Methotrexate osteopathy is manifested by (53):

- Severe lower extremity bone pain
- Osteopenia
- Dense provisional zones of calcification
- Metaphyseal insufficiency fractures

Both steroids and methotrexate may directly inhibit skeletal growth. Ifosfamide is an alkylating agent used in children for the treatment of soft tissue and bone sarcomas. It has a known nephrotoxic effect and may cause hypophosphatemic rickets (54). A single case of periosteal new bone formation along the ulnar shafts was reported in a four-year-old boy with neuroblastoma, who was treated with 13-cis-retinoic acid, a vitamin A analogue (55).

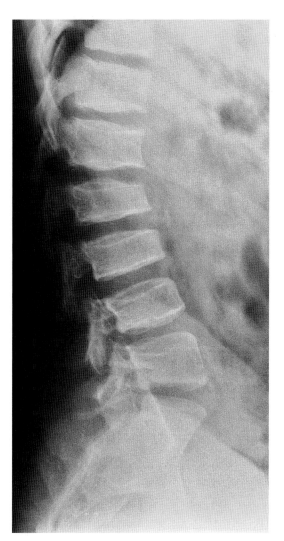

Figure 55.8 Loss of vertebral body height and irregularities of vertebral endplates. Lateral radiograph of the lumbar spine of a 17-year-old man who received radiation therapy for Wilms' tumor at the age of two years. *Source*: Courtesy of H I Libshitz.

Key Points: Effects of Chemotherapy on the Growing Skeleton

- Prolonged steroid therapy may induce osteopenia and fractures, especially in the spine
- Methotrexate osteopathy may develop in children on maintenance therapy for acute lymphoblastic leukemia
- Ifosfamide is nephrotoxic and may induce hypophosphatemic rickets

EFFECTS OF RADIATION ON THE BONE MARROW

MR imaging has provided a means of recording *in vivo* the changes that occur in the irradiated bone marrow. Immediately after initiation of radiotherapy, the signal intensity of the bone marrow on T1-weighted MR images decreases. This drop in the signal intensity of the marrow reflects an increase in free water that occurs because of edema and necrosis of the marrow. Early short tau inversion recovery (STIR) images show areas of increased signal intensity with a peak at nine days (56). As early as two weeks into therapy, and with doses as low as 8 Gy, the signal intensity of the bone marrow on T1-weighted MR imaging begins to rise as the number of adipocytes within the irradiated bone marrow grows (Fig. 55.9) (8,9,56). Conversion of the irradiated red marrow to fatty marrow is completed

before the end and about six to eight weeks after the start of radiation therapy in 90% of patients (57). This "bright" marrow is due to the short T1 value of adipose tissue and it is sharply delineated from bone marrow outside the radiation portals. Regeneration of the hematopoietic elements of the bone marrow has been reported to occur with doses lower than 30 Gy, 2 to 23 years after radiotherapy (10). With higher doses, however, conversion to fatty marrow appears to be irreversible (7,9,10). Bone marrow regeneration is affected by age, with patients under 18 years of age showing marrow recovery independent of radiation dose (45,57). Blomlie et al. reported changes on MR of non-irradiated bone marrow as well, during radiation therapy (58). These changes consist of an increase in fatty marrow and, according to the authors' conclusions, they are probably due to an indirect effect of radiation therapy rather than to scattered radiation. A significant, gradual decrease in contrast enhancement of non-irradiated bone marrow during and after the end of radiation therapy was observed with dynamic MR, and was considered to be suggestive of the effect of low radiation doses on the microvasculature of bone marrow outside the radiation portals (59).

EFFECTS OF CHEMOTHERAPY ON THE BONE MARROW

During the first days after the administration of chemotherapy regimens, a drop in the signal intensity of the bone marrow is

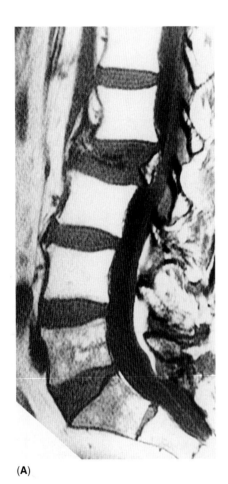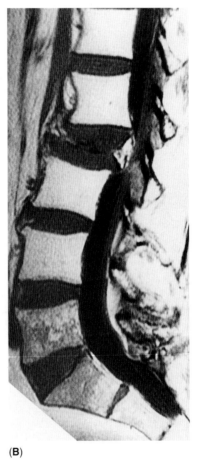

(A)   **(B)**

Figure 55.9 Postradiation MR changes of the spine. Sagittal T1-weighted (A) and enhanced T1-weighted (B) MR images of the lumbosacral spine of a 56-year-old man who received radiotherapy for Ewing's tumor at L2. Note high signal intensity of postradiation change (T12–L4) which is sharply delineated from red marrow outside the radiation field; there is no perceptible enhancement of the intact red marrow or of the affected, compressed L2 vertebra.

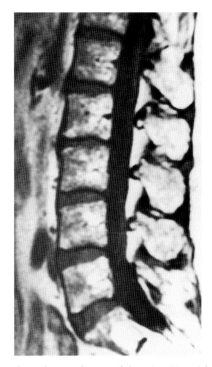

Figure 55.10 Postchemotherapy changes of the spine. T1-weighted sagittal MR image of the lumbar spine shows islands of regenerating red marrow in a 50-year-old man who is receiving chemotherapy for melanoma.

observed on spinal T1-weighted MR images together with increased brightness on T2-weighted images. The changes that occur in the bone marrow immediately after initiation of chemotherapy reflect an increase in free water in the congested bone marrow and vary, depending on the effect of chemotherapy on the bone marrow (12). Later, an increase in fatty signal intensity is observed within the bone marrow on MR. When hematopoietic recovery occurs, about three to four weeks into chemotherapy, the marrow becomes dark again on T1-weighted MR images due to the presence of regenerating red marrow (Fig. 55.10). At this stage, differentiation of regenerating bone marrow from malignant infiltration may be difficult. Absence of a marked increase in signal intensity on T2-weighted images and minimal or no enhancement on enhanced T1-weighted images, favor the presence of red marrow recovery. Signal intensity-time curves obtained on dynamic contrast-enhanced MR imaging have been shown to differ for normal and neoplastic marrow; recognition of enhancement patterns of red marrow adjusted for age and sex may assist in the differential diagnosis (60). Also, hematopoietic bone marrow can be distinguished from bone marrow infiltrated with malignant cells on "out-of-phase" gradient recalled echo MR imaging. A signal drop on "out-of-phase" gradient recalled echo images is seen in hematopoietic bone marrow whereas no change in signal is seen on "out-of-phase" images of bone marrow which is infiltrated by malignant cells (Figs. 55.11 and 55.12) (61,62). Ultra small superparamagnetic iron oxide

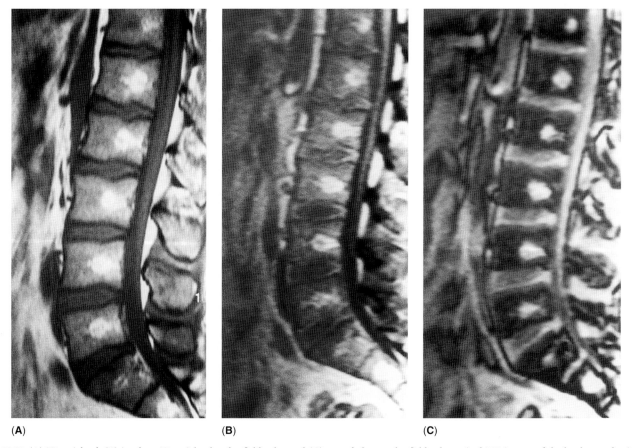

(A) (B) (C)

Figure 55.11 (A) T1-weighted, (B) in-phase T1-weighted turbo field-echo, and (C) out-of-phase turbo field-echo sagittal MR images of the lumbosacral spine in a 25-year-old healthy individual. Note drop of signal intensity of red marrow on the out-of-phase image (C) relative to the in-phase image (B) because of coexistence of water and fat protons.

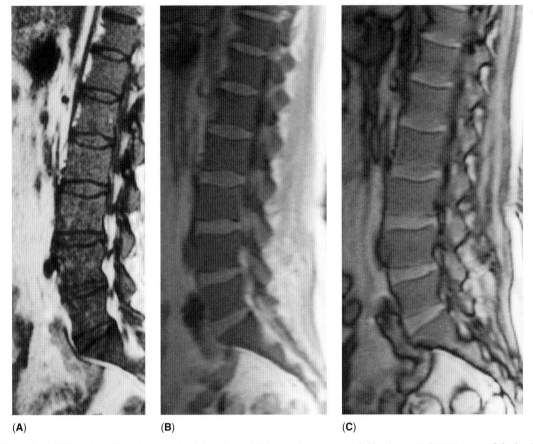

(A)   **(B)**   **(C)**

Figure 55.12 (A) T1-weighted, (B) in-phase T1-weighted turbo field-echo and (C) out-of-phase turbo field-echo sagittal MR images of the lumbosacral spine in a 54-year-old woman with diffuse large cell lymphoma. Note absence of signal intensity drop of abnormal marrow on out-of-phase image (C).

particles (USPIO) extravasate through the blood-bone marrow barrier, are phagocytised by reticuloendothelial cells and cause a drop in the signal intensity of normal or hypercellular red marrow on relatively T2-weighted MR images of the bone marrow (63). Changes are more pronounced on STIR images obtained 45 to 60 minutes after iron oxide infusion (64). USPIO-enhanced MR studies may aid the differential diagnosis of regenerated hypercellular red marrow from malignant infiltration of the bone marrow (63–65). However even with all currently available MR techniques, early (<20%) infiltration may be difficult to detect.

Reconversion of fatty to red marrow occurs in the opposite direction to marrow conversion, that is, from the axonal skeleton to the periphery. When there is an increased need for additional hematopoiesis, red marrow will appear in the proximal metaphyses of the femur and humerus. In extreme cases, red marrow may appear at other parts of the peripheral skeleton, which are occupied by fatty marrow in healthy adults. Reconversion of epiphyseal fatty marrow to hematopoietic marrow is very rare and occurs only after all other sites of red marrow have been activated and the demand for hematopoiesis has not been met.

Changes related to increased hematopoiesis are accentuated on MR images of the bone marrow when granulocyte colony-stimulating factor (G-CSF) is administered during chemotherapy to prevent neutropenia (66). Fletcher et al. reported changes of reconversion in the femoral diaphyses of children receiving hematopoietic growth factors in addition to chemotherapy for musculoskeletal tumors (67). No such changes were observed in children who did not receive

growth factors. In adults, red marrow reconversion was reported in 40% of patients who received G-CSF in conjunction to chemotherapy for treatment of primary musculoskeletal neoplasms with no obvious relationship between the extent of bone marrow reconversion and the number of G-CSF courses (68). Hematopoietic activity induced by growth factors may be asymmetric and it may simulate malignant dissemination to the bone marrow (69). Awareness of the treatment regimens is necessary for the accurate interpretation of post-therapy MR images.

MR imaging has also been applied to the evaluation of bone marrow after transplantation. Patients who have undergone stem cell transplantation are currently assessed with serial bone marrow biopsies and aspirations. Prospective MR studies are being carried out in an attempt to introduce a potential non-invasive means of following the changes that occur in the marrow of these patients. Stevens and his colleagues reported a characteristic band pattern, which was present on T1-weighted images of all but one of 15 patients who received bone marrow transplants (56). This band pattern consisted of a bright central zone of fatty marrow and a peripheral dark zone of hematopoietic cells. The band-like distribution of red and fatty marrow in the vertebral body may be explained by the pattern of vascular flow into the vertebra, which in turn determines the distribution of the proliferating blood cells. Iron overload has been reported to occur in about 40% of patients treated with bone marrow transplantation and may cause a drop in bone marrow signal intensity, more obvious on relatively T2-weighted images (70).

MR imaging is the most accurate imaging modality for the evaluation of large volumes of bone marrow and provides information complementary to the bone marrow biopsy. Detailed knowledge of the expected changes in the bone marrow under different conditions and close collaboration between the radiologist and the clinician is important if complex bone marrow changes are to be interpreted correctly and appropriate action taken.

Key Points: Bone Marrow Changes Following Treatment

- Changes in the bone marrow can be seen on T1-weighted MR images immediately after initiation of radiotherapy due to an increase in free water
- Within two weeks of the start of radiotherapy, fat starts to replace the red marrow; these changes can be irreversible with high doses
- Chemotherapy results in an increase in water within the bone marrow within days; within a week, there is an increase in fat; about three to four weeks later, regenerating marrow appears. All these changes can be monitored on MR images

Summary

- Radiation therapy results in an immediate inflammatory reaction and hypocellularity in the bone marrow. Endarteritis occurs later and results in bone necrosis
- Local demineralization is the earliest, most often the only radiographic change following radiotherapy. Lytic foci may grow and simulate neoplastic lesions
- Radiation-induced fractures are seldom seen less than two to three years after therapy, are most common in the pelvis and are best detected on MR
- Avascular necrosis occurs years after radiation treatment. It is important to recognize its presence before the development of subchondral fractures
- In the growing skeleton subjected to radiotherapy, slipped epiphysis is a serious complication and is made more likely by the addition of chemotherapy
- Both radiotherapy and chemotherapy produce serial changes in the bone marrow that can be monitored on MR images
- Within two weeks of the start of radiotherapy, fat starts to replace the red marrow
- Chemotherapy results in an increase in water within the bone marrow within days

REFERENCES

1. Ewing J. Radiation osteitis. Acta Radiol 1926; 5: 399–412.
2. Howland WJ, Loeffler RK, Starchman DE, Johnson RG. Post-irradiation atrophic changes of bone and related complications. Radiology 1975; 117: 677–85.
3. Rubin P, Gasarett GW. Clinical Radiation Pathology, Vol. II. Philadelphia: Saunders, 1968: 557–608.
4. Fajardo LF. Locomotive system. In: Pathology of Radiation Injury. New York: Masson, 1982: 176–86.
5. Knospe WH, Blom J, Crosby WH. Regeneration of locally irradiated bone marrow. I. Dose dependent, long-term changes in the rat, with particular emphasis upon vascular and stromal reaction. Blood 1966; 28: 398–415.
6. Sykes MP, Savel H, Chu FC, et al. Long-term effects of therapeutic irradiation upon bone marrow. Cancer 1964; 17: 1144–8.
7. Kauczor H-U, Dieti B, Brix G, et al. Fatty replacement of bone marrow after radiation therapy for Hodgkin disease: quantification with chemical shift imaging. J Magn Reson Imaging 1993; 3: 575–80.
8. Remedios PA, Colletti PM, Raval JK, et al. Magnetic resonance imaging of bone after radiation. Magn Reson Imaging 1988; 6: 301–4.
9. Yankelevitz DF, Henschke CI, Knapp PH, et al. Effect of radiation therapy on thoracic and lumbar bone marrow: evaluation with MR imaging. AJR Am J Roentgenol 1991; 157: 87–92.
10. Casamassima F, Ruggiero C, Caramella D, et al. Hematopoietic bone marrow recovery after radiation therapy: MRI evaluation. Blood 1989; 73: 1677–81.
11. Sacks EL, Goris ML, Glatstein E, Gilbert E, Kaplan HS. Bone marrow regeneration following large field radiation: influence of volume, age, dose, and time. Cancer 1978; 42: 1057–65.
12. Islam A, Catovsky D, Galton DA. Histological study of bone marrow regeneration following chemotherapy for acute myeloid leukemia and chronic granulocytic leukemia in blast transformation. Br J Haematol 1980; 45: 535–40.
13. de Santos LA, Libshitz HI. Adult bone. In: Libshitz HI, ed. Diagnostic Radiology of Radiotherapy Change. Baltimore, MD: Williams and Wilkins, 1979; 137–50.
14. Paling MR, Herdt JR. Radiation osteitis: a problem of recognition. Radiology 1980; 137: 339–42.
15. Libshitz HI. Radiation changes in bone. Semin Roentgenol 1994; 29: 15–37.
16. Baensch W. Knochenschädigung nach Röntgenbestrah lung. Fortschr Geb Roentgenstr 1927; 36: 1245–7.
17. Ikushima H, Osaki K, Furutani S, et al. Pelvic bone complications following radiation therapy of gynecologic malignancies; clinical evaluation of radiation-induced pelvic insufficiency fractures. Gynecol Oncol 2006; 103: 1100–4.
18. Abe H, Nakamura M, Takahashi S, et al. Radiation-induced insufficiency fractures of the pelvis: evaluation with ^{99m}Tc-methylene diphosphonate scintigraphy. AJR Am J Roentgenol 1990; 158: 599–602.
19. Blomlie V, Rofstad EK, Talle K, et al. Incidence of radiation-induced insufficiency fractures of the female pelvis: evaluation with MR imaging. AJR Am J Roentgenol 1996; 167: 1205–10.
20. Oh D, Huh SJ, Nam H, et al. Pelvic insufficiency fracture after pelvic radiotherapy for cervical cancer: analysis of risk factors. Int J Radiat Oncol Biol Phys 2008; 70: 1183–8.
21. Lundin B, Bjorkholm E, Lundell M. Jacobsson H. Insufficiency fractures of the sacrum after radiotherapy for gynaecological malignancy. Acta Oncol 1990; 29: 211–15.
22. Ries T. Detection of osteoporotic sacral fractures with radionuclides. Radiology 1983; 146: 783–5.
23. Cooper KL, Beabout JW, Swee RG. Insufficiency fractures of the sacrum. Radiology 1985; 156: 15–20.

24. Blomlie V, Lien HH, Iversen T, Winderen M, Tvera K. Radiation-induced insufficiency fractures of the sacrum: evaluation with MR imaging. Radiology 1993; 188: 241–4.

25. Pierce SM, Recht A, Lingos TI, et al. Long-term radiation complications following conservative surgery (CS) and radiation therapy (RT) in patients with early stage breast cancer. Int J Radiat Oncol Biol Phys 1992; 23: 915–23.

26. Iyer RB, Libshitz HI. Late sequelae after radiation therapy for breast cancer: imaging findings. AJR Am J Roentgenol 1997; 168: 1335–8.

27. Levine DS, Navarro OM, Chaudry G, Doyle JJ, Blaser SI. Imaging the complications of bone marrow transplantation in children. Radiographics 2007; 27: 307–24.

28. Griffith JF, Antonio GE, Kumta SM, et al. Osteonecrosis of hip and knee in patients with severe acute respiratory syndrome treated with steroids. Radiology 2005; 235: 168–75.

29. Bieber E, Hungerford DS, Lennox DW. Factors in diagnosis of avascular necrosis of the femoral head. Adv Orthop Surg 1985; 9: 93–6.

30. Mitchell DG, Rao VM, Dalinka MK, et al. Femoral head avascular necrosis: correlation of MR imaging, radiographic staging, radionuclide imaging, and clinical findings. Radiology 1987; 162: 709–15.

31. Koo KH, Ahn IO, Kim R, et al. Bone marrow edema and associated pain in early stage osteonecrosis of the femoral head: prospective study with serial MR images. Radiology 1999; 213: 715–22.

32. Cook AM, Dzik-Jurasz AS, Padhani AR, Norman A, Huddart RA. The prevalence of avascular necrosis in patients treated with chemotherapy for testicular tumours. Br J Cancer 2001; 85: 1624–6.

33. Jiang CC, Shih TT. Epiphyseal scar of the femoral head: risk factor of osteonecrosis. Radiology 1994; 191: 409–12.

34. Lafforgue P, Dahan E, Chagnaud C, et al. Early-stage avascular necrosis of the femoral head: MR imaging for prognosis in 31 cases with at least 2 years of follow-up. Radiology 1993; 187: 199–204.

35. Janssens AM, Offner FC, Van Hove WZ. Bone marrow necrosis. Cancer 2000; 88: 1769–80.

36. Tang YM, Jeavons S, Stuckey S, Middleton H, Gill D. MRI features of bone marrow necrosis. AJR Am J Roentgenol 2007; 188: 509–14.

37. Dickerman JD, Newberg AH, Moreland MD. Slipped capital femoral epiphysis (SCFE) following pelvic irradiation for rhabdomyosarcoma. Cancer 1979; 44: 480–2.

38. Edeiken BS, Libshitz HI, Cohen MA. Slipped proximal humeral epiphysis: a complication of radiotherapy to the shoulder in children. Skeletal Radiol 1982; 9: 123–5.

39. Probert JC, Parker BR. The effects of radiation therapy on bone growth. Radiology 1975; 114: 155–62.

40. Heaston DK, Libshitz HI, Chan RC. Skeletal effects of megavoltage irradiation in survivors of Wilms' tumor. AJR Am J Roentgenol 1979; 133: 389–95.

41. Riseborough EJ, Grabias SL, Burton RI, Jaffe N. Skeletal alterations following irradiation for Wilms' tumor: with particular reference to scoliosis and kyphosis. J Bone Joint Surg Am 1976; 58: 526–36.

42. Libshitz HI, Cohen MA. Radiation-induced osteochondromas. Radiology 1982; 142: 643–7.

43. Taitz J, Cohn RJ, White L, Russell SJ, Vowels MR. Osteochondroma after total body irradiation: an age-related complication. Pediatr Blood Cancer 2004; 42: 225–9.

44. Faraci M, Barra S, Cohen A, et al. Very late nonfatal consequences of fractionated TBI in children undergoing bone marrow transplant. Int J Radiat Oncol Biol Phys 2005; 63: 1568–75.

45. Hwang S, Panicek DM. Magnetic resonance imaging of bone marrow in oncology, Part 2. Skeletal Radiol 2007; 36: 1017–27.

46. Inoue YZ, Frassica FJ, Sim FH, et al. Clinicopathologic features and treatment of postirradiation sarcoma of bone and soft tissue. J Surg Oncol 2000; 75: 42–50.

47. Shaheen M, Deheshi BM, Riad S, et al. Prognosis of radiation-induced bone sarcoma is similar to primary osteosarcoma. Clin Orthop Relat Res 2006; 450: 76–81.

48. Kuttesch JF, Wexler LH, Marcus RB, et al. Second malignancies after Ewing's sarcoma: radiation dose-dependency of secondary sarcomas. J Clin Oncol 1996; 14: 2818–25.

49. Roebuck DJ. Skeletal complications in pediatric oncology patients. Radiographics 1999; 19: 873–85.

50. Ragab AH, Frech RS, Vietti TJ. Osteoporotic fractures secondary to methotrexate therapy of acute leukemia in remission. Cancer 1970; 25: 580–5.

51. Ecklund K, Laor T, Goorin AM, Connollyy LP, Jaramillo D. Methotrexate osteopathy in patients with osteosarcoma. Radiology 1997; 202: 543–7.

52. Meister B, Gassner I, Streif W, Dengg K, Fink FM. Methotrexate osteopathy in infants with tumors of the central nervous system. Med Pediatr Oncol 1994; 23: 493–6.

53. Schwartz AM, Leonidas JC. Methotrexate osteopathy. Skeletal Radiol 1984; 11: 13–16.

54. Skinner R, Pearson AD, Price L, Cunningham K, Craft AW. Hypophosphataemic rickets after ifosfamide treatment in children. Br Med J 1989; 298: 1560–1.

55. Grissom LE, Griffin GC, Mandell GA. Hypervitaminosis A as a complication of treatment for neuroblastoma. Pediatr Radiol 1996; 26: 200–2.

56. Stevens SK, Moore SG, Kaplan ID. Early and late bone-marrow changes after irradiation: MR evaluation. AJR Am J Roentgenol 1990; 154: 745–50.

57. Sacks EL, Goris ML, Glatstein E, Gilbert E, Kaplan HS. Bone marrow regeneration following large field radiation: influence of volume, age, dose, and time. Cancer 1978; 42: 1057–65.

58. Blomlie V, Rofstad EK, Skjonsberg A, Tvera K, Lien HH. Female pelvic bone marrow: serial MR imaging before, during and after radiation therapy. Radiology 1995; 194: 537–43.

59. Otake S, Mayr NA, Ueda T, Magnotta VA, Yuh WT. Radiation-induced changes in MR signal intensity and contrast enhancement of lumbosacral vertebrae: do changes occur only inside the radiation therapy field? Radiology 2002; 222: 179–83.

60. Savvopoulou V, Maris TG, Vlahos L, Moulopoulos LA. Differences in perfusion parameters between upper and lower lumbar vertebral segments with dynamic contrast-enhanced MRI (DCE MRI). Eur Radiol 2008; 18: 1876–83.

61. Disler DG, McCauley TR, Ratner LM, Kesack CD, Cooper JA. In-phase and out-of-phase MR imaging of bone marrow: prediction of neoplasia based on the detection of coexistent fat and water. AJR Am J Roentgenol 1997; 169: 1439–47.

62. Zampa V, Cosottini M, Michelassi C, et al. Value of opposed-phase gradient-echo technique in distinguishing benign and malignant vertebral lesions. Eur Radiol 2002; 12: 1811–18.

63. Metz S, Lohr S, Settles M, et al. Ferrumoxtran-10-enhanced MR imaging of the bone marrow before and after conditioning therapy in patients with non-Hodgkin lymphomas. Eur Radiol 2006; 16: 598–607.

64. Daldrup-Link HE, Rummeny EJ, Ihssen B, Kienast J, Link TM. Iron-oxide-enhanced MR imaging of bone marrow in patients with non-Hodgkin's lymphoma: differentiation between tumor infiltration and hypercellular bone marrow. Eur Radiol 2002; 12: 1557–66.

65. Daldrup-Link HE, Henning T, Link TM. MR imaging of therapy-induced changes of bone marrow. Eur Radiol 2007; 17: 743–61.

66. Saadate-Arab M, Troufleau P, Stines J, et al. MR imaging findings of bone marrow reconversion induced by growth factors in three patients. J Radiol 2002; 83: 147–52.

67. Fletcher BD, Wall JE, Hanna SL. Effect of hematopoietic growth factors on MR images of bone marrow in children undergoing chemotherapy. Radiology 1993; 189: 745–51.

68. Hartman RP, Sundaram M, Okuno SH, Sim FH. Effect of granulocyte-stimulating factors on marrow of adult patients with musculoskeletal malignancies: incidence and MRI findings. AJR Am J Roentgenol 2004; 183: 645–53.

69. Ryan SP, Weinberger E, White KS, et al. MR imaging of bone marrow in children with osteosarcoma: effect of granulocyte colony-stimulating factor. AJR Am J Roentgenol 1995; 165: 915–20.

70. Kornreich L, Horev G, Yaniv I, et al. Iron overload following bone marrow transplantation in children: MR findings. Pediatr Radiol 1997; 27: 869–72.

INTRODUCTION

Modern treatment of abdomino-pelvic malignancy is complex. Surgery, radiotherapy, biological therapies, and local ablative treatments can be used alone or in combination. Each mode of therapy produces specific and non-specific post-treatment appearances. Awareness of the pathophysiological processes including post-therapy imaging changes and expected time following treatment for their development enables them to be differentiated from other important pathology such as recurrent tumor or infection. Because of this it is very important for the radiologist to have a record of the patient's previous treatment, such as details of surgery including the operation note, the radiotherapy dose and fields, and prescribed chemotherapy.

Following surgery the imaging findings are typical and predictable. Tissue trauma and changes in blood supply induce inflammatory changes usually leading to fibrosis. In the absence of post-operative infection and with a few exceptions, such as anastomotic stricture, adhesions and hernias, late affects are unusual.

Conversely, late affects are common after radiotherapy and are recognized following chemotherapy and biological therapy. Local therapies produce specific post-treatment imaging appearances.

Cross-sectional imaging using computed tomography (CT), magnetic resonance (MR), and ultrasound (US) is ideal for assessing the treated patient by demonstrating anatomical alterations in bones, hollow organs, and other viscera including intra-organ anatomy and connective tissue changes. Advanced MR and nuclear medicine techniques including positron emission tomography CT (PET-CT) are invaluable for assessing damage in treated tissue by displaying disordered function, particularly prior to the development of altered anatomy.

RADIATION AND CHEMOTHERAPY INJURY

Radiation affects those tissues with the most rapid cell turnover. Disruption of intracellular DNA prevents cellular replication and results in depletion in stem cell populations. Local cytokine and chemokine release causes inflammation and early tissue damage. Subsequently, damage to microvasculature develops resulting in ischemia, tissue necrosis, and fibrosis. Chemotherapy also affects tissues with rapid cell turnover, resulting in parenchymal cell depletion, but damage to microvasculature and fibro-connective tissue is absent (1).

Radiation and drugs administered concurrently can act additively or synergistically to produce late tissue injury. When administered consecutively, they can each reveal pre-existing subclinical therapeutic damage. They may also aggravate the effects of infection, trauma, and other physical stresses.

Organs and tissues have been accorded tolerance doses of radiation. The minimum tolerance dose $(TD_{5/5})$ and maximum tolerance dose $(TD_{50/5})$ are defined by severe life-threatening complications occurring within five years of treatment, in 5% and 50% of treated populations, respectively. For example, the ovary has a $TD_{5/5}$ to $TD_{50/5}$ of 2 to 6 Gy and the gastro-intestinal tract has a $TD_{5/5}$ to $TD_{50/5}$ of 2 to 10 Gy for a single dose. The tissue or organ with the lowest tolerance dose determines dose limits in a particular body area (2).

As well as the total radiation dose, the following treatment factors affect the risk of radiation damage:

- Size, number, and frequency of radiation fractions
- Volume of irradiated tissue
- Duration of treatment
- Method of radiation delivery (e.g., brachytherapy)
- Combination with chemotherapy and/or surgery
- Use of biological response modifiers (e.g., hypothermia radiosensitizers, radio-protectors)

Patient factors increasing the risk of radiation injury are:

- Hypertension, atherosclerosis, and diabetes mellitus (3,4)
- Pelvic inflammatory disease and infection (5,6)
- Adhesions from prior surgery causing prolonged radiation exposure to immobile small bowel fixed in the treatment field (7)

Key Points: Radiation and Chemotherapy Injury

- Knowledge of treatment details helps differentiate post-therapy changes from recurrent tumor and infection
- Radiation and chemotherapy initially affects tissues with the most rapid cell turnover
- Late effects are most common after radiotherapy and are due to ischemia, tissue necrosis and fibrosis
- Treatment and patient factors influence radiation injury
- Radiation damages multiple organs and body systems in the abdomen and pelvis
- Tolerance doses of radiation are defined by severe life-threatening complications occurring within five years of treatment

Classification of Treatment Injury

Adverse effects following treatment are categorized as:

- Acute (occurring in the first three months)
- Subacute (occurring from three months to one year)
- Chronic (occurring later than one year)

There is considerable overlap between the groups; for example, acute effects characterized clinically and pathologically can occur after a delay of several months. Patients with severe acute radiation reactions are more likely to progress to serious chronic radiation damage. In 15% to 30% of patients (8), multiple organs are involved, resulting in increased morbidity and mortality.

There have been many systems devised for scoring the clinical severity of treatment injury. The LENT/SOMA (Late Effects

Normal Tissues/Subjective Objective Medical Management Analytic) system, agreed in 1995 by the RTOG (Radiation Therapy Oncology Group) and EORTC (European Organization for the Research and Treatment of Cancer) (9), allows a comprehensive record of subjective and objective clinical side-effects, but does not usually include imaging findings.

Treatment Effect Vs. Residual/Recurrent Tumor

A frequent problem in oncological imaging is the distinction between residual or recurrent tumor and treatment effect, particularly radiotherapy-induced changes. Cross-sectional imaging relies on the failure of tumor resolution, the enlargement or appearance of a mass, or evidence of metastases to identify malignant disease. More infiltrative tumor recurrence can be particularly difficult to distinguish from treatment effect.

Because of its superior contrast resolution MR has the advantage over CT of identifying persistent or new abnormal signal intensity within an organ and can sometimes differentiate between tumor and fibrosis. Tumor usually demonstrates intermediate signal intensity on T1W images, intermediate to high signal intensity on T2W images, and enhancement after intravenous (IV) contrast (10,11). Fibrosis returns low-signal intensity on both T1 and T2W images, and shows little or no enhancement after IV contrast injection. However, there is considerable overlap between tumor and fibrosis so that desmoplastic tumors (e.g., breast, carcinoid and rectal tumors) may have similar signal intensity characteristics to fibrosis. Radiation therapy effect, with edema and inflammation in the acute phase and capillary neovascularity in the chronic phase, may have MR features indistinguishable from tumor (12).

When diagnostic difficulty occurs it has been customary, until recently, to adopt a wait-and-watch approach, rescanning the patient at regular intervals to identify disease outside of the treatment field or the appearance or enlargement of a mass lesion. This approach has been largely superseded by using advanced imaging techniques, principally dynamic contrast-enhanced MR and [18]FDG PET-CT. For example, in bladder cancer, on MR, tumor enhances earlier and to a greater degree than radiation therapy effect following administration of IV contrast (13). In colorectal cancer [18]FDG PET-CT has become the imaging modality of choice to differentiate between the presacral fibrosis present as a consequence of abdomino-perineal resection of the rectum and recurrent rectal cancer in this location (14). MR diffusion-weighted imaging has been reported to differentiate between residual or recurrent tumor and post-chemoradiation changes in laryngeal cancer (15), which is promising for its use in the abdomen and pelvis. Occasionally percutaneous CT-guided biopsy will be required. In this instance, [18]FDG PET-CT is valuable in reducing sampling errors by directing the biopsy to the most likely site of active disease.

Key Points: Treatment Effect Vs. Residual/ Recurrent Tumor

- T2-weighted MR is superior to CT in its differentiation
- Contrast-enhanced MR is valuable but can cause confusion
- [18]FDG PET-CT is the investigation of choice for evaluation of post-surgery changes in the presacral region
- CT-guided biopsy maybe required

For ease of reference, discussion in this chapter has been divided into the effects of surgery, chemotherapy, and radiotherapy on the hepato-spleno-pancreatico-biliary, gastro-intestinal, genitourinary, and musculoskeletal systems. However, late effects, particularly following radiotherapy, are seldom limited to one organ or body system.

HEPATO-SPLENO-PANCREATICO-BILIARY SYSTEM

Surgical Change

Hepatic resection is most commonly performed for hepatocellular carcinoma or colorectal metastases. Hepatic resection may be anatomical (conforming to Couinaud's system of segmental anatomy) or non-anatomical (wedge resection). Metallic surgical clips are usually seen at the resection margin on CT. Perihepatic fluid collections are commonly seen immediately following surgery, but usually resolve within the first month. Post-operative complications include hepatic failure, perihepatic abscess, and biliary leak. In the months following resection, the remaining liver regenerates and may recover to its original volume, making the previous resection difficult to appreciate; so attention should be paid to the portal and hepatic venous anatomy (Fig. 56.1). The liver is the most common site of recurrence and, if this is isolated, further surgery may be possible (16).

Local tumor ablation is increasingly being used in the treatment of malignant liver tumors (see also chap. 51). Cryotherapy (the use of low temperature to destroy tumor) is usually performed at laparotomy and may be used alone or as an adjunct to surgery. Radiofrequency ablation (RFA) is usually performed percutaneously under imaging guidance. Cryotherapy and RFA both produce a rounded non-enhancing defect on CT or MR. A thin, enhancing hyperemic halo is commonly seen soon after ablation, which subsides over the first three months. Local tumor recurrence is diagnosed when there is nodular or irregular enhancement at the margin of the ablated area (17–19).

Following pancreato-duodenectomy (Whipple's procedure), radiology is valuable in the identification and percutaneous drainage of abdominal abscesses. These may occur within the retroperitoneum or throughout the peritoneal cavity and, therefore, post-operative CT should include the entire abdomen and pelvis. The bile ducts are susceptible to damage at the time of surgery, which may lead to biloma, hepatic abscess, or biliary stricture (20).

Splenectomy may be necessary to achieve full surgical clearance of a gastric or pancreatic tail tumor or other retroperitoneal mass. Occasionally, splenectomy is performed for symptom control in patients with hematological malignancy. Following splenectomy, adjacent structures will prolapse into the subphrenic space and may be mistaken for tumor. The pancreatic tail, unopacified stomach, and small bowel are most commonly misidentified.

Patients who undergo upper abdominal surgery for malignancy are at risk of portal venous system thrombosis; the risk following splenectomy is around 10%. Thrombosis may be recognized at post-operative CT or US; it is usually managed conservatively with anticoagulation and complications are rare (21).

Chemotherapy Change

A large number of chemotherapy agents may induce elevation of liver enzymes, which is commonly associated with hepatic steatosis.

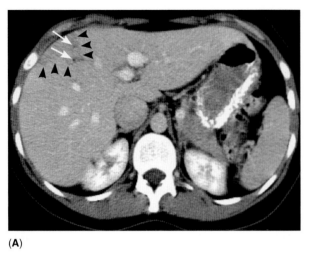
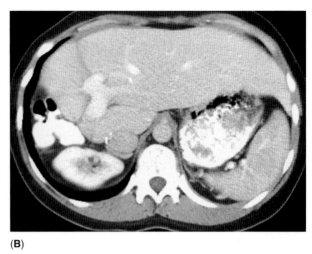

(A)   **(B)**

Figure 56.1 (**A**) Transaxial contrast-enhanced CT image of the liver in a patient with colorectal carcinoma. There is a small metastasis centrally within Segment VIII (not visible), causing a wedge-shaped peripheral perfusion defect (arrowheads) and localized dilatation of the biliary radicals (arrows). (**B**) Transaxial CT image of the same patient following right hemihepatectomy, showing marked hypertrophy of the caudate lobe (Segment I) and Segments II and III.

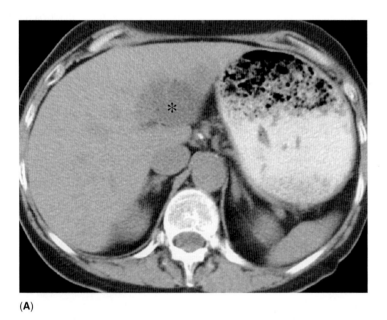
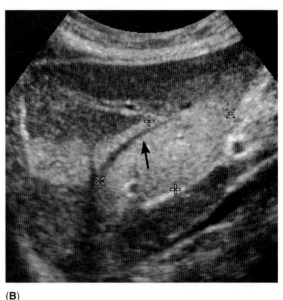

(A)   **(B)**

Figure 56.2 (**A**) Transaxial non-contrast-enhanced CT of the liver in a patient with ovarian cancer. There is a low-density lesion posteriorly within the left lobe of the liver, which mimics a metastasis (*). The attenuation value of the lesion was 18 Hounsfield units. (**B**) Longitudinal ultrasound image of the same patient shows a well-defined hyperechoic area within the liver. The liver contour is not distorted and a hepatic vein branch is seen passing through the lesion (arrow); these are features of focal fat deposition.

Radiologists should be aware of the appearance of focal fat deposition and focal fatty sparing to avoid erroneous diagnosis of metastasis. Focal fat deposition commonly occurs adjacent to the falciform ligament or anterior to the porta hepatis and is typically visible as a well-demarcated hyperechoic region on US and as an area of low density on CT, with a Hounsfield value close to that of water. Focal fat may occur in other areas of the liver and is recognized by its geographical margins and absence of mass effect (Fig. 56.2) (22,23). Areas of normal liver within an otherwise diffusely fatty liver are seen on US as hypoechoic lesions within a generally hyperechoic liver. These areas are commonly rounded and may easily be mistaken for tumor. When such a lesion is seen at a typical site (adjacent to the gallbladder or anterior to the porta

hepatis), focal fatty sparing must be considered (Fig. 56.3) (24,25). Diagnosis is often difficult on US or CT, and MR may be required to confirm the diagnosis. The most reliable MR technique is chemical-shift imaging, in which areas of fatty liver show loss of signal on "out-of-phase" images (Fig. 56.4) (26,27).

The most common pattern of hepatic steatosis is diffuse change throughout the liver, seen as diffuse heterogeneous increased echogenicity on US and reduced liver attenuation on CT. On US, this makes identification and measurement of metastases difficult on follow-up studies. An additional problem is calcification of liver metastases, which is particularly common in colorectal carcinoma, and may occur as a result of chemotherapy. The presence or absence of calcification in metastases is not a prognostic indicator (28).

Calcifications are often irregular and cause disruption of the US beam, making lesions extremely difficult to define.

Patients with liver metastases from breast cancer may rarely develop a striking "pseudocirrhosis" appearance following chemotherapy

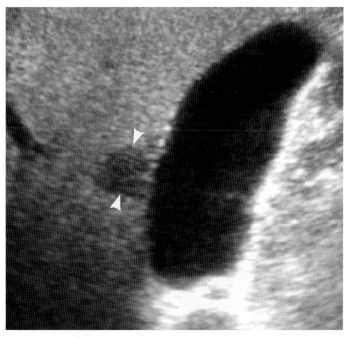

Figure 56.3 Ultrasound image showing focal fatty sparing adjacent to the gallbladder, mimicking a liver metastasis (arrowheads). The surrounding liver shows increased echogenicity due to fatty infiltration. The typical position and absence of a hypoechoic halo favor the diagnosis of focal fatty sparing.

(Fig. 56.5). The CT features are retraction of the liver surface at the site of previous metastases, resulting in a lobular hepatic contour, segmental volume loss and enlargement of the caudate lobe, all of which are signs seen in cirrhosis. Pathologically, there is nodular regenerative hyperplasia and absence of cirrhosis (29). The irregular appearance of the liver makes detection of residual tumor difficult.

Hepatic fibrosis, sclerosing cholangitis, and cirrhosis are rare complications of chemotherapy. Causative agents include methotrexate, chlorambucil, 5-fluorouracil, and floxuridine. The incidence of hepatic toxicity is higher if direct hepatic artery infusion of chemotherapy is performed. Very rarely, hepatic necrosis and liver failure may occur. Concurrent hepatic radiotherapy may increase the toxicity of vincristine and doxorubicin (30).

Patients undergoing bone marrow transplant (BMT) who receive myeloablative treatment, with either high-dose chemotherapy or whole-body irradiation, are prone to the specific complications of hepatic veno-occlusive disease (VOD) and graft-versus-host disease (GVHD). Hepatic VOD usually occurs in the first 20 days following BMT and presents clinically with tender hepatomegaly, ascites, and jaundice. Hepatic GVHD typically presents later, it has no specific imaging features, but is commonly associated with ascites. US can assist in the early diagnosis of hepatic VOD and differentiation from GVHD. Ascites and gallbladder wall thickening >6 mm detected on US have a high positive and negative predictive value for VOD, whereas Doppler evidence of reduced portal vein flow and presence of paraumbilical vein flow are the criteria with the highest specificity for the diagnosis (31).

Immunocompromised patients, particularly those with previous BMT, are also liable to systemic opportunistic infection, which

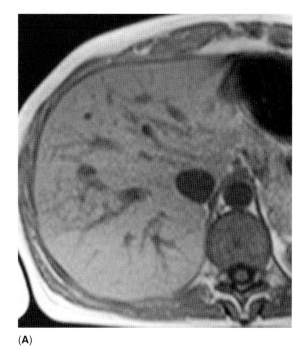

(A)

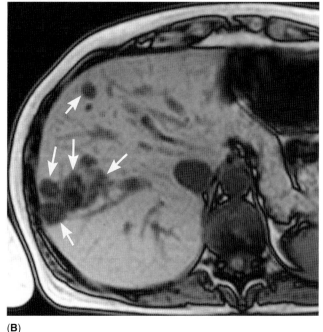

(B)

Figure 56.4 (A) In-phase and (B) out-of-phase T1-weighted MR images in a patient with colorectal cancer. Previous contrast-enhanced CT (not shown) had identified multiple soft tissue density liver lesions which had been diagnosed as metastases. The lesions cannot be clearly identified on the in-phase image, but show marked signal loss on the out-of-phase image (arrows), indicating that they are fat containing. The lesions have remained stable on long-term follow-up and are considered to represent focal fat deposition.

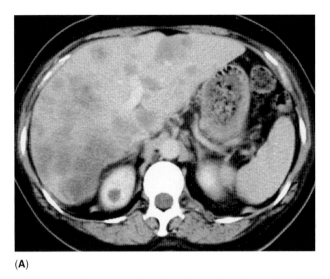
(A)

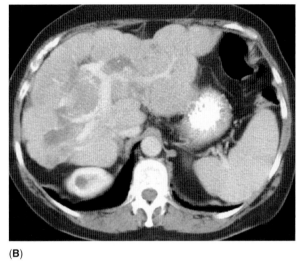
(B)

Figure 56.5 (**A**) Transaxial contrast-enhanced CT image of a patient with multiple hypodense liver metastases from breast carcinoma. (**B**) Transaxial CT image of the same patient following systemic chemotherapy. The liver metastases have reduced in size, causing retraction of the liver surface and a lobulated liver surface. The right lobe of the liver has atrophied and the caudate lobe and areas of the left lobe have hypertrophied. This appearance is known as pseudocirrhosis.

may affect the liver and spleen. The most common pathogens are fungi, particularly Candida, and tuberculosis, which may present as microabscesses within the abdominal organs (32).

Radiation Therapy Change

Liver
Primary radiotherapy to the whole liver is uncommon, but the liver is commonly partially irradiated when treatment is directed at adjacent structures. Radiation-induced liver disease (RILD) occurs in whole liver irradiation with a threshold dose of 20 to 30 Gy, but the liver will tolerate doses of over 70 Gy if only partially irradiated using conformal treatment. Patients with pre-existing liver disease, particularly chronic hepatitis, and patients receiving concurrent chemotherapy are more prone to toxicity (33,34).

Radiotherapy may also be delivered selectively to the liver by hepatic arterial embolization of Y90 microspheres (Selective Internal Radiation Therapy—SIRT), this technique delivers a high dose of β-radiation, which is primarily directed at metastases, but also affects the adjacent normal liver. RILD is more likely in the liver which is heavily infiltrated with metastases and is clinically apparent in 5% to 10% of cases (35).

Radiation-induced liver disease typically occurs four to eight weeks following radiotherapy treatment resulting in ascites, hepatomegaly, and elevation of liver enzymes, although jaundice is unusual. Pathologically, there is VOD with fibrinous obliteration of the central veins resulting in marked hepatic congestion. Most cases resolve within six months, although there may be residual fibrosis histologically (36,37).

In the subacute phase, RILD typically causes reduced attenuation on non-contrast CT within the treated area, thought to be due to liver edema. The treated area is normally clearly demarcated and corresponds to the radiotherapy field. Following administration of IV contrast medium, the irradiated area may enhance to a greater degree than the normal liver on arterial and portal-phase CT. This exaggerated enhancement is thought to be a consequence of occlusion of the small hepatic veins, which results in increased portal pressure and an

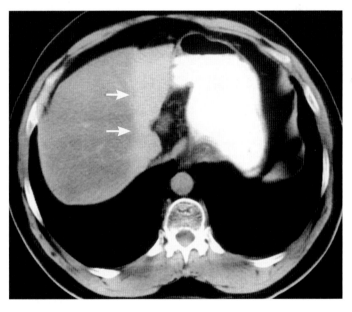

Figure 56.6 Transaxial CT image of a patient several months following radiotherapy for a lymphomatous nodal mass. There is a clear, straight line of demarcation (arrows) between the irradiated liver and the hypodense, unirradiated liver. The unirradiated liver shows evidence of fatty infiltration. The straight line represents the right lateral edge of the treatment field and is the hallmark of previous radiotherapy.

increase in hepatic arterial flow, together with delayed clearance of the contrast medium. Occasionally, if the liver is diffusely infiltrated with fat, the density pattern is reversed with fatty sparing of the irradiated liver resulting in increased attenuation (Fig. 56.6). No specific imaging features have been described for RILD following SIRT, although a reduction in volume of the normal hepatic parenchyma has been noted 12 months after treatment (38).

Corresponding changes occur on liver MR, with increased water within the irradiated liver causing reduced signal intensity on T1-weighted images and increased signal intensity on T2-weighted images (39–42).

Spleen

The spleen may be included in the radiotherapy field in the treatment of lymphoma. Direct splenic irradiation is occasionally performed to control symptoms of splenomegaly or hypersplenism. The spleen is very radiosensitive and a dose of 4 to 8 Gy will destroy the lymphoid tissue within hours. The effects of splenic radiotherapy are not usually clinically significant, although functional hyposplenism and fulminant pneumococcal sepsis have been reported. Higher radiation doses, in the region of 35 to 40 Gy, may result in splenic fibrosis and atrophy (42,43).

Pancreas

The pathological changes in the irradiated pancreas are similar to those of chronic pancreatitis, resulting in necrosis and fibrosis. The acinar epithelium is more radiosensitive than the islet cells. Imaging features are non-specific and similar to chronic pancreatitis (44,45).

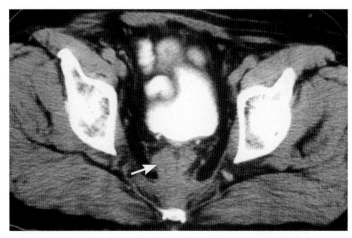

Figure 56.7 Transaxial CT image of the pelvis in a patient who has had a previous APR and perioperative radiotherapy. The seminal vesicles (right vesicle arrowed) are retracted posteromedially and there is a large presacral soft tissue mass. The mass was unchanged in appearance over several years and is due to post-treatment fibrosis.

Key Points: Liver, Spleen, and Pancreas

- Characteristic findings occur following hepatic surgery or local therapy
- Hepatic fatty change and focal fatty sparing cause confusion on US and CT; MR may be required to confirm the diagnosis
- Hepatic VOD usually occurs in the first 20 days following BMT and myeloablative therapy; hepatic GVHD presents later
- Following splenectomy, unopacified stomach, pancreatic tail and small bowel can be confused with tumor
- Changes in the irradiated pancreas cannot be differentiated from recurrent tumor without biopsy

GASTRO-INTESTINAL SYSTEM

Surgical Change

Early post-operative complications include anastomotic leak, abscess formation, bowel obstruction, hematoma, wound infection, and pancreatitis.

CT is the investigation of choice in the evaluation of abdominal abscess, pneumo-peritoneum, and anastomotic leak. Use of oral contrast is unnecessary in high-grade small bowel obstruction, but is of value in diagnosing anastomotic leak. CT helps to distinguish mechanical bowel obstruction from post-operative ileus; a transition point between proximal dilated and distal collapsed bowel should be sought (46).

In the upper abdomen, gastric surgery often results in anatomical changes, which cause difficulty in follow-up imaging. Local recurrence of gastric carcinoma may be subtle and manifest as localized bowel wall thickening or nodular peritoneal thickening. Adjacent loops of bowel may become obstructed due to tumor infiltration, and biliary obstruction may develop due to porta hepatis or peripancreatic nodes (47).

In the pelvis, the radiological appearance following abdomino-perineal resection (APR) for rectal or anal carcinoma causes particular difficulty. Following APR in the male, the bladder, seminal vesicles, and prostate are retracted posteriorly into the rectal bed. Fibrosis in the presacral space may surround and tether the seminal vesicles. The vesicles are often indistinct on CT and may be difficult to distinguish from fibrosis or recurrent tumor; however, they are usually well seen on T2-weighted MR (Figs. 56.7 and 56.8). In the female, the uterus and ovaries prolapse posteriorly into the presacral space and can easily be mistaken for a soft tissue mass on CT (Fig. 56.9). On MR, the uterus and ovaries are more readily identified.

Presacral fibrosis varies in appearance on CT or MR from thin band-like strands to a rounded mass, making differentiation from recurrent tumor difficult. MR morphology and signal characteristics can help in making this distinction as tumor is more commonly of high signal intensity on T2-weighted images. However, fibrosis can also show high signal intensity on T2-weighted images, particularly following radiotherapy (10). Dynamic contrast-enhanced MR is reported as being more accurate than non-enhanced imaging, with early enhancement suggesting tumor (48–50), although it has not been widely adopted in clinical practice for this purpose. Invasion of adjacent structures can also be difficult to assess as presacral fibrosis often involves the piriformis and levator ani muscles; however, sacral invasion indicates tumor. In practice, follow-up imaging and sometimes biopsy is necessary for confident diagnosis.

[18]FDG PET-CT is now established as the technique of choice for detection of pelvic tumor recurrence and for the characterization of indeterminate pelvic masses. The fusion of functional imaging using [18]FDG with anatomical imaging of CT is of particular value in the post-surgical pelvis where anatomy may be grossly distorted. However, false positive results do occur as a result of inflammation from recent surgery or radiotherapy, so [18]FDG PET-CT should not be performed for four months after surgery or radiotherapy. False negative results may also occur

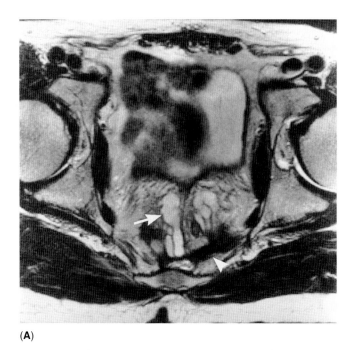

(A)

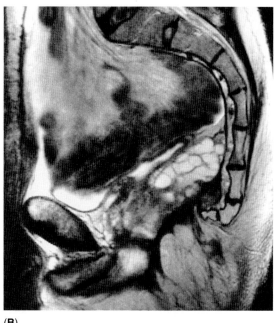

(B)

Figure 56.8 (**A**) Transaxial and (**B**) sagittal T2-weighted MR images of the pelvis in a patient who has had a previous APR. The seminal vesicles (right vesicle arrowed) have been retracted posteromedially by a band of fibrous tissue (arrowhead). In (**B**) the base of the prostate is seen to be displaced posteroinferiorly, with the prostate and seminal vesicles being fixed to the pelvic floor. Note the bladder is also being distorted. These T2-weighted images enable discrimination between anatomical structures, bands of fibrosis, and/or soft tissue "masses."

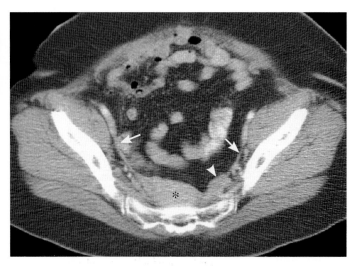

Figure 56.9 Transaxial contrast-enhanced CT image of the pelvis in a female patient who has undergone previous abdomino-perineal resection (APR). There is an apparent soft tissue mass with a smooth lobulated contour (arrowhead) in the presacral space due to the left ovary. Close inspection shows the round ligaments (arrows) extending from the mass, anteriorly along the pelvic walls. The uterus (*) and ovaries have prolapsed posteriorly following surgery.

with ^{18}FDG PET-CT, mainly in patients currently or recently treated with chemotherapy, and a minimum of six weeks without treatment is advised before imaging (Figs. 56.10 and 56.11) (51–57).

Chemotherapy Change

Chemotherapy effects on bowel mainly occur in the early phase following treatment. These include typhlitis (neutropenic enterocolitis), GVHD, and pseudomembranous colitis and are discussed in chapter 53.

Radiation Therapy Change

Although the small bowel is more radiosensitive than the large bowel, radiation damage is seen more commonly in the rectum and distal sigmoid colon. This is because the pelvis is commonly irradiated for carcinomas of the cervix, rectum, bladder, and prostate. The rectum and sigmoid are relatively fixed within the pelvis and therefore receive the largest dose. Conversely, the small bowel is mobile on a long mesentery with active peristalsis and receives a lower dose. However, adhesions from previous surgery can fix small bowel loops in the pelvis and make radiation damage more likely. Occasionally, surgical measures are taken to move the small bowel out of the radiotherapy field by packing the pelvis with either omentum or an absorbable synthetic mesh.

Stomach and Duodenum

Damage to the stomach and duodenum most commonly occurs as a result of radiotherapy for retroperitoneal lymph node metastases or pancreatic carcinoma. Initial changes affect the mucosa, causing ulceration indistinguishable from benign peptic ulcer disease on barium studies. Chronic changes result in fibrosis of the stomach wall, causing narrowing and rigidity of the gastric lumen, often with gastric outlet obstruction. The gastric wall may be indurated on barium studies, making differentiation from gastric carcinoma difficult. Changes in the duodenum include ulceration, thickened mucosal folds, and strictures (41,58).

Chronic changes are manifest on CT as deformity of the stomach, with wall thickening and inflammatory stranding into the adjacent fat.

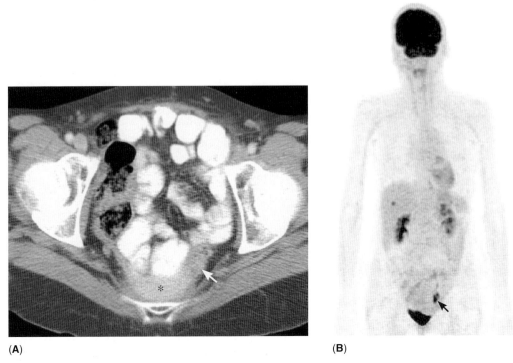

(A) **(B)**

Figure 56.10 (**A**) Transaxial contrast-enhanced CT image of a female patient who had undergone APR for anal carcinoma. The presacral mass (*) and left posterior pelvic soft tissue mass (arrow) were initially interpreted as being due to the uterus and left ovary. (**B**) Coronal ¹⁸FDG-PET image of the same patient shows a focus of increased activity in the left pelvis (arrow) corresponding to the left pelvic mass, which is in fact recurrent tumor. A further focus is seen in the liver. This was not visible on CT but was presumed to represent a small metastasis.

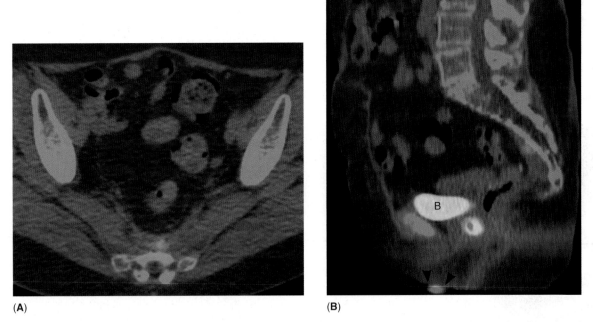

(A) **(B)**

Figure 56.11 (**A**) Transverse and (**B**) sagittal fused ¹⁸FDG-PET-CT images through the pelvis in a patient treated with anterior resection for colorectal carcinoma. The CT images show a band of soft tissue within the presacral space. Superiorly within this soft tissue is a focus of high FDG uptake which is consistent with presacral tumor recurrence. Also note FDG activity within the bladder (B), within the vagina, and on the perineum (arrowheads in **B**), due to urine contamination.

Small Bowel

Radiation damage to the small bowel most commonly occurs following radiotherapy for cervical and prostatic carcinoma. The pelvic small bowel loops and terminal ileum are particularly affected. In the early phase following radiotherapy there may be acute small bowel obstruction due to edema, which usually resolves spontaneously. Late effects present with chronic abdominal pain, diarrhea and, less commonly, malabsorption. There may be recurrent attacks of subacute small bowel obstruction, rarely progressing to complete obstruction. On barium studies, one of

the earliest changes of radiation damage is fixity of the small bowel loops within the pelvis, which is easily overlooked unless the bowel is palpated and compressed at fluoroscopy. Mucosal changes include thickening of the valvulae conniventes and nodular filling defects ("thumbprinting") due to submucosal edema. Mucosal ulceration, which may be evident microscopically, is rarely seen radiologically. The bowel loops may be separated due to wall thickening and are commonly fixed and angulated. On fluoroscopy, the bowel shows reduced peristalsis with pooling of barium within the loops. Small bowel strictures and fistulae are late features, which may be difficult to demonstrate (58–60). These radiological features are not specific for radiation damage and are particularly difficult to distinguish from Crohn's disease.

The role of CT in a previously irradiated patient with small bowel obstruction is to identify whether there is a single site or multiple sites of obstruction, to determine the anatomical level(s), and to identify whether obstruction is due to recurrent tumor. If a transition point between proximal dilated and distal collapsed bowel can be identified with no evidence of tumor, then the main differential diagnosis lies between radiation stricture and postoperative adhesions. Bowel wall thickening and mucosal abnormalities are pointers towards radiation damage, but often these conditions cannot be distinguished (Figs. 56.12 and 56.13) (46). CT is also useful in identifying fistulae, particularly if gas or oral contrast medium is identified outside the bowel.

MR enteroclysis has a similar sensitivity to conventional enteroclysis for detection of small bowel strictures. However, when used in combination with cross-sectional MR imaging, it has the advantage of showing the extent of bowel wall thickening and of excluding any associated mass lesion (61).

Colon and Rectum

Following pelvic radiotherapy, damage to the large bowel is usually confined to the rectum and sigmoid colon. Double-contrast barium enema (DCBE) is usually performed to assess the extent and severity of the disease. The earliest sign on DCBE is bowel spasm. Established disease most commonly manifests as a long smooth stricture with tapered margins involving the mid or distal sigmoid or proximal rectum. There may be shorter segments of more severe stenosis within the affected area and there may be multiple strictures (Fig. 56.14) (62). Characteristically, the mucosa is smooth and featureless, but ulceration and mucosal edema may occur, producing a "cobblestone" pattern. More rarely, there may be deep ulceration with the development of sinus tracts, pericolic or perirectal collections, or fistulae. Lateral views of the rectum often show widening of the presacral space.

Changes seen on CT include thickening of the rectal wall, increased attenuation of the perirectal fat and thickening of the perirectal fascia, resulting in widening of the presacral space (Fig. 56.15). In addition, presacral fibrosis may develop and can mimic a soft-tissue mass (63,64).

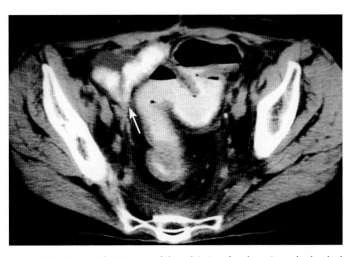

Figure 56.13 Transaxial CT image of the pelvis in a female patient who has had previous radiotherapy. The distal ileal loop in the right iliac fossa is tethered, causing an acute angulation (arrow) in the loop. The valvulae conniventes are irregularly thickened and there is a small amount of ascites lying anterior to the loop. The sigmoid colon is abnormal, being dilated with an irregularly thickened wall. In addition, there is soft tissue stranding in the pelvic fat and a presacral soft tissue band. All these findings are due to previous radiotherapy.

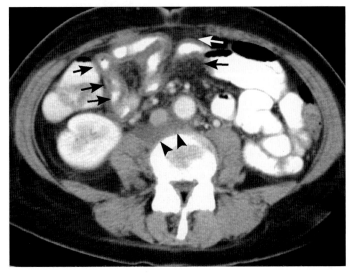

Figure 56.12 Transaxial contrast-enhanced CT image of the mid-abdomen of a patient who has received radiotherapy to the para-aortic region for retroperitoneal lymphoma (arrowheads). The small bowel loops in the central abdomen are thick-walled with narrowing of the lumen and abnormal angulation. The adjacent mesentry shows linear stranding. The area of abnormal bowel has clearly defined linear margins, corresponding to the radiotherapy field (arrows).

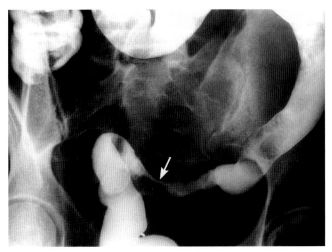

Figure 56.14 Barium enema demonstrating a variable calibre stricture in the sigmoid colon. Overall, there is a long segmental stricture within which there is a short-segment, very tight stricture (arrow). This area of the sigmoid colon received a greater dose then the more proximal sigmoid stricture.

The earliest changes of radiotherapy on MR are of increased signal intensity of the submucosa and inner (circular) muscle layer on T2-weighted images. Initially the outer muscle layer retains its normal low signal intensity. As the radiation damage progresses, there is thickening of the rectal wall (greater than 6 mm), high signal intensity within the outer muscle layer, and loss of differentiation of the rectal wall layers. There is high-signal intensity on T2-weighted images within the perirectal fat due to edema and thickening of the perirectal fascia to greater than 3 mm (65). If IV gadolinium (Gd) is administered, there is non-specific enhancement of the rectal wall.

In severe radiation bowel disease, there is necrosis and breakdown of the bowel wall due to ischemia, which can result in the development of sinus tracts or fistulae. Fistulation most commonly occurs between the rectum and vagina, but fistulae to the bladder, between loops of small and large bowel, and to skin may occur. Complex fistulae, involving the rectum, vagina, and bladder are not uncommon, particularly in patients treated for cervical carcinoma. Contrast studies of the rectum using either barium or water-soluble iodinated contrast are sensitive for detection of rectovaginal or colovesical fistula (Fig. 56.16). MR is highly accurate in demonstrating pelvic fistulae (66–68). These are normally well seen on spin-echo T2-weighted images, particularly if thin sections and a phased-array surface coil are employed (Fig. 56.17). Fat-suppressed T2-weighted and short tau inversion recovery (STIR) sequences have a higher sensitivity, but demonstrate the pelvic anatomy less well. MR has the added advantage of demonstrating extraluminal pelvic collections and recurrent tumor, which commonly coexist with radiation damage. Knowledge of the fistulous anatomy and likely sites of recurrence assists the surgeon in planning examination under anesthesia (EUA) and biopsy, and in deciding whether surgery is likely to be of value.

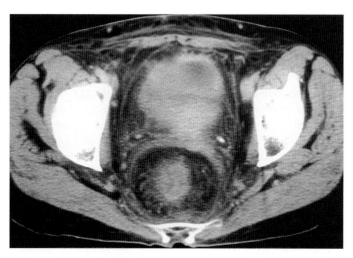

Figure 56.15 Transaxial CT image of the pelvis in a patient who has received pelvic radiotherapy. There is extensive soft tissue stranding in the perirectal space, together with thickening of the perirectal fascia. Edema is present in the anterior abdominal wall and there is a general increase in density of the pelvic fat.

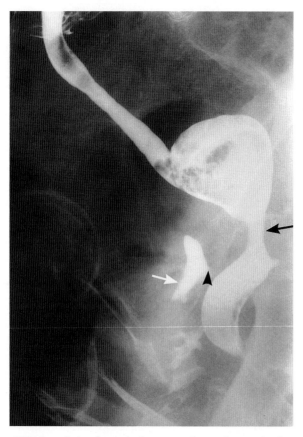

Figure 56.16 Lateral view from a barium enema in a patient previously treated with pelvic radiotherapy for carcinoma of the cervix. The left hemicolon has been defunctioned and an antegrade barium enema performed via a Foley catheter. There is a radiation stricture in the rectum (black arrow) and a fistula between the rectum and vagina. Contrast is present in the vagina (white arrow) and a small fistulous tract (arrowhead) can be identified.

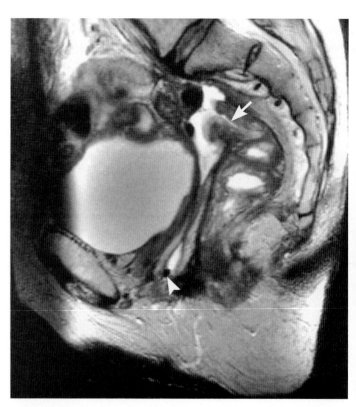

Figure 56.17 Sagittal T2-weighted MR image of a patient with recurrent cervical tumor on the left side of the pelvis involving the bladder and pelvic sidewall. The recurrent tumor is associated with a cavity containing fluid and air and there is a fistulous tract between the rectosigmoid junction through the recurrent tumor to the vault of the vagina. The communication with the large bowel is clearly seen (arrow). The vagina is clearly defined with a small amount of air being present at the introitus (arrowhead).

Key Points: Gastro-Intestinal System

- Radiation injury is most commonly seen in the rectum, sigmoid colon and pelvic small bowel
- Acute bowel reaction to radiotherapy is frequently reversible
- Chronic radiation damage is irreversible
- Barium study features in the small bowel are non-specific with mucosal abnormalities, angulated fixed loops and strictures; in the large bowel, smooth tapered strictures are characteristic
- Pelvic irradiation causes widening of the presacral space and thickening of the perirectal fascia
- MR is sensitive for detection of early radiation changes in the bowel wall and is valuable in the investigation of pelvic fistulae

THE GENITO-URINARY SYSTEM

The identification of treatment effects in the genito-urinary system requires rigorous interpretation of conventional imaging modalities such as CT and MR, as well as the adoption of newer techniques such as dynamic contrast-enhanced MR imaging. The genito-urinary tract is variably affected by cancer therapy, with the kidney and testis being more susceptible and the ureters relatively resistant. Onset of treatment effect is sometimes insidious, its diagnosis can be difficult, and multimodality treatments (often administered concurrently) can compound the problem since their effect is synergistic and produces more severe effects on normal tissue or a new pattern of organ toxicity.

Post-surgical Change

Standard genito-urinary surgical procedures and their complications should be recognizable on cross-sectional imaging. Difficulties occur when an organ has been incompletely resected, the post-surgical anatomy is altered, there are post-surgical complications simulating masses, or significant inflammatory change and fibrosis has developed. Consequently, it is extremely important to have detailed information about the exact procedure performed and, where possible, to allow time for acute post-surgical change to resolve before imaging the patient.

Partial Organ Resection

Radical resection for gynecological cancer requires a total hysterectomy. Occasionally, and particularly in benign disease, the cervix is left *in situ* and can be difficult to identify on CT, whereas its zonal anatomy is usually discernible on MR imaging (Fig. 56.18).

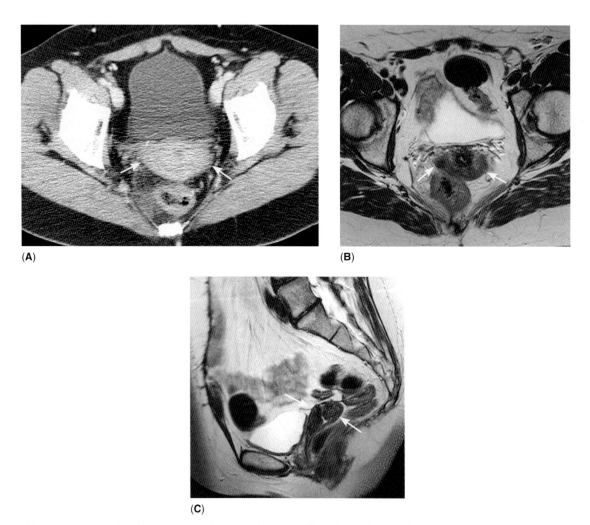

(A)

(B)

(C)

Figure 56.18 Partial organ resection. Subtotal hysterectomy. (**A**) Transaxial contrast-enhanced CT, (**B**) T2-weighted transaxial, and (**C**) T2-weighted sagittal MR images of the pelvis. There is a central pelvic mass (arrows) in a patient who had undergone a subtotal hysterectomy. The endocervical canal and zonal anatomy of the cervix can be seen on the MR images.

Partial cystectomy with bladder augmentation can result in unusual imaging appearances, again more easily interpretable on MR than CT.

Unusual Post-surgical Anatomy

Ovarian transposition can be performed during a modified radical hysterectomy to preserve ovarian function in patients about to receive post-operative radiotherapy (69). The transposed ovaries are usually moved into the iliac fossae and may be mistaken for a tumor mass on both CT and MR imaging (Fig. 56.19). The presence of follicular cysts and a vascular supply from the gonadal vessels may be helpful identifying features.

Retroperitoneal bladder hitches or flap formation for ureteric reimplantation cause unusual imaging appearances and the flaps can simulate a mass.

Postsurgical Complications (Fig. 56.20)

Lymphoceles, hematomata, and post-surgical collections can simulate residual tumor masses. Lymphoceles and hematomata have typical imaging appearances (70,71) but the latter can occur sporadically in unexpected positions such as the postorchidectomy retracted spermatic cord. Since the round ligaments are resected more laterally in ovarian than in cervical cancer surgery, a round ligament hematoma is more frequently observed in ovarian cancer patients (72).

Normal Post-operative Scarring

During a hysterectomy the vaginal vault is oversewn to give a "bow tie" appearance with a flattened central portion and bulbous lateral margins representing the sutured fornices (Fig. 56.21). If asymmetrical, the forniceal pseudomass may be mistaken for residual tumor. After a radical prostatectomy there may be extensive post-surgical fibrosis at the anastomotic site between the bladder base and membranous urethra mimicking residual tumor.

Chemotherapy Change

Chemotherapy has a direct toxic effect on the genito-urinary system, particularly the kidneys and the bladder, as well as indirect effects secondary to pancytopenia which predisposes the patient to infection or hematuria. Direct nephrotoxicity may be acute or chronic. The acute form is reversible and causes rapid onset renal failure. In this circumstance, imaging is performed to exclude renal obstruction. US may demonstrate enlarged kidneys with increased cortical echogenicity and lack of cortico-medullary differentiation. Chronic nephrotoxicity results in atrophic kidneys with loss of cortical substance. Bladder mucosal chemotoxicity is most marked in cyclophosphamide and ifosfamide-induced hemorrhagic cystitis (73), which produce a thickened bladder wall with intravesical clots. Intravesical chemotherapy or immunotherapy directly affects the bladder wall and ultimately produces a contracted, fibrosed bladder (Fig. 56.22).

Chemotherapy has an adverse permanent effect on fertility. In women the ovaries may atrophy with reduction or absence of follicles and the uterus then adopts a postmenopausal appearance with a reduction in size, endometrial atrophy, and decrease in myometrial signal intensity. There are no overt imaging findings in the male.

Radiation Therapy Change

The bladder is the most radiation sensitive organ in the urinary tract (74) and radiation bladder injury occurs in up to 20% of patients, half of whom go on to suffer severe long-term effects. In the acute phase, mucosal edema, hemorrhage, and necrosis may cause cystitis and hematuria. Subsequent fibrosis results in a small volume, non-distensible bladder producing symptoms of frequency and incontinence. Mucosal telangiectasia and ulceration may cause troublesome hematuria.

US, CT, and MR all demonstrate radiation-induced acute changes and more chronic bladder wall thickening (Fig. 55.23). Adjacent perivesical fibrosis can be identified on CT and MR, but MR can also identify a spectrum of radiation change within the bladder wall which corresponds with the severity of clinical symptoms. The earliest detectable abnormality is mucosal high signal intensity on T1- and T2-weighted images, probably reflecting hemorrhage and edema. Initially this is often localized to the posterior wall and trigone (65), but eventually the entire bladder mucosa may become involved. More severe radiation effect causes

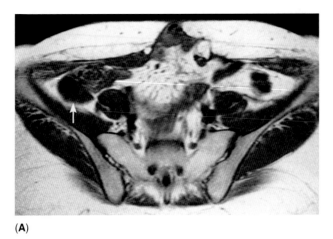

(A)

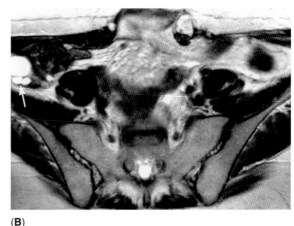

(B)

Figure 56.19 Unusual postsurgical anatomy. Ovarian transposition. Transaxial (A) T1-weighted and (B) T2-weighted MR images showing a transposed ovary (arrows) in the right iliac fossa.

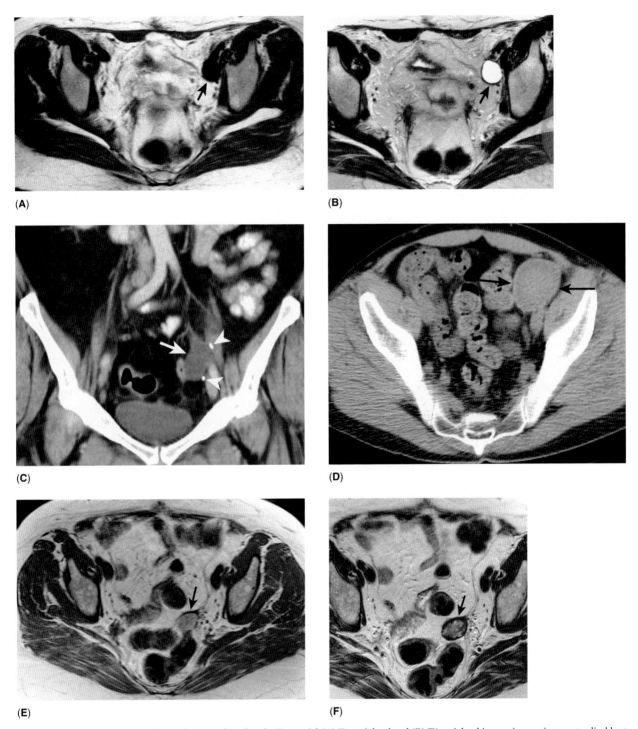

Figure 56.20 Complications of the surgical procedure. MR lymphocele. Transaxial (**A**) T1-weighted and (**B**) T2-weighted images in a patient postradical hysterectomy for cervical cancer demonstrating a left pelvic sidewall lymphocele (arrows) which is unilocular and of fluid signal intensity. (**C**) CT lymphocele. Contrast-enhanced coronal CT image demonstrating a left external iliac lymphocele (arrow) in a patient who had undergone a pelvic lymph node dissection with surgical clips (arrowheads) directly adjacent to the lymphocele. Lymphoceles are typically unilocular and of fluid attenuation. (**D**) Postorchidectomy pelvic hematoma. Non-contrast-enhanced CT examination demonstrating a left pelvic sidewall hematoma (arrows) secondary to bleeding from the retracted spermatic cord. Note the slight increase in attenuation in the centre of the hematoma due to increased electron density of the retracted clot. (**E** and **F**) Round ligament hematoma. Transaxial (**E**) T1-weighted and (**F**) T2-weighted MR images demonstrating a well rounded mass at the medial end of the left round ligament (arrows) which has T2-weighted signal intensity characteristics of a hematoma. A round ligament hematoma may resolve, decrease in size, or persist unaltered for up to one to two years.

T2-weighted high-signal intensity of the outer bladder wall, increased radial diameter of the wall and poor distensibility. Intravenous gadolinium DTPA injection may reveal enhancement of the bladder mucosa and patchy or diffuse enhancement of the outer wall, sometimes with variations in signal intensity between different layers of the bladder wall to give a banded or lamellated appearance (12). This enhancement may persist for several years.

With extreme radiation toxicity, fistula formation occurs between the bladder and the vagina or bowel. This diagnosis is usually clinically apparent, and cross-sectional imaging may reveal

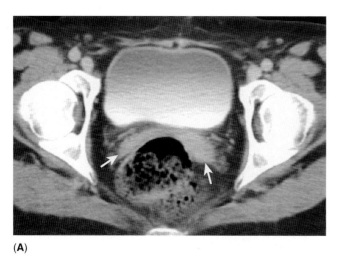

(A)

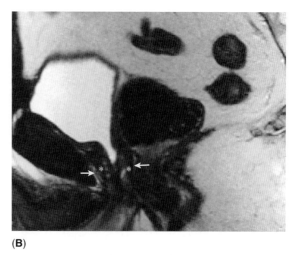

(B)

Figure 56.21 Normal postoperative scarring. (**A**) Vaginal appearances after hysterectomy. Transaxial CT scan demonstrating the normal appearance of the posthysterectomy vaginal vault. The central portion is apposed with rather bulbous but symmetrical oversewn fornices (arrows). (**B**) MR after prostatectomy. Sagittal T2-weighted image demonstrating the anastomosis (arrows) between the bladder base and the membranous urethra. There is a thick rind of low signal intensity surgical scarring (*) present.

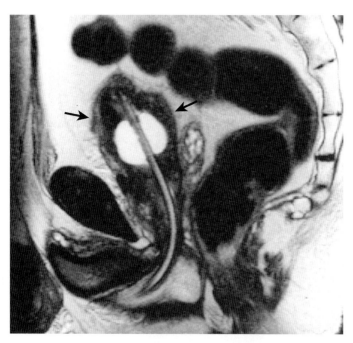

Figure 56.22 Bladder fibrosis after intravesical chemotherapy. Sagittal T2-weighted images demonstrating that the wall of the bladder is irregular, thickened and of uniform low signal intensity (arrows). The patient is catheterized because of intolerable frequency arising from the reduced bladder capacity.

the site of the fistula, particularly when a high-resolution thin-section MR technique is employed. Increasingly, MR is being used to delineate more complex fistulae involving multiple organs and fat-suppressed sequences may be valuable. Dynamic contrast-enhanced MR imaging is helpful when there is a more focal residual bladder wall abnormality of uncertain significance. Mural radiation change enhances gradually and persistently, whereas residual tumor enhances rapidly and intensely (Fig. 56.24).

The kidney is radiosensitive and is often the dose-limiting organ during treatment of abdominal malignancies, with the risk of nephrotoxicity increased by prior or concurrent chemotherapy.

Every effort is made to exclude all or most of the kidneys from the radiation field and it is only the irradiated portions which undergo atrophy (Fig. 56.25). When one kidney is irradiated, loss of renal function is evident on serial renograms as early as six months after treatment, with a 15% decrease in left kidney relative function in patients treated for stomach cancer by gastric bed irradiation progressing to up to 50% loss of function by a year (75). If both kidneys are irradiated, radiation nephropathy appears from months to years after treatment with an inverse relationship between the time-interval and renal dose (76). Ultimately radiation nephrotoxicity results in small, poorly functioning, non-obstructed kidneys.

Radiation-induced ureteric injury is uncommon, occurring in less than 5% of those sustaining complications from radiotherapy and there are two types of injury: stricture formation and vesicoureteric reflux. Stricture formation may cause renal failure but remain clinically silent. Radionuclide renography and glomerular filtration rate are useful since sequential studies will often reveal deterioration in renal performance before clinical or biochemical abnormalities occur. Strictures occur most frequently in the distal ureter immediately above the vesico-ureteric junction (Fig. 56.26), but occasionally they are found where the pelvic ureters cross anterior to the iliac vessels (77). Radiation strictures typically have a smoothly tapering, distal margin but the appearances are non-specific and may be seen in patients with tumor recurrence. Multislice CT urography with image reformation is useful to identify strictures, which may also be well demonstrated on MR imaging. Occasionally, it may be necessary to perform antegrade pyelography.

Vesico-ureteric reflux may occur secondary to distortion of the vesico-ureteric junction by bladder wall fibrosis. This predisposes the patient to infection and reflux nephropathy.

Radiotherapy affects the prostate and seminal vesicles in a similar fashion to any other irradiated organ but the acute edematous phase is usually unrecognized and it is long-term fibrosis which becomes apparent on imaging, with atrophy of both organs. On MR imaging the peripheral zone of the prostate becomes of

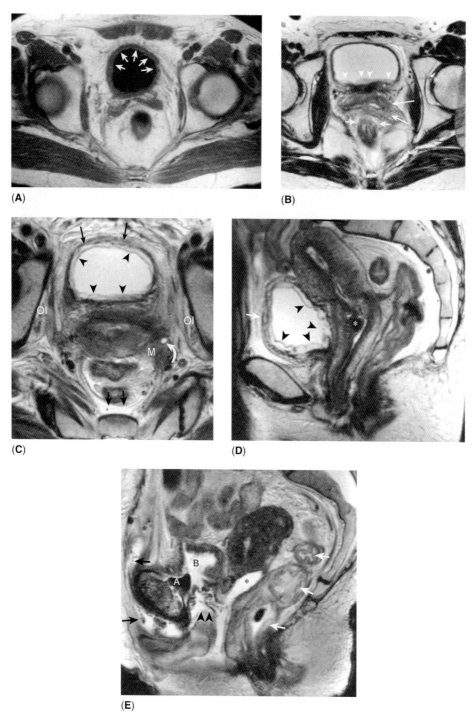

Figure 56.23 Radiation therapy effect on the bladder. (A) Acute radiotherapy change with hemorrhage. Transaxial T1-weighted image demonstrating a fine, high-signal intensity rind (arrows) on the inner margins of the bladder wall. This is due to hemorrhage within the mucosa. (B) Acute radiation change in the central pelvis. Transaxial T2-weighted image demonstrating radiotherapy change in a patient treated for cancer of the cervix. The posterior bladder wall demonstrates high signal mucosal thickening (arrowheads) as well as intermediate to low signal thickening of the muscle layer (*). Note that the anterior bladder wall retains its normal low signal intensity muscle layer. The vaginal vault is also abnormal with mucosal and submucosal thickening particularly on the left (long arrows). The anterior portion of the rectum demonstrates high signal intensity of the wall due to inclusion in the field (short arrows). Severe radiation change in the pelvis. (C) Transaxial and (D) sagittal T2-weighted sequences demonstrating severe acute radiation change. The mucosa of the bladder is markedly thickened (arrowheads), the muscle layer is thickened and demonstrates abnormal high signal intensity with some preservation of portions of the low signal intensity muscle to give a lamellated appearance particularly anteriorly (white arrows). The posterior bladder wall is retracted towards the cervix on the sagittal view. The vagina and rectum demonstrate abnormal high signal intensity mural thickening due to the radiation therapy effect. There is a radiation marker seed within the anterior lip of the cervix (*). More generalized changes are seen with edema in the presacral space (black arrows in C), generalized increase in stranding within the pelvic fat and abnormal high signal intensity of the obturator internus muscles (OI) due to an edematous reaction. An abnormal intermediate to low-signal intensity mass (M) is seen around the lateral margin of the uterus enveloping the distal left ureter (curved arrow in C). This represents incomplete resolution of tumor. (E) Severe radiation change with fistula formation and abscess. Sagittal T2-weighted image in a patient treated with radiation therapy for carcinoma of the cervix. The vagina is fluid-filled (*) and there is a fistula (arrowheads) communicating with the bladder (B) and a large retropubic abscess cavity (A). The abscess extends to the prepubic space (black arrows). Note the abnormal signal intensity within the recto-anus (white arrows) due to treatment effect.

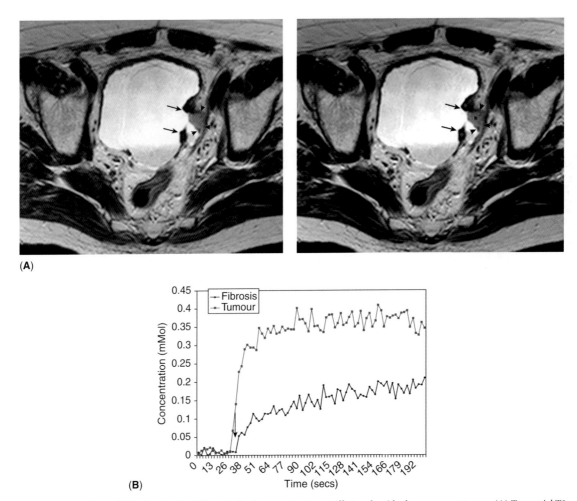

Figure 56.24 Dynamic contrast-enhanced MR showing the differentiation between treatment effect and residual or recurrent tumor. (**A**) Transaxial T2-weighted image of a bladder cancer patient treated with radical radiotherapy for stage T3 adenocarcinoma arising within a bladder diverticulum. There is low signal intensity (arrows) at the mouth of the diverticulum consistent with fibrosis and an intermediate to high-signal intensity lesion (arrowheads) within the diverticulum, consistent with recurrent tumor. Regions of interest for enhancement curves have been selected in the fibrosis (◆) and in the tumor (■). (**B**) Enhancement curves for the same patient. The fibrotic lesion demonstrates gradual and delayed enhancement with a relatively small area under the curve. The tumor mass demonstrates more rapid and intense enhancement. Vertical arrow—time of dynamic intravenous contrast injection.

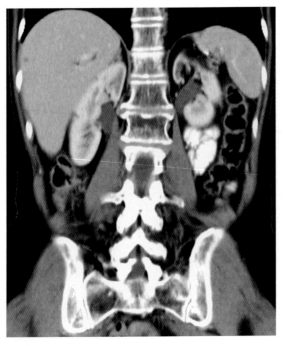

Figure 56.25 Radiation effect on the left kidney. Coronal contrast-enhanced CT scan in a patient with gastric cancer who had received irradiation to the superior portion of the left kidney during a course of radiotherapy to the surgical bed. Note the superior pole renal cortical loss with a straight margin and no underlying caliectasis.

uniformly low signal intensity on T2-weighted sequences (Fig. 56.27), making the diagnosis of recurrent tumor difficult, since most prostate tumors are also of low or intermediate signal intensity on T2-weighted images. The seminal vesicles shrink and demonstrate uniform low signal intensity on T2-weighted sequences (78).

The male urethra is sensitive to radiotherapy, especially after prior trans-urethral resection of the prostate (79). In severe cases, stricture formation occurs, usually in the prostatic or membranous portion of the urethra. This complication occurs more frequently after prostate brachytherapy unless the radiation dose is restricted in the periurethral region.

The adult male testis is an extremely radiosensitive organ and a dose of as little as 0.15 Gy can cause a significant drop in the sperm count (80). Consequently, treatment fields are designed to keep testicular doses to an absolute minimum consistent with adequate tumor coverage. Where testicular exposure is inevitable, sperm banking should be considered. There is no recognizable imaging finding apart from atrophy and this is not invariably present even with severe azoospermia.

In women of child-bearing age, radiotherapy effect on the uterus results in atrophy, best appreciated on T2-weighted MR images, where the normal zonal anatomy is lost and the myometrium becomes of uniform low signal intensity with a slit-like endometrium (81) (Fig. 56.28A). Rarely, radiation-induced cervical stenosis produces hydro- or hematometria and an increase in uterine size (82). The vagina demonstrates low signal intensity of its wall in the chronic phase after radiotherapy, although in the first three months after treatment, high signal intensity edema may be seen within the vaginal sub-mucosa on T2-weighted images (Fig. 56.28B) and there may be enhancement after IV Gadolinium DTPA injection.

After radiation therapy the ovaries shrink, lose their follicular cysts and eventually become fibrotic (Fig. 56.29). The effect of radiation on ovarian function depends on the radiation dose and the age of the patient. Relatively small doses can induce menopause

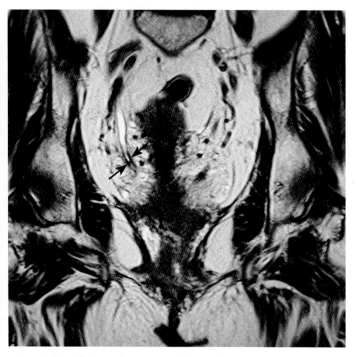

Figure 56.26 Radiation stricture of the right distal ureter. Coronal T2-weighted image demonstrating a smoothly tapered lower right ureteric stricture (arrows) in a patient who had been treated for cervical cancer three years previously. Note the uniform low signal intensity fibrous thickening of the wall at the stricture site.

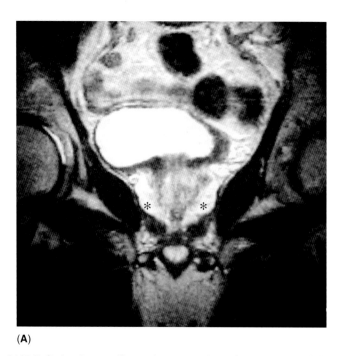

(A)

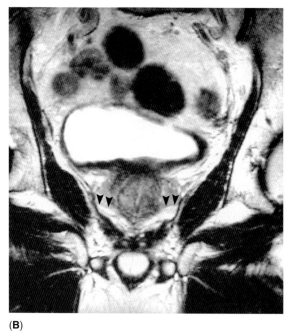

(B)

Figure 56.27 Radiation therapy effect on the prostate. Coronal MR images (A) before treatment and (B) after treatment for a bladder tumor. The normal high signal intensity of the peripheral zone is apparent in (A) (*) but in (B) there is a well demarcated low signal intensity component to the superior aspect of the peripheral zone bilaterally (arrowheads) which corresponds to the inferior aspect of the radiotherapy field used to treat the bladder.

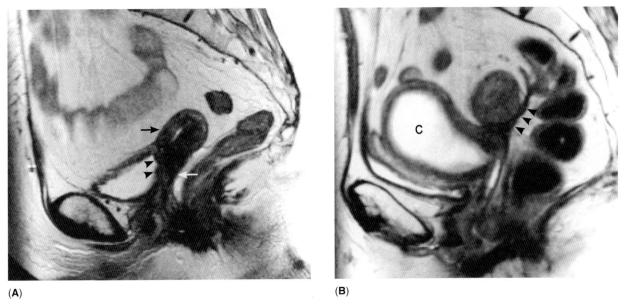

(A)

(B)

Figure 56.28 Radiation effect on the uterus. (A) Sagittal T2-weighted sequence demonstrating a small low signal intensity uterus (black arrow) with loss of its junctional anatomy. The upper vagina (white arrow) is of similar low signal intensity and the posterior wall of the bladder is tethered to the uterus and upper vagina (arrowheads). (B) Hydrometria in a patient treated for carcinoma of the cervix. The uterine cavity (C) is distended and filled with high signal intensity material due to a radiation-induced stenosis of the cervix. Note band-like signal intensity extending from the posterior vaginal fornix along the line of the peritoneal reflection (arrowheads). This is not a typical radiotherapy finding and may have occurred secondary to previous inflammation or surgery, or represent the fibrotic residuum of tumor infiltration.

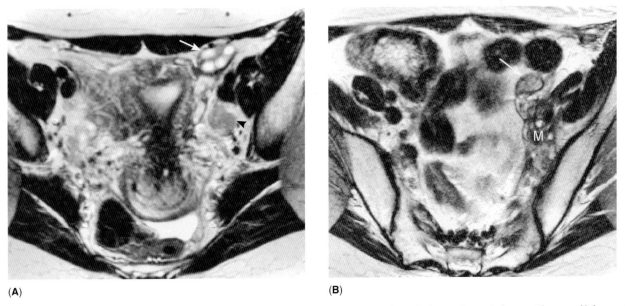

(A)

(B)

Figure 56.29 Radiation effect on the ovary. Transaxial T2-weighted images (A) before and (B) 18 months after radiotherapy for cervical cancer. The normal left ovary (arrow) is well seen in (A). After radiotherapy the ovary (arrow in B) has decreased in size and signal intensity with atrophy of the ovarian follicles. Also note the left obturator lymph node metastasis (arrowhead in A). On follow-up there is an ill-defined mass (M) on the left pelvic sidewall. This was confirmed to be residual/recurrent tumor.

in middle-aged women, whereas young women require a higher total exposure to induce ovarian failure.

Premenarchal girls treated with high-dose abdominal radiation (in the order of 20–30 Gy) will experience premature ovarian failure (83) and the uterus may remain of infantile proportions. In the long-term, radiotherapy causes decreased distensibility of the uterus and abdomino-pelvic connective tissue, both of which contribute to the high incidence of miscarriage and premature birth.

Chemoradiotherapy for Pelvic Cancer

The prescription of concurrent chemotherapy and radiotherapy results in new patterns of treatment effect. Pelvic ascites occurs almost invariably and persists for several years, usually unaltered in volume. In cervical cancer, the primary tumor site may markedly atrophy leaving a distorted uterus with a relatively large fundus and shrunken cervix. The chemotherapy prescribed may affect the timing, distribution, or severity of normal tissue effects (Fig. 56.30).

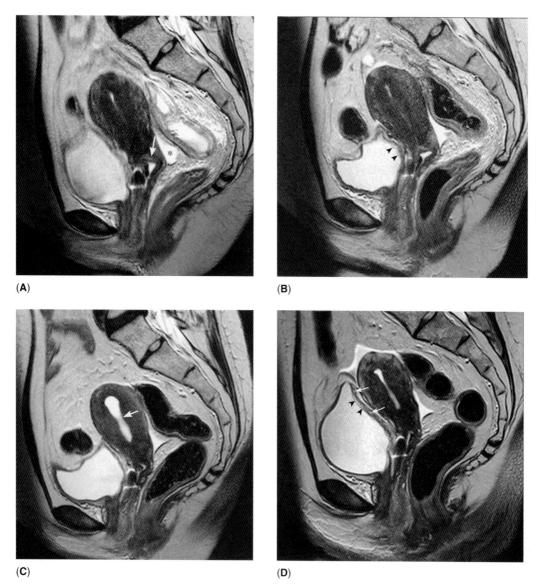

Figure 56.30 Chemoradiation effect. Sagittal T2-weighted images in a patient treated with chemoradiotherapy for carcinoma of the cervix. (A) Six months post-treatment. There is some residual intermediate signal intensity within the posterior cervix (arrow). A small volume of pelvic ascites has developed (*). There is high signal intensity of the bladder wall and rectum involving both the mucosa and muscle layer of each organ. (B) One year after treatment. The slightly altered signal intensity within the posterior cervix persists, as does the small volume of ascites. There has been incomplete restoration of the normal low signal intensity muscle layer of the bladder, which remains slightly abnormal posteriorly and is associated with small volume mucosal edema (arrowheads). The signal of the rectum has returned towards normal. (C) Two years after treatment. The cervix is now considerably atrophied with only a small indistinct area of slight increase in signal intensity within the posterior lip. Ascites is unaltered in volume. There is now slight distension of the endometrial cavity (arrow) due to high signal intensity retained secretions. The rectal wall is essentially normal. The posterior bladder wall has further improved with resolution of the mucosal edema. (D) Three years post-treatment. There has been no change in the cervix though the low signal intensity of the uterine myometrium is less uniform than on previous scans. Again ascites persists but has increased in volume with a small amount above the uterine fundus. Some mucosal high signal intensity is demonstrable within the rectum but the most pronounced change is in the posterior wall of the bladder where there is again abnormal high signal intensity within the outer portion of the muscle layer (arrows). Some mucosal edema is again seen (arrowheads). Sometimes normal tissue effects can become more severe after an initial improvement. Note there has been decompression of the endometrial distension in comparison to (C) presumed due to the cervical stenosis being incomplete.

Key Points: Genito-Urinary System

- Lymphoceles are common following radical lymph node dissection and are readily recognized as unilocular, thin-walled, fluid-filled lesions
- Chemotherapy is often nephrotoxic; US is useful for excluding renal obstruction
- The kidney is radiosensitive and is often the dose-limiting organ during treatment of abdominal malignancy
- The bladder is the most radiation-sensitive organ in the urinary tract, bladder injury occurring in up to 20% of patients following pelvic radiation
- The gynecological organs, prostate and seminal vesicles show fibrosis and atrophy following radiotherapy
- Semiquantitative dynamic contrast-enhanced MR improves the differentiation between treatment effect and recurrence in the bladder
- [18]FDG PET-CT has a role in the differentiation of radiation damage and tumor recurrence

MUSCULOSKELETAL SYSTEM

Of the cancer treatment modalities, radiation therapy is principally responsible for treatment-induced injury of the normal musculoskeletal tissues, nerves, and blood vessels of the abdomen and pelvis. Chemotherapy and corticosteroids can also have deleterious effects.

Bone (see also chap. 55)

After therapeutic radiation there is damage to the cellular elements of bone marrow and to cortical and trabecular bone.

Understanding the normal pattern of conversion of hemopoietic (red) to fatty (yellow) marrow with ageing is key to the interpretation of MR imaging after chemoradiotherapy. Conversion happens in an orderly pattern from distal to proximal, from the appendicular to the axial skeleton, and from the diaphyses towards the metaphyses of the long bones (84).

Appearances in the pelvic bones can cause confusion. Marrow conversion occurs later than in the long bones and hemopoietic marrow is more patchily distributed. Concentrations of fatty marrow are found around the sacro-iliac joints, acetabulae, and symphysis pubis (85–87). The normal bilateral and symmetrical appearance helps differentiate islands of hemopoietic tissue from tumor infiltration on T1-weighted images (Figs. 56.31 and 56.32).

Changes on MR of the lumbar spine and sacrum may be seen as early as the second week after radiotherapy, when STIR sequences demonstrate an increase in signal intensity of the bone marrow due to edema and cell necrosis (88). In addition, there is an early transient increase in contrast enhancement following Gd-DTPA at two weeks after radiotherapy, followed by a progressive decrease in contrast enhancement after four weeks (89). Subsequently, the signal intensity of the marrow on T1-weighted MR gradually increases as the hemopoietic marrow is replaced by fat. The bright appearance of irradiated lumbar vertebrae is irreversible when doses exceed 30 Gy (90). For lower doses, marrow regeneration may occur one year after radiotherapy (91). The boundary of these changes normally corresponds closely with the radiation field (92), although minor changes can be detected outside the field attributable to low-dose scattered radiation (89).

When therapeutic radiation is followed by high-dose chemotherapy and bone marrow or stem cell transplantation with or without the use of hemopoietic growth factors such as granulocyte-colony stimulating growth factor (G-CSF), differentiating regenerating hemopoietic marrow from metastatic disease in the pelvis and lumbar spine using conventional MR sequences can be problematic. Both regenerative marrow and metastatic infiltration have heterogeneous intermediate signal intensity on T1-weighted images and increased signal intensity on T2-weighted and STIR images. Metastatic disease replaces the various marrow constituents and changes the morphology of the vertebral body with loss of the conspicuity of the basivertebral vein; regenerating marrow does not, leaving some fatty elements. This phenomenon can be exploited using opposed-phase gradient-echo imaging when the fat elements of regenerating marrow have lower signal intensity than metastatic disease on out-of-phase imaging (93). Alternatively, IV contrast can be employed. Normal marrow does not perceptibly enhance with gadolinium-DTPA whereas diseased marrow does. However the highly cellular marrow of infants and children may enhance and cause confusion (94). The superparamagnetic iron oxide is

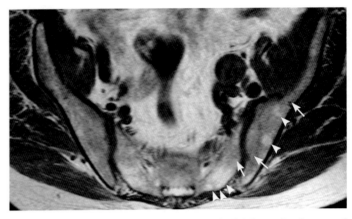

Figure 56.31 Transaxial T1-weighted MR image of pelvic bones showing normal patchy but symmetrical distribution of hemopoietic (arrows) and fatty (arrowheads) marrow.

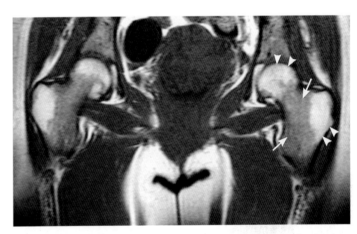

Figure 56.32 Coronal T1-weighted MR image of proximal femora showing normal but strikingly symmetrical distribution of hemopoietic (arrows) and fatty (arrowheads) marrow.

metabolized by hemopoietic cells of the reticulo-endothelial system, so that there is loss of signal on T1, T2, and STIR images in normal hemopoietic marrow but no loss of signal in marrow infiltrated by tumor (95). Following radiotherapy there is progressive ischemia that affects the cortical and trabecular bone, rendering it vulnerable to fracture, infection, and impaired healing. The appearances on plain radiographs reflect the initial resorption of dead bone and necrotic tissue followed by the deposition of new bone on unresorbed trabeculae, a process described as "creeping substitution" (96). A similar mixed lytic and sclerotic appearance is also seen on CT, but the superior contrast resolution of CT allows more subtle change to be appreciated, particularly in the pelvic bones. As a rule, post-radiation atrophy can be differentiated from infiltrative metastatic disease by noting the absence of abnormality outside the radiation field, the lack of a radiographically recognizable periosteal reaction (97), and the time delay before the development of an abnormality as metastases tend to occur earlier in the course of the disease.

Insufficiency fractures of the sacrum, and less commonly the pubis, occur in patients irradiated for gynecological malignancy in whom post-menopausal osteoporosis, steroid therapy and other metabolic bone diseases may be additional risk factors (98,99) (see chap. 55).

Subcapital fractures of the femoral neck previously occurred in approximately 2% of patients receiving pelvic radiation (100).

However, with the abandonment of lateral radiation fields, the change from orthovoltage to supervoltage or megavoltage treatment, and shielding of the femoral neck, these are now seldom seen.

Vertebral bodies that have their osseous matrix replaced by malignant tissue can collapse following chemotherapy or radiotherapy, as tumor resolves leaving little supporting bony substrate (101). Differentiating between benign post-treatment collapse, osteoporotic collapse, and collapse due to malignant disease is very difficult using plain radiography or CT, so MR is the modality of choice. Diffusion-weighted imaging has been employed with variable success (102,103). Findings supporting malignant fractures on MR are:

- Abnormality involving the entire vertebra
- Extension to the pedicles
- A bulging vertebral contour
- An epidural mass
- A cervical or lumbosacral location (104)
- Inhomogeneous enhancement following IV contrast (105)

Osteomyelitis is most likely to occur in the pelvis where radiation damage to pelvic bowel loops and surgical intervention increase the risk. The symphysis pubis is most commonly affected and there are usually symmetrical lytic and sclerotic changes in the pubic bones. On CT, an associated pelvic abscess is usually seen and a soft tissue mass, fistulae and gas in the symphysis pubis itself are possible additional findings (106).

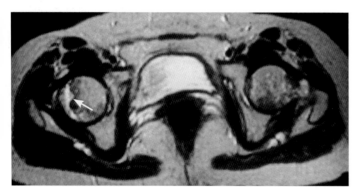

Figure 56.33 Transaxial T2-weighted MR image showing bilateral avascular necrosis of the femoral head following corticosteroid treatment and chemotherapy for Hodgkin's disease. Note "double line" sign in right femoral head (arrow) (see text).

Avascular necrosis (AVN) occurs as a complication of chemotherapy (107), radiotherapy, or corticosteroid therapy, either alone or in combination. Weight-bearing and trauma are possible additional risk factors accounting for the higher incidence in the femoral than humeral head (108). Early diagnosis is critical to allow surgical intervention and modification of therapy. MR is the modality of choice in demonstrating AVN as it is more sensitive than plain radiographs or radioisotope scans (109,110) and has the ability to identify any associated joint effusion or cartilage abnormality. Initially, on T1-weighted images there are diffuse areas of reduced signal intensity in the high-signal intensity fatty marrow of the femoral head. Subsequently, low-signal intensity bands or lines occur within the antero-superior aspect of the femoral head on both T1- and T2-weighted images. On T2-weighted images, an additional band of high signal intensity representing the interface between normal and infarcted marrow is seen ("double line" sign) (109) (Fig. 56.33). Progressive bone necrosis appears as high-signal intensity on T2-weighted images and low-signal intensity on T1-weighted images, and subsequent fibrosis as low-signal intensity on both T1-weighted and T2-weighted images. Radiographically, the first sign of AVN is a patchy increase in the density of the femoral head followed by development of a subchondral lucency, mirroring the MR appearances. The joint space is usually preserved, but may be reduced if there is eventual collapse and fragmentation of the femoral head.

Radiotherapy may produce changes in and around joints: for example, the sacro-iliac joints may be wide and irregular following radiotherapy. Plain radiography shows sclerosis of the adjacent joint surfaces, often in a bilateral and symmetrical pattern resembling osteitis condensans ilii (111). Similar sclerotic changes in the pubis resemble osteitis pubis.

Skeletal Muscle

Injury to skeletal muscle in the radiation field results from vascular damage and may progress for many years following treatment (112), with muscles undergoing necrosis with edema, atrophy, and eventual fibrosis. Sugimura et al. (65) noted changes on MR from three weeks to longer than 12 months after irradiation for pelvic malignancy. The homogeneous increase in signal intensity on T2-weighted images in a unilateral or bilateral distribution was seen in the pelvic sidewall muscles (Fig. 56.34). Chronic atrophic changes are also evident on CT with asymmetry or loss of muscle bulk.

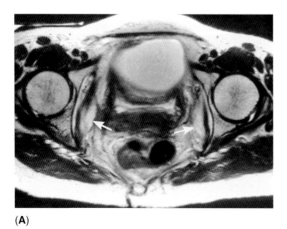

(A)

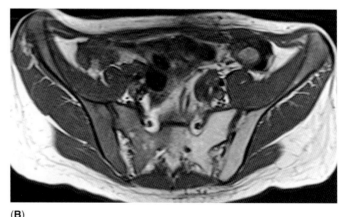

(B)

Figure 56.34 (A) Transaxial T2-weighted MR image of the pelvis demonstrating bilateral homogeneous increase in signal intensity in the obturator internus muscles (arrows) following pelvic radiotherapy. (B) Transaxial T1-weighted MR of pelvic bones in 30-year-old female following radiotherapy to the left hemipelvis for recurrent cervical cancer. There is a well-demarcated boundary between the normal hemopoietic marrow on the right side and the radiation-induced fatty marrow on the left.

Peripheral Nerves

Radiation change to the lumbosacral plexus is uncommon, but has been reported in patients with gynecological cancer who receive radiation doses in excess of 70 Gy to the whole pelvis (112). The imaging features have not been clearly defined.

Blood Vessels

Radiation damage to blood vessels occurs predominantly in the intimal layer with changes that are indistinguishable from atherosclerosis (113). The irradiated artery shows focal or diffuse irregularity, stenosis, or occlusion angiographically. Aneurysm formation and rupture may occur. Venous changes are infrequently reported but mesenteric venous occlusion has been noted following pelvic irradiation (114).

Treatment Effects on the Growing Skeleton

In children, skeletal abnormalities result not only from external beam radiation for solid tumors but also from total body irradiation in preparation for BMT (115). The most striking effect is on growth and may result from damage to nerves, blood vessels, muscles, and bones, either alone or in combination.

Radiation-induced interruption of vertebral body growth gives typical radiographic features. The vertebral body height is reduced and there may be anterior beaking resembling the appearance of the mucopolysaccharidoses. Dense, sometimes multiple, growth arrest lines occur parallel to the vertebral end plates and occasionally there is a "bone within a bone" appearance. The trabecular pattern is coarsened and the end plates are irregular. Asymmetrical vertebral development results in kyphosis and scoliosis, particularly when the spine and paravertebral muscles have been unevenly irradiated. The convexity of the scoliosis points away from the irradiated side (Fig. 56.35).

Changes evident in the pelvis are hypoplasia of the iliac blade and acetabulum predisposing to hip dislocation. The risk of slipped femoral capital epiphysis is increased and tends to occur at an earlier age than the idiopathic type (96). Associated rib hypoplasia may also be observed.

Children treated with long-term methotrexate in low dose for acute lymphoblastic leukemia and those treated with high-dose methotrexate for brain tumors (116) and osteosarcoma (117) are prone to methotrexate osteopathy; a syndrome of bone pain, osteopenia, and pathological fracture. The radiographic features of osteopenia, dense provisional zones of calcification, pathological fractures (frequently metaphyseal), and sharply outlined epiphyses resemble those of scurvy (119), but marked subperiosteal hemorrhage is absent.

The alkylating agent ifosfamide is nephrotoxic and can precipitate clinical and radiological hypophosphatemic rickets, particularly in patients with previous nephrectomy or pre-existing renal disease (119).

Key Points: Musculoskeletal System

- Understanding the normal distribution of hemopoietic and fatty bone marrow is key to the interpretation of MR after chemoradiotherapy
- Radiotherapy renders bone vulnerable to fracture, infection, and impaired healing
- Insufficiency fractures of the sacrum, pubis, femoral neck and vertebral body can occur following chemoradiotherapy
- Avascular necrosis results from radiotherapy, chemotherapy and corticosteroids used alone or in combination
- Radiotherapy affects skeletal muscle, peripheral nerves and blood vessels
- There are characteristic changes in the growing skeleton following radiotherapy

---

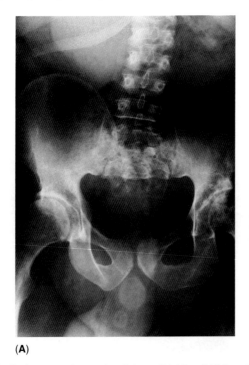
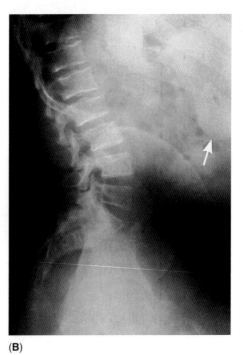

(A)   **(B)**

Figure 56.35 Effects of radiotherapy on the growing skeleton. (A) AP and (B) lateral radiographs of a 26-year-old man, treated with radiotherapy at aged two years for Wilms' tumor. There is kyphoscoliosis and hypoplasia of the left ribs and left iliac blade. Characteristic vertebral body changes are seen (see text). The sacro-iliac joints are fused. Avascular necrosis of the left femoral head has occurred and there is secondary dysplasia of the acetabulum. Degenerative changes are present in the right hip joint. The left kidney is absent and there is compensatory hypertrophy of the right kidney (arrow).

SECOND MALIGNANT NEOPLASMS (SEE ALSO CHAP. 7)

Some long-term survivors of cancer are already genetically predisposed to further malignancy; for example, women who have suffered from ovarian cancer have a higher risk of breast, thyroid, endometrial, and lung cancers. There is also a recognized risk of treatment-induced second malignancies (120,121). This is highest after treatment for childhood cancer and the overall risk varies between 2% and 12% in survivors at 20 years (122). Most tumors are musculoskeletal sarcomas, lymphomas, or leukemia (123,124). In the abdomen, hepatomas can occur in patients who have undergone upper abdominal radiation therapy (Fig. 56.36) and, in the pelvis, at-risk organs are the bladder and rectum (125). Patients who have had solid-organ transplantation are prone to post-transplantation lymphoproliferative disorder consisting of Epstein–Barr virus-induced B cell proliferation. The pattern of disease differs from other lymphomas, with extranodal and extrasplenic involvement (liver, small bowel, kidney, and mesentery) being common (126).

Radiation-induced sarcomas arise more frequently in soft tissues than in bone (127), usually more than 10 years after radiotherapy, but with a wide time range of 3 to 55 years (94). The most common cell types are malignant fibrous histiocytoma and osteosarcoma (128,129) (Fig. 56.37). The cardinal imaging feature is the presence of a new soft tissue mass within the radiation field. Therefore, it is necessary to obtain a histological diagnosis of any abnormal mass, particularly when there is a long time interval between the treatment of the primary lesion and the development of new symptoms. In bone, focal loss of the expected post-radiation high signal intensity fatty marrow on T1-weighted images is an early finding. On plain radiographs or CT, a lytic destructive lesion is identified which may extend beyond the area of pre-existing post-radiation atrophy (94). Differentiation from post-radiation osteomyelitis can be difficult and require biopsy. The presence of additional lesions outside the radiation field and a short latent period to the development of the lesion are indicative of metastatic disease.

Osteochondroma is the only benign radiation-induced bone neoplasm. It is relatively common, occurring in approximately 12% of treated children (130) and is not known to undergo malignant degeneration. The imaging features are indistinguishable from the idiopathic type.

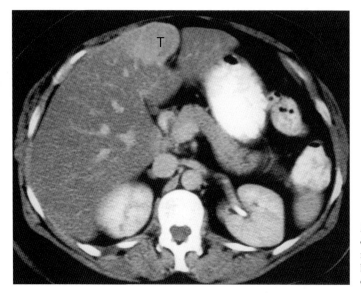

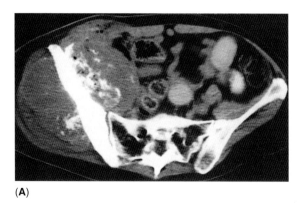

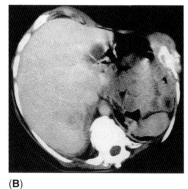

Figure 56.36 Second malignant neoplasm. Transaxial contrast-enhanced CT image of the liver in a patient with Hodgkin's disease who received chemotherapy and radiotherapy 10 years previously. There is a large mass (T) within the left lobe of the liver, which shows some enhancement on CT within an otherwise fatty liver. Biopsy of this lesion revealed hepatoma.

(A) **(B)**

Figure 56.37 Radiation-induced sarcoma. (A) Transaxial CT image of the pelvis showing a chondrosarcoma of the right iliac blade following radiotherapy for cervical carcinoma. (B) Postcontrast transaxial CT image of the upper abdomen showing an osteosarcoma of the left 12th rib in an adult irradiated in childhood for Wilms' tumor. (Also note the absent left kidney, vertebral body changes, and rib changes.)

Summary

- Surgery, chemotherapy and radiation all induce changes in normal tissues
- Significant radiation damage occurs in 5% to 10% of patients and is divided into acute, subacute and chronic reactions
- Clinically significant damage most frequently occurs in the gastro-intestinal and genito-urinary tracts
- Radiation damage to bowel includes mucosal lesions, fixation of bowel loops, motility disturbance, strictures and fistulae
- The bladder is the most radiation-sensitive organ in the urinary tract. Damage is seen in 20% of patients. Edema, hemorrhage and necrosis lead to fibrosis
- Distinction of radiation damage from recurrent tumor relies on morphological appearances on CT, US and MR. Signal intensity changes and use of IV contrast on MR may be helpful but considerable overlap occurs
- [18]FDG PET-CT is the modality of choice in differentiating treatment effect from recurrent tumor in the presacral region
- Radiation injury to the musculoskeletal system results in bone marrow atrophy, fractures, osteomyelitis, avascular necrosis, muscle atrophy and injury to fat, nerves, and blood vessels
- Characteristic changes occur in the growing skeleton following radiotherapy
- The development of a second malignancy occurs in 2% to 12% of patients following treatment of childhood cancer and is usually musculoskeletal sarcoma, lymphoma or leukemia

REFERENCES

1. Fu KK. Biological basis for the interaction of chemotherapeutic agents and radiation therapy. Cancer 1985; 55(Suppl 9): 2123–30.
2. Rubin P. Law and order of radiation sensitivity. Absolute versus relative. In: Vaeth SM, Meyer JL, eds. Frontiers of Radiation Therapy and Oncology 1989; 23: 7–40.
3. DeCosse JJ, Rhodes RS, Wentz WB, et al. The natural history and management of radiation induced injury of the gastro-intestinal tract. Ann Surg 1969; 170: 369–84.
4. van Nagell RJ, Jr. Small bowel injury following radiation therapy for cervical carcinoma. Am J Obstet Gynecol 1974; 118: 163–7.
5. Graham JB, Abad RS. Ureteral obstruction due to radiation. Am J Obstet Gynecol 1967; 99: 409–15.
6. Stockbrine MF, Hancock JE, Fletcher GH. Complications in 831 patients with squamous cell carcinoma of the intact uterine cervix treated with 3000 rads or more whole pelvis irradiation. Am J Roentgenol 1970; 108: 293–304.
7. Mason GR, Dietrich P, Friedland GW, Hagks GE. The radiological findings in radiation-induced enteritis and colitis. A review of 30 cases. Clin Radiol 1970; 21: 232–47.
8. Kimose HH, Fischer L, Spjeldnaes N, Wara P. Late radiation injury of the colon and rectum. Surgical management and outcome. Dis Colon Rectum 1989; 32: 684–9.
9. Pavy JJ, Denekamp J, Letschert J, et al. EORTC Late Effects Working Group. Late effects toxicity scoring: the SOMA scale. Radiother Oncol 1995; 35: 11–15.
10. Krestin GP, Steinbrich W, Friedman G. Recurrent rectal cancer: diagnosis with MR imaging versus CT. Radiology 1988; 168: 307–11.
11. Ebner F, Kresel HY, Mintz MC, et al. Tumor recurrence versus fibrosis in the female pelvis: differentiation with MR imaging at 1.5 T. Radiology 1988; 166: 333–40.
12. Hawnaur JM, Johnson RJ, Isherwood I, Jenkins JPR. Gadolinium–DTPA in magnetic resonance imaging of bladder carcinoma. In: Bydder G, Felix R, Bücheler E, et al., eds. Contrast Media in MRI. The Netherlands: Medicom, 1990: 357–63.
13. Dobson MJ, Carrington BM, Collins CD, et al. The assessment of the irradiated bladder carcinoma using dynamic contrast-enhanced MR imaging. Clin Radiol 2001; 56: 94–8.
14. Vogel WV, Wiering B, Corstens FH, Ruers TJ, Oyen WJ. Colorectal cancer: the role of PET/CT in recurrence. Cancer Imaging 2005; 5 Spec No. A: S143–8.
15. Vandecaveye V, de Keyzer F, Vander Poorten, et al. Evaluation of the larynx for tumour recurrence by diffusion-weighted MRI after radiotherapy: initial experience in four cases. Br J Radiol 2006; 79: 681–7.
16. Sasson AR, Sigurdson ER. Surgical treatment of liver metastases. Semin Oncol 2002; 29: 107–18.
17. Parikh AA, Curley SA, Fornage BD, Ellis LM. Radiofrequency ablation of liver metastases. Semin Oncol 2002; 29: 168–82.
18. Sottsky TK, Ravikumar TS. Cryotherapy in the treatment of liver metastases from colorectal cancer. Semin Oncol 2002; 29: 183–91.
19. Dromain C, de Baere T, Elias D, et al. Hepatic tumors treated with percutaneous radio-frequency ablation: CT and MR imaging follow-up. Radiology 2002; 223: 255–62.
20. Gervais DA, Fernandez-del Castillo C, O'Neill MJ, Hahn PF, MuellerPR. Complications after pancreatoduodenectomy: imaging and imaging-guided interventional procedures. Radiographics 2001; 21: 673–90.
21. Petit P, Bret PM, Atri M, et al. Splenic vein thrombosis after splenectomy: frequency and role of imaging. Radiology 1994; 190: 65–8.
22. Yoshikawa J, Matsui O, Takashima T, et al. Focal fatty change of the liver adjacent to the falciform ligament: CT and sonographic findings in five surgically confirmed cases. Am J Roentgenol 1987; 149: 491–4.
23. Halvorsen RA, Korobkin M, Ram PC, Thompson WM. CT appearance of focal fatty infiltration of the liver. Am J Roentgenol 1982; 139: 277–81.
24. White EM, Simeone JF, Mueller PR, et al. Focal periportal sparing in hepatic fatty infiltration: a cause of hepatic pseudomass on US. Radiology 1987; 162: 57–9.
25. Kissin CM, Bellamy EA, Cosgrove DO, Slcak N, Husband JE. Focal sparing in fatty infiltration of the liver. Br J Radiol 1986; 59: 25–8.
26. Hirohashi S, Ueda K, Uchida H, et al. Nondiffuse fatty change of the liver: discerning pseudotumor on MR images enhanced with ferumoxides—initial observations. Radiology 2000; 217: 415–20.

27. Martín J, Puig J, Falcó J, et al. Hyperechoic liver nodules: characterization with proton fat–water chemical shift MR imaging. Radiology 1998; 207: 325–30.

28. Hale HL, Husband JE, Gossios K, Norman AR, Cunningham D. CT of calcified liver metastases in colorectal carcinoma. Clin Radiol 1998; 53: 735–41.

29. Young ST, Paulson EK, Washington K, et al. CT of the liver in patients with metastatic breast carcinoma treated by chemotherapy: findings simulating cirrhosis. Am J Roentgenol 1994; 163: 1385–8.

30. King PD, Perry MC. Hepatotoxicity of chemotherapy. Oncologist 2001; 6: 162–76.

31. Lassau N, Leclère J, Auperin A, et al. Hepatic veno-occlusive disease after myeloablative treatment and bone marrow transplantation: value of gray-scale and Doppler US in 100 patients. Radiology 1997; 204: 545–52.

32. Shirkhoda A. CT findings in hepatosplenic and renal candidiasis. J Comput Assist Tomogr 1987; 11: 795–8.

33. Wharton JT, Delclos L, Gallager S, Smith JP. Radiation hepatitis induced by abdominal irradiation with the cobalt 60 moving strip technique Am J Roentgenol Radium Ther Nucl Med 1973; 117: 73–80.

34. Cheng JC, Wu JK, Huang CM, et al. Radiation-induced liver disease after three-dimensional conformal radiotherapy for patients with hepatocellular carcinoma: dosimetric analysis and implication. Int J Radiat Oncol Biol Phys 2002; 54: 156–62.

35. Jiao LR, Szyszko T, Al-Nahhas A, et al. Clinical and imaging experience with yttrium-90 microspheres in the management of unresectable liver tumours. Eur J Surg Oncol 2007; 33: 597–602.

36. Lawrence TS, Robertson, JM, Anscher MS, et al. Hepatic toxicity resulting from cancer treatment. Int J Radiat Oncol Biol Phys 1995; 31: 1237–48.

37. Unger EC, Lee JK, Weyman PJ. CT and MR imaging of radiation hepatitis. J Comput Assist Tomogr 1987; 11: 264–8.

38. Moroz P, Anderson JE, Van Hazel G, Gray BN. Effect of selective internal radiation therapy and hepatic arterial chemotherapy on normal liver volume and spleen volume. J Surg Oncol 2001; 78: 248–52.

39. Yamasaki SA, Marn CS, Francis IR, Robertson JM, Lawrence TS. High-dose localized radiation therapy for treatment of hepatic malignant tumors: CT findings and their relation to radiation hepatitis. Am J Roentgenol 1995; 165: 79–84.

40. Chiou SY, Lee RC, Chi KH, et al. The triple-phase CT image appearance of post-irradiated livers. Acta Radiol 2001; 42: 526–31.

41. Capps GW, Fulcher AS, Szucs RA, Turner MA. Imaging features of radiation-induced changes in the abdomen. Radiographics 1997; 17: 1455–73.

42. Dailey MO, Coleman CN, Fajardo LF. Splenic injury caused by theraputic irradiation for Hodgkin's disease. Ann Int Med 1982; 96: 44–7.

43. Weimann M, Becker G, Einsele H, Bamberg M. Clinical indications and biological mechanisms of splenic irradiation in chronic leukaemias and myeloproliferative disorders Radiother Oncol 2001; 58: 235–46.

44. Friedman NB. Effects of radiation on the gastrointestinal tract, including the salivary glands, the liver, and the pancreas. Arch Pathol 1942; 34: 749–87.

45. Lévy P, Menzelxhiu A, Paillot B, et al. Abdominal radiotherapy is a cause for chronic pancreatitis. Gastroenterology 1993; 105: 905–9.

46. Taourel PG, Fabre JM, Pradel JA, et al. Value of CT in the diagnosis and management of patients with suspected acute small-bowel obstruction Am J Roentgenol 1995; 165: 1187–92.

47. Kim KA, Park CM, Park SW, et al. CT findings in the abdomen and pelvis after gastric carcinoma resection Am J Roentgenol 2002; 179: 1037–41.

48. Muller-Scimpfle M, Brix G, Layer G, et al. Recurrent rectal cancer: diagnosis with dynamic MR imaging. Radiology 1993; 189: 881–9.

49. Kinkel K, Tardivon AA, Soyer P, et al. Dynamic contrast-enhanced subtraction versus T2-weighted spin-echo MR imaging in the follow-up of colorectal neoplasm: a prospective study of 41 patients. Radiology 1996; 200: 453–8.

50. Dicle O, Obuz F, Cakmacki H. Differentiation of recurrent rectal cancer and scarring with dynamic MR imaging. Br J Radiol 1999; 72: 1155–9.

51. Ito K, Kato T, Tadokoro M, et al. Recurrent rectal cancer and scar: differentiation with PET and MR imaging. Radiology 1992; 182: 549–52.

52. Johnson K, Bakhsh A, Young D, Martin TE, Jr, Arnold M. Correlating computed tomography and positron emission tomography scan with operative findings in metastatic colorectal cancer. Dis Colon Rectum 2001; 44: 334–7.

53. Ogunbiyi OA, Flanagan FL, Dehdashti F, et al. Detection of recurrent and metastatic colorectal cancer: comparison of positron emission tomography and computed tomography. Ann Surg Oncol 1997; 4: 613–20.

54. Whiteford MH, Whiteford HM, Ogunbiyi OA, et al. Usefulness of FDG-PET scan in the assessment of suspected metastatic or recurrent adenocarcinoma of the colon and rectum. Dis Colon Rectum 2000; 43: 759–70.

55. Saunders TH, Mendes Ribeiro HK, Gleeson FV. New techniques for imaging colorectal cancer: the use of MRI, PET and radioimmunoscintigraphy for primary staging and follow-up. Br Med Bull 2002; 64: 81–99.

56. Even-Sapir E, Parag Y, Lerman H, et al. Detection of recurrence in patients with rectal cancer: PET/CT after abdominoperineal or anterior resection. Radiology. 2004; 232: 815–22.

57. Avril NE, Weber WA. Monitoring responses to treatment in patients utilizing PET. Radiol Clin N Am 2005; 43: 189–204.

58. DuBrow RA. Radiation changes in the hollow viscera. Semin Roentgenol 1994; 24: 38–52.

59. Rogers LF, Goldstein HM. Roentgen manifestations of radiation injury to the gastrointestinal tract. Gastrointest Radiol 1977; 2: 281–91.

60. Mendelson RM, Nolan DJ. The radiological features of chronic radiation enteritis. Clin Radiol 1985; 36: 141–8.

61. Umschaden HW, Szolar D, Gasser J, Umschaden M, Haselbach H. Small-bowel disease: comparison of MR enteroclysis images with conventional enteroclysis and surgical findings Radiology 2000; 215: 717–25.

62. Taylor PM, Johnson RJ, Eddleston B, Hunter RD. Radiological changes in the gastrointestinal and genitourinary tract following radiotherapy for carcinoma of the cervix. Clin Radiol 1990; 41: 165–9.

63. Doubleday LC, Bernardino ME. CT findings in the perirectal area following radiation therapy. J Comput Assist Tomogr 1980; 4: 634–8.

64. Ohtomo K, Shuman WP, Griffin BR, et al. CT manifestation in the pararectal area following fast neutron radiotherapy. Radiol Medica 1987; 5: 198–201.

65. Sugimura K, Carrington BM, Quivey JM, Hricak H. Postirradiation changes in the pelvis: assessment with MR imaging. Radiology 1990; 175: 805–13.

66. Outwater E, Schieber ML. Pelvic fistulas: findings on MR images. Am J Roentgenol 1993; 160: 327–30.

67. Barker PG, Lunniss PJ, Armstrong P, et al. Magnetic resonance imaging of fistula in ano: technique, interpretation and accuracy. Clin Radiol 1994; 49: 7–13.

68. Spencer JA, Ward J, Beckingham IJ, Adams C, Ambrose NS. Contrast-enhanced MR imaging of perianal fistulas. Am J Roentgenol 1996; 167: 735–41.

69. Reed DH, Dixon AK, Williams MV. Ovarian conservation at hysterectomy: a potential diagnostic pitfall. Clin Radiol 1989; 40: 274–6.

70. Ilancheran A, Monaghan JM. Pelvic lymphocyst – a 10-year experience. Gynecol Oncol 1988; 29: 333–6.

71. van Sonnenberg E, Wittich GR, Casola G, et al. Lymphoceles: imaging characteristics and percutaneous management. Radiology 1986; 161: 593–6.

72. Razzaq R, Carrington BM, Hulse PA, Kitchener HC. Abdominopelvic CT scan findings after surgery for ovarian cancer. Clin Radiol 1998; 53: 820–4.

73. Marks LB, Carroll PR, Dugan TC, Anscher MS. The response of the urinary bladder, urethra and ureter to radiation and chemotherapy. Int J Radiat Oncol Biol Phys 1995; 31: 1257–80.

74. Johnson RJ, Carrington BM. Pelvic radiation disease. Clin Radiol 1992; 45: 4–12.

75. Jansen EP, Saunder MP, Boot H, et al. Prospective study on late renal toxicity following postoperative chemoradiotherapy in gastric cancer. Int J Radiat Oncol Biol Phys 2007; 67: 781–5.

76. Cassady JR. Clinical radiation nephropathy. Int J Radiat Oncol Biol Phys 1995; 31: 1249–56.

77. Parkin DE. Lower urinary tract complications of the treatment of cervical carcinoma. Obstet Gynecol Surveys 1989; 44: 523–9.

78. Taylor PM, Johnson RJ, Eddleston B, Hunter RD. Radiological changes in the gastrointestinal and genitourinary tract following radiotherapy for carcinoma of the cervix. Clin Radiol 1990; 41: 165–9.

79. Seymore CH, El-Mahdi AM, Schellhammer PF. The effect of prior transurethral resection of the prostate on post radiation urethral strictures and bladder neck contractures. Int J Radiat Oncol Biol Phys 1986; 12: 1597–1600.

80. Rowley MJ, Leach DR, Warner GA, Heller CG. Effect of graded doses of ionising irradiation on the human testis. Radiat Res 1974; 59: 665–78.

81. Arrivé L, Change YC, Hricak H, et al. Radiation-induced uterine changes: MR imaging. Radiology 1989; 170: 55–8.

82. Grigsby PW, Russell A, Bruner D, et al. Late injury of cancer therapy on the female reproductive tract. Int J Radiat Oncol Biol Phys 1995; 31: 1281–99.

83. Wallace WH, Shalet SM, Crowne EC, Morris-Jones PH, Gattamaneni HR. Ovarian failure following abdominal irradiation in childhood: natural history and prognosis. Clin Oncol 1989; 1: 75–80.

84. Andrews CL. Evaluation of the marrow space in the adult hip. Radiographics 2000; 20: 527–42.

85. Levine CD, Schweitzer ME, Ehrlich MS. Pelvic marrow in adults. Skeletal Radiol 1994; 23: 343–7.

86. Ricci C, Cova M, Kang YS, et al. Normal age-related patterns of cellular and fatty bone marrow distribution in the axial skeleton: MR imaging study. Radiology 1990; 177: 83–8.

87. Dawson KL, Moore SG, Rowland JM. Age related marrow changes in the pelvis: MR and anatomical findings. Radiology 1992; 183: 47–51.

88. Stevens SK, Moore SG, Kaplan ID. Early and late bone marrow changes after irradiation: MR evaluation. Am J Roentgenol 1989; 154: 745–50.

89. Otake S, Mayr NA, Ueda T, Magnotta VA, Yuh WT. Radiation induced changes in MR signal intensity and contrast enhancement of lumbosacral vertebrae: do changes occur only inside the radiation therapy field? Radiology 2002; 222: 179–83.

90. Casamassima F, Ruggiero C, Caramella D, et al. Hematopoietic bone marrow recovery after radiation therapy: MRI evaluation. Blood 1989; 73: 1677–81.

91. Yankelevitz DF, Henschke CI, Knapp PH, et al. Effect of radiation therapy on thoracic and lumbar bone marrow: evaluation with MR imaging. Am J Roentgenol 1991; 157: 87–92.

92. Remedios PA, Colletti PM, Raval JK, et al. Magnetic resonance imaging of bone after radiation. Magn Res Imag 1988; 6: 301–4.

93. Disler DG, McCauley TR, Ratner LM, Kesack CD, Cooper JA. In-phase and out-of-phase MR imaging of bone marrow: prediction of neoplasia based on the detection of coexistent fat and water. Am J Roentgenol 1997; 169: 1439–47.

94. Vanel D, Dromain C, Tardivon A. MRI of bone marrow disorders. Eur Radiol 2000; 10: 224–9.

95. Daldrup-Link HE, Rummeny EJ, Ihssen B, et al. Iron-oxide-enhanced MR imaging of bone marrow in patients with non-Hodgkin's lymphoma: differentiation between tumor infiltration and hypercellular bone marrow. Eur Radiol 2002; 12: 1557–66.

96. Libshitz HI. Radiation changes in bone. Semin Roentgenol 1994; 29: 15–37.

97. Bluemke DA, Fishman EK, Kuhlman JE, Zinreich ES. Complications of radiation therapy: CT evaluation. Radiographics 1991; 11: 581–600.

98. Rafii M, Firooznia H, Golimbu C, Horner N. Radiation induced fractures of sacrum: CT diagnosis. J Comput Assist Tomogr 1988; 12: 231–5.

99. Blomlie V, Lien HH, Iversen T, Winderen M, Tvera K. Radiation-induced insufficiency fractures of the sacrum: evaluation with MR imaging. Radiology 1993; 188: 241–4.

100. Bonfiglio M. The pathology of fracture of the femoral neck following irradiation. Am J Roentgenol 1953; 70: 449–59.

101. Moulopoulos LA, Dimopoulos MA. Magnetic resonance imaging of the bone marrow in hematologic malignancies. Blood 1997; 90: 2127–47.

102. Chan JH, Peh WC, Tsui EY, et al. Acute vertebral body compression fractures:discrimination between benign and malignant causes using apparent diffusion coefficients. Br J Radiol 2002; 75: 207–14.

103. Castillo M, Arbeleaz A, Smith JK, Fisher LL. Diffusion-weighted MR imaging offers no advantage over routine non-contrast imaging in the detection of vertebral metastases. Am J Neuroradiol 2000; 21: 948–53.

104. Moulopoulos LA, Yoshimitsu K, Libshitz HI. MR prediction of benign and malignant vertebral compression fractures. J Magn Res Imaging 1996; 6: 667–74.

105. Cuénod CA, Laredo JD, Chevret S, et al. Acute vertebral collapse due to osteoporosis or malignancy: appearance on unenhanced and gadolinium-enhanced MR images. Radiology 1996; 199: 541–9.

106. Wignall TA, Carrington BM, Logue JP. Post-radiotherapy osteomyelitis of the symphysis pubis: computed tomographic features. Clin Radiol 1998; 53: 126–30.

107. Harper PG, Trask C, Souhami RL. Avascular necrosis of bone caused by combination chemotherapy without corticosteroids. Br Med J 1984; 288: 267–8.

108. Mould JJ, Adam NM. The problem of avascular necrosis of bone in patients treated for Hodgkin's disease. Clin Radiol 1983; 34: 231–6.

109. Chan Lam D, Prentice AG, Copplestone JA, et al. Avascular necrosis of bone following intensified steroid therapy for acute leukaemia and high-grade malignant lymphoma. Br J Haematol 1994; 86: 227–30.

110. Gabriel H, Fitzgerald SW, Myers MT, Donaldson JS, Poznanski AK. MR imaging of hip disorders. Radiographics 1994; 14: 763–81.

111. Rubin P, Prabhasawat D. Characteristic bone lesions in post-irradiated carcinoma of the cervix. Metastases versus osteonecrosis. Radiology 1961; 76: 703–17.

112. Gillete EL, Mahler PA, Powers BE, Gillete SM, Vujaskovic Z. Late radiation injury to muscle and peripheral nerves. Int J Radiat Oncol Biol Phys 1995; 5: 1309–18.

113. Granmayeh M, Libshitz HI. Vascular system. In: Libshitz HI, ed. Diagnostic Roentgenology of Radiotherapy Change. Baltimore: Williams and Wilkins, 1979: 195–201.

114. Dencker H, Holmdahl KH, Lunderquist A, Olivecrona H, Tylén U. Mesenteric angiography in patients with radiation injury of the bowel after pelvis irradiation. Am J Roentgenol 1972; 114: 476–81.

115. Fletcher BD, Crom DB, Krance RA, Kun LE. Radiation-induced bone abnormalities after bone marrow transplantation for childhood leukemia. Radiology 1994; 191: 231–5.

116. Meister B, Gassner I, Streif W, Dengg K, Fink FM. Methotrexate osteopathy in infants with tumors of the central nervous system. Med Pediatr Oncol 1994; 24: 493–6.

117. Ecklind K, Laor T, Goorin AM, Connolly LP, Jaramillo D. Methotrexate osteopathy in patients with osteosarcoma. Radiology 1997; 2002: 543–7.

118. Roebuck DJ. Skeletal complications in pediatric oncology patients. Radiographics 1999; 19: 873–85.

119. Raney B, Ensign LG, Foreman J, et al. Renal toxicity of ifosfamide in pilot regimens of the intergroup rhabdomysarcoma study for patients with gross residual tumor. Am J Pediatr Hematol Oncol 1994; 16: 286–95.

120. Hutchison GB. Late neoplastic changes following medical irradiaton. Cancer 1976; 37: 1102–7.

121. Parker RG. Radiation-induced cancer as a factor in clinical decision-making (The 1989 Astro Gold Medal Address). Int J Radiat Oncol Biol Phys 1989; 18: 993–1000.

122. Tucker MA, d'Angio GJ, Boice JD, Jr, et al. Bone sarcomas linked to radiotherapy and chemotherapy in children. N Engl J Med 1987; 317: 588–93.

123. Messerschmidt GL, Hoover R, Young RC. Gynecologic cancer treatment: risk factors for therapeutically induced neoplasia. Cancer 1981; 48: 442–50.

124. Quilty PM, Kerr GR. Bladder cancer following low- or high-dose pelvic irradiation. Clin Radiol 1987; 38: 583–5.

125. Tucker MA, Frumeni JF. Treatment-related cancers after gynecologic malignancy. Cancer 1987; 60: 2117–22.

126. Pickhardt PJ, Seigel MJ. Post-transplantation lymphoproliferative disorder of the abdomen: CT evaluation in 51 patients. Radiology 1999; 213: 73–8.

127. Wiklund TA, Blomqvist CP, Räty I, et al. Postirradiation sarcoma. Analysis of nationwide cancer registry material. Cancer 1991; 68: 524–31.

128. Huvos AG, Woodard HQ, Cahan WG, et al. Postradiation osteogenic sarcoma of bone and soft tissues. A clinicopathological study of 66 patients. Cancer 1985; 55: 1244–55.

129. Sheppard DG, Libshitz HI. Post-radiation sarcomas: a review of the clinical and imaging features in 63 cases. Clin Radiol 2001; 56: 22–9.

130. Libshitz HI, Cohen MA. Radiation-induced osteochondromas. Radiology 1982; 142: 643–7.

57 The Immunocompromised Host: Clinical Considerations
Jacqueline M Parkin

INTRODUCTION

Immunocompromised individuals with increased risk of opportunist infection and malignancy comprise an increasing proportion of the patient population. There are several factors contributing to this. The broadening of indications for organ transplant, and improved management of transplant and rejection episodes has led to increased numbers and prolonged survival. Currently, 80% of renal transplant recipients may be expected to survive beyond 10 years. The advent of effective antiretroviral therapy for human immunodeficiency virus (HIV) infection has extended survival into decades. Management of malignancy with improved chemotherapy and biological treatment regimens, in addition to use of stem cell transplants or modified bone marrow transplants (BMTs) has led to prolonged survival of patients, but at the cost of long-term immune defects as a result of their therapies. A small but increasing population are those with congenital immunodeficiencies in whom BMT or even gene therapy is now possible, and who are surviving beyond early childhood and are at risk of malignancy.

The evolution in range and extent of immunosuppression in patients has significant implications for clinical care and diagnosis. Both the level of immunocompromise and time for which it is maintained are important factors predicting the development of tumors. The majority of patients receiving solid-organ transplant require lifelong immunosuppression. Malignancy is now the most significant factor in long-term morbidity and mortality, with a cumulative incidence of greater than 60% to 70% at 25 years post-renal transplant (1). Patients with HIV infection on highly active antiretroviral therapy (HAART) have persistent immunological abnormalities, meaning they may remain susceptible to cancers in the long term.

The understanding of the pathogenesis of tumors in the immunocompromised host is increasing. Predisposing factors for the development of certain malignancies, such as Epstein–Barr virus (EBV) associated with the development of post-transplant lymphoproliferative disorders (PTLD) or pretransplant seropositivity for human herpesvirus Type 8 (HHV-8) and development of Kaposi's sarcoma (KS), are being identified. This potentially leads to the targeted screening of high-risk individuals for early diagnosis and treatment of tumors, including reduction in iatrogenic immunosupression which can lead to tumor regression. Novel approaches to therapy have been developed, for example, clones of EBV-specific T-cells can be raised from bone marrow donors and stored in readiness to transfuse into the recipient should EBV-related lymphoproliferation develop. Understanding of the time-course of the development of tumors in relation to transplant enables appropriate monitoring to be put into place. The role of imaging in high-risk immunocompromised patients is crucial in this respect to enable the earliest diagnosis of neoplasms. Imaging also plays a central role in the monitoring of response to therapy and early detection of relapse, which is unfortunately a frequent occurrence in these diseases.

IMMUNE DYSREGULATION AND MALIGNANCY

In the beginning of the 20th century, even when understanding of the immune system was in its infancy, a potential function of the immune system in controlling carcinomas was recognized (2). Half a century later, Burnet and Thomas developed their hypothesis that the immune system was continually searching out and destroying premalignant and malignant cells to prevent the development of cancer—the immune surveillance theory (3–5).

Tumor Immunosurveillance—Immunoediting and Tumor Sculpture

Since its first description, there has been controversy over the clinical significance of the "immunosurveillance" concept in the elimination of malignant cells. There is no doubt that individuals with tumors mount specific antitumor responses to malignant cells, recognizing, for example, altered cell-surface molecules or re-expression of fetal antigens. This immune "pressure" leads to selection of tumor variants with reduced immunogenicity as these are not destroyed by the cytotoxic T cell response. For example, loss of HLA expression by malignant cells diminishes the ability of T cells to recognize the abnormal cells. This process, by which the immune system drives changes in the immunophenotype of tumor cells, has been termed "sculpting." The immunoediting hypothesis combines immunosurveillance and tumor-sculpting into one dynamic process of cancer–immune system interaction (6).

The evidence cited for a proactive role of the immune system in tumor control is as follows:

- It is not uncommon for post mortem examinations to show the presence of small foci of cancers that were not clinically apparent in life
- Cancers may resolve "spontaneously"
- Specific cytotoxic T cells are present in the blood and infiltrating tumor lesions in patients with established malignancy and the extent of this T cell response correlates with prognosis for some tumors
- There is an association of HLA-DR homozygosity suggesting a role of immune responsiveness
- Development of tumors is markedly enhanced in the immunosuppressed transplant population, this being documented very soon after the introduction of this technique (7,8), and also in patients with primary immunodeficiency (9)

However, although antitumor responses are often demonstrated in patients, the level of clinically relevant surveillance and protection is unclear. Understanding of the relationship of cancer to immunodeficiency (type, level, and duration) enables the hypothesis to be tested further. Cancer statistics within organ transplant registries and HIV studies enable this to be investigated with a relatively large number of individuals. Although it

Table 57.1 Major Tumors in Immunocompromised Patients

Skin cancer: non-melanomous	Squamous cell carcinoma, including oral and ano-genital disease
	Basal cell carcinoma
Skin cancer	Melanoma
Hepatic cancer	
Kaposi's sarcoma	
Lymphoma (mainly B cell)	Non-Hodgkin's lymphoma
	Body cavity-based lymphoma/primary effusion lymphoma
	Castleman's disease
	Post-transplant lymphoproliferative disorder (PTLD)
	MALToma

Table 57.2 Immunodeficiencies Associated with Tumor Development

Congenital	**T cell/T and B cell combined defects**
	Duncan's syndrome (EBV-associated lymphoproliferative disease)
	DiGeorge syndrome (skin cancer)
	DNA repair defects
	Ataxia telangiectasia
Acquired	**B cell**
	Common variable hypogamma-globulinemia (gut lymphoma)
	T cell
	Human T cell lymphoma Type 1 (HTLV-1) (T cell lymphoma/leukemia)
	HIV infection (Kaposi's sarcoma and lymphoma)
Immunodysregulation	**Autoimmune disease**
	Sjögren's syndrome (lymphoma)
Iatrogenic immunosuppression	**Solid-organ transplant**
	Immunosuppressive/cytotoxic treatment of inflammatory conditions and cancers

is certainly the case that malignancies are much more common, this rate varies from 3- to 500-fold as only some cancers are significantly affected.

The immunodeficiency states that are particularly susceptible to cancer development are those in which cell-mediated immunity (T cell and macrophage function) is affected. Macrophages function to present antigens to T cells, which then initiate the immune response; CD4 (helper) T cells orchestrate CD8 (cytotoxic) cells which destroy virally-infected and tumor cells. The tumors observed in those with cell-mediated defects are mainly those with underlying viral pathogenesis, where there is a manifold increase in tumor rate over the healthy population (Table 57.1). It is suggested that these represent the effects of opportunist infections and lack of control of viral replication leading to oncogenesis, rather than proof of the immunosurveillance theory. However, there is an increase, albeit much smaller, in other types of cancer. This suggests that the immune system may be playing a role, but that other factors are more prominent in the predisposition to these multifactorial diseases.

Association of Specific Tumors and Immunodeficiency

In the immunocompromised population, the greatest excess of tumors are those linked to viral infections (10). Particularly high incidence rates have been observed for non-Hodgkin's lymphoma (NHL), KS, and carcinomas of the skin, genito-urinary, oral, and ano-genital regions in patients with T cell defects, the major causes of which are listed in Table 57.2. The same types of cancers are seen regardless of the underlying cause of the immunodeficiency. The Cincinatti Tumor Transplant Registry (CTTR) shows skin and lip cancers making up 40% to 50% in transplant patients; PTLDs 17%; KS 4%; and renal, cervical and ano-genital (including prostate), hepato-biliary, and various sarcomas the remainder (11,12). There are similar findings in Scandinavian (13), Australian, and New Zealand registries (14). As discussed, many of these cancers have a viral etiology and are linked to infection with EBV, HHV-8 and human papilloma virus (HPV), respectively (15,16). In HIV infection there is increased risk of hepatic cancer linked to hepatitis B or C infection (17,18). The risks for other cancers, which are less closely linked to an infectious origin, are also increased in the immunocompromised, but to a much lower extent. Follow-up of 925 patients in Australia and New Zealand who received cadaveric renal transplants from 1965 to 1998 showed increased risk ratios for colon, pancreatic, lung, and endocrine neoplasms, in addition to malignant melanomas (14). Studies in Northern Europe have shown similar findings (13), with the addition of increased risk for cancers of the urinary tract. In addition to life-style (such as UV protection) vaccination may play a role in prevention of tumors and is available for hepatitis B and, more recently, for HPV. However, there are limitations: immunogenicity is reduced in patients on dialysis and those with HIV infection; vaccination prevents acquisition of infection with new HPV types, but does not affect pre-existing strains; the current HPV vaccines whilst offering protection against types (HPV-16/18) that cause cervical cancer, do not cover HPV 5 and 8 that are commonly found in cutaneous squamous cell dysplasia in transplant recipients.

The development of tumors in the immunocompromised is multifactorial and failure to control oncogenic viruses, although important, is not the only factor. The immune system in such individuals often shows signs of chronic activation in response to the barrage of infectious agents which gain entry, or reactivate, due to the underlying immunodeficiency. Continual activation makes lymphoid cells more prone to uncontrolled and/or malignant transformation, as shown in mucosa-associated lymphoid tissue lymphoproliferative disorders (MALTomas) thought to be caused by B cell activation in response to chronic *Helicobacter pylori* infection. Other important factors are decreased immunosurveillance against carcinogens; the failure of the immune system to eliminate malignant clones; environmental exposure, such as the rapid and profound effects of UV light exposure on the development of cutaneous squamous cell carcinoma in transplant recipients; genetic susceptibility; and potential carcinogenic effects of other drug or radiation therapies.

Key Points: Types of Tumor in Immunosuppressed Individuals

- Mainly tumors with viral etiology, especially:
  - Lymphoproliferative disorders, PTLD, NHL
  - Kaposi's sarcoma
  - Squamous cell carcinoma (SCC) of skin, mouth, and ano-genital region
- Melanoma

Table 57.3 Specific Immunosuppressive Agents

Inhibitors of lymphocyte proliferation	Corticosteroids Purine synthesis inhibitors: Azathioprine Mycophenolate mofetil Cyclophosphamide
IL-2 inhibitors	Calcineurin inhibitors: Cylosporin CD25 (receptor antibody) Sirolimus (Rapamycin) Tacrolimus
T lymphocyte antibodies/ inhibitors	Antithymocyte globulin (ATG) Campath-1 H (humanized) Anti-CD3, anti-CD4 CTLA4-Ig (Abatacept)
Lymphocyte trafficking	Anti-VLA/alpha 4 integrin (Natalizumab)
Anti-B lymphocyte antibodies	CD20
Anti-cytokines	Atumor necrosis factor/receptor Infliximab, enbrel, humira, Anti-IL6R (Actemra)

Drugs Used for Immunosuppression

An increasing range of immunosuppressive drugs is now available with effects on different elements of the immune system (Table 57.3). Regimens used in the control of transplant rejection target cell-mediated (T cell) responses, but most will have additional immunological effects. For example, corticosteroids reduce T cell proliferation and function, but also reduce adhesion molecule expression causing functional neutrophil defects; anti-T lymphocyte drugs such as anti-thymocyte globulin, mAbs to CD3 or CD4, or those that affect IL-2 production (cyclosporin A and tacrolimus), will also affect antibody production to some extent as T cell help is needed for B cell functioning.

Effects of Immunocompromise on the Clinical Presentation of Tumors

Not only is the spectrum of tumor types different in the immunocompromised host, but the clinical presentation is also affected. Immunocompromised patients will often be pediatric or young adults who will present with tumors normally associated with older individuals, such as SCCs or NHL. In the case of transplantation the malignancy may occasionally be of donor origin. The presentation is atypical compared with the immunocompetent population in several ways.

- Tumors are commonly multifocal or disseminated at presentation, e.g., many tens of skin cancers or KS lesions are not unusual
- The site of disease may be unexpected, e.g., lymphoma is frequently extranodal and there may be concurrent malignancies, even at the same anatomical site
- Disease is aggressive and survival lower than in those with a functioning immune response, e.g., cutaneous SCC, which is very common in young transplant patients, carries a mortality of 5% to 15%; skin cancers recur in 5% to 8% cases and metastasize often within two years of excision

Key Points: Presentation of Tumors in the Immunosuppressed

- Tumors are often disseminated at presentation
- Tumors develop at unusual sites
- Types of tumors usually observed mainly in the elderly occur in young immunosuppressed patients
- Progression and recurrence may be more aggressive than in immunocompetent patient
- Tumors can respond to reduction in immunosuppression

Factors Confounding Diagnosis

There needs to be a high index of suspicion of tumors as there may be a lack of the normal clinical symptoms of disease due to limited immune response to the tumor; for example, systemic "B" symptoms of fever and sweats may not be observed in patients with HIV infection and lymphoma. Concurrent opportunist infection is common and may confuse the diagnosis as this may be assumed to be the cause of the symptoms and signs, which are in reality due to the underlying tumor. This is further confounded as some of the therapies used for opportunist infections, such as rifampicin for tuberculosis, may also cause temporary shrinkage of lymphoma leading to an erroneous assumption of the lesion being mycobacterial. Steroids used in high dose for control of rejection may also cause shrinkage of lymphoma, confusing the picture. Previously unrecognized tumors are emerging, such as body cavity lymphomas, particularly in HIV-infected individuals. This underlines the importance of aggressive investigation and re-investigation, requiring tissue or body fluid sampling for diagnosis.

Key Points: Factors Confounding Diagnosis

- Tumors may occur with acute onset within weeks of immunosuppression mimicking infection
- Multiple tumors of different type can occur concurrently in the same site
- Co-existing opportunist infection may hinder diagnosis
- Drugs used for concurrent infection, e.g., rifampicin for tuberculosis or for suppression of graft rejection, and corticosteroids may cause temporary reduction in lymphoma lesions

FACTORS AFFECTING DEVELOPMENT OF TUMORS IN IMMUNOCOMPROMISED INDIVIDUALS

Degree of Immunosuppression

The development of malignancy appears to be dependent on both the level of immunosuppression and length of therapy. Cardiac transplant recipients tend to receive greater immunosuppression than other transplant patients and also show a greater incidence of tumor development, in particular NHL. There is a direct dose-dependent relationship between cyclosporin A therapy and development of skin cancers. The instigation of combination immunosuppressive therapies in transplant recipients was associated with an increased incidence of tumor development, which has been curtailed by better tailoring of the regimens. In addition, reduction of immunosuppressive therapy

in transplant recipients or improvement in immune function with antiretroviral therapy in HIV infection can directly lead to improvement/resolution of KS, PTLD, and MALTomas. The proliferation signal inhibitors (PSIs/mTOR inhibitors) sirolimus and everolimus, through inhibition of phosphatidy/inositil-3 kinase pathway have shown reduction in solid tumors (19) and KS (20) in the transplant setting.

Length of Immunosuppression

The time over which immunosuppression is maintained is also a significant risk factor for tumor development (21). Tumors that are clearly virally-driven (PTLDs and KS) develop rapidly post-transplant (median development within 12 months) or, for KS in HIV infection, when the CD4 count declines. Other cancers show a median time for development of 46 months post-transplant, with a continuing increase in incidence over subsequent years. For example, the cumulative risk of skin cancer in renal transplants is determined to be 13% to 18% at 10 years, 34% to 50% at 20 years, and 60% to 70% at 25 years (22). Therefore, unlike other settings where tumor-free time decreases the risk of recurrence of malignancy, in the chronically immunosuppressed time increases the risk.

Geographical Variation in Incidence of Tumors

The incidence of tumor types shows some difference geographically. This may reflect the use of different immunosuppressive regimens. The question has been raised as to whether some drugs are intrinsically more liable to increase susceptibility to tumors outside of the level of immunosuppression they induce. It is possible that the organ transplant type and/or the prophylactic antiviral therapies that are used affect the range and incidence of tumors that develop. Environmental co-factors also are involved, the level of UV exposure being reflected in the higher rate of sun and skin cancer in renal transplant recipients in Australia (45% at 10 years and 70% at 20 years) (23) compared to 30% to 40% at 20 years in Europe, and the rate of KS being reported more frequently in North African (Tunisia 41.6%), Middle East (Kuwait 19.7%), and Southern Europe (Italy 24.2%) compared to Northern Europe (France 2.9% and Hungary 8.4%) (24).

Key Points: Factors Affecting Development of Tumors

- The development of malignancy is dependent on the level of immunosuppression: cardiac transplant patients, who receive the greatest immunosuppression, show the greatest incidence of tumors
- The length of immunosuppression is a risk factor for tumor development
- The incidence of tumor types varies geographically

TUMORS COMMONLY OBSERVED IN SOLID-ORGAN TRANSPLANT RECIPIENTS

Post-Transplant Lymphoproliferative Disorder/Disease

This is the commonest cancer in the first year post-transplant, being overtaken by skin cancers at later stages. The incidence is 0.2% to 1% in renal, 2.5% in liver, and 1.2% to 3% in cardiac transplantation (25).

The proliferation develops relatively rapidly, 70% occurring in the first 12 months, then leveling in incidence at 0.03% to 0.4% in subsequent years. The allograft site is the most common focus of disease, but multiple organ involvement is also observed. The proliferations are predominantly B cell in type, but vary from benign lymphoid hyperplasia to the more common malignant lymphoma. The disease is patchy and may evolve rapidly requiring repeated sampling. The overall mortality is 35% (26), but varies from 9% to 50% (27) depending on whether disease is non-neoplastic or malignant. There are differences in reported incidences of PTLD and these are likely to be due to the variety of definitions used in the past. These have now been clarified by consensus definitions (28) of the American Society of Transplant Surgeons (ASTS) and the American Society of Transplant Physicians (ASTP).

The tumors are EBV-related in 70% of cases, tumor cells being positive for viral proteins. In addition to immunosuppression, particular risk factors are being EBV-seronegative pretransplant and receiving an organ from a seropositive donor (29). An additional risk is young age (less than 14 years) at transplant, with 6.3% to 20% in pediatric cases (27). However, young age may not be an independent risk factor, merely a surrogate for EBV seronegativity. To combat this disease there is development of EBV transfer regimens to protect recipients post-BMT, using EBV-specific T cell clones for adoptive transfer of immunity should PTLD emerge. Human herpes virus Type 8 may be responsible for some of the lymphomas that are not related to EBV (30).

There has been an increased incidence of PTLD since the introduction of heavily-immunosuppressive combination regimens and there is rapid development when OKT3 (T-cell-depleting mAb) is used in regimens with median time to PTLD of 53 days post-therapy. Tacrolimus, as primary immunosuppressive therapy, may also be an additional risk in children (27). Post-transplant lymphoproliferative disorder is clearly related to the level of immunosuppression and may resolve in up to 40% cases when drugs are stopped or reduced, depending on the level of malignant change.

MALTomas

MALTomas have been observed in heart, liver, and kidney transplant patients. Although one of the more rare tumors in the transplant population, the incidence is 10- to 100-fold higher than in the general population (31). The tumor may be most common in liver transplant recipients. Unlike the lymphoproliferative disorders, these tumors are usually EBV-negative, low-grade, and confined to the stomach or gastro-intestinal tract-associated tissue of pancreas or parotids. They occasionally metastasize. These tumors develop relatively late in the course of transplantation, with a median of 5.2 years. Clinical response has been documented using various regimens of antiHelicobacter treatment, reducing immunosuppressive regimen or local excision.

Skin Cancers

Overall, these are the most common cancers in transplant recipients with a year-on-year increase in incidence. Squamous cell and basal cell carcinomas account for >90% of all skin cancers (32–35). Of these, SCC is most common (5:1 SCC:BCC), with a 25- to 250-fold increased incidence over general population. The rate is

higher for men than women, but rare in those of Japanese origin. Basal cell cancer is increased by a factor of 10 (36).

Ultraviolet (UV) light exposure is critically important, the incidence being markedly higher in environments with high sunlight such as Australia (37), lesions mainly confined to sun-exposed areas, and a greater incidence in patients with pre-transplant high UV exposures. There appears to be no specific drug risk (a link between azathioprine and skin cancers has not been conclusively proven in extensive studies), although there may be very rapid development when OKT3 is used in the regimen. Most squamous cell cancers are associated with histological features of HPV infection in the lesions and can be associated with concurrent cutaneous warts. Lesions may contain multiple strains of wart virus, both oncogenic strains (16 and 18) and non-oncogenic strains are detected.

Genital or anal dysplasia and SCCs also show increased incidence in patients, with immunodeficiency of up to 100-fold (38). The risk is higher in men than woman, and in those with multiple sexual partners and a history of sexually-transmitted infection, including herpes simplex virus and HPV, suggesting that a sexually-transmitted agent, presumably HPV, is involved in the pathogenesis. Smoking, which is known to produce local immunosuppressive effect on genital mucosal immunity, is an additional risk factor in transplant as in immunocompetent individuals.

Kaposi's Sarcoma

The incidence of this tumor post-transplant is 84- to 500-fold that in the general population. This tumor is due to proliferation of vascular or lymphatic endothelial cells. The vascular cells create slit-like spaces that trap red cells, causing the typical purplish color of the lesions. Cutaneous disease is the most common initial presentation. The lower limbs are commonly affected by lymphedema due to local lymph node involvement. The tumor is usually multifocal, polyclonal in origin, and does not show characteristic features of malignancy in that metastasis does not occur. However, visceral involvement can cause life-threatening disease due to mechanical effects. Endobronchial lesions can cause bronchial obstruction and recurrent infection in the lung beyond the lesion; parenchymal involvement causes shortness of breath and chronic cough; pleural lesions may lead to significant pleural effusions. Disease in the gastro-intestinal tract may be a cause of protein-losing enteropathy. The brain is characteristically spared. Human herpesvirus Type 8 is thought to be the causative virus (39) and there is a very close association with pretransplant infection with HHV-8 (40). The incidence of KS parallels the carriage of HHV-8, highest in those from the Mediterranean, Middle East and Central/Sub-Saharan Africa.

Melanoma

There are conflicting data on the risk of melanoma, the rarity of the tumor requiring large numbers of patients to be studied. Estimates vary from no increase in risk up to a three- to four-fold higher incidence in transplant recipients than the age-matched population. As in the general population, it is observed mainly in those with fair skin, relatively more frequently in men and with increasing rate of risk with age. The median time to diagnosis is five years post-transplant.

Key Points: Tumors Common Following Solid-Organ Transplant

- PTLD is the commonest cancer in the first year post-transplant; tumors are EBV-related in 70% of cases and young patients are particularly at risk
- Skin cancers (squamous and basal cell) are the commonest cancers in transplant recipients
- MALTomas are 10- to 100-fold more common following transplantation than in the general population
- KS is up to 500 times more common post-transplant than in the general population
- Melanomas are three to four times more common in transplant recipients than in non-transplant recipients

CANCERS IN THE NON-TRANSPLANT PATIENT

Cancers in HIV Infection

The types of cancer observed in HIV-related immunodeficiency are very similar to those in transplant patients. In the North American population, the incidence rate in HIV infection over the matched general population is greater than 1000-fold and CNS NHL 250-fold increase in incidence (41). KS is particularly frequent in homosexual men and patients from sub-Saharan Africa, reflecting the higher rate of seropositivity to HHV-8 in these populations. A decrease in the incidence of new cases of KS in homosexual men was noted at the end of the 1980s/early 1990s. This was hypothesized to be due to reduced infection rate with HHV-8 due to changes in sexual practice. The success of combination antiretroviral therapy in reversing or preventing severe immunodeficiency in HIV-infected individuals has led to a marked decrease in the incidence of both KS and NHL, previously the two major cancers in this population. However, there are cases documented where lymphoproliferative disorders have emerged acutely during initiation of antiretroviral therapy. This may be an "immunoreconstitution" phenomenon due to intense stimulation of lymphocytes by infectious antigen within the host, as the immune system regenerates. The rapidity of onset can mimic an acute tuberculous or bacterial infection within lymph nodes.

However, despite the reduction in some AIDS-defining malignancies (NHL and KS) with highly active anti-retroviral therapy, ano-genital SCCs may be an increasing problem in patients with HIV infection, who like the transplant patients have long-term immunodeficiency. The natural history of intraepithelial neoplasia within the cervix or anus is not yet clear in this situation, and regular monitoring of patients and treatment of premalignant lesions is required. Several non-AIDS-defining cancers are emerging to show a two to nine times elevated risk in HIV-infected population, including cancers of the anus, oral cancer, liver, lung, and Hodgkin lymphoma, in particular Hodgkin disease. This reflects an association being more clearly detectable with the increasingly longer survival of HIV-infected individuals.

Other Conditions

There is a rapid expansion in use of biologicial immunomodulating therapies (targeting tumor necrosis factor, CD20+ B-cells, interleukin 6 receptor, CTLA4 T-cell co-stimulatory molecule,

and alpha-4 integrin) for autoimmune diseases, including those with a relatively high prevalence, such as rheumatoid arthritis, inflammatory bowel disease, psoriasis, and multiple sclerosis. The impact on tumor development of more widespread and long-term use of these disease modifying immunomodulating therapies is as yet uncertain. Some patients may commence therapy at a relatively young age and, therefore, have a high life-time exposure to immunosuppression. The association of anti-TNF agents, integrin inhibitors, and B-cell depleting therapies with opportunist infections such as re-activation of hepatitis B, mycobacteria, fungi, and JC polyoma virus, raises the concern that opportunist tumors may also emerge. Older patients in the transplant setting appear to be particularly susceptible to rapid development of skin cancers and the use of immunosuppressive regimens in conditions common in older patients, such as rheumatoid arthritis, may be associated with an increase in such tumors. To date the early concerns around increased risk of lymphoma have fortunately not been confirmed. However, the full effects of such drugs, when used over long periods of time, will not become clear for some years. Longer follow-up, through post-marketing surveillance and biologics registries is essential (42).

Summary

- Immunocompromised patients, especially those with T cell deficiencies, are highly susceptible to tumor development
- Immunocompromised patients are increasing in numbers due to improved management of primary and acquired immunodeficiency disorders, increasing numbers of solid-organ transplantations, and the application of an increasing number of immunosuppressive agents to a broadening population of patients with cancer and inflammatory diseases
- Although the level and length of time of immunosuppression are the main predictors for the development of malignancies, environmental and host factors also play a role
- The majority of tumors are related to failure to control oncogenic viruses such as EBV, HHV-8 and HPV
- The clinical presentation of cancer in these populations is atypical and usually aggressive
- Differentiation from opportunistic infections is challenging as tumors may mimic infection and multiple pathologies often occur concurrently
- Early diagnosis significantly improves outcome; some cancers may be detected when the proliferation is still polyclonal and when reduction in immunosuppression alone can lead to regression of the tumor

REFERENCES

1. Bouwes JN, Bavinck, Hardie DR, Green A, et al. The risk of skin cancer in renal transplant recipients in Queensland, Australia. A follow-up study. Transplantation 1996; 61: 715–21.
2. Ehrlich P. Ueber den jetzigen Stand der Karzinomforschung. Ned Tijdschr Geneeskd 1909; 5: 273–90.
3. Burnet FM. Cancer: a biological approach. Br Med J 1957; 1: 841–47.
4. Thomas L. Discussion to PB Medawar's paper. In: Lawrence HS, ed. Cellular and Humoral Aspects of the Hypersensitive States. New York: Hoeber-Harper, 1959: 529–32.
5. Burnet FM. The concept of immunological surveillance. Prog Exp Tumor Res 1970; 13: 1–27.
6. Dunn GP, Bruce AT, Ikeda H, et al. Cancer immunoediting: from immunosurveillance to tumor escape. Nat Immunol 2002; 3: 991–8.
7. Penn I. Malignant Tumors in Organ Transplant Recipients. New York: Springer-Verlag, 1970.
8. Bouwes Bavinck JN, Claas FH, Hardie DR, et al. Relation between HLA antigens and skin cancer in renal transplant recipients in Queensland Australia. J Invest Dermatol 1997; 108: 708–11.
9. Gatti RA, Good RA. Occurrence of malignancy in immunodeficiency diseases. A literature review. Cancer 1971; 28: 89–98.
10. Grulich AE, van Leeuwen MT, Falster MO, Vajdic CM, Incidence of cancers in people with HIV/AIDS compared with immunosuppressed transplant recipients: a meta-analysis. Lancet 2007; 370: 59–67.
11. Penn I. Post-transplant malignancies. Transplant Proc 1999; 31: 1260–2.
12. Penn L. Post-transplant malignancy. The role of immunosuppression. Drug Safety 2000; 23: 101–13.
13. Birkeland SA, Storm HH, Lamm LU, et al. Cancer risk after renal transplantation in the Nordic countries, 1964–86. Int J Cancer 1995; 60: 183–9.
14. Sheil AG. Cancer in dialysis and transplant patients. In: Morris PJ, ed. Kidney Transplantation. Philadelphia: WB Saunders, 2001: 558–70.
15. Boshoff C, Weiss R. AIDS-related malignancies. Nat Rev Cancer 2002; 2: 373–82.
16. Harward CA, Surentheran T, McGregor JM, et al. Human papillomavirus infection and non-melanomous skin cancer in immunosuppressed and immunocompetent individuals. J Med Virol 2000; 62: 289–97.
17. Engels EA, Frisch M, Lubin JH, et al. Prevalence of hepatitis C virus infection and risk for hepatocellular carcinoma and non-Hodgkin lymphoma in AIDS. J Acquir Immune Defic Syndr 2002; 31: 536–41.
18. El-Serag HB, Rudolph KL. Hepatocellular carcinoma: epidemiology and molecular carcinogenesis. Gastroenterology 2007; 132: 2557–76.
19. Kauffman HM, Cherikh WS, Cheng Y, Hanto DW, Kahan BD. Maintenance immunosuppression with target-of-rapamycin inhibitors is associated with a reduced incidence of de novo malignancies. Transplantation 2005; 80: 883–9.
20. Stallone G, Schena A, Infante B, et al. Sirolimus for Kaposi's sarcoma in renal-transplant recipients. N Engl J Med 2005; 352: 1317–23.
21. London N, Farmery S, Will E, et al. Risk of neoplasia in renal transplant patients. Lancet 1995; 346: 403–6.
22. Vial T, Descotes J. Immunosuppressive drugs and cancer. Toxicology 2003; 185: 229–40.
23. Bouwes Bavinck JN, Hardie DR, Green A, et al. The risk of skin cancer in renal transplant recipients in Queensland, Australia. A follow-up study. Transplantation 1996; 61: 715–21.

24. Harzallah K, Abderrahim E, Chareffedine K, et al. Cancers after renal transplantation: multicenter experience. Saudi J Kidney Dis Transpl 2008; 19: 825–30.

25. Opelz G, Henderson R. Incidence of non-Hodgkin's lymphoma in kidney and heart recipients. Lancet 1993; 342: 1514–16.

26. Niaudet P. Post-transplant lymphoproliferative disease following renal transplantation: a multicentre retrospective study of 41 cases observed between 1991 and 1996. French Speaking Transplantation Workshop. Transplant Proc 1998; 30: 2816–17.

27. Guthery SL, Heubi JE, Bucuvalas JC, et al. Determination for Epstein–Barr virus-associated post-transplant lymphoproliferative disorder in pediatric liver transplant recipients using objective case ascertainment. Transplantation 2003; 73: 989–93.

28. Paya CV, Fung JJ, Nalesnik MA, et al. Epstein–Barr virus-induced post-transplant lymphoproliferative disorders ASTS/ASTP EBV-PTLD Task Force and the Mayo Clinic organised International Consensus Development Meeting. Transplantation 1999; 68: 1517.

29. Newell KA, Alonso EM, Whitington PF, et al. Post-transplant lymphoproliferative disease in pediatric liver transplantation. Transplantation 1996; 62: 370–5.

30. Kapelushnik J, Ariad S, Benharroch D, et al. Post-renal transplantation human herpesvirus 8-associated lymphoproliferative disorder and Kaposi's sarcoma. Br J Haematol 2001; 113: 425–8.

31. Shehab TM, Hsi ED, Poterucha JJ, et al. *Helicobacter pylori*-associated gastric MALT lymphoma in liver transplant patients. Transplantation 2001; 71: 1172–5.

32. Webb MC, Compton F, Andrews PA, Koffman GC. Skin tumours post-transplantation: a retrospective analysis of 28 years' experience at a single centre. Transplantation Proc 1997; 29: 828–30.

33. Hiesse C, Rieu P, Kriaa F, et al. Malignancy after renal transplantation: analysis of incidence and risk factors in 1700 patients followed during a 25-year period. Transplant Proc 1997; 29: 831–3.

34. Winkelhorset JT, Brokelman WJ, Tiggeler RG, Wobbes T. Incidence and clinical course of de novo malignancies in renal allograft recipients. Eur J Surg Oncol 2001; 27: 409–13.

35. Sanchez EQ, Marubashi S, Jung G, et al. De novo tumours after liver transplantation: a single-institution experience. Liver Transplant 2002; 8: 285–91.

36. Euvrard S, Kanitakis J, Claudy A. Skin cancers after organ transplantation. N Engl J Med 2003; 348: 1681–91.

37. Carroll RP, Ramsay HM, Fryer AA, et al. Incidence and prediction of nonmelanoma skin cancer post-renal transplantation: a prospective study in Queensland, Australia. Am J Kidney Dis 2003; 41: 676–83.

38. Penn I. Cancers of the anogenital region in renal transplant recipients: analysis of 65 cases. Cancer 1986; 58: 611–16.

39. Jenkins FJ, Hoffmann LJ, Liegey-Dougall A. Reactivation of and primary infection with human herpesvirus 9 among solid-organ transplant recipients. J Infect Dis 2002; 185: 1238–43.

40. Catani P, Nanni G, Graffeo R, et al. Pretransplantion human herpesvirus 8 seropositivity as a risk factor for Kaposi's sarcoma in kidney transplant recipients. Transplant Proc 2000; 32: 526–7.

41. Engels AE, Biggar RJ, Hall HI, et al. Cancer risk in people infected with human immunodeficiency virus in the United States. Int J Cancer 2008; 123: 187–94.

42. Askling J; Bongartz T. Malignancy and biologic therapy in rheumatoid arthritis. Curr Opn Rheumatol 2008; 20: 334–9.

58 The Immunocompromised Host: Central Nervous System
Jane Evanson

INTRODUCTION

Immunocompromised patients are susceptible to the development of lymphoid neoplasms within the central nervous system (CNS). The patients at risk of these malignancies include those with congenital immunodeficiencies (e.g., Wiskott–Aldrich syndrome) as well as those with acquired immunodeficiency. Acquired immunodeficiency may be the result of illness, e.g., lupus, or infection, e.g., acquired immunodeficiency syndrome (AIDS), or iatrogenic immunosuppression, e.g., after transplantation. Two specific groups of patients are susceptible to these lymphoid malignancies: patients with AIDS and those who have received solid-organ transplants. In both these groups of patients the lymphoid proliferations are thought to be due to an Epstein–Barr virus (EBV)-induced B-cell proliferation, which is unopposed by the suppressed T cells [suppressed either as a result of immunosuppressive drugs or human immunodeficiency virus (HIV) infection]. Transplant patients most commonly develop post-transplant lymphoproliferative disorders within the first two years after transplantation. The lymphoid proliferations in these patients have some similarities in imaging appearances, which is not unexpected given their identical pathogenesis. These appearances are often distinct from those of primary central nervous system lymphoma (PCNSL) in the immunocompetent patient. There does not seem to be any documented increased risk of primary glial neoplasms of the CNS in these patients.

Key Points: General Features

- Immunosuppressed patients are susceptible to lymphoid neoplasms in the CNS
- The neoplasms are typically EBV-related B-cell lymphomas
- AIDS patients and solid-organ transplant patients are at particular risk
- Symptoms are variable and non-specific

PRIMARY CNS LYMPHOMA IN AIDS

It was recognized in the 1980s that patients with AIDS had an increased incidence of primary CNS lymphoma (PCNSL). Overall, there has been an approximately three-fold increase in the incidence of PCNSL in the last 20 years, most particularly in AIDS patients (1). It had been previously estimated that up to 3% of all patients with AIDS would develop PCNSL (1); however, since the introduction of highly active antiretroviral therapy (HAART), the risk of these patients developing PCNSL, or indeed any focal brain lesion, has reduced (2). Nonetheless, PCNSL remains the second most common cause of focal brain lesions in AIDS patients with neurological symptoms, after cerebral toxoplasmosis (2). Histologically, these PCNSLs are typically large cell B-cell non-Hodgkin's lymphomas; a minority are small cell

Burkitt's type. Presenting symptoms are variable and non-specific but seizures, focal neurological deficit, or headache are most common. The initial identification of focal brain abnormalities on imaging computed tomography (CT) or magnetic resonance (MR) imaging will not distinguish PCNSL from toxoplasmosis or other entities such as tuberculous (TB) granulomas or even progressive multifocal leuco-encephalopathy (PML). Commonly, a trial of treatment for toxoplasmosis is the initial management, whilst awaiting serological tests and cerebrospinal fluid (CSF) analysis (if safe). Detection of EBV DNA in the CSF has high sensitivity and specificity for PCNSL (3), whereas cytological examination of the CSF has a low sensitivity (4).

The prognosis remains poor, with only 10% of those treated surviving beyond a year (5). HAART treated patients have a longer survival than non-HAART treated patients (6). PCNSL is rare in children with AIDS although a few cases are reported (7) and they also seem to be related to EBV; the intracranial lesions are similar to those seen in adults.

Imaging Appearances of Primary CNS Lymphoma

Primary cerebral lymphomas in AIDS are commonly multifocal, 71% in a recent series (8). Therefore, the number of lesions will not reliably differentiate PCNSL from toxoplasmosis. The most common appearance is that of a ring-enhancing mass(es) (8) (Fig. 58.1), the peripheral enhancement after gadolinium reflecting central necrosis of the lesion, presumably related to the relatively rapid growth of these lesions. They can occur both in the deep grey matter of the basal ganglia or the periventricular region as well as more peripherally in the cerebral hemispheres, and the location of the lesion(s) is not a useful distinguishing feature in differentiating PCNSL from other pathologies. Posterior fossa involvement is uncommon but recognized (8). In the immunocompetent patient, PCNSL is typically solidly enhancing (9) (Fig. 58.2) but this is a less common, though recognized, appearance in the immunocompromised patient (10). The mass effect and edema with PCNSL is mild to modest and extensive edema is not common (8,10). It does seem there is an increased frequency of non-enhancing lymphoma in AIDS patients. Just over a quarter of lymphomatous lesions in a recent series did not show enhancement, and in some cases there were both enhancing and non-enhancing lesions present. It is well recognized that a small proportion of lymphomas will be non-enhancing (9) and it is important to remember that steroid administration can abolish enhancement in any CNS lymphoma. Small foci of hemorrhage, identified as high T1-weighted signal intensity prior to enhancement with contrast medium have been reported, as has a primary presentation with cerebral hemorrhage (11). T2-weighted signal characteristics are variable (8,10); the low T2-weighted signal intensity expected in very cellular neoplasms is not always striking.

MR is more sensitive than CT to the presence of PCNSL, but CT is often the first-line investigation in the acute setting (Fig. 58.3).

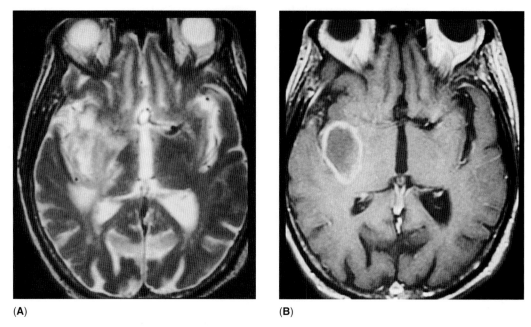

(A) **(B)**

Figure 58.1 (A) Primary CNS lymphoma in an AIDS patient. Axial T2-weighted image shows a mass in the right posterior temporal region. There is central high signal intensity compatible with necrosis and modest adjacent edema for the size of the mass. The periphery of the lesion is of relatively low T2 signal intensity—a variable feature of primary CNS lymphoma. This was a solitary lesion. (B) Axial T1-weighted image post-gadolinium. The mass shows ring enhancement with central necrosis.

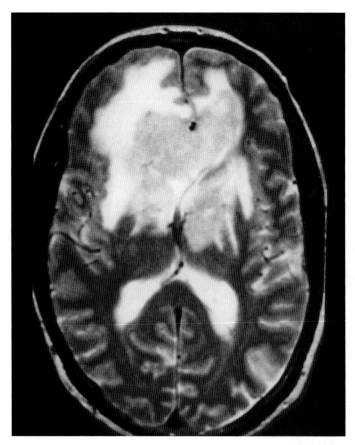

Figure 58.2 Primary CNS lymphoma in an immunocompetent patient. Axial T2-weighted MR image shows a solid mass extending across the genu of the corpus callosum and extending around the margins of the lateral ventricles with modest edema. There was homogeneous enhancement after contrast.

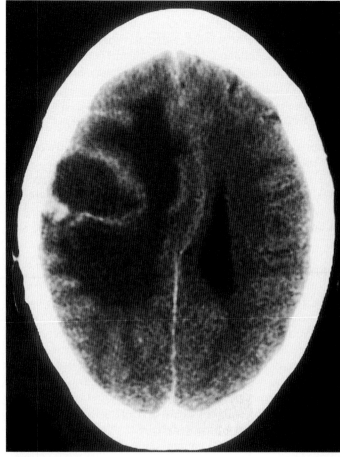

Figure 58.3 Enhanced CT of biopsy-proven primary CNS lymphoma in an AIDS patient. There is a large ring-enhancing mass in the right frontal region with prominent vasogenic edema.

Differential Diagnosis

Distinguishing between toxoplasmosis and PCNSL remains difficult (Fig. 58.4); whether the lesions are solitary or multiple will not allow accurate differentiation. Imaging findings should be correlated with results of other clinical investigations; examination of CSF for EBV DNA is a usefully sensitive and specific test for PCNSL (3). Thallium-201 brain single-photon emission computed tomography (SPECT) might be useful, if available. Increased thallium uptake is seen in lymphomas, with reported sensitivities of 100% and specificities of 93% (12), and may be more useful in lesions larger than 2 cm (13). However other groups have reported this technique as non-reliable (14) and the best option may be to be guided by local experience. Combining thallium SPECT and EBV DNA analysis shows a high diagnostic accuracy for AIDS-related primary cerebral lymphoma (15). The improved accuracy of CSF analysis has already reduced the requirement for cranial biopsy in these patients (5). Positron emission tomography scanning using 2-[F-18]fluoro-2-deoxy-D-glucose (^{18}FDG PET) is a promising technique, showing increased uptake in lymphoma compared with infective lesions (16,17).

Magnetic resonance spectroscopy (MRS) is a technique which produces information about the chemical metabolites present within either a single sampled voxel or multiple voxels (this multi voxel technique is also known as chemical shift imaging, CSI). The metabolite spectrum obtained from lymphoma should be distinct from that obtained from an infective lesion such as Toxoplasmosis, with a high Choline peak, reflecting active membrane turnover, and a moderate lipid peak (18). Correct positioning of the sampling voxel over the lesion is important because sampling the necrotic centre of a lesion rather than the solid periphery will not produce a spectrum that will help discriminate between lymphoma and an infective lesion (18).

Despite all these advances in non-invasive diagnostic techniques, there are still a significant proportion of these patients that will require a cranial biopsy to make the definitive diagnosis.

Other diagnoses to be considered include TB and PML. Multiple enhancing lesions of TB granulomata cannot be distinguished from toxoplasmosis or multifocal enhancing lymphoma solely on imaging grounds; CSF analysis may be contributory. Meningeal involvement suggests TB, cryptococcal meningitis or other infective processes. Progressive cranial radiological changes, due to the development of the Immune Reconstitution Inflammatory Syndrome (IRIS), are now recognized in patients being treated for such CNS infections who are also just starting HAART. Close correlation with the treatment history should suggest this possibility. The incidence of PML in AIDS patients has not declined despite the introduction of HAART therapy, unlike both toxoplasmosis and PCNSL (2). PML is a condition of demyelination due to JC polyoma virus and therefore manifests as areas of signal change within the white matter. Multifocal areas of low T1 and high T2 weighting are seen in the white matter without mass effect and without enhancement (Fig. 58.5) (19). The lack of local mass effect should be a helpful identifying feature. The parietal lobe is the most commonly involved; however, frontal, periventricular, brain stem, and posterior fossa involvement are all recognized (20). In a few cases, faint peripheral enhancement has been noted (19) and enhancement may develop after commencing treatment with HAART (21).Cerebrospinal fluid examination for the JC virus DNA has high specificity, in the order of 95% (22), but in negative or doubtful cases a brain biopsy may still be needed.

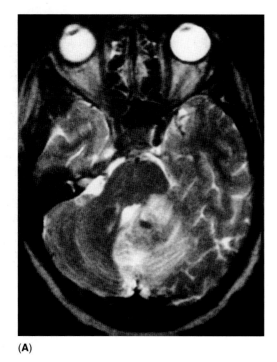

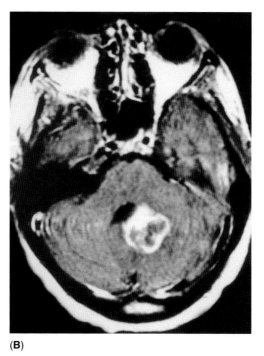

(A) (B)

Figure 58.4 Toxoplasmosis in an AIDS patient. (**A**) Axial T2-weighted MR image shows a relatively low signal intensity mass in the left cerebellar hemisphere with moderate edema. (**B**) Axial T1-weighted MR image post-gadolinium. Peripheral enhancement is evident; no other lesions were present. It is not possible to distinguish this from primary CNS lymphoma.

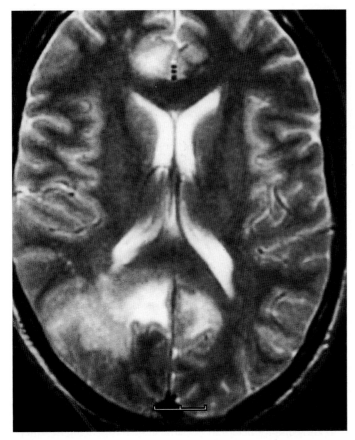

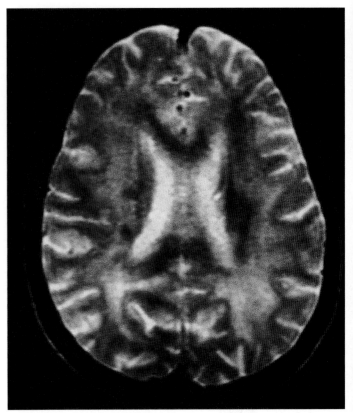

Figure 58.6 HIV encephalopathy. Axial T2-weighted MR image shows diffuse symmetrical high signal intensity in the hemispheric white matter.

Figure 58.5 Progressive multifocal leuco-encephalopathy. Axial T2-weighted MR image shows focal areas of high signal intensity change within the white matter of both occipital lobes and the right frontal lobe. The adjacent cortex is spared and there is minimal mass effect. There was no enhancement after contrast. Multifocal non-enhancing primary CNS lymphoma could have this appearance, but more mass effect would be expected.

The lesions of PML are typically asymmetrical, which should help to distinguish it from HIV encephalopathy, which produces extensive symmetrical high signal intensity throughout the supratentorial white matter (Fig. 58.6).

Key Points: Central Nervous System Lymphoma

- Ring-enhancing mass lesions are typical imaging findings of CNS lymphoma
- Differential diagnosis includes infections, toxoplasmosis, or TB
- AIDS patients are less at risk of CNS lymphoma since the introduction of HAART treatment
- Lymphoma is the second most common intracranial mass lesion in AIDS patients
- Lymphoma lesions are often multiple and show ring enhancement
- CSF analysis, SPECT, MR spectroscopy, or ^{18}FDG PET all aid diagnosis

POST-TRANSPLANTATION LYMPHOPROLIFERATIVE DISORDER

Post-transplantation lymphoproliferative disorder (PTLD) is a syndrome of uncontrolled lymphoid growth in the transplant patient. It occurs in approximately 2% to 3% of patients with solid-organ transplants (23). Transplanted children are particularly susceptible, with frequencies as high as 10% reported (24). Chronic immunosuppression in these patients allows an EBV-induced B-cell proliferation, and seronegativity for EBV at the time of transplantation is a risk factor (25). It has a propensity to involve extranodal sites, particularly the allografted organ, gastrointestinal tract, the thorax, and the CNS. CNS involvement is reported in between 10% and 25% of cases (26,27). The prevalence of PTLD is highest in patients after lung transplant, followed in decreasing order of frequency by kidney, pancreas, heart, and liver transplants (28). PTLD has been reported at any time between one month and 10 years after transplantation (29), although the majority occur within the first two transplant years. Definitive diagnosis of PTLD requires biopsy as it is vital to distinguish between the various histological types (30). There is a pathological classification subdividing PTLDs into polymorphic and monomorphic forms, most of the monomorphic forms being B-cell non-Hodgkin's lymphomas. Subsequent to biopsy, full clinical staging and imaging as for lymphomas is required. The treatment strategy is dependent upon the histology. A reduction in immunosuppression is the initial approach and, in a subgroup of patients, this alone may be successful. However monoclonal antibody therapy (rituximab) is now considered first line treatment (31). Chemotherapy and irradiation may be used if other treatment options have failed (30,32). Survival is best in pediatric patients and those with localized disease; five-year adult survival rates vary between 86% (24) and 50% (30).

The clinical presentation of PTLD has been grouped into three syndromes (33):

- Infectious mononucleosis-like
- Isolated or multiple tumors
- Widespread fulminant disease

PTLD in the CNS usually presents as part of the isolated/multiple tumor syndrome and may present with seizures, focal neurological deficit, or impaired mental state. It most commonly presents with isolated CNS involvement, rather than as part of diffuse systemic involvement with PTLD (34). Histologically the CNS PTLD is typically a high grade lymphoma of the monomorphic subtype which is histologically similar to the CNS lymphomas seen in the HIV population (34).

This would suggest a more aggressive clinical course in patients with CNS PTLD, as compared to the less aggressive PTLD histological subtypes. However a recent series reported variable survival with the worst outcomes in those who had received peripheral blood stem cell transplants (34).

Imaging Appearances of CNS Involvement

Ring-enhancing mass lesions are the typical imaging findings of CNS involvement with PTLD. The features are similar to those described above of AIDS-related PCNSL, namely, ring-enhancement, central necrosis, and location within both the deep or superficial structures of the cerebral hemispheres (Fig. 58.7). Posterior fossa involvement is less common but has been reported (34,35). Lesions may be solitary or, more frequently, multifocal (Fig. 58.8).

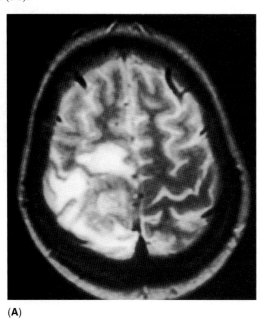

(A)

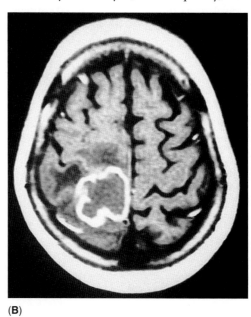

(B)

Figure 58.7 (A) PTLD in a transplant patient. Axial T2-weighted MR image shows a right parietal mass lesion with central necrosis and adjacent edema. The periphery of the lesion is of relatively low T2 signal intensity. (B) Axial T1-weighted MR image after gadolinium demonstrating ring enhancement.

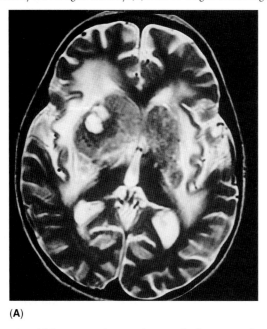

(A)

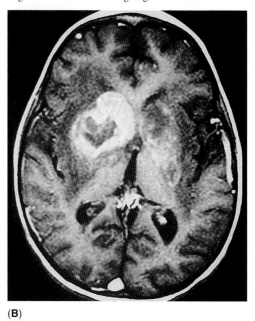

(B)

Figure 58.8 (A) PTLD in a child post-transplant. Axial T2-weighted MR image shows mass lesions in the periventricular region bilaterally; other lesions were present in the peripheral white matter (not shown). (B) Axial T1-weighted MR image show ring enhancement on the right and patchy enhancement on the left.

High T1 signal intensity on unenhanced images (representing hemorrhage) is recognized (35). The extent of associated vasogenic edema is variable. The dense cellularity of lymphoproliferative abnormalities is often associated with relatively low T2 signal intensity in the peripheral cellular part of the tumor. However, these signal characteristics are not a reliable discriminator between PTLD and other infectious lesions. Meningeal abnormalities or durally-based spinal lesions, which are typical of secondary lymphoma in immunocompetent patients, are unusual in PTLD but have been recognized (Fig. 58.9).

The differential diagnosis of a ring-enhancing mass lesion in the CNS of a transplant patient must include infection. Fungal infections, particularly Aspergillosis, should be considered, along with Candida, Nocardia, and histoplasmosis. Toxoplasmosis is less common in the transplant population than in the AIDS population. Ultimately, biopsy is necessary for diagnosis and to determine the appropriate treatment.

FDG-PET has been used in staging of PTLD (36–38) which is reported to be highly FDG avid, and this technique is likely to have an increasing role in the staging and monitoring of this condition.

Differential Diagnosis

A well-recognized complication of immunosuppressive therapies such as Cyclosporin A and Tacrolimus (FK506) is the posterior reversible encephalopathy syndrome (PRES) (39–41). PRES also usually presents with headaches, seizures, or altered mental state and hypertension is present in around 70% of patients (42). CT and MR imaging demonstrate symmetrical areas of vasogenic edema, predominantly in the white matter of the parietal and occipital regions. PRES is increasingly recognized as a syndrome of neurotoxicity associated with a diverse range of clinical situations comprehensively described in a recent review (42). It has been described in association with allogenic bone marrow transplantation (43), combination high dose chemotherapy as well as single agent chemotherapy such as cisplatin, cytarabine, Gemcitabine (42), intrathecal methotrexate (44), and in the treatment of acute lymphoblastic leukemia in children (45,46). PRES may also result from infection and sepsis.

The incidence of PRES after solid organ transplantation varies between 0.4% and 6% (43,47) and tends to occur earlier post-transplant in liver recipients than in renal recipients (42,43). In renal transplant patients PRES has been noted to be associated with transplant rejection and infection (42).

The underlying patho-physiological cause of the imaging appearances of PRES is not yet established, although evidence suggests that vasoconstriction and hypoperfusion produce brain ischemia and subsequent vasogenic edema (48). Diffusion imaging has confirmed that the signal intensity changes in this condition are due to vasogenic edema, which can be completely reversed with treatment. In severe cases, however, infarction and permanent damage may result (49).

MR imaging appearances are typically those of high signal intensity on T2-weighted images within the white matter of the parieto-occipital regions bilaterally (Fig. 58.10A). While PRES was initially considered to be a posterior lesion as described in its name, posterior reversible encephalopathy syndrome, frontal lobe, temporal lobe, and posterior fossa involvement are now increasingly recognized (50) but the parieto-occipital involvement is typically more severe. Brain stem involvement indicates severe PRES (Fig. 58.10B) (40,49). Mass effect is minimal and enhancement is usually absent, although faint, patchy enhancement has been reported (40). The lack of enhancement should help in distinguishing between this syndrome and PTLD where enhancement is typical. White matter involvement is dominant but cortical involvement is also recognized (51). Use of fluid attenuation inversion recovery (FLAIR) sequences increases the conspicuity of the cortical and subcortical involvement and should be used routinely in assessment of such cases (51). CT may show only minimal abnormality in the acute phase.

The MR changes and the symptoms of PRES are typically reversible, resolving fully after the adjustment of the immunosuppressant drugs, the treatment of hypertension or adjustment of chemotherapy (51–53). If severe or unrecognized, the prognosis can be poor. (See also chapters 31 and 53.)

Head and Neck Involvement with PTLD

Patients with PTLD affecting the extracranial head and neck may present with cervical lymphadenopathy or with focal masses in Waldeyer's ring. The lymphadenopathy may present as a large nodal mass or an excess number of relatively normal-sized nodes. Necrosis within the nodes appears to be more common than in immunocompetent patients with lymphoma (54). Sino-nasal and orbital masses may also be manifestations of PTLD (55). Head and neck PTLD is usually associated with disease in the thorax and abdomen (35).

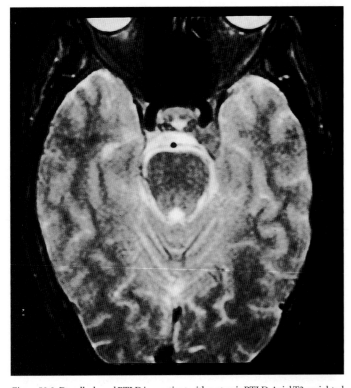

Figure 58.9 Durally-based PTLD in a patient with systemic PTLD. Axial T2-weighted MR image shows a subtle low signal intensity mass in the left carvernous sinus, which showed a little enhancement (not shown). These appearances are similar to those of secondary lymphoma seen in immunocompetent patients.

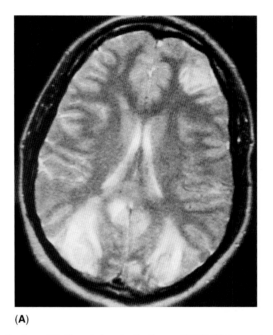

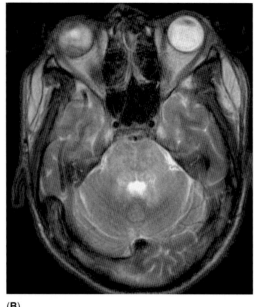

(A) **(B)**

Figure 58.10 Posterior Reversible Encephalopathy Syndrome (PRES) (**A**) in a patient with eclampsia. Axial T2-weighted MR image shows the high signal intensity in the white matter of the parieto-occipital regions bilaterally. The cortex is relatively spared. There is a little involvement of the left frontal white matter. (**B**) Axial T2-weighted MR image of a diabetic, septicemic patient with PRES. There is high T2 signal throughout the brainstem and extending into the cerebellar hemispheres.

Key Points: Post-Transplantation Lymphoproliferative Disorder

- PTLD occurs in 2% to 3% of organ transplant patients
- CNS involvement is seen in 10% to 25% of cases
- Imaging with CT and MR typically shows ring enhancement
- Differential diagnosis typically includes aspergillus and candidiasis
- Immunosuppressant drugs can cause imaging abnormalities in the white matter

- Post-transplantation lymphoproliferative disorder (PTLD) is a syndrome of uncontrolled lymphoid growth in the transplant patient
- PTLD has the highest incidence in lung-transplanted patients
- PTLD in the CNS usually presents as isolated involvement

Summary

- Immunocompromised patients are susceptible to the development of lymphoid neoplasms
- Patients with acquired immunodeficiency in AIDS and post-organ transplantation are susceptible to lymphoid malignancies
- There has been a threefold increase in primary CNS lymphoma (PCNSL) in the last 20 years
- Highly active anti-retroviral therapy has reduced the risk of PCNSL
- The prognosis of PCNSL is poor–10% one-year survival
- PCNSL is commonly multifocal
- Imaging of PCNSL with CT and MR usually shows a rim-enhancing mass(es)
- A small percentage of PCNSL masses are non-enhancing following injection of intravenous contrast medium
- Differential diagnosis of PCNSL includes toxoplasmosis, TB, and progressive multifocal leuco-encephalopathy (PML)

REFERENCES

1. Velasquez WS. Primary central nervous system lymphoma. J Neurooncol 1994; 20: 177–85.
2. Ammassari A, Cingolani A, Pezzotti P, et al. AIDS-related focal brain lesions in the era of highly active antiretroviral therapy. Neurology 2000; 55: 1194–200.
3. Bossolasco S, Cinque P, Ponzoni M, et al. Epstein-Barr virus DNA load in cerebrospinal fluid and plasma of patients with AIDS-related lymphoma. J Neurovirol 2002; 8: 432–8.
4. DeAngelis LM, Yahalom J, Heinemann MH, et al. Primary CNS lymphoma: combined treatment with chemotherapy and radiotherapy. Neurology 1990; 40: 80–6.
5. Sparano JA. Clinical aspects and management of AIDS-related lymphoma. Eur J Cancer 2001; 37: 1296–305.
6. Diamond C, Taylor TH, Im T, Miradi M, Anton-Culver H. Improved survival and chemotherapy response among patients with AIDS-related non-Hodgkin's lymphoma receiving highly active antiretroviral therapy. Hematol Oncol 2006; 24: 139–45.
7. Del Mistro A, Laverda A, Calabrese F, et al. Primary lymphoma of the central nervous system in two children with acquired immune deficiency syndrome. Am J Clin Pathol 1990; 94: 722–8.

8. Thurnher MM, Rieger A, Kleibl-Popov C, et al. Primary central nervous system lymphoma in AIDS: a wider spectrum of CT and MRI findings. Neuroradiology 2001; 43: 29–35.

9. Johnson B, Fram E, Johnson P, Jacobowitz R. The variable MR appearance of primary lymphoma of the central nervous system: comparison with histopathologic features. AJNR Am J Neuroradiol 1997; 18: 563–72.

10. Cordoliani YS, Derosier C, Pharaboz C, et al. [Primary brain lymphoma in AIDS. 17 cases studied by MRI before stereotaxic biopsies]. J Radiol 1992; 73: 367–76.

11. Fukui MB, Livstone BJ, Meltzer CC, Hamilton RL. Hemorrhagic presentation of untreated primary CNS lymphoma in a patient with AIDS. AJR Am J Roentgenol 1998; 170: 1114–5.

12. Kessler LS, Ruiz A, Post MJD, et al. Thallium-201 brain SPECT of lymphoma in AIDS patients: pitfalls and technique optimization. AJNR Am J Neuroradiol 1998; 19: 1105–9.

13. Young RJ, Ghesani MV, Kagetsu NJ, Derogatis AJ. Lesion size determines accuracy of thallium-201 brain single-photon emission tomography in differentiating between intracranial malignancy and infection in AIDS patients. AJNR Am J Neuroradiol 2005; 26: 1973–9.

14. Licho R, Litofsky NS, Senitko M, George M. Inaccuracy of Tl-201 brain SPECT in distinguishing cerebral infections from lymphoma in patients with AIDS. Clin Nucl Med 2002; 27: 81–6.

15. Antinori A, De Rossi G, Ammassari A, et al. Value of combined approach with thallium-201 single-photon emission computed tomography and Epstein-Barr virus DNA polymerase chain reaction in CSF for the diagnosis of AIDS-related primary CNS lymphoma. J Clin Oncol 1999; 17: 554–60.

16. Heald AE, Hoffman JM, Bartlett JA, Waskin HA. Differentiation of central nervous system lesions in AIDS patients using positron emission tomography (PET). Int J STD AIDS 1996; 7: 337–46.

17. Villringer K, Jäger H, Dichgans M, et al. Differential diagnosis of CNS lesions in AIDS patients by FDG-PET. J Comput Assist Tomogr 1995; 19: 532–6.

18. Kingsley PB, Shah TC, Woldenberg R. Identification of diffuse and focal brain lesions by clinical magnetic resonance spectroscopy. NMR Biomed 2006; 19: 435–62.

19. Whiteman ML, Post MJ, Berger JR, et al. Progressive multifocal leukoencephalopathy in 47 HIV-seropositive patients: neuroimaging with clinical and pathologic correlation. Radiology 1993; 187: 233–40.

20. Post MJ, Yiannoutsos C, Simpson D, et al. Progressive multifocal leukoencephalopathy in AIDS: are there any MR findings useful to patient management and predictive of patient survival? AIDS Clinical Trials Group, 243 Team. AJNR Am J Neuroradiol 1999; 20: 1896–906.

21. Thurnher MM, Post MJ, Rieger A, et al. Initial and follow-up MR imaging findings in AIDS-related progressive multifocal leukoencephalopathy treated with highly active antiretroviral therapy. AJNR Am J Neuroradiol 2001; 22: 977–84.

22. Fong IW, Britton CB, Luinstra KE, Toma E, Mahony JB. Diagnostic value of detecting JC virus DNA in cerebrospinal fluid of patients with progressive multifocal leukoencephalopathy. J Clin Microbiol 1995; 33: 484–6.

23. Nalesnik MA. Posttransplantation lymphoproliferative disorders (PTLD): current perspectives. Semin Thorac Cardiovasc Surg 1996; 8: 139–48.

24. Shapiro R, Nalesnik M, McCauley J, et al. Posttransplant lymphoproliferative disorders in adult and pediatric renal transplant patients receiving tacrolimus-based immunosuppression. Transplantation 1999; 68: 1851–4.

25. Ho M, Jaffe R, Miller G, et al. The frequency of Epstein-Barr virus infection and associated lymphoproliferative syndrome after transplantation and its manifestations in children. Transplantation 1988; 45: 719–27.

26. Chen JM, Michler RE. Heart xenotransplantation: lessons learned and future prospects. J Heart Lung Transplant 1993; 12: 869–75.

27. Lim GY, Newman B, Kurland G, Webber SA. Posttransplantation lymphoproliferative disorder: manifestations in pediatric thoracic organ recipients. Radiology 2002; 222: 699–708.

28. Walker RC, Paya CV, Marshall WF, et al. Pretransplantation seronegative Epstein-Barr virus status is the primary risk factor for posttransplantation lymphoproliferative disorder in adult heart, lung, and other solid organ transplantations. J Heart Lung Transplant 1995; 14: 214–21.

29. Basgoz N, Preiksaitis JK. Post-transplant lymphoproliferative disorder. Infect Dis Clin North Am 1995; 9: 901–23.

30. Nalesnik MA. Clinicopathologic characteristics of post-transplant lymphoproliferative disorders. Recent Results Cancer Res 2002; 159: 9–18.

31. Svoboda J, Kotloff R, Tsai DE. Management of patients with post-transplant lymphoproliferative disorder: the role of rituximab. Transpl Int 2006; 19: 259–69.

32. Benkerrou M, Durandy A, Fischer A. Therapy for transplant-related lymphoproliferative diseases. Hematol Oncol Clin North Am 1993; 7: 467–75.

33. Malatack JF, Gartner JC, Jr, Urbach AH, Zitelli BJ. Orthotopic liver transplantation, Epstein-Barr virus, cyclosporine, and lymphoproliferative disease: a growing concern. J Pediatr 1991; 118: 667–75.

34. Castellano-Sanchez AA, Li S, Qian J, et al. Primary central nervous system posttransplant lymphoproliferative disorders. Am J Clin Pathol 2004; 121: 246–53.

35. Pickhardt PJ, Wippold FJ, 2nd. Neuroimaging in posttransplantation lymphoproliferative disorder. AJR Am J Roentgenol 1999; 172: 1117–21.

36. Bakker NA, Pruim J, de Graaf W, et al. PTLD visualization by FDG-PET: improved detection of extranodal localizations. Am J Transplant 2006; 6: 1984–5.

37. Bianchi E, Pascual M, Nicod M, Delaloye AB, Duchosal MA. Clinical usefulness of FDG-PET/CT scan imaging in the management of posttransplant lymphoproliferative disease. Transplantation 2008; 85: 707–12.

38. von Falck C, Maecker B, Schirg E, et al. Post transplant lymphoproliferative disease in pediatric solid organ transplant patients: a possible role for [18F]-FDG-PET(/CT) in initial staging and therapy monitoring. Eur J Radiol 2007; 63: 427–35.

39. Hinchey J, Chaves C, Appignani B, et al. A reversible posterior leukoencephalopathy syndrome. N Engl J Med 1996; 334: 494–500.

40. Schwartz R, Bravo SM, Klufas RA, et al. Cyclosporine neurotoxicity and its relationship to hypertensive encephalopathy: CT and MR findings in 16 cases. Am J Roentgenol 1995; 165: 627–31.

41. Truwit C, Denaro C, Lake J, DeMarco T. MR imaging of reversible cyclosporin A-induced neurotoxicity. AJNR Am J Neuroradiol 1991; 12: 651–9.

42. Bartynski WS. Posterior reversible encephalopathy syndrome, part 1: fundamental imaging and clinical features. AJNR Am J Neuroradiol 2008; 29: 1036–42 .

43. Singh N, Bonham A, Fukui M. Immunosuppressive-associated leukoencephalopathy in organ transplant recipients. Transplantation 2000; 69: 467–72.

44. Yaffe K, Ferriero D, Barkovich A, Rowley H. Reversible MRI abnormalities following seizures. Neurology 1995; 45: 104–8.

45. Cooney MJ, Bradley WG, Symko SC, Patel ST, Groncy PK. Hypertensive Encephalopathy: complication in children treated for myeloproliferative disorders-report of three cases. Radiology 2000; 214: 711–16.

46. Shin RK, Stern JW, Janss AJ, Hunter JV, Liu GT. Reversible posterior leukoencephalopathy during the treatment of acute lymphoblastic leukemia. Neurology 2001; 56: 388–91.

47. Besenski N, Rumboldt Z, Emovon O, et al. Brain MR imaging abnormalities in kidney transplant recipients. AJNR Am J Neuroradiol 2005; 26: 2282–9.

48. Bartynski WS. Posterior reversible encephalopathy syndrome, part 2: controversies surrounding pathophysiology of vasogenic edema. AJNR Am J Neuroradiol 2008; 29: 1043–9.

49. Covarrubias DJ, Luetmer PH, Campeau NG. Posterior reversible encephalopathy syndrome: prognostic utility of quantitative diffusion-weighted MR images. AJNR Am J Neuroradiol 2002; 23: 1038–48.

50. Bartynski WS, Boardman JF. Distinct imaging patterns and lesion distribution in posterior reversible encephalopathy syndrome. AJNR Am J Neuroradiol 2007; 28: 1320–7 .

51. Casey SO, Sampaio RC, Michel E, Truwit CL. Posterior reversible encephalopathy syndrome: utility of fluid-attenuated inversion recovery MR imaging in the detection of cortical and subcortical lesions. AJNR Am J Neuroradiol 2000; 21: 1199–206.

52. Dillon WP, Rowley H. The reversible posterior cerebral edema syndrome. AJNR Am J Neuroradiol 1998; 19: 591.

53. Schwartz RB, Mulkern RV, Gudbjartsson H, Jolesz F. Diffusion-weighted MR imaging in hypertensive encephalopathy: clues to pathogenesis. AJNR Am J Neuroradiol1998; 19: 859–62.

54. Loevner LA, Karpati RL, Kumar P, et al. Posttransplantation lymphoproliferative disorder of the head and neck: imaging features in seven adults. Radiology 2000; 216: 363–9.

55. Gordon AR, Loevner LA, Sonners AI, Bolger WE, Wasik MA. Posttransplantation lymphoproliferative disorder of the paranasal sinuses mimicking invasive fungal sinusitis: Case report. AJNR Am J Neuroradiol 2002; 23: 855–7.

59 The Immunocompromised Host: Chest
Ioannis Vlahos

INTRODUCTION

The interactions of tumor, host immunity and infection are the subject of this chapter. The complex relationship between cancer and host immunity is multifactorial (Table 59.1). The current understanding of the pathogenesis of cancer suggests that tumor development and progression is frequently the result of tumor "escape" from the control of the immune system. This immune control is mediated by both cellular and molecular pathways (1,2). It is, therefore, not surprising that patients who are chronically immunosuppressed by means of primary immunosuppressive disease, notably by HIV infection, or by chronic iatrogenic immune suppression, especially transplant recipients, are particularly prone to tumor development.

The depressed immunity of these primarily immunosuppressed patients also results in opportunistic infections. Certain cancers, particularly lymphomas and leukemias, by means of their effect on the hemotopoietic system, may also result in clinical presentation with immunosuppression-induced infection. For most established cancers, treatment in both patients who were originally immune-competent or immune-compromised frequently involves chemotherapy or radiation treatment. Both these treatments may again secondarily induce further immunosuppression by inhibiting the bone marrow and hemotopoietic system.

Further complicating the interplay between tumor progression and immunity is the emergence and development of multiple new immunomodulatory therapies. These agents, which may target cellular or molecular signaling pathways, may be used in isolation or in combination with tumor vaccines, or synergistically with traditional chemotherapeutic or radiation regimes. The usage of such agents including interleukin-2, dendritic cell, and BCG vaccines is currently most common in melanoma, prostate, and bladder cancer but evolving to many other cancer, in particular lymphomas with unique cluster of differentiation cellular expression that may be targeted by monoclonal antibodies. The long-term effects of these agents are as yet unknown.

This chapter comprises the following major sections:

- Infection in the immune compromised host
- Complications of:
  - Immune-compromised recipients of bone marrow transplantation
  - Solid organ transplant recipients performed for, or resulting in, malignancy
- Cancer development in the human immunodeficiency syndrome

IMMUNE DEFICIENCY IN THE IMMUNE-COMPROMISED HOST

There are multiple mechanisms that may result in immune deficiency. The susceptibility of the immune-compromised host

(ICH) to infection varies according to the specific deficit in the immune system's protection against infective agents. Table 59.2 summarizes these potential deficiencies in patients with cancer, treated for cancer, or with a propensity to cancer development.

In addition to specific mechanisms of humoral or cellular immunity impairment, cancer patients may be further immune-compromised due to common co-existing conditions such as old age, diabetes mellitus, renal failure, steroid therapy, alcohol excess, or malnutrition.

INFECTIONS IN THE IMMUNE-COMPROMISED HOST

There are innumerable organisms that may result in infection in the immune-compromised host. An exhaustive description of all is, therefore, precluded. Fortunately, with the exceptions described below the radiological appearances of individual infections are similar, irrespective of the underlying immunosuppressive etiology. The most common clinically relevant infections have been described.

Fungal Infections
Pneumocystis jirovecii Infection

The infection previously termed *Pneumocystis carinii* has recently been taxonomically reclassified as *P. jirovecii*. Reflecting the clinical confusion that may arise from the reassignment of the carinii species, the term PCP has been retained for human infection now standing for Pneumocystis pneumonia.

PCP is a fungal infection that typically occurs in patients with depressed lymphocyte function and is, therefore, most common in HIV patients, bone marrow transplant recipients, and patients on chronic steroid therapy. In HIV patients there is a close relationship to the CD4 count, with increased risk below 200 cells/mm^3 and hence PCP infection is considered an AIDS-defining diagnosis. In non-HIV patients PCP infection mortality may be higher due to low clinical suspicion resulting in delayed diagnosis. The incidence of PCP infection in all patients has significantly reduced since the introduction of effective prophylaxis with trimethoprim/sulfamethoxazole (Septrin).

Clinical presentation includes dyspnea on exertion, nonproductive cough, fever, and weight loss. Hypoxia is often significantly more marked than clinical presentation would suggest.

The chest radiograph (CXR) may demonstrate perihilar airspace opacity or interstitial linear shadowing (3–5). Although this appearance is relatively typical, early subtle disease may be overlooked and is best appreciated on HRCT imaging (6,7) (Fig. 59.1). HCRT improves the sensitivity and specificity for the diagnosis (8) and a normal HRCT examination effectively excludes PCP (6,9). At HRCT the appearances can be very variable (Figs. 59.2–59.5). Multifocal bilateral perihilar opacity is initially ground-glass in appearance. With time, more confluent consolidative

Table 59.1 Cancer and Immunity

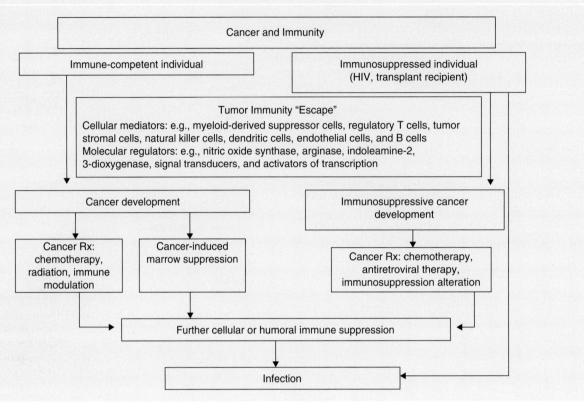

opacity may develop in untreated severe infection, although lobar consolidation is unusual (8,10). In severe infection the extreme subpleural lung surface appears to remain unaffected. Typically as PCP resolves there is progressive development of interlobular and intralobular septal reticulation (10,11). As this organizational retractile phase proceeds towards resolution, mild reversible airway tractional change may be seen. Comparable appearances of this phase may be seen also in atypical bacterial infections, drug reactions, and non-specific interstitial pneumonitis, which can also occur in HIV patients (12) (Fig. 59.2). Pneumatocele formation is unpredictable, occurring in up to one-third of patients, predominating in the upper and mid lungs and is unrelated to the severity of infection (13). The cause is unknown but thought perhaps to be due to either cytotoxic mediator-based cystic lung destruction, PCP cavitary micro-vessel infarction, or small airway obstruction. During the acute phase pneumothorax may occur as a result. Pneumatoceles may coalesce to simulate emphysema (Fig. 59.3) (13).

In general, the radiographic and CT resolution of findings may significantly lag behind clinical improvement (14). In patients who have resistant or recurrent infection, frequently due to inadequate treatment or prophylaxis, a granulomatoid nodular appearance may also occur (Fig. 59.4) (11,15–17). The appearance in HIV patients is possibly related to immune reconstitution syndrome (18), although may also occur in non-HIV patients (18–20). Effusions are unusual unless there are rare extrapulmonary manifestations. Nodal disease is also infrequent, although when it occurs calcification may develop. Similar calcification may be seen rarely in extrapulmonary abdominal visceral involvement (Fig. 59.5) (21,22).

Key Points: Radiological Features of PCP Infection

- CXR: perihilar airspace or interstitial opacity, often subtle, pneumatoceles
- HRCT: higher sensitivity, specificity, earlier diagnosis
  □ Early: perihilar ground-glass disease, upper, and mid lung pneumatoceles
  □ Progressive: consolidative disease, spares subpleural region
  □ Resolution: reticulation, mild tractional change, slow resolution of pneumatoceles
  □ Occasional: pneumothorax, nodal enlargement
  □ Rare: effusions, granumomatoid appearance, abdominal visceral and nodal calcification

Aspergillus Infection

Invasive pulmonary aspergillosis (IPA) infection is commonest in patients with marked neutropenia, namely patients who are immunocompromised due to lymphoproliferative disease or those in the early acute phase following chemotherapy, radiation treatment, or bone marrow transplantation. *Aspergillus fumigatus* is the commonest causative species. The risk of both fungal and bacterial infections is related to both the duration and severity of neutropenia. IPA is a common manifestation of severe neutropenia

Table 59.2 Immune Deficits, Effects, Causes and Infectious Susceptibility

Immune deficit	Effects	Causes	Pulmonary infectious susceptibility
Neutropenia or agranulocytosis	Impaired first line intravascular defense. Deficient phagocytosis of microorganisms and extravascular inflammatory response development	• Chemotherapy • Acute phase of bone marrow transplantation • Leukemia • Aplastic anaemia • Radiation • Secondary autoimmune neutropenia • Steroids	Bacterial • *Escherichia coli* • Staphylococcus • Pseudomonas • Klebsiella • Enterobacter • Legionella Fungal • Aspergillus • Mucormycosis
T-lymphocyte	Impaired-cell mediated immunity against obligate intracellular organisms and commensal organisms	• HIV • Lymphoma • Subacute/chronic phase of solid organ or marrow transplantation • Steroids • Chronic renal failure • Chemotherapy • Radiation	Fungal • Aspergillus • Pneumocystis • Cryptococcus Viral • CMV • HSV • HHV-6 • RSV Mycobacterial • *Mycobacterium tuberculosis* • Atypical mycobacteria Bacterial • Legionella • Nocardia • Protozoal • Toxoplasma
B-lymphocyte	Impaired antibody production and hence humoral response system	• Multiple myeloma • Leukemia • Lymphoma • Bone marrow transplantation • Chemotherapy	Bacterial • *Streptococcus pneumoniae* • *Haemophilus influenzae* • *E. coli* • Staphylococcus • Pseudomonas • Klebsiella Viral • RSV • HSV • CMV
Asplenia	Impaired humoral response, with increased susceptibility to encapsulated organisms	• Splenectomy	Bacterial • *S. pneumoniae* • *H. influenzae*

Abbreviations: CMV, cytomegalovirus; HHV-6, human herpes virus-6; HSV, herpes simplex virus; RSV, respiratory syncytial virus.

[AQ1]

($<$500 cells/mm^3). Semi-invasive aspergillosis, an intermediate form of disease, is not usually a clinical or radiological consideration as it occurs in a different subset of patients who are only mildly immune-compromised (23,24).

Patients with IPA typically present with fever, chest pain, cough, and dyspnea. The presence of concomitant sinusitis indicative of mucosal disruption increases the likelihood of aspergillus infection. Unlike viral infections, hemoptysis is not uncommon.

Typically, IPA results in small nodules or ill-defined early air-space opacities on CXR that progress to cavitation, particularly as the neutrophil count recovers. Pneumothoraces are not uncommon. HRCT imaging demonstrates disease at an earlier stage (25–27). Typical presentation features are of focal, solid, ill-defined nodules, usually greater than 1 cm in size that are surrounded by ground glass-opacity. This so-called "halo" appearance reflects hemorrhage from fungal angioinvasive infarction. Approximately two weeks later, the developing nodule may then develop early cavitation, the "air-crescent" sign (25,26,28,29). This "air-crescent" is also visible on CXR in upto 50% of cases (30) (Fig. 59.6). The development of the "air-crescent" sign or frank cavitation is associated with neutrophil recovery and is, therefore, an encouraging finding associated with improved survival (31–33). However, it must be noted

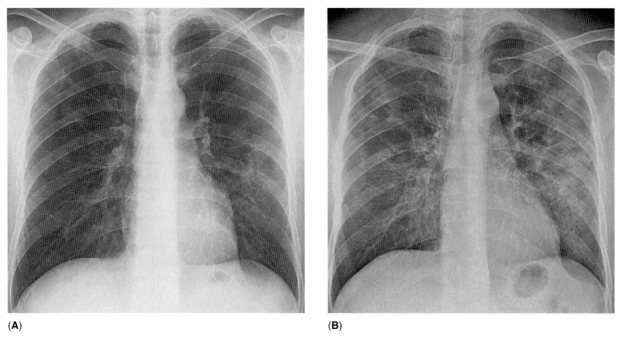

(A)   (B)

Figure 59.1 Early PCP infection in a dyspneic 34-year-old male patient with initial HIV presentation. (A) The CXR shows very subtle "ground-glass" bilateral perihilar air-space opacity resulting in loss of clarity of the underlying pulmonary vasculature. The diagnosis was confirmed by bronchoscopic lavage fluid examination. The findings on the CXR lag clinical presentation. (B) More prominent bilateral air-space opacity is present seven days later despite treatment initiation.

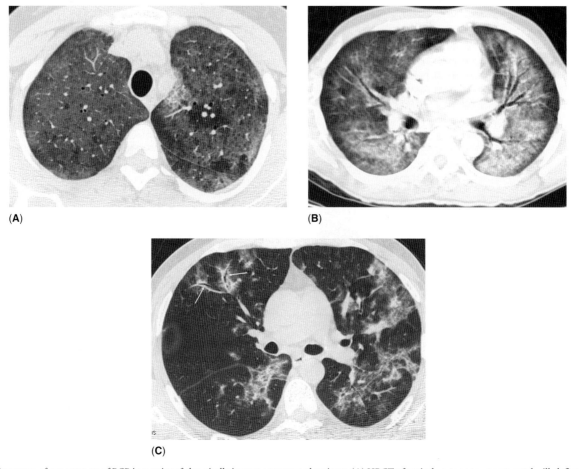

(A)   (B)

(C)

Figure 59.2 Spectrum of appearances of PCP in a series of chronically immunosuppressed patients. (A) HRCT of typical acute appearances, patchy ill-defined upper and mid-lung predominant ground-glass opacity. (B) In severe infection the ground-glass disease becomes confluent diffuse and a denser consolidative abnormality. Typically, as seen here, the subpleural lung is spared. (C) As the PCP infection resolves in the subacute phase the abnormality may become more reticular with retractile change and small residual peribronchial opacities with mild tractional dilatation of bronchi (arrows).

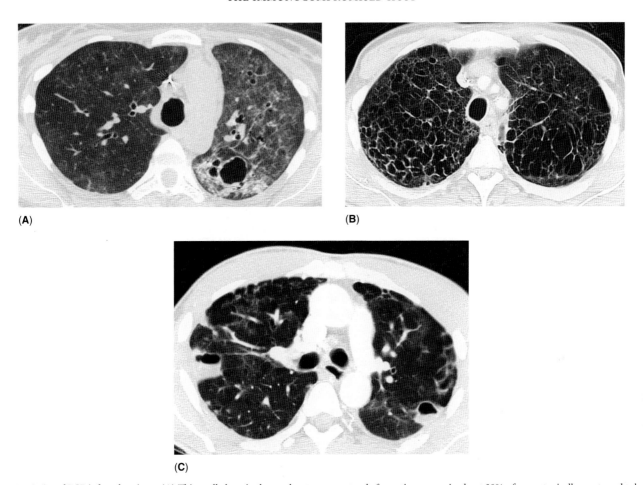

(A)

(B)

(C)

Figure 59.3 Series of PCP infected patients. (A) Thin-walled cystic change due to pneumatocele formation occurs in about 30% of cases, typically most resolve by 6 to 12 months. (B) Occasionally pneumatoceles can persist and become confluent mimicking confluent centrilobular emphysema. Note that compared to emphysema discrete walls are evident and there are no vessels coursing through the cystic spaces. (C) Occasionally pneumatoceles may become secondarily infected, as in this case, secondary to methicillin-resistant *Staphylococcus aureus*, resulting in air-fluid levels and thickened cyst walls.

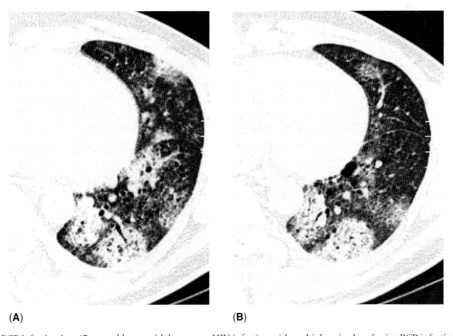

(A)

(B)

Figure 59.4 Granulomatoid PCP infection in a 47-year-old man with long-term HIV infection with multiple episodes of prior PCP infection and poor compliance with prophylaxis therapy. (A, B) The nodular ground glass and consolidative peribronchial appearances are typical of chronic granulomatoid pneumocystis infection. Background emphysema and chronic reticular change are also present. The diagnosis was confirmed by transbronchial biopsy to exclude fungal infection. Granulomas and evidence of PCP infection were evident without other organisms on stain or culture.

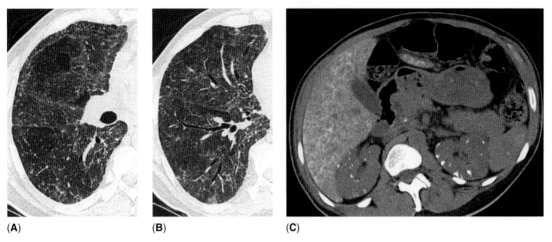

Figure 59.5 Chronic PCP infection with extranodal visceral calcification. (**A**, **B**) Target HRCT reconstructions of the right lung demonstrate diffuse patchy ground glass disease with a fine reticular pattern and small nodules. (**C**) There are peripheral renal calcifications but also a diffuse reticular hepatic and focal nodular splenic calcification. Since the widespread inception of PCP prophylaxis these appearances are rare unless, as in this case, there is poor PCP prophylaxis compliance.

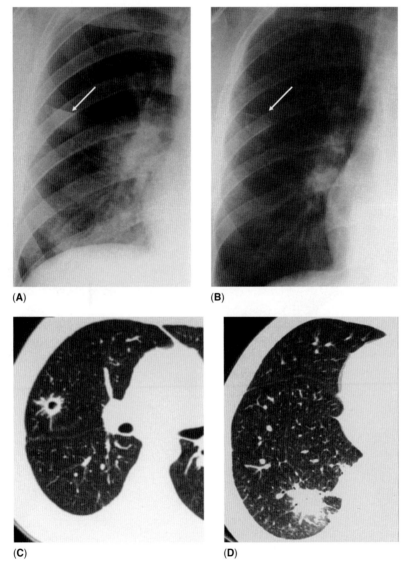

Figure 59.6 Invasive pulmonary aspergillosis. Acute myelogenous leukemia in a 34-year-old with severe neutropenia, fever, and cough. The initial film (**A**) demonstrates right perihilar air-space consolidation and a focal ill-defined nodule adjacent to the minor fissure (arrow). (**B**) 12 days later, an "air-crescent" has formed at the superior margin of the lesion (arrow). This feature is highly suggestive of invasive fungal disease. The lesion went on to frank cavitation seen on accompanying HRCT on day 14 (**C**). Note also the hemorrhagic ground glass surrounding the larger right lower lobe abnormality, (**D**) also reflecting invasive aspergillosis.

that frequently the air-crescent sign develops long after presumptive treatment is initiated or definitive diagnosis has already been established (32). This pattern of radiographic and CT evolution is, however, not unique to aspergillus species and has been described in less common fungal infections such as mucormycosis. However, in a series of 111 patients evaluated with HRCT, Escuissato et al. determined that nodules greater than 1 cm in size and a halo sign were significantly more common in fungal disease than other bacterial or viral infection (34) (Fig. 59.7).

In approximately 30% of patients, airway invasion occurs resulting in multiple peribronchial nodules or larger focal mass-like areas of air-space disease that may exceed 5 cm in size (35). In these patients "tree-in-bud" is not uncommon and more likely related to airways-invasive aspergillus disease than endobronchial mycobacterial disease (Fig. 59.8) (36). Sinuses to the airways are occasionally visible. Despite the extent of disease, hilar adenopathy and effusions are unusual in angioinvasive or airway invasive disease.

As IPA depends on profound neutropenia it is uncommon in HIV patients unless the marrow is suppressed (particularly by zidovudine) or the CD4 count is <50 cells/mm³. In this group of patients the radiographic appearances are comparable to non-HIV patients, although an additional infection of the central airways has also been described—obstructing bronchopulmonary aspergillosis (37,38). This may be difficult to differentiate from AIDS-related airway disease.

Key Features: Features of Invasive Aspergillosis

- Severe neutropenia: commonly lymphoproliferative disorders, chemotherapy or BMT induced
- HIV association unusual: consider CD4 <50, zidovudine marrow-suppression
- CXR: initial nodules; ill defined, air-crescent development in 50%; cavitation, pneumothorax
- HRCT: higher sensitivity, specificity, earlier diagnosis
  - Early: focal nodules, focal ground glass opacity
  - Angio-invasive disease: "halo" appearance, subsequent "air-crescent"; cavitation associated with neutropenic recovery and better survival
  - Airway-invasive disease: erosion into airways, centrilobular nodules, tree-in-bud, air-space opacification, rarely sinuses
  - HIV association: obstructing bronchopulmonary aspergillosis

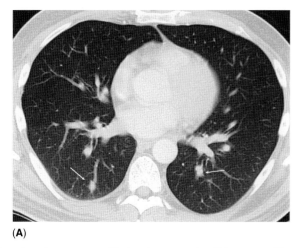

(A)

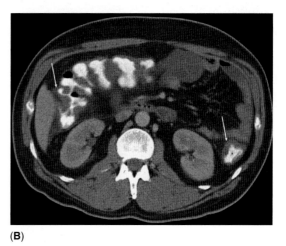

(B)

Figure 59.7 Invasive pulmonary aspergillosis and neutropenic colitis. 28-year-old presenting with lymphoma. Marked chemotherapy induced neutropenia and diarrhea. (A) Pulmonary basilar images of a CT examination demonstrate ill-defined nodules measuring more than 1 cm and highly suggestive of fungal infection (arrows). (B) Diffuse bowel edema is present (arrows), most marked in the hepatic flexure, consistent with neutropenic infectious colitis.

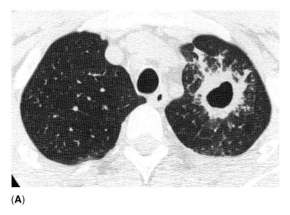

(A)

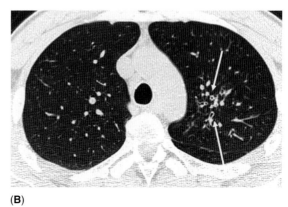

(B)

Figure 59.8 Invasive pulmonary aspergillosis in AIDS. (A) HIV-infected patient with a CD4 count of 60 cells/mm³. IPA is unusual in HIV unless the CD4 count is severely depressed, usually <50 cells/mm³. Cavitation has occurred in the left upper lobe which demonstrates a "halo" of peripheral ground glass. More inferiorly (B) the airways are asymmetrically thickened with regard to the right side with small clustered centrilobular nodules (arrows) consistent with airway invasive aspergillosis.

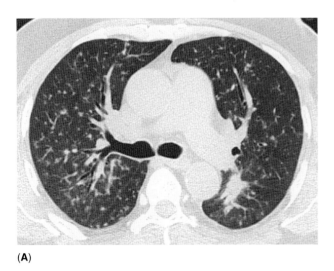

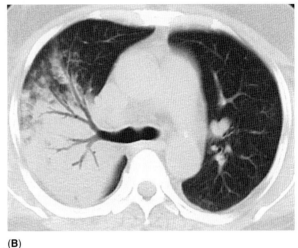

(A) **(B)**

Figure 59.9 Miliary histoplasmosis and *Streptococcus pneumoniae*. Forty-five-year-old immunosuppressed renal transplant recipient with fever under investigation for post-transplant lymphoproliferative disorder. (**A**) Multiple randomly distributed micronodules are present consistent with miliary infection. Larger focal irregular nodular density in left lower lobe. Transbronchial biopsy confirmed miliary histoplasmosis. (**B**) Six months later following treatment the same patient presented with lobar pneumonia due to *S. pneumoniae*, reflecting the wide range of infectious susceptibility in the ICH.

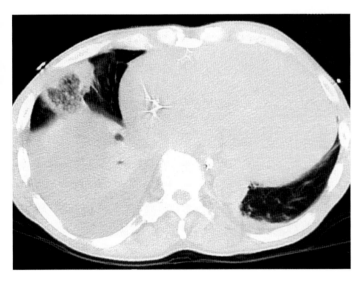

Figure 59.10 Mucormycosis infection in a chronically immunosuppressed renal transplant recipient. The lesion demonstrates a peripheral rind of consolidation with central ground glass. This appearance is variably described as a "reverse halo," "atoll," or "bird's nest" sign. Similar appearances could reflect infarction or organizing pneumonia.

Other Fungal Infections

Other rarer fungal infections may also occasionally occur in the immunocompromised host depending on the level of immunosuppression at presentation and whether the infection is due to primary exposure or re-activation. Some fungi such as histoplasmosis may present as miliary nodules identical to tuberculosis (Fig. 59.9), others such as mucormycosis as large masses or evolving cavities indistinguishable from aspergillosis (Fig. 59.10). Cryptococcosis may have an appearance that resembles either of these appearances but, most typically, results in mass-like consolidation (Fig. 59.11). The diagnosis of these rarer infections frequently requires a combination of serology, transbronchial and percutaneous biopsy, and empiric therapy.

Bacterial Infection

The immunocompromised host (ICH) is predisposed to a variety of bacterial infections throughout their period of immunosuppression.

The particular susceptibility will depend on the level and type of immunosuppression at the time of presentation (39). In most cases the radiological appearances of infection by different bacterial organisms are comparable to those of infection in non-immune compromised hosts. The majority, therefore, present with non-specific focal air-space disease (Fig. 59.12) or nodular ill-defined opacities (Fig. 59.13). Compared to immune-competent hosts, infections in the ICH are more likely to be multifocal or associated with cavitation (Figs. 59.14 and 59.15) (40,41). In addition to common bacterial infections, unusual bacterial species are also more common in the ICH (Figs. 59.16 and 59.17). For example, infection with Nocardia, Rhodococcus, and some legionella species are unusual in immune-competent individuals. Bartonella infection contracted from cats and cats' lice and fleas results in bacillary angiomatosis in AIDS patients. The infection may mimic Kaposi's sarcoma with pulmonary nodules, endobronchial lesions, enhancing mediastinal and

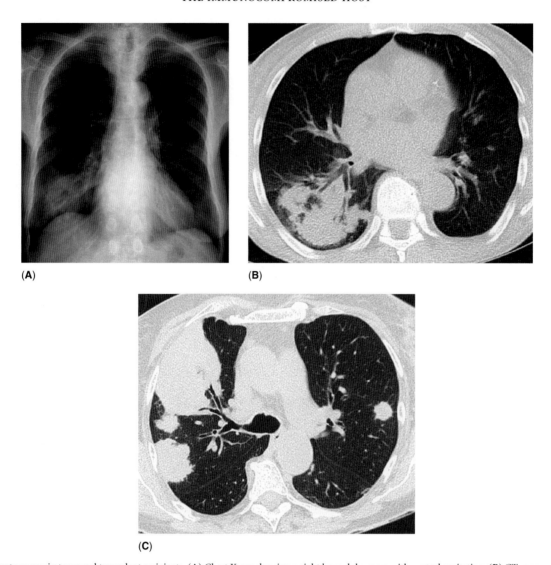

(A)　　　　　　**(B)**

(C)

Figure 59.11 Cryptococcus in two renal transplant recipients. (**A**) Chest X-ray showing a right lower lobe mass with central cavitation. (**B**) CT: mass appears as densely consolidated lung with nodular margins corresponding to acinar filling. The absence of ground glass helps to divert away from a diagnosis of aspergillus infection. (**C**) Cryptococcus infection in a separate patient demonstrates mass-like opacities initially thought to reflect PTLD due to their mass-like density. Diagnosis in both cases was confirmed by bronchoscopy performed to exclude post-transplant lymphoproliferative disorder.

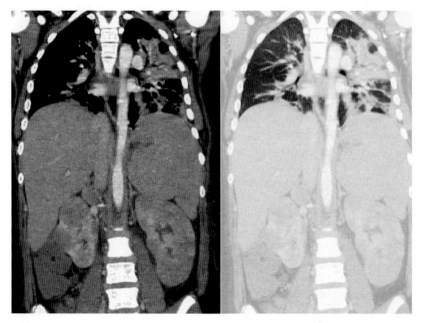

Figure 59.12 Presumed multifocal bacterial pneumonia in an eight-year-old girl with diffuse infiltrative pre-B ALL. Lobar and segmental consolidative pattern. The patient's fever and dyspnea rapidly improved following a standard community-acquired infection antibiotic regimen. Note the leukemic renal infiltration. The precise organism is often not isolated as antibiotic therapy is started early following imaging demonstration of infection.

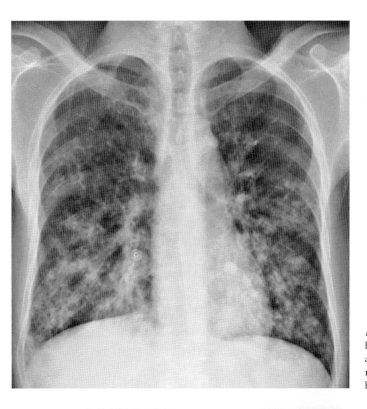

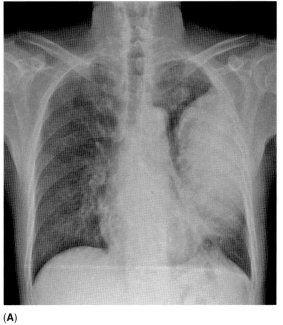

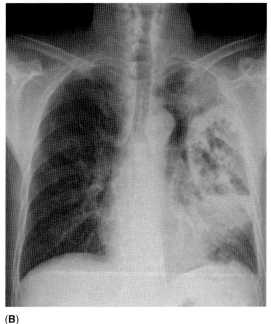

Figure 59.13 AIDS-related airway disease. Recurrent airway infection presents as a bronchopneumonic pattern with peribronchial nodular consolidation. Appearances in this case were due to recurrent *Streptococcus pneumoniae* infection, a common causative organism along with recurrent PCP that ultimately may result in bronchiectatic chronic airway inflammation.

(A)
(B)

Figure 59.14 CLL and bacterial infection. (A) sixty-four-year-old patient with immunosuppression secondary to CLL developed expansile left upper lobe pneumonia with (B) later cavitation at seven days. Blood cultures grew penicillin-sensitive *Streptococcus pneumoniae*. Multifocal or cavitary *S. pneumoniae* infection is occasionally present in immune-competent individuals. However, these features are more commonly seen in the ICH.

hilar nodes, and pleural effusions (42,43). Infections in the ICH may also demonstrate involvement of unusual thoracic locations such as the trachea and chest wall (Figs. 59.16 and 59.17).

In patients with neutropenic bacterial sepsis, the radiographic appearances of pulmonary airspace disease may be significantly less dense than that of a non-neutropenic host and may be more delayed in development (44,45). Evaluation by HRCT significantly increases the sensitivity for detection of infection and may detect ground glass or consolidative opacity earlier in up to 60% of

patients with a clinical suspicion of infection but a normal CXR (44,46,47). In this neutropenic patient subset pleural effusions and empyema are less common.

Septic Emboli
Both septic emboli and secondarily infected pulmonary emboli are not infrequent in immunocompromised individuals, particularly in HIV-infected patients with HIV contracted through IV drug abuse (Fig. 59.18). The radiographic and CT appearances of

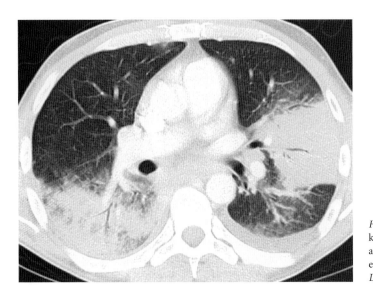

Figure 59.15 CLL and bacterial infection. Seventy-one-year-old patient with known CLL and immunosuppression presented with dyspnea, fever, headache, and systemic malaise. CT confirmed multifocal consolidation with a small left effusion. Subcarinal adenopathy was previously present. Cultures confirmed *Legionella pneumophila*.

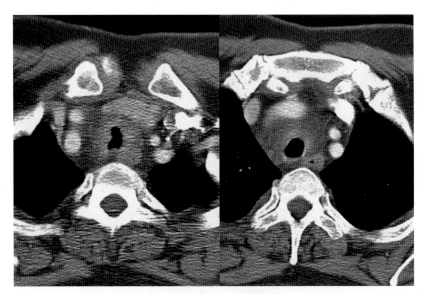

Figure 59.16 Acute bacterial tracheitis. Twenty-four-year-old male patient with nasopharyngeal midline Natural Killer cell lymphoma recently treated aggressively with chemotherapy and now profoundly pancytopenic with stridor. CT examination shows circumferential ill-defined thickening of the trachea. The margins are ill-defined and the mediastinal fat is edematous, differentiating this from the far more unusual occurrence of primary tracheal lymphoma. The findings responded within one week to systemic antibiotic therapy. However, the patient died within a month due to a combination of later systemic sepsis and disease progression.

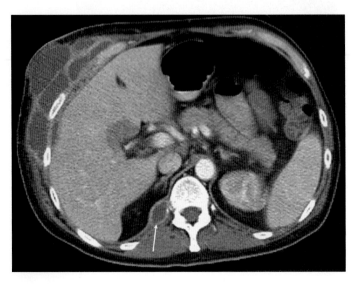

Figure 59.17 Fifty-three-year-old with HIV and *Nocardia* infection. The infection likely originated in the thorax and subsequently extended through fascial planes to the pleura, diaphragm, and chest wall. Multilocular fluid collection with wall enhancement extends through fascial planes to involve the right anterior chest and abdominal wall. Posteriorly (arrow) the right diaphragmatic crus is separately involved. *Source*: Courtesy of Dr. M. Godoy, New York.

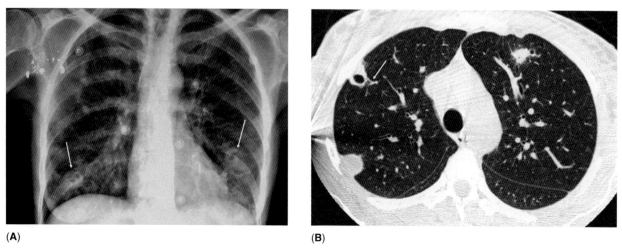

(A) **(B)**

Figure 59.18 Septic emboli. Thirty-eight-year-old female patient with HIV secondary to intravenous drug abuse. (**A**) Chest X-ray demonstrates multifocal ill-defined parenchymal nodular and consolidative opacities with suspected cavitation in the lower zones (arrows). Bullet fragments are present in the right axilla from a prior untoward incident. (**B**) HRCT images demonstrate multiple peripheral nodules, some in close relationship to vessels (arrow) indicating their hematogenous distribution. The nodules are in various phases of evolution, including ill-defined solid, well-defined cystic, and cavitary nodules.

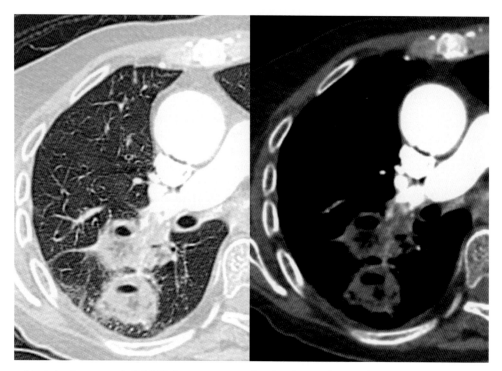

Figure 59.19 Pseudomonas-infected pulmonary emboli. Mildly immunosuppressed patient due to a history of abdominal malignancy. Chest X-ray (not shown) performed for fever and dyspnea demonstrated nodules suspicious for metastases. CT for staging confirms multiple air-fluid levels secondary to unsuspected pulmonary emboli in the right main pulmonary artery. Blood cultures grew *Pseudomonas aeruginosa*.

septic emboli include multiple peripheral pulmonary nodules of varying sizes (48). These are frequently basilar and in close proximity to the pleural surface or to small peripheral vessels indicating their hemotogenous distribution. The nodules may be either well defined or ill-defined and typically develop cavitation. In distinction to other neoplastic diseases such as metastatic squamous cell carcinoma, or other mycobacterial or fungal infections, the distribution of disease is predominantly basilar but also appears to be in different phases of evolution, reflecting that the nodules are the result of multiple phases of pulmonary embolization (49–51).

Pulmonary embolism is also relatively common in patients with neoplasia (52,53). Up to 10% of routine enhanced CT studies may demonstrate incidental pulmonary emboli and the detected incidence may be higher with MDCT systems capable of routine acquisition at 1 mm collimation (54,55). Larger pulmonary emboli may result in infarction and may become secondarily infected. This appearance is most common in patients who are immune-compromised. Pulmonary infarcts most typically present as peripheral areas of ground glass or consolidative opacity, occasionally wedge-shaped in appearance. In contrast to air-space opacity due to infection, air-bronchograms are absent with a more mottled appearance of the lung parenchyma. In ICH with infected emboli cavitary appearances are common, but are an uncommon appearance for sterile infarcts (Fig. 59.19).

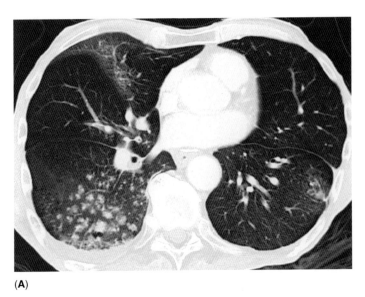

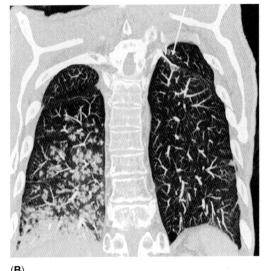

(A)　　　　　　　　　　　　　　　　　　　　　　　　　　**(B)**

Figure 59.20 Prior lung cancer—endobronchial tuberculosis. Seventy-six-year-old with left upper lobe wedge resection for lung cancer 18 months prior, presented with indolent chronic malaise and weight loss thought to be due to poor operative recovery or subclinical recurrent disease. (A) HRCT demonstrates ill-defined acinar nodular consolidation and tree-in-bud opacity consistent with infectious bronchiolitis. The extent of endobronchial disease is better demonstrated on (B) the coronal MIP rendering. Note wedge sutures in the left apex (arrow). Cultures confirmed tuberculosis. Cancer immunosuppressed patients are not particularly susceptible to tuberculosis. However, lung cancer patients are perhaps more so due to immunosuppression related to elderly state, prior smoking, and operative history.

Key Points: Bacterial Infection in the ICH

- Radiographic appearance comparable to non-ICH, although multifocal and cavitary disease are more common
- Neutropenic patients may have delayed and less dense parenchymal opacity
- Pleural disease is unusual
- Septic emboli and secondary infection of pulmonary emboli are common
- Unusual infections may resemble malignancy, for example, bacillary angiomatosis

Mycobacterial Disease

Both *Mycobacterium tuberculosis* infection and atypical mycobacterial infection are uncommon in the ICH other than in the context of HIV. In non-HIV patients the presentation is comparable to non-immune compromised hosts with a typical post-primary disease appearance due to reactivation of prior disease (Fig. 59.20).

In HIV infection active *M. tuberculosis* is more common than in the background population. The disease may reflect reactivation disease or primary infection. Most typically the radiographic appearances are of the latter characterized by parenchymal air-space disease and marked nodal enlargement (Fig. 59.21). However, a combination of primary disease, progressive or post-primary disease is common. Miliary infection may also be present (Fig. 59.22) (56). CT may demonstrate endobronchial disease characterized by centrilobular nodules and tree-in-bud opacity. More fulminant disease demonstrates widespread air-space consolidation (57). At CT, associated large mediastinal and hilar nodes frequently demonstrate peripheral enhancement and low-density centers (58). Patients with CD4 counts >200 cells/mm³ tend to present with appearances more suggestive of post-primary disease; lower CD4 counts result in more atypical

appearances overall more suggestive of primary disease (59). Paradoxically, as the CD4 count falls, cavitation becomes less frequent and even normal CXR appearances are reported (59). Radiological diagnosis of *M. tuberculosis* is particularly important in these patients as skin-mediated tests of infection and acid-fast analysis of bronchoalveolar lavage (BAL) and sputum fluid are falsely negative in at least 50% of HIV patients with culture proven *M. tuberculosis* (60–62).

Non-tuberculous "atypical" mycobacterial disease is not particularly common in HIV patients (58). The most common organism, *Mycobacterium avium*-intracellulare complex (MAC) is commonly isolated to the thorax in immune-compromised hosts; however, gastrointestinal and abdominal visceral infection is more common in HIV infection (63). *Mycobacterium abscessus* and *Mycobacterium kansasii* may occur in the thorax but are less common overall (64,65).

Key Points: Mycobacterial Disease in ICH

Non-HIV infection:
- *M. tuberculosis* unusual, usually post-primary disease
HIV patients:
- *M. tuberculosis* common, usually primary disease
- Progressive primary, post-primary, and miliary disease also common
- Lower CD4 counts result in more atypical appearances
- Tuberculin, and acid-fast evaluation false negative in >50%
- Atypical mycobacteria not common

Viral Infection

Cytomegalovirus

The most common viral pneumonia in immune-compromised individuals is due to cytomegalovirus (CMV). Latent CMV

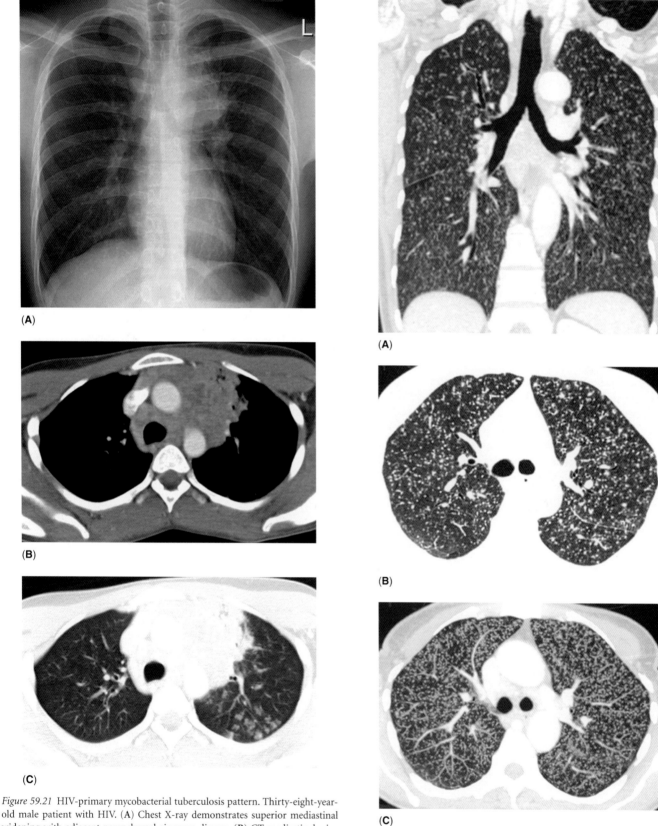

Figure 59.21 HIV-primary mycobacterial tuberculosis pattern. Thirty-eight-year-old male patient with HIV. (A) Chest X-ray demonstrates superior mediastinal widening with adjacent parenchymal air-space disease. (B) CT mediastinal windows confirm extensive adenopathy with central low attenuation centers and peripheral enhancement. (C) Lung windows demonstrate contiguity with parenchymal consolidation with areas of parenchymal acinar consolidation and tree-in-bud opacity posteriorly. The primary pattern of disease in this patient likely reflects the low CD4 count (160 cells/mm³).

Figure 59.22 HIV and miliary TB. Forty-two-year-old patient with HIV and CD4 count of 260 cells/mm³. (A) Coronal HRCT MPR from MDCT dataset. Innumerable small nodules are present. Both this and (B) the axial HRCT image confirm a random distribution of micronodules contacting the pleural and fissural surfaces. A slight basilar predominance as in this case is common. (C) The extent of disease is further demonstrated by a 3 mm thin MIP image.

infection is common and as the infection frequently co-exists with other opportunistic infections such as PCP, it is not always clinically clear whether CMV is clinically pathogenically significant. This poses a clinical problem as pathogenic CMV has a very high mortality in the ICH. Only small series describe the isolated appearances of CMV. In one series, solitary or multiple pulmonary nodules of varying size were the commonest feature in 57% (66). In other studies diffuse air-space opacification was common (67,68). However, it is likely that earlier infection may present with mild interstitial shadowing or a normal CXR. At HRCT these earlier appearances appear as ground glass opacities with innumerable small, centrilobular, ground glass nodules (Fig. 59.23). With time, more consolidative opacity and features of mild organization with interlobular septal thickening, reticular density and early tractional change develop. These organizational appearances are common in CMV as well as other atypical or viral infections. Additionally, these appearances may be similar to edema or in particular to drug-toxicity, which is an important differential diagnosis.

Key Points: CMV Infection in ICH

- Common in both HIV and transplant recipients
- Frequent co-existence with PCP
- Frequently latent, high mortality when pathogenic
- CXR—nodules or airspace disease
- HRCT—small centrilobular nodules, ground glass, tending to confluence, and reticular organization
- Appearances of other viral infections, edema, or drug toxicity may be similar

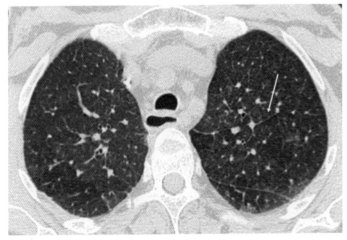

Figure 59.23 CMV pneumonia. Breast cancer patient with dyspnea and cough following right mastectomy and gemcitabine chemotherapy commencement 12 days earlier. Representative HRCT image demonstrates subtle patchy ground glass opacity and centrilobular nodularity. There is mild interlobular septal thickening most notable in the left upper lobe (arrow). These appearances while typical of early viral infection are not radiologically diagnostic. The leading diagnoses to be considered include edema, chemotoxicity, and viral infection. CMV was confirmed at bronchoscopy.

IMAGING THE IMMUNE COMPROMISED HOST: INTERPRETIVE CONSIDERATIONS

The imaging of the ICH with infection is particularly complex due to the multiple potential pathologies that may have similar clinical and overlapping radiological presentation. As indicated above, the mechanism of immunosuppression may indicate particular susceptibilities to infection, narrowing the differential. In certain conditions such as HIV infection, this infective predisposition will vary according to the severity of immunosuppression, expressed as the CD4 count. Even within a single patient, however, multiple co-existing infective pathologies may complicate the interpretative task. There are, however, additionally several other non-infective pathological processes that may mimic the clinical presentation or imaging findings of infection that should be considered when imaging the ICH.

Many immune-compromised patients are cancer patients; immune-compromised either by the disease process itself or the treatment for the cancer. Therefore, progressive primary disease, disease recurrence or metastatic disease should always be considered.

Chronically immunosuppressed patients due to primary immunosuppressive disease without cancer are also predisposed to the development of a new malignancy. The two main instances of these are in HIV infection and chronic iatrogenic immunosuppression for transplantation. In thoracic imaging of these patients the key determination is to differentiate findings of neoplastic disease from immunosuppressive infection or therapy complications. Integral to this assessment is the immunosuppressive impact of any new lymphoproliferative disorder or any further immune modulation induced by treatment for the immunosuppression-associated malignancy.

In HIV infection, imaging is particularly complex as both AIDS-defining cancer diagnoses, such as Kaposi's sarcoma and non-Hodgkin's lymphoma, primarily occur in the thorax, but there may also be metastatic disease from many non-AIDS-defining malignancies more common in HIV. Knowledge of the particular risks of these patients to primary, metastatic, or recurrent disease aids interpretation. The utilization of highly active antiretroviral therapy (HAART) for HIV may be a further complicating factor. This treatment significantly reduces the viral load and partially restores the inflammatory response to infection. This partial immune reconstitution syndrome (IRS) may result in a flare-up of subclinical infective disease appearances, with worsening parenchymal disease, effusions, and significant nodal enlargement that may simulate malignant disease (Fig. 59.24).

Diffuse pulmonary ground glass or consolidative opacity in radiation pneumonitis may mimic bacterial or PCP infection. The appearances occur six weeks to six months following irradiation and may be potentiated by chemotherapy (Fig. 59.25). With time, the margins of the pneumonitis become more sharply demarcated, aiding interpretation. Interestingly, there is anecdotal evidence to suggest radiation therapy may have a protective effect on PCP infection.

The development of chemotherapeutic agent toxicity is not uncommon and may frequently mimic opportunistic infection. There are many different mechanisms for the development of drug toxicity including diffuse alveolar damage, hypersensitivity, usual or non-specific interstitial pneumonitis, eosinophilia, organizing

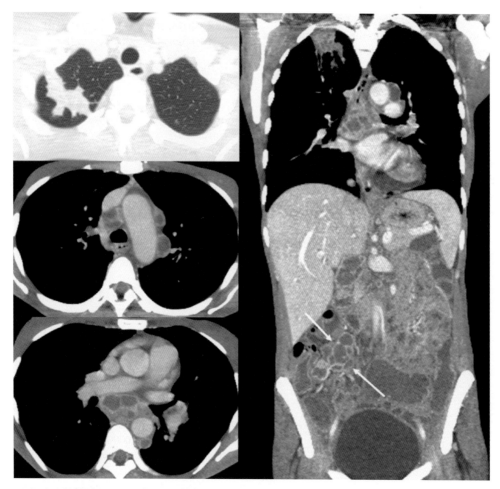

Figure 59.24 Immune reconstitution and TB. Twenty-eight-year-old female HIV patient with fever and weight loss three weeks following initiation of HAART therapy. Previous chest X-ray two months earlier (not shown) was unremarkable. Current axial CT images demonstrate right upper lobe consolidation and extensive rim-enhancing, centrally necrotic, mediastinal, and hilar lymph nodes consistent with TB. The off-axis coronal MPR demonstrates the parenchymal consolidation and multiple mesenteric nodes in the abdomen (arrows) demonstrate similar characteristics. These features are due to a flare-up of subclinical TB by the partially reconstituted immune system following HAART therapy and can be confusing in HIV patients with suspected malignancy.

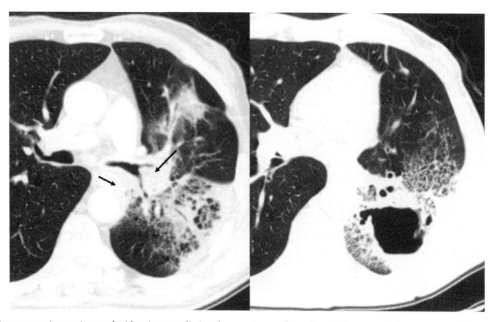

Figure 59.25 Left hilar lung cancer (arrows) treated with primary radiation therapy six months earlier. Diffuse ground glass appearance is secondary to radiation pneumonitis. The central cavity is sterile; an unusual complication of radiation pneumonitis. Both post-radiation and chemotherapy appearances can be confused with opportunistic infection in an ICH. In this case appearances were improving from prior imaging.

pneumonia, and fibrosis (Figs. 59.26 and 59.27). Knowledge of the mechanism, distribution and timelines for the development of pulmonary manifestations of chemotherapy toxicity aids in the differentiation from cancer progression or infection. For example, drug toxicity is common in breast cancer BMT recipients and in patients receiving gemcitabine or paclitaxel therapies, described in up to 30% of patients. These complications typically occur following the first or second dose and usually in the second week of treatment, with similar clinical symptoms to infection (69).

Bone marrow transplant recipients and solid organ transplant recipients are susceptible to a unique distribution of infectious and non-infectious complications, and are discussed in the next section of this chapter.

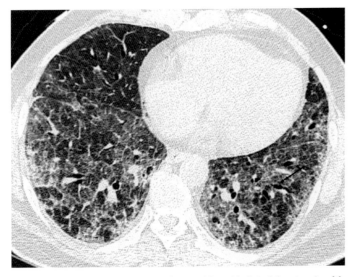

Figure 59.26 Bleomycin toxicity. Lymphoma with rapid clinical deterioration following bleomycin therapy. HRCT imaging demonstrates bilateral ground glass opacity with reticular change and mild tractional airway change (arrow) suggestive of organizational mild fibrosis. Open lung biopsy confirmed diffuse alveolar damage due to bleomycin resulting in ARDS-like HRCT appearances. Radiologically these appearances resemble subacute PCP, an important differential in this population. Bleomycin may also cause peripheral pneumonitis.

Key Points: Imaging Considerations in Immunosuppression

Differentiate imaging appearances due to:
Neoplasia:
- Progressive primary, metastatic, or recurrent disease
- Immunosuppression-induced malignancy
Infection:
- Opportunistic infection
  □ secondary to HIV, transplantation immunosuppression
  □ secondary to marrow suppression by cancer
  □ secondary to marrow suppression by treatment
- Bacterial or Mycobacterial infection
Drug effects:
- Chemotherapeutic toxicity
- Immune reconstitution syndrome in HIV treated with HAART
- Specific complications of bone marrow transplantation

COMPLICATIONS OF TRANSPLANTATION

Bone Marrow Transplantation

Bone marrow transplantation (BMT) is a common therapy utilized not only for a wide variety of hematological and solid neoplastic etiologies but also for several non-neoplastic hematological, metabolic, and genetic conditions. Bone marrow may either be harvested from the patient themselves (autologous), from an HLA-matched donor (allogeneic), or purified to contain only stem cells (stem cell transplant) (Table 59.3). Autologous transplantation permits higher chemotherapeutic or radiation doses to be administered prior to re-introduction of the bone marrow. Allogeneic transplantation requires chemotherapy or radiation conditioning regimens to ablate the native marrow prior to infusion of the BMT. In both cases, compared to other cancer patients, the use of higher radiation or chemotherapeutic doses may result in increased pulmonary toxicity

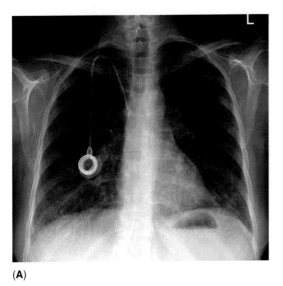

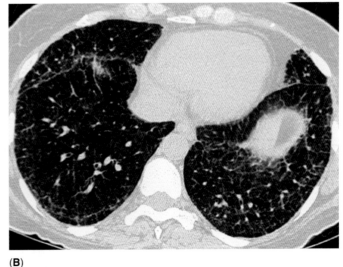

(A)   **(B)**

Figure 59.27 Methotrexate toxicity. Forty-three-year-old patient with breast cancer treated by indwelling central venous catheter. (A) Basilar increased interstitial reticular markings are present on chest X-ray. (B). At HRCT, peripheral subpleural basilar ground glass and reticular densities are present. This peripheral distribution is typical in methotrexate toxicity and common in many other chemotoxicities, and should help differentiate from opportunistic infection.

Table 59.3 Differences Between Autologous and Allogeneic Transplant Complications

Disease	Autologous and stem cell	Allogeneic
Infectious		
Bacterial	+++	+++
Fungi	+++	+++
Pneumocystis jiroveci	++	+++
Cytomegalovirus and other viruses	+	+++
Non-infectious		
Pulmonary edema	+++	+++
Diffuse alveolar hemorrhage	++	++
Idiopathic pneumonia syndrome	+	+++
Bronchiolitis obliterans	+	+++
Impaired pulmonary function tests	++	+++
Graft-versus-host disease	Rare	+++

Source: Adapted from Ref. 72.

themselves or immunosuppressive sequelae. BMT itself is also associated with a unique spectrum of pulmonary complications, many of which have immune-mediated mechanisms (70,71).

Pulmonary complications are divided into infectious or non-infectious, and occur in 40% to 60% of patients resulting in significant morbidity and mortality (72,73). In children, pulmonary complications as a cause of death (9%) are second only to disease progression (74). At autopsy, pulmonary complications are the sole or contributory cause of death in three quarters of cases (75).

Pulmonary complications are dependent on the type and duration of immunosuppression induced by the disease itself, its treatment, the BMT conditioning regime, and the possible development of graft versus host disease (GVHD). The frequency of these complications also varies according to the type of BMT (36,70,72). Although infection remains a major cause of death in these patients, infection morbidity and mortality varies significantly according to age, the original disease, and BMT modality. Recently, a very low infectious mortality (2%) has been described for stem cell transplants in breast cancer patients (76).

BMT complications are divided into early (less than 100 days from transplantation) or late (greater than 100 days). This chronological division, although arbitrary, reflects the different types of complications that are pre-eminent during these periods (35,77). These different susceptibilities reflect the varying immunological deficits: during the first two to three weeks, the "engraftment period," BMT recipients are pancytopenic. Infections suffered relate to profound neutropenia and moderate lymphopenia. This deficit takes approximately one month to recover and is more profound in allogeneic BMT. Total immune function gradually improves over the remainder of the first year (77,78).

Early Non-infectious Complications
Pulmonary Edema
Pulmonary edema is relatively common in the early period, usually in the second to third week post-BMT. Edema may be due to cardiogenic or non-cardiogenic causes or a combination of both (72,79). The clinical and radiological manifestations are comparable to those of pulmonary edema in patients without prior BMT. Cardiogenic edema is possibly contributed to by cardiac or renal chemotoxicity from

chemotherapeutic or immunosuppressive toxicity, particularly doxorubicin (adriamycin), cyclophosphamide, cisplatin, or cyclosporine. Fluid overload may also result due to attempted reduction of toxicity by fluid dilution of administered toxic chemotherapies, antibiotics, total parenteral nutrition, or blood products. Non-cardiogenic edema is precipitated by increased capillary permeability, which may be due to the use of cyclophosphamide or total body irradiation used as part of a conditioning regime or subsequent infection (72,77).

Idiopathic Pneumonia Syndrome
Idiopathic pneumonia syndrome (IPS) is defined as an acute lung injury following BMT for which no infectious etiology is identified (70,72,77,79). This complication occurs in about 12% of cases throughout the first 100 days following BMT (80). Pathologically it is likely to be secondary to an interstitial mononuclear cell infiltrate associated with diffuse alveolar damage. It is more common in patients with a poor performance status before BMT, high-dose total body irradiation, and the presence of GVHD. The severity of IPS is reduced in patients who are receiving cyclosporine or immunoglobulin prophylaxis for GVHD, suggesting an immune basis for the disease (81). The mortality of IPS exceeds 70%; however, only about one-third die of progressive respiratory failure, the remainder die from recurrent IPS or infections that may occur despite an initial improvement of IPS in up to 44% of patients (72,75,82).

The radiographic and CT features of IPS are similar to ARDS with multilobar airspace opacity that may become more reticular or fibrotic with time. The radiological appearances also form part of the diagnostic criteria that include the imaging features, the clinical features of a pneumonia (dyspnea, fever, non-productive cough, hypoxia) but without infective organism identified on at least two separate bronchoalveolar lavage (BAL) specimen (70,72). Pneumomediastinum is not infrequently associated with IPS, particularly in those receiving high doses of conditioning radiation, but rarely requires management (72,79).

Diffuse Alveolar Hemorrhage
Diffuse alveolar hemorrhage (DAH) occurs in up to 21% of patients, peaking in incidence at two weeks post-BMT (72,74,75,77,79). The incidence is higher in older patients, patients with solid tumors, and in patients treated with total body irradiation. The incidence is particularly high in those in whom there is pre-existing airway inflammation as the pathological process is suspected to result from an influx of neutrophils into the lung parenchyma (72,79). The clinical presentation is similar to that of IPS. Notably, however, hemoptysis is uncommon and there are no detectable coagulation abnormalities (72).

Radiographically the presentation is of multifocal parenchymal consolidation although the initial appearance is frequently of non-specific interstitial shadowing (83). At HRCT, lobular ground glass opacification is demonstrated, sometimes associated with reticular interlobular and intralobular septae as the hemorrhage becomes more organized. The appearances appear more consolidative in the dependent portions of the lung parenchyma (Fig. 59.28). Diagnosis is confirmed by BAL which reveals progressively more blood stained specimens. Determination of the specific diagnosis is important because the untreated mortality exceeds 50% but, unlike IPS, DAH can be successfully treated with high-dose steroids (74,79).

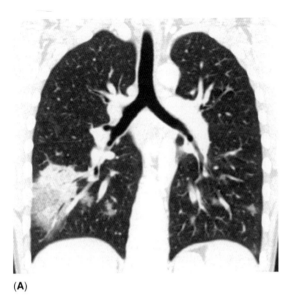
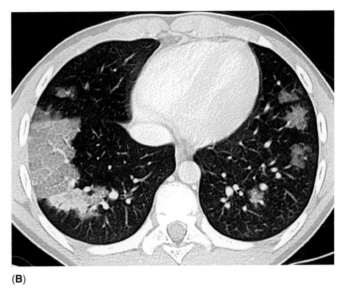

(A) (B)

Figure 59.28 BMT with diffuse alveolar hemorrhage. Adolescent patient treated for leukemia with allogeneic bone marrow transplant. (A) Coronal MPR and (B) axial CT images. Typical appearances of patchy parenchymal ground-glass with prominence of the intralobular septae are demonstrated resulting in a "crazy-paving" appearance. More consolidative opacity is also present. Unusually the patient presented with hemoptysis which paradoxically is not a common feature. However, this presentation differentiated these appearances from secondary alveolar proteinosis which may appear similar.

Key Points: Early Non-infectious Complications of BMT

- Edema, DAH, IPS, and drug toxicity are common and frequently immune-mediated
- All are more common with stronger conditioning chemotherapy or total body irradiation
- All may present with diffuse airspace abnormality at CXR or CT
- IPS requires exclusion of infection by BAL on at least two occasions
- DAH typically demonstrates patchy dependent ground-glass and possible "crazy-paving" at HRCT; hemoptysis is uncommon
- Unlike IPS, DAH is steroid-responsive

Early Infectious Complications
Bacterial Infections

Bacterial infections are most common during the first two weeks following BMT when the patient is neutropenic prior to marrow grafting (72,77). Rates of infection as high as 75% have been reported, although the incidence and severity of these have significantly reduced due to the introduction of prophylactic antibiotics (84–87). The organisms most responsible are gram negative organisms from the GI tract or oral mucosal surfaces. The use of central IV catheters also predisposes to gram-positive staphylococcal and streptococcal infections. Pain management with opiates predisposes to aspiration of anaerobes and gram-negative bacteria. Outbreaks of atypical infections such as *Legionella pneumophila* disease have also been described with high mortality in BMT recipients (72,77,88). The radiological appearances are as described above for other immune-compromised hosts.

Viral Infections

Multiple different viral agents are responsible for infection during the early post-BMT period. These include cytomegalovirus (CMV), herpes simplex virus (HSV), human herpes virus-6

(HHV-6), respiratory syncytial virus (RSV), and parainfluenza virus (72). Of these the most virulent associated with mortality rates reported to be as high as 85% is CMV (72,77). Seronegative CMV patients may contract CMV from a seropositive BMT and, therefore, this is eliminated by restricting seronegative BMT to seronegative recipients (87). The vast majority of CMV infection, therefore, is the result of reactivation of latent CMV in seropositive patients who are profoundly immune compromised during BMT. The incidence of CMV pneumonia is approximately 15% and increased in the elderly and in those with GVHD or marked immunosuppression, particularly those who receive whole body irradiation. CMV infection typically peaks during the second half of the early post-BMT period (50–100 days) but can occur at any time during the first six months (72,89). Clinically, patients present with non-specific features including fever, dyspnea, non-productive cough, and hypoxemia. The diagnosis of CMV pneumonia is frequently confirmed by demonstrating typical macrophage inclusion bodies at BAL (84,90). However, although both CMV-positive BAL and detectable serum CMV viremia do not definitively imply CMV pneumonia, both are considered significant risk factors meriting treatment. The incidence and course of CMV pneumonia are influenced by the usage of prophylactic high-dose acyclovir and treatment by ganciclovir or human immunoglobulin. Despite these treatments relapse occurs in one-third of cases and if respiratory failure ensues death is likely (72).

HSV infection is the most common infection in BMT recipients but is usually limited to infection of the mucosal surfaces of the oral cavity. Pulmonary involvement is a rare but highly dangerous complication that occurs by direct extension into the bronchopulmonary tree and hence the lung parenchyma (72). This resembles the early stages of CMV infection, described above, but can become a more diffuse pneumonia in the presence of a marked viremia. HHV-6, RSV, and parainfluenza virus infection are less frequent pathogens in BMT patients presenting with fever and parenchymal ill-defined interstitial opacities representing pneumonitis.

Fungal Infections

Fungal infections are common and reported to occur in up to 45% of BMT recipients (72,77). Following the introduction of prophylaxis for bacterial infections and PCP, fungal disease and CMV pneumonia are now the commonest infection in BMT recipients (67,74). Typically, fungal infection occurs in the first 30 days after BMT when neutropenia is most marked. Although candidal infection is most likely the commonest cause of fungal infection overall, this is a rare cause of isolated pneumonia. Invasive Aspergillus infection accounts for 90% of pulmonary fungal infections, with involvement in up to 20% of patients (34,72). This is commoner in patients with prolonged neutropenia or prior steroid therapy (72,91). Fungal infection remains difficult to diagnose and, therefore, the use of antifungal agents is common in patients with persistent fever non-responsive to broad spectrum antibiotics (75). The untreated mortality of IPA in BMT recipients approaches 85%. Early radiological detection is imperative as the high mortality is likely in part due to delayed diagnosis and treatment implementation.

The incidence of PCP in patients with BMT since the advent of Septrin prophylaxis is currently less than 10%, usually in patients who could not receive prophylaxis or in those who have GVHD. Although the yield of BAL is thought to be over 90% in HIV this is much lower in BMT recipients, likely due to the lower overall PCP burden but also the interstitial location early in the course of disease. In these patients transbronchial biopsy significantly increases yield (72).

Key Points: Early Infectious Complications of BMT

- Bacterial infections and PCP are now less common due to effective prophylaxis
- CMV pneumonia and Aspergillus fungal infection are the current commonest infections
- The untreated mortality of both is very high
- Early infection (neutropenic engraftment period) is likely for fungal or bacterial disease
- Later infection, post first month (lymphocyte dysfunction) is commoner for viral infection
- Delayed presentation of any infection is usually in the context of GVHD

Delayed Complications
Bronchiolitis Obliterans

The incidence of obstructive airways disease following BMT has been described as between 2% and 13%, almost exclusively in allogeneic BMT (72,79). The main cause of this obstructive airways disease is thought to be due to bronchiolitis obliterans (BO). Although obstructive airways disease without histological evidence of BO does occur, at least part of these cases may reflect sampling variation at biopsy. BO typically occurs after the first 100 days. The risk is higher in patients with chronic GVHD and in those with depressed immunoglobulin levels following BMT. These factors may reflect the pathogenetic mechanism, which remains unknown but thought possibly to be due to small airway GVHD or autoimmune airways disease, perhaps precipitated by viral airway infection (92). Although BO has a poor response to current treatment regimens, early diagnosis is considered important as approximately two-thirds of patients will be dead three years' post-BMT (72).

Clinically patients present with symptoms that initially resemble upper airway infection. However, with time, there is persistent cough, dyspnea, and non-productive cough with marked wheezing. Pulmonary function tests demonstrate marked non-reversible obstructive physiology with mild diffusion capacity reduction. The definitive diagnosis requires confirmation with open lung biopsy. Characteristic imaging findings in conjunction with pulmonary function tests and BAL and transbronchial biopsy confirming the absence of infection are considered a clinically acceptable surrogate.

Chest radiographic findings include hyperinflation with possible bronchial wall thickening in the perihilar region. Interstitial or airspace opacity is conspicuous by its relative absence. At HRCT the pathological findings are more apparent. There is frequently marked hyperinflation with mosaic attenuation present with marked variation of vascular size in the areas of increased and reduced opacity. Segmental and subsegmental airway dilatation may be present with mild bronchial wall thickening. Mild areas of focal peripheral atelectasis or ground glass opacity may be present. The mosaic attenuation is markedly accentuated in expiration reflecting air-trapping secondary to small airway inflammation (Fig. 59.29) (93,94). These findings may be so characteristic as to permit a clinical diagnosis in the absence of pulmonary function

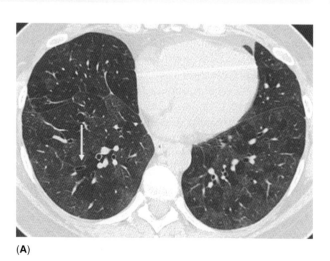
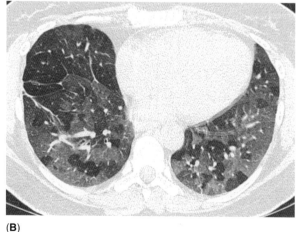

(A)   **(B)**

Figure 59.29 Typical bronchiolitis obliterans (BO) in a BMT recipient. (A) The inspiratory HRCT image demonstrates mosaic lung attenuation with geographic areas of reduced and increased opacity. The vessel size is mildly reduced in the "blacker" lung and there is mild subsegmental airway dilatation (arrow), a feature of BO. (B) The mosaic attenuation is markedly accentuated in the expiration image confirming diffuse small airway inflammation and air-trapping.

tests; these may not always be obtainable in very young children (93). More unusual described features include occasional pneumothoraces and pneumomediastinum (95). The presence of small apical bullae with small recurrent pneumothoraces has also been reported as a late sequela of BMT-related BO (96).

Key Points: Bronchiolitis Obliterans in BMT

- Occurs after first 100 days
- Irreversible obstructive physiology is common
- Possible mechanisms include GVHD, autoimmune airway disease, and viral infection
- HRCT findings include hyperinflation, mosaic attenuation accentuated in expiration, central airway thickening, segmental and subsegmental airway dilatation

Graft Vs. Host Disease

Graft versus host disease (GVHD) occurs as a result of an immune reaction in which donor T-cells recognize the host's tissues as foreign. According to the severity grade of GVHD the mortality may be as high as 50%. Acute GVHD is defined as occurring in the first 100 days, and occurs in between 25% and 75% of BMT recipients. This is a systemic illness that affects the skin, liver, and gastrointestinal tract but rarely affects the lung parenchyma. Conversely, pulmonary involvement in chronic GVHD occurring after the first 100 days is common. Two-thirds of these cases will have had prior acute GVHD (72,79). Chronic GVHD presents as a diffuse autoimmune disease resulting in a Sjogren's like syndrome, pan-serositis, autoimmune hepatitis, malabsorption, and immune deficiency. The thoracic involvement is, therefore, varied and includes manifestations of autoimmune disease such as lymphoid interstitial pneumonia, bronchiolitis obliterans, pleural and pericardial effusions, but also infections related to immune defects; in particular to encapsulated bacteria, PCP, and aspergillus. The radiological manifestations may reflect a combination of these pathologies. Late infection with bacteria, pneumocystis, or viral agents, particularly systemic varicella, most commonly occur in the setting of chronic GVHD (34). Nearly 30% of patients will experience such infections later than six months post-BMT (97). Bronchiectasis has been rarely described in BMT recipients, possibly a sequela of chronic GVHD (98).

Key Points: Graft Vs. Host Disease in BMT

- Acute GVHD occurs <100 days; systemic illness, pulmonary involvement rare
- Chronic GVHD occurs >100 days; pulmonary involvement common
- Graft donor T-cells attack host tissues as foreign
- Irreversible obstructive physiology common
- Pulmonary manifestations of chronic GVHD include lymphoid interstitial pneumonia, bronchiolitis obliterans, pleural or pericardial effusions, and persistent infections, particularly with encapsulated bacteria, PCP, and aspergillus

Less Frequent Complications

Secondary malignancy is well described in BMT recipients with a relative frequency of seven times the general population. Risk factors include conditioning total body irradiation and acute GVHD. The median presentation time is at one year following BMT and most typically these are lymphoproliferative disorders, especially NHL. However, solid tumors are also described (72).

Vascular complications are relatively uncommon in BMT but may affect both arterial and venous vessels of all sizes resulting in vascular endothelial thickening. Transient arterial thrombi, including fat marrow embolism, are also not infrequent (99,100). Rarely, pulmonary veno-occlusive disease can occur (72,77,100).

Organizing pneumonia has also been described in BMT recipients (77,101–103). Unlike its previous confusing misnomer, BOOP (bronchiolitis obliterans organizing pneumonia) suggested there is no evidence radiologically or histologically in these cases of bronchiolitis obliterans. The radiological manifestations are similar to organizing pneumonia in patients without BMT, namely peripheral multifocal ground glass or consolidative opacity, sometimes triangular in appearance, associated with mild focal tractional airway change indicating its chronic organizational nature (101,103).

Long-term restrictive physiology with possible associate fibrotic lung disease have been described in children and adults, and may not entirely be related to prior chemotoxicity or radiation (70,87, 104–106).

Secondary pulmonary alveolar proteinosis (PAP) with HRCT appearances comparable to primary PAP have been described in multiple hematological malignancies and in BMT recipients. The significance of this underappreciated diagnosis is that occasionally reversible respiratory failure may result (72). Radiological suspicion should prompt periodic acid-Schiff-positive testing at BAL which might not otherwise be performed. Secondary PAP appears to improve with recovery of neutropenia (79).

Imaging Evaluation of Bone Marrow Transplant Recipients

Chest radiography is an essential initial evaluation tool in patients with pulmonary complications of BMT. Although many of the radiographic appearances overlap, chest radiography and evaluation of the time course of serial change assist in narrowing the diagnostic possibilities (107,108).

Focal lobar or sublobar air-space opacity is most likely due to infection, including the possibility of bacterial or fungal disease. However, the CXR sensitivity for pulmonary infiltrates may be poor, particularly for neutropenic patients. Nodules, particularly if they evolve to cavitation, are more suggestive of fungal disease or septic emboli. Diffuse bilateral air-space opacity is more indicative of edema, IPS, DAH, CMV infection, radiation, or chemotoxicity. Of these, infection, edema and DAH may evolve over a period of hours, whereas, the remainder have a more indolent course changing gradually over days (Fig. 59.30). The presence of CXR-detectable adenopathy is most suggestive of recurrence of the original disease (72).

The utilization of CT and, in particular, HRCT has a high clinical impact on patient management (72). CT, especially HCRT, detects subtle abnormalities earlier, identifying disease in patients with normal radiographs, characterizing the distribution and extent of disease. In one study, clinically significant additional findings not apparent on chest X-ray were identified in over half the cases (109). In a different representative study the negative predictive value of the chest X-ray for infection in BMT recipients was approximately 50% but much higher, nearer 80%, for HRCT. As a result, the use of CT after chest X-ray altered clinical management in 25% of cases (110). HRCT increases the specificity with which diagnoses may be established, especially

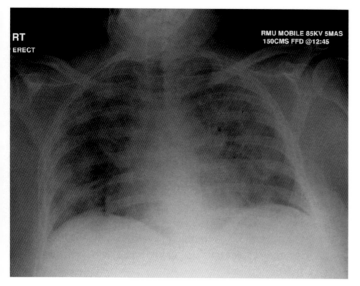

Figure 59.30 Diffuse air-space opacification occurring one year after allogeneic bone marrow transplantation. In the early post-BMT phase these appearances are commonly due to edema, idiopathic pneumonia syndrome, diffuse alveolar hemorrhage, or infection. In this chronic phase the appearances are likely infective, occurring in the context of graft versus host disease. Diagnosis in BMT recipients requires knowledge of the typical complications, their timelines for development and their evolution. PCP was cultured in this case.

fungal disease, PCP, bronchiolitis, pneumonia, radiation pneumonitis, and recurrent or new neoplastic disease (35,109,111). CT also may be useful in guiding sites for BAL, transbronchial biopsy, open lung biopsy, or planning CT-guided bronchoscopy, particularly for focal nodular disease (47,84,85,109,112,113).

Key Points: Time-Course of Bone Marrow Transplantation Complications

Early phase (<30 days: engraftment period, neutropenia predominates)

- Bacterial infections
- Fungal infections
- Diffuse alveolar hemorrhage
- Pulmonary edema
- Idiopathic pneumonia syndrome
- Drug reactions

Early phase (30–100 days: neutropenic recovery, persistent lymphocyte dysfunction)

- Viral infections (CMV, RSV)
- Pneumocystis infection
- Idiopathic pneumonia syndrome

Late phase (>100 days: gradual recovery of overall immunity to one year)

- Chronic GVHD manifesting as
  □ Obstructive lung disease (bronchiolitis obliterans)
  □ Infections—PCP, bacterial
- Bronchiolitis obliterans independent of known GVHD
- Organizing pneumonia
- Disease recurrence
- Rarely restrictive lung disease ± fibrosis

Solid Organ Transplantation

Solid organ transplantation is well established, predominantly for the treatment of organ failure. In the context of immunosuppression and cancer imaging, two areas are of specific interest: the pulmonary complications of patients with hepatocellular carcinoma (HCC) treated with liver transplantation, and the development of secondary malignancy in solid organ transplant recipients.

Recipients of Liver Transplantation for HCC

As with other solid organ transplant recipients, the necessary immunosuppression results in a propensity to opportunistic infection. However, compared to bone marrow recipients it must be noted that the degree of immunosuppression is significantly less as there is no attempt to ablate native bone marrow and the potentiating effects of conditioning radiation therapy are not encountered.

Thoracic disease is common, occurring in at least half of patients manifesting as effusions, atelectasis or diffuse airspace abnormality (114). Indeed, right diaphragmatic elevation and a right transudative effusion are invariable in the first week. Persistence of significant pleural fluid beyond the first week may reflect infection or rejection (115,116). Similar to other solid organ transplant recipients the main differential diagnosis for diffuse parenchymal air space disease is ARDS, edema, or adjuvant chemotherapy drug toxicity. However, the primary immunosuppressive agents used in transplantation are relatively rarely implicated in pulmonary drug toxicity. Rare instances of reversible hypersensitivity are described with azathioprine and diffuse interstitial pneumonitis, organizing pneumonia or alveolar proteinosis with sirolimus (117).

Infection remains the main mortality risk in immunosuppressed HCC liver transplant recipients. The overall incidence of pneumonia is low (10–15%); however, the mortality of those with infection appears high (40%), particularly those with fungal pneumonia (up to 90%). The incidence of infection appears related to the incidence of prior rejection, the complexity of the surgery itself, and the presence of hepatic or renal impairment (114,118). Living related recipients appear at higher risk than cadaveric hepatic recipients (119).

In initial studies, the predominant reported cause of early infection was bacterial in at least two thirds of patients; infection with CMV or PCP was commoner a few months after transplantation (118,120). The use of PCP and CMV prophylaxis, coupled with the progressive use of the more potent rescue or primary immunosuppressive agents such as tacrolimus (FK506) has resulted in an adjustment of the profile of infections. The incidence of PCP and CMV prophylaxis according to some series is now completely eliminated (121,122). Currently, approximately just over half of cases are due to acute bacterial infection, predominantly *Staphylococcus aureus* or gastrointestinal tract-derived gram negative bacilli (122). Fungal pneumonia, particularly aspergillus, is increasingly common, resulting in approximately one-third of infections. The small remainder of infections is accounted for by later onset mycobacterial or protozoal (toxoplasma) infections. As immunosuppression tapers beyond six months the risk of Aspergillus infection and gram-negative bacterial infection diminishes. The risk of bacterial infection persists throughout the post-transplant period; however, beyond six months the susceptibility changes to community-acquired organisms such as pneumococcus and

hemophilus influenzae; legionella is described to account for up to a quarter of cases (120,121,123).

A persistent concern in this patient group is the development of interval pulmonary metastatic nodular disease. In general, nodular disease is relatively uncommon in liver transplant recipients, occurring in less than 10% of patients (124). The discrimination of metastatic nodules from other etiologies may be difficult as their CT appearances may overlap significantly. The timing of development of nodules may be of assistance. Although metastatic nodules may occur at any time they are unusual in the first two to three months following transplantation. In this period Aspergillus fungal infection is the commonest cause, the remainder likely to be due to bacterial infection. In the period from 3 to 24 months other fungal infections (cryptococcosis, coccidioidomycosis), bacterial nocardia infection, and mycobacterial disease are commonest (124). Although metastatic disease may be associated with recurrent alpha-fetoprotein elevation, ultimately focal nodules often require image-guided percutaneous or open-lung biopsy for definitive characterization.

Secondary Malignancy

The rate of malignancy is significantly elevated in chronically immunosuppressed transplant recipients as opposed to the general population (125–127). Postulated etiologies include decreased lymphocytic surveillance of early malignant lesions, chronic transplant organ antigenic stimulation, chronic viral oncogene stimulation, and possible mutagenic effects of immunosuppressive agents such as azathioprine (116).

The most common malignant manifestation of transplantation is skin cancer followed by post-transplant lymphoproliferative disorder (PTLD). However, other cancers also occur with lesser frequency, including squamous cell head and neck tumors and all subtypes of non-small cell primary lung cancer (128). The risk of lung cancer is probably highest in heart or lung transplant recipients (116). Lung cancers in transplant recipients are frequently more aggressive and present at an advanced stage (129).

Post-Transplant Lymphoproliferative Disorder (PTLD)

PTLD is the commonest systemic malignancy in solid organ transplant recipients. PTLD refers to a wide range of lymphoproliferative disorders of varying clonality and differentiation. Although mild hyperplasia alone may occur, an aggressive multifocal disease pattern with poor prognosis is most common (130,131). The vast majority of PTLD tumors are B-cell tumors (90%) and at least 95% are EBV positive (130,132). EBV infection of immunosuppressed EBV-negative transplant recipients appears to be the major causative factor. The impact of immunosuppression is revealed by the higher incidence of PTLD in patients immunosuppressed with the very powerful agent OKT3, an anti-CD3 murine antibody. Moreover, these lesions are frequently poorly responsive to standard lymphoma treatments, responding instead to reduction of immunosuppression and antiviral therapy (132).

There are multiple risk factors for PTLD development (132,133). The disease is commoner in children compared to adults. In part the incidence also depends on the type of organ transplant. While the incidence in liver transplant recipients is approximately 2% to 3% (123,124), in renal transplant recipients it is significantly higher (4–7%) (123). In renal transplantation, the commonest

organ recipients, the relative risk of PTLD compared to the general population is particularly high (×8) (123). It is even higher in cardiac transplant recipients (×25) (134).

At least 50% of patients with PTLD present within the first year, with 90% within the first five years. Thereafter a constant lesser risk persists, particularly for non-EBV related cases (132,135). Patients may present with a viral illness, particularly an infectious mononucleosis-like presentation, as a lymphoma with adenopathy or an extranodal mass, or with fulminant sepsis (132). The presentation symptoms are also dependent in part on the organs of involvement. Of all the cases of PTLD approximately 7% involve the lung parenchyma, although multiple organ involvement is common. Other organs involved include the gastro-intestinal tract, liver, kidneys, and spleen.

Radiologically most pulmonary cases present as well-defined nodules or masses measuring up to 5 cm, although occasional solitary pulmonary nodules or patchy air-space disease are also recognized presentations (124) (Fig. 59.31). The distribution is predominantly peribronchovascular and involves the mid and lower lungs. A "halo" appearance around nodules has been described; however, frank cavitation would suggest infection which is a common alternative diagnosis in this patient group. The presence of well defined or of a single focus of pulmonary disease has been associated with a more benign disease course. Mediastinal nodes are common; pleural and pericardial effusions may also occur (132).

Key Points: Secondary Malignancy in Solid Transplant Recipients

- Skin cancer is commonest, followed by PTLD, head and neck, and lung cancers
- PTLD tumors vary in clonality and aggression but nearly all are B-cell and EBV-related
- PTLD risk is highest in renal and cardiac transplants
- Pulmonary involvement occurs in 7% of PTLD
- Pulmonary PTLD manifests as solitary or multiple nodules with adenopathy and occasional effusions
- In PTLD ill-defined nodules or multifocal parenchymal disease are associated with a worse prognosis

CANCER IN HIV-INFECTION

The chronic immunosuppression of HIV is associated with the pathogenesis of cancer. Immune dysfunction, concomitant infection with other oncogenes [hepatitis B and C, Ebstein-Barr virus, and human papilloma viruses (HPV)], and smoking (137,138), are thought to be co-variables in oncogenesis. Kaposi's sarcoma, non-Hodgkin's lymphoma, and cervical cancer are considered AIDS-defining diagnoses and may be the first clinical presentation of HIV infection. Although AIDS-defining infections in general have a CD4 cell count threshold above which they do not occur, the relationship of immunosuppression to cancer expression is more complex. Although the development of an AIDS-defining cancer confirms the severity of HIV infection and immunosuppression, this may not be directly related to the CD4 count. Comparing AIDS-defining diagnoses, Maiman and

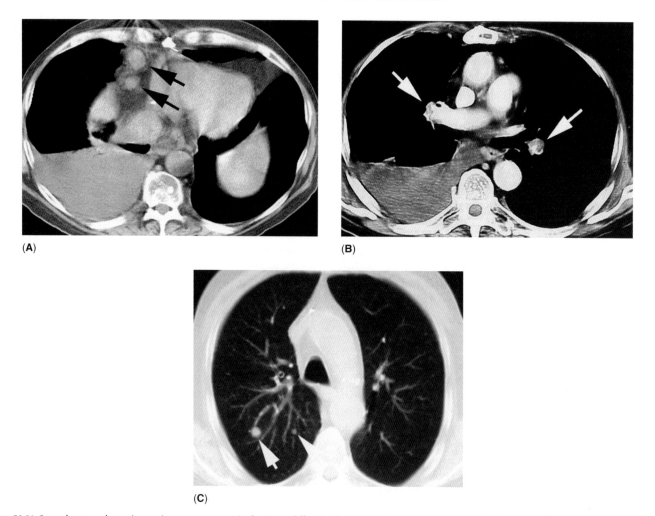

(A)   (B)

(C)

Figure 59.31 Secondary neoplasms in two immunocompromised patients following heart transplantation—post-transplant lymphoproliferative disorder (PTLD) and lymphoma. (**A** and **B**) Thirteen months after cardiac transplantation, this 64-year-old man developed shortness of breath. CT shows a large right pleural effusion, bilateral pulmonary emboli (white arrows), and adenopathy in the right paracardiac region (black arrows). Cytology of the pleural effusion revealed monoclonal large cell lymphoma. (**C**) Eight months after cardiac transplantation, this 61-year-old man's CT shows new lung nodules (arrows). Open lung biopsy revealed PTLD. *Source*: Figure 59.31A from Ref. 136.

colleagues (139) demonstrated that the mean CD4 count in Kaposi's sarcoma and non-Hodgkin's lymphoma was significantly lower (153 cells/mm^3) than that of patients with cervical cancer (312 cells/mm^3), although the overall survival duration was not different in the two groups.

The advent of highly antiretroviral therapy (HAART) for HIV infection in the late 1990s has led to a significant extension of the life expectancy of patients with HIV (140–142) with a concomitant reduction in the incidence rate of AIDS-defining cancer diagnoses (143). Although these diagnoses still constitute 80% of new cancer diagnoses in HIV patients, several large registry studies from HIV patient populations in the United Kingdom (144), Australia (145), and the United States (146,147), have demonstrated that a significant incidence increase is also present for non-AIDS defining cancer diagnoses. A recent prospective study, incorporating data from over 54,000 HIV patients from 13 regional United States cancer centers over a 12-year observation period, compared new primary incidence tumors against matched demographic non-HIV infected patient data from SEER (Surveillance, Epidemiology, and End Results from the U.S. National Cancer Institute) (148). Increased cancer rates were corroborated for primary anal,

Table 59.4 Relative Incidence Risk for Non-AIDS Defining Cancer in HIV Infection[148]

Anal	42.9	Melanoma	2.6
Vaginal	21.0	Oropharyngeal	2.6
Hodgkin's lymphoma	14.7	Leukemia	2.5
Liver	7.7	Colorectal	2.3
Lung	3.3	Renal	1.8

[AQ3

vaginal, Hodgkin's lymphoma, leukemias, lung, melanoma, liver, oropharyngeal, colorectal, and renal cancer (Table 59.4). A chronological analysis demonstrated that the incidence of anal cancer demonstrated a four-fold incidence increase in HIV-patients from the pre-HAART era (1992–1995) to the recent HAART era (2000–2003). The incidences of Hodgkin's lymphoma, melanoma, liver cancer, colorectal, and prostate cancer are also increasing, whereas the incidence of lung cancer has remained relatively constant. These findings probably partially relate to the duration of immunosuppression and in part to the persistence of other oncogenes such as HPV-16 in anal cancer that are unaffected by HAART.

Lung Cancer in HIV

Incidence, Etiology, and Demographics

The increased incidence of lung cancer in HIV-infected individuals became apparent in the early years of the HIV epidemic as the initial infective complications became more manageable and the introduction of HAART extended the life expectancy of infected individuals (149–153). In this post-HAART period the relative risk of lung cancer compared to the non-infected population has increased, although this has predominantly reflected the reduced incidence in matched uninfected populations. Although lung cancer remains the commonest cause of non AIDS-defining cancer in HIV, the absolute incidence of lung cancer in HIV cases has remained relatively stable (85–170 cases/100,000 person years) (148,154). The incidence is now comparable to the increased incidence of anal and breast cancer; Hodgkin's lymphoma and colorectal cancer are only minimally less common. The relative risk remains between 3.3 and 4.7 more common than for matched non-HIV infected populations (148,154), with a higher relative risk in women.

The etiology of lung cancer in HIV remains unknown. A higher incidence in patients with AIDS rather than earlier HIV-infection suggests the disease might be related to the degree of immunosuppression (155). However, lung cancer does not have a threshold response related to the CD4 count, nor the HIV viral load (154–156). A relationship to the nadir of the CD4 count has been reported (148) but many cases occur in patients with only moderate immunosuppression with a mean CD4 count of 250/mm³ (157). Twenty-five to fifty percent of patients will have AIDS at diagnosis, but this proportion is falling (158).

HIV may, therefore, have a direct oncogenic effect. However, it is likely that the effect is multifactorial, incorporating environmental factors and possibly other viral oncogenes (157). Recent studies suggest that HIV predisposes to accelerated onset and more severe emphysema (159,160). Although the development of lung cancer in HIV is not predicated on the development of emphysema, this does

suggest that an altered humoral response to lung injury, particularly with regard to smoking may be contributory. Cytotoxic lymphocyte activation, lung capillary endothelial cell injury and apoptosis, sphingolipid imbalance, and oxidative stress in the lung are specific putative mechanisms suggested for the development of emphysema, and may also be implicated in cancer development (160,161). Although smoking remains the main risk factor for the development of lung cancer in HIV, HIV infection has been demonstrated to be a significant predictor of the development of both emphysema (161) and lung cancer (154–156), independent of smoking.

A meta-analysis of several studies suggests the mean age of development of lung cancer in HIV is younger (45 years) compared to that of the general population (62 years). Although this remains a disease predominantly of men (9:1 ratio), this male predominance is suspected to be diminishing due to the equalization of HIV incidence between the sexes and the notable significantly higher relative risk of lung cancer in women with HIV compared to the general population (157).

The clinical presentation of lung cancer in HIV is comparable to that of non-HIV infected patients, including cough, chest pain, dyspnea, hemoptysis, and metastatic disease. The majority (86–90%) of cases represent non-small cell lung cancer (NSCLC) with a preponderance of adenocarcinoma reflecting a similar distribution to non-HIV patients (153,158,162,163).

Radiological Appearance, Diagnosis, and Management

Studies of the radiological appearances of lung cancer in HIV patients have included only small series of up to 30 patients (149,164–167). The histological distribution is similar to non-HIV patients; adenocarcinoma is the commonest tumor histology in up to 50% of cases followed by squamous cell carcinoma (33%) (157,168).

Radiographic presentation is typically of a nodule or mass on chest radiograph or CT in two-thirds of patients. Most lesions (60–75%) are peripheral, of which the vast majority (>90%) are in the upper lobes (165,166) (Figs. 59.32 and 59.33). Similar to

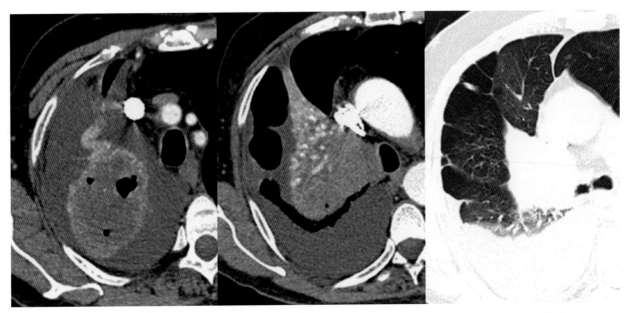

Figure 59.32 HIV infection and lung cancer. Fifty-eight-year-old male with HIV; CD4 > 500 cells/mm³. A large right hilar mass is present occluding the right upper lobe bronchus. Cystic change is present in the right upper lobe consistent with postobstructive infective liquefaction. The lung windows also demonstrate advanced emphysema, a common feature in HIV-infected patients. Lung cancer often occurs with normal or only mildly depressed CD4 counts.

non-HIV infected patients, enlarged lymph nodes occurred in 60% of patients and pleural effusion or metastases in approximately one-third of patients (164–166). Cavitation occurs in nearly a quarter of patients (165).

There are differences from lung cancer in the general community. HIV-related bronchogenic carcinoma is typically larger at presentation (usually T2 or greater, >4.5 cm) and occurs in significantly younger patients (165). The upper lobe preponderance of tumors is perhaps more marked than in the general population (165,166). In one series, nearly 70% of tumors were poorly differentiated (164). Therefore, poorly differentiated, rapidly growing tumors in young smoking patients should raise the suspicion of HIV infection (Fig. 59.34) (164).

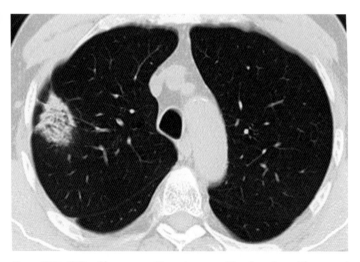

Figure 59.33 HIV and lung cancer. Sixty-nine-year-old male patient with a ground glass right upper lobe lesion, initially thought to be infective. The lesion was persistent and eventually resected. Histopathology demonstrated an adenocarcinoma, the commonest subtype in HIV patients. Partial bronchoalveolar cell features likely accounted for ground glass appearances. A high clinical suspicion is warranted in long-term HIV patients, particularly if they continue to smoke.

Late stage presentation of bronchogenic carcinoma in HIV patients is common (169) with 75% to 90% presenting with Stage III/IV disease (153,158,162,163). In a study of 15 AIDS patients with lung carcinoma, Bazot and colleagues found no correlation between the CD4 count and the staging of malignancy. This late presentation is likely due to a combination of factors including delayed presentation, the failure to suspect lung cancer in a younger patient, the aggressive course of the malignancy, and the presence or suspicion of other opportunistic or AIDS-defining malignancy (166) (Fig. 59.35). The predominantly peripheral location of lesions also makes lesions less amenable to bronchoscopic biopsy and lavage, which are usually helpful in the routine management of HIV patients. Particularly as many lesions are imperceptible on CXR, CT screening has been advocated to increase early diagnosis, although this has not yet had widespread implementation (170).

Traditionally the outcome of HIV-related lung cancer has been considered dismal. Early series suggested that regardless of TNM staging, one-year survival was only 10% compared to 40% in control populations. Median survival was only 4.5 months compared to approximately 10 months, respectively. However, this earlier data in large part precedes the advent of HAART. Previously, patients who developed lung cancer died predominantly of infective complications, whereas now mortality is usually related to the lung cancer itself. The poor performance status of HIV patients presenting with HIV previously often precluded curative surgical treatment, chemotherapy, or radiation treatment (153,158,162,163). More recent data, however, suggests this trend may be changing. In more recent sample studies, patients with Stage 3b/IV lung cancer with CD4 counts above 200 were able to receive chemotherapy and achieved comparable survival to non-HIV historical controls (171). In the small proportion of patients presenting with Stage I or II disease encouraging successful surgical treatment, limited data has been described and remains the first option (158,165,172). Analysis of mortality in these patient groups remains confounded by the coexistence of other significant infective and malignant co-factors of morbidity and mortality.

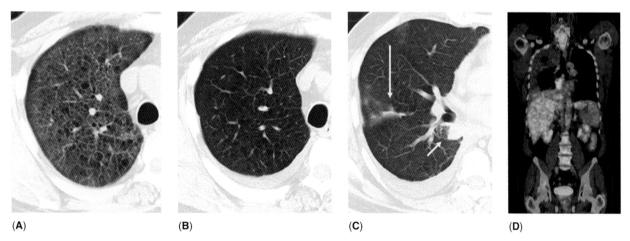

(A) (B) (C) (D)

Figure 59.34 Advanced lung cancer and HIV. (A) Initial presentation CT demonstrated PCP on a background of premature emphysema in this 50-year-old patient. (B, C) Six months later following treatment the PCP has resolved. However, a new lesion has evolved in the azygo-esophageal recess (short arrow) with new nodular fissural thickening (long arrow). Findings were due to an aggressive, poorly differentiated, rapidly developing lung adenocarcinoma with pleural metastases. (D) Fused PET-CT image demonstrates right infrahilar increased FDG activity.

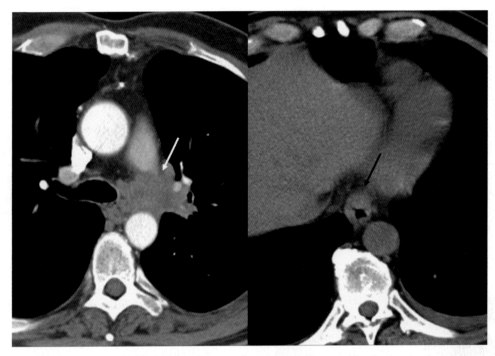

Figure 59.35 HIV and multiple malignancy. A central left upper lobe squamous cell carcinoma (white arrow) has developed and resulted in presentation for weight loss and cough. However, CT images also demonstrate eccentric distal esophageal thickening (black arrow). Esophageal and lung carcinoma were confirmed by bronchoscopy and esophagoscopy. Although both lung cancer and gastrointestinal tumors are significantly more common in chronic HIV infection, neither is considered an AIDS-defining illness.

Current management guidelines suggest that lung cancer treatment should be the same as for non-HIV infected individuals and, therefore, early accurate diagnosis and staging is paramount. Percutaneous needle biopsy should be performed early in patients in whom there is a delayed or absent response to opportunistic infection treatment (173). The value of percutaneous needle biopsy in patients with HIV discriminating opportunistic infection from lung cancer has been determined in several studies (165,174,175) without significant increased risk compared to the general population. It must be recalled that a benign diagnosis in these cases should be treated with circumspection as benign infectious diagnoses may coexist in up to 20% to 30% of cases (164,165).

The radiological definition of mediastinal nodal status is problematic on CT in view of persistent adenopathy in many patients with HIV. As with non-HIV patients, a combination of PET imaging, transbronchial needle aspiration, or mediastinoscopy may be required for complete mediastinal staging.

HIV patients on chemotherapy or radiation regimens for lung cancer require careful radiological monitoring. In particular, interactions between antiretroviral agents and chemotherapy may result in further immunosuppression. This is particularly important for patients treated with zidovudine (azidothymidine) in whom the marrow toxicity effects may be potentiated by chemotherapy (176,177). Radiation sequela, particularly early esophagitis with stricture formation, may be potentiated in HIV infection. This effect, first demonstrated in initial attempts to treat Kaposi's sarcoma (178,179), may be due to impaired mucosal repair mechanism in conjuction with the presence of pre-existing infection such as yeasts, CMV, or herpes (180).

The use of conformal therapy is believed to reduce the incidence of these complications.

Key Points: Lung Cancer in HIV

- Commonest non-AIDS defining cancer in HIV
- NSCLC predominates, especially adenocarcinoma (50%)
- Relative risk ratio is 3.3–4.7 × that of the general population
- M:F ratio 9:1 but decreasing because of more female HIV cases and higher female relative risk
- Radiology comparable to non-HIV lung cancers
- Peripheral upper lobe lesions are common
- Early age onset lung cancer with undifferentiated histology, rapidly progressive lesions non-responsive to opportunistic treatment should raise the possibility of HIV
- Chemotherapy may potentiate immunosuppression
- Radiotherapy may precipitate early and severe esophageal strictures

Kaposi's Sarcoma in HIV

Kaposi's sarcoma remains the commonest AIDS defining cancer diagnosis in HIV, nearly exclusively sexually transmitted in homosexual males. However, the incidence has dramatically reduced from 1800 to 2500 cases/100,000 person years in the pre-HAART era to 330–350 in the post-HAART era (1996 onwards) (146–148). The degree of immunosuppression is severe with CD4 counts at presentation <50 cells/mm³ (146). The disease progression of pulmonary KS is more rapid and aggressive than the rare instances of pulmonary KS unassociated

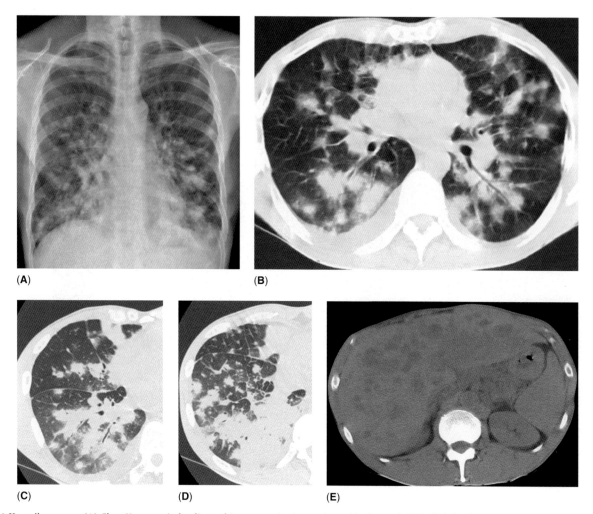

Figure 59.36 Kaposi's sarcoma. (**A**) Chest X-ray: typical radiographic presentation in a patient with advanced AIDS. Ill-defined symmetric perihilar peribronchial nodu-lar opacities extend in to the lower lobes. (**B**) CT demonstrates the "flame-shaped" peribronchial opacities that typically are larger than 1 cm and an associated right effusion. (**C,D**) HRCT images of the right lung demonstrate typical associated interlobular septal thickening and more confluent consolidative opacity. (**E**) Non-contrast images of the liver demonstrate multiple Kaposi's sarcoma hepatic lesions, a recognized extrapulmonary manifestation.

with HIV (181). The disease is thought probably to be related to co-infection with the human herpes virus HHV-8, although the causality of this viral infection is contested (182–185). In AIDS patients with KS, up to one third will have pulmonary involve-ment and up to half of these patients will be symptomatic. Mucocutaneous involvement appears invariable. Clinically, patients with KS present with fever, recurrent pneumonia, hemoptysis, and dyspnea. Not all patients require treatment, although this may include intralesional therapy, chemotherapy, or radiation treatment (178,186,187).

Pathologically this highly vascular disease consists of a poly-clonal expansion of sheets of atypical spindle cells with interven-ing slit-like vascular and lymphatic endothelial spaces filled with hemosiderin-laden macrophages. These align themselves along the lymphatics of the axial interstitium and of the subpleural spaces (187). The pathological appearances of a perilymphatic distribution of a hemorrhagic disease result in relatively distinc-tive radiological features that permit differentiation from other infective and neoplastic disease entities.

On CXR ill-defined perihilar nodular air-space opacities are identified tending towards confluence. Although superficially this appearance resembles air-space infection the symmetry and nodularity should alert to the possibility of KS (Fig. 59.36). Pleural effusions are common (20–30%) and occasional Kerley B lines may be seen. Hilar or mediastinal adenopathy is appreciable in 10% (188–192).

The appearances of KS at HRCT are relatively characteristic with ill-defined ("flame-shaped") perihilar peribronchovascular air-space opacities (Fig. 59.37). Genuinely endobronchial lesions may occur (193,194). On HRCT the nodules of KS are typically larger (1–2 cm) than those of other opportunistic infections. Air-space opacities may coalesce secondary to tumor infiltration, hemorrhage, or airway obstruction with postobstructive atelecta-sis (187). In addition to the opacities, a combination of CT and HRCT readily demonstrate the ancillary features of KS includ-ing the presence of adenopathy or effusions, each present in up to 50% of cases. HRCT imaging highlights associated interlobular septal thickening (40%) which may be thickened or nodu-lar (192,195,196). Extrathoracic manifestations such as osseous or hepatic involvement are also occasionally seen (197).

The HRCT appearances of Kaposi's sarcoma have been proven to be distinctive and usually obviate the need for confirmatory

transbronchial or transthoracic biopsy. In a series evaluating HIV patients with known KS diagnoses, KS was suggested as the first diagnosis in 83% of cases or in the top three in 92% (195). When a confident diagnosis is made, this is likely to be correct in over 90% of cases (198). In distinguishing KS from other causes of opportunistic infection a predominance of nodules larger than 1 cm significantly favors neoplastic disease over opportunistic infection. A peribronchovascular distribution of nodules is highly specific for KS (199). In more confluent non-nodular disease lymphoma is an alternative consideration.

The MRI appearances of KS have been described in a small series of patients (200). Typical findings are lesions characterized by high T1 and low T2 signal intensity, presumably reflecting their hemorrhagic nature. Recently a flare-up of KS has been described in patients with HIV and KS treated with HAART, resulting in immune reconstitution syndrome (Fig. 59.38) (201).

Key Points: CT/HRCT of Kaposi's Sarcoma in HIV

- Perihilar peribronchovascular nodules
- Axial interstitial involvment
- "Flame-shaped" 1 to 2 cm opacities
- Coalescent airspace disease
- Effusions (50%)
- Lymphadenopathy (50%)
- Interlobular septal thickening (40%)
- Extrathoracic involvement (hepatic)
- Size of nodules >1 cm with peribronchovascular distribution highly favors KS over other neoplastic disease or opportunistic infection
- Worsening appearances with immune reconstitution syndrome

Lymphoproliferative Disorders in HIV

The significantly higher incidence of lymphoma in HIV-infected patients compared to the general population was noted very early in the clinical evaluation of HIV patients. By 1985 non-Hodgkin's lymphoma had been classified as an AIDS-defining cancer. However, in subsequent years, our understanding, epidemiology, and clinical presentation of lymphoma in HIV-infected patients has changed significantly (143,146,148).

In the early years of the HIV pandemic the risk of non-Hodgkin's lymphoma in HIV patients was 60 to 200 times higher than the general population and for certain subtypes such as primary

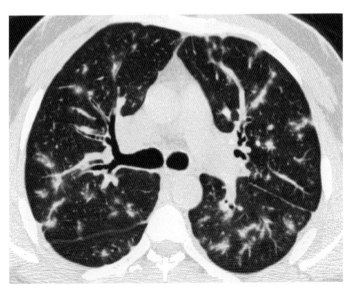

Figure 59.37 Kaposi's sarcoma. HRCT demonstrates characteristic appearances with multiple central peribronchovascular ill-defined nodular opacities. These appearances are referred to as "flame-shaped." Bronchoscopy confirmed multiple endobronchial bluish papules.

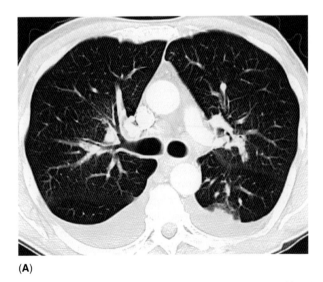

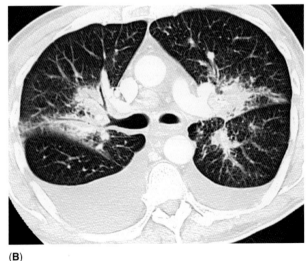

(A)   (B)

Figure 59.38 Kaposi's sarcoma immune reconstitution. Fifty-nine-year-old HIV positive man. (A) Initial scan depicts mild central peribronchovascular thickening and bilateral pleural effusions. (B) CT scan performed 14 days later shows a rapid increase in peribronchovascular thickening and pleural effusion enlargement, with development of bilateral perihilar consolidation. The findings are secondary to partial immune reconstitution following HAART therapy. *Source*: Courtesy of Dr. M. Godoy, New York.

CNS lymphomas as high as 1000 times (202,203). In this pre-HAART era the outcome of these patients with AIDS related lymphoma (ARL) was dismal. Patients presented with advanced stage, bulky disease with extensive extranodal disease. In order to balance the risks of further immunosuppression induced by chemotherapy, and chemotoxicity, variable dose regimens were developed. In studies evaluating low-dose versus standard combination regimen chemotherapy, no survival differences were demonstrated (204). Low-dose patients tended to die of ARL, high-dose patients of infection. The survival of patients in similar trials was uniformly poor compared to comparable NHL in non-HIV infected populations. Complete response rates of up to 50% and survival of only six to nine months were typical in these studies (204,205). Interestingly, the response of patients to ARL appeared more predicated on their CD4 count, any other AIDS defining illness, and their overall performance score rather than features more traditionally associated with evaluation of NHL prognosis (lactate dehydrogenase level, CNS or marrow involvement).

This dependence on the level of immunosuppression was underscored by the change in incidence of ARL following the introduction of HAART in the late 1990s. Several international studies demonstrated that concomitant with the improved CD4 counts and reduced viral loads in these patients the incidence of ARL fell by a factor of two to three (143,145,146,148). In one study the relative risk ratio compared to the general population decreased from 80 to 17, from the pre-HAART to the recent HAART era (148). The vast majority of ARL tumors are still classified as diffuse large B-cell (DLBCL) or Burkitt-type lymphomas but even within these groups significant variations have developed over the recent years (203). In one registry analysis, 38% of ARL pre-HAART was highly aggressive immunoblastic DLBCL. This proportion and primary CNS lymphoma halved following the introduction of HAART. Conversely, the proportion of centroblastic DLBCL and Burkitt's lymphoma in ARL has doubled (206). It appears that greater immunosuppression results in immunoblastic or CNS lymphoma, lesser in centroblastic DLBCL or Burkitt's lymphoma. The etiology for the development of ARL remains complex and multifactorial. For example, although Ebstein-Barr virus infection is common in AIDS-related Burkitt's, this type of lymphoma does not occur in other forms of chronic immunosuppression. This suggests that in this case the HIV oncogenic effects may be more important than the EBV oncogenic effect (203).

Although ARL still presents with extranodal disease and high LDH levels, the overall survival following chemotherapy and HAART is now significantly improved with reduction of opportunistic infections (207,208). A further impact of HAART has been the persistence of co-infection with other potential oncogenes such as HHV-8 and EBV. These have resulted in the increased incidence of new or previously rare tumors such as primary effusion lymphoma or oral plasmablastic lymphoma (204,209).

Recently it has also become apparent that other lymphomas such as Hodgkin's lymphoma are also more common in HIV, although are not AIDS-defining diagnoses presently. Longitudinal studies suggest that the relative risk of HIV-related Hodgkin's lymphoma (HIV-HL) is now between 11 and 18 times that of the general population (148,204). Compared to HIV-negative

Table 59.5 WHO Categories of HIV-Lymphoid Diseases

1. **Lymphoma also occurring in immunocompetent individuals**
   Diffuse large B-cell lymphoma (common)
      Centroblastic (increasingly common)
      Immunoblastic, including primary CNS (now less common)
   Burkitt's and Burkitt variants (common)
   Hodgkin's lymphoma (increasingly common)
   MALT-type lymphomas
   T-cell lymphomas
   Castleman's disease
2. **Lymphoma specific to HIV-infected patients**
   Plasmablastic lymphoma (oral rare)
   Primary effusion lymphoma
3. **Lymphoma also occurring in other immunosuppressed states**
   Polymorphic B-cell lymphomas (PTLD-like)

Abbreviations: CNS, central nervous system; MALT, mucosa-associated lymphoid tissue; PTLD, post-transplant lymphoproliferative disorder.
Source: Adapted from Refs. 203, 212.

individuals nearly all HIV-HL patients are infected with EBV. It has been suggested that HAART, via immune reconstitution, may increase B-cell stimulation and the number of EBV infected B-cells potentiating the oncogenic risk of EBV (210). Through the HAART era there has been a gradual decrease of the nodular sclerosing subtype, with a relative increase of the less favorable mixed cellularity or lymphocyte-depleted subtypes (203,211).

In recognition of the wide array of lymphomas that may occur in patients with HIV not limited to NHL the WHO has classified lymphoid tumors in HIV into three categories (Table 59.5).

Imaging Features of ARL
Clinically, intrathoracic disease occurs in only 10% to 30% of ARL; hepatosplenic, bone marrow, subcutaneous nodal tissue, and the CNS are commoner sites of involvement (213–215). At autopsy, however, the recognized incidence of subclinical pleuro-parenchymal disease is much higher and approaches 70% (216).

There appear to be no significant distinguishing features between the different subtypes of ARL. However, compared to non-HIV related lymphoma, thoracic ARL involvement is distinguished by typical appearances of advanced stage, markedly aggressive lymphomas with more frequent extranodal involvement (>90%) (Fig. 59.39) (213).

In an early small study of 11 patients with thoracic ARL, Sider and colleagues suggested that contrary to non-immunocompromised hosts, in ARL extranodal parenchymal lesions and pleural effusions were a commoner presentation than mediastinal adenopathy or a mass (Fig. 59.40) (214). Subsequent studies confirmed that the common plain radiographic appearances of ARL include unilateral or bilateral pleural effusions (50%), mediastinal adenopathy (25%), diffuse air-space infiltration with air-bronchograms or regional reticulonodular densities (25%). Single or pulmonary nodules or masses are a very common feature occurring in up to 50% of cases (216–218). Of these, the majority are large (>5 cm) and peripheral or pleural-based (217,219). In about half of the nodule presentations, the nodules are solitary, and cavitation is described in a quarter (217). Rapidly growing, single or multiple nodules that may double in size within four to six weeks have been described in up to 25% of cases (214,215).

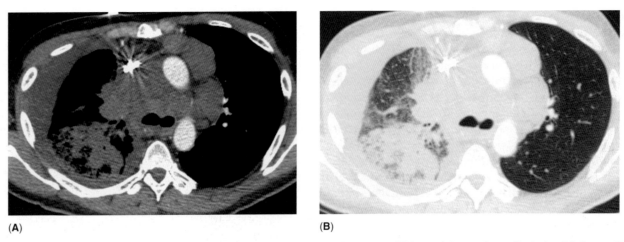

(A)   **(B)**

Figure 59.39 AIDS-related lymphoma. Advanced stage B-cell lymphoma in a patient with AIDS. In addition to (**A**) extensive mediastinal nodal disease, (**B**) pleural effusions and extensive right lung parenchymal involvement by lymphoma is demonstrated. The superior vena cava and, more inferiorly, the right pulmonary arteries (not shown) are significantly compressed.

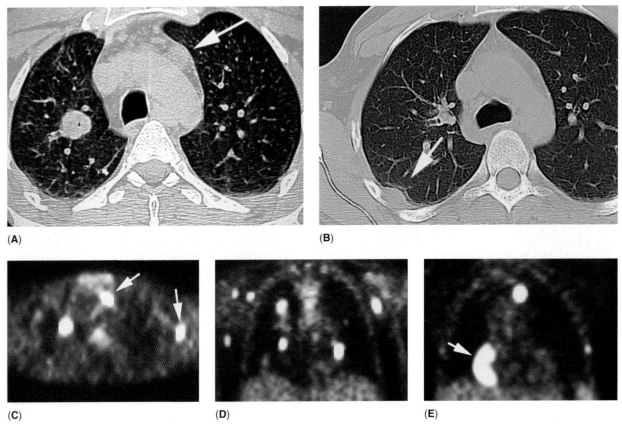

Figure 59.40 A 36-year-old man with AIDS, CD4 count of 45 and viral load of 431,200. (**A** and **B**) CT showed multiple new pulmonary nodules including one in the right upper lobe (**A**) and one abutting the right pleura (**B**, arrow). Also present were some mildly enlarged lymph nodes in the anterior mediastinum. (**A**, arrow). (**C**–**E**) An ¹⁸FDG PET scan was performed. (**C**) Axial ¹⁸FDG PET image shows intense abnormal uptake in the right upper lobe nodule and in lymph nodes (arrows) in the mediastinum and left axilla. (**D**) Coronal ¹⁸FDG PET image shows abnormal uptake in multiple other lesions in the lungs and lymph nodes. (**E**) Coronal ¹⁸FDG PET shows abnormal uptake in a pericardial effusion (arrow) as well as in the lymph node in the upper mediastinum. Bronchoscopy with transbronchial biopsy of the right upper lobe nodule revealed large cell lymphoma. The entire ¹⁸FDG PET scan showed multiple lesions in the head, chest, abdomen, and pelvis compatible with widely disseminated lymphoma. *Source*: Courtesy of Jannette Collins, MD, Med.

Pericardial effusions are not uncommon (13%) (Fig. 59.41) (213,217). More rarely, but still more common than non-AIDS related lymphoma, is a cardiac mass or chest wall invasion (214,220) (Figs. 59.42 and 59.43).

CT improves the detection of pleuroparenchymal abnormalities and identifies disease in patients in whom the CXR may appear normal (217,219), as such a higher proportion of patients demonstrate effusions (70%), or mediastinal or hilar adenopathy (50%).

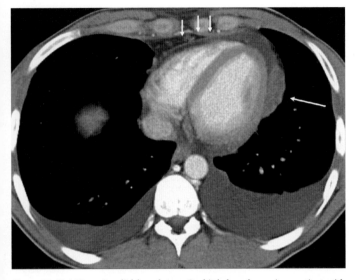

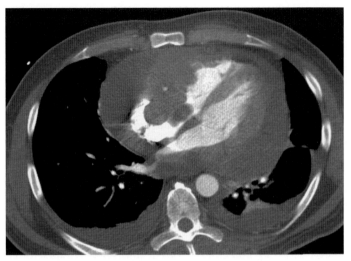

Figure 59.41 ARL pericardial lymphoma. Burkitt's lymphoma in a patient with AIDS. In addition to bilateral pleural effusions, a pericardial effusion with parietal pericardial enhancement (short arrows) and pericardial soft tissue (long arrow) is present. Cardiac and pericardial involvement is more common in ARL than non-HIV related lymphoma.

Figure 59.42 B-cell lymphoma in a patient with AIDS and cardiac invasion of the right-sided chambers. Bilateral effusions and a pericardial effusion are also present. Cardiac invasion is a rare manifestation of lymphomas but is seen with increased frequency in the aggressive B-cell lymphomas associated with AIDS and also in patients with post-transplantation lymphoproliferative disorder (PTLD).

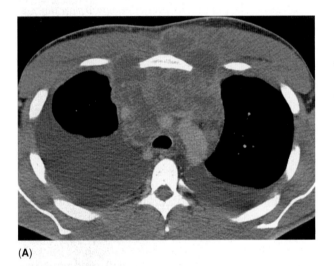

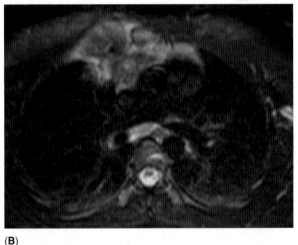

(A)   **(B)**

Figure 59.43 ARL with chest wall invasion, two patients. (A) CT image of a patient with a large B-cell lymphoma with mediastinal vascular encasement and anterior chest wall invasion seen best on these delayed-phase images. (B) In a different patient with ARL, T2-weighted MR image demonstrates chest wall invasion. The T2 signal intensity is correlated to the degree of aggression of the lymphoma.

Air-space mass-like opacities may be present which may show some minor tractional distortion of the contained airways indicative of chronicity. More pulmonary nodules are detected and cavitation may be more frequently and reliably determined. HRCT imaging, either prospectively acquired or retrospectively reconstructed from volumetric MDCT data sets, allows more definitive evaluation of CXR reticulonodular opacities. This may help demonstrate a typical perilymphatic peribronchiolar distribution of disease and any associated septal thickening. Pleural effusions are also more frequently detected, characterized and localized. Although autopsy series demonstrate frequent microscopic pleural nodularity (30%), less than 10% have pleural thickening or nodules at CT (216).

Perhaps the greatest value of CT imaging in ARL patients is its ability not only to detect and characterize ARL but also to differentiate it from other co-existent opportunistic pathologies (198). In this evaluation a knowledge of clinical parameters and image-guided intervention play integral roles.

Dilemmas in the Imaging of Thoracic AIDS-Related Lymphoma
Although post mortem analyses suggest a high level of thoracic involvement in ARL, in one retrospective review of 20 ARL autopsy cases with pulmonary involvement only one was diagnosed ante mortem (216). In a study of 116 patients with known ARL, retrospectively 52 had thoracic CXR or CT abnormalities. However, 32 of these related to opportunistic infection, KS, or other miscellaneous conditions, and only 20 were due to ARL itself (217). In only 13% was the thorax the predominant site of involvement (217).

The radiological task therefore requires not only identification of thoracic abnormalities in patients in whom the disease might be unsuspected but also in differentiating these appearances from co-existent opportunistic infection or other malignancy.

When thoracic involvement is the predominant site of presentation, thoracic symptoms of cough, dyspnea, and hemoptysis are common as opposed to patients in whom the chest is a secondary area of disease (216,217). In these instances of secondary involvement, it is typical for less than 20% of the overall tumor bulk to be intrathoracic.

Multiple sites of nodal enlargement is a common feature in patients with HIV. It is worthwhile to note that persistent generalized lymphadenopathy, a histological benign hyperplasia of nodes (clinically defined as persistent enlargement of lymph nodes at two or more extrainguinal sites for more than three months), does not frequently involve the mediastinal or hilar region. Therefore, enlarged mediastinal nodes in HIV should not be considered reactive as they are likely to be secondary to one of the common causes of adenopathy: mycobacterial disease, Kaposi's sarcoma, or ARL (215). Although massive adenopathy does occur in ARL, markedly enlarged lymph node enlargement is not a common feature of this entity. Even though CT does exhibit more nodal enlargement than seen on CXR, still only 25% are significantly large. This contrasts with marked nodal enlargement common in non-AIDS related lymphoma. Very large nodes, particularly if necrotic, should raise the possibility of mycobacterial disease (214,221,222). Hypervascular nodes can occur in both KS and Castleman's disease. Calcified nodes are not common and more indicative of chronic PCP infection.

Pulmonary ARL nodules remain difficult to characterize despite CT (223). The nodules of lymphoma are typically well defined, differentiating them from the ill-defined nodules of Kaposi's sarcoma (214). Large nodules, which may cavitate, do however overlap in appearance with mycobacterial and fungal disease. Indeed these cases are not infrequently initially misdiagnosed as invasive aspergillosis (217).

A factor that is perhaps contributory to the poor early detection of ARL is the very poor diagnostic yield of bronchoalveolar lavage and bronchial brushings which are commonly used to evaluate patients with HIV (216,224). Conversely, transbronchial biopsy and especially percutaneous needle biopsy or open lung biopsy are frequently diagnostic (174,216,224). CT evaluation is helpful in either directly guiding biopsy or identifying the best site for non-radiological intervention. Pleural effusions in ARL are always exudative, frequently bloody and with very high LDH levels. In contrast to the reported very low diagnostic rates for pleural aspiration (11%) and non-thoracoscopic pleural biopsy (15%) in non-HIV patients with lymphoma, in ARL these procedures have high diagnostic yields (75% and 100%, respectively) (216).

In summary, the diagnosis of ARL requires a high index of suspicion. Lymphoma should be considered in patients when there is an unexplained pleural effusion or a persistent diffuse interstitial or alveolar air-space process. These cases may be initially confused for PCP or bacterial infection which also frequently co-exist (214).

Key Points: Imaging of AIDS-Related Lymphoma

- Aggressive disease with extranodal involvement is common (>90%)
- Pulmonary involvement: nodules, masses, consolidation, and effusions are common
- Large rapidly enlarging peripheral masses >5 cm are common, 25% cavitate
- Massive mediastinal adenopathy is less common than non-HIV related lymphoma
- Chest wall, pericardial, and cardiac involvement is more common
- Co-existence of opportunistic infections is present in 20% to 30%
- Delayed diagnosis is common; failure to respond to infection regimens requires early biopsy

Imaging of Other HIV-Related Lymphomas
Hodgkin's Disease
Although it is now appreciated that Hodgkin's disease is more common in HIV, there are few studies describing the imaging features of this disease specifically in HIV. Compared to Hodgkin's lymphoma, in the general population patients with HIV-HL have an advanced stage at presentation, frequent B symptoms, frequent extranodal disease, and an aggressive course. The skin, lung, and gastrointestinal tract are frequently involved by extranodal disease, whereas these would be only rarely involved in non-HIV Hodgkin's lymphoma (203).

Castleman's Disease
The appearances of some of the rarer lymphomas occurring only in HIV have been described as case reports or small series. The appearances of multicentric Castleman's disease in HIV have been described as resulting in hepatosplenomegaly with peripheral adenopathy (225). Pulmonary involvement is unusual but similar to lymphocytic interstitial pneumonitis with reticulonodular appearances. One of the hallmarks of this disease is the development of acute onset exacerbation of disease that may resolve spontaneously or in response to chemotherapy within a few days. These MCD "attacks" are characterized by rapid clinical deterioration with concomitant rapid onset radiographic abnormalities. CT demonstrates small volume lymph nodes measuring up to 3 cm with associated effusions. The pulmonary appearances are varied and include both micronodular disease in a perilymphatic distribution, inter- and intralobular septal thickening but also ground glass or consolidative areas (225). These appearances also resolve rapidly matching clinical improvement.

The appearances of *MALTomas* and PTLD-like disease are described as small peribronchovascular nodules measuring 2 to 4 mm or larger discrete nodules. In MALTomas focal areas of ground glass nodules may also occur (226). The presence of an isolated pleural or pericardial effusion without other soft-tissue mass or nodal disease appears to be a typical appearance of rare *primary effusion lymphoma* (227,228).

Lymphocytic Interstitial Pneumonitis (LIP)
The entity of LIP is often confusing and merits mention for purposes of clarification. The disease has several clinical and

pathological presentations. In children, LIP presents with reticulonodular opacities and under the age of 13 is an AIDS-defining diagnosis. The disease usually presents earlier, at age two to three years, and pathologically is a lymphoproliferative response of the bronchial-associated lymphatic tissue (BALT) to HIV infection with or without concomitant EBV infection (215,229). Typical appearances include chronic miliary nodular appearances frequently initially confused with miliary tuberculous infection (226). On both CXR and CT more reticulonodular or ground glass opacities may develop (230).

In adults, the disease has two forms. A pathologically similar disease to children may rarely be seen in HIV-infected adult patients in whom this is not classified as an AIDS-defining diagnosis. Most adult patients with LIP have a disease identical to LIP in patients with autoimmune disease, particularly Sjögren's disease. Although these appearances may be miliary, more typically diffuse peribronchiolar ground glass appearances resembling NSIP, smooth interlobular septal thickening or a combination of thin-walled cysts with small nodules occur (187). In these cases LIP is the result of a polyclonal expansion. Although the literature has previously been confused on this issue, all cases of LIP appear to be due to a polyclonal lymphoid response to a viral or unknown stimulus. There is no risk of transformation to a monoclonal lymphoma in HIV-related LIP (226) and case reports of lymphomatous transformation in non-HIV-related LIP appear to be related to original misclassification of low-grade lymphoma (187,230). As such, the entity is now considered a benign disease entity.

Key Points: Lymphocytic Interstitial Pneumonitis

- AIDS defining in children under age 13 usually presents as miliary nodules
- Not AIDS-defining in adults, identical to autoimmune LIP
- In adults, diffuse or peribronchial ground glass, nodules, and cysts are common
- Polyclonal expansion—no malignant potential in adults with LIP

Summary

- Immune compromise can occur as a result of primary immunosuppressive disease, cancer, or treatments for either
- Infection is the commonest complication in the ICH and is predetermined by the type of immune-deficit and the severity of underlying immunosuppression. In HIV-infection there is a strong predictive relationship to CD4 counts
- BMT is associated with increased risk of opportunistic infection but also other immune-mediated non-infectious complications. Complications are characterized as early (<100 days) or late (>100 days)
- CMV and invasive aspergillosis have surpassed bacterial and PCP infection as the commonest infections in BMT-recipients due to improved antibiotic prophylaxis. The time course of infections is predictable, except when GVHD is present
- Long-term immunosuppression by HIV or in transplant recipients is associated with secondary cancer. The commonest thoracic manifestation in solid organ transplantation is PTLD presenting as pulmonary nodules and adenopathy

- Cancer development in HIV is widespread and not limited to the current AIDS-defining diagnoses of NHL, Kaposi's sarcoma, cervical carcinoma, and LIP in <13 years of age. Lung cancer, Hodgkin's lymphoma, and other multiple tumors are also commoner
- Kaposi's sarcoma has radiologically distinctive features obviating biopsy requirement
- Lung cancer in HIV occurs earlier and is more aggressive with late stage presentation and an upper lobe predominance
- The appearances of immunosuppressive infection, recurrence of original neoplastic disease, development of new malignant disease, and the specific complications of tumor treatment frequently overlap. Radiological interpretation requires a working knowledge of the likely timelines and appearances of these entities, in association with an understanding of the varying clinical factors and presentations

REFERENCES

1. Herber DL, Nagaraj S, Djeu JY, Gabrilovich DI. Mechanism and therapeutic reversal of immune suppression in cancer. Cancer Res 2007; 67: 5067–9.
2. Herber DL. Molecular Targets in Cancer Therapy—Fourth Biennial Meeting. Mechanism and therapeutic reversal of immune suppression in cancer. Idrugs 2007; 10: 227–9.
3. Forrest JV. Radiographic findings in Pneumocystis carinii pneumonia. Radiology 1972; 103: 539–44.
4. Gedroyc WM, Reidy JF. The early chest radiographic changes of Pneumocystis pneumonia. Clin Radiol 1985; 36: 331–4.
5. Seigel R, Wolson AH. The radiographic manifestations of chronic Pneumocystis carinii pneumonia. Am J Roentgenol 1977; 128: 150–2.
6. Opravil M, Marincek B, Fuchs WA, et al. Shortcomings of chest radiography in detecting Pneumocystis carinii pneumonia. J Acq Immune Defic Syndr 1994; 7: 39–45.
7. Gruden JF, Huang L, Turner J, et al. High-resolution CT in the evaluation of clinically suspected Pneumocystis carinii pneumonia in AIDS patients with normal, equivocal, or nonspecific radiographic findings. Am J Roentgenol 1977; 169: 967–75.
8. Crans CA Jr, Boiselle PM. Imaging features of Pneumocystis carinii pneumonia. Crit Rev Diagn Imaging 1999; 40: 251–84.
9. Richards PJ, Riddell L, Reznek RH, et al. High resolution computed tomography in HIV patients with suspected Pneumocystis carinii pneumonia and a normal chest radiograph. Clin Radiol 1996; 51: 689–93.
10. Kuhlman JE, Kavuru M, Fishman EK, Siegelman SS. Pneumocystis carinii pneumonia: spectrum of parenchymal CT findings. Radiology 1990; 175: 711–14.
11. Travis WD, Pittaluga S, Lipschik GY, et al. Atypical pathologic manifestations of Pneumocystis carinii pneumonia in the acquired immune deficiency syndrome. Review of 123 lung biopsies from 76 patients with emphasis on cysts, vascular invasion, vasculitis, and granulomas. Am J Surg Pathol 1990; 14: 615–25.
12. Vogel MN, Brodoefel H, Hierl T, et al. Differences and similarities of cytomegalovirus and pneumocystis pneumonia in

HIV-negative immunocompromised patients thin section CT morphology in the early phase of the disease. Br J Radiol 2007; 80: 516–23.

13. Chow C, Templeton PA, White CS. Lung cysts associated with Pneumocystis carinii pneumonia: radiographic characteristics, natural history, and complications. Am J Roentgenol 1993; 161: 527–31.

14. Datta D, Ali SA, Henken EM, et al. Pneumocystis carinii pneumonia: the time course of clinical and radiographic improvement. Chest 2003; 124: 1820–3.

15. Klein JS, Warnock M, Webb WR, Gamsu G. Cavitating and noncavitating granulomas in AIDS patients with Pneumocystis pneumonitis. Am J Roentgenol 1989; 152: 753–4.

16. Kadakia J, Kiyabu M, Sharma OP, Boylen T. Granulomatous response to Pneumocystis carinii in patients infected with HIV. Sarcoidosis 1993; 10: 44–9.

17. Moran CA, Angritt P. Granulomatous Pneumocystis carinii in AIDS patients. Mil Med 1993; 158: 633–5.

18. Otahbachi M, Nugent K, Buscemi D. Granulomatous Pneumocystis jiroveci Pneumonia in a patient with chronic lymphocytic leukemia: a literature review and hypothesis on pathogenesis. Am J Med Sci 2007; 333: 131–5.

19. Bondoc AY, White DA. Granulomatous Pneumocystis carinii pneumonia in patients with malignancy. Thorax 2002; 57: 435–7.

20. Kester KE, Byrd JC, Rearden TP, et al. Granulomatous Pneumocystis carinii pneumonia in patients with low-grade lymphoid malignancies: a diagnostic dilemma. Clin Infect Dis 1996; 22: 1111–12.

21. Feuerstein IM, Francis P, Raffeld M, Pluda J. Widespread visceral calcifications in disseminated Pneumocystis carinii infection: CT characteristics. J Comp Assist Tomogr 1990; 14: 149–51.

22. Mayor B, Schnyder P, Giron J, et al. Mediastinal and hilar lymphadenopathy due to Pneumocystis carinii infection in AIDS patients: CT features. J Comput Assist Tomogr 1994; 18: 408–11.

23. Gefter WB, Weingrad TR, Epstein DM, Ochs RH, Miller WT. "Semi-invasive" pulmonary aspergillosis: a new look at the spectrum of aspergillus infections of the lung. Radiology 1981; 140: 313–21.

24. Tsukada G, Stark P. Radiographic findings in semi-invasive pulmonary aspergillosis. Semin Respir Infect 1998; 13: 274–6.

25. Kuhlman JE, Fishman EK, Siegelman SS. Invasive pulmonary aspergillosis in acute leukemia: characteristic findings on CT, the CT halo sign, and the role of CT in early diagnosis. Radiology 1985; 157: 611–14.

26. Kuhlman JE, Fishman EK, Burch PA, et al. Invasive pulmonary aspergillosis in acute leukemia. The contribution of CT to early diagnosis and aggressive management. Chest 1987; 92: 95–9.

27. Blum U, Windfuhr M, Buitrago-Tellez C, et al. Invasive pulmonary aspergillosis. MRI, CT, and plain radiographic findings and their contribution for early diagnosis. Chest 1994; 106: 1156–61.

28. Hruban RH, Meziane MA, Zerhouni EA, et al. Radiologic-pathologic correlation of the CT halo sign in invasive pulmonary aspergillosis. J Comput Assist Tomogr 1987; 11: 534–6.

29. Kuhlman JE, Fishman EK, Burch PA, et al. CT of invasive pulmonary aspergillosis. Am J Roentgenol 1988; 150: 1015–20.

30. Kim MJ, Lee KS, Kim J, et al. Crescent sign in invasive pulmonary aspergillosis: frequency and related CT and clinical factors. J Comput Assist Tomogr 2001; 25: 305–10.

31. Greene RE, Schlamm HT, Oestmann JW, et al. Imaging findings in acute invasive pulmonary aspergillosis: clinical significance of the halo sign. Clin Infect Dis 2007; 44: 373–9.

32. Gefter WB, Albelda SM, Talbot GH, et al. Invasive pulmonary aspergillosis and acute leukemia. Limitations in the diagnostic utility of the air crescent sign. Radiology 1985; 157: 605–10.

33. Brodoefel H, Vogel M, Hebart H, et al. Long-term CT follow-up in 40 non-HIV immunocompromised patients with invasive pulmonary aspergillosis: kinetics of CT morphology and correlation with clinical findings and outcome. Am J Roentgenol 2006; 187: 404–13.

34. Escuissato DL, Gasparetto EL, Marchiori E, et al. Pulmonary infections after bone marrow transplantation: high-resolution CT findings in 111 patients. Am J Roentgenol 2005; 185: 608–15.

35. Worthy SA, Flint JD, Muller NL. Pulmonary complications after bone marrow transplantation: high-resolution CT and pathologic findings. Radiographics 1997; 17: 1359–71.

36. Gosselin MV, Adams RH. Pulmonary complications in bone marrow transplantation. J Thorac Imag 2002; 17: 132–44.

37. Miller WT Jr, Sais GJ, Frank I, et al. Pulmonary aspergillosis in patients with AIDS. Clinical and radiographic correlations. Chest 1994; 105: 37–44.

38. Staples CA, Kang EY, Wright JL, Phillips P, Muller NL. Invasive pulmonary aspergillosis in AIDS: radiographic, CT, and pathologic findings. Radiology 1995; 196: 409–14.

39. Carratalà J, Rosón B, Fernández-Sevilla A, Alcaide F, Gudiol F. Bacteremic pneumonia in neutropenic patients with cancer: causes, empirical antibiotic therapy, and outcome. Arch Intern Med 1998; 158: 868–72.

40. Heussel CP, Kauczor HU, Ullmann AJ. Pneumonia in neutropenic patients. Eur Radiol 2004; 14: 256–71.

41. Maschmeyer G. Pneumonia in febrile neutropenic patients: radiologic diagnosis. Curr Opin Oncol 2001; 13: 229–35.

42. Baron AL, Steinbach LS, LeBoit PE, et al. Osteolytic lesions and bacillary angiomatosis in HIV infection: radiologic differentiation from AIDS-related Kaposi sarcoma. Radiology 1990; 177: 77–81.

43. Moore EH, Russell LA, Klein JS, et al. Bacillary angiomatosis in patients with AIDS: multiorgan imaging findings. Radiology 1995; 197: 67–72.

44. Heussel CP, Kauczor HU, Heussel G, et al. Early detection of pneumonia in febrile neutropenic patients: use of thin-section CT. Am J Roentgenol 1997; 169: 1347–53.

45. Jochelson MS, Altschuler J, Stomper PC. The yield of chest radiography in febrile and neutropenic patients. Ann Intern Med 1986; 105: 708–9.

46. Heussel CP, Kauczor HU, Heussel GE, et al. Pneumonia in febrile neutropenic patients and in bone marrow and blood stem-cell transplant recipients: use of high-resolution computed tomography. J Clin Oncol 1999; 17: 796–805.

47. Barloon TJ, Galvin JR, Mori M, Stanford W, Gingrich RD. High-resolution ultrafast chest CT in the clinical management of febrile bone marrow transplant patients with normal or nonspecific chest roentgenograms. Chest 1991; 99: 928–33.

48. Mrose HE, DeLuca SA. Septic emboli. Am Fam Physician 1987; 35: 147–8.

49. Kuhlman JE, Fishman EK, Teigen C. Pulmonary septic emboli: diagnosis with CT. Radiology 1990; 174: 211–13.

50. Kwon WJ, Jeong YJ, Kim KI, et al. Computed tomographic features of pulmonary septic emboli: comparison of causative microorganisms. J Comput Assist Tomogr 2007; 31: 390–4.

51. Huang RM, Naidich DP, Lubat E, et al. Septic pulmonary emboli: CT-radiographic correlation. Am J Roentgenol 1989; 153: 41–5.

52. Gomez ML, Gomez-Raposo C, Lobo Samper F. Frequency, risk factors, and trends for venous thromboembolism among hospitalized cancer patients. Cancer 2008; 113: 223–4.

53. Khorana AA, Francis CW, Culakova E, Kuderer NM, Lyman GH. Frequency, risk factors, and trends for venous thromboembolism among hospitalized cancer patients. Cancer 2007; 110: 2339–46.

54. Engelke C, Manstein P, Rummeny EJ, Marten K. Suspected and incidental pulmonary embolism on multidetector-row CT: analysis of technical and morphological factors influencing the diagnosis in a cross-sectional cancer centre patient cohort. Clin Radiol 2006; 61: 71–80.

55. Paddon AJ. Incidental pulmonary embolism detected by routine CT in patients with cancer. Cancer Imaging 2005; 5: 25–6.

56. Gutierrez J, Miralles R, Coll J, et al. Radiographic findings in pulmonary tuberculosis: the influence of human immunodeficiency virus infection. Eur J Radiol 1991; 12: 234–7.

57. de Albuquerque Mde F, Albuquerque SC, Campelo AR, et al. Radiographic features of pulmonary tuberculosis in patients infected by HIV: is there an objective indicator of co-infection? Rev Soc Bras Med Trop 2001; 34: 369–72.

58. Laissy JP, Cadi M, Cinqualbre A, et al. Mycobacterium tuberculosis versus nontuberculous mycobacterial infection of the lung in AIDS patients: CT and HRCT patterns. J Comput Assist Tomogr 1997; 21: 312–17.

59. Keiper MD, Beumont M, Elshami A, Langlotz CP, Miller WT Jr. CD4 T lymphocyte count and the radiographic presentation of pulmonary tuberculosis. A study of the relationship between these factors in patients with human immunodeficiency virus infection. Chest 1995; 107: 74–80.

60. Stanley MW, Horwitz CA, Burton LG, Weisser JA. Negative images of bacilli and mycobacterial infection: a study of fine-needle aspiration smears from lymph nodes in patients with AIDS. Diagn Cytopathol 1990; 6: 118–21.

61. Ahmed AJ, Gateley A, D'Alonzo G. Diagnosis of pulmonary tuberculosis complicating HIV infection: superiority of sputum smear over bronchoalveolar lavage. South Med J 1992; 85: 444–5.

62. Kvale PA, Hansen NI, Markowitz N, et al. Routine analysis of induced sputum is not an effective strategy for screening persons infected with human immunodeficiency virus for Mycobacterium tuberculosis or Pneumocystis carinii. Pulmonary Complications of HIV Infection Study Group. Clin Infect Dis 1994; 19: 410–16.

63. Cathebras PJ, Bouchou K, Rousset H. Pulmonary Mycobacterium avium intracellulare with transient CD4+ T-lymphocytopenia without HIV infection. Eur J Med 1993; 2: 509–10.

64. Levine B, Chaisson RE. Mycobacterium kansasii: a cause of treatable pulmonary disease associated with advanced human immunodeficiency virus (HIV) infection. Ann Intern Med 1991; 114: 861–8.

65. Fishman JE, Schwartz DS, Sais GJ. Mycobacterium kansasii pulmonary infection in patients with AIDS: spectrum of chest radiographic findings. Radiology 1997; 204: 171–5.

66. McGuinness G, Scholes JV, Garay SM, et al. Cytomegalovirus pneumonitis: spectrum of parenchymal CT findings with pathologic correlation in 21 AIDS patients. Radiology 1994; 192: 451–9.

67. Leung AN, Gosselin MV, Napper CH, et al. Pulmonary infections after bone marrow transplantation: clinical and radiographic findings. Radiology 1999; 210: 699–710.

68. Wilczek B, Wilczek HE, Heurlin N, Tydén G, Aspelin P. Prognostic significance of pathological chest radiography in transplant patients affected by cytomegalovirus and/or pneumocystis carinii. Acta Radiol 1996; 37: 727–31.

69. Patz EF Jr, Peters WP, Goodman PC. Pulmonary drug toxicity following high-dose chemotherapy with autologous bone marrow transplantation: CT findings in 20 cases. J Thorac Imaging 1994; 9: 129–34.

70. Folz RJ. Mechanisms of lung injury after bone marrow transplantation. Am J Resp Cell Mol Biol 1999; 20: 1097–9.

71. Leiper AD. Non-endocrine late complications of bone marrow transplantation in childhood: part I. Br J Haematol 2002; 118: 3–22.

72. Soubani AO, Miller KB, Hassoun PM. Pulmonary complications of bone marrow transplantation. Chest 1996; 109: 1066–77.

73. Eikenberry M, Bartakova H, Defor T, et al. Natural history of pulmonary complications in children after bone marrow transplantation. Biol Blood Marrow Transplant 2005; 11: 56–64.

74. Benya EC, Goldman S. Bone marrow transplantation in children. Imaging assessment of complications. Pediatr Clin North Am 1997; 44: 741–61.

75. Roychowdhury M, Pambuccian SE, Aslan DL, et al. Pulmonary complications after bone marrow transplantation: an autopsy study from a large transplantation center. Arch Pathol Lab Med 2005; 129: 366–71.

76. Barton T, Collis T, Stadtmauer E, Schuster M. Infectious complications the year after autologous bone marrow transplantation or peripheral stem cell transplantation for treatment of breast cancer. Clin Infect Dis 2001; 32: 391–5.

77. Levine DS, Navarro OM, Chaudry G, Doyle JJ, Blaser SI. Imaging the complications of bone marrow transplantation in children. Radiographics 2007; 27: 307–24.

78. Wah TM, Moss HA, Robertson RJ, Barnard DL. Pulmonary complications following bone marrow transplantation. Br J Radiol 2003; 76: 373–9.

79. Khurshid I, Anderson LC. Non-infectious pulmonary complications after bone marrow transplantation. Postgrad Med J 2002; 78: 257–62.

80. Clark JG, Hansen JA, Hertz MI, et al. NHLBI workshop summary. Idiopathic pneumonia syndrome after bone marrow transplantation. Am Rev Respir Dis 1993; 147: 1601–6.

81. Sullivan KM, Kopecky KJ, Jocom J, et al. Immunomodulatory and antimicrobial efficacy of intravenous immunoglobulin in bone marrow transplantation. N Engl J Med 1990; 323: 705–12.

82. Crawford SW, Hackman RC. Clinical course of idiopathic pneumonia after bone marrow transplantation. Am Rev Respir Dis 1993; 147: 1393–400.

83. Witte RJ, Gurney JW, Robbins RA, et al. Diffuse pulmonary alveolar hemorrhage after bone marrow transplantation: radiographic findings in 39 patients. Am J Roentgenol 1991; 157: 461–4.

84. Feinstein MB, Mokhtari M, Ferreiro R, Stover DE, Jakubowski A. Fiberoptic bronchoscopy in allogeneic bone marrow transplantation: findings in the era of serum cytomegalovirus antigen surveillance. Chest 2001; 120: 1094–100.

85. Dunagan DP, Baker AM, Hurd DD, Haponik EF. Bronchoscopic evaluation of pulmonary infiltrates following bone marrow transplantation. Chest 1997; 111: 135–41.

86. Busca A, Saroglia EM, Giacchino M, et al. Analysis of early infectious complications in pediatric patients undergoing bone marrow transplantation. Support Care Cancer 1999; 7: 253–9.

87. Griese M, Rampf U, Hofmann D, et al. Pulmonary complications after bone marrow transplantation in children: twenty-four years of experience in a single pediatric center. Pediatr Pulmonol 2000; 30: 393–401.

88. Kugler JW, Armitage JO, Helms CM, et al. Nosocomial Legionnaires' disease. Occurrence in recipients of bone marrow transplants. Am J Med 1983; 74: 281–8.

89. Saavedra S, Jarque I, Sanz GF, et al. Infectious complications in patients undergoing unrelated donor bone marrow transplantation: experience from a single institution. Clin Microbiol Infect 2002; 8: 725–33.

90. Sakamaki H, Yuasa K, Goto H, et al. Comparison of cytomegalovirus (CMV) antigenemia and CMV in bronchoalveolar lavage fluid for diagnosis of CMV pulmonary infection after bone marrow transplantation. Bone Marrow Transplant 1997; 20: 143–7.

91. Soubani AO, Qureshi MA. Invasive pulmonary aspergillosis following bone marrow transplantation: risk factors and diagnostic aspect. Haematologia 2002; 32: 427–37.

92. Yokoi T, Hirabayashi N, Ito M, et al. Broncho-bronchiolitis obliterans as a complication of bone marrow transplantation: a clinicopathological study of eight autopsy cases. Nagoya BMT Group. Virchows Arch 1997; 431: 275–82.

93. Sargent MA, Cairns RA, Murdoch MJ, et al. Obstructive lung disease in children after allogeneic bone marrow transplantation: evaluation with high-resolution CT. Am J Roentgenol 1995; 164: 693–6.

94. Ooi GC, Peh WC, Ip M. High-resolution computed tomography of bronchiolitis obliterans syndrome after bone marrow transplantation. Respiration 1998; 65: 187–91.

95. Kumar S, Tefferi A. Spontaneous pneumomediastinum and subcutaneous emphysema complicating bronchiolitis obliterans after allogeneic bone marrow transplantation—case report and review of literature. Ann Hematol 2001; 80: 430–5.

96. Sverzellati N, Zompatori M, Poletti V, Geddes DM, Hansell DM. Small chronic pneumothoraces and pulmonary parenchymal abnormalities after bone marrow transplantation. J Thorac Imag 2007; 22: 230–4.

97. Cunningham I. Pulmonary infections after bone marrow transplant. Semin Resp Infect 1992; 7: 132–8.

98. Morehead RS. Bronchiectasis in bone marrow transplantation. Thorax 1997; 52: 392–3.

99. Gulbahce HE, Manivel JC, Jessurun J. Pulmonary cytolytic thrombi: a previously unrecognized complication of bone marrow transplantation. Am J Surg Pathol 2000; 24: 1147–52.

100. Pihusch R, Salat C, Schmidt E, et al. Hemostatic complications in bone marrow transplantation: a retrospective analysis of 447 patients. Transplantation 2002; 74: 1303–9.

101. Kanda Y, Takahashi T, Imai Y, et al. Bronchiolitis obliterans organizing pneumonia after syngeneic bone marrow transplantation for acute lymphoblastic leukemia. Bone Marrow Transplant 1997; 19: 1251–3.

102. Baron FA, Hermanne JP, Dowlati A, et al. Bronchiolitis obliterans organizing pneumonia and ulcerative colitis after allogeneic bone marrow transplantation. Bone Marrow Transplant 1998; 21: 951–4.

103. Dodd JD, Muller NL. Bronchiolitis obliterans organizing pneumonia after bone marrow transplantation: high-resolution computed tomography findings in 4 patients. J Comput Assist Tomogr 2005; 29: 540–3.

104. Wilczynski SW, Erasmus JJ, Petros WP, Vredenburgh JJ, Folz RJ. Delayed pulmonary toxicity syndrome following high-dose chemotherapy and bone marrow transplantation for breast cancer. Am J Respir Crit Care Med 1998; 157: 565–73.

105. Cerveri I, Zoia MC, Fulgoni P, et al. Late pulmonary sequelae after childhood bone marrow transplantation. Thorax 1999; 54: 131–5.

106. Cerveri I, Fulgoni P, Giorgiani G, et al. Lung function abnormalities after bone marrow transplantation in children: has the trend recently changed? Chest 2001; 120: 1900–6.

107. Clark JG, Crawford SW. Diagnostic approaches to pulmonary complications of marrow transplantation. Chest 1987; 91: 477–9.

108. McLoud TC, Naidich DP. Thoracic disease in the immunocompromised patient. Radiol Clin North Am 1992; 30: 525–54.

109. Graham NJ, Muller NL, Miller RR, Shepherd JD. Intrathoracic complications following allogeneic bone marrow transplantation: CT findings. Radiology 1991; 181: 153–6.

110. Schueller G, Matzek W, Kalhs P, Schaefer-Prokop C. Pulmonary infections in the late period after allogeneic bone marrow transplantation: chest radiography versus computed tomography. Eur J Radiol 2005; 53: 489–94.

111. Mori M, Galvin JR, Barloon TJ, Gingrich RD, Stanford W. Fungal pulmonary infections after bone marrow transplantation: evaluation with radiography and CT. Radiology 1991; 178: 721–6.

112. Ben-Ari J, Yaniv I, Nahum E, et al. Yield of bronchoalveolar lavage in ventilated and non-ventilated children after bone marrow transplantation. Bone Marrow Transplant 2001; 27: 191–4.

113. Snyder CL, Ramsay NK, McGlave PB, Ferrell KL, Leonard AS. Diagnostic open-lung biopsy after bone marrow transplantation. J Pediatr Surg 1990; 25: 871–7.

114. Hong SK, Hwang S, Lee SG, et al. Pulmonary complications following adult liver transplantation. Transplantation Proc 2006; 38: 2979–81.

115. O'Brien JD, Ettinger NA. Pulmonary complications of liver transplantation. Clin Chest Med 1996; 17: 99–114.

116. Kotloff RM. Noninfectious pulmonary complications of liver, heart, and kidney transplantation. Clin Chest Med; 26: 623–9.

117. Jimenez Perez M, Olmedo Martin R, Marin Garcia D, et al. Pulmonary toxicity associated with sirolimus therapy in liver transplantation. Gastroenterol Hepatol 2006; 29: 616–18.

118. Golfieri R, Giampalma E, Morselli Labate AM, et al. Pulmonary complications of liver transplantation: radiological appearance and statistical evaluation of risk factors in 300 cases. Eur Radiol 2000; 10: 1169–83.

119. Saner FH, Olde Damink SW, Pavlakovic G, et al. Pulmonary and blood stream infections in adult living donor and cadaveric liver transplant patients. Transplantation 2008; 85: 1564–8.

120. Knollmann FD, Mäurer J, Bechstein WO, et al. Pulmonary disease in liver transplant recipients. Spectrum of CT features. Acta Radiol 2000; 41: 230–6.

121. Singh N, Gayowski T, Wagener M, Marino IR, Yu VL. Pulmonary infections in liver transplant recipients receiving tacrolimus. Changing pattern of microbial etiologies. Transplantation 1996; 61: 396–401.

122. Singh N, Gayowski T, Wagener MM, Marino IR. Pulmonary infiltrates in liver transplant recipients in the intensive care unit. Transplantation 1999; 67: 1138–44.

123. Fishman JE, Rabkin JM. Thoracic radiology in kidney and liver transplantation. J Thorac Imaging 2002; 17: 122–31.

124. Paterson DL, Singh N, Gayowski T, Marino IR. Pulmonary nodules in liver transplant recipients. Medicine 1998; 77: 50–8.

125. Grulich AE, van Leeuwen MT, Falster MO, Vajdic CM. Incidence of cancers in people with HIV/AIDS compared with immunosuppressed transplant recipients: a meta-analysis. Lancet 2007; 370: 59–67.

126. Sheil AG. Cancer in organ transplant recipients: part of an induced immune deficiency syndrome. Br Med J (Clin Res Ed) 1984; 288: 659–61.

127. Birkeland SA. Malignant tumors in renal transplant patients. The Scandia transplant material. Cancer 1983; 51: 1571–5.

128. Ahmed Z, Marshall MB, Kucharczuk JC, Kaiser LR, Shrager JB. Lung cancer in transplant recipients: a single-institution experience. Arch Surg 2004; 139: 902–6.

129. Jimenez C, Marqués E, Manrique A, et al. Incidence and risk factors of development of lung tumors after liver transplantation. Transplant Proc 2005; 37: 3970–2.

130. Andreone P, Gramenzi A, Lorenzini S, et al. Posttransplantation lymphoproliferative disorders. Arch Intern Med 2003; 163: 1997–2004.

131. Leblond V, Dhedin N, Mamzer Bruneel MF, et al. Identification of prognostic factors in 61 patients with posttransplantation lymphoproliferative disorders. J Clin Oncol 2001; 19: 772–8.

132. Nalesnik MA. Posttransplantation lymphoproliferative disorders (PTLD): current perspectives. Semin Thorac Cardiovasc Surg 1996; 8: 139–48.

133. Tsao L, Hsi ED. The clinicopathologic spectrum of posttransplantation lymphoproliferative disorders. Arch Pathol Lab Med 2007; 131: 1209–18.

134. Roithmaier S, Haydon AM, Loi S, et al. Incidence of malignancies in heart and/or lung transplant recipients: a single-institution experience. J Heart Lung Transplant 2007; 26: 845–9.

135. Saadat A, Einollahi B, Ahmadzad-Asl MA, et al. Posttransplantation lymphoproliferative disorders in renal transplant recipients: report of over 20 years of experience. Transplant Proc 2007; 39: 1071–3.

136. Kuhlman JE. Thoracic imaging in heart transplantation. J Thorac Imaging 2003; 17: 113–121.

137. Smith C, Lilly S, Mann KP, et al. AIDS-related malignancies. Ann Med 1998; 30: 323–44.

138. Wistuba II, Behrens C, Gazdar AF. Pathogenesis of non-AIDS-defining cancers: a review. AIDS Patient Care STDS 1999; 13: 415–26.

139. Maiman M, Fruchter RG, Clark M, et al. Cervical cancer as an AIDS-defining illness. Obstet Gynecol 1997; 89: 76–80.

140. Lohse N, Hansen AB, Pedersen G, et al. Survival of persons with and without HIV infection in Denmark, 1995–2005. Ann Intern Med 2007; 146: 87–95.

141. Moore RD, Chaisson RE. Natural history of HIV infection in the era of combination antiretroviral therapy. AIDS 1999; 13: 1933–42.

142. Palella FJ Jr, Delaney KM, Moorman AC, et al. Declining morbidity and mortality among patients with advanced human immunodeficiency virus infection. HIV Outpatient Study Investigators. N Engl J Med 1998; 338: 853–60.

143. Brodt HR, Kamps BS, Gute P, et al. Changing incidence of AIDS-defining illnesses in the era of antiretroviral combination therapy. AIDS 1997; 11: 1731–8.

144. Newnham A, Harris J, Evans HS, Evans BG, Moller H. The risk of cancer in HIV-infected people in southeast England: a cohort study. Br J Cancer 2005; 92: 194–200.

145. Grulich AE, Li Y, McDonald A, et al. Rates of non-AIDS-defining cancers in people with HIV infection before and after AIDS diagnosis. AIDS 2002; 16: 1155–61.

146. Biggar RJ, Chaturvedi AK, Goedert JJ, Engels EA, Study HACM. AIDS-related cancer and severity of immunosuppression in persons with AIDS. J Natl Cancer Inst 2007; 99: 962–72.

147. Engels EA, Pfeiffer RM, Goedert JJ, et al. Trends in cancer risk among people with AIDS in the United States 1980-2002. AIDS 2006; 20: 1645–54.

148. Patel P, Hanson DL, Sullivan PS, et al. Incidence of types of cancer among HIV-infected persons compared with the general population in the United States, 1992–2003. Ann Intern Med 2008; 148: 728–36.

149. Braun MA, Killam DA, Remick SC, Ruckdeschel JC. Lung cancer in patients seropositive for human immunodeficiency virus. Radiology 1990; 175: 341–3.

150. Bagheri K, Connell RK, Safirstein BH. Lung cancer in a drug addict seropositive for human immunodeficiency virus. Am J Roentgenol 1992; 158: 210.

151. Fraire AE, Awe RJ. Lung cancer in association with human immunodeficiency virus infection. Cancer 1992; 70: 432–6.

152. Remick SC. Lung cancer. An HIV-related neoplasm or a coincidental finding? Chest 1992; 102: 1643–4.

153. Sridhar KS, Flores MR, Raub WA Jr, Saldana M. Lung cancer in patients with human immunodeficiency virus infection compared with historic control subjects. Chest 1992; 102: 1704–8.

154. Engels EA, Brock MV, Chen J, et al. Elevated incidence of lung cancer among HIV-infected individuals. J Clin Oncol 2006; 24: 1383–8.

155. Chaturvedi AK, Pfeiffer RM, Chang L, et al. Elevated risk of lung cancer among people with AIDS. AIDS 2007; 21: 207–13.

156. Kirk GD, Merlo C, O'Driscoll P, et al. HIV infection is associated with an increased risk for lung cancer, independent of smoking. Clin Infect Dis 2007; 45: 103–10.

157. Lavole A, Wislez M, Antoine M, et al. Lung cancer, a new challenge in the HIV-infected population. Lung Cancer 2006; 51: 1–11.

158. Spano JP, Massiani MA, Bentata M, et al. Lung cancer in patients with HIV Infection and review of the literature. Med Oncol 2004; 21: 109–15.

159. Sahebjami H. Emphysema-like changes in HIV. Ann Intern Med 1992; 116: 876.

160. Diaz PT, King MA, Pacht ER, et al. Increased susceptibility to pulmonary emphysema among HIV-seropositive smokers. Ann Intern Med 2000; 132: 369–72.

161. Petrache I, Diab K, Knox KS, et al. HIV associated pulmonary emphysema: a review of the literature and inquiry into its mechanism. Thorax 2008; 63: 463–9.

162. Vyzula R, Remick SC. Lung cancer in patients with HIV-infection. Lung Cancer 1996; 15: 325–39.

163. Alshafie MT, Donaldson B, Oluwole SF. Human immunodeficiency virus and lung cancer. Br J Surg 1997; 84: 1068–71.

164. Gruden JF, Webb WR, Yao DC, Klein JS, Sandhu JS. Bronchogenic carcinoma in 13 patients infected with the human immunodeficiency virus (HIV): clinical and radiographic findings. J Thorac Imag 1995; 10: 99–105.

165. Bazot M, Cadranel J, Khalil A, et al. Computed tomographic diagnosis of bronchogenic carcinoma in HIV-infected patients. Lung Cancer 2000; 28: 203–9.

166. Fishman JE, Schwartz DS, Sais GJ, Flores MR, Sridhar KS. Bronchogenic carcinoma in HIV-positive patients: findings on chest radiographs and CT scans. Am J Roentgenol 1995; 164: 57–61.

167. Karp J, Profeta G, Marantz PR, Karpel JP. Lung cancer in patients with immunodeficiency syndrome. Chest 1993; 103: 410–13.

168. Cadranel J, Garfield D, Lavole A, et al. Lung cancer in HIV infected patients: facts, questions and challenges. Thorax 2006; 61: 1000–8.

169. Brock MV, Hooker CM, Engels EA, et al. Delayed diagnosis and elevated mortality in an urban population with HIV and lung cancer: implications for patient care. J Acquir Immune Defic Syndr 2006; 43: 47–55.

170. James JS. Lung cancer: very high death rate with HIV, huge reduction possible with CT screening for early diagnosis. AIDS Treat News 2006; 420: 5–6.

171. Hakimian R, Fang H, Thomas L, Edelman MJ. Lung cancer in HIV-infected patients in the era of highly active antiretroviral therapy. J Thorac Oncol 2007; 2: 268–72.

172. Powles T, Thirwell C, Newsom-Davis T, et al. Does HIV adversely influence the outcome in advanced non-small-cell lung cancer in the era of HAART? Br J Cancer 2003; 89: 457–9.

173. Tenholder MF, Jackson HD. Bronchogenic carcinoma in patients seropositive for human immunodeficiency virus. Chest 1993; 104: 1049–53.

174. Gruden JF, Klein JS, Webb WR. Percutaneous transthoracic needle biopsy in AIDS: analysis in 32 patients. Radiology 1993; 189: 567–71.

175. Scott WW Jr, Kuhlman JE. Focal pulmonary lesions in patients with AIDS: percutaneous transthoracic needle biopsy. Radiology 1991; 180: 419–21.

176. Tan B, Ratner L. The use of new antiretroviral therapy in combination with chemotherapy. Curr Opin Oncol 1997; 9: 455–64.

177. Richman DD, Fischl MA, Grieco MH, et al. The toxicity of azidothymidine (AZT) in the treatment of patients with AIDS and AIDS-related complex. A double-blind, placebo-controlled trial. N Engl J Med 1987; 317: 192–7.

178. Cooper JS, Fried PR, Laubenstein LJ. Initial observations of the effect of radiotherapy on epidemic Kaposi's sarcoma. JAMA 1984; 252: 934–5.

179. Chak LY, Gill PS, Levine AM, et al. Radiation therapy for acquired immunodeficiency syndrome-related Kaposi's sarcoma. J Clin Oncol 1988; 6: 863–7.

180. Leigh BR, Lau DH. Severe esophageal toxicity after thoracic radiation therapy for lung cancer associated with the human immunodeficiency virus: a case report and review of the literature. Am J Clin Oncol 1998; 21: 479–81.

181. Kadri Altundag M, Celik I. Human immunodeficiency virus negative Kaposi sarcoma and lymphoproliferative disorders. Cancer 2000; 88: 708–9.

182. Du MQ, Bacon CM, Isaacson PG. Kaposi sarcoma-associated herpesvirus/human herpesvirus 8 and lymphoproliferative disorders. J Clin Pathol 2007; 60: 1350–7.

183. Lambert M, Gannage M, Karras A, et al. Differences in the frequency and function of HHV8-specific CD8 T cells between asymptomatic HHV8 infection and Kaposi sarcoma. Blood 2006; 108: 3871–80.

184. Guttman-Yassky E, Dubnov J, Kra-Oz Z, et al. Classic Kaposi sarcoma. Which KSHV-seropositive individuals are at risk? Cancer 2006; 106: 413–19.

185. O'Brien TR, Engels EA, Rosenberg PS, Goedert JJ. Relationship between Kaposi sarcoma-associated herpesvirus and HIV. JAMA 2002; 287: 1525–8.

186. Cheung MC, Pantanowitz L, Dezube BJ. AIDS-related malignancies: emerging challenges in the era of highly active antiretroviral therapy. Oncologist 2005; 10: 412–26.

187. Muller NL, Fraser RS, Soo Lee K, Johkoh T. Diseases of the Lung. Radiologic and Pathologic Correlations. Philadelphia: Lippincott Williams & Wilkins, 2003.

188. Davis SD, Henschke CI, Chamides BK, Westcott JL. Intrathoracic Kaposi sarcoma in AIDS patients: radiographic-pathologic correlation. Radiology 1987; 163: 495–500.

189. McCauley DI, Naidich DP, Leitman BS, Reede DL, Laubenstein L. Radiographic patterns of opportunistic lung infections and Kaposi sarcoma in homosexual men. Am J Roentgenol 1982; 139: 653–8.

190. Brown RK, Huberman RP, Vanley G. Pulmonary features of Kaposi sarcoma. Am J Roentgenol 1982; 139: 659–60.

191. Naidich DP, Garay SM, Leitman BS, McCauley DI. Radiographic manifestations of pulmonary disease in the acquired immunodeficiency syndrome (AIDS). Semin Roentgenol 1987; 22: 14–30.

192. Naidich DP, McGuinness G. Pulmonary manifestations of AIDs. CT and radiographic correlations. Radiol Clin North Am 1991; 29: 999–1017.

193. Gruden JF, Huang L, Webb WR, et al. AIDS-related Kaposi sarcoma of the lung: radiographic findings and staging system with bronchoscopic correlation. Radiology 1995; 195: 545–52.

194. Miller RF, Tomlinson MC, Cottrill CP, et al. Bronchopulmonary Kaposi's sarcoma in patients with AIDS. Thorax 1992; 47: 721–5.

195. Hartman TE, Primack SL, Muller NL, Staples CA. Diagnosis of thoracic complications in AIDS: accuracy of CT. Am J Roentgenol 1994; 162: 547–53.

196. Wolff SD, Kuhlman JE, Fishman EK. Thoracic Kaposi sarcoma in AIDS: CT findings. J Comput Assist Tomogr 1993; 17: 60–2.

197. Luburich P, Bru C, Ayuso MC, Azon A, Condom E. Hepatic Kaposi sarcoma in AIDS: US and CT findings. Radiology 1990; 175: 172–4.

198. Kang EY, Staples CA, McGuinness G, Primack SL, Müller NL. Detection and differential diagnosis of pulmonary infections and tumors in patients with AIDS: value of chest radiography versus CT. Am J Roentgenol 1996; 166: 15–19.

199. Edinburgh KJ, Jasmer RM, Huang L, et al. Multiple pulmonary nodules in AIDS: usefulness of CT in distinguishing among potential causes. Radiology 2000; 214: 427–32.

200. Khalil AM, Carette MF, Cadranel JL, et al. Magnetic resonance imaging findings in pulmonary Kaposi's sarcoma: a series of 10 cases. Eur Resp J 1994; 7: 1285–9.

201. Godoy MC, Rouse H, Brown JA, et al. Imaging features of pulmonary Kaposi sarcoma-associated immune reconstitution syndrome. Am J Roentgenol 2007; 189: 956–65.

202. Beral V, Peterman T, Berkelman R, Jaffe H. AIDS-associated non-Hodgkin lymphoma. Lancet 1991; 337: 805–9.

203. Grogg KL, Miller RF, Dogan A. HIV infection and lymphoma. J Clin Pathol 2007; 60: 1365–72.

204. Navarro WH, Kaplan LD. AIDS-related lymphoproliferative disease. Blood 2006; 107: 13–20.

205. Kaplan LD, Straus DJ, Testa MA, et al. Low-dose compared with standard-dose m-BACOD chemotherapy for non-Hodgkin's lymphoma associated with human immunodeficiency virus infection. National Institute of Allergy and Infectious Diseases AIDS Clinical Trials Group. N Engl J Med 1997; 336: 1641–8.

206. Diamond C, Taylor TH, Aboumrad T, Anton-Culver H. Changes in acquired immunodeficiency syndrome-related non-Hodgkin lymphoma in the era of highly active antiretroviral therapy: incidence, presentation, treatment, and survival. Cancer 2006; 106: 128–35.

207. Oriol A, Ribera JM, Brunet S, et al. Highly active antiretroviral therapy and outcome of AIDS-related Burkitt's lymphoma or leukemia. Results of the PETHEMA-LAL3/97 study. Haematologica 2005; 90: 990–2.

208. Oriol A, Ribera JM, Esteve J, et al. Lack of influence of human immunodeficiency virus infection status in the response to therapy and survival of adult patients with mature B-cell lymphoma or leukemia. Results of the PETHEMA-LAL3/97 study. Haematologica 2003; 88: 445–53.

209. Ortega KL, Arzate-Mora N, Ceballos-Salobreña A, Martin-Rico P. Images in HIV/AIDS. Oral plasmablastic lymphoma. AIDS Read 2007; 17: 446–7.

210. Righetti E, Ballon G, Ometto L, et al. Dynamics of Epstein-Barr virus in HIV-1-infected subjects on highly active antiretroviral therapy. AIDS 2002; 16: 63–73.

211. Biggar RJ, Jaffe ES, Goedert JJ, et al. Hodgkin lymphoma and immunodeficiency in persons with HIV/AIDS. Blood 2006; 108: 3786–91.

212. Raphael M, Borisch B, Jaffe ES. Lymphomas associated with infection by the human immunodeficiency virus (HIV). In: Jaffe ES, Harris NL, Stein H, Vardiman JW, eds. World Health Organization Classification of Tumours, Pathology and Genetics of Haematopoietic and Lymphoid Tissues. Lyon, France: IARC Press, 2001: 620–3.

213. Goodman PC. Non-Hodgkin's lymphoma in the acquired immunodeficiency syndrome. J Thorac Imag 1991; 6: 49–52.

214. Sider L, Weiss AJ, Smith MD, VonRoenn JH, Glassroth J. Varied appearance of AIDS-related lymphoma in the chest. Radiology 1989; 171: 629–32.

215. Oldham SA, Barron B, Munden RF, Lamki N, Lamki L. The radiology of the thoracic manifestations of AIDS. Crit Rev Diagn Imaging 1998; 39: 259–338.

216. Eisner MD, Kaplan LD, Herndier B, Stulbarg MS. The pulmonary manifestations of AIDS-related non-Hodgkin's lymphoma. Chest 1996; 110: 729–36.

217. Blunt DM, Padley SP. Radiographic manifestations of AIDS related lymphoma in the thorax. Clin Radiol 1995; 50: 607–12.

218. Collins J, Muller NL, Leung AN, et al. Epstein-Barr-virus-associated lymphoproliferative disease of the lung: CT and histologic findings. Radiology 1998; 208: 749–59.

219. Shin MS, McElvein RB, Listinsky CM, Ho KJ. CT manifestation of non-Hodgkin's lymphoma as a solitary pulmonary nodule in a patient with acquired immunodeficiency syndrome. Clin Imaging 1993; 17: 279–81.

220. Townsend RR. CT of AIDS-related lymphoma. Am J Roentgenol 1991; 156: 969–74.

221. Haramati LB, Choi Y, Widrow CA, Austin JH. Isolated lymphadenopathy on chest radiographs of HIV-infected patients. Clin Radiol 1996; 51: 345–9.

222. Jasmer RM, Gotway MB, Creasman JM, et al. Clinical and radiographic predictors of the etiology of computed tomography-diagnosed intrathoracic lymphadenopathy in HIV-infected patients. J Acquir Immune Defic Syndr 2002; 31: 291–8.

223. Jasmer RM, Edinburgh KJ, Thompson A, et al. Clinical and radiographic predictors of the etiology of pulmonary

nodules in HIV-infected patients. Chest 2000; 117: 1023–30.

224. Bazot M, Cadranel J, Benayoun S, et al. Primary pulmonary AIDS-related lymphoma: radiographic and CT findings. Chest 1999; 116: 1282–6.

225. Guihot A, Couderc LJ, Rivaud E, et al. Thoracic radiographic and CT findings of multicentric Castleman disease in HIV-infected patients. J Thorac Imaging 2007; 22: 207–11.

226. McGuinness G, Scholes JV, Jagirdar JS, et al. Unusual lymphoproliferative disorders in nine adults with HIV or AIDS: CT and pathologic findings. Radiology 1995; 197: 59–65.

227. Ferrozzi F, Tognini G, Mulonzia NW, Bova D, Pavone P. Primary effusion lymphomas in AIDS: CT findings in two cases. Eur Radiol 2001; 11: 623–5.

228. Oza UD, Munn S. Imaging HIV/AIDS. Body cavity-based lymphoma. AIDS Patient Care STDS 2003; 17: 129–32.

229. Heitzman ER. Pulmonary neoplastic and lymphoproliferative disease in AIDS: a review. Radiology 1990; 177: 347–51.

230. Oldham SA, Castillo M, Jacobson FL, Mones JM, Saldana MJ. HIV-associated lymphocytic interstitial pneumonia: radiologic manifestations and pathologic correlation. Radiology 1989; 170: 83–7.

60 The Immunocompromised Host: Abdomen and Pelvis
Roger Chinn and Simon Padley

INTRODUCTION

The immune system is invoked in the prevention of and response to neoplasia (1). Thus any compromise to the immune system may result in an increased risk of malignancy and greater subsequent morbidity.

Congenital immunodeficiency syndromes are very rare. They are not generally associated with increased risk of malignancy. They usually present in childhood or early adulthood with increased infection risk (2). There are a few rare exceptions such as X-linked immunodeficiency with hyper-IgM syndrome in which liver and gastrointestinal malignancies are more common (3).

In contrast, acquired immunodeficiency is relatively common. From a global perspective, malnutrition and infection with tuberculosis are the commonest causes of compromise to the immune system. However, in the context of induction of malignancy, the causes with the biggest impact are infection with human immunodeficiency virus (HIV) and treatment-induced immunodeficiency. It is these two scenarios that will be discussed further in this chapter.

Drug-induced immunodeficiency is utilized to prevent rejection following organ transplantation. However, immunosuppression is an undesirable side-effect of many chemotherapy regimens. Both during and after chemotherapy the risk of malignancy is increased. However the relative risk may return to normal some time after cessation of treatment (4).

The HIV is a retrovirus that infects and destroys or impairs the function of cells of the immune system. Initially asymptomatic, as infection progresses the immune system becomes weaker, creating susceptibility to opportunistic infections and to neoplasia. HIV infection may progress after a variable interval to acquired immunodeficiency syndrome (AIDS). The natural history is for up to 10 to 15 years to pass before an HIV-infected person develops AIDS. With the newer highly active antiretroviral therapy (HAART) this process may well take even longer (5).

In July 2008, the Joint United Nations Programme on HIV/AIDS (UNAIDS) estimated that 33 million people are living with HIV infection (6). The vast majority (22.5 million) live in sub-Saharan Africa; a further 4.9 million in South, East, and South-East Asia; 2.3 million in Europe and Central Asia; 1.9 million in the Caribbean and Latin America; and 1.2 million in North America. Half of these people are women. In 2007, there were an estimated 2.7 million new infections and there were two million deaths attributable directly to the disease.

The vast majority of new HIV infections and AIDS-related deaths have occurred where access to prevention and treatment is inadequate in low or middle income countries. Despite this, the total number of people in North America and Western and Central Europe living with HIV is increasing. This is due to the effects of highly active antiretroviral therapy (HAART) and an increase in the number of new HIV diagnoses in Western Europe since 2002. There is also an important contribution from nationals of low or middle income countries, typically in sub-Saharan Africa, acquiring HIV and then migrating to Europe or the United States.

HIV represents a pandemic which is continuing to grow in importance. Prevalence in adults ranges from 0.1% in East Asia to 5% in sub-Saharan Africa. The epidemic is generalized and sustained in many southern sub-Saharan African countries. In contrast, and excluding this largest patient group, the rest of the world is seeing new infection concentrated primarily among populations most at risk, such as men who have sex with men, injecting drug users, sex workers and their sexual partners.

INCREASED RISK OF MALIGNANCY AND ITS CAUSE IN IMMUNOCOMPROMISED HOSTS

There are three tumors so closely associated with HIV that their presence in the context of HIV infection confers a diagnosis of AIDS upon the patient. These AIDS-defining tumors are Kaposi sarcoma, carcinoma of the uterine cervix, and non-Hodgkin lymphoma (NHL) (7). Recently, several studies have provided longitudinal data and detailed meta-analysis of the literature related to risk of malignancy in immunocompromised patients (8–11). Overall, malignancy occurs at an increased standardized incidence ratio (SIR) of 9.8 in immunocompromised people with HIV/AIDS and a SIR of 2.2 in transplant recipients. When Kaposi sarcoma and NHL are excluded, the SIRs are similar at 1.9 in the HIV group and 1.4 in the transplant group. The pattern of increased risk is much the same in both populations. Increased incidence of tumors in both groups includes Hodgkin's lymphoma, hepatocellular carcinoma, stomach carcinoma, vulval carcinoma, penile carcinoma, anal canal carcinoma, renal carcinoma, leukemia, myeloma, and both non-melanoma and melanoma skin cancers (Figs. 60.1 and 60.2).

It has not been conclusively proven that these increased rates of malignancy deficiency are truly related to immune compromise. Indeed it has been postulated that alternative causes could include lifestyle and other risk factors (12). Increased medical surveillance in immunocompromised people could also result in increased detection of malignancy. However, this suggestion is not borne out by a higher incidence rate of prostate or breast carcinoma; two tumors most commonly diagnosed through screening programs.

Many of the tumors that are more common in immunocompromised populations have a confirmed or putative association with an infectious agent (13). Epstein Barr virus (EBV) has been causally linked with non-Hodgkin and Hodgkin's lymphoma (14). *Helicobacter pylori* are the cause of 60% of stomach cancers (15). Hepatitis B and C viruses (HBV and HCV) are both causes of hepatocellular carcinoma (16). Human herpes virus 8 (HHV8) is a necessary factor in the etiology of Kaposi sarcoma (17). Human papilloma virus (HPV) is the causative agent for cancer of the cervix and for other anogenital tumors (18).

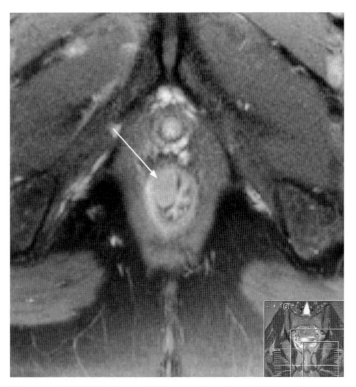

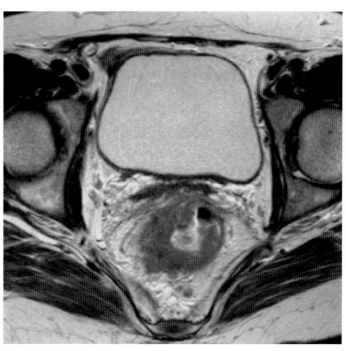

Figure 60.1 Axial MR T1 image with fat saturation after gadolinium enhancement demonstrating a small anal squamous cell carcinoma (arrow) in a patient with AIDS.

Figure 60.2 Axial MR T2 image of a locally invasive rectal adenocarcinoma with mesorectal nodal involvement in a renal transplant recipient. *Source*: Image courtesy of Dr. D Blunt.

Overall there is little variation between the types of malignancy occurring at greater rates in HIV infection compared to other causes of immunodeficiency. However, in HIV infection, there is an increased rate of Kaposi sarcoma, anogenital tumors, and hepatocellular carcinoma which can be explained by lifestyle differences (9).

Whilst the majority of HIV-related malignancies have shown a reduction of incidence in the post-HAART era, an increasing rate of anal carcinoma has been recorded (10). This may be explained by lack of effect of HAART upon the causative role of HPV in anal intraepithelial neoplasia (AIN). When coupled with the improved survival that HAART confers there has been a consequent increase in the numbers progressing from AIN to anal carcinoma.

In HIV patients there is conflicting evidence regarding the risk of colo-rectal carcinoma (8–11). It may well be that the incidence will increase with longer survival. In contrast to virally mediated tumors, other common epithelial cancers, such as prostate or ovarian tumors, do not occur with greater frequency in either group. Currently these tumors are not believed to have a causative infectious agent.

THE CLINICAL AND IMAGING FEATURES SPECIFIC TO IMMUNODEFICIENCY RELATED MALIGNANCY WITHIN THE ABDOMEN AND PELVIS

The manifestations of most malignant tumors in patients with immunocompromise do not generally differ from patterns described in patients with a competent immune system. This is particularly true of metastatic disease occurring in the abdomen or pelvis.

The majority of tumors types are therefore discussed adequately within dedicated chapters. In the remainder of this chapter consideration is given to the two most common malignancies seen in immunocompromise: Kaposi sarcoma and lymphoma.

Kaposi Sarcoma

Kaposi sarcoma (KS) is worthy of specific focus because of its relative rarity in the general population. Kaposi sarcoma is a malignant neoplasm originating in vascular endothelium and so may affect a wide variety of anatomical sites. Most frequently it presents as a skin lesion. In all cases it is associated with infection with human herpes virus 8 (HHV8). It is the most common malignancy in AIDS. Standardized incidence ratios in HIV-infected patients are 3640 and in the transplant population 208 (9). This greatly increased risk in HIV infection correlates further with the severity of immune deficiency and increasing risk of exposure to HHV8. In the most frequently affected group (men who have sex with men) the strongest correlates of risk are the number of sexual partners followed by the degree of immune deficiency (19). Mucous membranes and lymph nodes may also be involved at the time of presentation.

Usually later on in disease progression and immune decline, Kaposi sarcoma may involve any part of the gastrointestinal tract (20). This is often asymptomatic but may result in anemia from hemorrhage or bowel obstruction (21). A single case of jejunal perforation has been reported (22).

In the stomach, small and large bowel, discrete submucosal nodules will be present. These may be identified and, if required, biopsied at endoscopy. As disease progresses lesions may develop central umbilication. Eventually focal and then more diffuse wall

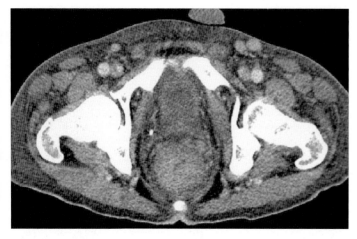

Figure 60.3 CT Scan of Kaposi sarcoma in the rectum with enhancing nodes in inguinal regions in a patient with AIDS.

thickening will occur. Lymph node involvement is often present within the mesentery, retroperitoneum, pelvis, and inguinal region (Fig. 60.3).

Solid organ involvement does occur in about one third of patients with skin disease. Kaposi sarcoma represents the most common intrahepatic neoplasm in AIDS found in 32% of patients at autopsy (23).

If the cause of immune deficiency can be removed or treated, there may be regression of lesions. HIV-infected patients yet to be treated will benefit from HAART. If immune reconstitution is achieved, the lesions may undergo spontaneous regression or at least stabilize. Immunocompromised transplant patients with KS may benefit from a change of the immune suppressant agent (24,25). Chemotherapeutic regimens and immunotherapy with interferon have to be carefully tailored to the individual's response. The combination of the disease, the toxic effects of the agents, the cause of immune suppression, and the effect of primary treatments such as HAART can be debilitating.

Imaging Investigation of Kaposi Sarcoma
Imaging provides a mechanism for localization and staging of disease as well as aiding characterization of disease type. Identification of common co-morbid conditions and possible differential diagnoses is important. Treatment-related conditions may also co-exist. For example, both renal stones and benign pancreatic disease have been linked to various antiretroviral therapies. The most common non-malignant causes of abdominal symptoms, together with associated imaging findings, are described in Table 60.1 (26).

Contrast luminal studies are of more limited utility in the immunocompromised population than in the general population due to a wide differential diagnosis and high levels of co-morbidity. Ultrasound (US) is often utilized as a preliminary investigation, but in our practice CT scanning is most frequently utilized and provides the means to assess solid and hollow organs in both abdomen and pelvis in a single rapid examination. Multidetector technology with multiplanar reconstruction of datasets has increased diagnostic yield further. MR is reserved as an important problem-solving tool.

Imaging Findings in Kaposi Sarcoma
Barium meal and follow-through studies may demonstrate focal nodular or diffuse wall thickening in the stomach or small bowel wall. Larger lesions may develop central punctuate ulceration and have a target appearance (27).

US is rarely useful since focal lesions in solid organs are not common. If visible on US they will appear as small non-specific hyperechoic foci.

Multidetector CT scanning will usually demonstrate bowel wall thickening, when present, most effectively if water or positive oral contrast has been utilized to define the bowel lumen. In this case it can even demonstrate more focal nodular lesions (Fig. 60.4). Lymph node enlargement is usually readily appreciated even allowing for the relatively scant amount of visceral related fat in these patients. The nodes tend to be hypervascular and consequently enhance avidly on CT after administration of IV contrast medium (28) (Fig. 60.5). It should be remembered that while nodal enhancement is a useful sign it is not specific, and nodal enhancement may be seen in other conditions including multicentric Castleman's disease (MCD).

Hepatosplenomegaly, when present, is usually not associated with focal lesions. Periportal edema may be evident. When focal lesions are present in these organs they are usually in the 5 to 12 mm range, closely associated with portal vein tracts when in the liver and hypoattenuating after contrast enhancement (28,29). On delayed scans enhancement of lesions can occur which can render them indistinguishable from hemangiomata. MRI does not usually provide added value in the characterization of either gut lesions or solid organ disease.

Monitoring response to treatment is usually undertaken with CT. On occasion, despite an early clinical response, there may be subsequent paradoxical increase in disease load. This can be seen if there is significant improvement in the immune status after the initiation of HAART. This process is one manifestation of immune reconstitution inflammatory syndrome (IRIS), which may influence the presentation and progress of a variety of HIV-related conditions (30). For example, IRIS occurs as a response to the antigens of latent infection such as mycobacteria or cytomegalovirus whether the organism is alive or dead. When IRIS occurs in Kaposi sarcoma, an aggressive form of disease may result in significant symptomatic decline (31) and, should this occur, chemotherapy may be required but HAART need not be halted. Imaging appearances may deteriorate.

While much less frequent, Kaposi sarcoma in transplant recipients has features similar to those already described. In addition, there may be involvement of the allograft organ (32).

Table 60.1 Differential Diagnoses and Causes of Co-morbidity in the Abdomen in HIV

Causes	Imaging findings in the abdomen and pelvis
Mycobacterium tuberculosis	• Lymphadenopathy with low attenuation centrally • Hepatomegaly • Splenomegaly • Focal lesions in liver, spleen, or kidney • Ascites and/or peritoneal thickening • Terminal ileal or diffuse small bowel wall thickening
Mycobacterium avium-intracellulare complex	• Lymphadenopathy • Hepatomegaly • Splenomegaly • Focal lesions in liver, spleen, or kidney • Proximal small bowel wall thickening • Ascites and/or peritoneal thickening
Cytomegalovirus	• Ulcerated large bowel mucosa seen on barium enema • Focal or diffuse colitis on computed tomography with transmural and pericolic edema • Lymphadenopathy is not seen • Stomach or small bowel involvement cause mural thickening and rarely a polypoidal mass simulating neoplasia • May cause biliary ductal fibrosis with intrahepatic and extrahepatic ductal stenoses
Histoplasmosis	• Distal ileal or ascending colon has mural thickening and pericolic inflammation which resembles carcinoma • Other features similar to *M. tuberculosis*
Cryptosporidiosis	• Small bowel wall thickening • Cholangiopathy with papillary, intrahepatic, and extrahepatic ductal stenoses • Acalculous cholecystitis
Bacillary angiomatosis	• Associated with skin lesions • Focal liver lesions • Enhancing lymphadenopathy
Pneumocystis carinii	• Rarely causes diffuse focal hepatic and splenic lesions with rim calcification and lymphadenopathy that may calcify
Renal calculus	• Urolithiasis is often related to treatment with protease inhibitors
Pancreatitis	• Protease inhibitors can cause hyperlipidemia-related pancreatitis
Lipodystrophy	• Some antiretroviral therapy will cause central visceral adipose deposition and wasting of the extremities with hyperlipidemia and insulin resistance

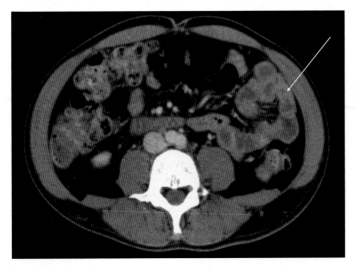

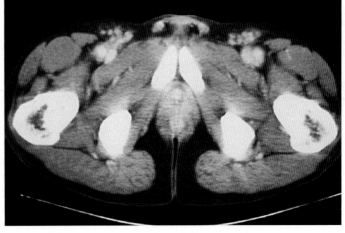

Figure 60.4 Contrast-enhanced CT scan demonstrating Kaposi sarcoma causing nodular thickening of small bowel wall in left flank (arrow).

Figure 60.5 Contrast-enhanced CT scan demonstrating Kaposi sarcoma causing avid enhancement of inguinal lymphadenopathy. The nodes are isodense with the adjacent common femoral vessels.

Key Points: Kaposi Sarcoma

- Gastrointestinal involvement is rare without skin Kaposi sarcoma
- Nodular or diffuse bowel wall thickening is the most likely finding in gastrointestinal Kaposi sarcoma
- Lymphadenopathy involved with Kaposi sarcoma usually displays intense enhancement
- Although solid organ involvement with Kaposi sarcoma is common, it is rarely demonstrated radiologically
- Immune reconstitution may result in clinical and radiological deterioration (IRIS)
- Kaposi sarcoma may infiltrate allograft organs

Lymphoma in the Immunocompromised Host

There is a clear increase in the standardized incidence ratio (SIR) for all forms of lymphoma in the AIDS and non-AIDS groups (8–10). Estimates of the degree of increased risk suggest a SIR for Hodgkin's lymphoma of approximately 11 in the HIV population and 3.9 in the transplant population. For non-Hodgkin lymphoma the figures are 75 and 8, respectively. These numbers are derived from meta-analysis of the available literature (9) and span the pre-HAART and the HAART eras. Overall the majority of clinical cases of lymphoma associated with immunocompromise occur in HIV infection. Whilst there are a mixed group of lymphoma subtypes, 95% are B-cell lymphomas (33,34). Currently the World Health Organization has classified AIDS-related lymphomas (ARL) into three groups. These are:

- Lymphomas that also occur in the immunocompetent population such as Burkitt's lymphoma and diffuse large B-cell lymphoma (DBCL)
- Lymphomas that occur particularly in the HIV-infected patients such as primary effusion lymphoma (PEL) and plasmablastic lymphoma
- Lymphomas that also occur in other immunodeficiency states such as post-transplant lymphoproliferative disorder-like B-cell lymphoma associated with HIV infection (35).

Multicentric Castleman's disease (MCD) is a further rare form of lymphoproliferation that is more commonly encountered in the context of HIV. The pathology of MCD indicates a chronic antigen stimulation response and a close association with human herpes virus 8 (HHV8) has been found in cases of HIV-related MCD. Diagnosis is made on the clinical presentation of a lymphoproliferative disorder with multisystem involvement and typical lymph node biopsy results. The prognosis of MCD is poor with a median survival of 48 months from diagnosis, and a greatly increased risk of the development of classic AIDS related non-Hodgkin's lymphoma. Whatever the sub-type of lymphoma may be, there is considerable overlap in imaging appearances.

In contrast to the immune-competent population, in the HIV population lymphoma tends to be advanced at the time of diagnosis, is more likely to produce B symptoms, and typically is extra nodal. In AIDS patients ARL is the second most common malignancy overall and occurs in all AIDS groups. There is no direct relationship with CD4 count and incidence (36).

Influence of HAART on Incidence and Treatment

Before the advent of HAART, treatment of lymphoma was fraught with the difficulties inherent in achieving a balance between the likely success of treatment and the risks of further chemotherapy-related immunocompromise. As a result, a number of approaches were investigated ranging from low dose to escalated dose regimens (37–40). Outcomes for all methods were disappointing compared to the non-HIV population with median survivals of between five and eight months (37–39). Traditional predictors of outcome for lymphoma were found to be less important than factors related to the HIV infection, including CD4 count, AIDS-defining illness and performance scores (37). One trial demonstrated that patients on low-dose therapy were likely to die of recurrence, while patients on standard therapy were likely to die from infection and that both limbs of the trial did equally badly with a median survival of less than 36 weeks (40). Re-examination of the relative risk of lymphoma following widespread introduction of HAART (9,41) suggests that the incidence of all subtypes of lymphoma has reduced slightly to approximately 50% to 80% of the pre-HAART incidence. The exception to this reduction is Burkitt lymphoma where the incidence has increased by a factor of 3.8. As a result of the sustained evidence that HAART therapy improves outcome in AIDS-related lymphoma, and despite complexities of polypharmacy, chemotherapy has become a central component of therapy for ARL (41).

Imaging Investigation of Lymphoma

When US has been undertaken as the initial investigation (42), abnormality is frequently detected. In a review from the pre-HAART era, in 38 patients undergoing US as the initial radiological investigation, the commonest finding was of a focal liver lesion. Most of these lesions were hypoechoic, in some cases mimicking fluid. Nodal masses in the retroperitoneum, mesentery, or porta hepatis were described in 15 patients, with bowel or other organ involvement evident in the majority of the remainder.

In our practice CT scanning with IV contrast medium forms the mainstay of radiological investigation after disease is suspected clinically or detected on US, and also forms the basis for radiological follow-up. MRI is reserved for problem-solving in specific situations or for local staging, especially in pelvic disease. Barium contrast studies are now rarely undertaken, reflecting a more general change in practice.

Imaging Findings in Lymphoma Associated with Immunocompromise

In a number of reviews of CT appearances of non-CNS NHL in the HIV population, the abdomen and pelvis were the most commonly involved regions (43–45). The largest review found intra-abdominal disease in 64% of patients at one or more sites (44). In 36% of patients there was no evidence of disease in the abdomen or only mild hepatic or splenic enlargement.

Gastrointestinal Tract

Overall, the gastrointestinal tract has been reported as the most common site of intra-abdominal involvement in all immunocompromised patients, with more than 50% of patients with abdominal lymphoma demonstrating evidence of bowel disease on CT. The stomach is the most frequently involved region, followed by

small bowel, rectum, perianal disease, duodenum, and colon (44). In 20% of patients more than one area of the gastrointestinal tract was involved by non-contiguous disease.

Gastric Lymphoma

Radiological findings in the stomach include diffuse gastric wall thickening, focal gastric wall thickening, or a discrete mass with or without ulceration (44) (Fig. 60.6). Generalized gastric wall thickening is relatively less common than in the non-immunocompromised population. Of the 15 patients with stomach involvement in the series reported by Radin et al. (44), 13 also had disease detected in solid viscera, nodes, or both.

Small Bowel

Disease may be localized to the small bowel, with or without nodal enlargement, but without other evidence of disease elsewhere; a pattern observed in 36% of one series of 22 patients

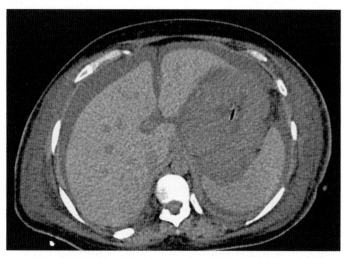

Figure 60.6 CT scan of Burkitt's lymphoma of the stomach demonstrating extensive intramural involvement and luminal compression.

with small bowel involvement (45). The most common segment involved is the terminal ileum and this may extend to involve the cecum in one third of patients. Small bowel disease may be evident as one of two main patterns. The first is circumferential wall thickening which may vary from 1.5 to 7 cm from lumen to serosal surface (Fig. 60.7). This wall thickening is usually of uniform soft tissue density although areas of low attenuation reflecting necrosis have been described (45). The wall thickening may involve a single contiguous segment of bowel, or less commonly two or more non-contiguous segments, on occasion involving almost all of the small intestine. The mean length of involved segments in the series of Balthazar et al. (45) was 10 cm, and overall there was no significant difference in appearance between the immunocompromised and immunocompetent patient groups. Usually the bowel lumen was normal or narrowed rather than dilated, and some patients may present with small bowel obstruction. The second broad pattern of radiological appearance was that of aneurysmal dilatation of the small bowel, involving single or multiple segments of bowel, and in some cases associated with segments of diffuse wall thickening as described above. These areas of dilatation have the radiological appearance of cavities with thick nodular walls. There have also been occasional cases presenting as an intraluminal polyp without other features of bowel wall thickening, dilatation or obstruction.

In summary, small bowel involvement is the sole pathology in one third of cases and associated with more widespread disease in two thirds of cases. In either case the pattern of annular wall thickening of one or more segments or a focal cavitating mass should strongly suggest small bowel lymphoma and prompt tissue diagnosis.

Large Bowel

Large bowel involvement is a rare manifestation of lymphoma in the non-HIV group. Bulky perirectal lymphomas are recognized as a rare but characteristic presentation of ARL and may cause a large central pelvic mass resulting from massive

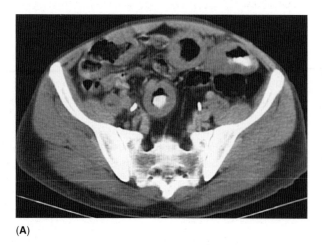 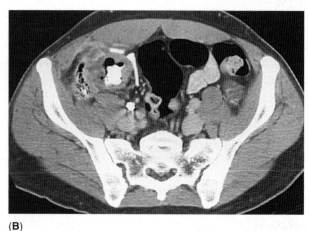

(A)   **(B)**

Figure 60.7 ARL: small bowel. (A and B) Images from CT studies in two different patients reveal focal, variable, segmental, soft tissue attenuating wall thickening indicative of enteric ARL. No barium correlation is necessary to establish the etiology. Note the lack of peritumoral adenopathy frequently accompanying similar lesions in non-ARL cases.

thickening of the rectal wall displacing the lower pelvic viscera (46) (Fig. 60.8).

Liver and Spleen

Diffuse enlargement of the liver in the absence of focal disease is relatively rare and, when present, is usually only moderate in degree, less than 20 cm in craniocaudal dimension. The presence of one or more focal hepatic masses, from 1 to 15 cm in diameter, is associated with more marked hepatomegaly (Fig. 60.9). These lesions are usually hypodense on contrast-enhanced CT (Fig. 60.10). As masses get larger, CT appearances become more varied, with diffuse or heterogeneous enhancement centrally and rim enhancement peripherally reported. Lesions may calcify following treatment. There is usually evidence of involvement of other abdominal viscera of lymph nodes, isolated liver involvement being rare. Isolated splenic enlargement is also rare and, when present, is usually moderate at most (up to 20 cm) (44). Marked isolated splenomegaly should raise the possibility of Castleman's disease as the cause of lymphoproliferation. As splenomegaly becomes more pronounced, it is more likely to be in association with hepatomegaly, ascites, and nodal enlargement. Focal low attenuation splenic lesions are rare and may be single or multiple and from one to several centimeters in diameter.

Pancreatic Disease

Pancreatic involvement is rare, usually mimicking a pancreatic neoplasm with a mass in the head or body of the gland, and distal duct dilatation and parenchymal atrophy. In almost all cases there is involvement of bowel elsewhere and nodal enlargement (47). There may be contiguous extension into the pancreas from adjacent disease, again mimicking pancreatic carcinoma (Fig. 60.11).

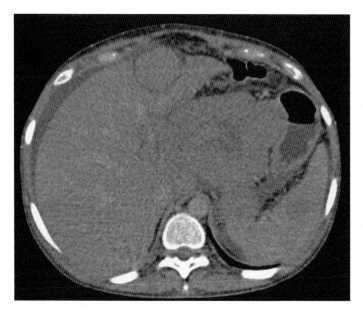

Figure 60.8 ARL: rectum. This is a typical appearance of ARL involving rectum on CT with lateral spread throughout the pelvis.

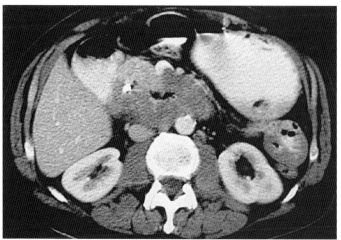

Figure 60.10 Contrast-enhanced CT scan demonstrating focal liver involvement with Burkitt's lymphoma.

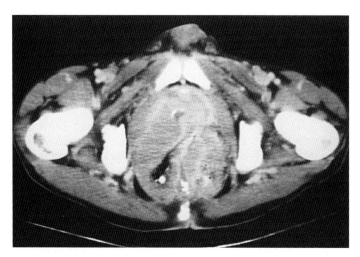

Figure 60.9 Burkitt's lymphoma. The CT demonstrates marked hepatomegaly and a more focal lesion in the left lobe of the liver. There is also diffuse gastric wall thickening.

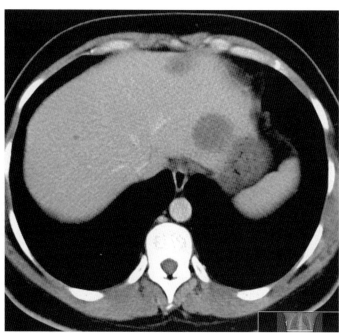

Figure 60.11 ARL: duodenum. The patient had presented with obstructive jaundice. On the contrast-enhanced CT scan a bulky low attenuation mass surrounds the irregular, ulcerated duodenal lumen. The mass invades the superior mesenteric vein. Notice the discretely defined borders of the enhanced pancreatic parenchyma.

Renal and Adrenal Lymphoma

Focal renal involvement by lymphoma is well recognized in the context of immune compromise, but is relatively uncommon, occurring in 10% to 15% of cases in the HIV population. Isolated renal disease due to lymphoma is distinctly uncommon (48,49). The most usual description of renal disease is of one or more focal low attenuation renal masses on contrast-enhanced CT (Fig. 60. 12), with lesions usually being denser than renal parenchyma prior to contrast administration. As with disease in other intra-abdominal solid organs there is usually involvement at one or more other intra-abdominal sites. Perirenal disease has also been described, either unilateral or bilateral, as nodular deposits or more diffusely infiltrating tumor. Unilateral or bilateral adrenal gland enlargement has also been described, larger masses demonstrating central

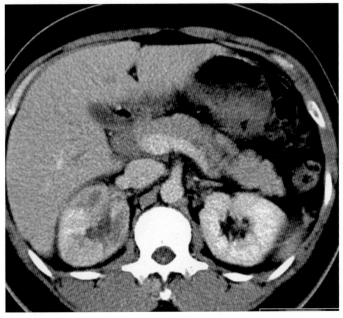

Figure 60.12 Contrast-enhanced CT scan demonstrating patchy focal involvement of the right kidney by Burkitt's lymphoma in HIV infection.

low attenuation thought to be necrosis. In almost all cases focal disease in the bowel, liver, or both was also present (44). Although lymphomas may affect any portion of the genitourinary tract, focal masses along transitional epithelium are rare. Lower genitourinary involvement, when seen, manifests as sheet-like infiltration of the lower pelvic viscera. The fat planes between the bladder, seminal vesicles, and prostate are blurred by the dense soft tissue sheets of infiltrating neoplasm. As the disease is treated, follow-up imaging will show the normal visceral contours emerging from the pelvic infiltration.

Lymph Nodes

Although extranodal involvement is the hallmark of ARL, nodal disease does occur and may be of significant bulk (Fig. 60.13). Lymph node involvement was described in more than 50% of patients in the series by Radin et al. (44), usually in association with other intra-abdominal disease. Nodes were often hyperdense compared to muscle and there may be central nodal necrosis especially as nodal size increases. Avid nodal enhancement is a feature that has been particularly associated with multicentric Castleman's disease, often in association with splenomegaly (50) (Fig. 60.14). Small volume nodal disease, especially in the absence of visceral abnormality, should be interpreted with caution since there are many other reasons why patients with HIV in particular may have nodal enlargement.

Peritoneal Cavity

Whilst diffuse peritoneal and omental disease is most commonly seen as a manifestation of metastatic carcinoma, occasionally this radiological pattern of involvement is due to lymphoma (51). Peritoneal lymphomas are a rare subtype of AIDS-associated NHL, occurring with less severe immune deficiency than for other NHLs. The increased frequency among persons with prior KS suggests a common etiology, presumably infection with KS-associated herpes virus, as found in primary effusion lymphoma. Large peritoneal masses are a feature of Burkitt lymphoma in the HIV population, usually in association with bowel or solid organ involvement (Fig. 60.15).

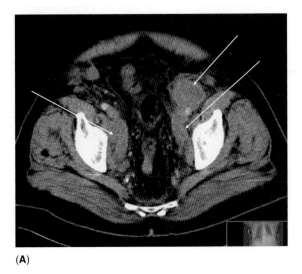

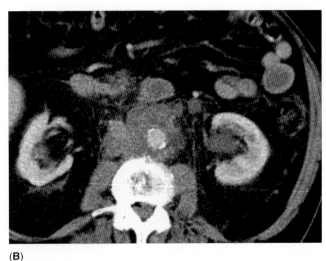

(A)   **(B)**

Figure 60.13 (A) Contrast-enhanced CT scan demonstrating bulky nodal involvement in the pelvic side-wall by AIDS related lymphoma (arrows). (B) Contrast-enhanced CT scan demonstrating circumferential lymphadenopathy surrounding the aorta in a patient with AIDS-related lymphoma.

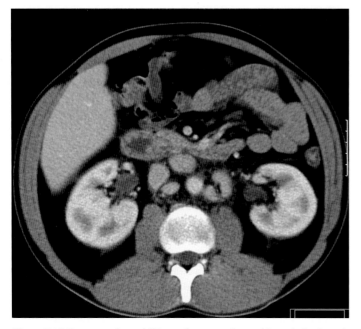

Figure 60.14 Contrast-enhanced CT scan demonstrating multicentric Castleman's disease causing enhancing retroperitoneal nodal enlargement in an HIV-infected patient.

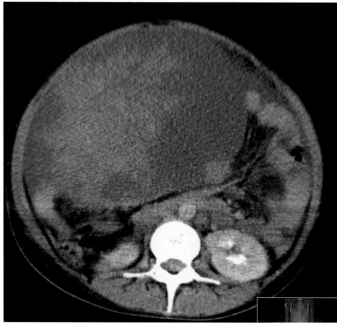

Figure 60.15 Contrast-enhanced CT scan demonstrating bulky peritoneal disease caused by Burkitt's lymphoma in a patient with AIDS.

Key Points: AIDS-Related Lymphoma

- Intrabdominal disease is the most common site of non-CNS NHL
- The bowel is involved in 50% of patients with abdominal lymphoma
- In order of involvement, stomach is most frequent, then small bowel, rectum, perianal disease, duodenum, and colon
- Non-contiguous bowel involvement is frequently described
- The main patterns of bowel involvement are of transmural thickening or aneurysmal dilatation
- Isolated hepatosplenomegaly is relatively rare in the absence of focal lesions

Summary

- Human immunodeficiency virus (HIV) and treatment-induced immunodeficiency are the most significant causes of immunodeficiency in terms of induction of malignancy. Malignancy occurs at an increased standardized ratio of approximately 10 in immunocompromised people with HIV/AIDS and of two in transplant recipients
- The particular tumor types encountered with increased frequency include Hodgkin's lymphoma, hepatocellular carcinoma, stomach carcinoma, vulval carcinoma, penile carcinoma, anal canal carcinoma, renal carcinoma, leukemia, myeloma, and both non-melanoma and melanoma skin cancers
- There are three AIDS-defining tumors: Kaposi sarcoma, carcinoma of the uterine cervix, and non-Hodgkin lymphoma
- In immunocompromised patients, most malignant tumors have patterns of disease that do not differ from those described in patients with a competent immune system

- Many of the more common tumors in immunocompromised populations have a confirmed or putative association with an infectious agent such as Herpes group viruses, *H. pylori*, and hepatitis B and C viruses
- In order of frequency, HIV-related Kaposi sarcoma involves skin, mucous membranes, lymph nodes, and the luminal gastrointestinal tract
- In HIV, lymphoma tends to be extranodal and is advanced at the time of diagnosis, usually with B symptoms. NHL most commonly involves the abdomen and pelvis, where the bowel is involved in 50% of cases
- In HIV infection, identification of common co-morbid conditions is important. For example, immune reconstitution following HAART may result in clinical and radiological deterioration

REFERENCES

1. Burnet FM. The concept of immunological surveillance. Prog Exp Tumor Res 1970; 13: 1–27.
2. Shyur SD, Hill HR. Immunodeficiency in the 1990s. Pediatr Infect Dis J 1991; 10: 595–611.
3. Winkelstein JA, Marino MC, Ochs H, et al. The X-linked hyper-IgM syndrome: clinical and immunologic features of 79 patients. Medicine 2003; 82: 373–84.
4. Kinlen LJ. Immunosuppression and cancer. In: Vainio H, Magee PN, McGregor DB, McMichael AJ, eds. Mechanisms of Carcinogenesis in Risk Identification. Lyon: International Agency for Research on Cancer, 1992: 237–53.
5. Moore RD, Chaisson RE. Natural history of HIV infection in the era of combination antiretroviral therapy. AIDS 1999; 13: 1933–42.

6. UNAIDS. Report on the global HIV/AIDS epidemic 2008: executive summary. (UNAIDS, Geneva 2008). [Available from: http://www.unaids.org/en/KnowledgeCentre/Resources/Publications/].

7. Centers for Disease Control: 1993 revised classification system for HIV infection and expanded surveillance case definition for AIDS among adolescents and adults. Morb Mortal Wkly Rep 1992; 41: 1–19.

8. Engels EA, Biggar RJ, Hall HI, et al. Cancer risk in people infected with human immunodeficiency virus in the United States. Int J Cancer 2008; 123: 187–94.

9. Grulich AE, van Leeuwen MT, Falster MO, Vajdic CM. Incidence of cancers in people with HIV/AIDS compared with immunosuppressed transplant recipients: a meta-analysis. Lancet 2007; 370: 59–67.

10. Patel P, Hanson DL, Sullivan PS, et al. Adult and Adolescent Spectrum of Disease Project and HIV Outpatient Study Investigators. Incidence of types of cancer among HIV-infected persons compared with the general population in the United States, 1992-2003. Ann Intern Med 2008; 148: 728–36.

11. Serraino D, Piselli P, Busnach G, et al. For the Immunosuppression and Cancer Study Group. Risk of cancer following immunosuppression in organ transplant recipients and in HIV-positive individuals in southern Europe. Eur J Cancer 2007; 43: 2117–23.

12. Frisch M, Biggar RJ, Engels EA, Goedert JJ. Association of cancer with AIDS-related immunosuppression in adults. JAMA 2001; 285: 1736–45.

13. Parkin DM. The global health burden of infection-associated cancers in the year 2002. Int J Cancer 2006; 118: 3030–44.

14. IARC Monographs on the Evaluation of Carcinogenic Risks to Humans. Infections with Epstein-Barr Virus and Human Herpes Viruses, Vol. 70. Lyon: IARC, 1997.

15. Eurogast Study Group. An international association between Helicobacter pylori infection and gastric cancer. Lancet 1993; 341: 1329–62.

16. IARC Monographs on the Evaluation of Carcinogenic Risks to Humans. Hepatitis Viruses, Vol. 59. Lyon: IARC, 1994.

17. Boshoff C, Weiss RA. Epidemiology and pathogenesis of Kaposi's sarcoma-associated herpesvirus. Phil Trans Roy Soc Lond B 2001; 356: 517–34.

18. IARC Monographs on the Evaluation of Carcinogenic Risks to Humans. Human Papillomaviruses, Vol. 90. Lyon: IARC, 2007.

19. Martro E, Esteve A, Schulz TF, et al. Risk factors for human Herpesvirus 8 infection and AIDS associated Kaposi's sarcoma among men who have sex with men in a European multicentre study. Int J Cancer 2007; 120: 1129–35.

20. Krown SE, Testa MA, Huang J. AIDS-related Kaposi sarcoma prospective validation of the AIDS Clinical Trials Group staging classification. J Clin Oncol 1997; 15: 3085–92.

21. Ioachim HL, Adsay V, Giancotti FR, Dorsett B, Melamed J. Kaposi's sarcoma of internal organs. A multiparameter study of 86 cases. Cancer 1995; 75: 1376–85.

22. Yoshida EM, Chan NH, Chan-Yan C, Baird RM. Perforation of the jejunum secondary to AIDS-related gastrointestinal Kaposi sarcoma. Can J Gastroenterol 1997; 11: 38–40.

23. Niedt GW, Schinella RA. Acquired immunodeficiency syndrome: clinicopathologic study of 56 autopsies. Arch Pathol Lab Med 1985; 109: 727–34.

24. Stallone G, Schena A, Infante B, et al. Sirolimus for Kaposi's sarcoma in renal-transplant recipients. N Engl J Med 2005; 352: 1317–23.

25. Lebbe C, Euvrard S, Barrou B, et al. Sirolimus conversion for patients with posttransplant Kaposi's sarcoma. Am J Transplant 2006; 6: 2164–8.

26. Koh DM, Langroudi B, Padley SPG. Abdominal CT in patients with AIDS. Imaging 2002; 24: 24–34.

27. Pantongrag-Brown L, Nelson AM, Brown AE, Buetow PC, Buck JL. Gastrointestinal manifestations of acquired immunodeficiency syndrome: radiologic-pathologic correlation. RadioGraphics 1995; 15: 1155–78.

28. Herts BR, Megibow AJ, Birnbaum BA, Kanzer GK, Noz ME. High-attenuation lymphadenopathy in AIDS patients: significance of findings at CT. Radiology 1992; 185: 777–81.

29. Restrepo CS, Martinez S, Lemos JA, et al. Imaging manifestations of Kaposi sarcoma. RadioGraphics 2006; 26: 1169–85.

30. Behrens GM, Meyer D, Stoll M, Schmidt RE. Immune reconstitution syndromes in HIV infection following effective antiretroviral therapy. Immunobiology 2000; 202: 186–93.

31. Bower M, Nelson M, Young AM, et al. Immune reconstitution inflammatory syndrome associated with Kaposi's sarcoma. J Clin Oncol 2005; 23: 5224–8.

32. Diaz-Candamio MJ, Pombo F, Lorenzo MJ, Alonso A. Kaposi's sarcoma involving a transplanted kidney: CT findings. Am J Roentgenol 1998; 171: 1073–4.

33. Levine AM, Seneviratne L, Espina BM, et al. Evolving characteristics of AIDS-related lymphoma. Blood 2000; 96: 4084–90.

34. Knowles DM. Etiology and pathogenesis of AIDS-related non-Hodgkin's lymphoma. Hematol Oncol Clin North Am 2003; 17: 785–820.

35. Raphael M, Borisch B, Jaffe ES. Lymphomas associated with infection by the human immunodeficiency virus (HIV). In: Jaffe ES, Harris NL, Stein H, eds. World Health Organization Classification of Tumours: Pathology and Genetics Tumours of Haematopoietic and Lymphoid Tissues. Lyon: IARC Press, 2001.

36. Redvanly RD, Silverstein JE. Intra-abdominal manifestations of AIDS. Radiol Clin North Am 1997; 35: 1083–125.

37. Kaplan LD, Abrams DI, Feigal E, et al. AIDS-associated non-Hodgkin's lymphoma in San Francisco. JAMA 1989; 261: 719–24.

38. Kaplan LD, Kahn JO, Crowe S, et al. Clinical and virologic effects of recombinant human granulocyte-macrophage colony-stimulating factor in patients receiving chemotherapy for human immunodeficiency virus-associated non-Hodgkin's lymphoma: results of a randomized trial. J Clin Oncol. 1991; 9: 929–40.

39. Levine AM. Acquired immunodeficiency syndrome-related lymphoma: clinical aspects. Semin Oncol 2000; 27: 442–53.

40. Kaplan LD, Straus DJ, Testa MA, et al. Low-dose compared with standard-dose m-BACOD chemotherapy for non-Hodgkin's lymphoma associated with human immunodeficiency virus infection. National Institute of Allergy and

Infectious Diseases AIDS Clinical Trials Group. N Engl J Med 1997; 336: 1641–8.

41. Navarro WH, Kaplan LD. AIDS-related lymphoproliferative disease. Blood 2006; 107: 13–20.

42. Townsend RR, Laing FC, Jeffrey RB Jr, Bottles K. Abdominal lymphoma in AIDS: evaluation with US. Radiology 1989; 171: 719–24.

43. Townsend RR. CT of AIDS-related lymphoma. Am J Roentgenol 1991; 156: 969–74.

44. Radin DR, Esplin JA, Levine AM, Ralls PW. AIDS-related non-Hodgkin's lymphoma: abdominal CT findings in 112 patients. Am J Roentgenol 1993; 160: 1133–9.

45. Balthazar EJ, Noordhoorn M, Megibow AJ, Gordon RB. CT of small-bowel lymphoma in immunocompetent patients and patients with AIDS: comparison of findings. Am J Roentgenol 1997; 168: 675–80.

46. Ioachim HL, Weinstein MA, Robbins RD, et al. Primary ano-rectal lymphoma. A new manifestation of the acquired immune deficiency syndrome (AIDS). Cancer 1987; 60: 1449–53.

47. Jones WF, Sheikh MY, McClave SA. AIDS-related non-Hodgkin's lymphoma of the pancreas. Am J Gastroenterol 1997; 92: 335–8.

48. Eisenberg PJ, Papanicolaou N, Lee MJ, Yoder IC. Diagnostic imaging in the evaluation of renal lymphoma. Leuk Lymphoma 1994; 16: 37–50.

49. Tsang K, Kneafsey P, Gill MJ. Primary lymphoma of the kidney in the acquired immunodeficiency syndrome. Arch Pathol Lab Med 1993; 117: 541–3.

50. Hillier JC, Shaw P, Miller RF, et al. Imaging features of multi-centric Castleman's disease in HIV infection. Clin Radiol 2004; 59: 596–601.

51. Lynch MA, Cho KC, Jeffrey RB Jr, Alterman DD, Federle MP. CT of peritoneal lymphomatosis. Am J Roentgenol 1988; 151: 713–15.

61 Clinical Applications in Molecular Targeted Therapy

Timothy A Yap, Debashis Sarker, Stan B Kaye, and Johann S de Bono

INTRODUCTION

The Advent of Molecular Targeted Anticancer Agents

Historically, strategies in the treatment of cancer have involved the use of empirically-based chemotherapeutic agents. Although these cytotoxic drugs represent potent anticancer therapies, their inability to differentiate between malignant and non-malignant cells has meant inevitable toxicities and safety concerns for cancer patients. This has led to limitations in their use as well as clinical development, and has resulted in the search for novel rationally designed and molecular targeted agents (1,2).

There is evidence that certain cancers contain multiple genetic and epigenetic abnormalities, which remain dependent on one or a few genes for both maintenance of the malignant phenotype and cell survival, resulting in "oncogene addiction." Thus, inhibition of one or a few of these abnormalities through the pharmacological ablation of related signaling pathways may block cancer cell growth and be used as a therapeutic strategy for selectively killing cancer cells (2–4). The success of agents such as imatinib mesylate (Gleevec) and erlotinib (Tarceva) have provided an important proof-of-principle that molecular targeted inhibitors can have a major impact against various cancers (2).

Conventional evaluation of a drug in clinical trial relies on careful study of its pharmacokinetic (PK) and pharmacodynamic (PD) properties. The pharmacokinetic properties of a drug relate to its absorption, distribution, metabolism, and excretion, while the pharmacodynamic properties are linked to the mechanism of drug action in the body, as well as the relationship between drug dosage and effects. In essence, PD biomarkers assess "what the drug does to the body," while PK endpoints are concerned with "what the body does to the drug." The pharmacokinetic-pharmacodynamic evaluation of, and clinical trial design for novel targeted inhibitors require a different approach to that used for cytotoxic chemotherapies. These targeted agents may require the identification of a biologically effective dose range, in addition to the determination of the maximum tolerated dose. The former may be achieved through the use of a pharmacological audit trail, which employs a combination of appropriate diagnostic, pharmacokinetic, pharmacodynamic, predictive, and response biomarkers to enable the safe and effective dose of such therapies to be established in different molecular contexts, thus addressing the key issues in molecular targeted drug discovery and development (Fig. 61.1) (5–7).

Current Issues with Drug Development

Despite recent successes with several molecular targeted agents, drug development of novel anticancer agents remains slow, typically taking between 8 to 10 years from initial preclinical drug discovery studies to regulatory approval (2,8,9). It is also a costly process, averaging between US $700 to 1700 million for the approval of a single compound. Analyses of data obtained from the 1990s demonstrated that drug development is also a high-risk enterprise, with only 5% of cancer drugs entering clinical trials gaining regulatory approval (9). This also implies that large numbers of oncology patients are enrolled into clinical trials of ineffective drugs.

Several reasons have been cited for these inadequacies, and efforts have been made to address these issues (2,9). For example, problems with pharmacokinetics and poor bioavailability of drugs were the main reasons for failures in drug development in the past. These issues have now largely been avoided through the preclinical optimization of these properties. The main reasons for failure have now shifted to drug toxicity and inadequate therapeutic activity, each making up approximately a third of all causes of drug developmental failures.

In 2006, the Food and Drug Administration (FDA) developed a Critical Path Opportunities List to modernize and increase efficiency, predictability, and productivity in the development of new medicinal compounds. Crucially, biomarker development and streamlining clinical trials were identified as the two most important areas for improving drug development (10). It was postulated that novel biomarkers could improve the efficiency of product development, rapidly identify safety issues in preclinical and early clinical testing, minimize costly late drug attrition, and facilitate the advancement of modern clinical trials to produce better data faster.

Biomarkers in Drug Development

A biomarker may be defined as a characteristic that is objectively measured and evaluated as an indicator of normal biological or pathogenic processes, or of pharmacological responses to a therapeutic intervention (11). Biomarkers should be analytically validated and clinically qualified, and developed in tandem with novel molecular therapies. They may be classified as either pre-treatment or post-treatment biomarkers. Pre-treatment biomarkers may be prognostic or predictive in aiding patient selection. Post-treatment biomarkers may be used as pharmacological endpoints to measure the effect of a drug on target modulation. Rarely, a post-treatment biomarker may also function as a surrogate or "intermediate" endpoint, becoming a substitute for a clinical endpoint and in predicting clinical benefit, harm, or a lack of benefit or harm (11).

Predictive Biomarkers: Selecting Appropriate Patients

Solid tumors demonstrate significant inter- and intra-tumoral heterogeneity and possess distinct genetic abnormalities and

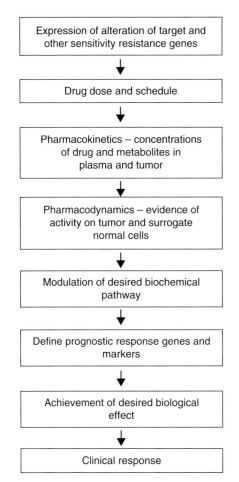

Figure 61.1 The pharmacological audit trail for molecular cancer therapeutics. The pharmacological audit trail provides a rational basis for assessing the risk of failure of the development of a novel compound at any particular stage, with the likelihood of failure decreasing as the hierarchy of sequential questions are successfully answered. It also provides the basis for making key informed decisions, including which patients to treat, what the optimum dose and schedule of a novel compound is, and whether to continue or terminate a drug development program. *Source*: Adapted from Ref. 7.

treatment responses (12). In this era of targeted therapies, it may be time for a paradigm shift away from the traditional management of cancer based on anatomical and histological parameters to one involving a more "target-specific" strategy. For example, biomarkers that predict "addiction" to a particular signaling pathway should be used to match patients with inhibitors. These biomarkers can be monitored post-therapy, and if required, repeated following disease relapse to revise the personalized treatment strategy (12).

Pharmacodynamic Biomarkers: Proof of Target Modulation
Both PK and PD biomarkers must be rigorously validated and their relationship defined during the preclinical drug discovery phase, so that the best candidate can be selected for clinical development (2).

- PK governs drug delivery, availability, and exposure, and is crucial to the drug development process since adequate drug exposure is required for the compound to have the desired biological effect
- PD biomarkers, which are critically dependent on drug PK, provide proof of principle that the proposed target is being modulated and ideally this would also correlate with anti-tumor activity

Robust PD endpoints will therefore confirm that any anti-tumor effects of a drug are due to target inhibition, and in the presence of tumor shrinkage they indicate the nature of that drug target is critical for tumor cell proliferation and survival, that is, these PD studies validate both the drug target and drug development process (5,6).

The use of PK and PD markers and demonstration of anti-tumor activity together enable the construction of a framework that allows all key stages in drug development to be monitored, linked, and interpreted (5,6). The linkage of information on the status of the molecular target, PD and PK endpoints, to measures of biological and clinical anti-tumor effects constitutes a pharmacological audit trail (Fig. 61.1) (2). This framework systematically traces all phases of drug development, from target identification to clinical outcome and permits rational decisions to be made in a hypothesis-testing fashion, aiding in the successful development of modern therapeutics (2). Such studies are key to 'troubleshooting' the drug development process.

PD biomarkers may also be used to identify "on" and unplanned, and potentially undesired "off" target effects of a drug, and to assess drug effects on tumor and surrogate normal tissue. They may also be utilized for selecting the optimal dose and schedule of drug administration, understanding mechanisms of response and resistance, designing rational drug combinations, and predicting treatment outcome. It is thus crucial to identify robust PD biomarkers in preclinical models, so that these can be employed in assessing biological activity and treatment response in clinical studies (2,5,6).

Nevertheless, the real value of such detailed biomarker studies remains controversial. A recent meta-analysis of the use of biomarkers in Phase I oncology trials conducted between 1991 and 2002 concluded that while biomarkers have made a limited and mainly supportive contribution to the selection of a Phase II dose in 11 of 87 studies, they regularly provided evidence supporting the proposed mechanism of drug action (in 34 of 87 published trials) (13). However, the primary determinants of Phase II dose and schedule were toxicity and/or efficacy in all but one of the 87 studies analyzed. These studies indicated that the proportion of trials utilizing biomarkers has increased over time, from 14% in 1991 to 26% in 2002 (p < 0.02) although the data on the analytical validity of these assays were not available. With the increased discovery, development, and validation of novel biomarkers, including functional imaging, it is expected that an even greater number of appropriate, fit-for-purpose biomarkers will be implemented in clinical studies of new cancer agents, and will ultimately have a greater impact on key decision-making. Evidence that these biomarker studies are cost-effective in the long run is nonetheless now required.

Key Points: Drug Development

- Drug development of novel molecular targeted compounds takes between 8 to 10 years from initial preclinical drug discovery studies to regulatory approval
- Solid tumors demonstrate significant inter- and intra-patient tumor heterogeneity and possess distinct genetic abnormalities and treatment responses
- Pre-treatment predictive biomarkers may support patient selection for novel therapies
- Post-treatment biomarkers may be used as pharmacological endpoints to measure the effect of a drug on target modulation
- PK and PD biomarkers need to be rigorously validated and their relationship defined during the preclinical drug discovery phase
- Clinically qualified intermediate endpoint or surrogate endpoint biomarkers are urgently needed to accelerate anti-cancer drug approval

FUNCTIONAL IMAGING: CLINICAL IMPLICATIONS

The Need for Non-invasive Functional Imaging in the Clinic

In recent years, great progress has been made in improving our understanding of tumor biology and the molecular basis of malignant progression (14). The temporal and spatial heterogeneity of malignant tumors is well described (15). This occurs not just as a result of disease natural history, but also following the selective pressure of effective anti-cancer therapy (16). It is also due to a constant interaction between cancer cells and their microenvironment, including the extracellular matrix, host immune cells, and tumor vasculature. This results in an interdependence of tumor genotype, oxygen tension, tumor pH, and metabolic status. This continuous interaction allows the continued survival of tumors, despite pressure from the host immune response and anti-cancer therapy (16).

Non-invasive imaging has traditionally been employed to detect and stage disease, but advances over the past decade have revolutionized the role of imaging in cancer through the use of faster and more sensitive technology (17). Traditionally, tumor growth and efficacy of therapies have been assessed through the use of tumor volume measurements employing structural imaging methods, including computed tomography (CT), magnetic resonance (MR) imaging, or ultrasound (US). Although these techniques are well established in the clinic, their structural readouts are poor indicators of treatment response. This is undesirable for patients who may be exposed to potentially ineffective therapies for prolonged periods of time, and also for clinical drug developers, since an early and accurate readout is necessary for optimal clinical development (18).

Novel imaging probes and genetic engineering systems have now been developed, including functional imaging techniques capable of tracking specific molecular pathways, and cell or tissue function. These may be utilized in the assessment and monitoring of certain "hallmarks of cancer" including angiogenesis, metabolism, cell proliferation, and apoptosis (14,18).

The combination of non-invasive and functional imaging, with either single- or multi-modality approaches, potentially allows the accurate assessment and monitoring of precancerous lesions to malignancy, and that of tumor progression after malignant transformation, through the visualization of cancer-specific molecules, signaling pathways, and functional parameters. Such imaging technology holds the promise of changing the face of drug discovery and development, especially in the determination of PK and PD endpoints.

In addition to functional imaging, there exists a large number of molecular assays and techniques for the accurate determination of PK and PD endpoints in cancer drug development (2). Although the use of invasive techniques like tumor biopsies in clinical trials remain vital, they can pose challenging ethical and logistical issues for both patients and medical staff during the routine procurement of tumor tissue in early phase clinical trials of molecularly targeted agents (2). Functional imaging techniques by contrast are non-invasive biomarkers and are a safer and more acceptable option for patients. Other alternative sources for such biomarker studies include the evaluation of circulating tumor cells from the blood of cancer patients. There is thus now an increased focus on the development and use of such biomarkers in the clinic.

This chapter will now trace the clinical experience of the main functional imaging modalities from the perspective of cancer biology and will also discuss the clinical implications of functional imaging in assessing PK and PD endpoints in drug development, and in particular, focus on the strengths and weaknesses of individual technologies in the development of novel agents. The detailed technical and practical aspects of these imaging methodologies are beyond the scope of this review and are discussed in chapters 62 to 65.

Role of Functional Imaging in the Drug Development Process

Following chemical and biological development in the laboratory, novel therapies typically proceed through stringent phases of clinical testing before eventually gaining regulatory approval for a given labeled indication, if successful. Each clinical trial phase is designed to answer specific questions and accordingly, functional imaging plays a different role in each of these distinct phases as outlined below (19).

Phase I Clinical Trials

These are first-in-human dose escalation studies involving patients with a range of advanced or refractory malignancies who have exhausted all forms of established therapies or for which no standard treatments exist (19). Such studies typically involve a small patient population of 20 to 100 patients. The primary endpoints are to assess the safety and tolerability of novel therapies and to recommend a Phase II dose and schedule, traditionally through the establishment of the maximum tolerated dose. Evaluation of preliminary anti-tumor effects is usually included as a secondary endpoint. A recent study however concluded that the demonstration of efficacy in Phase I studies is significantly predictive of FDA regulatory approval (20). With the advent of novel molecularly targeted agents, PK and PD measurements are gaining increasing importance in demonstrating proof of principle of drug action in the tumor, and in the estimation of the optimum biological dose range to aid in the selection of a Phase II dose (13).

Novel imaging techniques, including both novel MR imaging modalities and positron emission tomography (PET) may therefore increasingly play important roles in Phase I trials by demonstrating functional or metabolic responses in these small cohorts of patients. For example, dynamic contrast-enhanced MR imaging (DCE-MRI) studies have been shown to provide additional insight into the biological action of novel anti-angiogenic agents and to facilitate dose-relationship analyses across studies (21). [18F]-FDG-PET may also be used with relative ease to obtain whole-body scans in Phase I trial patients, thus allowing the monitoring of total disease burden in order to understand differential disease responses (19). Radiolabeled drug analogues may also be utilized to study PK distribution of novel compounds at this stage of development (22). This is key to evaluating drug penetration into tumor, an underestimated cause of drug resistance particularly in for example the management of diseases like glioblastoma or large necrotic masses. Functional imaging may play increasingly important roles in these early stage trials to address crucial mechanistic and efficacy issues to optimize the subsequent development of these novel agents. The additional imaging costs involved in the small studies may limit the broader applicability of these technologies but are relatively minor compared to the risk of taking forward suboptimal dosing schedules of novel compounds.

Phase II Clinical Trials

Phase II studies focus on evaluating drug anti-tumor activity, traditionally for a specific disease type but also for specific molecular indications (e.g., loss of BRCA function), but also continue to assess patient safety in a larger population, usually up to several hundred patients. In addition to providing objective measurements of tumor response in Phase II trials, functional imaging is also vital in interrogating tumor-specific drug mechanisms, evaluating mixed responses due to biological disease heterogeneity, improving dose scheduling, and developing combination therapies. Improved functional imaging could also become key to improving patient selection and as a robust predictor of clinical benefit, thereby accelerating drug approval (19). A recent statistical study, however, has suggested that up to 20 Phase II clinical trials of different novel therapies may be required to prove that a PD biomarker, including functional imaging biomarkers, will aid the drug development process (23).

Phase III Clinical Trials

Once efficacy and safety have been demonstrated for novel agents in Phase II studies, these are usually compared against the current standard treatment in Phase III trials prior to regulatory submission. This typically involves randomized double-blind trials with several hundreds to thousands of patients in multiple centers. Typical endpoints of Phase III studies include survival, time to disease progression, and symptom and quality of life assessments, although for many diseases overall survival is the primary approvable endpoint. The role of imaging is currently limited to objective tumor response criteria, usually with MR imaging or CT, and can define time to disease progression (24).

The limited utilization of functional imaging endpoints in Phase III trials to date has largely been because of poorly validated data, lack of standardized methodologies across multiple centers, and cost. It is expected that with increased experience and availability, techniques such as PET may potentially be utilized to deliver robust efficacy endpoints in the near future (19). Clinical qualification of such functional imaging techniques in Phase III trials as a surrogate endpoint in the future may be utilized to obtain regulatory approval for novel therapies. However, further clinical trials will be required to explore this possibility.

Implementing Functional Imaging in Clinical Trials

Prior to employing functional imaging endpoints in clinical studies, there are a number of important factors to establish. These include ensuring the reproducibility of imaging techniques, utilizing robust image processing and analysis methodologies, biomarker validation and qualification, and standardization of protocols and technologies in multicenter studies (19).

Reproducibility of imaging techniques will greatly impact on the statistical significance of any detected changes induced by a specific therapy. Thus, efforts might be made to minimize any possibilities for variability that may arise during a clinical study. Strategies may include scanner calibration and quality assurance (QA) procedures, utilizing standardized and well-designed scanner-specific acquisition protocols, operator training, and operational consistency of the assigned operator (19,25). Following this, it will be necessary to acquire reproducibility data from a representative patient cohort, for example through a pilot study by performing test and re-test scanning to provide representative data, from which statistical powering for a particular study can be obtained. If possible, two baseline scans should be carried out, although this may pose logistical and practical issues for both patients and staff.

Robust image processing and analyses are essential for the accurate measurement and interpretation of biomarker data (19). Objective analysis tools will permit fully automated extraction of quantitative image parameters in clinical trials. To develop new image analysis techniques, large high-quality datasets are required to test improved image analysis techniques and validate them against clinical indices, such as outcome. For example, the RIDER (Reference Image Database to Evaluate Response) project initiated by the National Cancer Institute (NCI) aims to collate imaging data from CT and PET-CT to facilitate the development of new tools to study lung cancer.

The imaging methodology must also be appropriately validated so that it can be implemented in a timely way to maximize its value for decision-making (19,25). Currently, there is no agreed framework that broadly covers the validation of imaging biomarkers for regulatory use, although some general principles have been proposed (26,27). Biomarker validation or qualification is a graded, "fit-for-purpose" process, linking a biomarker with biological and clinical endpoints (27). Vital issues associated with this may be addressed in separate methodology-focused studies, prior to implementation in a clinical trial. It is also important to weigh the risk of using data from an insufficiently validated biomarker in decision-making in a clinical trial, against the cost of not incorporating such a biomarker.

To maximize recruitment, it is not uncommon for early clinical trials to be carried out in multiple sites. As such, it will be crucial to standardize acquisition and analysis protocols, nomenclature, and methodologies prior to commencing any clinical trial (19,25). This standardization aims to reduce the various factors that contribute to multisite imaging variability. An initial comprehensive review of available manpower and imaging hardware across study sites will be essential to determine the feasibility of a particular imaging study.

Key Points: Functional Imaging Markers

■ Novel imaging probes may be utilized in the assessment and monitoring of certain "hallmarks of cancer" including angiogenesis, metabolism, cell proliferation, and apoptosis

■ Functional imaging has the potential to determine PK and PD endpoints in drug development

■ Phase I clinical trials are first-in-human dose escalation studies involving patients with a range of advanced or refractory malignancies

■ Imaging techniques, for example dynamic contrast-enhanced MR imaging (DCE-MRI) and [18F]-FDG-PET may have an important role in Phase I trials by demonstrating functional or metabolic responses

■ Phase II studies focus on evaluating drug anti-tumor activity

■ Phase III trials compare the new drug against the current standard treatment

■ Robust image processing and analyses are essential for the accurate measurement and interpretation of biomarker data

This includes reviewing the scanner manufacturer, model and software versions to ensure that any possibility for variability is excluded (28). It will also be important to implement specific QA procedures throughout the study. An initial pilot study prior to commencement of a clinical trial should be also incorporated to ensure data quality and protocol compliance across study centers (19).

IMAGING APPROACHES IN CLINICAL TRIALS

Angiogenesis Inhibitors and Functional Imaging

Over 30 years after the first experiments by Judah Folkman and colleagues, the critical role of angiogenesis to the oncogenic process is now regarded as one of the "hallmarks of cancer," and the development of molecular agents targeting this pathway remains one of the undoubted successes of the modern cancer therapeutic era (14,29). The approval of the angiogenic inhibitors bevacizumab (colorectal cancer), sunitinib (renal cancer), and sorafenib (renal and hepatocellular cancer) has clearly validated this approach; however, to date, these successes have occurred in patients with advanced disease and are often associated with short response durations and drug resistance.

The mechanism of action of angiogenic inhibitors—prevention of tumor growth and metastases—often limits the validity of conventional cross-sectional imaging in response assessments. The development of functional imaging could potentially optimize the appropriate development and use of antiangiogenics by the appropriate selection of patients likely to respond, selection of dose and schedule, evaluation of biological activity, and determination of clinical resistance mechanisms (30).

The functional assessment of tumor vasculature and cellular density are key angiogenic parameters that can be assessed using functional imaging. Although there are many potential imaging modalities available for measuring tumor vasculature, the three which have been extensively investigated in the clinic are dynamic contrast-enhanced (DCE)-MRI, diffusion-weighted MR imaging (DWI), and DCE-CT. Dynamic contrast-enhanced ultrasound (DCE-US) also has the potential to assess tumor vasculature but remains in the research arena.

Dynamic Contrast-Enhanced MR Imaging (DCE-MRI)

DCE-MRI is a non-invasive quantitative method of investigating microvascular structure and function by tracking the pharmacokinetics of injected low-molecular weight contrast agents as they pass through the tumor vasculature (21). The most commonly used agent is gadolinium diethyltriaminepentaacetic acid (Gd-DTPA). The technique is sensitive to alterations in vascular permeability, extracellular extravascular and vascular volumes, and in blood flow.

The most commonly measured parameters are those pertaining to tumor microvasculature. Signal changes measured during a dynamic enhancement acquisition can be used to estimate contrast agent concentrations *in vivo* (31). Concentration-time curves can then be fitted using recognized pharmacokinetic models (32). Examples of these parameters include:

- K^{trans} (permeability-surface area product per unit volume of tissue)—this is the volume transfer constant of the contrast agent
- V_e—leakage space as a percentage of unit volume of tissue
- K_{ep}—rate constant
- IAUC—initial area under the contrast agent-time curve

The degree of signal enhancement is dependent on physiological and physical factors, including tissue perfusion, arterial input function (AIF) (AIF: the concentration-time course of the contrast agent in the artery supplying the vascular bed), capillary surface area, capillary permeability, and volume of the extracellular extravascular leakage space (EES) (21). The choice of model has often varied significantly in the published literature, and has led to recent recommendations by a United Kingdom consensus group for the use of MRI in the assessment of novel antivascular and antiangiogenic agents (33). Among their recommendations were that simple models describing the volume transfer coefficient of contrast between the blood plasma and the EES (K^{trans}) and the size of the EES (V_e) should be used along with IAUC.

The effects of many antiangiogenic and vascular disrupting agents have been investigated in a range of Phase I and II clinical trials (Fig. 61.2). In an early important study, Morgan and colleagues performed a Phase I study of the vascular endothelial growth factor receptor (VEGFR) inhibitor vatalanib (PTK/ZK) to investigate the use of DCE-MRI as a potential PD biomarker (34). Scans were performed at baseline, after two days, and at the end of a 28-day cycle in patients with liver metastases from colorectal cancer. It was found that patients with stable disease (SD) by RECIST (Response Evaluation Criteria in Solid Tumors) had a greater reduction in Ki (unidirectional influx constant) at Day 2 and after Cycle 1 compared with patients with progressive disease (19). Only reductions in Ki of >40% were associated with reductions in tumor size. However, this Phase I study did not indicate if patients with RECIST SD or progressive disease, but with smaller reductions in Ki, benefited from anti-angiogenic therapy in terms of prolonged survival (30).

In other DCE-MRI studies of vatalanib, Mross et al. (35) and Thomas et al. (36) demonstrated clearly that cross-study standardization of the imaging (including technique, endpoints, and timing) can enable important comparisons to be made between studies. However, despite the promise of DCE-MRI as a PD biomarker in these early phase trials, and its use in helping to define dosing, the placebo-controlled Phase III trials of vatalanib

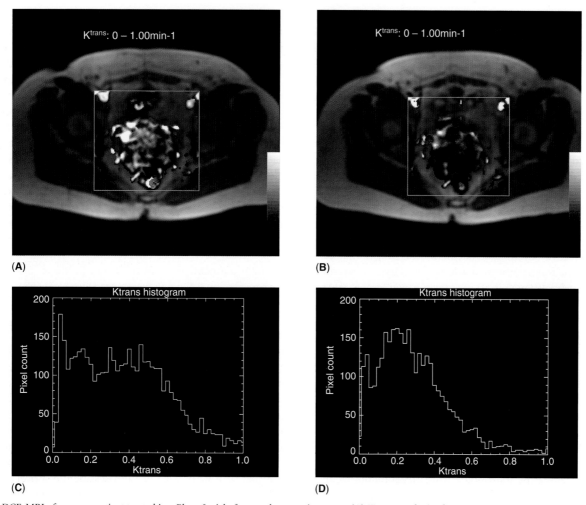

Figure 61.2 DCE-MRI of a cancer patient treated in a Phase I trial of a vascular targeting agent. (**A**) K^{trans} map obtained pre-treatment in a cancer patient with a pelvic lesion. (**B**) is a K^{trans} map in the same patient four hours after treatment with a vascular targeting agent. The mean reduction in K^{trans} is greater than 30%, with some regions achieving a reduction of 100%. The vascular parameter K^{trans} is the forward rate constant obtained from pharmacokinetic modeling of the distribution of a paramagnetic contrast agent following administration using DCE-MRI. (**C**) and (**D**) show the histograms obtained from the image data, demonstrating a clear left shift in K^{trans} values. *Source*: Courtesy of Dr. David Collins, Royal Marsden Hospital, U.K.

combined with chemotherapy for first or second line therapy in metastatic colorectal cancer have proved chastening for the oncology research community, with both studies failing to achieve their primary endpoint of improvement in overall survival (37,38). One potential explanation offered is the utilization of a suboptimal dosing regime, since similar trials with bevacizumab and chemotherapy have revealed a survival advantage. Studies using other small molecule oral VEGFR inhibitors are now ongoing.

These include a study by Liu et al. (39) in which 26 patients were treated with the oral angiogenesis inhibitor AG-013736 and imaged at baseline and two days after initiation of treatment. A relationship between key MR-derived vascular parameters (K^{trans} and IAUC) and exposure to AG-013736 was identified. The study also demonstrated the ability of DCE-MRI to be sufficiently standardized for limited multicenter application. Unfortunately, valid DCE-MRI data were only available for one of three patients who achieved durable partial responses by RECIST. Thus, no conclusions could be made as to an association between vascular response and clinical response. In the single patient with a clinical response and evaluable DCE-MRI data, a significant decrease in K^{trans} (47%) and IAUC (53%) was observed.

Similar reductions in K^{trans} were shown with BIBF1120 and cediranib (AZD2171) without demonstrating clinical responses by RECIST (40,41). However, Flaherty et al. recently reported a small trial where a reduction in K^{trans} correlated with response rate and progression-free survival in patients treated with the multi-kinase inhibitor sorafenib (42). The study included 17 metastatic renal cell carcinoma (RCC) patients who underwent DCE-MRI studies as part of a pilot evaluation. Four patients achieved partial responses by WHO criteria following sorafenib treatment, with a median time to progression of 12.9 months. K^{trans} significantly declined by 60.3% (CI 46.1–74.6%) post sorafenib therapy, while the percentage decline in K^{trans} and change in tumor size determined by CT scans were significantly associated with progression-free survival (p = 0.01 and 0.05 respectively). K^{trans} at baseline was also significantly associated with progression-free survival (p = 0.02). This study thus showed that in RCC patients, baseline tumor vascular permeability was a predictive marker of favorable response to sorafenib, while its inhibition following treatment was associated with improved outcome.

DCE-MRI has also been utilized as a PD marker for the evaluation of vascular targeting agents such as combretastatin-A4 phosphate (CA4P) and 5,6,-dimethylxanthenone-4-acetic acid (DMXAA).

In these studies, the observed decrease in the kinetics of contrast agent uptake was interpreted in terms of tumor perfusion reduction (25). In the Phase I trial of CA4P (43), DCE-MRI contributed to the appropriate selection of a recommended Phase II dose and schedule. This was in part due to extensive preclinical work comparing dose-response with DCE-MRI to a technique for the measurement of absolute blood flow in the same animal model (44).

The use of DCE-MRI in the Phase I trial of the human anti-VEGF antibody HuMV833 highlighted problems associated with tumor heterogeneity in early phase clinical trials. Although this agent resulted in a median decrease of 44% in K_{fp} (first pass permeability), the heterogeneity of response in those cohorts with three or fewer patients was such that discrimination of one level from another was difficult (45).

In conclusion, DCE-MRI parameters may be subject to random error, biological variation, and systematic inaccuracies that cause day-to-day variation in measured values. The choice of parameter still varies widely, although most investigators would now regard a change in K^{trans} of >40% as likely to represent a true difference correlating with disease stability and response. It remains essential to know the intra-patient variability for the study population to have confidence that a change in parameters is due to drug effect. Therefore, many (though not all) centers perform two baseline scans to measure reproducibility for each trial dataset, in accordance with published guidelines (43,46). Recommendations for increasing the statistical power of these studies include the use of larger cohorts of patients, perhaps at two to three dose levels close to the maximum tolerated dose in Phase I trials, with patients bearing a single tumor type (47). As discussed, the practical aspects of conducting these studies require the appropriate standardization of machines, protocols, and quality assurance over multiple sites to ensure production of the highest quality data (25).

Diffusion-Weighted MR Imaging (DW-MRI) (see Chapter 65)

DWI differs from conventional MR imaging in that it measures the mobility of water within tissues in addition to reflecting tumor shape and size (48). DWI is non-invasive and has advantages over DCE-MRI in that it can be performed in patients with poor venous access, can be repeated at short intervals if necessary, is cheaper and has a shorter examination time. Therefore, these images can be appended to existing imaging protocols without a significant increase in examination time (49). The disadvantages are its lower spatial resolution and small distortion artefacts, which make the exact localization of different areas more challenging. In addition, DWI MR images may be more significantly impacted than DCE-MRI images by partial volume effects and movement artefacts. DWI has potential utility in determining changes in tumor cellularity following antiangiogenic therapy. This parameter is strongly affected by molecular viscosity and membrane permeability between intra- and extracellular compartments, active transport and flow, and directionality of tissue/cellular structures that impede water mobility (50). Thus DWI can be used to characterize highly cellular regions of tumors, distinguishing cystic regions from solid ones, and in detecting treatment response, manifested as a change in cellularity within the tumor over time. DWI has been initiated recently as a potential non-invasive technique to monitor the anti-tumoral effects of

radiotherapy and chemotherapy with the aim of predicting therapy outcome. In contrast to conventional MR imaging, viable tumor can be differentiated from tumor necrosis with DWI (51). In a series of preclinical studies utilizing rats implanted with rhabdomyosarcomas, a comparison between DCE-MRI and DWI was performed using CA4P. Although both modalities allowed monitoring of perfusion changes, DWI imaging provided additional information about intra-tumoral cell viability versus necrosis following the administration of CA4P (52). High cellular density related to a low apparent diffusion co-efficient (ADC) value, reflecting the lack of mobility of water protons, whereas high ADC values relate to necrotic tissue with inherent diffusion of water protons due to the loss of cell membrane integrity (53,54). Although the use of DWI in antiangiogenic Phase I trials has been limited to date, small studies have evaluated DWI in distinguishing recurrent or residual disease from post-treatment changes, making it a potentially important tool in the monitoring of disease progression following treatment (Fig. 61.3) (55).

Dynamic contrast-enhanced CT (DCE-CT)

Although MR imaging has historically been the modality of choice for DCE-imaging, recent advances in CT technology (faster imaging, higher resolution, more robust data processing) have led to it being increasingly investigated as a potential biomarker tool for the evaluation of antiangiogenic agents (Fig. 61.4). DCE-CT is relatively simple to perform, is widely available, and reproducible (56,57). A significant potential advantage over DCE-MRI is that the quantification measurements are simpler since the relationship between signal and contrast concentration is more linear than that seen with MR imaging, despite the reduced sensitivity (58). However, CT has the major disadvantage of ionizing radiation dosage, which potentially limits the number of scans that may be performed in patients.

In a small study of six patients with locally advanced rectal cancer using the VEGF-specific antibody bevacizumab, the effects of tumor perfusion were examined (59). Twelve days after the single dose, DCE-CT showed a significant decrease in tumor blood perfusion (40–44%) and blood volume (16–39%). In addition, this was accompanied by a reduction in microvascular density and interstitial fluid pressure (biopsies obtained by flexible sigmoidoscopy). At our institution, we performed a similar study investigating the potential effects of cediranib on DCE-CT vascular parameters (22). There was evidence of reductions in DCE-CT parameters post-treatment, particularly perfusion, permeability surface product (PSP). Changes were evident on DCE-CT as soon as 24 hours after the initiation of treatment. For each of these parameters, a decrease from baseline levels beyond the baseline reference range was reported for three patients (including two with RECIST stable disease) at one month after the start of daily dosing of cediranib. Overall, within-patient variability (W-PV) was generally low for all DCE-CT parameters measured and was consistently lower than between-patient variability. The W-PV was largest for PSP (18%) and lowest for mean transit time (7%). These data indicate high technical reproducibility, and we are now planning to compare the reproducibility and dynamism of response directly with DCE-MRI.

A study conducted by Fournier and colleagues investigated post-treatment changes in tumor vascular parameters in patients with metastatic renal cancer utilizing DCE-CT (60). Twenty-six

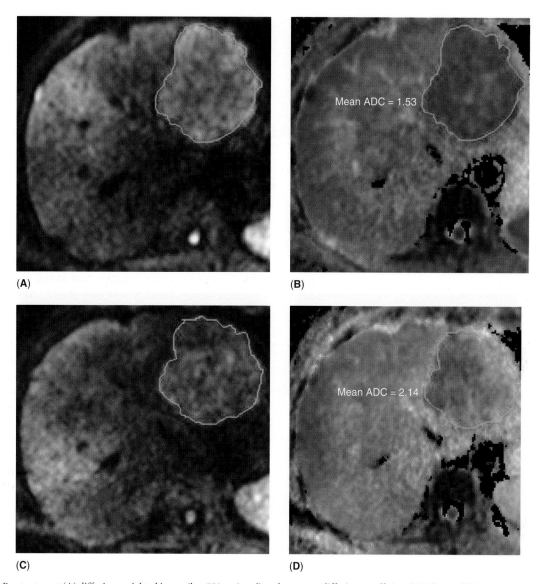

Figure 61.3 DWI. Pre-treatment (**A**) diffusion-weighted image (b = 750 sec/mm²) and apparent diffusion co-efficient (ADC) map (**B**) showing a cancer metastasis in the left lobe of the liver. The metastasis returned a mean ADC of 1.53×10^{-3} mm²/sec. Following one cycle of anti-vascular treatment, the diffusion-weighted image (**C**) and ADC map (**D**) reveal a significant increase in the mean ADC (2.14×10^{-3} mm²/sec) of the metastasis in keeping with treatment response. *Source*: Courtesy of Dr. Dow-Mu Koh, Royal Marsden Hospital, U.K.

patients were treated with sorafenib (N = 9) versus placebo (N = 13), or sunitinib (N = 17) versus interferon (N = 5). There was a statistically significant drop in tumor blood flow (TBF) and tumor blood volume (TBV) as early as the first cycle of treatment compared to pre-treatment, showing the biological effect of the drug on tumor vascularity. There was a significantly higher drop in TBF and TBV in patients who would be later classified as responders (N = 16) versus non-responders (N = 10) after the first cycle of treatment (−66% vs. −6%, p = 0.02; −60% vs. −26.5%, p = 0.04). The changes in mean transit time (MTT) and vascular permeability (VP) were not correlated to the best response.

Dynamic Contrast-Enhanced Ultrasound (DCE-US)

There is increasing evidence that recent advances in functional ultrasonography, using contrast agent and perfusion software allow the detection of microvascularization and perfusion for superficial and deep malignant tumors. It is therefore possible to provide information on the state of tumor vascularity and response to therapy.

The addition of contrast agents significantly improves spatial resolution of conventional US, potentially increasing the intensity of color doppler signal by 800% (61). The commonest contrast agents used involve the use of IV injections of small (typically 3 μ) air or gas bubbles ("microbubbles") that boost the doppler signal from blood vessels (62). Microbubble air contrast has potential advantages over the contrast agents used for DCE-MRI and CT in that these provide information on both intravascular and interstitial space, potentially measuring the intravascular volume of tumors.

Treatment response can be predicted earlier according to modifications of this vascularization before any changes in tumor volume. The acquisition of raw linear data affords the precise quantification of the perfusion, in particular using time tracking of the region of interest.

One of the biggest challenges facing conventional US imaging is that of operator dependency, which can influence reproducibility in longitudinal studies of drug effects. The major advantage of DCE-US, with perfusion software (Vascular Recognition Imaging) and contrast

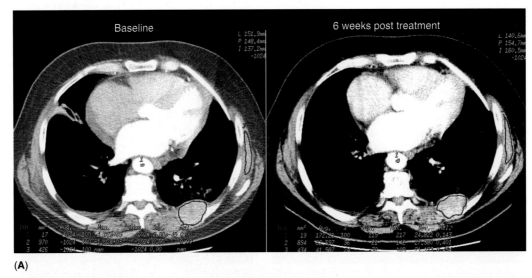

(A)

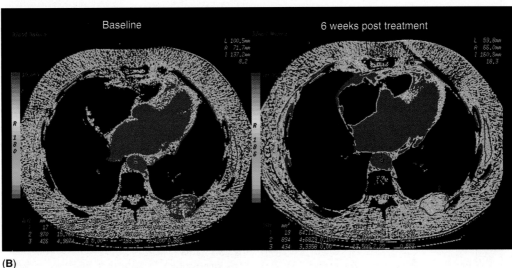

(B)

Figure 61.4 CT and DCE-CT images after six weeks of treatment with a VEGFR inhibitor. (**A**) Conventional CT: No change in size of rib metastasis (circled in image). (**B**) Parameter maps of blood volume show significant reduction post-treatment. RECIST assessment alone would not be sensitive to this functional response. *Source*: Courtesy of Dr. Alison Reid and Dr. Adrian Tang, Royal Marsden Hospital, U.K.

agent injection, for the evaluation of new anti-tumor treatments, is that the examination is inexpensive and is always rapidly feasible and repeatable without adverse effects. In addition, it has been demonstrated that this technique may be less operator dependent.

In a study involving 30 advanced renal cell cancer patients treated with sorafenib, DCE-US was evaluated using perfusion software (Vascular Recognition Imaging) and contrast agent injection (63). Changes in tumor vasculature were found to correlate with tumor response, progression-free survival (PFS), and overall survival (OS), supporting DCE-US as a novel non-invasive imaging technique which might be an effective tool for evaluating antiangiogenic drugs in renal cancer (63).

Positron Emission Tomography (PET)

PET has been increasingly used over the last decade to assess the response of tumors to chemotherapy in patients with a range of malignancies. PET allows dynamic measurement of the three-dimensional distribution of a positron-labeled compound within the body (25). The most commonly used isotope in oncology is 2-[^{18}F]-fluoro-2-deoxyglucose (FDG) (Fig. 61.5). The use of FDG-PET in monitoring the treatment of gastrointestinal stromal

tumor (GIST) with the c-kit inhibitor imatinib has exemplified the significant advantages it possesses over conventional cross-sectional imaging, and suggests the key role this technology may play in aiding the drug development process (Fig. 61.6) (64). In initial studies, high levels of FDG uptake were demonstrated in patients with untreated GIST (65). PET was subsequently shown to be superior to CT imaging in the detection of the earliest functional parameters indicating tumor response induced by imatinib (66). These changes were shown to occur as early on as 24 hours post-imatinib dose (67). Current studies using FDG-PET are assessing the development of imatinib resistance and the efficacy of salvage therapy with second generation c-kit inhibitors (68).

The utility of PET in performing PD biomarker analyses can be separated into those employing generic or specific biological endpoints (2,25,69).

Generic Endpoints

Cellular Proliferation. The most commonly used isotopes have been ^{11}C-thymidine and [^{18}F]-fluorothymidine (FLT) (70,71). FLT-PET has been shown to effectively image the induction of G1 arrest by MEK inhibitors in mutant BRAF tumors, potentially

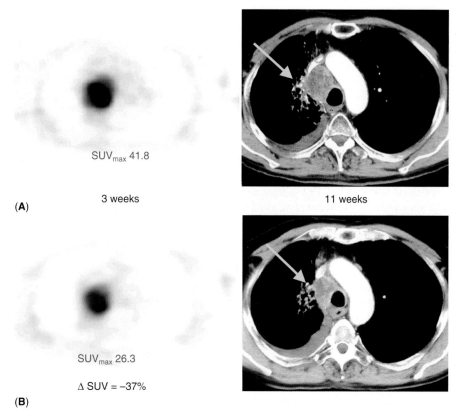

Figure 61.5 FDG-PET of a NSCLC patient treated with an mTOR inhibitor. (**A**) Mediastinal lymph node metastasis from NSCLC showing a 37% reduction in standardized uptake value (SUV) three weeks after commencing an mTOR inhibitor. This was subsequently confirmed at 11 weeks by a reduction in volume on CT scans (**B**). *Source*: Courtesy of Dr. Gary Cook, Royal Marsden Hospital, U.K.

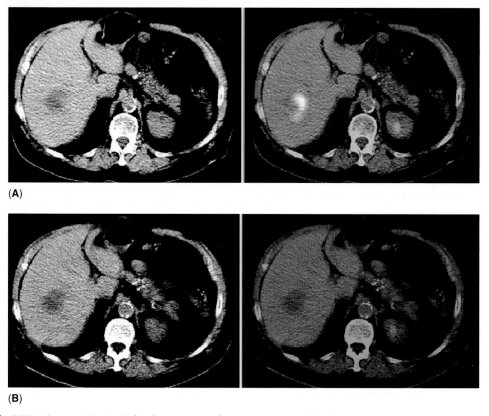

Figure 61.6 FDG PET of a GIST patient receiving imatinib. A liver metastasis from a gastric GIST (**A**) before and (**B**) one week after commencing imatinib therapy. FDG PET/CT scans, unenhanced CT (left), fused FDG PET and CT (right). Although there has been no morphological change in the metastasis, the abnormal baseline metabolic activity (color scale) has rapidly resolved indicating sensitivity to the drug. The SUV fell from 5.0 to 1.8. *Source:* Adapted from Ref. 64.

providing a useful non-invasive method for assessing the early biological response to this class of drugs (72). In a study of 19 patients with recurrent malignant glioma undergoing therapy with bevacizumab and irinotecan, a decrease of >25% in FLT uptake has been defined as a metabolic response (73). FLT changes were compared with response determined by MR imaging and patient survival. There were nine responders (47%) and 10 non-responders (53%). Metabolic responders survived three times as long as non-responders, and both early and later FLT-PET responses were significantly superior predictors of overall survival, compared with the MR imaging responses. Studies are now being conducted to investigate whether FLT-PET performed as early as one to two weeks after starting treatment is as predictive, as this preliminary study indicates, at six weeks.

Tumor Glycolysis. Significant changes in tumor glycolysis, as described above with imatinib, may also occur following treatment with other kinase inhibitors. In particular, drugs which inhibit the phosphoinositide 3-kinase (PI3K)-AKT-mammalian target of rapamycin (mTOR) pathway have particular relevance for the use of FDG-PET. Signaling through the insulin receptor activates PI3K and AKT, stimulating glucose uptake through activation of mTOR and hypoxia induced factor-1-alpha (HIF-1α) (74). The same glycolytic enzymes that are regulated by the pathway are responsible for the uptake and retention of FDG, thus offering the potential for FDG-PET in providing a non-invasive readout of PI3K pathway inhibition (75). Preclinical studies have demonstrated the utility of this approach with mTOR inhibitors in renal cancer, and clinical trials are now underway (76).

Tissue Perfusion. Oxygen-15 (^{15}O)–labeled water PET has been used to assess tissue perfusion. ^{15}O-water is a short-lived tracer with a two-minute half-life. In view of this, the tracer has to be made at a cyclotron in close proximity to the PET scanner. Cyclotrons are however costly and thus the utility of this tracer has been limited to research centers. In Phase I trials of the vascular targeting agents CA4P and endostatin, both studies showed a dose-dependent reduction in tumor perfusion, with a non-linear relation in the endostatin study. CA4P caused a rapid perfusion reduction in solid tumors after 30 minutes, which remained significant after 24 hours (77).

More specific PET endpoints are being validated to provide proof of principle for the proposed mechanism of action of novel molecular targeted therapeutics. These include (25):

- Detection of apoptosis with [^{124}I]-annexin V (78)
- VEGF/VERGFR expression with [^{124}I]-labeled antibodies and peptides (79)
- Measurement of ErBB2 receptor degradation with [^{68}Ga]-labeled anti-ErBB2 antibody fragment after treatment with heat shock protein 90 (HSP90) inhibitors (80). This technology has also been found to be superior to FDG-PET in predicting early response to the HSP90 inhibitor 17-AAG (81).
- 16β-^{18}F-fluoro-5α-dihydrotestosterone (^{18}F-FDHT) PET in patients with metastatic prostate cancer to assess androgen receptor expression (82).

Despite significant advances in the use of PET studies, a number of concerns remain regarding their use as a biomarker of tumor response. One of the biggest issues has been variation in the methodology for PET data collection, analysis, and standardization of scanner technologies. The NCI has recently published guidelines for conducting clinical trials with PET in an attempt to standardize protocols across different institutions (83). This should facilitate clinical trials using PET and ensure reliability of data. In addition, the Oncology Biomarkers Qualification Initiative, a collaboration between the NCI, FDA, and Centers for Medicare and Medicaid Services, are producing standardized protocols for specific cancer types. Aside from FDG-PET, the technologies discussed above have not been standardized or validated, and are therefore best explored in hypothesis-testing Phase I drug development programs.

Another important area for development in the future is the co-registration of PET with other technologies such as MRI. This would potentially provide the ability to determine the extent to which drug distribution influences changes in principal vascular parameters and vice versa (31).

Magnetic Resonance Spectroscopy (see Chapter 65)

Magnetic resonance spectroscopy (MRS) describes the ability of nuclear magnetic resonance to investigate the metabolism of endogenous compounds, tracers, or drugs and their metabolites (25,84). Different chemicals containing the same type of nucleus (e.g., ^{1}H, ^{31}P, ^{13}C) exhibit characteristic chemical shifts in resonance frequency (RF), allowing the chemical form of the element to be identified and so providing a minimally-invasive window on metabolism within the body. The data produced are visualized in the form of spectra with individual peaks representing different chemicals (Fig. 61.7). Endogenous metabolites that can be utilized as pharmacodynamic biomarkers include phosphocholine, phosphomonoesters, or inorganic phosphate using ^{31}P-MRS, or lactate, choline, or inositol compounds using ^{1}H-MRS (Figs. 61.8–61.10). Clinical studies

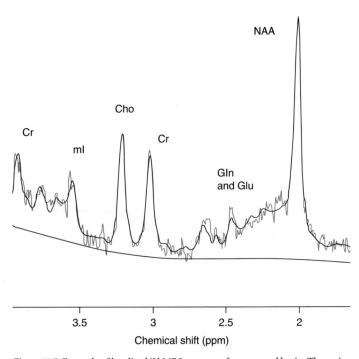

Figure 61.7 Example of localized ^{1}H MRS spectrum from normal brain. The major peaks are creatine (Cr), myo-Inositol (mI), total choline (Cho), glutamine and glutamate (Gln and Glu), N-acetyl aspartate (NAA). *Source*: Courtesy of Dr. Geoffrey Payne, Royal Marsden Hospital, U.K.

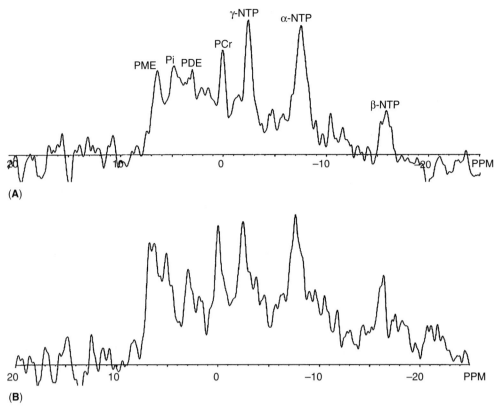

Figure 61.8 In vivo ^{31}P-MRS of HT29 xenografts treated with 17AAG. In vivo ^{31}P-MRS of an HT29 tumor xenograft (**A**) pre-17-allylamino, 17-demethoxygeldanamycin (17AAG) and (**B**) post-17AAG treatment. Peak assignments were as follows: phosphomonoester (PME), inorganic phosphate (Pi), phosphodiester (PDE), phosphocreatine (PCr), nucleoside triphosphate (α-, β-, and γ-NTP). Results were confirmed by 14 separate experiments, and representative spectra are shown. *Source:* Adapted from Ref. 87.

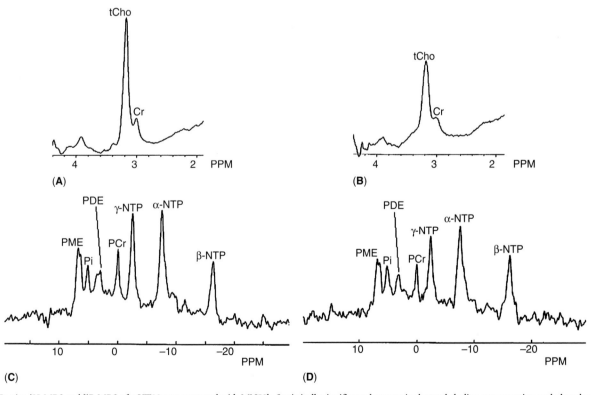

Figure 61.9 In vivo ^{1}H-MRS and ^{31}P-MRS of a HT29 tumor treated with MN58b. Statistically significant decreases in the total choline concentration and phosphomonoesters/total phosphorus signal ratio were found in HT29 xenografts following MN58b treatment. In vivo proton ^{1}H-MRS of a HT29 tumor (**A**) before and (**B**) after MN58b treatment. In vivo phosphorus ^{31}P-MRS of a HT29 tumor (**C**) before and (**D**) after MN58b treatment. Peak assignments were as follows: phosphomonoesters (PME), phosphodiesters (PDE), inorganic phosphate (Pi), phosphocreatione (PCr), nucleoside triphosphate (α-NTP, β-NTP, γ-NTP), total choline (tCho), creatine (Cr). *Source:* Adapted from Ref. 88.

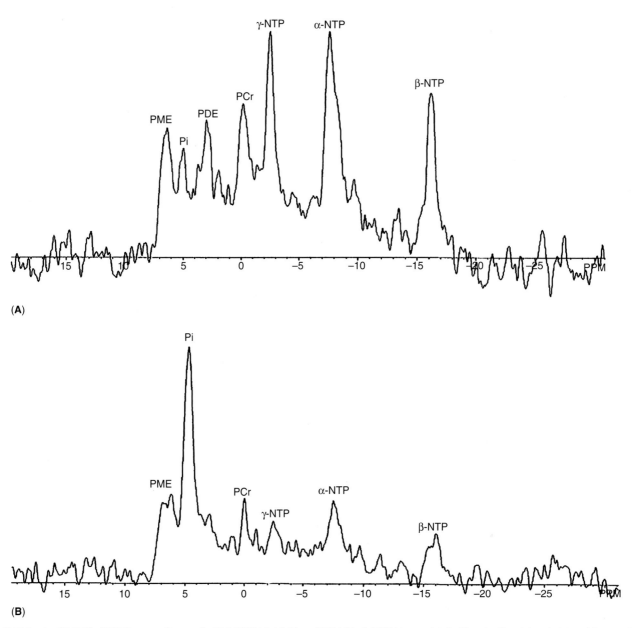

Figure 61.10 In vivo ³¹P-MRS of HT29 xenografts treated with LAQ824. Inhibition of HDAC by LAQ824 is associated with a significant drop in tumor bioenergetics and increase in phosphomonoesters and phosphocholine levels. In vivo ³¹P MR spectra of a HT29 tumor (A) before and (B) after LAQ824 treatment (25 mg/kg i.p. for two days) are shown. Peak assignments: phosphomonoesters (PME), phosphodiesters (PDE), inorganic phosphate (Pi), phosphocreatine (PCr), and nucleoside triphosphates (α-, β-, γ-NTP). *Source*: Adapted from Ref. 89.

have predominantly used ¹H-MRS (particularly looking at changes in total choline in brain, prostate, and breast lesions), since this utilizes the same hardware as conventional ¹H MRI, and to a lesser extent ³¹P-MRS in a range of tumor types. For example, a reduction in the phosphomonoester peak has been shown in patients with breast cancer treated with chemotherapy; these changes may be a marker for changes in tumor proliferation (85). ¹H-MRS has also recently been used to demonstrate that changes in permeability and tumor size correlate with a fall in choline in glioma patients treated with temozolomide (86).

The demonstration of changes in phospholipids using ³¹P-MRS with the HSP90 inhibitor 17-AAG has shown the potential utility of MRS as a pharmaocodynamic biomarker (Fig. 61.8) (87). Using

HT29 human colorectal cancer cells and xenografts, treatment with 17-AAG led to both increases in phosphocholine and phosphomonoesters. In addition, the ratio of phosphomonoester to phosphodiester was increased after 17-AAG treatment relative to the pre-treatment ratio.

MRS has also been used to investigate the PD effects of MN58b, a novel choline kinase inhibitor and LAQ824, a histone deacetylase (HDAC) inhibitor in preclinical studies (Figs. 61.9 and 61.10) (88,89). Treatment with both targeted agents resulted in altered phospholipid metabolism both in cultured tumor cells and *in vivo*. MRS may thus potentially be utilized as a noninvasive PD tool for monitoring tumor response following treatment with both choline kinase and HDAC inhibitors.

One of the issues in the use of MRS is specificity for molecularly targeted agents. For example, both MEK and PI3K inhibitors have been shown to reduce phosphocholine levels in preclinical models (90,91). If MRS is therefore to be used as a PD marker, it is likely that this is a downstream biomarker for several mitogenic and oncogenic signaling cascades. It is hoped that specificity will be improved with improvements in biologically targeted contrast agents (92).

Other potential issues with MRS are low sensitivity and poor resolution of signals, which may be improved with higher field MR systems (2.0–8.0 T). Standardization of protocols across different institutions has been addressed by an international workshop with recommendations published (93), and by large-scale multicenter trials, such as the Interpret study of ^{1}H MRS to develop a classification tool of spectra from brain tumors (94).

Key Points: Functional Imaging Methods for Assessing Molecular Therapy

- Functional imaging may be able to optimize the development and use of antiangiogenics by the appropriate selection of patients likely to respond to treatment
- DCE-MRI is sensitive to alterations in vascular permeability, extracellular extravascular and vascular volumes, and in blood flow
- Using DCE-MRI the choice of parameters for measurement varies widely, although most investigators now regard a change in K^{trans} of >40% as likely to represent a true difference correlating with disease stability and response
- DWI has the potential to determine changes in tumor cellularity following angiogenic therapy
- High tumor cellularity relates to a low apparent diffusion coefficient
- DCE-CT has the ability to quantify vascular parameters such as tumor blood volume, perfusion, and permeability surface product
- DCE-Ultrasound using contrast agents and perfusion software is an evolving technique for evaluating antiangiogenic drugs
- PET is evolving as an important functional imaging technique in the assessment of generic and specific biological endpoints in evaluating therapeutic response
- Generic endpoints include cellular proliferation and tumor glycolysis
- VEGF/VERGFR expression with [^{124}I]-labeled antibodies and peptides is an example of a specific endpoint
- ^{1}H MRS and ^{31}P MRS have been studied in a range of tumors including the brain, breast, and prostate
- MRS has the potential to be a useful PD marker

CHALLENGES FOR FUNCTIONAL IMAGING IN THE CLINIC

Currently, many issues exist that hinder the broader use of functional imaging techniques in the clinic. As discussed, the uptake of functional imaging in Phase III trials remains poor, while questions still remain about its impact on key decision-making in earlier phase clinical trials.

The clinical development of functional imaging techniques is still in its infancy, and more work is required to identify new strategies to detect novel molecular targets and pathways. In view of the low concentration of molecular receptors and targets, coupled with the relative insensitivity of imaging techniques, it is likely that amplification strategies to increase the sensitivity of detection will be required (17). Also, cellular internalization of reporter molecules is likely to be necessary to image certain key pathways. The increased implementation of integrated multi-modular approaches in functional imaging will result in new technical and computational challenges and may be limited by increased costs.

The costs involved with functional imaging are compounded by the need for serial acquisition of images. However, it may be argued that the potential benefits of such biomarkers in providing vital information in early phase trials may prove to be more cost-effective in the long term development of a novel anticancer agent. For example, if imaging can be used to more accurately identify patients who will respond to a certain therapy, then the savings can be redistributed in ways that will benefit all stakeholders involved. Thus, it is vital to ensure that any added benefits of functional imaging biomarkers exceed their potential negative impact on costs, logistics, and speed of clinical trial completion. Given the high attrition rate of individual drugs, it makes sense to prioritize the development of generic imaging assays that measure the biological processes that are generally more applicable to a wide range of drug classes, especially angiogenesis, proliferation, cell cycle status, apoptosis, and invasion (25).

Important technical issues including reproducibility and poor image processing and analysis have limited the clinical development of functional imaging. These are essential factors that should be addressed prior to implementation in clinical trials and appropriately validated. Once a new imaging technique has been validated and qualified, a strategy will still be required to develop this from a technique of interest to a quantitative biomarker that can inform the clinical trial process. In multicenter trials, QA is critical to standardize acquisition and analysis protocols and methodologies to limit variability to a minimum (19).

Greater investment by funding bodies and industry is required, especially in the development, validation, and standardization of minimally invasive techniques and the development of instrumentation (25). Collaborations and communication of data between academic, pharmaceutical, and regulatory communities need to continue to develop, in order to advance the use of functional imaging in clinical studies. Finally, for novel (and expensive) drugs which have proved to be efficacious, the issue of affordability is causing increasing concern. Robust preclinical imaging techniques for selecting at an early stage those patients for whom continued costly treatment is justified must remain a major priority for such collaboration, as will the development of robust surrogate or intermediate imaging endpoints that can be used to support accelerated regulatory drug approval. Such accelerated approval may make the regulatory process less expensive and these novel agents more affordable to cancer patients.

FUTURE DIRECTION

The sequencing of the human genome and the efforts of the Cancer Genome Project, together with novel technological and biological advances in bioinformatics, microarray analysis, and

high throughput screening, have improved our understanding of the molecular basis of cancer (16,95–97). Despite several high-profile successes in the development of novel biological therapies, drug development has remained a slow process. It is envisioned that biomarkers, including functional imaging ones, will play a vital role in the dissection of molecular pathways critically important to cancer, as well as in patient selection and in the development of PK and PD endpoints in clinical trials. These will allow prioritization of drugs that are most likely to succeed, accelerating their regulatory approval, and reducing late and expensive drug attrition, reducing the overall risks and costs of pharmaceutical development (25). An important advantage of functional imaging biomarkers is that these are non-invasive; thus they overcome many ethical and logistical issues associated with invasive assays involving tumor and surrogate tissue in clinical trials (25).

There is an urgent need for a paradigm shift away from the use of anatomical imaging, to clinical functional visualization of specific molecular pathways and cellular functions in tumors. As functional imaging technologies become increasingly available, they need to be utilized in the construction of a pharmacological audit trail that would allow key questions in drug discovery and development to be addressed. Ultimately, this will enable effective drugs to be developed more quickly, for the benefit of all patients during their cancer journey.

Summary

- Certain cancers contain multiple genetic and epigenetic abnormalities, which remain dependent on one or a few genes for both maintenance of the malignant phenotype and cell survival. Inhibition of one or a few of these abnormalities may be used as a therapeutic strategy for selectively killing cancer cells
- Conventional evaluation of a drug in early clinical trial relies on careful study of its pharmacokinetic (PK) and pharmacodynamic (PD) properties
- Drug development of novel anticancer agents remains slow, typically taking between 8 and 10 years from initial pre-clinical drug discovery studies to regulatory approval
- A biomarker may be defined as a characteristic that is objectively measured and evaluated as an indicator of normal biological or pathogenic processes, or of pharmacological responses to a therapeutic intervention
- Biomarkers are classified as either pre-treatment or post-treatment biomarkers. Pre-treatment biomarkers may be prognostic or predictive in aiding patient selection. Post-treatment biomarkers may be used as pharmacological endpoints to measure the effect of a drug on target modulation
- Novel imaging probes and genetic engineering systems have now been developed, These may be utilized in the assessment and monitoring of certain "hallmarks of cancer" including angiogenesis, metabolism, cell proliferation, and apoptosis
- Functional imaging technology holds the promise of changing the face of drug discovery and development, especially in the determination of PK and PD endpoints
- Functional imaging may provide unique information in Phase I trials based on efficacy, thus enabling further development to optimize drugs
- In Phase II trials functional imaging may improve patient selection and provide a robust predictor of clinical benefit
- Improving reproducibility of functional imaging endpoints will have a major impact on the statistical significance of detected changes associated with a specific therapy
- DCE-MRI is sensitive to alterations in vascular permeability, extracellular-extravascular and vascular volumes, and in blood flow. The choice of parameters for measurement varies widely, although most investigators now regard a change in K^{trans} of greater than 40% as likely to represent a true difference correlating with disease stability and response
- DCE-CT has the ability to quantify vascular parameters such as tumor blood volume, perfusion, and permeability surface product
- DCE-Ultrasound using contrast agents and perfusion software is an evolving technique for evaluating antiangiogenic drugs
- PET is evolving as an important functional imaging technique. Generic endpoints include cellular proliferation and tumor glycolysis. VEGF/VERGFR expression with [^{124}I]-labeled antibodies and peptides is an example of a specific endpoint
- ^{1}H MRS and ^{31}P MRS measurements have potential in a range of tumors including the brain, breast, and prostate
- As functional imaging technologies become increasingly available, they need to be utilized in the construction of a pharmacological audit trail that would allow key questions in drug discovery and development to be addressed

REFERENCES

1. George D, Verweij J. Introduction to "A multitargeted approach: clinical advances in the treatment of solid tumours." Ann Oncol 2007; 18 (Suppl 10): x1–12.
2. Sarker D, Workman P. Pharmacodynamic biomarkers for molecular cancer therapeutics. Adv Cancer Res 2007; 96: 213–68.
3. Weinstein IB. Cancer. Addiction to oncogenes—the Achilles heal of cancer. Science 2002; 297: 63–4.
4. Weinstein IB, Joe AK. Mechanisms of disease: Oncogene addiction—a rationale for molecular targeting in cancer therapy. Nat Clin Pract Oncol 2006; 3: 448–57.
5. Workman P. Auditing the pharmacological accounts for Hsp90 molecular chaperone inhibitors: unfolding the relationship between pharmacokinetics and pharmacodynamics. Mol Cancer Ther 2003; 2: 131–8.
6. Workman P. How much gets there and what does it do?: The need for better pharmacokinetic and pharmacodynamic endpoints in contemporary drug discovery and development. Curr Pharm Des 2003; 9: 891–902.
7. Workman P. Challenges of PK/PD measurements in modern drug development. Eur J Cancer 2002; 38: 2189–93.
8. Kelloff GJ, Sigman CC. New science-based endpoints to accelerate oncology drug development. Eur J Cancer 2005; 41: 491–501.
9. Kola I, Landis J. Can the pharmaceutical industry reduce attrition rates? Nat Rev Drug Discov 2004; 3: 711–15.
10. http://www.fda.gov/oc/initiatives/criticalpath/reports/opp_report.pdf

11. Biomarkers Definitions Working Group Bethesda MD. Biomarkers and surrogate endpoints: preferred definitions and conceptual framework. Clin Pharmacol Ther 2001; 69: 89–95.

12. Thomas GV. mTOR and cancer: reason for dancing at the crossroads? Curr Opin Genet Dev 2006; 16: 78–84.

13. Goulart BH, Clark JW, Pien HH, et al. Trends in the use and role of biomarkers in phase I oncology trials. Clin Cancer Res 2007; 13: 6719–26.

14. Hanahan D, Weinberg RA. The hallmarks of cancer. Cell 2000; 100: 57–70.

15. Vaupel P, Kallinowski F, Okunieff P. Blood flow, oxygen and nutrient supply, and metabolic microenvironment of human tumors: a review. Cancer Res 1989; 49: 6449–65.

16. Dzik-Jurasz AS. Molecular imaging in oncology. Cancer Imaging 2004; 4: 162–73.

17. Glunde K, Pathak AP, Bhujwalla ZM. Molecular-functional imaging of cancer: to image and imagine. Trends Mol Med 2007; 13: 287–97.

18. Rudin M. Imaging readouts as biomarkers or surrogate parameters for the assessment of therapeutic interventions. Eur Radiol 2007; 17: 2441–57.

19. Murphy PS, McCarthy TJ, Dzik-Jurasz AS. The role of clinical imaging in oncological drug development. Br J Radiol 2008; 81: 685–92.

20. Roberts TG, Jr, Goulart BH, Squitieri L, et al. Trends in the risks and benefits to patients with cancer participating in phase 1 clinical trials. JAMA 2004; 292: 2130–40.

21. O'Connor JP, Jackson A, Parker GJ, Jayson GC. DCE-MRI biomarkers in the clinical evaluation of antiangiogenic and vascular disrupting agents. Br J Cancer 2007; 96: 189–95.

22. Reid A, Tang A, Spicer J, et al. An open, pharmacokinetic (PK) and mass balance study of 14C-AZD2171, incorporating DCE-CT evaluations. J Clin Oncol (ASCO Annual Meeting Proceedings Part I) 2007; 25(June 20 Suppl): 14140.

23. Holmgren E. Quantifying the usefulness of PD biomarkers in Phase 2 screening trials of oncology drugs. Stat Med 2008; 27: 4928–38.

24. Johnson JR, Williams G, Pazdur R. End points and United States Food and Drug Administration approval of oncology drugs. J Clin Oncol 2003; 21: 1404–11.

25. Workman P, Aboagye EO, Chung YL, et al. Minimally invasive pharmacokinetic and pharmacodynamic technologies in hypothesis-testing clinical trials of innovative therapies. J Natl Cancer Inst 2006; 98: 580–98.

26. Williams SA, Slavin DE, Wagner JA, Webster CJ. A cost-effectiveness approach to the qualification and acceptance of biomarkers. Nat Rev Drug Discov 2006; 5: 897–902.

27. Wagner JA, Williams SA, Webster CJ. Biomarkers and surrogate end points for fit-for-purpose development and regulatory evaluation of new drugs. Clin Pharmacol Ther 2007; 81: 104–7.

28. Prentice RL. Surrogate endpoints in clinical trials: definition and operational criteria. Stat Med 1989; 8: 431–40.

29. Folkman J. Angiogenesis: an organizing principle for drug discovery? Nat Rev Drug Discov 2007; 6: 273–86.

30. Jubb AM, Oates AJ, Holden S, Koeppen H. Predicting benefit from anti-angiogenic agents in malignancy. Nat Rev 2006; 6: 626–35.

31. Atri M. New technologies and directed agents for applications of cancer imaging. J Clin Oncol 2006; 24: 3299–308.

32. Tofts PS. Modeling tracer kinetics in dynamic Gd-DTPA MR imaging. J Magn Reson Imaging 1997; 7: 91–101.

33. Leach MO, Brindle KM, Evelhoch JL, et al. The assessment of antiangiogenic and antivascular therapies in early-stage clinical trials using magnetic resonance imaging: issues and recommendations. Br J Cancer 2005; 92: 1599–610.

34. Morgan B, Thomas AL, Drevs J, et al. Dynamic contrast-enhanced magnetic resonance imaging as a biomarker for the pharmacological response of PTK787/ZK 222584, an inhibitor of the vascular endothelial growth factor receptor tyrosine kinases, in patients with advanced colorectal cancer and liver metastases: results from two phase I studies. J Clin Oncol 2003; 21: 3955–64.

35. Mross K, Drevs J, Muller M, et al. Phase I clinical and pharmacokinetic study of PTK/ZK, a multiple VEGF receptor inhibitor, in patients with liver metastases from solid tumours. Eur J Cancer 2005; 41: 1291–9.

36. Thomas AL, Morgan B, Horsfield MA, et al. Phase I study of the safety, tolerability, pharmacokinetics, and pharmacodynamics of PTK787/ZK 222584 administered twice daily in patients with advanced cancer. J Clin Oncol 2005; 23: 4162–71.

37. Hecht J, Trarbach T, Jaeger E, et al. A randomized, double-blind, placebo-controlled, phase III study in patients (Pts) with metastatic adenocarcinoma of the colon or rectum receiving first-line chemotherapy with oxaliplatin/5-fluorouracil/leucovorin and PTK787/ZK 222584 or placebo (CONFIRM-1). J Clin Oncol (ASCO Annual Meeting Proceedings Part I of II) 2005; 23(June 1 Suppl): LBA3.

38. Koehne C, Bajetta E, Lin E, et al. Results of an interim analysis of a multinational randomized, double-blind, phase III study in patients (pts) with previously treated metastatic colorectal cancer (mCRC) receiving FOLFOX4 and PTK787/ZK 222584 (PTK/ZK) or placebo (CONFIRM 2). J Clin Oncol (ASCO Annual Meeting Proceedings Part I) 2006; 24(June 20 Suppl): 3508.

39. Liu G, Rugo HS, Wilding G, et al. Dynamic contrast-enhanced magnetic resonance imaging as a pharmacodynamic measure of response after acute dosing of AG-013736, an oral angiogenesis inhibitor, in patients with advanced solid tumors: results from a phase I study. J Clin Oncol 2005; 23: 5464–73.

40. Mross K, Gmehling D, Frost A, et al. A clinical Phase I, pharmacokinetic (PK), and pharmacodynamic study of twice daily BIBF 1120 in advanced cancer patients. J Clin Oncol (ASCO Annual Meeting Proceedings Part I of II) 2005; 23(June 1 Suppl): 3031.

41. Drevs J, Medinger M, Mross K, et al. Phase I clinical evaluation of AZD2171, a highly potent VEGF receptor tyrosine kinase inhibitor, in patients with advanced tumors. J Clin Oncol (ASCO Annual Meeting Proceedings Part I of II) 2005; 23(June 1 Suppl): 3002.

42. Flaherty KT, Rosen MA, Heitjan DF, et al. Pilot study of DCE-MRI to predict progression-free survival with sorafenib therapy in renal cell carcinoma. Cancer Biol Ther 2008; 7: 496–501.

43. Galbraith SM, Maxwell RJ, Lodge MA, et al. Combretastatin A4 phosphate has tumor antivascular activity in rat and man as demonstrated by dynamic magnetic resonance imaging. J Clin Oncol 2003; 21: 2831–42.

44. Maxwell RJ, Wilson J, Prise VE, et al. Evaluation of the antivascular effects of combretastatin in rodent tumours by dynamic contrast enhanced MRI. NMR Biomed 2002; 15: 89–98.

45. Jayson GC, Zweit J, Jackson A, et al. Molecular imaging and biological evaluation of HuMV833 anti-VEGF antibody: implications for trial design of antiangiogenic antibodies. J Natl Cancer Inst 2002; 94: 1484–93.

46. Jayson GC, Parker GJ, Mullamitha S, et al. Blockade of platelet-derived growth factor receptor-beta by CDP860, a humanized, PEGylated di-Fab', leads to fluid accumulation and is associated with increased tumor vascularized volume. J Clin Oncol 2005; 23: 973–81.

47. Galbraith SM. Antivascular cancer treatments: imaging biomarkers in pharmaceutical drug development. Br J Radiol 2003; 76 Spec No. 1: S83–S6.

48. Hamstra DA, Rehemtulla A, Ross BD. Diffusion magnetic resonance imaging: a biomarker for treatment response in oncology. J Clin Oncol 2007; 25: 4104–9.

49. Koh DM, Collins DJ. Diffusion-weighted MRI in the body: applications and challenges in oncology. AJR Am J Roentgenol 2007; 188: 1622–35.

50. Ross BD, Moffat BA, Lawrence TS, et al. Evaluation of cancer therapy using diffusion magnetic resonance imaging. Mol Cancer Ther 2003; 2: 581–7.

51. Thoeny HC, De Keyzer F, Chen F, et al. Diffusion-weighted magnetic resonance imaging allows noninvasive in vivo monitoring of the effects of combretastatin a-4 phosphate after repeated administration. Neoplasia 2005; 7: 779–87.

52. Thoeny HC, De Keyzer F, Vandecaveye V, et al. Effect of vascular targeting agent in rat tumor model: dynamic contrast-enhanced versus diffusion-weighted MR imaging. Radiology 2005; 237: 492–9.

53. Herneth AM. Diffusion weighted imaging: have we found the "Holy Grail" of diagnostic imaging or is it still a game of numbers? Eur J Radiol 2003; 45: 167–8.

54. Herneth AM, Guccione S, Bednarski M. Apparent diffusion coefficient: a quantitative parameter for in vivo tumor characterization. Eur J Radiol 2003; 45: 208–13.

55. Goshima S, Kanematsu M, Kondo H, et al. Hepatic hemangioma: Correlation of enhancement types with diffusion-weighted MR findings and apparent diffusion coefficients. Eur J Radiol 2008.

56. Gillard JH, Antoun NM, Burnet NG, Pickard JD. Reproducibility of quantitative CT perfusion imaging. Br J Radiol 2001; 74: 552–5.

57. Atri M, McGregor C, McInnes M, et al. Multidetector helical CT in the evaluation of acute small bowel obstruction: Comparison of non-enhanced (no oral, rectal or IV contrast) and IV enhanced CT. Eur J Radiol 2009; 71: 135–40.

58. Miles KA, Charnsangavej C, Lee FT, et al. Application of CT in the investigation of angiogenesis in oncology. Acad Radiol 2000; 7: 840–50.

59. Willett CG, Boucher Y, di Tomaso E, et al. Direct evidence that the VEGF-specific antibody bevacizumab has antivascular effects in human rectal cancer. Nat Med 2004; 10: 145–7.

60. Fournier L, Thiam R, Cuenod C, et al. Dynamic contrast-enhanced CT (DCE-CT) as an early biomarker of response in metastatic renal cell carcinoma (mRCC) under anti-angiogenic treatment. J Clin Oncol (ASCO Annual Meeting Proceedings Part I) 2007; 25(June 20 Suppl): 14003.

61. Iordanescu I, Becker C, Zetter B, Dunning P, Taylor GA. Tumor vascularity: evaluation in a murine model with contrast-enhanced color Doppler US effect of angiogenesis inhibitors. Radiology 2002; 222: 460–7.

62. Blomley MJ, Eckersley RJ. Functional ultrasound methods in oncological imaging. Eur J Cancer 2002; 38: 2108–15.

63. Lamuraglia M, Escudier B, Chami L, et al. To predict progression-free survival and overall survival in metastatic renal cancer treated with sorafenib: pilot study using dynamic contrast-enhanced Doppler ultrasound. Eur J Cancer 2006; 42: 2472–9.

64. Castell F, Cook GJ. Quantitative techniques in [18]FDG PET scanning in oncology. Br J Cancer 2008; 98: 1597–601.

65. Antoch G, Kanja J, Bauer S, et al. Comparison of PET, CT, and dual-modality PET/CT imaging for monitoring of imatinib (STI571) therapy in patients with gastrointestinal stromal tumors. J Nucl Med 2004; 45: 357–65.

66. Stroobants S, Goeminne J, Seegers M, et al. 18FDG-Positron emission tomography for the early prediction of response in advanced soft tissue sarcoma treated with imatinib mesylate (Glivec). Eur J Cancer 2003; 39: 2012–20.

67. Demetri GD, von Mehren M, Blanke CD, et al. Efficacy and safety of imatinib mesylate in advanced gastrointestinal stromal tumors. N Engl J Med 2002; 347: 472–80.

68. Weber WA, Grosu AL, Czernin J. Technology Insight: advances in molecular imaging and an appraisal of PET/CT scanning. Nat Clin Pract 2008; 5: 160–70.

69. Kelloff GJ, Krohn KA, Larson SM, et al. The progress and promise of molecular imaging probes in oncologic drug development. Clin Cancer Res 2005; 11: 7967–85.

70. Eary JF, Mankoff DA, Spence AM, et al. 2-[C-11]thymidine imaging of malignant brain tumors. Cancer Res 1999; 59: 615–21.

71. Shields AF, Grierson JR, Dohmen BM, et al. Imaging proliferation in vivo with [F-18]FLT and positron emission tomography. Nat Med 1998; 4: 1334–6.

72. Solit DB, Santos E, Pratilas CA, et al. 3'-deoxy-3'-[18F]fluorothymidine positron emission tomography is a sensitive method for imaging the response of BRAF-dependent tumors to MEK inhibition. Cancer Res 2007; 67: 11463–9.

73. Chen W, Delaloye S, Silverman DH, et al. Predicting treatment response of malignant gliomas to bevacizumab and irinotecan by imaging proliferation with [18F] fluorothymidine positron emission tomography: a pilot study. J Clin Oncol 2007; 25: 4714–21.

74. Thompson JE, Thompson CB. Putting the rap on Akt. J Clin Oncol 2004; 22: 4217–26.

75. Mellinghoff IK, Sawyers CL. TORward AKTually useful mouse models. Nat Med 2004; 10: 579–80.

76. Thomas GV, Tran C, Mellinghoff IK, et al. Hypoxia-inducible factor determines sensitivity to inhibitors of mTOR in kidney cancer. Nat Med 2006; 12: 122–7.

77. Anderson HL, Yap JT, Miller MP, et al. Assessment of pharmacodynamic vascular response in a phase I trial of combretastatin A4 phosphate. J Clin Oncol 2003; 21: 2823–30.

78. Collingridge DR, Glaser M, Osman S, et al. In vitro selectivity, in vivo biodistribution and tumour uptake of annexin V radiolabelled with a positron emitting radioisotope. Br J Cancer 2003; 89: 1327–33.

79. Collingridge DR, Carroll VA, Glaser M, et al. The development of [(124)I]iodinated-VG76e: a novel tracer for imaging vascular endothelial growth factor in vivo using positron emission tomography. Cancer Res 2002; 62: 5912–19.

80. Smith-Jones PM, Solit DB, Akhurst T, et al. Imaging the pharmacodynamics of HER2 degradation in response to Hsp90 inhibitors. Nat Biotechnol 2004; 22: 701–6.

81. Smith-Jones PM, Solit D, Afroze F, Rosen N, Larson SM. Early tumor response to Hsp90 therapy using HER2 PET: comparison with 18F-FDG PET. J Nucl Med 2006; 47: 793–6.

82. Larson SM, Morris M, Gunther I, et al. Tumor localization of 16beta-18F-fluoro-5alpha-dihydrotestosterone versus 18F-FDG in patients with progressive, metastatic prostate cancer. J Nucl Med 2004; 45: 366–73.

83. Shankar LK, Hoffman JM, Bacharach S, et al. Consensus recommendations for the use of 18F-FDG PET as an indicator of therapeutic response in patients in National Cancer Institute Trials. J Nucl Med 2006; 47: 1059–66.

84. Leach MO. Magnetic resonance spectroscopy (MRS) in the investigation of cancer at The Royal Marsden Hospital and The Institute of Cancer Research. Phys Med Biol 2006; 51: R61–S82.

85. Leach MO, Verrill M, Glaholm J, et al. Measurements of human breast cancer using magnetic resonance spectroscopy: a review of clinical measurements and a report of localized 31P measurements of response to treatment. NMR Biomed 1998; 11: 314–40.

86. Murphy PS, Viviers L, Abson C, et al. Monitoring temozolomide treatment of low-grade glioma with proton magnetic resonance spectroscopy. Br J Cancer 2004; 90: 781–6.

87. Chung YL, Troy H, Banerji U, et al. Magnetic resonance spectroscopic pharmacodynamic markers of the heat shock protein 90 inhibitor 17-allylamino,17-demethoxygeldanamycin (17AAG) in human colon cancer models. J Natl Cancer Inst 2003; 95: 1624–33.

88. Al-Saffar NM, Troy H, Ramirez de Molina A, et al. Noninvasive magnetic resonance spectroscopic pharmacodynamic markers of the choline kinase inhibitor MN58b in human carcinoma models. Cancer Res 2006; 66: 427–34.

89. Chung YL, Troy H, Kristeleit R, et al. Noninvasive magnetic resonance spectroscopic pharmacodynamic markers of a novel histone deacetylase inhibitor, LAQ824, in human colon carcinoma cells and xenografts. Neoplasia 2008; 10: 303–13.

90. Beloueche-Babari M, Jackson LE, Al-Saffar NM, et al. Magnetic resonance spectroscopy monitoring of mitogen-activated protein kinase signaling inhibition. Cancer Res 2005; 65: 3356–63.

91. Beloueche-Babari M, Jackson LE, Al-Saffar NM, et al. Identification of magnetic resonance detectable metabolic changes associated with inhibition of phosphoinositide 3-kinase signaling in human breast cancer cells. Mol Cancer Ther 2006; 5: 187–96.

92. Lanza GM, Winter P, Caruthers S, et al. Novel paramagnetic contrast agents for molecular imaging and targeted drug delivery. Curr Pharm Biotechnol 2004; 5: 495–507.

93. Leach MO, Arnold D, Brown TR, et al. International Workshop on Standardization in Clinical Magnetic Resonance Spectroscopy Measurements: proceedings and recommendations. Acad Radiol 1994; 1: 171–86.

94. Tate AR, Majos C, Moreno A, et al. Automated classification of short echo time in in vivo 1H brain tumor spectra: a multicenter study. Magn Reson Med 2003; 49: 29–36.

95. Futreal PA, Kasprzyk A, Birney E, et al. Cancer and genomics. Nature 2001; 409: 850–2.

96. Lander ES, Linton LM, Birren B, et al. Initial sequencing and analysis of the human genome. Nature 2001; 409: 860–921.

97. Venter JC, Adams MD, Myers EW, et al. The sequence of the human genome. Science 2001; 291: 1304–51.

62 Positron Emission Tomography: Principles and Clinical Applications
Niklaus G Schaefer, Thomas F Hany, and Gustav K von Schulthess

INTRODUCTION

The definitions of functional imaging and molecular imaging are relatively vague (1). Functional imaging encompasses functional magnetic resonance (MR) imaging (e.g., using BOLD technology, macroscopic and microscopic motion imaging and imaging of any molecular biological phenomenon); molecular imaging is best defined as "a new discipline that unites molecular biology and in vivo imaging. It enables visualization of cellular function and following the molecular process in living organisms without perturbing them" (2). Nuclear medicine (NM) methods are more suitable for this purpose than the other imaging methods. This is because of the exquisite sensitivity of NM detection devices for radioactivity. While x-ray contrast agents change image contrast perceptibly in the millimolar range and MR contrast agents change them in the 10-μM range, radiopharmaceuticals can be detected in nano- or even picomolar concentration. Further enhancement of the MR signal by using ultrasmall superparamagnetic iron oxide (USPIO) agents at concentrations less than micromolar is possible in principle, but in practice the mobility in the human body of such agents is greatly impeded by their size. This makes targeting difficult and USPIO agents usually are not suitable as clinical molecular imaging agents. An increase in MR field strength improves the signal-to-noise ratio (SNR) approximately in proportion, but going from a 1.5 to a 7 T magnet improves the SNR by no more than a factor of five. The improved sensitivity of radiopharmaceuticals over MR contrast agents is a factor of 10,000 to 1 million. As a result, the radiotracer imaging methods, positron emission tomography (PET) and single photon emission computed tomography (SPECT) are currently the only techniques which permit true molecular imaging. Indeed, NM has been a molecular imaging modality since its conception. Radioactive iodine and its molecular properties were used to image and treat benign and malignant thyroid disease using basic molecular biological mechanisms of uptake and iodination of thyroglobulin (3) (see chap. 30).

While PET had been invented before the early days of computed tomography (CT), its clinical breakthrough is the result of three sequential developments. First, the insight, that ^{18}F–fluorodeoxyglucose is avidly taken up into most malignant tumors, but only in very few normal tissues. Second, equipment manufacturers began producing PET machines, which were capable of providing extended body examinations in less than 60 minutes, thereby permitting efficient staging. Third, the introduction of clinical PET-CT in early 2001. In particular, the last development has now resulted in PET-CT scanners and true 3D reconstruction algorithms, which consistently provide attenuation corrected PET images with anatomic reference and scan times less than 15 minutes. All current literature points out the fact that PET-CT is a better test than PET, CT, or PET and CT analyzed side-by-side (4,5). As the CT component in a PET-CT can be chosen to be a high end

CT, a full one-stop shop PET-CT with contrast enhancement can be performed, provided that the NM physicians and radiologists solve their local turf battles in this area. Although SPECT-CT also has some useful applications in clinical practice, it is largely limited to bone SPECT, iodine SPECT in thyroid malignancies, in somatostatin receptor SPECT positive tumors such as carcinoids and in noradrenaline tracer SPECT, which permits imaging of tumors such as pheochromocytoma and neuroblastoma. Since FDG PET dominates NM oncologic imaging at this time, most of this chapter is devoted to summarizing the experience to date with this tracer.

THE NORMAL FDG-PET SCAN: ARTEFACTS AND PITFALLS

It is well known that imaging specialists unfamiliar with FDG PET will be overly sensitive in lesion detection, thus generating too many false positive findings. It is therefore relevant for the cancer radiologist to be familiar with some of the most frequent pitfalls. Only a brief summary is given here and for data acquisition techniques and for a more extensive discussion of normal findings, the reader is referred to textbooks specifically discussing PET-CT (6).

Using PET-CT, artefacts on PET images are mainly due to CT artefacts, as a result of attenuation correction with CT data. Problems noted are due mainly to mis-registration between the two scans due to patient motion (7), but are also due to the fact that CT is acquired in respiratory arrest, while PET is acquired during free-breathing. We have found that with modern fast multidetector CT (MDCT) the best way to proceed is to acquire a low dose CT attenuation scan during free breathing in a similar way to the PET scan. This low dose CT scan is also clinically evaluated. If a contrast-enhanced CT examination is required it can be done at the end of the study. PET artefacts due to CT attenuation correction occur mainly around the diaphragm. A high density contrast agent from a previous study and metallic implants, for example, in the dental region, will also cause artefacts, which on the PET scans appear as increased tracer accumulations (8). Whether a finding is real or not can be diagnosed easily if the PET scans not corrected for attenuation are also viewed: if an artefact is present, it will not show up on these scans.

A normal PET scan obtained after a minimum of four hours of fasting in a non-diabetic will demonstrate FDG uptake in the brain, the kidney, renal collecting system, bladder, and sometimes the heart (Fig. 62.1). Some patients show FDG-uptake in brown fatty tissue, which is distributed along the neck, axial skeleton, mediastinum, and down to around the upper abdominal organs (Fig. 62.1) (9). Normal breast tissue and ovaries (10) can exhibit FDG-uptake and finally, statically or dynamically exercised muscle will frequently take up FDG. Both these findings are usually easily detectable on a PET-CT study. A notable finding is FDG accumulation in muscles around the larynx. If recurrent nerve palsy is

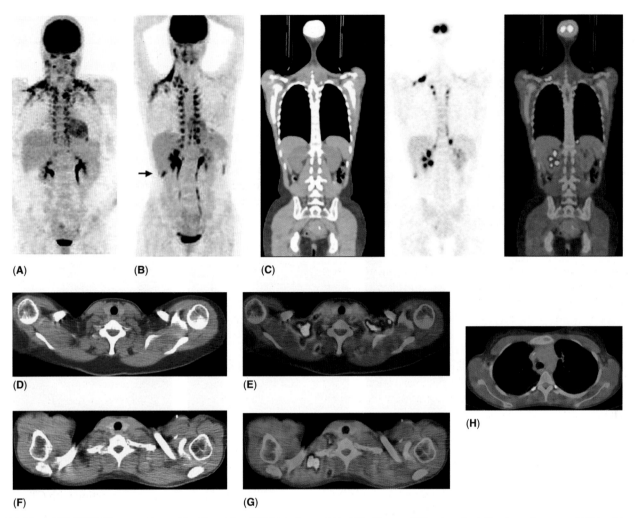

Figure 62.1 Normal ¹⁸F-FDG PET scans with considerable uptake of FDG into brown fat in (**A**) a 35-year-old female patient after chemotherapy and (**B**) in a 24-year-old female patient after chemoradiation. In this patient there is asymmetric uptake of tracer into the brown fat of the neck. There is lack of uptake to the left side of the neck due to previous radiotherapy. In both patients there is intense symmetric FDG accumulation in the paraspinous region well shown in images (**A**) and (**B**). In addition there is a focus of fat below the right lobe of the liver (arrow) (**B**), and a further focus superomedial to the spleen, best shown on the PET-CT image (**C**). Uptake of FDG in fat can be correlated with areas of hypodensity on corresponding CT images (**D**) to (**H**).

present, for example due to an aorto-pulmonic window tumor or after radical neck surgery, these globular muscles may appear as FDG foci which are easily confused with metastatic scalene lymph nodes. However their anatomic location on PET-CT again resolves this diagnostic pitfall (11).

Frequently, FDG is taken up by bowel. If extensive areas of large bowel show uptake the findings usually require no further investigation, but it should be remembered that inflammatory bowel disease will also show increased uptake; focal lesions in the large bowel require a colonoscopy, as two-thirds of those lesions are cancerous or precancerous (12).

Mild or chronic inflammation in the musculoskeletal system will also show FDG uptake as activated inflammatory cells are strongly FDG avid. Hence, osteoarthritic changes, mainly in the acromio-clavicular joints, tendinoses, and inflammatory changes around joint prostheses will all demonstrate increased uptake of FDG. Gastroesophageal reflux,

gastritis, diverticulitis, and mild inflammatory reaction to any foreign material such as vascular grafts will show mild to moderate FDG uptake and this must be recognized. Acute fractures, for example, in the ribs, will also be revealed as FDG foci. Scrutiny of the bone window CT images allows differentiation from bone metastases.

There are some benign lesions which show avid FDG uptake. The most frequently identified is a Warthin's tumor in the parotid gland (13). Villonodular sinovitis is known to take up FDG and in our experience, other rare benign tumors also sometimes avidly take up FDG. In general, if a lesion clearly identified as pathological takes up FDG, this is a poor prognostic sign and if a lesion continues to take up FDG after therapy, the prognosis is worse. There is ample evidence in the literature that a metabolic response to therapy as demonstrated by FDG PET correlates well with survival in patients with many different malignant tumors.

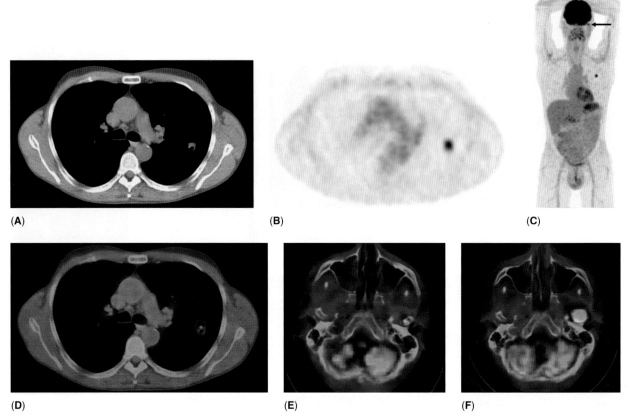

Figure 62.2 A 62-year-old male patient with a pulmonary nodule demonstrated on axial CT (**A**). Axial PET (**B**) and coronal FDG PET MIP (**C**) images demonstrate that the nodule takes up FDG. This is confirmed on (**D**) a PET-CT scan. A small focus of avid FDG-uptake is noted in the left temporal bone in the coronal MIP image (**C**, arrow) This is also seen on the corresponding PET-CT image (**E**). Follow-up study three months later (**F**) shows that the lesion in the temporal bone has increased in size indicating progression.

Key Points: General

- PET and SPECT are currently the only techniques which permit true molecular imaging
- All current literature points out the fact that PET-CT is a better test than PET, CT, or PET and CT analyzed side-by-side
- A normal PET scan obtained after a minimum of four hours of fasting will demonstrate FDG uptake into the brain, the kidneys, renal collecting system, bladder, and sometimes the heart
- Occasionally uptake is seen in the normal breast and ovaries
- Some patients show FDG-uptake in brown fatty tissue
- Mild or chronic inflammation in the musculoskeletal system shows FDG uptake because activated inflammatory cells avidly take up FDG
- Metabolic response to therapy as demonstrated by a decline in FDG PET uptake in the tumor correlates well with survival in many different malignant tumors

INDICATIONS FOR FDG-PET IN CLINICAL ONCOLOGY

The vast majority of patients referred for PET scanning are cancer patients, and most examinations are performed using FDG either with FDG PET scanning or FDG PET-CT. For simplicity in this section we refer to FDG PET(CT).

FDG (F-18 fluorodeoxyglucose), a derivative of glucose, has proven to be a successful tracer because most malignant tumors take up much more FDG than their surrounding tissue. Tumors either express more glucose transporter molecules, or use more glucose or both. These pathophysiological mechanisms enable ready identification of primary tumors and their metastases (Fig. 62.2).

As the use of PET in various tumors is discussed in other chapters in this book, this chapter summarizes the clinical settings in which PET is indicated in oncology on a tumor-by-tumor basis. The impact of PET on the management of different types of malignancy is indicated as follows:

- 0 none
- + low
- ++ moderate
- +++ high
- ++++ very high

Hodgkin's Lymphoma and Aggressive Non-Hodgkin's Lymphoma

Staging: Impact ++++

FDG PET(CT) detects significantly more extranodal sites of lymphoma (bone, liver, spleen) than anatomic imaging alone. This leads to improved staging in all subtypes of Hodgkin's diseases and aggressive non-Hodgkin's lymphoma (14).

Mid-Term Assessment: Impact ++++
FDG PET(CT) predicts progression-free survival after one to four cycles of chemotherapy in Hodgkin's disease and aggressive non-Hodgkin's lymphoma. Large studies are underway in which chemotherapy is altered after early restaging with FDG PET (15,16).

End of Chemotherapy Assessment: Impact ++++
Similar results have been achieved after mid-term assessment with FDG PET(CT). FDG PET(CT) is also used in the assessment of residual masses after therapy. FDG active residual masses after induction chemotherapy have a worse prognosis compared with inactive masses or in patients in whom a mass has completely resolved on anatomical imaging. Patients with active residual tumor require further treatment (17,18).

Follow-Up: Impact +
As yet, there is only very limited data on the value of FDG PET(CT) in patients who have achieved a complete response after induction therapy. The technique is therefore not recommended as routine follow-up. However, in patients with clinically suspected recurrence (e.g., increased LDH, night sweat) FDG PET(CT) appears to be useful (19).

Response to Salvage Chemotherapy: Impact ++++
Several studies have shown that FDG PET(CT) prior to and after salvage chemotherapy predicts the risk of failure to high dose chemotherapy and autologous stem cell support. These studies have shown shorter progression-free survival in patients with persistent FDG uptake in lymphoma lesions prior to high dose chemotherapy and autologous stem cell support (20,21).

Planning Radiotherapy: Impact ++++
Lesions seen on the FDG PET(CT) prior to chemotherapy must be included in planning the radiation field in patients who are undergoing additional radiotherapy for residual disease after the end of induction chemotherapy (22).

Indolent Non-Hodgkin's Lymphoma
General Indications: Impact 0 to +
There is still limited data on FDG PET(CT) in patients with low grade lymphomas. There is evidence that nodal marginal zone lymphoma, MALT type lymphoma, follicular lymphoma Grade I/II, and mantle cell lymphoma are well depicted by FDG PET(CT). Therapy response assessment is also valid for these types of lymphoma. However, limited data shows that FDG PET(CT) is not useful in small lymphocytic lymphoma. FDG PET(CT) may also have a role in directing biopsy in patients with low-grade non-Hodgkin's lymphoma suspected of transformation into more aggressive disease (23,24).

Myeloma
General Indications: Impact +
There is very limited data of FDG PET(CT) in myeloma. However, small series show that FDG PET(CT) is able to detect osseous lesions in myeloma. Whole-body CT and MR imaging of the spine and pelvis still remain the gold standard imaging techniques for the detection of bone marrow involvement in myeloma and no imaging modality can replace bone marrow biopsy. The role of FDG

PET(CT) needs to be clarified but at present it appears that the technique only provides additional information for the assessment of osseous myeloma in areas not covered by MR imaging (25,26).

Melanoma
Staging: Impact ++
FDG PET(CT) is of proven value in the staging of malignant melanoma and should be added to conventional imaging routinely in high-risk patients (melanoma thicker than 4 mm, proven loco-regional or distant metastases). FDG PET(CT) has a role in depicting distant metastases and its greatest impact is on the detection of extranodal metastases. FDG PET(CT) cannot replace sentinel node biopsy, and brain metastases are not accurately identified with FDG PET(CT). Furthermore, FDG PET(CT) is not useful for staging loco-regional lymph nodes (27).

Follow-Up: Impact ++++
FDG PET(CT) seems valuable in the follow-up of high-risk patients and/or patients with rising tumor markers (S-100) (28).

Lung Cancer (Non-Small Cell)
Solitary Pulmonary Nodule: Impact ++++
FDG PET(CT) accurately discriminates between malignant and benign lesions, but due to FDG accumulation in inflammatory lesions, there can be false positive lesions (29).

Primary Tumor Staging: Impact ++++
FDG PET(CT) has a better diagnostic performance in T staging than PET alone. However, there are some lung cancers such as bronchioloalveolar cell carcinoma, which can have little or no FDG-uptake (27).

Local Metastases: Impact ++++
Patients with Stage I disease and negative mediastinal lymph nodes on FDG PET(CT) usually do not need further mediastinoscopy. However, this strategy should be used with caution in patients with central tumors and those with primary tumors with low FDG uptake such as bronchioloalveolar cell carcinoma. In the case of a positive mediastinal FDG PET(CT), a biopsy/mediastinoscopy is recommended to confirm mediastinal involvement (false positive lesions due to inflammation have to be excluded) (30).

Distant Metastases: Impact ++++
FDG PET(CT) has a high sensitivity and specificity for the detection of extrathoracic disease compared to conventional imaging. Therefore FDG PET(CT) can obviate the need for surgical procedures in patients with metastasis from non-small-cell lung cancer (31).

Recurrence: Impact ++++
FDG PET(CT) should routinely be added to the conventional work-up in detecting recurrent disease in patients with clinically suspected recurrence.

Lung Cancer (Small Cell)
General: Impact +
Only small studies in patients with small cell lung cancer address the use of FDG PET(CT). This tumor type is often FDG-positive. Current staging only classifies the disease status as limited-stage

or extensive-stage, and this information can also be obtained by CT imaging. Thus, the value of FDG PET-CT is limited (27).

Pleural Mesothelioma
General: Impact +
In most cases pleural mesothelioma demonstrates FDG-uptake and may be used in the assessment of therapy response (32,33).

Breast Cancer
Primary Tumor: Impact 0
FDG PET(CT) should not be used in the work-up of suspected breast cancer (34).

Local Metastases: Impact 0
FDG PET(CT) has little or no additional value compared to axillary lymph node dissection and sentinel node biopsy (34).

Distant Metastases: Impact +++
FDG PET(CT) has the potential to detect distant metastases in high-risk patients and may replace conventional work-up (34).

Recurrence: Impact ++
FDG PET(CT) has only limited value in the evaluation of a histologically proven local recurrence but is valuable in detection of distant metastases and replaces conventional imaging like bone scanning in such cases (34).

Cervical Cancer
Staging: Impact +
FDG PET(CT) for primary staging has a promising role in locally advanced previously untreated cervical cancer. FDG PET-CT has only limited value in the detection of additional locoregional lymph node metastases. FDG PET-CT has additional value for the detection of distant metastasis (35–37).

Recurrence: Impact +
FDG PET(CT) may be beneficial in the detection of locoregional recurrence and detection of distant metastases; FDG PET should be performed only when equivocal findings result from the conventional work-up (38,39).

Ovarian Cancer
Staging: Impact +
FDG PET(CT) can depict tumor deposits and metastases greater than 1 cm in diameter as well as nodal infiltration and distant metastasis. However, peritoneal infiltration is often missed and therefore surgical staging remains the gold standard (40–42).

Recurrence: Impact +
FDG PET(CT) may be helpful in the detection of recurrent disease in patients with rising cancer antigen (CA125) and equivocal findings on conventional work-up (43–45).

Endometrial Cancer
Staging: Impact 0
Very limited information of FDG PET in the management of endometrial cancer is available. Therefore FDG PET(CT) for staging or restaging of endometrial cancer is not routinely performed at this time (46,47).

Vulval Cancer
General: Impact 0
There is only limited data in case series; FDG PET(CT) is not recommended (48).

Head and Neck Cancer
Cancer of Unknown Origin: Impact +++
FDG PET(CT) is able to identify unknown primary tumors in more than 20% of the patients with positive cervical lymph nodes and an unknown primary tumor (49).

Primary Tumor Staging: Impact +
FDG PET-CT has only limited additional value compared to CT or MR imaging in the evaluation and staging of the primary tumor (50).

Nodal Staging: Impact +
FDG PET(CT) has only limited additional value compared to CT or MR imaging in the evaluation of loco-regional lymph node metastases (51).

Distant Metastases: Impact ++
FDG PET(CT) should routinely be added to further imaging modalities to improve staging of distant metastasis in node positive, advanced head and neck cancer (52).

Recurrence: Impact +
FDG PET(CT) is more accurate than CT or MR imaging in the detection of local recurrence and should be added when findings are unequivocal (53).

Esophageal Cancer
Primary Tumor Staging: Impact +
Primary staging of esophageal cancer is performed by endoscopic ultrasonography as the standard of reference. FDG PET(CT) does delineate advanced T-stage (T3-T4) in esophageal cancer with a sensitivity ranging from 69% to 97%, but small tumors (Stage T1-T2) are difficult to depict and false negative examinations can occur (54).

Nodal Staging: Impact +
FDG PET(CT) has only a limited value in locoregional lymph node staging (sensitivity 20–50%). Lymph node staging remains the domain of endoscopic ultrasonography (55).

Distant Metastases: Impact ++
FDG PET(CT) provides useful information in the detection of distant metastasis in approximately 5% of patients. The major role of FDG PET(CT) is in the avoidance of unnecessary surgical procedures in patients with inoperable disease (56).

Recurrence: Impact ++
FDG PET(CT) has a high sensitivity in the detection of recurrence of esophageal cancer. FDG PET(CT) may be used as an adjunct and, if available, should routinely be added to conventional imaging in the diagnostic work-up of patients with suspected recurrent esophageal cancer (57).

Gastric Cancer

Primary Tumor Staging: Impact +
FDG PET(CT) plays only a minor role in staging gastric cancer. The intestinal type is depicted with a sensitivity of 44%, the signet cell type and the diffuse type have even lower sensitivities for detection (58).

Nodal Staging: Impact +
FDG PET(CT) has variable sensitivity in detection of lymph node metastases (up to 70%). However, due to variable uptake patterns of the primary tumor, the overall sensitivity is probably lower (59).

Distant Metastases: Impact ++
There is insufficient data on FDG PET(CT) in the staging of distant metastasis in patients with gastric cancer.

Recurrence: Impact ++
The role of FDG PET(CT) in recurrent gastric cancer is under investigation. Sensitivities of up to 70% have been described in the few studies reported (60).

Colorectal Carcinoma

Primary Tumor: Impact 0
FDG PET(CT) plays no role in the detection of primary colorectal cancer. Screening of asymptomatic patients for colorectal cancer with FDG PET(CT) is not recommended (27).

Nodal Staging: Impact 0
FDG PET(CT) has a low sensitivity in the detection of lymph node metastasis in patients with unresected primary colorectal cancer. Thus FDG PET(CT) is not recommended in lymph node staging of primary colorectal carcinoma (61).

Distant Metastases (Hepatic): Impact ++++
FDG PET(CT), preferably in conjunction with contrast-enhanced CT, should be used routinely in addition to conventional imaging in the pre-operative diagnostic work-up of patients with potentially resectable hepatic metastases from colorectal cancer. The detection of liver metastasis is the most useful information to be gained by FDG PET(CT) (62).

Distant Metastases (Extra Hepatic): Impact ++++
The use of FDG PET(CT) in conjunction with contrast-enhanced CT is beneficial for evaluating recurrence of colorectal carcinoma if contrast-enhanced CT is inconclusive, if carcinoembryonic antigen levels (CEA) are increased, or if local relapse is clinically suspected. Most of the benefit is attributable to detection of extra-hepatic metastases, which generally preclude resection of liver metastases. FDG PET(CT) can avoid unnecessary surgery and help to determine other appropriate treatment (63).

Recurrence: Impact ++++
In patients with a clinical suspicion of recurrence and/or an increased CEA level, FDG PET is recommended. FDG PET(CT) can discriminate between a post-operative scar and active tumor recurrence. In patients with rising CEA, FDG PET(CT) can localize the site of disease in many cases. In patients with suspected recurrence FDG PET(CT) finds more hepatic and extrahepatic lesions than conventional imaging studies (64).

Pancreatic Cancer

Primary Diagnosis: Impact +
FDG PET(CT) improves detection rates in patients with equivocal contrast-enhanced CT findings (65).

Primary Tumor Staging: Impact +
FDG PET(CT) in conjunction with dedicated contrast-enhanced CT improves decision-making regarding local resectability (66).

Nodal Staging: Impact 0
Due to low sensitivity in the detection of loco-regional lymph node metastases, FDG PET(CT) plays no significant role in the lymph node staging of pancreatic cancer (67).

Distant Metastases: Impact ++
FDG PET(CT) improves detection of distant metastases, for example, in the neck (68).

Recurrence: Impact ++
FDG PET(CT) may delineate scar from active tumor tissue in patients with rising tumor markers (69).

Hepatocellular Cancer (HCC)

General: Impact 0
FDG-uptake in HCC is related to tumor grade (low grade tumor/histological Grade I does not demonstrate distinguishable FDG-uptake compared with normal liver tissue) (70,71).

Cholangiocarcinoma

General: Impact +
FDG PET can be used to assess mass-forming cholangiocellular carcinoma. The sensitivity of FDG PET in these patients is 85%. In infiltrating type cholangiocarcinoma, FDG PET(CT) has a sensitivity lower than 20%. A certain advantage may be seen in the detection of distant metastases (e.g., mediastinal lymph node metastases) (72).

Gallbladder Cancer

General: Impact +
The role of FDG PET has been described in a small series. The sensitivity of FDG PET in staging of the primary tumor is 78%. Extrahepatic metastases have been found with a sensitivity of 50% (73).

Gastrointestinal Stromal Tumor (GIST)

General: Impact +++
GIST demonstrate high FDG-uptake, the major utility for FDG PET(CT) is in the assessment of early therapeutic response (74).

Renal Cell Cancer

General: Impact 0
The detection of renal cell carcinoma with FDG PET(CT) is hampered because FDG is excreted through the kidneys. Therefore FDG PET(CT) plays no role in the staging of primary renal cancer. However, FDG PET(CT) may play a role in the detection of nodal and distant metastasis from renal cancer (75,76).

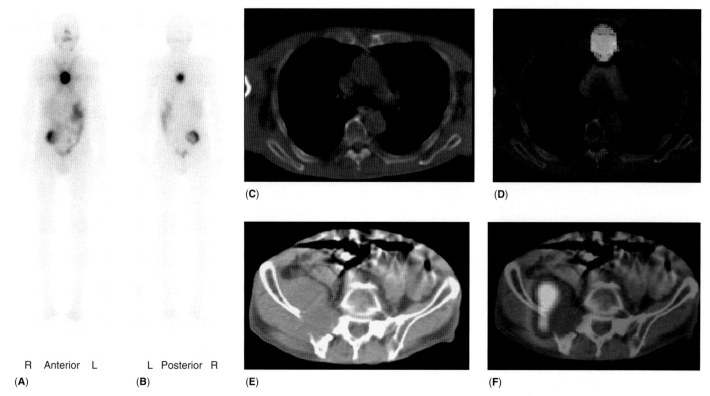

R   Anterior   L   L   Posterior   R
(A)   (B)   (E)   (F)

Figure 62.3 A 65-year-old patient with metastatic follicular thyroid cancer. (A) and (B) I-131 scans after I-131 therapy with 7400 MBq in the AP and PA projection showing lesions in the upper chest and in the right pelvis. These lesions are well-demonstrated on the fused SPECT-CT images (C), (D), (E), and (F).

Prostate Cancer

Staging: Impact 0
Studies have shown that FDG PET(CT) is generally not suitable for staging prostate cancer. FDG PET(CT) does not reliably delineate bone metastases (77).

Recurrence: Impact 0
In patients with rising PSA after prostatectomy, FDG PET(CT) does not reliably differentiate between scar tissue and local recurrence (78).

Bladder Cancer

General: Impact +
Urinary excretion of ^{18}F-FDG through the kidneys into the urinary tract hampers the evaluation of the pelvic region and in particular the bladder. For this reason, FDG PET(CT) has not been useful in local staging. However, FDG PET(CT) may have a role in detection of nodal and distant metastases (79).

Thyroid Cancer

Staging: Impact 0
FDG PET(CT) is not beneficial in the initial staging of follicular or papillary thyroid cancer.

Recurrence: Impact ++
FDG PET(CT) is beneficial in patients who have previously been treated for thyroid cancer when the findings of ^{131}-Iodine whole-body scintigraphy are negative but the level of thyroglobulin serum marker is elevated (80,81).

Soft Tissue Sarcoma

General: Impact 0
The evidence is insufficient to support the use of FDG PET(CT) in patients with soft tissue sarcoma (82).

Unknown Primary Tumor

General: Impact ++++
FDG PET(CT) should routinely be added to the conventional work-up of patients with unknown primary cancer (83).

SPECT AND SPECT-CT

As stated, for some tumors, SPECT-CT scanning is well established, but will only be mentioned briefly here. Established applications encompass bone SPECT, mainly used in osseous tumors and in the differentiation of metastases from degenerative joint disease in the spine, Iodine SPECT-CT, mainly used after radioiodine therapy (Fig. 62.3), and Indium Octreotide SPECT-CT used for endocrine tumors. It is beyond the scope of this section to describe details of the normal SPECT-CT scans in these disease entities.

OTHER TRACERS USED IN TUMOR IMAGING WITH PET

There are a large number of other tracers that have been used in tumor imaging with PET or are currently being investigated. None of them have reached importance comparable to that of FDG. The applications are summarized in tabular form in Table 62.1. A brief discussion of the tracers most widely used is given here.

Table 62.1 New PET Tracers in Oncology—a Tabulated Overview

Tracer	Biology	Tumor types	PET studies	References
^{18}F-DOPA	^{18}F-fluoro-l-dihydroxyphenyl-alanine is useful for the evaluation of the in vivo activity of aromatic l-amino acid decarboxylase. NET arise from the APUD system and are able to take up, accumulate and decarboxylate amine precursors, so they are characterized by high ^{18}F-DOPA uptake on PET scans	Neuroendocrine tumors (NET)	^{18}F-DOPA PET provides sensitive localization of primary tumors, lymph node staging and metastatic disease in patients with neuroendocrine tumors.	84,85
^{68}Ga-DOTATOC	NET can heterogeneously overexpress somatostatin receptors (SSTR). [1,4,7,10-tetraazacy-clododecane-N,N'N",N-tetraacetic-acid-d-Phe1-Tyr3]-octreotide binds the somatostatin receptor 2.	Neuroendocrine tumors (NET)	^{68}Ga-DOTATOC uptake is higher than ^{18}F-FDG uptake in neuroendocrine tumor lesions. ^{68}Ga-DOTATOC predicts response to SSTR directed therapy. Consequently ^{68}Ga-DOTATOC could be a promising tool for the accurate evaluation of patients with metastatic NETs	86
[11]C- or ^{18}F choline derivatives	Phosphatidylcholine is an essential element of phospholipids of the cell membrane and choline is its precursor. Neoplastic tissue has elevated levels of phosphatidylcholine. Choline kinase, which catalyses the phosphorylation of choline, is also elevated in neoplastic tissue	Prostate cancer	^{11}C-choline PET is superior to ^{18}F-FDG PET and complementary to conventional imaging in restaging prostate cancer in patients with increasing PSA levels.	87, 88
^{18}F-MISO	Hypoxia is a known prognostic factor in oncology. Hypoxic tumors are more resistant to chemotherapy and radiotherapy. Fluorine-18-Misonidazole is a nitromidazole compound which undergoes an intracellular chemical reaction in hypoxic tissue when pO_2 is lower than 10 mmHg. The reaction product binds covalently to intracellular macromolecules. ^{18}F-MISO is not retained in necrosis.	Non-small-cell lung cancer, breast cancer, gliomas, head and neck cancer	^{18}F-MISO PET is able to monitor the changing hypoxia status of lung tumors during radiotherapy. Studies in sarcoma and head and neck cancer have demonstrated a correlation of ^{18}F-FMISO uptake with poor outcomes to radiation and chemotherapy.	89–93
[60]Cu-ATSM	Cu-diacetyl-bis (N4-methylthiosemicarbazone) shows retention in hypoxic tumor tissue due to the altered redox environment in hypoxic tumors by increased NADH levels.	Cervical cancer, lung cancer	In human studies of lung and cervical cancers, encouraging evidence has emerged that [60]Cu-ATSM can act as a prognostic indicator for response to therapy.	94,95
^{18}F-DHT	16β-Fluoro-5-dyhidrotestosterone (FDHT) is a structural analogue of 5-dyhidrotestosterone, the primary ligand of the androgen receptors. Androgen receptors play a role in the biologic behavior of prostate cancer. ^{18}F-FDHT has binding affinity and selectivity for androgen receptors.	Prostate cancer	^{18}F-FDHT could be a sensitive tracer for the detection of prostate metastases. ^{18}F-FDHT determines the level and the activity of androgen receptors. This may be helpful to initiate or suspend hormonal therapy. At present time, there is little data and the clinical value of ^{18}F-FDHT PET remains unknown	96,97
^{18}F-FLT	^{18}F-3-fluoro-3-deoxy-thymidine (^{18}F-FLT) is a pyrimidine analogue and reflects the activity of a thymidine kinase-1 during the S phase of DNA synthesis. Therefore ^{18}F-FLT is a radiotracer for in vivo evaluation of the cell proliferation rate. Due to these biological characteristics, ^{18}F-FLT is considered a promising radiotracer for treatment monitoring of cancers.	Lung cancer, colorectal cancer, melanoma, soft tissue sarcoma, breast cancer, brain tumors	There is strong correlation between FLT uptake and the proliferation rate by the Ki-67 index. FLT is a surrogate marker of proliferation, and it is considered to be a potential tool for monitoring anti-cancer treatment. It may offer more in vivo capability than FDG to evaluate the patient's response to new drugs and to predict clinical outcome. More preclinical and clinical studies are needed to validate this application	98–104
[11]C-acetate	Acetate is a metabolic substrate of β-oxidation for synthesis of cholesterol and of lipids. ^{11}C-acetate is incorporated into the lipid-soluble fraction of tumor cells and reflects the high-growth activity. ^{11}C-acetate is not eliminated through urination and therefore may be a good tracer for the imaging of prostate and kidney tumors.	Renal cell carcinoma (RCC), Prostate cancer, Hepatocellular carcinoma (HCC)	The imaging of renal cell carcinoma was the initial purpose for the introduction of ^{11}C-acetate. However, recent reports do not support the use of ^{11}C-acetate in RCC. In prostate cancer, ^{11}C-acetate-PET depicts neoplasms in 59% of the patients. FDG PET is mostly unsuitable for imaging prostate cancer. ^{11}C-acetate is more sensitive than FDG PET for detection of HCC	105–109
[18]F–fluoride	The fluoride ions are exchanged with the hydroxyl group in bone crystals and form fluoroapatite. Increased ^{18}F–fluoride PET uptake in bone lesions reflects both an increased blood flow and an increased bone accretion.	Bone metastases of various tumors	^{18}F–fluoride PET is more accurate for detection of osteolytic and osteoblastic lesions compared to scintigraphy and MRI. ^{18}F–fluoride PET-CT is highly sensitive and specific for detection of bone metastases, and is superior to ^{18}F–fluoride PET as well as planar and SPECT bone scintigraphy.	110–113

(Continued)

Table 62.1 New PET Tracers in Oncology—a Tabulated Overview (*Continued*)

Tracer	Biology	Tumor types	PET studies	References
[11]C-methionine	^{11}C-methionine has been developed as a PET tracer for imaging of gliomas, which overexpress amino acid transporters. In contrast to FDG it does not accumulate in normal brain tissue.	Glioma	^{11}C-methionine has been investigated in several settings; for detection of primary or suspected recurrence of glioma, as a prognostic marker, as guidance for stereotactic brain biopsy, as a predictor of histopathologic grading, as a predictor of radiosensitivity in gliomas, for delineating radiotherapy target volume and for predicting treatment response	114–120
EGFR—Imaging	EGFR is a tyrosine kinase receptor that plays a role in the control of cell proliferation, differentiation, apoptosis, and angiogenesis. Currently mutational status of EGFR predicts response to certain tyrosine kinase inhibitors. Today, EGFR status is evaluated by biopsy. In the future, EGFR-PET may have a role in non-invasive, whole body assessment of patients who could possibly profit of tyrosine kinase inhibitor therapy.	Lung Cancer	In a recent study presented at ASCO 2008 the authors used ^{11}C based PET EGFR imaging in patients with lung cancer (NSCLC). The SUV of the suspected lesions correlated well with the score of the immunohistochemistry but not with tumor size. This data indicates that ^{11}C-based EGFR imaging may play a vital role for non-invasive assessment of EGFR expression and could determine the efficacy of costly EGFR-targeted therapy	121–123
HER-2 imaging	HER-2 is a member of the erB receptors family. It is overexpressed in about 25–30% of breast cancers and other malignancies. HER-2 gene amplification is widely studied with IHC and FISH and its expression levels are correlated to the responsiveness to Herceptin™ (Trastuzumab™, ROCHE, Basel, Switzerland), a specific anti-HER-2 monoclonal antibody	Breast Cancer	HER-2 imaging may provide information about potential use of Herceptin™ and maybe also separate early responders from non-responders. [89]Zr-trastuzumab shows excellent and specific tumor uptake and is suitable for clinical use.	124–126
c-Kit imaging	c-KIT is a tyrosine kinase receptor for the stem cell factor. The downstream signaling includes the control of cell proliferation.	Various Tumors	There is often heterogeneous response to tyrosine kinase inhibitors of c-KIT and PDGFR, and new radiotracers directed to c-KIT may predict their therapy response. A recently synthesized PET tracer labeling imatinib with ^{11}C may be useful in monitoring the drug response and assessing possible drug resistance	127,128
Angiogenesis imaging	Angiogenesis occurs in hypoxic tissue and is a complex biological process. The most important regulator of angiogenesis comes from the VEGF signaling pathway. VEGF is a growth factor that promotes endothelial cell migration and growth in hypoxic tumors. There is currently no predictor of response to antiangiogenic therapy. PET could play a vital role in identifying patients who may benefit from this costly therapy	Various Tumors	There is Phase I data of an iodine bound anti-angiogenic humanized mouse antibody (HuMV833). The antibody distribution and clearance were markedly heterogeneous between and within patients and individual tumors. Larger trials are needed to evaluate the possible advantage of angiogenesis imaging in PET.	129
Gene expression imaging	Gene therapy-based approaches have been considered interesting anti-cancer strategies. Molecular imaging is a good candidate for imaging gene expression in vivo non-invasively. The most studied approach is the imaging of reporter genes using a specific PET reporter probe.	Various Tumors	Several experimental studies have been carried out. The value of PET ^{18}F-FHBG uptake in liver cancer as a predictor of response to gene therapy HSV1-tk treatment has been described. PET imaging of gene expression in humans seems to be feasible, but more studies are clearly needed in order to really improve the clinical application of gene therapy in cancer treatments.	130–132

F-Ethyl tyrosine (FET) and *C-11 methionine*, both amino acids. The former is preferable as it is F-18 rather than C-11 based which makes its distribution easier. In general terms, amino acids seem to be more specific for inflammatory foci than FDG, but are less sensitive in tumor detection. This is a disadvantage except for tumor detection and therapy monitoring of brain tumors, as FDG is also avidly taken up by the normal cortex, thus giving relatively poor lesion to background contrast (Fig. 62.4).

F-Thymidine (FLT) is a thymidine analogue labeling DNA synthesis. Thymidine is a marker of cellular proliferation. Indications for its use are limited, probably because there is something resembling a metabolic cascade in the tumors imaged: tumors which proliferate rapidly will take up FLT, but they also utilize FDG as a major energy source and thus are well demonstrated by FDG PET. This is true for initial staging and also for therapy monitoring applications. Therefore, no striking advantages have been found over FDG in most clinical studies.

F-DOPA and *[68]Ga DOTATOC* and similar compounds. These tracers are useful in neuroendocrine tumors, but respond to different "receptor" sets. The Ga compounds are somatostatin receptor markers and can be used as a replacement of In-octreotide scans. These tracers appear quite useful, as the tumors imaged

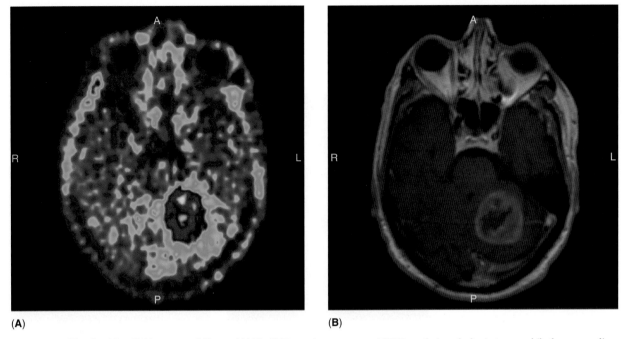

(A)　　　　　　　　　　　　　　　**(B)**

Figure 62.4 A 72-year-old male with a glioblastoma multiforme. (A) The FET scan demonstrates avid FET uptake into the brain tumor, while the surrounding cortex has no uptake. (B) The corresponding T1-weighted gadolinium-enhanced MR image demonstrates the morphology of the lesion. Central necrosis is seen on FET-PET as well as MR.

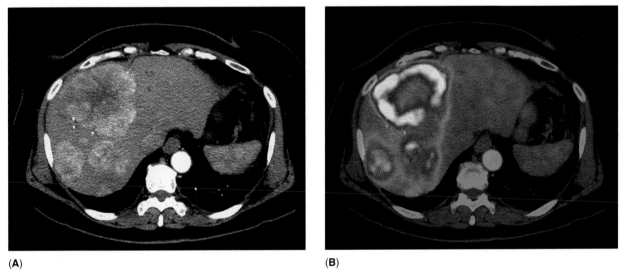

(A)　　　　　　　　　　　　　　　**(B)**

Figure 62.5 A 73-year-old female with neuroendocrine tumor metastases in the liver. (A) The metastases are well demonstrated on a diagnostic contrast-enhanced CT. (B) PET-CT was performed to provide a whole-body survey to document the full extent of metastatic disease.

with these compounds typically are not FDG-avid and FDG PET is therefore not recommended (Fig. 62.5).

F-Choline and *analogues, C-11 acetate.* These compounds have proven to be useful in the imaging of recurrent prostate cancer. The former compounds are preferable because they are F-18 based and thus lend themselves better to widespread application and can also be used in PET centers without cyclotron facilities (Fig. 62.6).

F-18 misonidazole and others. These compounds are used for hypoxia imaging. Their clinical value is sparsely documented.

F-18 fluoride. F-18 fluoride is an excellent and highly sensitive bone scanning agent, which has the potential to produce superior bone scans compared to the Tc-based bone scanning agents. Whether its use has the incremental value of being cost-effective in addition to improved sensitivity is under investigation currently (Fig. 62.7).

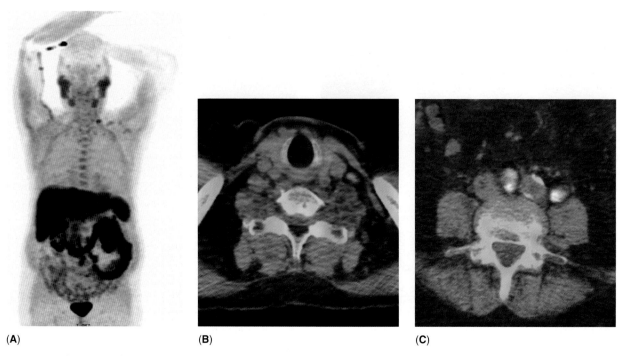

(A)   **(B)**   **(C)**

Figure 62.6 A 73-year-old patient with prostate cancer and rising PSA despite antihormonal treatment. (A) ¹⁸F-Choline scan shows typical normal choline distribution with increased activity in the liver and gut but no cerebral uptake. (B) There is ¹⁸F-Choline uptake into the left supraclavicular lymph node, and (C) into an interaorto-caval lymph node and left paraaortic lymph node.

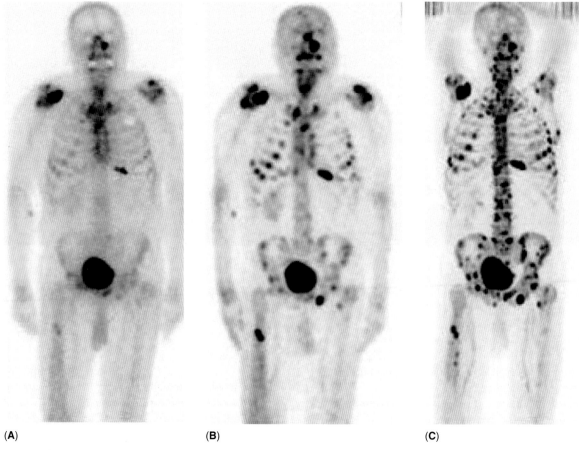

(A)   **(B)**   **(C)**

Figure 62.7 A 68-year-old patient with breast cancer. (A) The planar ⁹⁹ᵐTc-MDP bone scan shows only a few bone metastases. (B) Using a two FOV bone SPECT data acquisition technique many bone lesions become visible, and (C) even more lesions are visible on ¹⁸F-Fluoride PET. Bone scanning with PET is very sensitive and many osteoarticular degenerative lesions are seen as well. ¹⁸F-Fluoride PET-CT will clearly differentiate osteoarticular from metastatic disease.

FUTURE DEVELOPMENTS: TECHNICAL AND RADIOPHARMACEUTICAL

While FDG PET-CT has been well adopted worldwide for many indications, this is not the case for other PET tracers used for oncologic applications or for SPECT-CT in tumor imaging. Developments of imaging technology and future developments of radiopharmaceuticals will occur rapidly and the likely clinical developments are outlined below.

Technology

PET Technology

PET scanners with improved spatial resolution are likely to appear on the market. Speed and spatial resolution are closely linked for both PET and MR. A short time acquisition results in poor resolution. Higher resolution requires a longer acquisition time. Since substantial increases in spatial resolution through time-of-flight imaging methods can only be achieved if the speed of electronics is increased four-fold or more, clinical applications of time-of-flight technology is not likely to become relevant over the next few years.

SPECT technology may undergo rapid changes in the next few years, as solid state based imaging systems promise a substantially higher spatial resolution in the 5 mm range, which is comparable with PET. If systems that are currently under discussion for cardiology become available for applications in oncology, the use of many single photon radiopharmaceuticals may have to be revisited. As no FDG analogue is currently available for single photon based nuclear medicine, such cameras will not have an impact on current PET tumor staging.

CT scanners become more rapid and efficient with time. Current scanners cover axial fields of view of 4 to 16 cm. This allows CT perfusion measurements of whole organs, thus enabling one to perform FDG-PET-perfusion-CT scanning. The clinical value of such procedures has yet to be demonstrated.

PET-MR scanners are currently under discussion and head systems are available as research scanners. A full integration of PET and MR into a machine which simultaneously acquires body data is unlikely to appear in the clinical arena in the next five years because reduced work flow and technical issues make such technology very expensive. More likely, systems with the two scanners a few meters apart and a patient shuttled between them, will be implemented. These systems are then essentially similar to PET-CT. Such PET-MR scanners may have some advantages over PET-CT, but these have to be defined first for any potential application.

Radiopharmaceuticals

The development of new clinical radiopharmaceuticals is a much longer process than the development of new technology. Therefore, it is unlikely, that new tumor imaging agents either for PET or SPECT will become available clinically other than those highlighted in Table 62.1 (84–132). There is a large array of potential compounds, but the most likely and exciting development will be that of labelled drugs where a combination of imaging and therapy is possible. Such agents may appear in the time frame of the next five years, but it is too early to identify good candidates. If such candidates are identified, then this may be seen as a revival of the successful iodine imaging and therapy paradigm, on which clinical nuclear medicine was founded.

Summary

- A normal PET scan shows uptake of FDG in the brain, kidney, renal collecting system, and bladder. The heart, breast, ovaries, and brown fat also show uptake in some patients
- Mild or chronic inflammation in the musculoskeletal system may show FDG uptake
- Metabolic response to therapy as demonstrated by changes in FDG PET-CT correlates well with survival in many different malignant tumors
- FDG PET-CT detects significantly more extranodal sites of lymphoma (bone, liver, spleen) than anatomic imaging leading to improved staging in Hodgkin's disease and aggressive non-Hodgkin's lymphoma
- FDG PET-CT predicts progression-free survival after one to four cycles of chemotherapy in Hodgkin's disease and aggressive non-Hodgkin's lymphoma
- FDG PET-CT is used in the assessment of residual masses after therapy. FDG active residual masses after induction chemotherapy have a worse prognosis compared to inactive masses
- FDG PET-CT accurately discriminates between malignant and benign lesions, but due to FDG accumulation in inflammatory lesions, there can be false positive results
- FDG PET-CT has a useful role in staging lung cancer, particularly in the detection of distant metastases. It is also indicated in the detection of recurrence
- PET-CT is beneficial for evaluating recurrence of colorectal carcinoma if contrast-enhanced CT is inconclusive, if carcinoembryonic antigen (CEA) levels are increased, or if local relapse is clinically suspected. Most of the benefit is attributable to detection of extrahepatic metastases, which generally preclude resection of liver metastases
- In patients with a clinical suspicion of colorectal cancer recurrence, FDG PET can discriminate between post-operative scar and active tumor recurrence. In patients with rising CEA, FDG PET can localize the site of disease in many cases
- FDG PET(CT) should routinely be added to the conventional work-up of patients with unknown primary cancer
- There are a large number of tracers, which have been used in tumor imaging with PET in addition to FDG. As yet none have reached clinical importance comparable to that of FDG. They include ^{18}F-ethyl tyrosine (FET), ^{11}C methionine, ^{18}F-DOPA, and ^{68}Ga DOTATOC

REFERENCES

1. Massoud TF, Gambhir SS. Molecular imaging in living subjects: seeing fundamental biological processes in a new light. Genes Dev 2003; 17: 545–80.
2. http://en.wikipedia.org/wiki/Molecular_imaging
3. Dohán O, De la Vieja A, Paroder V, et al. The sodium/iodide Symporter (NIS): characterization, regulation, and medical significance. Endocr Rev 2003; 24: 48–77.

4. Hany TF, Steinert HC, Goerres GW, Buck A, von Schulthess GK. PET diagnostic accuracy: improvement with in-line PET-CT System: In results. Radiology 2002; 225: 575–81.

5. Lardinois D, Weder W, Hany Th, et al. Staging of non-small-cell lung cancer with integrated positron-emission tomography and computed tomography. N Engl J Med 2003; 348: 2500–7.

6. von Schulthess GK, ed. Clinical Molecular Anatomic Imaging: PET, PET/CT and SPECT/CT, 2nd edn. Philadelphia: Lippincott Williams & Wilkins, 2006.

7. Goerres GW, Burger C, Kamel E, et al. Respiration-induced attenuation artifact at PET/CT: technical considerations. Radiology 2003; 226: 906–10.

8. Dizendorf E, Hany TF, Buck A, von Schulthess GK, Burger C. Cause and magnitude of the error induced by oral CT contrast agent in CT-based attenuation correction of PET emission studies. J Nucl Med 2003; 44: 732–8.

9. Hany TF, Gharehpapagh E, Kamel EM, et al. Brown adipose tissue: a factor to consider in symmetrical tracer uptake in the neck and upper chest region. Europ J Nucl Med 2002; 29: 1393–8.

10. Lerman H, Metser U, Grisaru D, et al. Normal and abnormal 18F-FDG endometrial and ovarian uptake in pre- and post-menopausal patients: assessment by PET/CT. J Nucl Med 2004; 45: 266–71.

11. Kamel EM, Goerres GW, Burger C, von Schulthess GK, Steinert HC. Recurrent laryngeal nerve palsy in patients with lung cancer: detection with PET-CT image fusion – Report of six cases. Radiology 2002; 224: 153–8.

12. Kamel EM, Thumshirn M, Truninger K, et al. Significance of incidental 18F-FDG accumulations in the gastrointestinal tract in PET/CT: Correlation with endoscopic and histo-pathologic results. J Nucl Med 2004; 45: 1804–10.

13. Goerres GW, Hany ThF, von Schulthess GK. PET and PET/CT of the head and neck: FDG uptake in normal anatomy, benign lesions and treatment effects. AJR Am J Roentgenol 2002; 179: 1337–43.

14. Schaefer NG, Hany TF, Taverna C, et al. Non-Hodgkin lymphoma and Hodgkin disease: coregistered FDG PET and CT at staging and restaging—do we need contrast-enhanced CT? Radiology 2004; 232: 823–9.

15. Haioun C, Itti E, Rahmouni A, et al. [18F]fluoro-2-deoxy-D-glucose positron emission tomography (FDG-PET) in aggressive lymphoma: an early prognostic tool for predicting patient outcome. Blood 2005; 106: 1376–81.

16. Hutchings M, Loft A, Hansen M, et al. FDG-PET after two cycles of chemotherapy predicts treatment failure and progression-free survival in Hodgkin lymphoma. Blood 2006; 107: 52–9.

17. Jerusalem G, Beguin Y, Fassotte MF, et al. Whole-body positron emission tomography using 18F-fluorodeoxyglucose for posttreatment evaluation in Hodgkin's disease and non-Hodgkin's lymphoma has higher diagnostic and prognostic value than classical computed tomography scan imaging. Blood 1999; 94: 429–33.

18. Spaepen K, Stroobants S, Dupont P, et al. Prognostic value of positron emission tomography (PET) with fluorine-18 fluorodeoxyglucose ([18F]FDG) after first-line chemotherapy in non-Hodgkin's lymphoma: is [18F]FDG-PET a valid alternative to conventional diagnostic methods? J Clin Oncol 2001; 19: 414–19.

19. Jerusalem G, Beguin Y, Fassotte MF, et al. Early detection of relapse by whole-body positron emission tomography in the follow-up of patients with Hodgkin's disease. Ann Oncol 2003; 14: 123–30.

20. Spaepen K, Stroobants S, Dupont P, et al. Prognostic value of pretransplantation positron emission tomography using fluorine 18-fluorodeoxyglucose in patients with aggressive lymphoma treated with high-dose chemotherapy and stem cell transplantation. Blood 2003; 102: 53–9.

21. Cremerius U, Fabry U, Wildberger JE, et al. Pre-transplant positron emission tomography (PET) using fluorine-18-fluoro-deoxyglucose (FGD) predicts outcome in patients treated with high-dose chemotherapy and autologous stem cell transplantation for non-Hodgkin's lymphoma. Bone Marrow Transpl 2002; 30: 103–11

22. Specht L.2-[18F]fluoro-2-deoxyglucose positron-emission tomography in staging, response evaluation, and treatment planning of lymphomas. Semin Radiat Oncol. 2007; 17: 190–7.

23. Jerusalem G, Beguin Y, Najjar Fet al. Positron emission tomography (PET) with 18F-fluorodeoxyglucose (18F-FDG) for the staging of low-grade non-Hodgkin's lymphoma (NHL). Ann Oncol 2001; 12: 825–30.

24. Najjar F, Hustinx R, Jerusalem G, Fillet G, Rigo P. Positron emission tomography (PET) for staging low-grade non-Hodgkin's lymphomas (NHL). Cancer Biother Radiopharm 2001; 16: 297–304.

25. Bredella MA, Steinbach L, Caputo G, Segall G, Hawkins R. Value of FDG PET in the assessment of patients with multiple myeloma. AJR Am J Roentgenol 2005; 184: 1199–204.

26. Zamagni E, Nanni C, Patriarca F, et al. A prospective comparison of 18F-fluorodeoxyglucose positron emission tomography-computed tomography, magnetic resonance imaging and whole-body planar radiographs in the assessment of bone disease in newly diagnosed multiple myeloma. Haematologica 2007; 92: 50–5.

27. Fletcher JW, Djulbegovic B, Soares HP, et al. Recommendations on the use of 18F-FDG PET in oncology. J Nucl Med 2008; 49: 480–508.

28. Friedman KP, Wahl RL. Clinical use of positron emission tomography in the management of cutaneous melanoma. Semin Nucl Med 2004; 34: 242–53.

29. Gould MK, Maclean CC, Kuschner WG, Rydzak CE, Owens DK. Accuracy of positron emission tomography for diagnosis of pulmonary nodules and mass lesions: a meta-analysis. JAMA 2001; 285: 914–24.

30. De Leyn P, Lardinois D, Van Schil PE, et al. ESTS guidelines for preoperative lymph node staging for non-small cell lung cancer. Eur J Cardiothorac Surg 2007; 32: 1–8.

31. van Tinteren H, Hoekstra OS, Smit EF, et al. Effectiveness of positron emission tomography in the preoperative assessment of patients with suspected non-small-cell lung cancer: the PLUS multicentre randomised trial. Lancet 2002; 359: 1388–93.

32. Ceresoli GL, Chiti A, Zucali PA, et al. Early response evaluation in malignant pleural mesothelioma by positron emission

tomography with [18F]fluorodeoxyglucose. J Clin Oncol 2006; 24: 4587–93.

33. Francis RJ, Byrne MJ, van der Schaaf AA, et al. Early prediction of response to chemotherapy and survival in malignant pleural mesothelioma using a novel semiautomated 3-dimensional volume-based analysis of serial 18F-FDG PET scans. J Nucl Med 2007; 48: 1449–58.

34. Hodgson NC, Gulenchyn KY. Is there a role for positron emission tomography in breast cancer staging? [Review]. J Clin Oncol 2008; 26: 712–20.

35. Wong TZ, Jones EL, Coleman RE. Positron emission tomography with 2-deoxy-2-[(18)F]fluoro-D-glucose for evaluating local and distant disease in patients with cervical cancer. Mol Imaging Biol 2004; 6: 55–62.

36. Tran BN, Grigsby PW, Dehdashti F, Herzog TJ, Siegel BA. Occult supraclavicular lymph node metastasis identified by FDG-PET in patients with carcinoma of the uterine cervix. Gynecol Oncol 2003; 90: 572–6.

37. Spottswood SE, Lopatina OA, Fey GL, Boardman CH. Peritoneal carcinomatosis from cervical cancer detected by F-18 FDG positron emission tomography. Clin Nucl Med 2005; 30: 56–9.

38. Havrilesky LJ, Wong TZ, Secord AA, et al. The role of PET scanning in the detection of recurrent cervical cancer. Gynecol Oncol 2003; 90: 186–90.

39. Unger JB, Ivy JJ, Connor P, et al. Detection of recurrent cervical cancer by whole-body FDG PET scan in asymptomatic and symptomatic women. Gynecol Oncol. 2004; 94: 212–16.

40. Hubner KF, McDonald TW, Niethammer JG, et al. Assessment of primary and metastatic ovarian cancer by positron emission tomography (PET) using 2-[18F]deoxyglucose (2-[18F]FDG). Gynecol Oncol 1993; 51: 197–204.

41. Schroder W, Zimny M, Rudlowski C, Bull U, Rath W. The role of 18-F-flurorodeoxyglucose position imaging tomography 18-F-FGD PET in ovarian carcinoma. Int J Gynecol Cancer 1999; 9: 117–22.

42. Yoshida Y, Kurokawa T, Kawahara K, et al. Incremental benefits of FDG positron emission tomography over CT alone for the preoperative staging of ovarian cancer. AJR 2004; 182: 227–33.

43. Kim S, Chung JK, Kang SB, et al. [18F]FDG PET as a substitute for second-look laparotomy in patients with advanced ovarian carcinoma. Eur J Nucl Med Mol Imaging 2004; 31: 196–201.

44. Takekuma M, Maeda M, Ozawa T, Yasumi K, Torizuka T. Positron emission tomography with 18F-fluoro-2-deoxyglucose for the detection of recurrent ovarian cancer. Int J Clin Oncol 2005; 10: 177–81.

45. Unger JB, Ivy JJ, Connor P, et al. Detection of recurrent cervical cancer by whole-body FDG PET scan in asymptomatic and symptomatic women. Gynecol Oncol 2004; 94: 212–16.

46. Nakahara T, Fujii H, Ide M, et al. F-18 FDG uptake in endometrial cancer. Clin Nucl Med 2001; 26: 82–3.

47. Belhocine T, De Barsy C, Hustinx R, Willems-Foidart J. Usefulness of (18)F-FDG PET in the post-therapy surveillance of endometrial carcinoma. Eur J Nucl Med Mol Imaging 2002; 29: 1132–9.

48. Pandit-Taskar N. Oncologic Imaging in Gynecologic Malignancies. J Nucl Med 2005; 46: 1842–50.

49. Miller FR, Hussey D, Beeram M, et al. Positron emission tomography in the management of unknown primary head and neck carcinoma. Arch Otolaryngol Head Neck Surg 2005; 131: 626–9.

50. Vermeersch H, Loose D, Ham H, Otte A, Van de Wiele C. Nuclear medicine imaging for the assessment of primary and recurrent head and neck carcinoma using routinely available tracers. Eur J Nucl Med Mol Imaging 2003; 30: 1689–700.

51. Yen TC, Chang JT, Ng SH, et al. Staging of untreated squamous cell carcinoma of buccal mucosa with 18F-FDG PET: comparison with head and neck CT/MRI and histopathology. J Nucl Med 2005; 46: 775–81.

52. Schmid DT, Stoeckli SJ, Bandhauer F, et al. Impact of positron emission tomography on the initial staging and therapy in locoregional advanced squamous cell carcinoma of the head and neck. Laryngoscope 2003; 113: 888–91.

53. Périé S, Hugentobler A, Susini B, et al. Impact of FDG-PET to detect recurrence of head and neck squamous cell carcinoma. Otolaryngol Head Neck Surg 2007; 137: 647–53.

54. Kato H, Miyazaki T, Nakajima M, et al. The incremental effect of positron emission tomography on diagnostic accuracy in the initial staging of esophageal carcinoma. Cancer 2005; 103: 148–56.

55. von Rahden BH, Stein HJ. Staging and treatment of advanced esophageal cancer. Curr Opin Gastroenterol 2005; 21: 472–7.

56. Liberale G, Van Laethem JL, Gay F, et al. The role of PET scan in the preoperative management of oesophageal cancer. Eur J Surg Oncol 2004; 30: 942–7.

57. Kato H, Miyazaki T, Nakajima M, et al. Value of positron emission tomography in the diagnosis of recurrent oesophageal carcinoma. Br J Surg 2004; 91: 1004–9.

58. Yamada A, Oguchi K, Fukushima M, Imai Y, Kadoya M. Evaluation of 2-deoxy-2-[18F]fluoro-D-glucose positron emission tomography in gastric carcinoma: relation to histological subtypes, depth of tumour invasion, and glucose transporter-1 expression. Ann Nucl Med 2006; 20: 597–604.

59. Kim SK, Kang KW, Lee JS, et al. Assessment of lymph node metastases using 18F-FDG PET in patients with advanced gastric cancer. Eur J Nucl Med Mol Imaging 2006; 33: 148–55.

60. De Potter T, Flamen P, Van Cutsem E, et al. Whole-body PET with FDG for the diagnosis of recurrent gastric cancer. Eur J Nucl Med Mol Imaging 2002; 29: 525–9.

61. Abdel-Nabi H, Doerr RJ, Lamonica DM, et al. Aging of primary colorectal carcinomas with fluorine-18 fluorodeoxyglucose whole-body PET: correlation with histopathologic and CT findings. Radiology 1998; 206: 755–60

62. Wiering B, Krabbe PF, Jager GJ, Oyen WJ, Ruers TJ. The impact of fluor-18-deoxyglucose-positron emission tomography in the management of colorectal liver metastases. Cancer 2005; 104: 2658–70.

63. Staib L, Schirrmeister H, Reske SN, Beger HG. Is (18) F-fluorodeoxyglucose positron emission tomography in recurrent colorectal cancer a contribution to surgical decision making? Am J Surg 2000; 180: 1–5.

64. Huebner RH, Park KC, Shepherd JE, et al. A meta-analysis of the literature for whole-body FDG PET detection of recurrent colorectal cancer. J Nucl Med 2000; 41: 1177–89.

65. Papos M, Takacs T, Tron L, et al. The possible role of F-18 FDG positron emission tomography in the differential diagnosis of focal pancreatic lesions. Clin Nucl Med 2002; 27: 197–201.

66. Inokuma T, Tamaki N, Torizuka T, et al. Evaluation of pancreatic tumours with positron emission tomography and F-18 fluorodeoxyglucose: comparison with CT and US. Radiology 1995; 195: 345–52.

67. Diederichs CG, Staib L, Vogel J, et al. Values and limitations of 18F-fluorodeoxyglucose-positron-emission tomography with preoperative evaluation of patients with pancreatic masses. Pancreas 2000; 20: 109–16.

68. Reske SN, Kotzerke J. FDG-PET for clinical use. Results of the 3rd German Interdisciplinary Consensus Conference, "Onco-PET III," 21 July and 19 September 2000. Eur J Nucl Med 2001; 28: 1707–23.

69. Ruf J, Lopez Hanninen E, Oettle H, et al. Detection of recurrent pancreatic cancer: comparison of FDG-PET with CT/MRI. Pancreatology 2005; 5: 266–72.

70. Trojan J, Schroeder O, Raedle J, et al. Fluorine-18 FDG positron emission tomography for imaging of hepatocellular carcinoma. Am J Gastroenterol 1999; 94: 3314–19.

71. Khan MA, Combs CS, Brunt EM, et al. Positron emission tomography scanning in the evaluation of hepatocellular carcinoma. J Hepatol 2000; 32: 792–979.

72. Anderson CD, Rice MH, Pinson CW, et al. Fluorodeoxyglucose PET imaging in the evaluation of gallbladder carcinoma and cholangiocarcinoma. J Gastrointest Surg 2004; 8: 90–7.

73. Kluge R, Schmidt F, Caca K, et al. Positron emission tomography with [(18)F]fluoro-2-deoxy-D-glucose for diagnosis and staging of bile duct cancer. Hepatology 2001; 33: 1029–35.

74. Gayed I, Vu T, Iyer R, et al. The role of 18F-FDG PET in staging and early prediction of response to therapy of recurrent gastrointestinal stromal tumours. J Nucl Med 2004; 45: 17–21.

75. Powles T, Murray I, Brock C, et al. Molecular positron emission tomography and PET/CT imaging in urological malignancies. Eur Urol 2007; 51: 1511–20.

76. Kang DE, White RL, Jr, Zuger JH, Sasser HC, Teigland CM. Clinical use of fluorodeoxyglucose F 18 positron emission tomography for detection of renal cell carcinoma. J Urol 2004; 171: 1806–9.

77. Effert PJ, Bares R, Handt S, et al. Metabolic imaging of untreated prostate cancer by positron emission tomography with 18fluorine-labeled deoxyglucose. J Urol 1996; 155: 994–8.

78. Schoder H, Herrmann K, Gonen M, et al. 2-[18F]fluoro-2-deoxyglucose positron emission tomography for the detection of disease in patients with prostate-specific antigen relapse after radical prostatectomy. Clin Cancer Res 2005; 11: 4761–9.

79. Drieskens O, Oyen R, Van Poppel H, et al. FDG-PET for preoperative staging of bladder cancer. Eur J Nucl Med Mol Imaging 2005; 32: 1412–17.

80. Salvatore B, Paone G, Klain M, et al. Fluorodeoxyglucose PET/CT in patients with differentiated thyroid cancer and elevated thyroglobulin after total thyroidectomy and (131)I ablation. Q J Nucl Med Mol Imaging 2008; 52: 2–8.

81. Alzahrani AS, Abouzied ME, Salam SA, et al. The role of F-18-fluorodeoxyglucose positron emission tomography in the postoperative evaluation of differentiated thyroid cancer. Eur J Endocrinol 2008; 158: 683–9.

82. Bastiaannet E, Groen H, Jager PL, et al. The value of FDG-PET in the detection, grading and response to therapy of soft tissue and bone sarcomas: a systematic review and meta-analysis. Cancer Treat Rev 2004; 30: 83–101

83. Delgado-Bolton RC, Fernandez-Perez C, Gonzalez-Mate A, Carreras JL. Meta-analysis of the performance of 18F-FDG PET in primary tumour detection in unknown primary tumours. J Nucl Med 2003; 44: 1301–14.

84. Ambrosini V, Tomassetti P, Rubello D, et al. Role of 18F-dopa PET/CT imaging in the management of patients with 111In-pentetreotide negative GEP tumours. Nucl Med Commun 2007; 28: 473–7.

85. Koopmans KP, de Vries EG, Kema IP, et al. Staging of carcinoid tumours with 18F-DOPA PET: a prospective, diagnostic accuracy study. Lancet Oncol 2006; 7: 728–34.

86. Koukouraki S, Strauss LG, Georgoulias V, et al. Comparison of the pharmacokinetics of 68Ga DOTATOC and [18F] FDG in patients with metastatic neuroendocrine tumours scheduled for 90Y-DOTATOC therapy. Eur J Nucl Med Mol Imag 2006; 33: 1115–22.

87. Ramirez De Molina A, Rodriguez-Gonzalez A, Gutierrez R, et al. Overexpression of choline kinase is a frequent feature in human tumour-derived cell lines and in lung, prostate and human colorectal cancers. Biochem Biophys Res Commun 2002; 296: 580–3.

88. Picchio M, Messa C, Landoni C, et al, Value of [11C]choline-positron emission tomography for re-staging prostate cancer: a comparison with [18F] fluorodeoxyglucose-positron emission tomography. J Urol 2003; 169: 1337–40.

89. Koh WJ, Bergman KS, Rasey JS, , et al. Evaluation of oxygenation status during fractionated radiotherapy in human nonsmall cell lung cancers using [F-18]fluoromisonidazole positron emission tomography. Int J Radiat Oncol Biol Phys 1995; 33: 391–8.

90. Rajendran JG, Wilson DC, Conrad EU, , et al. [(18)F]FMISO and [(18)F]FDG PET imaging in soft tissue sarcomas: correlation of hypoxia, metabolism and VEGF expression. Eur J Nucl Med Mol Imaging 2003; 30: 695–704.

91. Ng P, Rajendran JG, Schwartz DL, et al. Can [F-18] fluoromisonidazole PET imaging predict treatment response in head and neck cancer? J Nucl Med 2003; 44: 128P.

92. Rajendran JG, Mankoff DA, O'sullivan F, et al. Hypoxia and glucose metabolism in malignant tumours: evaluation by [18F]fluoromisonidazole and [18F]fluorodeoxyglucose positron emission tomography imaging. Clin Cancer Res 2004; 10: 2245–52.

93. Hicks RJ, Rischin D, Fisher R, et al. Utility of FMISO PET in advanced head and neck cancer treated with chemoradiation incorporating a hypoxia-targeting chemotherapy agent. Eur J Nucl Med Mol Imaging 2005; 32: 1384–91.

94. Dehdashti F, Mintun MA, Lewis JS, et al. In vivo assesment of tumour hypoxia in lung cancer with 60Cu-ATSM. Eur J Nucl Med Mol Imaging 2003; 30: 844–50.

95. Dehdashti F, Grigsby PW, Mintun MA, et al. Assessing tumour hypoxia in cervical cancer by positron emission tomography with 60Cu-ATSM: relationship to therapeutic

response-a preliminary report. Int J Radiat Oncol Biol Phys 2003; 55: 1233–8.

96. Larson SM, Morris M, Gunther I, et al. Tumour localization of 16β-18F-fluoro-5-dyhidrotestosterone versus 18F-FDG in patients with progressive, metastatic prostate cancer. J Nucl Med 2004; 45: 366–73.

97. Dehdashti F, Picus J, Michalski JM, et al. Positron tomographic assessment of androgen receptors in prostatic carcinoma. Eur J Nucl Med Mol Imag 2005; 32: 344–50.

98. Rasey JS, Grierson JR, Wiens LW, Kolb PD, Scwartz JL. Validation of FLT uptake as a measure of thymidine kinase-1 activity in A549 carcinoma cells. J Nucl Med 2002; 43: 1210–17.

99. Vesselle H, Grierson J, Muzi M, et al. In vivo validation of 3′deoxy-3′-[(18)F]fluorothymidine ([(18)F]FLT) as a proliferation imaging tracer in humans: correlation of [(18)F]FLT uptake by positron emission tomography with Ki-67 immunohistochemistry and flow cytometry in human lung tumours. Clin Cancer Res 2002; 8: 3315–23.

100. Francis DL, Visvikis D, Costa DC, et al. Potential impact of [18F]-3-fluoro-3-deoxy-thymidine versus [18F]-fluoro-2-deoxy-d-glucose in positron emission tomography for colorectal cancer. Eur J Nucl Med Mol Imag 2003; 30: 988–94.

101. Cobben DC, Jager PL, Elsinga PH, et al. 18F-3-fluoro-3-deoxy-l-thymidine: a new tracer or staging of metastatic melanoma? J Nucl Med 2003; 44: 1927–32.

102. Cobben DC, Elsinga PH, Suurmeijer AJ, et al. Detecion and grading od soft tissue sarcomas of the extremities with 18F-3-fluoro-3-deoxy-l-thymidine. Clin Cancer Res 2004; 10: 1685–90.

103. Smyczek-Gargya B, Fersis N, Dittmann H, et al. PET with [18F]fluorothymidine for imaging of primary breast cancer: a pilot study. Eur J Nucl Med Mol Imaging 2004; 31: 720–4.

104. Chen W, Cloughesy T, Kamdar N, et al. Imaging proliferation in brain tumours with 18-FLT PET: comparison with 18F-FGD. J Nucl Med 2005; 46: 945–52.

105. Yoshimoto M, Waki A, Yonekura Y, et al. Characterisation of acetate metabolism in tumour cells in relation to cell proliferation: acetate metabolism in tumour cells. Nucl Med Biol 2001; 28: 117–22.

106. Kotzerke J, Linné C, Meinhardt M, et al. [1-(11)C] Acetate uptake is not increased in renal cell carcinoma. Eur J Nucl Med Mol Imag 2007; 34: 884–8.

107. Oyama N, Miller TR, Dehdashti F, et al. 11C acetate PET imaging of prostate cancer: detection of recurrent disease at PSA relapse. J Nucl Med 2003; 44: 549–55.

108. Ho CL, Chen S, Yeung DW, Cheng TK. Dual-tracer PET/CT imaging in evaluation of metastatic hepatocellular carcinoma. J Nucl Med2007; 48: 902–9.

109. Ho CL, Yu SC, Yeung DW. 11C-acetate PET imaging in hepatocellular carcinoma and other liver masses. J Nucl Med 2003; 44: 213–21.

110. Schirrmeister H, Glatting G, Hetzel J, et al. Prospective evaluation of clinical value of planar bone scans, SPECT, and 18F-labeled NaF PET in newly diagnosed lung cancer. J Nucl Med 2001; 42: 1800–4.

111. Hetzel M, Arslandemir C, Konig HH, et al. F-18 NaF PET for detection of bone metastases in lung cancer: accuracy, cost-effectiveness and impact on patient management. J Bone Min Res 2003; 18: 2206–14.

112. Even-Sapir E, Metser U, Flusser G, et al. Assessment of malignant skeletal disease: initial experience with 18F–fluoride PET/CT and comparison between 18F–fluoride PET and 18F–fluoride PET/CT. J Nucl Med 2004; 45: 272–8.

113. Even-Sapir E, Metser U, Mishani E, et al. The detection of bone metastases in patient with high-risk prostate cancer: 99mTc-MDP planar bone scintigraphy, single- and -field-of-view SPECT, 18F–fluoride PET, and 18F–fluoride PET/CT. J Nucl Med 2006; 47: 287–97.

114. Jacobs AH, Thomas A, Kracht LW, et al. 18F-fluoro-l-thymidine and 11C-Methylmetionine as markers of increased transport and proliferation in brain tumours. J Nucl Med 2005; 46: 1948–58.

115. Kaschten B, Stevenaert A, Sadzot B, et al. Preoperative evaluation of 54 gliomas by PET with fluorine-18-fluorodeoxyglucose and/or carbon-11-methionine. J Nucl Med 1998; 39: 778–85.

116. Buck AK, Halter G, Schirrmeister H, et al. Imaging of proliferation in lung tumours with PET: 18FLT versus 18FDG. J Nucl Med 2003; 44: 1426–31.

117. Ceyssens S, Van Laere K, de Groot T, et al. [11C]methionine PET, histopathology, and survival in primary brain tumours and recurrence. AJNR 2006; 27: 1432–7.

118. Ribom D, Engler H, Blomquist E, Smits A. Potential significance of (11)C-methionine PET as marker for the radiosensitivity of low-grade gliomas. Eur J Nucl Med Mol Imag 2002; 29: 632–40.

119. Nuutinen J, Sonninen P, Lehikoinen P, et al. Radiotherapy treatment planning and long-term follow-up with [(11)C] methionine PET in patients with low-grade astrocytoma. Int J Rad Oncol Biol Phys 2000; 48: 43–52.

120. Galldiks N, Kracht LW, Burghaus L, et al. Use of 11C-methionine PET to monitor the effects of temozolomide chemotherapy in malignant gliomas. Eur J Nucl Med Mol Imag 2006; 33: 516–24.

121. Baselga J. The EGFR as a target for anticancer therapy – focus on cetuximab. Eur J Cancer 2001; 37: S16–S22.

122. Cai W, Chen K, He L, et al. Quantitative PET of EGFR expression in xenograft-bearing mice using (64)Cu-labeled cetuximab, a chimeric anti-EGFR monoclonal antibody. Eur J Nucl Med Mol Imag 2007; 34: 850–8.

123. Yu JM, Liu N, Yang G, et al. 11C-PD153035 PET/CT for molecular imaging of EGFR in patients with non-small cell lung cancer (NSCLC). J Clin Oncol 2008; 26(May 20 Suppl): abstract 3503.

124. Slamon DJ, Leyland-Jones B, Shak S, et al. Use of chemotherapy plus a monoclonal antibody against HER2 for metastatic breast cancer that overexpresses HER2. New Engl J Med 2001; 344: 783–92.

125. Smith-Jones PM, Solit DB, Akhurst T, et al. Imaging the pharmacodynamics of HER-2 degradation in response to Hsp90 inhibitors. Nat Biotechnol 2004; 22: 701–6.

126. Dijkers E, Lub-de Hooge MN, Kosterink JG, et al. Characterization of ^{89}Zr-trastuzumab for clinical HER2 immunoPET imaging. J Clin Oncol (ASCO Annual Meeting Proceedings Part I) 2007; 25(June 20 Suppl): 3508.

127. Heinrich MC, Corless CL, Demetri GD, et al. Kinase mutations and imatinib response in patients with metastatic gastrointestinal stromal tumour. J Clin Oncol 2003; 21: 4342–9.

128. Kil KE, Ding YS, Lin KS, et al. Synthesis and positron emission tomography studies of carbon-11-labeled imatinib (Gleevec). Nucl Med Biol 2007; 34: 153–63.

129. Jayson GC, Zweit J, Jackson A, et al. Molecular imaging and biological evaluation of HuMV833 anti-VEGF antibody: implications for trial design of anti-angiogenic antibodies. J Natl Cancer Inst 2002; 94: 1484–93.

130. Penuelas I, Haberkorn U, Yaghoubi S, Gambhir SS. Gene therapy imaging in patients for oncological applications. Eur J Nucl Med Mol Imag 2005; 32: S384–S403.

131. Alauddin MM, Conti PS. Synthesis and preliminary evaluation of 9-(4-[18F]-Fluoro-3-hydroxymethylbutyl)guanine ([18F]-FHBG): a new potential imaging agent for viral infection and gene therapy using PET. Nucl Med Biol 1998; 25: 175–80.

132. Gambhir SS, Barrio JR, Wu L, et al. Imaging of adenoviral-directed herpes simplex virus type 1 thymidine kinase reporter gene expression in mice with radiolabelled ganciclovir. J Nucl Med 1998; 39: 2003–11.

63 Measurement of Angiogenesis: MRI Principles and Practice
Tristan Barrett, Anwar Padhani, and Peter L Choyke

INTRODUCTION

Angiogenesis, the sprouting of new capillaries from existing blood vessels, and vasculogenesis, the de novo generation of blood vessels, are the two primary methods of vascular expansion by which nutrient supply to tissues is adjusted to match physiological needs. Angiogenesis is an essential component of several normal physiological processes that include menstrual cycle changes in the ovaries and uterus, organ regeneration, wound healing, and the spontaneous growth of collateral vessels in response to ischemia (1). Pathological angiogenesis is an integral part of a number of disease states (e.g., rheumatoid arthritis, age-related macular degeneration, proliferative retinopathy, psoriasis) and is critical for growth of primary malignant tumors and for the development of metastases (2). This chapter describes the process of tumor angiogenesis and features unique to tumor microvasculature. Emphasis will be placed on the technique of dynamic contrast-enhanced magnetic resonance imaging (DCE-MRI) (3–5). Comparisons of DCE-MRI with other imaging techniques that are able to depict the angiogenic status of tumors in situ, including macromolecular contrast media (MMCM)-enhanced MR (6), endothelial stem-cell imaging, diffusion-weighted MR imaging, and functional multidetector computed tomography (fMDCT) (7) are made. Additionally, the potential of positron emission tomography (PET) to image angiogenesis is briefly discussed. The clinical potential of angiogenesis imaging will be highlighted and the ongoing challenges of functional imaging techniques as clinical and research tools will be explored.

TUMOR ANGIOGENESIS

Angiogenesis involves a cascade of events in which mature, resting host endothelial cells are stimulated to form new blood vessels. The angiogenic phenomenon is a complex multistep process involving many growth factors (cytokines) and interactions between varieties of cell types (Fig. 63.1). A detailed review of the processes initiating and controlling both regulated and unregulated neoangiogenesis is beyond the scope of this chapter and interested readers are directed to other comprehensive texts where further information can be found (8,9). However, a few pertinent observations are in order.

It is well established that diffusion distances for oxygen and other nutrients in tissues are of the order of 80 to 100 µm, with necrosis occurring approximately 150 µm from vessels (10). As tumors grow, an initial avascular phase is followed by neovascularization which permits further tumor growth. Although some tumors co-opt native vessels from the start and are apparently well vascularized (11), it is clear that tumor growth beyond 1 to 2 mm³ requires vascular in-growth. The primary stimulus for new vessel formation is presumed to be hypoxia. In tumors, areas of high angiogenic activity are found adjacent to regions of hypoxia caused by the disparity between blood flow, actual nutrient delivery

at a cellular level, and oxygen consumption (12,13). Tissue angiogenesis is stimulated by a complex cascade of proangiogenic growth factors (cytokines) and by suppression of antiangiogenic factors; this is known as the balance hypothesis for the "angiogenic switch" (Fig. 63.2) (14). Expression of angiogenic cytokines can be induced as responses to hypoxic stress, by hormone stimulation, but can also result from the activation of oncogenes.

The process of angiogenesis in normal tissues is well organized and self-regulated (15,16) and therefore differs from that in tumors in which the process is disorganized and deregulated. This is probably due to imbalances between pro- and antiangiogenic cytokines. The precise nature of these imbalances is not completely understood and is probably multifactorial with significant variation between different tumors and their microenvironments. It is clear that "normal" stromal cells, such as macrophages, also take part in angiogenesis. The factors involved in angiogenesis can be classified according to the role they play in the process (17). Many tumors secrete high levels of proangiogenic cytokines, including vascular endothelial growth factor (VEGF) and fibroblast growth factor (FGF). Importantly, proangiogenic factors serve as survival factors for proliferating endothelial cells and the developing immature vasculature. Tumors also produce anti-angiogenic factors (e.g., angiostatin, endostatin, and thrombospondins), many of which suppress angiogenesis at metastatic sites but not of the primary tumor (18,19). Apoptosis (programmed cell death) is important in angiogenesis. Anti-angiogenesis factors are pro-apoptotic for proliferating endothelial cells. It is the net balance of positive (proliferative and anti-apoptotic) and negative regulators of angiogenesis (pro-apoptotic) that determine the state of angiogenesis at the local level.

The angiogenic process in tumors (Fig. 63.3) begins when normal vessels become activated by VEGF; within minutes, vasodilatation and increased permeability to macromolecular serum proteins occurs. Extravasation of plasma proteins leads to deposition of a provisional extracellular matrix (ECM), which will facilitate endothelial cell migration. In response to angiogenic stimuli such as VEGF and FGF, endothelial cells at first proliferate and degrade their basement membrane. Prior to endothelial proliferation and migration, activated vessels show local shedding of pericytes and smooth muscle cells. These perivascular cells are essential for maintaining vascular integrity but also further suppress endothelial cell proliferation. Proliferation, migration, and elongation of endothelial capillaries requires degradation of the ECM, and activated endothelial cells release a number of proteolytic enzymes, including matrix metalloproteinases (MMPs). The sprouting and migration of endothelial cells is mediated by vascular cell adhesion molecules such as integrins. Tube formation follows, leading to the generation of a functional but immature endothelial plexus. The final stages of angiogenesis include stabilization, remodeling, and maturation of the new vessels by recruitment of pericytes and smooth muscle cells (20). Angiopoietin-I (AngI) plays important

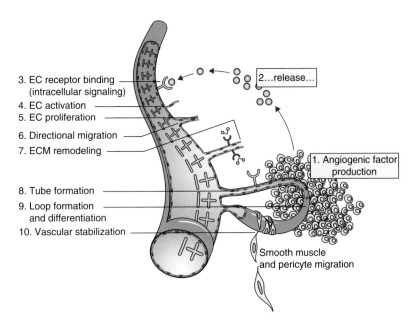

3. EC receptor binding
   (intracellular signaling)
4. EC activation
5. EC proliferation
6. Directional migration
7. ECM remodeling

8. Tube formation
9. Loop formation
   and differentiation
10. Vascular stabilization

2…release…

1. Angiogenic factor
   production

Smooth muscle
and pericyte migration

Figure 63.1 Angiogenesis, the cascade of events. Activation of host endothelium cells by angiogenic stimuli results in a series of events leading to the formation of a vascular plexus that supplies oxygen and nutrients to tumors. *Abbreviations*: EC, endothelial cell; ECM, extracellular matrix. *Source*: Adapted from The Angiogenesis Foundation (www.angio.org).

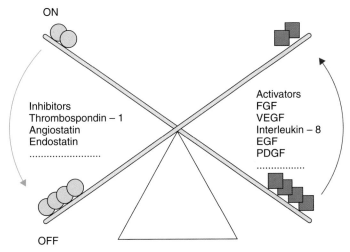

ON

Inhibitors
Thrombospondin – 1
Angiostatin
Endostatin
………………………

Activators
FGF
VEGF
Interleukin – 8
EGF
PDGF
……………….

OFF

Figure 63.2 The balance hypothesis for the angiogenic switch. It is the balance of proliferative (antiapoptotic) and proapoptotic factors that determines the state of angiogenesis at this level. *Abbreviations*: EGF, epidermal growth factor; FGF, fibroblast growth factor; PDGF, platelet-derived growth factor; VEGF, vascular endothelial growth factor. *Source*: Adapted from Ref. 14.

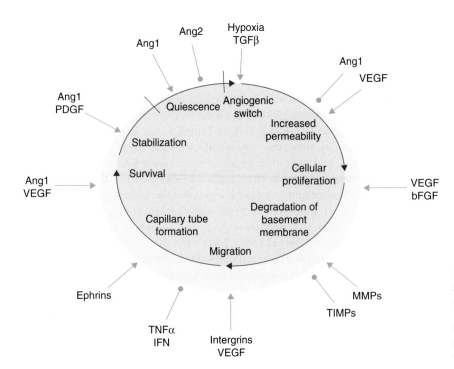

Ang1
Ang2
Hypoxia
TGFβ
Ang1
VEGF

Ang1
PDGF

Quiescence
Angiogenic
switch
Increased
permeability
Stabilization
Cellular
proliferation
VEGF
bFGF

Ang1
VEGF
Survival

Capillary tube
formation
Degradation of
basement
membrane
Migration

Ephrins

TNFα
IFN
Intergrins
VEGF
MMPs
TIMPs

Figure 63.3 The angiogenic cascade and major mediators of angiogenesis. Stimulators ↑, inhibitors !. *Abbreviations*: Ang, angiopoietin; bFGF, beta fibroblast growth factor; IFN, interferon; PDGF, platelet-derived growth factor; TIMP, tissue inhibitor of matrix metaloproteinases (MMP); TGF, transforming growth factor; TNF, tumor necrosis factor; VEGF, vascular endothelial growth factor. *Source*: Adapted from Ref. 17.

roles in the recruitment of smooth muscle cells and pericytes, while Ephrins enable the fusion of smooth muscle cells and pericytes to endothelial cell tubes.

Key Points: Tumor Angiogenesis

- Angiogenesis is critical for tumor growth
- The primary stimulus for angiogenesis in tumors is hypoxia
- Tumors cannot grow beyond the size of 1 to 2 mm^3 without blood supply
- Angiogenesis is invoked by proangiogenic (e.g., VEGF and FGF) and suppressed by antiangiogenic factors (e.g., angiostatin and endostatin)
- New vessels develop as a result of proliferation and elongation of endothelial cells to form tube-like structures. These become remodeled, mature and stabilize by recruitment of pericytes and smooth muscle cells

TUMOR VASCULAR CHARACTERISTICS

The uncoordinated, disorganized nature of neo-angiogenesis within tumors is in contradistinction to the growth of normal blood vessels where pericytes or smooth muscle cells form a well-constructed monolayer of tightly joined endothelial cells. However, it should be noted that many of these features are not unique to tumor tissues and may also be found in areas of reparative tissue or inflammation. The structural and functional characteristics of malignant tumor vessels (Fig. 63.4) include:

- Tumor vessels are disorganized, tortuous, irregular, and have a variable branching pattern (21). They lack the highly specialized features of normal arterioles, capillaries, or venules
- No hierarchy is observed, there are abrupt changes in diameter and blind-ending vessels, particularly within the center, and the endothelial cells often lack intercellular

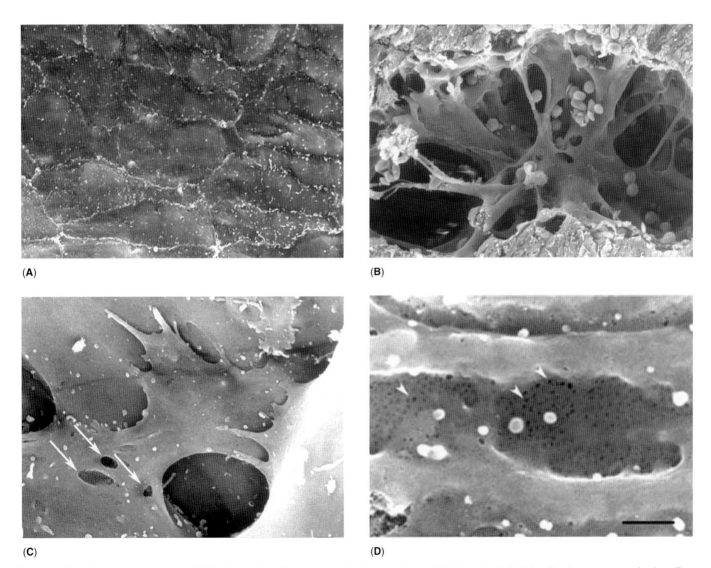

(A)

(B)

(C)

(D)

Figure 63.4 Scanning electon microscopy (SEM) of normal, and neo-angiogenic microvasculature. (**A**) Normal endothelial surface in a mouse venule; the cells are smooth and flat, with no gaps between them. (**B**) to (**D**) Endothelial cells in a murine breast carcinoma. (**B**) The cells have bizarre shapes and some even project into the lumen where they can obstruct blood flow. (**C**) Higher magnification shows holes which can result in leakage through and between the cells (arrows). (**D**) Collections of 80-nm fenestrae (arrowheads) are located in some regions of the endothelium (bar = 1 μm). *Source:* Adapted from Ref. 24.

junctions. Furthermore, the functional relationships between these cells are disturbed (22)

- Endothelial cells are laid down erratically, they may overlap, form multiple layers, and have cytoplasmic processes that project into or across the vascular lumen (23) (Fig. 63.4)
- All components of the tumor vessel wall are abnormal with a lack of pericytes or smooth muscle associations with endothelial cells, or incomplete basement membranes and innervations
- Gaps between or through endothelial cells, with fenestrations of up to 80 nm in diameter make the tumor vessels leaky to plasma proteins and prone to hemorrhage (23,24). Caveoli, small transcytoplasmic vesicles, also transport proteins across the endothelial cell (25)
- Arteriovenous shunting, vascular tortuosity, and vasodilation lead to an intermittent or unstable blood flow and areas of spontaneous hemorrhage (26)
- Marked heterogeneity of vascular density with areas of high angiogenic activity interspersed with regions of low vessel density
- High interstitial pressure results from extravasation of proteins and fluid into the tumor and is aggravated by the relative paucity of functional lymphatic vessels for drainage of extravasated fluid (27). Interstitial pressure becomes progressively greater toward the tumor center. Despite vessel hyperpermeability, this raised interstitial pressure is sufficient to impair diffusion of macromolecules and drugs thereby contributing to therapy resistance (28)

BIOLOGICAL AND CLINICAL IMPORTANCE OF TUMOR ANGIOGENESIS

The recognition that angiogenesis is essential for the growth and spread of tumors has prompted research into novel therapeutic agents that specifically target the tumor vasculature. Oncologists have focused on developing antiangiogenic agents that target the developing tumor neovasculature and vascular disruptive agents that target the established microvasculature. Antiangiogenic drugs fall into two categories: inhibitors of proangiogenic factors (e.g., anti-VEGF monoclonal antibodies) or analogues of endogenous angiogenesis inhibitors (e.g., endostatin) (29). Recent interest has centered on angiogenic markers that are preferentially expressed or upregulated by tumor cells, for instance: VEGF receptors, prostate specific membrane antigen (PSMA), platelet derived growth Factor (PDGF-R)-β, and $\alpha_v\beta_3$ integrin. This promising area of oncologic research has brought with it an urgent need to accurately quantify tumor angiogenesis. Unlike standard cytotoxic chemotherapy regimes, antiangiogenic agents are frequently cytostatic. Any reductions in tumor size or growth rate are likely to occur over a longer time period (18), thus imaging methods which are based only on gross anatomic changes may be insensitive to early changes in vascularity due to therapy. Furthermore, antiangiogenic agents are often very expensive and accurate biomarkers may make it possible to predict treatment failure long before definitive tumor progression can be measured, based on change in tumor volume, thus allowing other management options to be considered at an earlier stage.

Key Points: Tumor Vascular Characteristics

- Tumor vessels are disorganized, tortuous, irregular, with non-hierarchical structures
- Arteriovenous shunting, vascular tortuosity, and gaps between endothelial cells render tumor vessels leaky and prone to hemorrhage
- Interstitial pressure is increased in tumors, and becomes progressively greater toward the center; this may impair diffusion of macromolecules for imaging or treatment
- The structural abnormalities within tumor neovasculature form the basis of the differential contrast enhancement seen in malignancy
- The angiogenic switch has been shown to be an important step in the process of tumor invasion and metastasis
- Recent oncological research has lead to the development of a number of antiangiogenic and vascular disruptive agents, making accurate imaging of angiogenesis a necessity for the assessment of therapeutic efficacy
- Antiangiogenic induced reductions in tumor size or growth rate are likely to occur over a long time period, thus traditional anatomic imaging methods may be insensitive to early changes

METHODS TO ASSESS ANGIOGENESIS

Ideally, a diagnostic method should offer accuracy whilst being minimally invasive, demonstrating function and sampling the whole tumor. The traditional "gold standard" method of measuring angiogenesis involves sampling the tumor tissue and examining it under a microscope to provide an estimate of the microvessel density (MVD). MVD employs immunohistochemistry to stain for angiogenic surface markers such as CD31 (PECAM-1), CD34, or antibodies against factor VIII and is a measure of the average number of positively stained endothelial cells within a high power microscopy field. Biopsy specimens on which MVD determinations are made are information-rich but are inherently invasive. Furthermore, as the specimens are ex vivo they cannot determine if blood flow is present within each vessel, or whether the vessel is hyperpermeable. Tumors are heterogeneous with angiogenesis often being maximal in the periphery; this renders MVD prone to sampling bias. Depending on the tumor area biopsied MVD may under- or overestimate the extent of angiogenesis in another tumor region.

Other potential diagnostic tests include measurement of serum levels of angiogenic markers, such as VEGF, or circulating endothelial progenitor cells (30), and imaging techniques. Angiogenic serum markers currently lack sufficient sensitivity and specificity, do not give any indication of tumor location, but clearly hold potential as monitoring tools. However, functional dynamic imaging methods are non-invasive, provide localization of the entire tumor burden, and have the potential to combine anatomical information with quantitative, non-invasive functional depiction of the microvasculature.

Functional imaging of angiogenesis may be targeted or non-targeted. Targeted imaging uses contrast agents directed to specific endothelial markers of angiogenesis. Non-targeted imaging methods rely on the physiologic properties of neo-angiogenic vessels

within the tumor microenvironment, such as flow and permeability, in order to provide insights into the angiogenic status of a tumor.

Key Points: Methods to Assess Angiogenesis

- Ideally a diagnostic method should offer accuracy while being minimally invasive, demonstrating tumor function and sampling the whole tumor
- MVD uses immunohistochemistry to stain for angiogenic surface markers, thus deriving the average number of microvessels within the selected microscopy field
- MVD estimates are information rich but are inherently invasive, non-functional assays and may suffer from sampling bias
- Indirect methods of assessing angiogenic status include measuring serum levels of angiogenic markers and imaging techniques

IMAGING OF ANGIOGENESIS

Technological advances have made imaging at a molecular level a realistic possibility. Thus, contrast agents targeted to markers of angiogenesis such as $\alpha_v\beta_3$ integrin may enable in vivo monitoring of dynamic cellular processes. However, in practice, targeted imaging remains a challenge. Difficulties arise from the fact that the agents must be delivered intravascularly and that there are few targets, thus non-specific background signal from the unbound agent which remains in the blood pool predominates. Indeed, it is usually necessary to allow the blood pool to clear before it is even possible to do targeted imaging of the vasculature. Additionally, vessels comprise only a small (<10%) percentage of the total mass of a typical tumor, further reducing sensitivity (31). To overcome these problems binding needs to be both highly specific and efficient and the washout of unbound conjugates must be rapid. Unlike other areas of molecular imaging accessibility to targets is an advantage for

angiogenesis imaging: cell surface markers of angiogenesis are located on the vessel walls, which is convenient for intravenously administered contrast agents. Nevertheless, imaging modalities need to be sensitive enough to detect very low concentrations of the agent (32). Modalities with sufficiently high sensitivity to enable targeted imaging include optical imaging, positron emission tomography (PET), and single photon emission computed tomography (SPECT) but these modalities suffer from reduced spatial resolution. MR imaging offers good spatial resolution, but has relatively poor sensitivity on a molar basis, thus substantial gains in sensitivity are necessary. Such improvements may be achieved in the future through technological advances in coils and pulse sequences and the use of compounds containing hyperpolarized Carbon-13.

Comparison of Imaging Methods

Various modalities have been used to demonstrate the physiology of tumor angiogenesis including MR imaging, CT, PET, SPECT, ultrasound (US), and optical imaging; however, each modality brings its own advantages and disadvantages (Table 63.1). Both CT and MR imaging have the advantage of good spatial resolution, they are minimally invasive, and are more widely available than PET or SPECT scanners. CT, PET, and SPECT all expose patients to ionizing radiation, which is particularly problematic when follow-up studies are needed to monitor treatment response.

CT has the advantage of producing images in which the attenuation (measured in Hounsfield units) is directly proportional to the iodine concentration of the contrast medium, which allows accurate quantification and facilitates comparisons between centers. Dynamic CT can be used for imaging angiogenesis and has basic principles in common with dynamic MR imaging. It sequentially images an anatomical region as contrast media passes through it and information on blood flow/volume, mean transit time, and capillary permeability are derived from the enhancement patterns

Table 63.1 Comparison of the Advantages and Disadvantages of the Functional Imaging Techniques that Can Be Used to Evaluate Angiogenesis

Modality	Advantages	Disadvantages
Dynamic contrast-enhanced (DCE) MRI	Good spatial resolution Availability Good toxicity profile for low-molecular weight agents Good sensitivity Quantitative analysis	Movement artefacts Susceptibility artifact Patient unsuitability: Claustrophobia/metallic implants Potential toxicity of macro-molecular contrast agents Skilled interpretation required for quantitative techniques Reproducibility between centers Non-linear relationship between contrast concentration and signal intensity
Dynamic CT	Excellent spatial resolution Availability Quantitative analysis Linear relationship of contrast dose to attenuation	Ionizing radiation Nephrotoxicity of iodinated contrast media
Contrast-enhanced ultrasound	Expense Availability Portable Potential for targeted agents Non-invasive	Operator dependent Spatial Resolution Limited anatomical access Relatively large size of ultrasound microbubbles
PET	High Sensitivity Targetable contrast agents Quantification Linearity of contrast uptake values	Ionizing radiation Availability (Radiochemistry, cyclotrons, etc.) Spatial Resolution Production of contrast agent isotopes with a short half-life

observed. To date there has only been limited research involving dynamic CT to study angiogenesis, in part due to the concerns over radiation exposure related to repeated CT imaging; furthermore, some studies have demonstrated a poor correlation with the histological measure of angiogenesis, MVD (33).

US, depending on the technique used, can image vascular structures down to a size of 40 μm in diameter (34). Contrast-enhanced US is becoming more widely used (35). The technique involves microbubbles which are generally several microns in diameter. Their relatively large size compared to conventional CT or MR contrast media means that they remain confined within the vascular space, allowing measurement of perfusion and blood volume. Additionally, the microbubbles can be destroyed by US energy, enabling vessel refill rates to be assessed. However, there are certain anatomical regions such as the lung and brain that are poorly accessible by US, and the technique remains highly operator-dependent.

PET has many highly desirable properties of high sensitivity and whole body 3D display. PET studies require cyclotron-produced radioisotopes which decay by positron emission and annihilation to produce an electron pair of opposite 512 keV gamma rays. The isotopes have short half lives, that is, oxygen-15 (~2 minutes), nitrogen-13 (10 minutes), carbon-11 (20 minutes), and Fluorine-18 (110 minutes). These isotopes act as tracers which are incorporated into molecules. Examples relevant to angiogenesis imaging include ^{15}O-water and ^{11}C-carbon monoxide for estimating bulk tumor blood flow and red cell blood flow, respectively. However, oxygen-15 is particularly difficult to use because its short half-life necessitates an onsite cyclotron with a radiopharmaceutical laboratory. Fluorine-18, due to its prolonged half-life, is more widely used, particularly in the form of ^{18}FDG to measure metabolic activity within tumors. Recent research has centered on the use of fluorine-18 labeled targets of angiogenic markers such as ^{18}F-labeled RGD glycopeptides to target endothelial cells expressing the $\alpha_v\beta_3$ integrin (36). The fact that PET tracers have the ability to measure picomolar concentrations of molecules (37) makes them suitably sensitive to detect markers of angiogenesis within tumors; however, the poor spatial resolution, expense, limited availability of radiochemistry, cyclotrons and scanners, and radiation dose are significant barriers to the routine use of PET for angiogenesis imaging.

Combining more than one modality in the same imaging session may help to overcome the disadvantages of the individual techniques, thus maximizing the information obtained. The most pertinent current example of this is PET-CT which combines the sensitive, functional imaging of PET with the anatomical information and spatial resolution of CT. The problem of aligning data sets from separate PET and CT scans is in part overcome by dual PET-CT scanners; additionally, CT can be used for attenuation correction of the PET data (38). However, such combination scans are not without problems, not least the higher radiation exposure. Furthermore, PET-CT scans are often acquired with a PET agent alone, without the benefit of either IV or oral CT contrast, thus, soft tissue differentiation may prove difficult with unenhanced CT scans. Multimodality contrast probes are a possible means of overcoming this in the future. Macromolecular nanoprobes are ideally suited for the incorporation of multiple imaging beacons on each carrier molecule, but their development remains in research phase. PET-MRI offers a reduction in the overall radiation exposure and affords excellent soft-tissue contrast; additionally it can provide functional

MR assessments. PET scanners, as currently designed, are affected by the presence of an external magnetic field; however, the latest PET-MRI developments using solid-state detectors allow operation in high magnetic fields and prototype PET-MRI units are now being delivered to animal research institutes and hospitals (39).

Of all the modalities available, *MRI* offers the greatest practical potential for imaging angiogenesis. It is widely accessible, is already used to assess size and stage for a number of primary tumors, and does not involve radiation exposure.

Magnetic Resonance Methods of Assessing Angiogenesis

Broadly speaking, MR imaging techniques can be divided into two groups: those that use extrinsic contrast agents and those that do not.

Contrast-enhanced methods for imaging angiogenesis:

- Dynamic contrast-enhanced (DCE) MRI using low molecular weight agents (<1000 Da) that rapidly diffuse in the extracellular fluid space (ECF agents)
- DCE-MRI using large-molecular agents (>30,000 Da) designed for prolonged intravascular retention [also known as macromolecular (MMCM), or blood pool agents]
- MR imaging utilizing contrast agents targeted to markers of angiogenesis, including stem cell imaging, where endothelial cells are tracked as they migrate to areas of neo-angiogenesis

Non contrast-enhanced methods for imaging angiogenesis:

- Arterial spin labeling (ASL) imaging, where radiofrequency pulses are used for magnetic labeling of blood to provide a measure of tissue perfusion
- Blood oxygenation level dependent (BOLD) imaging, using heavily T2*-weighted sequences to measure the differences in the magnetic properties of hemoglobin relating to its oxygenation state to derive estimates of hypoxia and blood flow
- Diffusion-weighted MR imaging, based on the motion of water molecules within tissues

Dynamic Contrast-Enhanced MRI (DCE-MRI)

DCE-MRI involves the acquisition of serial MR images before, during, and after the injection of IV contrast agent. MR contrast agents leak at variable rates through the vasculature, with leakage rates being dependent on the size of the contrast medium molecules relative to the size of vascular pores. The temporal resolution of DCE-MRI techniques are related to how quick the contrast medium leaves the vascular spaces. Thus, temporal resolution for small molecular weight contrast media are relatively fast (in the order of 5–20 seconds), whereas for larger contrast agents temporal resolutions in the order of one to two minutes are usually adequate.

Dynamic Contrast-Enhanced MRI: Low Molecular Weight DCE-MRI

Clinical DCE-MRI can be performed with low molecular weight gadolinium-chelate-based contrast agents (LMCM, weight <1000 Da). When these contrast agents are used two distinct phenomena can be observed, depending on the experimental setup. Dynamic relaxivity-based contrast techniques use a rapid series of T1-weighted

images to observe the passage of contrast media, usually resulting in tissue "brightening"; by default, this technique is typically referred to as DCE-MRI. This technique is sensitive to the presence of contrast medium both within vessels and in the extravascular, extracellular space – the latter predominates due to the low blood volumes in tissues and tumors (approximately 5–10%). Conversely, if T2*-weighted sequences are used to monitor the effects of contrast medium passage, "darkening" of the tissue occurs because the technique is sensitive to the presence of concentrated contrast medium within the vascular space. This technique is usually referred to as dynamic susceptibility-weighted MR imaging (DSC-MRI). These two distinct techniques are compared in Table 63.2.

For full data quantification (see below), it is usually necessary to obtain, or estimate, an arterial input function (AIF). This can be achieved by measuring signal changes in arteries near to the anatomical location of the organ/tissue or tumor being studied. This can be performed before or at the same time as the dynamic data acquisition. If accurately measured, the AIF helps to compensate for changes related to the rate of injection and the cardiac status of the patient. Baseline "T1 maps" are also acquired prior to injection, which effectively allows conversion of the MR signal intensity into gadolinium concentration.

Quantification

Dynamic contrast scans can be analyzed by quantitative or semi-quantitative means; these parameters provide an assessment of vascularization by providing information on blood flow, and/or permeability, and have been shown to correlate with the degree of angiogenesis within tumors (40). The physiological parameters of these methods are presented in Table 63.3.

Pharmacokinetic quantitative analysis of DCE-MRI is the most widely used method of measuring vessel permeability changes, analysis typically being derived from a variation of the Toft's two-compartment kinetic model which, in turn, has its roots in Kety's dynamic model (Fig. 63.5) (41). In the model, an injected contrast agent leaks into the extravascular extracellular space (EES) and assessments of tissue perfusion and permeability can be derived from the shape of the tumor wash-in and wash-out curves. Angiogenic vessels would be expected to be very leaky and thus have a rapid forward leakage rate (represented by the term K^{trans}). In tumors, K^{trans} represents both blood flow and permeability; it predominantly represents blood flow when there is a high first-pass extraction fraction, or permeability surface area product when the concentration of contrast agent within the vascular space exceeds that in the interstitial space. Following extravasation from vessels, the contrast agent

Table 63.2 Comparison of the Different Dynamic Contrast Enhanced MRI and Perfusion CT Techniques

	T1-weighted DCE-MRI 2D/3D	T2*-weighted DSE-MRI 2D	Perfusion CT Single level (2D)	Perfusion CT Volume (3D)
Contrast	0.5 mmol/mL gadolinium	0.5 mmol/mL gadolinium	>300 mg/mL iodine	>300 mg/mL iodine
• Dose	0.1 mmol/kg	≥0.2 mmol/kg	0.5 mL/kg	1.0 mL/kg
• Typical volume	10–15 mL	25–35 mL	40 mL	100 mL
• Injection rate	3 mL/sec bolus	4–6 mL/sec bolus	5–7 mL/sec bolus	2 mL/sec infusion
Acquisition type	Single level	Single level	Single level	Multiple helical
Typical Z-axis coverage	$12-15 \times 5-8$ mm	3×8 mm	8×5 mm	Whole tumor
Data sampling	5–12 sec for 5–7 min	1–2 sec for 1–2 min	1 sec for 1–2 min	5 sec for 1–2 min
SNR of technique	Very high	Low	Low	Low
Signal change observed/ magnitude of effect	Increase/large	Decrease/small	Increase/small	Increase/small
Analysis technique	General multi-compartment model	Central volume theorem	Uni-compartmental analysis Deconvolution Distributed parameter model	Patlak analysis
Parameter measured	Transfer constant (K^{trans}) Leakage space (v_e) Rate constant (k_{ep}) Fractional blood volume (v_p)	Relative blood flow, Relative blood volume, Mean transit time	Blood flow Blood volume Mean transit time Permeability surface area product	Permeability surface area product Blood volume
Advantages	No radiation burden	No radiation burden	Straightforward quantification	Straightforward quantification
Disadvantages	Complex quantification	Complex quantification	Radiation burden	Radiation burden

Table 63.3 MRI Based Measures of Angiogenesis

Quantitative
- Transfer constant (K^{trans}; units min^{-1}): the inflow rate of contrast agent transfer from blood to interstitium; represents both blood flow and permeability surface area
- Rate constant (k_{ep}; units min^{-1}): the reverse rate constant, representing backflow of the contrast agent from the extravascular extracellular space into the vasculature
- fpV (units %): the fraction of plasma volume, related to whole tissue volume
- Leakage space (v_e; units %): the fractional extravascular, extracellular leakage volume

Semi-quantitative
- Initial area under the gadolinium concentration curve (IAUGC; units mmol/sec). Usually measured to a particular time point (e.g., 30–90 sec), indicating the amount of contrast agent reaching a tissue and being retained
- The slope of the wash-in and washout concentration curves
- The time to maximal enhancement
- Perfusion measures derived from DSC-MRI are usually semi-quantitatively assessed and based on the relationship rBF = rBV/MTT, where rBF = relative blood flow, rBV = relative blood volume, and MTT = mean transit time of the contrast agent

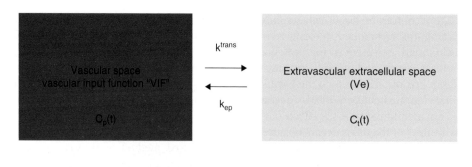

$$C_t(t) = k^{trans}[C_p(t) \otimes e^{(k_{ep}\ast t)}]$$

Figure 63.5 Schema representing the two-compartmental pharmacokinetic model for quantitative analysis of DCE-MRI. The data is fitted by a nonlinear algorithm to the above equation describing the contrast agent concentration in the region of interest $[C_t(t)]$ as a function of the arterial input $[C_p(t)]$ and three standard fit parameters. K^{trans} (representing both blood flow and permeability), k_{ep} (the reverse rate constant), and v_e (fractional extravascular, extracellular leakage volume).

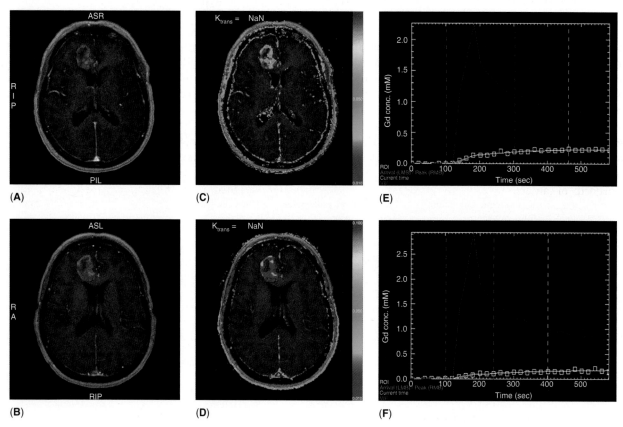

Figure 63.6 DCE-MRI in a patient with glioblastoma multiforme. *Top* row = baseline images, *bottom* row = following four weeks' treatment with an anti-VEGF monoclonal antibody. Despite relatively little change in lesion size T1-weighted images (**A**) and (**B**), the K^{trans} color-encoded permeability maps (**C**) and (**D**) show a significant decrease, also reflected by a reduction in the semi-quantitative measure of the area under the gadolinium curve (**E**) and (**F**).

then leaks back from the EES to the vascular space at another rate, also increased in tumor vessels (k_{ep}, the reverse rate constant) (5,42).

Semi-quantitative parameters are simple to acquire, but tend to be more dependent on the exact injection protocol and acquisition variables used in the study, making accurate comparison between institutions difficult. Moreover, semi-quantitative measures have less intrinsic physiologic meaning.

Validation and Clinical Applications
LMCM gadolinium-based DCE-MRI has been evaluated widely in the last decade. Validation of the technique has come from pre-clinical and clinical work where correlations with diverse

histopathological features have been shown, including tumor proliferation rate and microvessel density (43). Importantly, strong positive correlations have been found with independent measurements of tissue blood flow. Clinical validation has come from the use of the technique in a variety of applications including screening women at high genetic risk for breast cancer (44), for lesion characterization in a variety of anatomical locations, for the assessment of residual disease, and when disease relapse is suspected. DCE-MRI has also been used to monitor treatment response in a number of primary malignancies including breast (45,46), prostate (47,48), brain (49), and head and neck (50) tumors (Fig. 63.6). Furthermore, DCE-MRI of the breast

provides a supplemental problem-solving tool for the diagnosis of breast cancer (Figs. 63.7 and 63.8). Semi-quantitative measurements are typically used in clinical practice based on the contrast uptake, plateau, and washout patterns within lesions.

An important new application of the technology has been the evaluation of antivascular anticancer drugs. For example, initial pre-clinical experiments using antiangiogenic agents in tumor models have shown reductions in tumor vessel permeability as early as one day after the start of treatment (51). Furthermore, DCE-MRI has been successfully used to monitor treatment in a number of Phase I clinical trials of angiogenic inhibitors or antivascular therapies, including Combretastatin A4 phosphate (52), a microtubule inhibitor, and PTK/ZK (53), a VEGF tyrosine kinase inhibitor. Studies have shown that change from baseline measurements significantly correlates with dose-dependent drug responses (54). Furthermore, reductions in DCE-MRI parameters become apparent at time points as early as 4-6 hours after administration of vascular disruptive agents. Although anti-VEGF agents can cause DCE-MRI changes as early as 24 to 48 hours, it is more usual to see consistent changes after 10 to 12 days possibly because of the effects of vascular normalization (55). Thus, DCE-MRI can be used as a monitoring pharmacodynamic parameter in drug development. However, from an efficacy perspective, DCE-MRI does not appear to do well in predicting which patients will benefit from long-term antiangiogenic therapy (with the possible exceptions of renal cell cancer and hepatoma), probably because, at this stage, antiangiogenic drugs are still not given as monotherapies for the majority of cancers.

Key Points: Dynamic Contrast-Enhanced MRI

- Serial MR images are acquired following the contrast agent as it passes through a tumor region-of-interest
- Pre-scanning needs to include careful selection of the target region, acquisition of an arterial input function and a T1 map
- Breath-hold techniques and anti-peristaltic medication where appropriate can help to minimize motion artefacts
- Assessment can be quantitative or semi-quantitative
- Quantitative measures are typically based on a variation of the "two-compartment" pharmacokinetic model
- Reductions in DCE-MRI parameters typically become apparent at early time points, making these results potentially useful for early selection of treatment responders
- DCE-MRI may help in selecting the optimal dose for anti-angiogenic drugs
- DCE-MRI has been used in the research setting to monitor treatment in prostate, brain, and head and neck tumors. DCE-MRI is starting to be used more routinely, when clinically indicated, for the diagnosis of breast cancer

Limitations

Inevitably with a complex technique such as DCE-MRI, there are limitations to its application. These are related to both the technological limitation of machines, which affects the rate and volume of the data acquired, and to the methods used in data quantification.

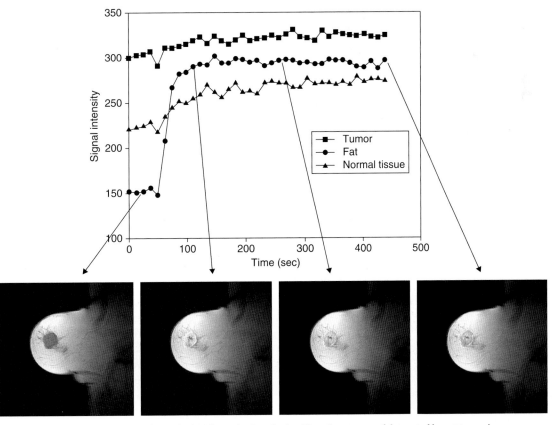

Figure 63.7 Example of a T1-weighted DCE-MRI study. Marked, and sustained, early ring-like enhancement of the central breast tumor is seen compared to the gradual increase in signal intensity of fibroglandular breast parenchyma and fat.

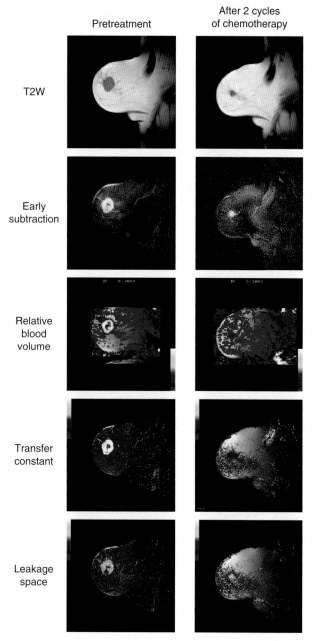

Figure 63.8 Monitoring chemotherapy response of breast cancer with DCE-MRI. A 52-year-old post menopausal woman with a Grade III invasive ductal cancer of the breast. Columns depict sample images at identical slice positions before and after two cycles of 5-fluorouracil, epirubicin, and cyclophosphamide chemotherapy. Rows depict T2-weighted anatomical images, subtraction images (obtained by subtracting the MR image acquired 100 seconds after contrast agent administration from the baseline image), relative blood volume map, transfer constant map (color range 0–1/min), and the leakage space (maximum v_e 100%), respectively. With treatment, the number of enhancing pixels is seen to decrease on the subtraction images, with a reduction in relative blood volume and transfer constant. Leakage space changes are least marked. This patient had a complete clinical and radiological response to treatment after six cycles of chemotherapy.

There are well known uncertainties over the reliability of the kinetic parameter estimates derived from kinetic modeling of the DCE-MRI data. These are due either to assumptions implicit in the kinetic model, or the accuracy of tissue contrast agent measurements. For example, the Tofts' model uses a standard description of the time-varying blood concentration of the contrast agent (the arterial input function), and assumes that the supply of contrast medium is not flow limited. Additionally this model presumes that the tissue blood volume contributes negligibly to signal intensity changes as compared with signal arising from contrast medium in the interstitial space. Furthermore, the methods used to calculate native and changing T1-relaxation rates vary in the literature. Indeed, there have been three international consensus meetings which have recognized these issues and have sought not to be prescriptive with regard to these issues, while acknowledging that tissue contrast agent modeling remains a controversial area (56). Despite these complexities, quantitative DCE-MRI kinetic parameters can provide insights into the underlying tissue pathophysiological processes and they are useful tools for making treatment decisions both in the clinic and in pharmaceutical drug development.

Key Points: Limitations of DCE-MRI

- Standardization of acquisition and analysis protocols is necessary to allow accurate inter and intra-patient comparison
- Problems related to pharmacokinetic modeling: simplification of terms within the model and AIF acquisition
- Quantification of changes, which may need to be substantial in order to reach significance
- Specificity of findings: certain benign conditions may mimic malignant findings on DCE-MRI
- Availability of software, technologist, and clinician training

Dynamic Contrast-Enhanced MRI: Macromolecular Weight DCE-MRI

Macromolecular contrast media (MMCM) have a molecular weight >30,000 Da and are either inherently paramagnetic, or incorporate paramagnetic transition metals, such as gadolinium. Inherently paramagnetic MMCMs include superparamagnetic iron oxide particles (SPIOs) and ultrasmall superparamagnetic iron oxides (USPIOs), which have additional potential for imaging the reticuloendothelial and lymphatic systems, respectively. Examples of gadolinium containing MMCMs that have been developed include albumin-(Gd-DTPA), liposomes, dextran compounds, dendrimers, and viral particles (57). Few of these have been approved for human use outside of clinical trials.

MMCMs were initially designed for use as MR angiography agents (Fig. 63.9) due to their prolonged intravascular retention time. However, they possess characteristics that also make them suitable for imaging angiogenesis. Low molecular weight contrast media (LMCM) diffuse quickly into the extracellular fluid space, leading to large first-pass fractions and may even pass non-selectively through normal vessels. Conversely, MMCMs do not pass through normal endothelial walls, potentially making them more selective for the imaging of tumor neovasculature, which tends to be selectively hyperpermeable to larger molecules. Furthermore, their different pharmacokinetic properties may represent angiogenesis-related tissue change more accurately. As previously mentioned, the extent to which K^{trans} represents blood flow or permeability-surface area product varies. The larger diameter MMCMs diffuse less freely than LMCMs, resulting

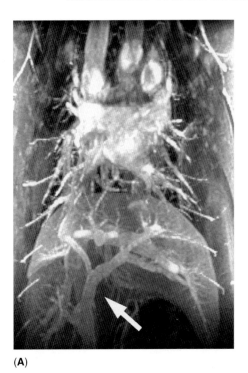

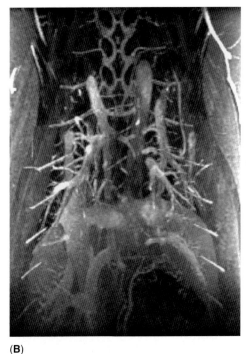

(A)   **(B)**

Figure 63.9 Blood pool imaging with a macromolecular agent. T1-weighted image (**A**) pre-contrast and (**B**) after administration of a Generation-6 dendrimer in a murine model. The vascular enhancement demonstrates the potential of macromolecular agents for use in MR angiography. *Source*: From Dr. C A Boswell, National Institutes of Health, Bethesda, U.S.A.

in a relatively "permeability limited" state. Therefore, provided blood flow is adequate, the derived K^{trans} values may more accurately reflect permeability within tumors. Additionally, their potential as blood pool agents may enable more accurate estimates of tumor blood volume. The slower diffusion rate of MMCMs leads to reduced concentration of contrast within tumor tissue. This apparent decrease in enhancement is partially compensated for by the larger number of (for example) gadolinium atoms and slower rate of rotation, resulting in a higher relaxivity value. This slower diffusion also means the tumor-to-background contrast gradually increases with time—making imaging timing less important when compared to LMCMs, but with the cost of longer data acquisition times and increased background signal.

Concerns remain over the safety profile of MMCMs, and this has limited their use in humans. The prototype agent, albumin-(Gd-DTPA) has prolonged retention of the agent due to its molecular size and subsequent potential for toxicity. This is particularly true of gadolinium containing compounds and the risk of gadolinium ion-chelate dissociation.

In late 2005, the macromolecular agent MS-325 (Vasovist, Gadofosveset Trisodium) was approved for human use for MR angiography in European Union states, and was more recently licensed for use in Australia, Switzerland, and Canada. MS-325 binds strongly but reversibly to serum albumin, only the bound form can be considered a macromolecular contrast agent. The equilibrium between free and bound forms depends on the concentrations of the MS-325 and the plasma albumin, and the albumin-binding affinity constant of the bound form (58). To date MS-325 has been used as a contrast agent for aorto-iliac

MR angiography in Phase II and III clinical trials, with results comparable to those obtained by conventional angiography (Fig. 63.10) (59–61). MS-325 has potential as an angiogenesis-imaging agent; however, pre-clinical studies have so far proven disappointing, a proposed obstacle being the successful differentiation of the pharmacokinetics of the free and bound forms of MS-325, as well as the induced increase in relaxivity after protein binding (62).

Key Points: Macromolecular Weight DCE-MRI

- MMCM have a molecular weight >30,000 Da
- MMCMs are inherently paramagnetic, or incorporate MR contrast agents such as gadolinium
- MMCMs do not pass through normal endothelial pores, potentially making them more selective for the imaging of tumor neovasculature
- Quantitative K^{trans} values may more accurately reflect permeability within tumors when compared to LMCM
- Concerns remain over the safety profile of MMCMs, due to their prolonged intravascular retention
- The majority of agents are still in the research phase; however, MS-325 has recently been approved for human use in MR angiography

Endothelial Stem Cell Imaging

Another novel approach for MR angiogenesis imaging is the tracking of endothelial progenitor stem cells as they migrate to regions of neovascularization. Prior to injection, the stem cells are labeled with an MR contrast agent to enable in vivo monitoring. They can

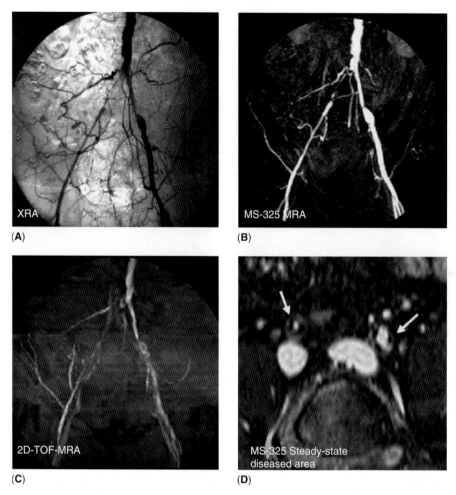

(A)   (B)

(C)   (D)

Figure 63.10 Macromolecular contrast-enhanced MR arteriography in a patient. Comparable coronal projections of (**A**) conventional angiography, (**B**) MS-325 enhanced MR angiography, (**C**) two-dimensional TOF MR angiography, and (**D**) a transverse reconstruction of a steady-state MS-325 dataset showing stenoses (arrows) in both right and left common iliac arteries. *Source*: Adapted from Ref. 59.

continue to be imaged for the life-span of the cell, provided the MR contrast agent remains within the cell. Toxicity concerns remain over gadolinium ions, which may be more likely to dissociate from their chelate in the lower intracellular pH environment of lysosomes or endosomes. Conversely, when cells are labeled with iron it is naturally processed by the body. Remarkably, even single cells loaded with iron particles can be demonstrated with MR imaging (63), making it an ideal labeling agent. Iron may induce hypersensitivity reactions and, while unlikely at the doses administered, there remains the potential for iron overload. Furthermore, intracellular iron may theoretically induce production of free radicals and reactive oxygen species (64); however, initial results show cell survival to be unaffected (65). Importantly, the iron particles do not affect the ability of the stem cells to function or differentiate (65). One important issue is whether the iron stays within the stem cells or is taken up by macrophages and macrophage-like cells, thus separating the imaging "tag" from the stem cell. Pre-clinical results are promising. Following injection of iron-loaded endothelial precursor cells into murine glioma models, MR imaging can demonstrate migration of these cells towards, and their incorporation into, the tumor neovasculature, which can be confirmed by histology (66). Iron, however,

is a negative MR contrast agent, making it difficult to differentiate from normal areas of signal void such as from blood vessels and calcification. Additional scans, such as T2* mapping can help to distinguish the presence of iron for correlation. Although at a relatively early stage, this research offers the potential to image angiogenesis and to monitor its progression during the life span of the stem cell (Fig. 63.11).

Key Points: Endothelial Stem Cell Imaging

- Endothelial stem cells can be labeled ex vivo with an MR contrast agent
- Following IV injection, the cells can be monitored by MR imaging as they track to areas of neoangiogenesis
- Iron can be naturally processed by the body; furthermore, even single cells loaded with iron particles can be demonstrated with MR imaging
- Labeling does not affect survival of cells or their ability to function and differentiate
- Iron produces "negative" contrast-enhancement, thus additional sequences may be necessary to confirm its presence

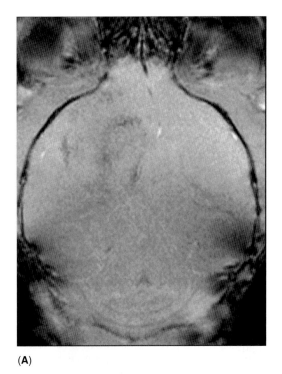

(A)

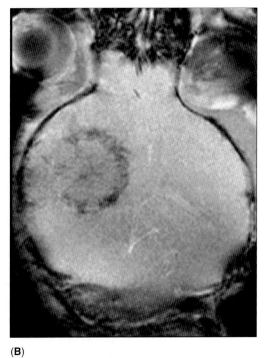

(B)

Figure 63.11 MR imaging of iron-labeled endothelial precursor cells in a murine glioma model. Images acquired following implantation, in separate mice, of either (**A**) unlabeled or (**B**) iron-labeled stem cells. Darker signal is seen in (**B**) due to "negative" enhancement of the tumor by iron within the stem cells, as later confirmed by histology. *Source*: Adapted from Ref. 32.

Other MRI Techniques for Microvessel Imaging

Arterial Spin Labeled (ASL) Imaging

ASL is a non-invasive MR imaging technique that does not require an extrinsic contrast agent to provide measures of tissue perfusion. Radiofrequency (RF) pulses are used to invert the nuclear spin of protons of arterial blood upstream of the area of interest (67). This "magnetically labelled" blood then exchanges with the local protons, changing their magnetization. Subtraction images of tagged from untagged images are used to produce perfusion maps. The RF "tag" can be pulsed or applied continuously (68). ASL techniques have mainly been used in brain imaging, where it is easier to isolate and tag the carotid vessels. Whilst the technique has traditionally been used for functional imaging of cerebral blood flow, it can also be adapted to quantify blood flow within tumors, thus providing estimates of blood flow, presumptively related to angiogenesis. It is essential that the distance from "tagging" to imaging is small to minimize the ensuing T1 relaxation which can result in a loss of the magnetic labeling (69). This is more of a problem for non-brain imaging and particularly for more peripheral lesions, or indeed liver imaging, due to the dual blood supply of the organ. These problems have limited the use of ASL outside the brain. However, newer techniques such as velocity-encoded ASL, where arterial spins can be distinguished according to their speed, may provide a solution (70). ASL-MRI has been shown to be a quantitative, reproducible method for measuring blood flow. The fact that ASL does not necessitate contrast agent administration may make it a particularly useful method for monitoring angiogenesis in patients with impaired renal function, or renal failure.

Key Points: Arterial Spin Labeling

- ASL imaging uses RF pulses to "magnetically label" blood to enable exchanges with the local protons
- Subtraction images of tagged from untagged images are necessary to produce perfusion maps
- ASL is mainly used for brain imaging and is technically challenging elsewhere in the body
- Intrinsic contrast imaging suffers from low contrast-to-noise ratios

Diffusion MRI

Diffusion-weighted MRI (DW-MRI) displays information on the random (Brownian) motion of water molecules in tissues. Water movement in tissues is not entirely random: it is modified by flow within conduits and by interactions with lipophilic cellular membranes, intracellular organelles, and macromolecules (71). Diffusion-weighted images can be sensitive to large or small displacements of water, to different tissue microenvironments due to macroscopic flows (i.e., within ducts and blood vessels) or microscopic extracellular space, and even intracellular water displacements. It is the experimental setup that determines whether the measured apparent diffusion coefficient (ADC) is dominated by macroscopic or microscopic water movements (72–75).

There is limited direct evidence that ADC values are related proportionally to blood flow, or that the changes induced by therapies are correlated with alterations in tumor blood flow. However, strong indirect pre-clinical and clinical data show that low b-value

ADC maps can be used to evaluate the functioning of organs such as the kidneys and salivary glands and might be useful for evaluating the most hypervascular of tumors, as well as some extremity sarcomas (71). Similarly, low b-value ADC maps can assess treatments that alter tumor vascularity (e.g., chemotherapy and vascular disruptive agents), and observed changes correlate to DCE-MRI parameters (76).

CHALLENGES FOR ANGIOGENESIS IMAGING TECHNIQUES

The imaging of angiogenesis still presents the radiologist with a number of challenges, either relating to the nature of the disease process at a microscopic and macroscopic level, or the limitations of current imaging modalities. Additionally, the accurate assessment of imaging techniques is hindered by the lack of a comparable and accurate "gold standard" measure of angiogenesis; the widely used histological measure MVD suffers from sampling bias and is non-dynamic in its representation. However, it should be noted that, from an efficacy point of view, disease-free and long-term survival are ultimately the most clinically relevant endpoints. As previously mentioned consensus needs to be reached on acquisition protocols and the kinetic model used for analysis in order to allow accurate intra-patient and inter-site comparison. Furthermore, problems with the kinetic model itself and selected arterial input function need to be ironed out.

The nature of the process of angiogenesis and the mechanism of action of anti-angiogenic agents makes treatment efficacy difficult to quantify. Reductions in tumor size, the traditional measure of therapy response, are insufficient to monitor the effects of angiogenic inhibition, and changes at the molecular level need to be demonstrated. Imaging at the molecular level requires high sensitivity (due to the low number of targets) and specificity (to avoid increased background signal). Changes at such a microscopic level make patient movement a particular problem and can invalidate functional parameter estimates. The reduced spatial resolution of PET imaging exacerbates the problem of movement; mis-registration of signal can lead to an overestimation of lesion size and heterogeneity with lesions cannot be properly assessed. Indeed, appreciation of heterogeneity within tumors may be diagnostically important and relevant to treatment monitoring (77). Semi-quantitative MR imaging measurements or those that derive mean values from the whole tumor will also fail to appreciate this diversity. Recent advances in quantitative DCE-MRI using pixel-by-pixel analysis helps emphasize lesion heterogeneity. Herein, multiple small, individual parameter measurements are performed within a defined region-of-interest, which can then be displayed as color-encoded maps. In addition, such analysis improves standardization, helps to correctly delineate the tumor outline, and may minimize partial volume averaging errors and more accurately represent pathophysiological processes within the tumor. However, pixel-by-pixel analysis requires specialized software for analysis, takes longer to process, and suffers from a reduced signal-to-noise ratio.

At present these problems mean that changes in pharmaco-kinetic parameters need to be substantial in order to overcome intra and inter-observer error and reach significance. RECIST criteria that rely on changes in size may be insufficient for the assessment of anti-angiogenic agents and the degree of parameter changes equivalent to the status of "stable disease," "partial response," "complete response," and "progressive disease" will need to be re-defined. The above challenges will need to be overcome in order to produce a valid, accurate, reproducible, and clinically relevant imaging method of quantifying tumor angiogenesis and measuring response to treatment.

Summary

- Tumors cannot grow beyond the size of 1 to 2 mm^3 without a blood supply
- Angiogenesis is invoked by proangiogenic (e.g., VEGF and FGF) and suppressed by antiangiogenic factors (e.g., angiostatin and endostatin)
- Tumor vessels are disorganized, tortuous, irregular, with non-hierarchical structures. Arteriovenous shunting, vascular tortuosity, and gaps between endothelial cells render tumor vessels leaky and prone to hemorrhage
- Traditional anatomic imaging methods may not be appropriate for assessing response to treatment of anti-angiogenic drugs
- Direct measurement of angiogenesis is performed by MVD counting using immuno-staining techniques
- Dynamic contrast-enhanced MR techniques use either low molecular weight agents, or macromolecular contrast media
- DCE-MRI analysis can be either quantitative or semi-quantitative. Quantitative measures are typically based on a variation of the "two-compartmental" pharmacokinetic model
- Quantitative parameters include K^{trans} (representing both blood flow and permeability), k$_{ep}$ (the reverse rate constant), fpV (fraction of plasma volume), and v$_e$ (fractional extravascular extracellular leakage volume)
- Non-contrast MR techniques rely on intrinsic contrast and suffer from low signal-to-contrast ratios. Examples include diffusion-weighted and arterial spin labeling (ASL) imaging
- DCE-MRI parameters may help in selecting the optimal dose for anti-angiogenic drugs in early phase clinical trials. Changes typically become apparent at early time points, potentially making DCE-MRI useful for early selection of treatment responders
- Potential obstacles to the widespread use of DCE-MRI include accuracy of the pharmacokinetic model, lack of specificity, sampling bias, availability of software, and establishing how to ascertain treatment response
- MMCM have a molecular weight >30,000 Da. They are starting to gain approval for human use: MS-325 has recently been approved for human use in MR angiography; however, its usefulness as an angiogenesis imaging method has not been established
- Endothelial stem cells labeled with an MR contrast agent offer future potential for angiogenesis imaging. Following IV injection the cells can be monitored by MR imaging as they track to areas of neoangiogenesis

REFERENCES

1. Conway EM, Collen D, Carmeliet P. Molecular mechanisms of blood vessel growth. Cardiovasc Res 2001; 49: 507–21.
2. Folkman J. Angiogenesis in cancer, vascular, rheumatoid and other disease. Nat Med 1995; 1: 27–31.
3. Parker GJ, Tofts PS. Pharmacokinetic analysis of neoplasms using contrast-enhanced dynamic magnetic resonance imaging. Top Magn Reson Imaging 1999; 10: 130–42.
4. Padhani AR. Dynamic contrast-enhanced MRI in clinical oncology: current status and future directions. J Magn Reson Imaging 2002; 16: 407–22.
5. Knopp MV, Giesel FL, Marcos H, von Tengg-Kobligk H, Choyke P. Dynamic contrast-enhanced magnetic resonance imaging in oncology. Top Magn Reson Imaging 2001; 12: 301–8.
6. Brasch R, Turetschek K. MRI characterization of tumors and grading angiogenesis using macromolecular contrast media: status report. Eur J Radiol 2000; 34: 148–55.
7. Miles KA. Functional computed tomography in oncology. Eur J Cancer 2002; 38: 2079–84.
8. Figg WD, Folkman J, eds. Angiogenesis: An Integrative Approach from Science to Medicine. New York: Springer, 2008.
9. Voest VV, D'Amore PA. Tumor Angiogenesis and Microcirculation. New York: Marcel. Dekker, 2001.
10. Gray LH, Conger AD, Ebert M, Hornsey S, Scott OC. The concentration of oxygen dissolved in tissues at the time of irradiation as a factor in radiotherapy. Br J Radiol 1953; 26: 638–48.
11. Holash J, Wiegand SJ, Yancopoulos GD. New model of tumor angiogenesis: dynamic balance between vessel regression and growth mediated by angiopoietins and VEGF. Oncogene 1999; 18: 5356–62.
12. Secomb TW, Hsu R, Braun RD, et al. Theoretical simulation of oxygen transport to tumors by three-dimensional networks of microvessels. Adv Exp Med Biol 1998; 454: 629–34.
13. Raleigh JA, Calkins-Adams DP, Rinker LH, et al. Hypoxia and vascular endothelial growth factor expression in human squamous cell carcinomas using pimonidazole as a hypoxia marker. Cancer Res 1998; 58: 3765–8.
14. Hanahan D, Folkman J. Patterns and Emerging Mechanisms of the Angiogenic Switch during Tumorigenesis. Cell 1996; 86: 353–64.
15. Lawrence WT. Physiology of the acute wound. Clin Plast Surg 1998; 25: 321–40.
16. Benjamin LE, Golijanin D, Itin A, Pode D, Keshet E. Selective ablation of immature blood vessels in established human tumors follows vascular endothelial growth factor withdrawal. J Clin Invest 1999; 103: 159–65.
17. Kaban K, Herbst RS. Angiogenesis as a target for cancer therapy. Hematol Oncol Clin North Am 2002; 16: 1125–71.
18. Hahnfeldt P, Panigrahy D, Folkman J, Hlatky L. Tumor development under angiogenic signaling: a dynamical theory of tumor growth, treatment response, and postvascular dormancy. Cancer Res 1999; 59: 4770–5.
19. Folkman J. New perspectives in clinical oncology from angiogenesis research. Eur J Cancer 1996; 32A: 2534–9.
20. Darland DC, D'Amore PA. Blood vessel maturation: vascular development comes of age. J Clin Invest 1999; 103: 157–8.
21. Baluk P, Hashizume H, McDonald DM. Cellular abnormalities of blood vessels as targets in cancer. Curr Opin Genet Dev 2005; 15: 102–11.
22. Armulik A, Abramsson A, Betsholtz C. Endothelial/pericyte interactions. Circ Res 2005; 97: 512–23.
23. Hashizume H, Baluk P, Morikawa S, et al. Openings between defective endothelial cells explain tumor vessel leakiness. Am J Pathol 2000; 156: 1363–80.
24. Ocak I, Baluk P, Barrett T, McDonald DM, Choyke P. The biologic basis of in vivo angiogenesis imaging. Front Biosci 2007; 12: 3601–16.
25. Carver LA, Schnitzer JE. Caveolae: mining little caves for new cancer targets. Nat Rev Cancer 2003; 3: 571–81.
26. Braun RD, Lanzen JL, Dewhirst MW. Fourier analysis of fluctuations of oxygen tension and blood flow in R3230Ac tumors and muscle in rats. Am J Physiol 1999; 277: H551–68.
27. Padera TP, Kadambi A, di Tomaso E, et al. Lymphatic metastasis in the absence of functional intratumor lymphatics. Science 2002; 296: 1883–6.
28. Ruoslahti E. Specialization of tumour vasculature. Nat Rev Cancer 2002; 2: 83–90.
29. Folkman J. Role of angiogenesis in tumor growth and metastasis. Semin Oncol 2002; 29: 15–8.
30. Hoar FJ, Lip GY, Belgore F, Stonelake PS. Circulating levels of VEGF-A, VEGF-D and soluble VEGF-A receptor (sFIt-1) in human breast cancer. Int J Biol Markers 2004; 19: 229–35.
31. Miller JC, Pien HH, Sahani D, Sorensen AG, Thrall JH. Imaging angiogenesis: applications and potential for drug development. J Natl Cancer Inst 2005; 97: 172–87.
32. Barrett T, Brechbiel M, Bernardo M, Choyke PL. MRI of tumor angiogenesis. J Magn Reson Imaging 2007; 26: 235–49.
33. Li ZP, Meng QF, Sun CH, et al. Tumor angiogenesis and dynamic CT in colorectal carcinoma: radiologic-pathologic correlation. World J Gastroenterol 2005; 11: 1287–91.
34. Ferrara KW, Merritt CR, Burns PN, et al. Evaluation of tumor angiogenesis with US: imaging, Doppler, and contrast agents. Acad Radiol 2000; 7: 824–39.
35. Ellegala DB, Leong-Poi H, Carpenter JE, et al. Imaging tumor angiogenesis with contrast ultrasound and microbubbles targeted to alpha(v)beta3. Circulation 2003; 108: 336–41.
36. Zhang X, Xiong Z, Wu Y, et al. Quantitative PET imaging of tumor integrin alphavbeta3 expression with 18F-FRGD2. J Nucl Med 2006; 47: 113–21.
37. Rohren EM, Turkington TG, Coleman RE. Clinical applications of PET in oncology. Radiology 2004; 231: 305–32.
38. Blodgett TM, Meltzer CC, Townsend DW. PET/CT: form and function. Radiology 2007; 242: 360–85.
39. Pichler BJ, Judenhofer MS, Wehrl HF. PET/MRI hybrid imaging: devices and initial results. Eur Radiol 2008; 18: 1077–86.
40. Padhani AR, Husband JE. Dynamic contrast-enhanced MRI studies in oncology with an emphasis on quantification, validation and human studies. Clin Radiol 2001; 56: 607–20.
41. Tofts PS, Brix G, Buckley DL, et al. Estimating kinetic parameters from dynamic contrast-enhanced T(1)-weighted MRI of a diffusable tracer: standardized quantities and symbols. J Magn Reson Imaging 1999; 10: 223–32.

42. Brix G, Kiessling F, Lucht R, et al. Microcirculation and microvasculature in breast tumors: pharmacokinetic analysis of dynamic MR image series. Magn Reson Med 2004; 52: 420–9.

43. Schlemmer HP, Merkle J, Grobholz R, et al. Can pre-operative contrast-enhanced dynamic MR imaging for prostate cancer predict microvessel density in prostatectomy specimens? Eur Radiol 2004; 14: 309–17.

44. Lord SJ, Lei W, Craft P, et al. A systematic review of the effectiveness of magnetic resonance imaging (MRI) as an addition to mammography and ultrasound in screening young women at high risk of breast cancer. Eur J Cancer 2007; 43: 1905–17.

45. Pickles MD, Lowry M, Manton DJ, Gibbs P, Turnbull LW. Role of dynamic contrast enhanced MRI in monitoring early response of locally advanced breast cancer to neoadjuvant chemotherapy. Breast Cancer Res Treat 2005; 91: 1–10.

46. Eliat PA, Dedieu V, Bertino C, et al. Magnetic resonance imaging contrast-enhanced relaxometry of breast tumors: an MRI multicenter investigation concerning 100 patients. Magn Reson Imaging 2004; 22: 475–81.

47. Padhani AR, Gapinski CJ, Macvicar DA, et al. Dynamic contrast enhanced MRI of prostate cancer: correlation with morphology and tumour stage, histological grade and PSA. Clin Radiol 2000; 55: 99–109.

48. Ocak I, Bernardo M, Metzger G, et al. Dynamic contrast-enhanced MRI of prostate cancer at 3 T: a study of pharmacokinetic parameters. AJR Am J Roentgenol 2007; 189: 849.

49. Aronen HJ, Perkio J. Dynamic susceptibility contrast MRI of gliomas. Neuroimaging Clin N Am 2002; 12: 501–23.

50. Baba Y, Furusawa M, Murakami R, et al. Role of dynamic MRI in the evaluation of head and neck cancers treated with radiation therapy. Int J Radiat Oncol Biol Phys 1997; 37: 783–7.

51. Marzola P, Degrassi A, Calderan L, et al. In vivo assessment of antiangiogenic activity of SU6668 in an experimental colon carcinoma model. Clin Cancer Res 2004; 10: 739–50.

52. Anderson HL, Yap JT, Miller MP, et al. Assessment of pharmacodynamic vascular response in a phase I trial of combretastatin A4 phosphate. J Clin Oncol 2003; 21: 2823–30.

53. Lee L, Sharma S, Morgan B, et al. Biomarkers for assessment of pharmacologic activity for a vascular endothelial growth factor (VEGF) receptor inhibitor, PTK787/ZK 222584 (PTK/ZK): translation of biological activity in a mouse melanoma metastasis model to phase I studies in patients with advanced colorectal cancer with liver metastases. Cancer Chemother Pharmacol 2006; 57: 761–71.

54. Mross K, Drevs J, Muller M, et al. Phase I clinical and pharmacokinetic study of PTK/ZK, a multiple VEGF receptor inhibitor, in patients with liver metastases from solid tumours. Eur J Cancer 2005; 41: 1291–9.

55. Jain RK, Tong RT, Munn LL. Effect of vascular normalization by antiangiogenic therapy on interstitial hypertension, peritumor edema, and lymphatic metastasis: insights from a mathematical model. Cancer Res 2007; 67: 2729–35.

56. Leach MO, Brindle KM, Evelhoch JL, et al. The assessment of antiangiogenic and antivascular therapies in early-stage clinical trials using magnetic resonance imaging: issues and recommendations. Br J Cancer 2005; 92: 1599–610.

57. Barrett T, Kobayashi H, Brechbiel M, Choyke PL. Macromolecular MRI contrast agents for imaging tumor angiogenesis. Eur J Radiol 2006; 60: 353–66.

58. Cavagna FM, Maggioni F, Castelli PM, et al. Gadolinium chelates with weak binding to serum proteins. A new class of high-efficiency, general purpose contrast agents for magnetic resonance imaging. Invest Radiol 1997; 32: 780–96.

59. Rapp JH, Wolff SD, Quinn SF, et al. Aortoiliac Occlusive Disease in Patients with Known or Suspected Peripheral Vascular Disease: Safety and Efficacy of Gadofosveset-enhanced MR Angiography—Multicenter Comparative Phase III Study. Radiology 2005; 236: 71–8.

60. Bluemke DA, Stillman AE, Bis KG, et al. Carotid MR angiography: phase II study of safety and efficacy for MS-325. Radiology 2001; 219: 114–22.

61. Goyen M, Edelman M, Perreault P, et al. MR angiography of aortoiliac occlusive disease: a phase III study of the safety and effectiveness of the blood-pool contrast agent MS-325. Radiology 2005; 236: 825–33.

62. Turetschek K, Floyd E, Helbich T, et al. MRI assessment of microvascular characteristics in experimental breast tumors using a new blood pool contrast agent (MS-325) with correlations to histopathology. J Magn Reson Imaging 2001; 14: 237–42.

63. Arbab AS, Yocum GT, Wilson LB, et al. Comparison of transfection agents in forming complexes with ferumoxides, cell labeling efficiency, and cellular viability. Mol Imaging 2004; 3: 24–32.

64. Emerit J, Beaumont C, Trivin F. Iron metabolism, free radicals, and oxidative injury. Biomed Pharmacother 2001; 55: 333–9.

65. Arbab AS, Yocum GT, Kalish H, et al. Efficient magnetic cell labeling with protamine sulfate complexed to ferumoxides for cellular MRI. Blood 2004; 104: 1217–23.

66. Anderson SA, Glod J, Arbab AS, et al. Noninvasive MR imaging of magnetically labeled stem cells to directly identify neovasculature in a glioma model. Blood 2005; 105: 420–5.

67. Silva AC, Kim SG, Garwood M. Imaging blood flow in brain tumors using arterial spin labeling. Magn Reson Med 2000; 44: 169–73.

68. Detre JA, Alsop DC. Perfusion magnetic resonance imaging with continuous arterial spin labeling: methods and clinical applications in the central nervous system. Eur J Radiol 1999; 30: 115–24.

69. Detre A, Alsop DC. Perfusion fMRI with arterial spin labeling (ASL). In: Moonen CTW, Bandettini PA, eds. Functional MRI. Heidelburg: Springer, 1999: 47–62.

70. Golay X, Hendrikse J, Lim TC. Perfusion imaging using arterial spin labeling. Top Magn Reson Imaging 2004; 15: 10–27.

71. Patterson DM, Padhani AR, Collins DJ. Technology insight: water diffusion MRI—a potential new biomarker of response to cancer therapy. Nat Clin Pract Oncol 2008; 5: 220–33.

72. Parker GJ. Analysis of MR diffusion weighted images. Br J Radiol 2004; 77: S176–85.

73. Turner R, Le Bihan D, Maier J, et al. Echo-planar imaging of intravoxel incoherent motion. Radiology 1990; 177: 407–14.

74. Niendorf T, Dijkhuizen RM, Norris DG, van Lookeren Campagne M, Nicolay K. Biexponential diffusion attenuation in various states of brain tissue: implications for diffusion-weighted imaging. Magn Reson Med 1996; 36: 847–57.

75. Mulkern RV, Vajapeyam S, Haker SJ, Maier SE. Magnetization transfer studies of the fast and slow tissue water diffusion components in the human brain. NMR Biomed 2005; 18: 186–94.

76. Jordan BF, Runquist M, Raghunand N, et al. Dynamic contrast-enhanced and diffusion MRI show rapid and dramatic changes in tumor microenvironment in response to inhibition of HIF-1alpha using PX-478. Neoplasia 2005; 7: 475–85.

77. Pastorino F, Brignole C, Marimpietri D, et al. Vascular damage and anti-angiogenic effects of tumor vessel-targeted liposomal chemotherapy. Cancer Res 2003; 63: 7400–9.

64 Measurement of Angiogenesis: CT Principles and Practice
Vicky Goh

INTRODUCTION

Dynamic contrast-enhanced computed tomography (CT) techniques have been the subject of resurgent interest in recent years due to an evolving need for in vivo assessment of tumor angiogenesis on an individual patient basis. CT has many advantages over other imaging methods. It is widely available, provides excellent anatomical detail and quantification of tumor perfusion, blood volume and vascular leakage by Food and Drug Administration (FDA) approved user-friendly commercial software is straightforward (Table 64.1). Vascular estimates have been correlated with histological angiogenesis markers. The latest high-end multidetector row CT systems are capable of rapid scanning and large volume coverage enabling entire tumors to be evaluated.

QUANTIFICATION OF VASCULAR PARAMETERS

Tumor perfusion, blood volume and vascular leakage can be estimated via kinetic modeling of the changes in tumor enhancement following intravenous (IV) CT contrast agent administration.

Perfusion reflects the flow rate of whole blood through the vasculature of a defined tissue volume or mass (F; *mL/min/100 mL or mL/min/100g tissue*). At CT this encompasses flow in arteries, arterioles, capillaries, venules, and veins.

Blood volume (BV; *mL/100mL or mL/100g tissue*) reflects the volume of flowing whole blood within the functioning vasculature of a defined tissue volume or mass. Again this encompasses arteries, arterioles, capillaries, venules, and veins at CT.

Vascular leakage may be expressed as extraction fraction (EF); or *capillary permeability surface area product* (PS; *mL/min/100mL or mL/min/100g tissue*). The extraction fraction is the fraction of whole blood contrast agent that is transferred to the extravascular–extracellular space during a single passage of the contrast agent. The capillary permeability surface area product represents the product of permeability and total surface area of capillary endothelium in a unit volume or mass of tissue and reflects the total diffusional flux across the capillaries.

CT CONTRAST AGENTS

CT contrast agents used in clinical practice are low molecular weight contrast agents (<1 kDa), typically derivatives of iodobenzoic acid with negligible serum protein binding, thus their distribution is similar to extracellular fluid. CT contrast agents show simple two compartment kinetics: the injected contrast agent initially remains within the intravascular compartment during the first few cardiac cycles. It then diffuses from the intravascular into the extravascular-extracellular compartment (with the exception of some sites, e.g., brain, testis, and retina) at a rate determined by the rate of delivery, vessel surface area, and vessel leakiness. There is negligible transfer into the intracellular compartment (<1%). Contrast agent then passes back from the extravascular-extracellular compartment into the intravascular compartment, and is excreted rapidly by the kidneys, though there can be some hepato-biliary excretion. Up to half of the administered dose is recovered within the first two hours of dosing.

Macromolecular CT contrast agents have not yet been licensed for clinical use but potentially permit more specific assessment of vascular blood volume and leakage. Unlike low molecular weight contrast agents that have a relatively high first pass extraction fraction for both normal tissue and tumor, macromolecular first pass extraction is low, in the order of <1% for normal vasculature. As a higher proportion of intravascular contrast agent remains during the first pass, vascular volume measurement will be more accurate. Tumor microvessels are also hyperpermeable to macromolecules in contrast to normal vessels, a specific property of the tumor neovasculature that macromolecular contrast agents can assess. However to date there has been little data on macromolecular contrast-enhanced perfusion CT, and no published human studies. In rats, imaging with PEG12000-Gen4-triiodo in experimental breast cancer has shown that quantitative estimation of vascular permeability is possible (1). Similarly early changes in hepatic flow have been demonstrated with chemically-induced primary liver tumors using a blood pool macromolecular agent demonstrating its potential for tumor detection prior to development of overt lesions (2).

Key Points: Quantification of Vascular Parameters

Contrast enhancement at CT reflects:

- Rate of delivery, volume, and concentration of the contrast agent
- Vessel surface area
- Vessel leakiness, that is, vascular permeability
- Rate of contrast agent backflux from the extravascular-extracellular into the intravascular compartment
- Rate of contrast agent excretion

THE RELATIONSHIP BETWEEN CT ENHANCEMENT AND CONTRAST AGENT CONCENTRATION

The relationship between contrast agent concentration and CT enhancement is straightforward. There is a direct linear relationship between enhancement and iodine concentration (Fig. 64.1). For example, at 80 kV an enhancement change of 54 Hounsfield units (HU) is equivalent to 1 mg/mL of iodine, while at 120 kV an enhancement change of 37 HU is equivalent to 1 mg/mL of iodine. Thus quantification by kinetic modeling can be simplified as, in practice, contrast concentration may be substituted by the CT Hounsfield unit number. This is a major advantage over magnetic

Table 64.1 Comparison of the Different Imaging Modalities for Quantification of Tissue Vascularity

	MDCT	DCE-MRI	PET	US
Tracer	Iodine based contrast agent	Gadolinium based contrast agent	^{15}labeled H_2O or ^{14}CO	Microbubbles
Z-axis coverage	2D: up to 125 mm 3D: up to 280 mm	2D: up to 48 mm 3D: up to 60 mm	Whole body	Whole tumor
Measured Parameters	2D: BF, BV, PS 3D: BF, BV, PS	K^{trans}, k_{ep}, v_e Relative BF, BV	BF, BV	BF, BV, MTT
Analysis technique	Slope method Mullani Gould Patlak analysis Modified distributed parameter analysis	Generalized kinetic model Central volume theorem	Mullani-Gould First pass analysis	Central volume theorem
Advantage	Straightforward quantification Good spatial resolution Relatively cheap and widely available	Good contrast resolution No radiation burden	Direct quantification	No radiation burden Relatively cheap and widely available
Disadvantage	Radiation burden	Quantification challenging Limited availability	Radiation burden Limited availability Expensive	Limited to superficial sites Unable to assess microvasculature: regional perfusion only

Abbreviations: BF, blood flow; BV, blood volume; k_{ep}, rate constant; K^{trans}, transfer constant; MTT, mean transit time; PS, permeability surface area product; v_e, extravascular-extracellular volume for a given tissue volume.

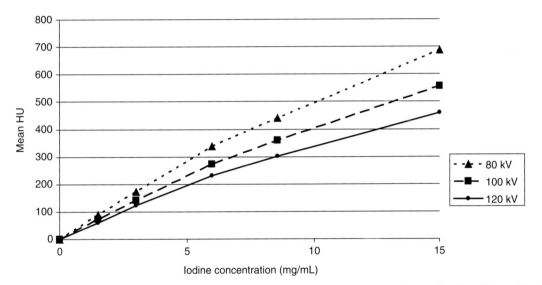

Figure 64.1 The linear relationship between CT enhancement change (Hounsfield units) and iodine concentration (mg/mL) at three different kilovoltages: 80 kV, 100 kV, and 120 kV.

resonance (MR) imaging where the relationship between signal intensity change and contrast agent concentration is not so easily defined and may be non-linear.

KINETIC MODELING

Different models have been applied in order to obtain more physiologically based vascular measurements. Those commonly applied include methods based on:

- Fick principle, for example, Mullani-Gould (peak method) or "Slope" method
- Patlak analysis
- Distributed parameter analysis

Fick Principle

Methods based on the Fick principle (Fig. 64.2) have been most commonly used to assess tissue or organ "perfusion" (blood flow per unit volume of tissue) (3,4). The tissue of interest is treated as a single well-stirred compartment incorporating both intra- and extravascular-extracellular compartments. The amount of contrast within tissue per unit time is equivalent to the arterial concentration minus the venous concentration multiplied by blood flow.

Patlak Analysis

Methods based on Patlak analysis provide estimates of blood volume and vascular leakage (expressed as extraction fraction, K_1) only. Patlak analysis has been used previously to model tracer kinetics in nuclear medicine studies (5,6), but has been adapted

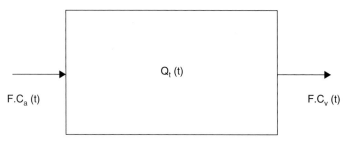

Figure 64.2 Fick principle. *Abbreviations*: F, flow; C_a, arterial contrast agent concentration; C_v, venous contrast agent concentration; Q_t, tissue contrast agent mass.

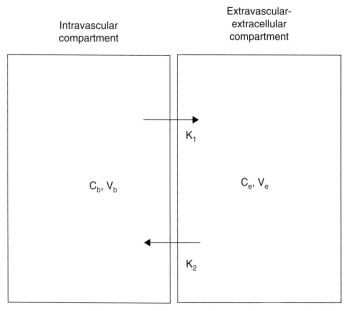

Figure 64.3 Modified Patlak analysis. The relationship between the intravascular and extravascular-extracellular compartments is shown. *Abbreviations*: C_b, whole blood contrast concentration; C_e, extravascular-extracellular compartment contrast concentration; K_1, extraction fraction; K_2, rate constant; V_b, blood volume; V_e, extravascular-extracellular compartment volume.

and simplified for CT analysis. The relationship between the intravascular and extravascular-extracellular compartments is shown in Figure 64.3. The intravascular and extravascular-extracellular compartments are assumed to be well-mixed. For the purposes of CT analysis, only the one-way transfer of freely diffusible contrast from the intravascular to the extravascular-extracellular compartment is considered. The return of contrast from the extravascular-extracellular compartment back to the intravascular compartment is assumed to be negligible. Clearly this assumption will only hold for a limited time period following contrast injection.

Distributed Parameter Analysis

The adiabatic approximation of the distributed parameter model is based on a two compartment model first proposed by Johnson and Wilson (7). This model depicts the capillary-tissue unit as two cylinders, the inner cylinder representing the intravascular compartment, and the outer cylinder representing the extravascular-extracellular compartment (Fig. 64.4). As the contrast agent enters the capillary, it begins to diffuse across the capillary membrane, thus the intravascular contrast agent concentration is a function of the position along the vessel and time. The extravascular-extracellular compartment is treated as a well-stirred compartment; the contrast agent concentration is a function of time only (Fig. 64.4).

Key Points: Kinetic Modeling

- The linear relationship between enhancement and iodine concentration simplifies quantification by kinetic modeling as iodine concentration can be substituted by the CT Hounsfield unit number
- Perfusion, blood volume, and vascular leakage (expressed as extraction fraction or permeability surface area product) can be estimated using CT
- Commonly applied kinetic models in commercial software platforms include Mullani-Gould and Slope methods for estimating perfusion; Patlak analysis for estimating blood volume and vascular leakage; and distributed parameter analysis for estimating perfusion, blood volume, and vascular leakage
- Parameters obtained by different models are not necessarily interchangeable unless experimental conditions are optimized

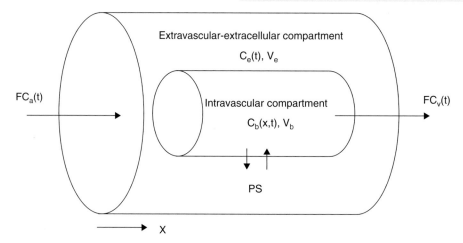

Figure 64.4 The capillary-tissue unit. The intravascular contrast agent concentration C_b (x,t) is dependent on the distance, x, along the capillary, decreasing from the arterial C_a (t) to venous side, C_v (t) as well as time, t. The extravascular-extracellular contrast agent concentration C_e (t) is a function of time, t, only. *Abbreviations*: F, flow; PS, permeability surface area product; V_b, blood volume; V_e, volume of extravascular-extracellular compartment.

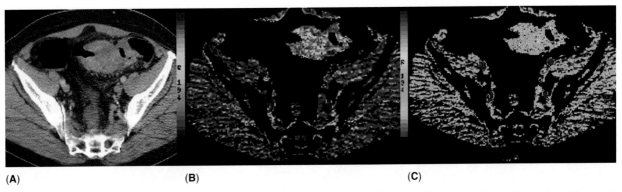

Figure 64.5 Single level perfusion CT of a sigmoid colon cancer. (A) Contrast-enhanced image of the cancer. (B) Corresponding perfusion (blood flow: mL/min/100g tissue) and (C) blood volume (mL/100g tissue) parametric maps are shown.

Table 64.2 Typical Acquisition Parameters for Axial Single Level and Volumetric Helical CT Techniques

	MDCT Single level	MDCT Single level	MDCT Volumetric
Kinetic model	Slope method Mullani Gould method Patlak analysis	Modified distributed parameter analysis	Patlak analysis Modified distributed parameter analysis
Vascular measures	F, BV, K_1	F, BV, PS	F, BV, K_1
Contrast agent	>300 mg/mL iodine	>300 mg/mL iodine	>300 mg/mL iodine
Dose	0.5 mL/kg	1.0–1.5 mL/kg	1.0 mL/kg
Typical volume	35–50 mL	70–100 mL	50–100 mL
Injection rate	5–10 mL/sec	3–5 mL/sec	3–6 mL/sec
Acquisition type	Axial	Axial	Helical
Slice thickness	5–10 mm	5–10 mm	5–10 mm
Z-axis coverage	Up to 125 mm	Up to 125 mm	Up to 280 mm
Sampling rate	1 acquisition/1–3 sec	1 acquisition/0.5–1 sec	1 acquisition/5 sec
Sampling duration	Up to 60 sec	Up to 120 sec	Up to 180 sec

Abbreviations: BV, blood volume; F, perfusion; K_1, Patlak extraction fraction; PS, permeability surface area product.

DATA ACQUISITION

Sequential data sampling following IV contrast administration is necessary to estimate perfusion, blood volume, and vascular leakage. The sampling rate and sampling duration depends on a number of factors including the type of vascular parameter to be estimated, for example, perfusion, blood volume, or permeability surface area product; kinetic model; and tumor site. Data acquisition can be broadly categorized into two types: axial single level and helical volumetric techniques. The radiation dose imposed by studies clearly depends on acquisition parameters (kV, mA), z-axis coverage, data sampling rate, and duration.

Axial Techniques

Axial single level techniques are commonly performed. Data is acquired at a single anatomical level – the z-axis coverage is dependent on the number and configuration of CT detectors, for example, up to 128 mm with 256-detector CT systems. Although acquisitions may be divided into the "first pass" and "delayed" phase studies, in practice acquisitions incorporate both phases to enable simultaneous determination of perfusion, blood volume, and vascular leakage (Fig. 64.5). At least one baseline unenhanced image has to be acquired to enable detection of enhancement change following IV contrast administration.

For first pass studies a small volume of CT contrast agent is injected as a rapid bolus, for example, 35 to 50 mL at 5 to 10 mL/ sec. Acquisitions are typically performed within 40 to 60 seconds of contrast agent administration (Table 64.2). A high data sampling rate (in the order of one acquisition per 0.5 or 1 second) is required for accurate determination of perfusion by some models, for example, deconvolution based modified distributed parameter analysis. The disadvantage of high sampling rates particularly for abdominal-pelvic tumors is the radiation burden to the patient. Vascular leakage may also be estimated from first pass data using Patlak analysis but the experimental conditions are important to prevent underestimation. For delayed phase studies less frequent data sampling may be employed (in the order of one acquisition every five seconds) to estimate vascular leakage. Durations ranging from 2 to 10 minutes have been utilized in the past (3).

Volumetric Helical Techniques

Recent technological improvements have enabled volumetric helical techniques to be developed (8,9). The latest state-of-the-art scanners are capable of high temporal resolution, thus perfusion

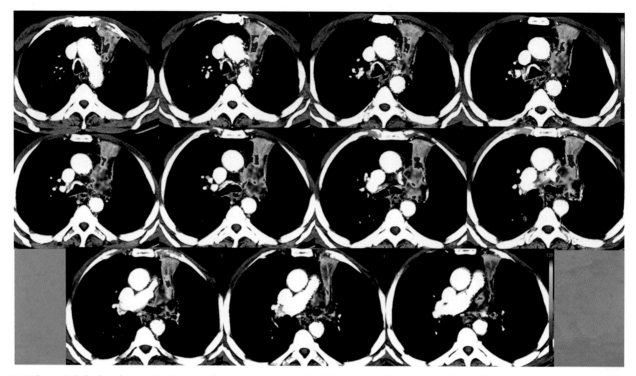

Figure 64.6 Volumetric helical perfusion CT of a central lung tumor involving the left upper lobe bronchus resulting in distal atelectasis. Multiple sequential helical acquisitions encompassing the entire lung tumor were obtained. The blood volume map is color coded such that areas of high blood volume are red, while areas of low blood volume are purple. The tumor shows relatively lower blood volume in comparison with adjacent atelectatic lung.

can be estimated in addition to blood volume and vascular leakage. Multiple helical acquisitions are performed (Table 64.1) permitting dynamic changes in enhancement over a large tissue volume, up to 28 cm can be assessed currently (Fig. 64.6). The advantages of such helical techniques is the volume coverage – the entire tumor (8) or organ, for example, liver (9) can be encompassed; the ability to reconstruct images to different slice thicknesses, and the ability to compensate for z-axis motion. This is pertinent particularly for therapeutic assessment and for heterogeneous tumors.

Key Points: Data Acquisition

- Sequential data sampling following IV contrast administration is necessary to estimate perfusion, blood volume, and vascular leakage
- Data sampling rate and sampling duration will vary depending on the vascular parameter to be estimated, kinetic model, and tumor site. Perfusion estimation requires high sampling rates and a short sampling duration
- Axial single level or helical volumetric techniques can be performed but a larger volume coverage can be achieved with helical volumetric techniques currently

VALIDATION

Comparison with Other Methods and Measurement Reproducibility

CT techniques have been validated in both animal and human studies. These have demonstrated that CT estimates lie within the documented physiological range, and are comparable to measurements obtained by other methods, including microspheres (10–12), xenon CT (13) and ^{15}O labeled-H_2PET (14,15), and Evans blue dye (16). Measurement reproducibility has been found to be acceptable. A coefficient of variation of 13.2% to 35% has been reported for the cranial circulation of both animals and humans (17,18), while co-efficients of variation ranging from 14% to 24% have been reported for perfusion, blood volume, and permeability surface area product in tumors (11,19). Studies of observer variability have demonstrated varying agreement, with better intra- than inter-observer agreement in general: coefficients of variation in studies have ranged from 2.5–9.5% (20) to 14–20.8% (21) in cranial studies, 3% to 13% in a study of squamous cancers of the extracranial head and neck (22), and 20% to 34% in a colorectal tumor study (23).

Assessment of Tumor Angiogenesis

The relationship between perfusion CT parameters and histological markers of angiogenesis (microvessel density and vascular endothelial growth factor expression) has been investigated in various tumors including lung (24–26), renal (27), and colorectal cancer (28,29). Results have been variable. Some studies have shown a positive correlation between CT measures (perfusion, blood volume, and permeability surface area product), and histological markers (24,27,29), while other studies have shown no relationship between perfusion and histological microvessel density (28,29) or vascular endothelial growth factor expression (29). This is in line with data from studies of dynamic contrast-enhanced MR imaging, and partially reflects the technical challenges of performing such studies, for example, ensuring the same tumor areas are compared.

Key Points: Validation

- Perfusion CT estimates lie within the expected physiological range and have been validated against techniques including labeled microspheres, Evans blue dye, xenon CT, and ^{15}labeled-H_2O PET
- Measurement reproducibility is acceptable for clinical practice but is variable
- Assessment of individual baseline reproducibility may be the most dependable process to assess whether therapeutic changes are significant on an individual patient basis
- Perfusion CT estimates correlate with histological markers of angiogenesis including microvessel density and vascular endothelial growth factor

APPLICATION IN CLINICAL PRACTICE

Until recently perfusion CT has been predominantly a research based technique. However clinical usage is increasing particularly for the evaluation of drugs targeted at the tumor vasculature, administered alone or in combination with standard therapy. Nonetheless perfusion CT also has other potential uses; it may

- Potentially improve lesion detection
- Facilitate differential diagnosis
- Provide information regarding tumor biology at tumor staging, especially in combination with ^{18}FDG PET, where perfusion CT techniques obviate the need for specific PET "blood flow" tracers, which are of limited availability in clinical practice
- Provide prognostic information

Assessment of Drugs Targeting the Tumor Vasculature

From a simplistic imaging perspective, drugs targeting the tumor vasculature can be broadly divided into anti-angiogenic and vascular disruptive agents (Table 64.3). The effects of these drugs on CT parameters are similar regardless of the mechanism of drug action. The dominant effect is a reduction in blood flow and vascular permeability. However the timing of the onset of vascular changes enables these two therapeutic strategies to be distinguished on imaging. Both xenograft and human imaging studies of antiangiogenic drugs (for example, bevacizumab, valatinib, ZD6474, SU11248, and BIBF1120) have shown that anti-vascular effects are not immediate, only arising 24 to 48 hours post drug administration. In contrast vascular disruptive agents (for example, CA4P, DMXAA, and ZD6126), which target the tumor endothelium cause rapid shutdown of the vasculature within minutes of drug administration, with secondary tumor cell death as a consequence. Anti-angiogenic drugs may also induce "normalization" of the vasculature which may be difficult to detect because the improvement in blood flow will not be distinguishable from non-responsiveness, although concomitant vascular pruning should be visible on morphological imaging.

Assessment of therapeutic response using standard response criteria, RECIST or WHO, has been problematic as these drugs do not necessarily result in tumor shrinkage despite conferring a survival advantage (30,31). For example, the addition of the anti-angiogenic vascular endothelial growth factor (VEGF)–directed antibody, Bevacizumab to chemotherapy as first- and second-line treatment of metastatic colorectal cancer prolonged progression-free survival by 4.4 months compared to chemotherapy alone, yet an objective reduction in tumor size was only noted in an additional 10% of cases. Similarly Sorafenib, a multikinase inhibitor of tumor cell proliferation and angiogenesis, prolonged progression-free survival by three months in patients with advanced renal cell cancer refractory to standard treatment but an objective reduction in tumor size was noted in 10% only. Perfusion CT may provide evidence of a vascular response (Figs. 64.7 and 64.8). For example, a reduction in blood flow (66–83%) was demonstrated in an animal tumor model with Sorafenib despite absence of size change (32), and a reduction in rectal tumor blood flow (40–44%) and blood volume (16–39%) with Bevacizumab (33).

In Phase I clinical trials perfusion CT may help define a biologically active dose. Drug toxicities are used widely in Phase I studies to define a dose to take forward for further evaluation, however, anti-angiogenic drugs have relatively low toxicity and a wider therapeutic window making this approach less valid (34). While not used routinely, imaging can define a biologically active dose that is lower than the dose limiting toxicity and maximum tolerated dose by demonstrating an anti-vascular effect during dose escalation (35).

Perfusion CT may also assist treatment scheduling by providing supportive mechanistic information of the interactions between antiangiogenic, vascular disruptive, cytotoxic therapies, and radiotherapy. As an example, radiotherapy given before but not after a

Table 64.3 Comparison of Antiangiogenic and Vascular Disruptive Agents

	Antiangiogenic drugs	Vascular disruptive agents
Mechanism of action	Inhibition of growth factor support of neovasculature Apoptosis of immature blood vessels	Collapse of proliferating vasculature Possible collapse of mature tumor vasculature
Duration of drug action	Long term vascular changes Normalization in short term	Short lived vascular effects Dose dependent
Toxicity	Less toxic but not like vascular disruptive agents or chemotherapy	More toxic than anti-angiogenic drugs but unlike chemotherapy
Physiologic effects assessed by imaging	Reduced permeability Reduced blood flow Reduced blood volume	Reduced blood flow Reduced blood volume Reduced vascular tortuosity
Onset of antivascular effects	24–48 hr	Minutes usually reversible after a single dose

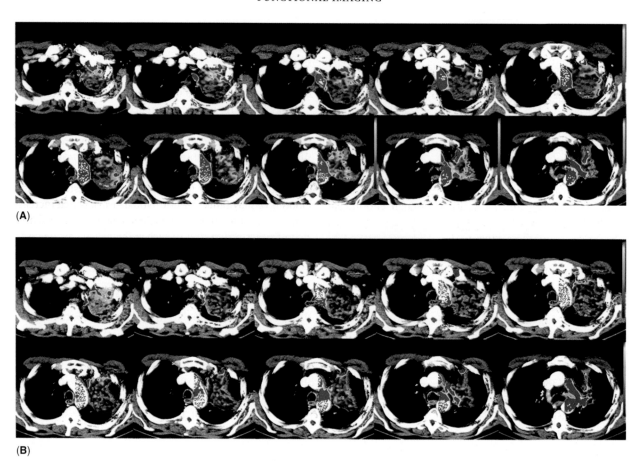

(A)

(B)

Figure 64.7 Volumetric helical perfusion CT technique performed in a lung cancer, (**A**) prior and (**B**) one hour following drug administration to assess the acute vascular changes of L-NNA, a nitric oxide synthase inhibitor. A marked reduction in tumor blood volume is seen following drug administration.

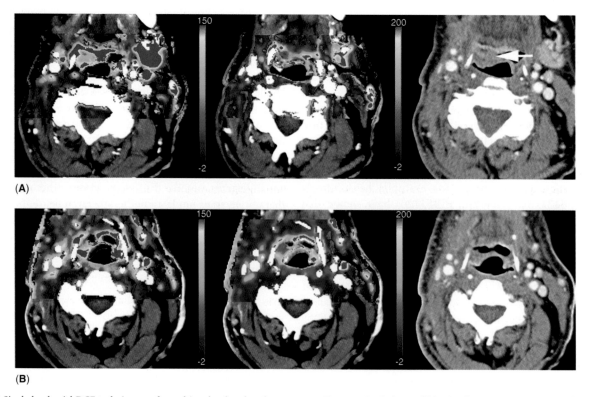

(A)

(B)

Figure 64.8 Single level axial DCE technique performed in a head and neck squamous cell cancer. Perfusion and blood volume parametric map and corresponding contrast-enhanced image of a right piriform fossa carcinoma, (**A**) prior and (**B**) following treatment with a combination of cetuximab, combretastatin, and radiotherapy. Following treatment the primary tumor has shrunk and decreased in vascularity.

vascular disrupting agent (VDA) appears to enhance its anti-vascular effect. Perfusion CT assessment of the interaction of the vascular disrupting agent, combretastatin-A4-phosphate with radiotherapy in advanced lung cancer has shown that an acute increase in vascular blood volume and permeability with radiotherapy prior to VDA administration appears to synergistically increase the VDA effect (36).

Nevertheless the relationship between vascular changes in early phase studies and efficacy endpoints of Phase III studies is a complex one. Some drugs that have showed promise in early phase studies have been disappointing in efficacy trials, for example, PTK787/ZK 222584 (Vatalanib); a multiple vascular endothelial growth factor receptor inhibitor that blocks the activity of all known VEGF receptor tyrosine kinases (37). The causes for negative clinical studies are complex and may relate to pharmacokinetics, mechanism of drug action, compliance issues, etc., and underlies the need to have effective techniques capable of monitoring anti-angiogenic effects in vivo.

Assessment of Standard Chemotherapy

Unlike drugs targeted at the tumor vasculature, there is little data to suggest that standard chemotherapeutic agents cause an acute anti-vascular effect (38). Few perfusion CT studies have assessed standard chemotherapy effect. Two studies have investigated if pre-treatment perfusion CT tumor measurements can predict for response, for example, to induction chemotherapy in advanced squamous cell carcinoma (39,40). These studies showed that a >20% reduction in blood volume correlated with endoscopic response and that a high initial tumor blood volume indicated likely response (39), with >50% reduction in tumor volume after chemotherapy (40).

Assessment of the Vascular Effects of Radiotherapy

In vitro studies of the acute effects of ionizing radiation on tumor vasculature have shown that the tumor response to radiation is regulated by tumor endothelial cell apoptosis. Acutely, an increase in vascular permeability and perfusion occurs as a consequence of endothelial cell damage and inflammation, and possibly due to further new vessel formation as up-regulation of vascular endothelial growth factor either directly or through activation of endothelium hypoxia inducible factor, has been reported in various cancer cell lines after ionizing radiation. In the longer term a decrease in vascular permeability is always seen due to basement membrane thickening, extracapillary fibrosis, and endothelial damage. A reduction in overall microvessel functionality from thrombosis and obliteration of the vessel lumen also occurs.

In vivo studies, for example, of prostate cancer have confirmed the initial hyperemic effect (41); in lung cancer have demonstrated a vascular effect as early as after 9 Gy (42), however the increase is vascular permeability and blood volume is not sustained with a subsequent reduction in tumor vascularity after 27 Gy (Fig. 64.9). Following completion of radiotherapy or chemoradiation a decrease in mean tumor vascularity has been reported in head and neck cancer (43) and colorectal cancer (44,45) though changes have not been homogeneous on an individual patient basis. For example, in a small colorectal cancer study of nine patients, before and two weeks following completion of chemoradiation, although mean blood flow decreased with treatment, two patients showed an increase in blood flow (44).

Prediction of therapeutic response has been assessed in these studies but numbers have been small and results have not been concordant, limiting the use of these techniques for this application currently. For example, in colorectal cancer while one study showed a higher baseline blood flow was suggestive of a poorer response to chemoradiation (45), another study of radiotherapy alone showed the converse (44). In head and neck cancer a lower initial blood flow was predictive of local relapse subsequent to radiotherapy (43). It has been suggested that low initial blood flow may reflect tumor hypoxia (43), which increases resistance to radiotherapy. Nevertheless data of the vascular effects of radiotherapy are useful as such information aids scheduling of radiotherapy in combination with targeted therapy.

Tumor Detection

Previous axial single level studies of the liver have demonstrated the potential of hepatic perfusion to detect metastases. Hepatic metastases are mostly arterially supplied and this arterial dominance can be observed in the surrounding hepatic parenchyma (46). Micrometastases also appear to alter hepatic perfusion patterns (reduction of portal flow) due to increases in hepatic resistance, which may be related to the presence of microthrombi within portal venules or to cytokine release (47). Areas of elevated arterial perfusion in otherwise "normal" livers have been shown to herald the development of overt metastatic disease (48). Axial single level studies of the liver have also been performed of hepatocellular cancer which have demonstrated the arterial dominance of such tumors (49,50).

To date the limited z-axis volume coverage and technical challenges of axial single level imaging have restricted its clinical utility for hepatic lesion detection. However the recent development of whole liver volume perfusion CT overcomes many of these issues, and usage in this clinical scenario is likely to increase. Initial data have been promising: one study has suggested that sensitivity and specificity for lesion detection is better than conventional four-phase imaging (9).

Lesion Characterization

Perfusion CT may also aid lesion characterization. Studies of pulmonary nodules have shown that additional vascular assessment, both semi-quantitative and quantitative, may improve lesion characterization. Studies that have examined semi-quantitative measures such as peak enhancement as a means of differentiating solitary pulmonary nodules (SPN) have shown that an enhancement threshold of 20 HU may potentially distinguish between benign and malignant nodules with a sensitivity and specificity of up to 99% and 70% respectively (25,51–54). Accuracies of up to 92% can be achieved if both wash in and wash out characteristics are taken into account (55).

Similarly perfusion is higher in malignant than benign SPNs. Sitartchouk et al. found that perfusion and blood volume were significantly different in malignant and benign nodules (56). Similarly Zhang and Kono found in 65 patients with SPNs (mean size 1.9 cm) that the mean perfusion value of malignant SPNs was significantly higher than benign nodules (70 vs. 10mL/min/100mL respectively), however inflammatory nodules also

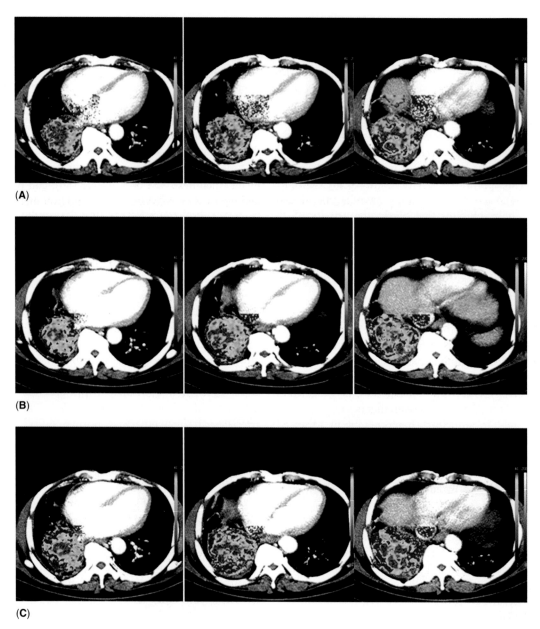

Figure 64.9 Volumetric perfusion CT of a lung cancer. Selected axial images (**A**) before and (**B**) after one and (**C**) after two fractions of radiotherapy demonstrate an acute increase in tumor vascularity with fractionated radiotherapy.

demonstrated elevated perfusion values in this study reducing specificity (54). More recently studies estimating permeability in addition to perfusion in solitary lung nodules have suggested that permeability measurements potentially aid differentiation of inflammatory nodules and cancer. Ma et al. found that permeability was significantly higher in cancer compared with inflammatory nodules (57). Combined assessment of perfusion/permeability and metabolism (by FDG PET) may further improve lesion characterization in the future (58).

Perfusion CT may facilitate the differentiation of patients with cancer and diverticular disease. Up to 30% of colon cancers are coincident with diverticular disease, and distinction can be difficult by clinical symptoms or morphological imaging alone. Vascular parameters such as blood flow, blood volume, and permeability surface area product are different between patients

with cancer, acute diverticulitis, and inactive diverticular disease with highest values in cancers. Blood flow and blood volume have a sensitivity of 80% and specificity of 75% and 70% respectively for differentiating cancer from acute diverticulitis and may be better than that achieved using established CT morphological criteria (59). Similarly perfusion measurements are different for benign and malignant extracranial head and neck lesions (60).

Tumor Staging
Preliminary data suggest that perfusion CT may have a role in tumor staging. Perfusion CT measurements may reflect tumor grade or stage in a number of tumor types including hepatocellular cancer (49), lymphoma (61), lung (24–26), and colorectal cancer (62) though not all published studies have found a consistent relationship. Perfusion is greater in higher than in lower grade

hepatocellular cancer (49); perfusion and permeability surface area product are increased in higher than in lower grade lymphoma (61), and permeability surface area product is increased in primary colorectal tumors with distant metastases compared with tumors without evidence of metastases at staging (62). Given the positive correlation between permeability surface area product and angiogenesis as assessed by microvessel density in colorectal cancer (63), this supports the notion that angiogenesis is linked to a greater likelihood of metastasis. Studies of lung cancer have been conflicting with some studies demonstrating higher perfusion in higher stage cancers, and other studies showing no relationship. Similarly no relationship has been demonstrated in cervical cancer (64).

In colorectal cancer perfusion measurements may supplement standard morphological staging (62). A study has suggested that baseline primary tumor perfusion is substantially lower in patients who develop subsequent metastases despite "curative" surgery, in comparison to patients who remain disease-free (62). While patient numbers were small (n = 35) one positive feature was the length of clinical follow up (>3 years). Such an association has been noted also for other cancers including extracranial head and neck cancers (43) and cervical cancer (65).

Perfusion CT in combination with FDG PET may provide valuable in vivo information of the tumor metabolic-flow relationship (Fig. 64.10). The metabolic-flow relationship is complex. A functioning vasculature is a pre-requisite for adequate glucose and oxygen delivery to support tumor metabolism yet inadequate tumor vascularization or a poorly functioning vasculature, resulting in hypoxia, may stimulate anaerobic glycolysis with an apparent increase in tumor metabolism. The balance between perfusion and metabolism may provide an indication of a tumor's potential biological behavior: uncoupling of perfusion and metabolism may indicate a tumor that is predisposed to aggressive behavior. Preliminary studies have been published in lung cancer (58), extracranial head and neck cancer (66), and breast cancer (67), and reported for colorectal cancer and liver metastases but further study is required to determine if this approach augments tumor staging in clinical practice.

Detection of Recurrent Disease and Surveillance

There is little published evidence to suggest that perfusion CT may be of use in the assessment of recurrent disease with the exception of extracranial head and neck tumors (68) where the increase in vascular permeability may reflect recurrent disease. However given the level of evidence, it is unlikely to supplant current imaging approaches. Similarly, in terms of disease surveillance there is little evidence that perfusion CT is currently of use, with the possible exception of hepatic metastases. Preliminary studies

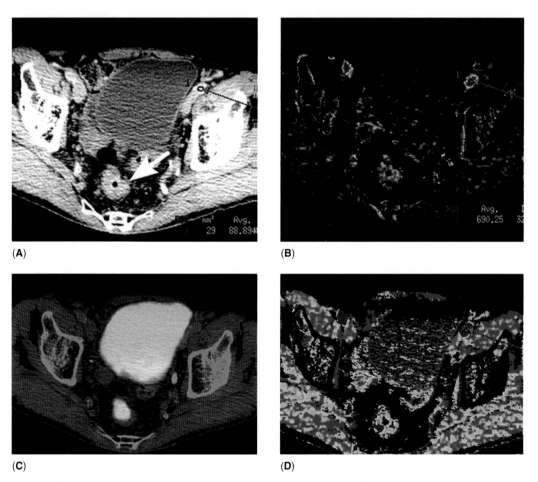

(A)

(B)

(C)

(D)

Figure 64.10 ¹⁸FDG PET-CT/perfusion CT study of a rectal cancer (arrow on CT) demonstrating a well-perfused metabolically active tumor. Region of interest on external iliac artery on CT to measure arterial input function. (**A**) Contrast-enhanced CT, (**B**) FDG PET-CT, (**C**) blood flow and (**D**) blood volume maps of the rectal cancer are shown.

have suggested that occult metastases may be predicted from areas of elevated hepatic perfusion (48), similar to data from Doppler US studies (69). However with the introduction of whole liver volume techniques, perfusion CT for surveillance for hepatic metastatic disease is more viable (9). Further study is needed to determine if there is indeed a role for perfusion CT.

Key Points: Clinical Applications

- The main application of perfusion CT is for therapeutic assessment particularly of anti-vascular drugs where vascular effect may be detected in advance of any size change
- Preliminary data supports the application of perfusion CT for characterization of lung nodules and for differentiation of colon cancer from diverticulitis with high sensitivities and specificities. There may also be a role for perfusion CT in tumor detection and staging but these techniques require further validation

Summary

- CT provides excellent anatomical detail and quantification of vascular parameters such as tumor perfusion, blood volume, and vascular leakage and is now a simple procedure
- The latest high-end multidetector row CT systems are capable of rapid scanning and large volume coverage enabling entire tumors to be evaluated
- Perfusion reflects the flow rate of whole blood through the vasculature of a defined tissue volume or mass. At CT this encompasses flow in arteries, arterioles, capillaries, venules, and veins
- Blood volume reflects the volume of flowing whole blood within the functioning vasculature of a defined tissue volume or mass
- Vascular leakage may be expressed as extraction fraction (EF); or capillary permeability surface area product
- Contrast enhancement at CT reflects the rate of delivery, volume and concentration of the contrast agent, vessel surface area, vessel leakiness, rate of contrast agent backflux from the extravascular-extracellular into the intravascular compartment, and the rate of contrast agent excretion
- Different models are applied to obtain physiologically based vascular measurements—Fick principle, Patlak analysis, distributed parameter analysis
- Data acquisition is usually achieved with axial single level techniques but recent developments allow volumetric helical techniques to be applied
- CT techniques have been validated in both animal and human studies. These have demonstrated that CT estimates lie within the documented physiological range, and are comparable to measurements obtained by other methods
- Perfusion CT estimates correlate with histological markers of angiogenesis including microvessel density and vascular endothelial growth factor
- The main application of perfusion CT is for therapeutic assessment of novel therapies, particularly anti-vascular drugs where vascular effect may be detected before any change in tumor size

ACKNOWLEDGMENTS

Thanks are due to Dr. Quan Sing Ng, Dr. Henry Mandeville, Professor Michele Saunders, Professor Peter Hoskin, Professor Gill Tozer, Professor Steve Halligan, Professor Clive Bartram, Dr. Stuart Taylor, Dr. Ashley Groves, and Professor Peter Ell for their collaboration with research studies. This chapter could not have been written without their input and expertise.

REFERENCES

1. Simon GH, Fu Y, Berejnoi K, et al. Initial computed tomography imaging experience using a new macromolecular iodinated contrast medium in experimental breast cancer. Invest Radiol 2005; 40: 614–20.
2. Fournier LS, Cuenod CA, de Balazaire C, et al. Early modifications of hepatic perfusion measured by functional CT in a rat model of hepatocellular carcinoma using a blood pool agent. Eur Radiol 2004; 4: 2125–33.
3. Miles KA, Griffiths MR. Perfusion CT: a worthwhile enhancement? Br J Radiol 2003; 76: 220–31.
4. Miles KA. Measurement of tissue perfusion by dynamic computed tomography. Br J Radiol 1991; 64: 409–12.
5. Patlak CS, Blasberg RG, Fernstmacher JD. Graphical evaluation of blood-to-brain transfer constants from multiple-time uptake data. J Cereb Blood Flow Metab 1983; 3: 1–7.
6. Patlak CS, Blasberg RG. Graphical evaluation of blood-to-brain transfer constants from multiple time uptake data. J Cereb Blood Flow Metab 1985; 5: 584–90.
7. Johnson JA, Wilson TA. A model for capillary exchange. Am J Physiol 1966; 210: 1299–303.
8. Ng QS, Goh V, Fichte H, et al. Lung cancer perfusion at multidetector-row CT: reproducibility of whole tumor quantitative measurements. Radiology 2006; 239: 547–53.
9. Meijerink MR, van Waesberghe JHTM, van der Weide L, et al. Total liver volume perfusion CT using 3D image fusion to improve detection and characterization of liver metastases. Eur Radiol 2008; 18: 2345–54.
10. Cenic A, Nabavi DG, Craen RA, et al. Dynamic CT measurement of cerebral blood flow: a validation study. AJNR Am J Neuroradiol 1999; 20: 63–73.
11. Purdie TG, Henderson E, Lee TY. Functional CT imaging of angiogenesis in rabbit VX2 soft-tissue tumor. Phys Med Biol 2001; 46: 3161–75.
12. Stewart EE, Chen X, HadwayJ, et al. Hepatic perfusion in a tumor model using DCE-CT: an accuracy and precision study. Phys Med Biol 2008; 53: 4249–67.
13. Wintermark M, Thiran JP, Maeder P, Schnyder P, Meuli R. Simultaneous measurement of regional cerebral blood flow by perfusion CT and stable xenon CT: a validation study. AJNR Am J Neuroradiol 2001; 22: 905–14.
14. Gillard JH, Minhas PS, Hayball MP, et al. Assessment of quantitative computed tomographic cerebral perfusion imaging with H2(15)O positron emission romography. Neurol Res 2000; 22: 457–64.
15. Bisdas S, Donnerstag F, Berding G, et al. Computed tomography assessment of cerebral perfusion using a distributed

parameter tracer kinetics model: validation with H(2)((15))0 positron emission tomography measurements and initial clinical experience in patients with acute stroke. J Cereb Blood Flow Metab 2008; 28: 402–11.

16. Pollard RE, Broumas AR, Wisner ER, Vekich SV, Ferrara KW. Quantitative contrast enhanced ultrasound and CT assessment of tumor response to antiangiogenic therapy in rats. Ultrasound Med Biol 2007; 33: 235–45.

17. Nabavi DG, Cenic A, Dool J, et al. Quantitative assessment of cerebral hemodynamics using CT: stability, accuracy, and precision studies in dogs. J Comput Assist Tomogr 1999; 23: 506–15.

18. Cenic A, Nabavi DG, Craen RA, et al. A CT method to measure hemodynamics in brain tumors: validation and application of cerebral flow maps. AJNR Am J Neuroradiol 2000; 21: 462–70.

19. Goh V, Halligan S, Hugill JA, Bartram CI. Quantitative assessment of tissue perfusion using MDCT: comparison of colorectal cancer and skeletal muscle measurement reproducibility. AJR Am J Roentgenol. 2006; 187: 164–9.

20. Sanelli PC, Nicola G, Tsiouris AJ, et al. Reproducibility of post-processing of quantitative CT perfusion maps. AJR Am J Roentgenol 2007; 188: 213–18.

21. Fiorella D, Heiserman J, Prenger E, Partovi S. Assessment of the reproducibility of postprocessing dynamic CT perfusion data. AJNR Am J Neuroradiol 2004; 25: 97–107.

22. Bisdas S, Surlan-Popovic K, Didanovich V, Vogl T. Functional CT of squamous cell carcinoma in the head and neck: repeatability of tumor and muscle quantitative measurements, inter- and intra-observer agreement. Eur Radiol 2008; 18: 2241–50.

23. Goh V, Halligan S, Hugill JA, et al. Quantitative assessment of colorectal cancer perfusion using MDCT: inter- and intraobserver agreement. AJR Am J Roentgenol. 2005; 185: 225–31.

24. Tateishi U, Kusumoto M, Nishihara H, et al. Contrast enhanced dynamic computed tomography for the evaluation of angiogenesis in patients with lung carcinoma. Cancer 2002; 95: 835–42.

25. Yi CA, Lee KS, Kim EA, et al. Solitary pulmonary nodules: dynamic enhanced multidetector row CT study and comparison with vascular endothelial growth factor and microvessel density. Radiology 2004; 233: 191–9.

26. Li Y, Yang ZG, Chen TW, et al. Peripheral lung carcinoma: correlation of angiogenesis and first-pass perfusion parameters of 64-detector row CT. Lung Cancer 2008; 61: 44–53.

27. Wang JH, Min PQ, Wang PJ, et al. Dynamic CT evaluation of tumor vascularity in renal cell carcinoma. AJR Am J Roentgenol 2006; 186: 1423–30.

28. Li ZP, Meng QF, Sun CH, et al. Tumor angiogenesis and dynamic CT in colorectal carcinoma: radiologic-pathologic correlation. World J Gastroenterol 2005; 11: 1287–91.

29. Goh V, Halligan S, Daley F, et al. Quantitative assessment of colorectal tumor vascularity at Perfusion CT: Do tumor vascular measurements reflect angiogenesis? Radiology 2008; 249: 510–7.

30. Hurwitz H, Fehrenbacher L, Novotny W, et al. Bevacizumab plus irinotecan, fluorouracil, and leucovorin for metastatic colorectal cancer. N Engl J Med 2004; 350: 2335–42.

31. Escudier B, Eisen T, Stadler WM, et al. Sorafenib in advanced renal cell carcinoma. N Engl J Med 2007; 356: 125–34.

32. Sabir A, Schor-Bardach R, Wilcox CJ, et al. Perfusion MDCT enables early detection of therapeutic response to antiangiogenic therapy. AJR Am J Roentgenol 2008; 191: 133–9.

33. Willett CG, Boucher Y, di Tomaso E, et al. Direct evidence that the VEGF-specific antibody bevacizumab has antivascular effects in human rectal cancer. Nat Med 2004; 10: 145–7.

34. Parulekar WR, Eisenhauer EA. Phase I trial design for solid tumour studies of targeted non-cytotoxic agents: theory and practice. J Natl Cancer Inst 2004; 96: 990–7.

35. McNeel DG, Eickhoff J, Lee FT, et al. Phase I trial of a monoclonal antibody specific for $\alpha_v\beta_3$ integrin (MEDI-522) in patients with advanced malignancies, including an assessment of effect on tumor perfusion. Clin Canc Res 2005; 11: 7851–60.

36. Ng QS, Goh V, Carnell D, et al. Tumor antivascular effects of radiotherapy combined with combretastatin a4 phosphate in human non-small-cell lung cancer. Int J Radiat Oncol Biol Phys 2007; 67: 1375–80.

37. Jain RK, Duda DG, Clark JW, Loeffler JS. Lessons from phase III clinical trials on anti-VEGF therapy for cancer. Nat Clin Prac Oncol 2006; 3: 24–30.

38. Lankester KJ, Taylor NJ, Stirling JJ, et al. Dynamic MRI for imaging tumor microvasculature: comparison of susceptibility and relaxivity techniques in pelvic tumors. J Magn Reson Imaging 2007; 25: 796–805.

39. Gandhi D, Chepeha DB, Miller T, et al. Correlation between initial and early follow-up CT perfusion parameters with endoscopic tumor response in patients with advanced squamous cell carcinomas of the oropharynx treated with organ-preservation therapy. AJNR Am J Neuroradiol 2006; 27: 101–6.

40. Zima A, Carlos R, Gandhi D, et al. Can pre-treatment CT perfusion predict response of advanced squamous cell carcinoma of the upper aerodigestive tract treated with induction chemotherapy? ANJR Am J Neuroradiol 2007; 28: 299–304.

41. Harvey C, Blomley MJ, Dawson P. Functional CT imaging of the acute hyperaemic response to radiation therapy of the prostate gland: early experience. J Comput Assist Tomogr 2001; 25: 43–9.

42. Ng QS, Goh V, Milner J, et al. Effect of nitric-oxide synthesis on tumour blood volume and vascular activity: a phase I study. Lancet Oncol 2007; 8: 111–18.

43. Hermans R, Meijerink M, Van den Bogaert W, et al. Tumor perfusion rate determined non-invasively by dynamic computed tomography predicts outcome in head-and-neck cancer after radiotherapy. Int J Radiat Oncol Biol Phys 2003; 57: 1351–6.

44. Sahani DV, Kalva SP, Hamberg LM, et al. Assessing tumor perfusion and treatment response in rectal cancer with multisection CT: initial observations. Radiology 2005; 234: 785–92.

45. Bellomi M, Petralia G, Sonzogni A, et al. CT perfusion for the monitoring of neo-adjuvant chemoradiation therapy in rectal carcinoma. Radiology 2007; 244: 486–93.

46. Miles KA, Leggett DA, Kelley BB, et al. In vivo assessment of the neovascularization of liver metastases using perfusion CT. Br J Radiol 1998; 71: 276–81.

47. Cuenod C, Leconte I, Siauve N, et al. Early changes in liver perfusion caused by occult metastases in rats: detection with quantitative CT. Radiology 2001; 218: 556–61.

48. Leggett DA, Kelley BB, Bunce IH, Miles KA. Colorectal cancer: diagnostic potential of CT measurements of hepatic perfusion and implications for contrast enhancement protocols. Radiology 1997; 205: 716–20.

49. Sahani DV, Holalkere NS, Mueller PR, Zhu AX. Advanced hepatocellular carcinoma: CT Perfusion of liver and tumor tissue- initial experience. Radiology 2007; 243: 736–43.

50. Ippolito D, Sirroni S, Pozzi M, et al. Hepatocellular carcinoma in cirrhotic liver disease: functional computed tomography with perfusion imaging in the assessment of tumor vascularization. Acad Radiol 2008; 15: 919–27.

51. Swensen SJ, Brown LR, Colby TV, Weaver AL, Midthun DE. Lung nodule enhancement at CT: prospective findings. Radiology 1996; 201: 447–55.

52. Swensen SJ, Brown LR, Colby TV, Weaver AL. Pulmonary nodules: CT evaluation of enhancement with iodinated contrast material. Radiology 1995; 194: 393–8.

53. Swensen SJ, Morin RL, Schueler BA, et al. Solitary pulmonary nodule: CT evaluation of enhancement with iodinated contrast material-a preliminary report. Radiology 1992; 182: 343–7.

54. Zhang M, Kono M. Solitary pulmonary nodules: evaluation of blood flow patterns with dynamic CT. Radiology 1997; 205: 471–8.

55. Jeong YJ, Lee KS, Jeong SY, et al. Solitary pulmonary nodule: characterization with combined wash in and wash out features at dynamic multidetector row CT. Radiology 2005; 237: 675–83.

56. Sitartchouk I, Roberts HC, Pereira AM, et al. Computed tomography perfusion using first pass methods for lung nodule characterization. Invest Radiol 2008; 43: 349–58.

57. Ma SH, Le HB, Jia BH, et al. Peripheral pulmonary nodules: relationship between multislice spiral CT perfusion imaging and tumor angiogenesis and VEGF expression. BMC Cancer 2008; 8: 186–204.

58. Miles KA, Griffiths MR, Keith CJ. Blood flow metabolic relationships are dependent on tumour size in non-small cell lung cancer: a study using quantitative contrast-enhanced computer tomography and positron emission tomography. Eur J Nucl Med Mol Imaging 2006; 33: 22–8.

59. Goh V, Halligan S, Taylor SA, et al. Diverticulitis versus colorectal cancer: Are CT perfusion measurements better discriminators than morphological criteria. Radiology 2007; 242: 456–62.

60. Bisdas S, Baghi M, Wagenblast J, et al. Differentiation of benign and malignant parotid tumours using deconvolution based perfusion CT imaging: feasibility of the method and intial results. Eur J Radiol 2007; 64: 258–65.

61. Dugdale PE, Miles KA, Bunce I, et al. CT measurement of perfusion and permeability within lymphoma masses and its ability to assess grade, activity, and chemotherapeutic response. J Comput Assist Tomogr 1999; 23: 540–7.

62. Goh V, Halligan S, Wellsted D, Bartram CI. Can perfusion CT assessment of primary colorectal adenocarcinoma blood flow at staging predict for subsequent metastatic disease? Pilot Study. Eur Radiol 2009; 19: 79–89.

63. Goh V, Halligan S, Daley FM, et al. Assessment of colorectal cancer vascularity: Quantitative assessment with MDCT—Do tumor perfusion measurements reflect angiogenesis? Radiology 2008; 249: 510–17.

64. Haider MA, Milosevic M, Fyles A, et al. Assessment of the tumor microenvironment in cervix cancer using dynamic contrast enhanced CT, interstitial fluid pressure and oxygen measurements. Int J Radiat Oncol Biol Phys 2005; 62: 1100–7.

65. Mayr NA, Yuh WT, Arnholt JC, et al. Pixel analysis of MR perfusion imaging in predicting radiation therapy outcome in cervical cancer. J Magn Reson Imaging 2000; 12: 1027–33.

66. Bisdas S, Spicer K, Rumboldt Z. Whole-tumor perfusion CT parameters and glucose metabolism measurements in head and neck squamous cell carcinomas: a pilot study using combined positron-emission tomography/CT imaging. AJNR Am J Neuroradiol. 2008; 29: 1376–81.

67. Groves AM, Wishart GC, Shastry M, et al. Metabolic-flow relationships in primary breast cancer: feasibility of combined PET/dynamic contrast enhanced CT. Eur J Nucl Med Mol Imaging 2009; 36: 416–21.

68. Bisdas S, Baghi M, Smolarz A, et al. Quantitative measurements of perfusion and permeability of oropharyngeal and oral cavity cancer, recurrent disease, and associated lymph nodes using first pass contrast enhanced computed tomography studies. Invest Radiol 2007; 42: 172–9.

69. Leen E, Goldberg JA, Angerson WJ, McArdle CS. Potential role of doppler perfusion index in selection of patients with colorectal cancer for adjuvant chemotherapy. Lancet 2000; 355: 34–7.

65 Magnetic Resonance: Emerging Technologies and Applications
Anwar R Padhani

INTRODUCTION

In this chapter, magnetic resonance (MR) functional techniques, which have the potential to make an important impact on future clinical practice, are considered. These imaging markers include blood oxygenation level-dependent MR imaging (BOLD-MRI) which can depict tissue oxygenation, diffusion-weighted imaging (DW-MRI) (tissue water motion), and magnetic resonance spectroscopic imaging (MRSI) (tumor metabolism). These imaging biomarkers focus on depicting critical pathophysiological processes and metabolic pathways within tumors and normal tissues. Thus these techniques are able to map key cancer hallmarks spatially, which include deregulated tumor cell proliferation, angiogenesis, metastasis, apoptosis and the consequences of altered metabolism (Fig. 65.1), and promise to provide critical information not only prior to treatment to stratify therapeutic choice, but also during therapy to assess the efficacy of treatment and to monitor subsequent changes in the biological characteristics of the tumor. A major advantage of functional imaging techniques is that they are non-invasive and therefore can be repeated readily during the course of the patient's disease.

HYPOXIA IMAGING

The fact that low tissue oxygen tension increases tumor resistance to radiotherapy has been known for decades. Tomlinson and Gray showed that hypoxia exists in human lung tumors and that necrosis occurs about 100 µm from the nearest blood vessel which is close to the diffusion distance of soluble oxygen (1). Decades of research in radiation biology, focusing on attempts to circumvent hypoxia-mediated radio-resistance, have met with only modest success. Over the last decade or so it has become evident that hypoxia changes the pattern of gene expression which in turn alters the malignant potential of tumors; this leads to more aggressive cell survival traits, which results in cancer cells becoming more difficult to treat by radiation and chemotherapy (2).

Hypoxia Overview

Oxygen is recognized as a sensitizer mediating the cytotoxic effects of ionizing radiation. Typically, well-oxygenated cells are three times more sensitive to radiation than the same cells when they are hypoxic as indicated by the Oxygen Enhancement Ratio (OER typically ranges between values of 2.5 and 3.0). The OER is the relative sensitivity of oxic cells/anoxic cells to the lethal effects of low linear-energy-transfer (LET) radiations (3). Hypoxia-induced radioresistance is multifactorial. The interaction of radiation with intracellular water leads to the formation of free radicals which, in the presence of cellular oxygen, results in fixed DNA damage. The effectiveness of radiotherapy becomes progressively limited as tumor pO_2 levels fall. Half maximal sensitivity to x-rays and gamma radiation occurs at oxygen tensions of approximately 2 to 5 mmHg; above pO_2 values of approximately 10 to 15 mmHg, near maximal oxygen effects are seen. However, it should also be recognized that the sensitivity of cells to radiation is dependent on the phase of the cell cycle. Evidence is accumulating that hypoxia-mediated proteomic and genomic changes also contribute to radioresistance by:

- Increasing the levels of heat shock proteins (HSPs), which are induced in response to environmental stresses like heat, cold, and oxygen deprivation (4)
- Increasing the number of tumor cells that can resist programmed cell death (apoptosis) by mutating the p53 gene (the slowing of cell division is dependent on a protein brake known as p53; the disruption of the functioning of this protein is associated with approximately 50–55% of human cancers)

The presence of hypoxia within human tumors before starting treatment has been observed in squamous cell carcinomas, gliomas, adenocarcinomas (breast and pancreas), and sarcomas. Studies with Eppendorf pO_2 histography, whereby oxygen sensing electrodes are directly implanted into tissues have shown that the normal cervix pO_2 is a median of 42 mmHg compared with a median of 10 mmHg in squamous carcinomas (5–7). In cervical cancer the oxygenation status is independent of size, stage, histopathological type, and grade of malignancy. Eppendorf pO_2 histography has also shown heterogeneity within and between the same tumor types, and that hypoxia contributes to poor prognosis; $pO_2 < 10$ mmHg results in poor local tumor control, poor disease-free survival and overall survival in squamous carcinomas of the head and neck, and of cervical cancers (8,9).

Three principle types of tumor hypoxia are recognized (Fig. 65.2) (10):

- Perfusion-related (acute) hypoxia resulting from inadequate blood flow in tumors occurring as a result of structural and functional abnormalities of tumor neovasculature (these are more fully described in chapters 63 and 64). Acute hypoxia is often intermittent as it is precipitated by transient rises in interstitial fluid pressure and affects all cells right up to vessel walls
- Diffusion-related (chronic) hypoxia caused by increased oxygen diffusion distances due to tumor growth, increases the distance between blood vessels. It affects cells greater than 70 to 100 µm from the nearest blood vessel (depending on their proximity to the arterial or venous end)
- Anemic hypoxia is related to the reduced O_2-carrying capacity of the blood

There are a number of ways in which tissue oxygenation status can be assessed in vivo, for example, using a tissue sensor

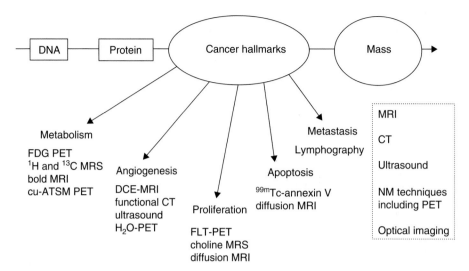

Figure 65.1 Imaging techniques that are able to map key cancer hallmarks spatially.

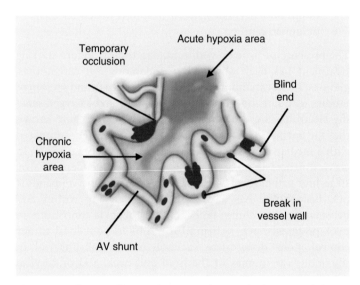

Figure 65.2 Schematic diagram showing perfusion related acute and chronic hypoxic area.

oxygenation probe, or in vitro using material from surgical biopsy. Non-imaging methods include histological appearances (specifically the presence of necrosis), immunohistochemical staining for intrinsic markers of hypoxia [e.g., carbonic anhydrase IX (CA-IX) and hypoxia inducible factor-1 (HIF-1)] and for the binding of externally-administered nitroimidazoles (11). Non-invasive imaging methods may play an important role in measuring hypoxia in the future by selecting cancer patients who would benefit from treatments that overcome, circumvent or take advantage of the presence of hypoxia. Key requirements of any method that evaluates tumor hypoxia routinely in clinical practice include non-invasive assessments which allow serial changes during treatment to be monitored and the ability to evaluate heterogeneity between and within tumors.

From an imaging perspective, an ideal test would:

- Distinguish normoxia/hypoxia/anoxia/necrosis
- Distinguish between perfusion-related (acute) and diffusion-related (chronic) hypoxia if possible
- Reflect cellular in preference to vascular pO_2
- Be applicable to any tumor site with complete loco-regional evaluation
- Be simple to perform, non-toxic, and allow repeated measurements
- Be sensitive at pO_2 levels relevant to tumor therapy

The challenge for hypoxia imaging is to create images showing low levels of tissue pO_2 demonstrating a phenomenon that occurs on a much smaller scale than can be achieved with conventional imaging techniques. ^{18}F-MISO and [60/64]Cu-ATSM PET, and BOLD-MRI are the lead contenders for human application based on their non-invasive nature, ease of use and robustness, measurement of hypoxia status, validity, ability to demonstrate heterogeneity, and general availability (12,13).

BOLD-MRI

Blood oxygenation level-dependent (BOLD) and intrinsic susceptibility-weighted MRI are interchangeable terms (14). The primary source of image contrast in BOLD MR images is endogenous paramagnetic deoxyhemoglobin which increases the transverse relaxation rate (R_2^*) of water in blood and surrounding tissues, thus BOLD-MRI is sensitive to pO_2 within vessels, and in tissues adjacent to perfused vessels (14). Fundamentally, image contrast observed on susceptibility-weighted MR images is dependent on tissue perfusion and levels of red blood cell oxygenation, as well as on static tissue components. Static tissue components include iron content (e.g., myoglobin found in muscle) and the presence of tissue collagen, fibrosis, or ligaments. In order to decouple the effects of flow from deoxyhemoglobin and static components, it is necessary to acquire multiple T2*-weighted images with increasing repetition times while maintaining all

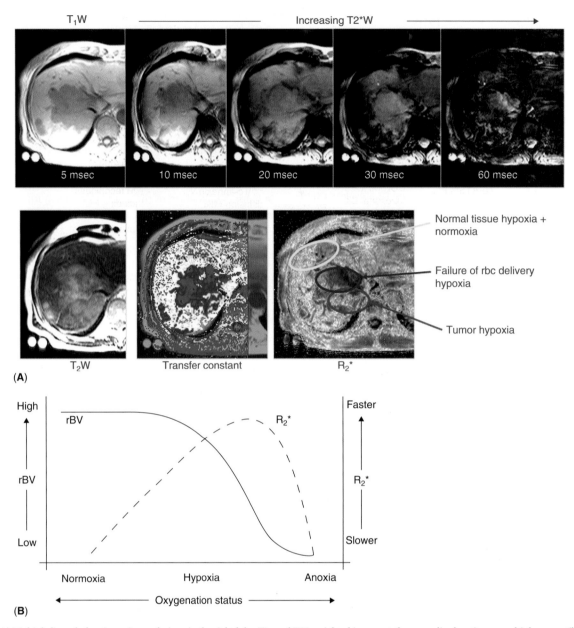

Figure 65.3 (**A**) Multiple liver cholangiocarcinoma lesions in the right lobe. T1- and T2*-weighted images at the same slice location as multiple susceptibility weighted T2* images. The repetition time of T2* images is maintained but increasing echo times are used to calculate the intrinsic relaxivity map (R2*) on a pixel-by-pixel basis. (**B**) Diagram to illustrate that correct interpretation of R2* data requires volume information in order to infer oxygenation status.

other measurement factors. From these the T_2^* relaxation rate R_2^* (=$1/T_2^*$) can be calculated and mapped (Fig. 65.3).

The observation that image contrast is related to the level of red blood cell oxygenation implies that:

- BOLD-MR images are more likely to reflect acute (perfusion-related) tissue hypoxia because low pO_2 levels extend to the level of the blood vessels and therefore affect the oxygenation status of red blood cells
- Chronic hypoxia can be depicted by BOLD-MRI (15). For BOLD-MRI to be able to provide information on tissue oxygenation status, it is important for red blood cells to be delivered to and reside within tissues at least for a time, for example, in the medulla of the kidney, so that deoxygenation can occur

Human and xenograft studies have shown that tumor perfusion varies widely (between and within tumors) and that red blood cell perfusion is not simply related to the presence or absence of vessels; that is, plenty of tumor vessels may be present but perfusion by red blood cells may not actually occur (16). Alternatively, if blood flow is relatively high and tissue residence times for red cells are relatively low (hyperdynamic circulation limiting oxygen exchange with tissue compartments remote from blood vessels), then R_2^* may only reflect blood volumes and not tissue oxygenation. The latter explains in part why there are no direct correlations between baseline R_2^* and tissue pO_2 in most tissues (that is, R_2^* does NOT measure tissue pO_2). Furthermore these complexities mean that it is necessary to know the distribution of blood volume in tissue in order to be able to correctly interpret R_2^* images, thereby permitting inference of oxygenation

status (Fig. 65.3). Thus, if a tissue is perfused but has a high R_2^* in one area/region compared with another area/region in the same tissue (i.e., the static components are the same), then it may be inferred that the higher R_2^* region is relatively more hypoxic; this hypothesis is supported by pre-clinical and clinical data (15,17). Figure 65.3 shows regional differences in liver R_2^* without differences in blood flow implying that higher R_2^* regions are more hypoxic than lower R_2^* regions.

As stated above, the use of BOLD-MRI for assessment of tissue hypoxia is predicated on the assumption that the oxygenation of hemoglobin is proportional to blood arterial pO_2 which is in equilibrium with oxygenation of surrounding tissues. For example, many studies have shown that changes in R_2^* in response to vasomodulation with carbogen (95% CO_2 : 5% O_2) inhalation, are temporally correlated with changes in tissue pO_2. Tumors differ in their responses to carbogen inhalation with only 50% to 60% of human tumors showing changes in R_2^* (18,19). The reasons for these heterogeneous responses are complex but undoubtedly include the fact that tumors have adapted to widely different perfusion characteristics.

The primary advantages of BOLD-MRI for hypoxia assessment are that there is no need to administer exogenous radioactive contrast material, and images with high temporal and high spatial resolution can be obtained rapidly and repeated if needed. It is possible to decouple the effects of inflow and deoxyhemoglobin which are seen in native BOLD images and so to demonstrate changes in oxygenation independent of changes in blood flow. Major limitations of BOLD-MRI include the fact that it does not measure tissue pO_2 directly (either in blood or tissues because of a non-linear relationship of R_2^* and tissue pO_2), the images obtained have low signal-to-noise ratio and clinical studies with carbogen vasomodulation are technically challenging (approximately 25–35% of patient examinations fail due to respiratory distress caused by an increased respiratory drive induced by carbogen) (18,19). Furthermore for correct interpretation of BOLD-MRI there is also a requirement to measure blood volume in tissue. This can now be achieved by using techniques described in MR imaging of angiogenesis (see chap. 63).

Other Methods of Measuring Hypoxia

Positron Emission Tomography
^{18}F-MISO (Fluoromisonidazole)
^{18}F-MISO is a hypoxia imaging agent whose uptake is homogeneous in most normal tissues, and whose delivery to tumors is not limited by perfusion due to its high partition coefficient (20). ^{18}F-MISO accumulates in tissues by binding to intracellular macromolecules when $pO_2 < 10$ mmHg. Useful and well-validated images can be achieved 75 to 150 minutes after injection and no arterial sampling or metabolite analysis is required.

[64]Cu-ATSM Copper (II) Diacetyl-di[N(4)-Methylthiosemicarbazone]
[64]Cu-ATSM also appears to be a promising new technique for delineating the extent of hypoxia within tumors with PET (21–28). In human studies of lung and cervical cancers, encouraging evidence is emerging that ^{64}Cu-ATSM can act as a prognostic indicator for response to therapy (29,30).

Key Points: Hypoxia

- Tumor hypoxia, leading to treatment resistance and enhanced tumor progression, represents a significant challenge to the curability of human tumors
- Tumor hypoxia can be detected by non-invasive and invasive techniques but the inter-relationships between these remains largely undefined
- F-MISO and Cu-ATSM-PET, and BOLD-MRI are the leading contenders for human application based on their non-invasive nature, ease of use and robustness
- Human validation of the utility of hypoxia imaging is sparse
- Hypoxia imaging may allow better selection of those cancer patients who may benefit from novel anti-hypoxia directed therapies

DIFFUSION-WEIGHTED MR IMAGING (DW-MRI)

Diffusion-weighted MR imaging (DW-MRI) displays information related to the thermally driven, random (Brownian) motion of water molecules in tissues. DW-MRI is the only imaging modality that can display this tissue property. Unlike in free fluids, water movement in tissues is not entirely random but instead is modified by flows within conduits and by interactions with lipophilic cellular membranes, intracellular organelles, and macromolecules. Recent technical advances have enabled DW-MRI to be applied for tumor evaluation extracranially and have led to the clinical development of whole body DW-MRI. There are now convincing data to support its use in the characterization of malignancy, including determination of lesion aggressiveness and for monitoring response to a variety of treatments (31,32).

Average water displacements in free water are usually across greater distances than the diameter of cells (typically a few micrometer); therefore, water diffusion in tissues is not unrestricted but attenuated, thus measured diffusion in tissue is termed the apparent diffusion coefficient (ADC; measured in mm²/sec). Intracellular and extracellular compartments will have their own unique water diffusion constants although intracellular diffusion makes an insignificant contribution to image contrast in routine body imaging protocols. Diffusion-weighted images can be made sensitive to macroscopic water movements (i.e., within ducts and blood vessels) or to smaller displacements of water (extravascular space) by the judicious adjustment of used b-values (Fig. 65.4).

Measurement and Quantification

The extent of water molecule motion in tissues can be assessed by applying one or more motion probing diffusion gradients to fat-suppressed T2-weighted spin-echo echo-planar sequences. This entails the application of balanced mono- or bipolar gradients placed symmetrically about a focusing 180° pulse (Fig. 65.4). Water molecules that have not moved over the period of time when the first set of gradients is applied will acquire phase shifts that are exactly cancelled out by the proceeding second gradient set; thus there is no net additional signal loss induced by the application of the paired motion probing gradients (aside from normal T2-decay). However, for water molecules that have moved during

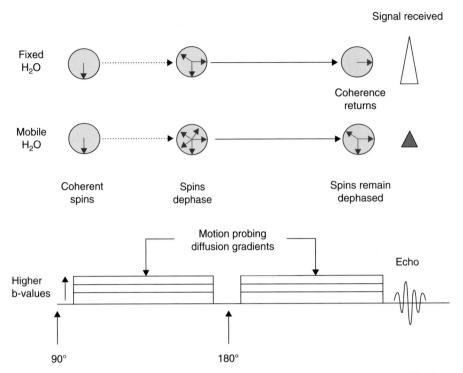

Figure 65.4 Schematic diagram to show the acquisition of diffusion-weighted images. Diffusion weighted images are produced by the application of two gradients on either side of the refocusing 180° pulse. Increasing gradient heights increases the b-values of images produced. Water molecules that have no net movement over the period of time when the first gradient is applied acquire phase shifts that are cancelled out by the second gradient and no additional signal is lost by the application of the diffusion gradients. Water molecules that have moved during the application of the first gradient, however, will experience greater phase shifts that will not be totally cancelled out by the second gradient; this results in a net loss of signal.

the application of the first gradient set, the acquired phase shifts will not be completely cancelled out by the second set of gradients, and residual phase incoherencies will result in losses of signal that are directly related to degree of water movement. The weighting of the applied diffusion gradients is indicated by their b-value (measured in sec/mm^2), which includes the amplitude and duration of the applied gradients and time between the paired gradients.

With increasing diffusion weighting there is a biexponential decrease of the measured signal; biexponential because the signal intensity changes observed with the application of low b-value diffusion gradients is dominated by physiological motions of greater magnitude, such as blood flow, cerebrospinal fluid (CSF), and ductal flows (this is termed intravoxel incoherent motion—IVIM). At higher b-values, bulk water motion plays less of a role in the continued signal attenuation observed and so signal decays become dominated by extravascular water diffusion components (this is the second exponential). Although the signal decay observed is biexponential, the usual practice is to assume monoexponential decay and therefore the gradient of a straight line plot of the natural logarithm of the signal intensity (at different b-values) yields the apparent diffusion coefficient (ADC) (Fig. 65.5).

Clinical Protocols

Initial clinical applications of DW-MRI focused on the evaluation of intracranial pathologies including imaging of stroke. Recently technological breakthroughs have led to the development of DW-MRI for extracranial assessment. These include combining echo-planar data collections with parallel imaging, both of which

have contributed to substantial reductions in data acquisition times thus enabling bulk motion induced signal losses to be substantially reduced. The ability to acquire images at very short echo times has resulted in improved signal-to-noise ratios of images. In practice, measurements are made by the application of motion probing gradients in at least three orthogonal directions with signal averaging to produce high quality trace images which can be used for lesion detection and/or to calculate ADC values.

Currently, several techniques are in use. Multiple averaged, free breathing techniques seem more robust with higher signal-to-noise ratio (SNR) than breath-hold techniques, although imaging times are relatively longer and some image blurring does occur. Multiple averaging applied over longer periods of time can be used to improve SNR enabling thinner slices to be acquired and this has permitted whole body DW-MRI to emerge as a clinically useful modality (31,33).

Whole body DW-MRI shows promise in identifying malignant disease on the basis of high signal intensity on high b-value images. In practice, only two b-values are required (usually b0–50 sec/mm^2 and b800–1000 sec/mm^2). Whole body volume is achieved by combining smaller contiguous body portions. The resultant combined dataset can be analyzed using three-dimensional multiplanar reformatted images and maximum intensity projections (MIPs) which even allows whole body ADC maps to be generated (Fig. 65.6). The main disadvantage of the whole body approach relates to long image acquisition times (usually 10–15 minutes for the torso). The technique is therefore more prone to bulk motion artefact and is also prone to artefact arising from soft tissue-air interfaces.

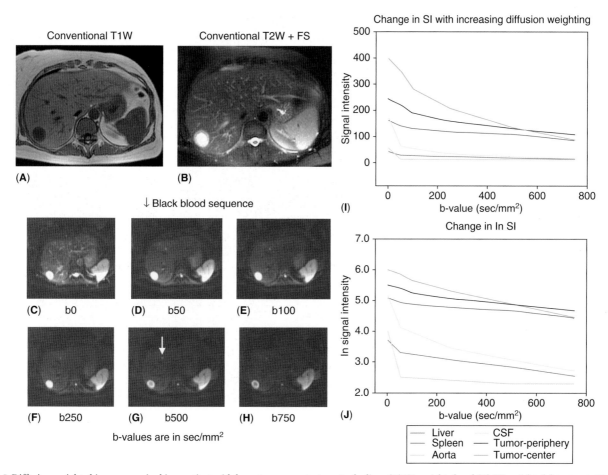

Figure 65.5 Diffusion-weighted images acquired in a patient with breast cancer metastases to the liver. (**A**) T1-weighted and (**B**) T2-weighted fat saturated MR images showing a large necrotic lesion in the liver. (**C**) to (**H**) diffusion-weighted images with b0 to b750 sec/mm². Note (**D**) b50 and (**E**) b100 images show blood as black (called black blood images). Also note loss of signal from the center of the large necrotic metastasis in the right lobe and another small metastasis visualized on (**G**) b500, (arrow) which is not visible on the T1-weighted and T2-weighted fat saturation images. (**I**) and (**J**) Graphs demonstrate the relationship between signal intensity and increasing b-values for normal liver, spleen, aorta, CSF, and the periphery and center of the large metastasis. This is the same patient as illustrated in Fig. 65.10.

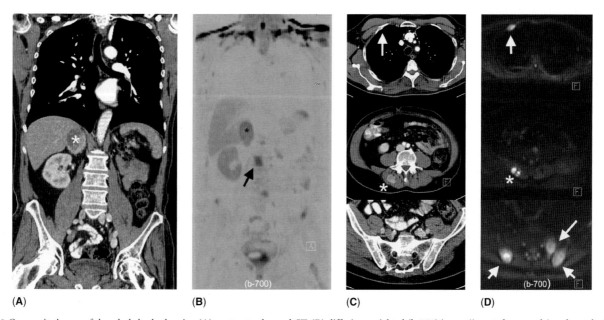

Figure 65.6 Composite image of the whole body showing (**A**) contrast enhanced CT, (**B**) diffusion-weighted (b-700) image (inverted grey scale) and matched (**C**) axial CT and (**D**) b-700 diffusion-weighted images in a patient with a resected left renal cancer. Note that soft tissue metastases to the right adrenal and muscle are well shown on both imaging modalities (*) whereas bony metastases are better shown on diffusion-weighted images (arrows). Artefacts along the shoulders on the diffusion-weighted coronal image are caused by poor fat supression at the soft tissue-air interface.

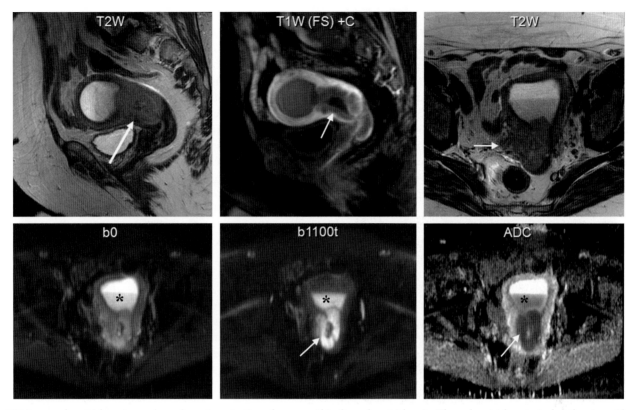

Figure 65.7 Large endometrial carcinoma (arrow) causing retention of mucus within the endometrial cavity. The endometrial contents show layering with marked hyperintensity on b1100 sec/mm² trace image associated with low ADC values in the dependent portion (*). Similar appearances are occasionally seen in abscesses.

Since DW-MRI is a low SNR technique that is prone to artefacts, image optimization strategies are needed. For instance, there is a need to minimize T1 contamination so long repetition times (TR) are normally used. Fat suppression is mandatory in order to reduce the chemical shift-induced ghosting commonly seen with echo-planar imaging and many fat suppression schemes are used. Fat suppression that incorporates short Tau inversion recovery (STIR) is often preferred when evaluating large volumes due to superior uniform fat suppression (unfortunately this has the effect of increasing imaging times). However, when analyzing smaller volumes, chemical fat selective saturation and selective water excitation are the techniques of choice due to the higher SNR of resultant images (33).

Interpretation Guidelines

Visual inspection of DW-MRI and co-registered anatomical images should always be undertaken together. b0 sec/mm² images are fat suppressed with water appearing bright. It is the higher b-value images that provide initial indications of the cellularity and tissue structure; areas retaining high signal intensity on b800 to b1000 sec/mm² images usually, but not always, indicate highly cellular tissues including some normal tissues such as the normal lymph nodes, nerves, normal endometrium, bowel mucosa, and testes (Fig. 65.7), whereas lower signal intensity regions are seen in most normal tissues, glandular formation, cystic spaces, necrosis, or fibrosis. However, high signal intensities on b800 to b1000 sec/mm² images are not always reliable indicators of cellularity (occasionally fluid/edema remain at a high signal intensity because of high proton density); this observation is called "*T2-shine through*" and corresponding ADC maps should always be inspected and interpreted according to the guidance given in Table 65.1.

Table 65.1 Interpretation of Tumor Diffusion-Weighted Images

Signal intensity on high b-value image (b800–b1000)	Relative value on apparent diffusion coefficient (ADC) maps	Interpretation
High	Low	Generally, high cellularity tumor; rarely high protein cavity, coagulative necrosis, or abscess
High	High	T_2-shine through; often proteinaceous fluid
Low	Low	Fibrous tissue with low water content with/ without viable tumor cells
Low	High	Fluid; liquefactive necrosis; lower cellularity/grade tumor; gland formation

It is important to remember that neither ADC maps nor high b-value images should be interpreted in isolation, as there are no unique cut-off ADC values that distinguish cancer from non-cancer/normal tissues. There are a number of reasons for a lack of an ADC cut-off including the fact that ADC values are dependent on the range of b-values used for calculations. Another important point to remember is the fact that both well-differentiated tumors and necrotic poorly-differentiated tumors can have overlapping high ADC values because DW-MRI does not distinguish reliably between water movements in cystic/glandular structures and areas of necrosis. Furthermore as already noted some normal tissues have low ADC values including the spleen, brain, and nerves.

Fibrosis (surgical, post therapy, benign prostatic hyperplasia) and smooth muscle hyperplasia (fibroids) may also have low ADC values. Thus diagnostic characterization requires integration of morphology, high b-value image signal appearances and ADC maps.

Potential Clinical Uses

The basic premise for enhanced tumor detection relates to the fact the malignant tissues are generally more cellular than benign tissues, with water diffusion being more restricted in tumors due to a combination of increased cell density, haphazard tissue organization, and increased extracellular space tortuosity. DW-MRI has been shown to be advantageous for the detection of liver metastases. In liver applications, detection is optimal on lower b-value images (<200 sec/mm²). Using this range of b-values, water in blood vessels exhibits marked signal attenuation, making vessels appear dark (black blood images), thus optimizing image contrast between lesions and liver parenchyma (Fig. 65.5).

DW-MRI is also able to differentiate between benign and malignant focal hepatic lesions in many cases (this is done by assessing signal intensity on high b-value images and corresponding ADC values), based on the higher ADC of benign lesions compared with malignant tumors (34). However, when cystic, necrotic, and treated metastases are included, results in the liver are less good (35). In line with these findings, reduced ADC values of malignant breast tumors compared with those of benign lesions and normal tissue have also been noted (36–38). Sumi et al. showed that lymphoma nodes had significantly lower ADC values than benign nodes (39). However metastatic cervical lymph nodes in patients with head and neck cancers had significantly higher ADC values than benign nodes (39). This apparently discrepant result is explained by the common occurrence of necrosis in nodes with metastatic squamous cell carcinomas. These and other studies have shown that false positive results occur with abscess and infective processes and false negatives occur with cystic, necrotic lesions and in well-differentiated neoplasms (particularly adenocarcinomas – Fig. 65.8), which again emphasizes the need to interpret DW-MRI with all other anatomic information.

DW-MRI may also play a role in determining the etiology of vertebral body collapse, a clinical scenario that often poses difficulty in the management of oncology patients. It has been shown that vertebral metastases can be distinguished from normal vertebrae by their significantly lower ADC values. Several groups have also observed that vertebral body collapse secondary to malignant infiltration often appears hyperintense on diffusion-weighted images and has a corresponding lower ADC value compared with benign osteoporotic vertebral body collapse, where the reverse is noted even when an acute fracture is present (40,41). However, significant overlaps in the ADC

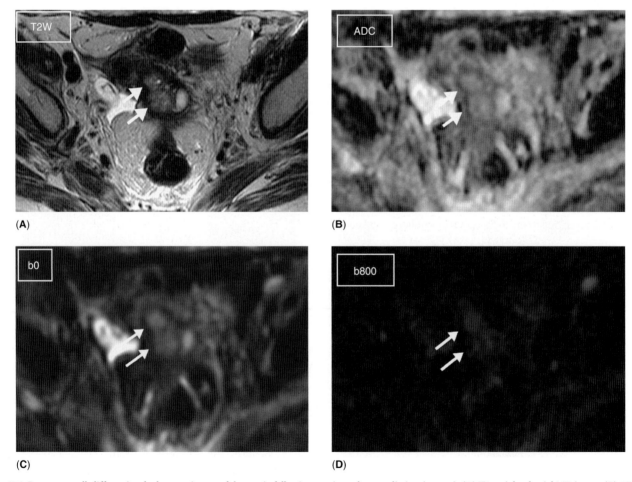

(A)

(B)

(C)

(D)

Figure 65.8 Recurrent well-differentiated adenocarcinoma of the cervix following previous chemoradiation (arrows). (A) T2-weighted axial MR image, (B) ADC map, (C) b0, (D) b800 sec/mm². Note the relatively high ADC value on the ADC map and the low signal intensity of b800 sec/mm² image. These appearances could be misinterpreted as necrosis, cyst formation, or well-differentiated cancer.

values of osteoporotic and malignancy-associated vertebral body collapse exists; moreover, infection can often mimic the appearances of metastatic vertebral body collapse on DW-MRI.

Since cellular death and vascular changes in response to treatment can both precede changes in lesion size, so changes in DW-MRI may be an effective early biomarker for treatment outcome for therapies that induce apoptosis (32,42). In most malignant tumors, successful treatment is reflected by increases in ADC values (Fig. 65.9). Rising ADC values with successful therapy have been noted in several anatomic sites, including breast cancers (43,44), primary and metastatic cancers to the liver (45–47), primary sarcomas of bone (48,49), and in brain malignancies (50).

As a caveat to the above observation of rising ADC values with successful treatment, it has been noted that soon after initiation of therapy transient decreases in ADC can also be observed; this appears to be related to cellular swelling, reductions in blood flow or due to reductions in extracellular space. For instance, it has been noted that anti-VEGF therapies in brain tumors lead to an initial reduction in vasogenic edema which lowers ADC values (51). The extent and duration of such ADC reductions is likely to depend on the type of treatment administered, tumor type, and the timing of imaging with respect to the treatment. Cellular swelling has also been noted to occur in the early phases of apoptosis in response to anticancer treatment (52).

Ultimately after successful therapy, ADC values can be reduced by fibrosis and dehydration as reported in rectal cancers (49) and

brain gliomas (51). This can be problematic because low ADC may also indicate the presence of residual active disease (Fig. 65.10). It is only by observing corresponding high b-value images that the distinction between post-therapy fibrosis and residual active disease can be made by applying the criteria given in Table 65.1. These additional observations indicate that ADC changes are dependent on complex interplays of biophysical processes in response to therapy, emphasizing the need to better understand tissue changes that are reflected in ADC maps.

Key Points: Diffusion-Weighted Imaging (DW-MRI)

- DW-MRI is sensitive to thermally-driven molecular water motion which in vivo is impeded by cellular packing, intracellular organelles, membranes, and macromolecules
- Sensitivity to diffusion-based image contrast is primarily controlled by the b-value with the appropriate b-value range dependent on tissue diffusion properties, signal-to-noise ratio and the need to suppress perfusion effects
- In general, tumors have lower ADC values whereas normal/benign/reactive tissues have correspondingly higher values
- ADC values for distinguishing malignancy from normal/reactive tissues and benign disease are dependent on histological characteristics such as tumor type, differentiation, and necrosis

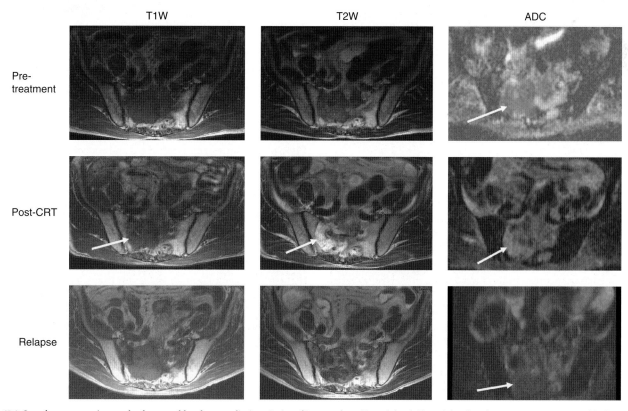

Figure 65.9 Sacral metastases incompletely treated by chemoradiation. Series of images show T1-weighted, T2-weighted, and ADC 0 to 1000 sec/mm² before and after completing chemoradiation therapy (CRT), and at the time of relapse (three months after completing therapy). Note the restricted diffusion on the ADC map of the sacral metastasis (arrow) before therapy which increases in response to chemoradiotherapy. There are focal areas of low ADC seen in the metastasis with residual active disease or fibrosis. The ADC image at relapse indicates that residual active disease was probably present at the end of chemoradiation. *Source*: From Ref. 52.

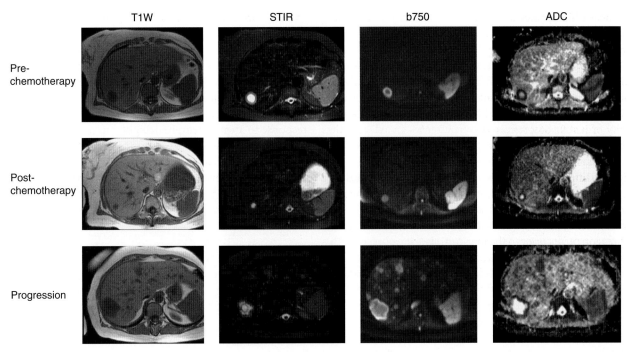

Figure 65.10 Liver metastases from breast cancer. Columns showing T1-weighted, STIR, diffusion-weighted (b750) and ADC MR images before chemotherapy, following completion of chemotherapy, and three months after chemotherapy at the time of disease progression. Note large necrotic metastasis in the posterior aspect of the right lobe has regressed on chemotherapy but there is persistent hyperintensity at the tumor edge on the high b-value (b750 sec/mm^2) image suggesting residual persistent active disease. Three months later progressive disease is detected on the basis of enlargement of the existing metastasis and the presence of multiple new lesions. This is the same patient as illustrated in Figure 65.5.

- DW-MRI may be an effective early biomarker for treatment outcome for therapies that induce tumor cell apoptosis with successful treatment generally causing increases in ADC values
- Rapid evolution of body imaging protocols and divergence amongst and between vendors on data measurements/analysis are impediments for widespread implementation of DW-MRI
- Incomplete validation and documentation of reproducibility in extracranial tissues is limited

MR SPECTROSCOPY

Magnetic resonance spectroscopy (MRS) and its multivoxel imaging counterpart (MRSI) is a non-invasive method for studying tumor biochemistry and metabolism; a method that does not require the administration of ionizing radiation or contrast medium. Although MRS has revealed that cancers have specific and unique biochemical characteristics, a full understanding of the metabolic alterations associated with carcinogenesis is still lacking. Thus, there is little knowledge as to how common the altered biochemical features seen in MRS are generalized across tumor types and at all stages of disease evolution. Furthermore, in general it is not known how a particular treatment affects the biochemical features that are seen with MRS.

Although there have been some large scale clinical trials to define the role of MRS in clinical practice, the technique has been adopted by very few centers because it is perceived by radiologists as being "hard to do," and there is, as yet, no single clinical application where only MRS alone provides unique information which addresses a clinical need. This section describes the technical background and limitations of MRS, as well as the metabolic derangements which can be depicted. A brief review of some of its potential clinical roles is presented. Detailed knowledge of the biochemistry relevant to the study of MRS is beyond the scope of this chapter. Interested readers are referred to reviews by Alger and Kwock et al. where good introductions can be found (53,54).

Technical Background

MRI and MRS both measure signals from the chemical compounds in tissues. For hydrogen (^{1}H) MR, this means any metabolite containing ^{1}H nuclei, of which water is the most common. A radiofrequency (rf) pulse at the start of any MR sequence gives energy to the protons, which is immediately given off in the form of a "free induction decay" (FID). In MRI, this signal is refocused and encoded to produce images of different contrasts depending on the timings of refocusing pulses or on the gradient schemes used. In MRS it is the "raw" FID that is used to provide metabolite information. One-dimensional Fourier transforms of the FID gives a spectrum, with peaks whose areas are proportional to the abundance of particular metabolites. Key problems with this approach are (*i*) seeing metabolites with low abundance, and (*ii*) using machines where the main magnetic field is not uniform or strong enough, such that peaks are broadened to the point where they vanish into the background noise. The latter can be improved by magnetic field shimming – tweaking the field in the volume of interest making it more uniform, and by improving the signal-to-noise ratio by using multiple repetitions of the sequence and by using higher field systems. Higher field MR systems inherently have a better signal-to-noise ratio and wider spectral peak separation because they are both proportional to field strength. Superconducting scanners with fields of 1.5T or higher and the ability to perform localized (high order) shims are recommended for spectroscopy.

Very few atomic nuclei (isotopes) of biological significance have magnetic properties suited to study by MRS (^{1}H, ^{31}P, ^{13}C, and ^{19}F).

Most clinical MRS studies in cancer are concerned with signals from ^{31}P or ^{1}H atoms in endogenous metabolites but occasionally ^{19}F signals from anticancer drugs appear in the literature. MRS signals from different nuclei can easily be distinguished from each other because they have very different resonance frequencies. For example, ^{1}H nuclei produce resonance signals at around 42.57 MHz T-1 and ^{31}P resonates at 17.23 MHz T-1 with a relative sensitivity of just 0.066 compared with ^{1}H. This creates technical difficulties in acquiring enough signal-to-noise in ^{31}P measurements, and the magnet hardware (transmitter, amplifiers, etc.) are also slightly different to that used for ^{1}H work. Metabolites of a given nucleus will have slightly different resonance frequencies because of the differing chemical structures of molecules.

To observe metabolites, ^{1}H-MRS sequences use complex water and fat-suppression pulses prior to the main acquisition, and in doing so only leave signals from metabolites. The separation of the resonance frequencies from individual molecules is termed the "chemical shift." The chemical shift of a given metabolite from the position of water is very small (Hz) compared with the resonance frequency of hydrogen

(MHz), and is thus usually described in parts per million (ppm). Advantages of expressing metabolite position as ppm include normalization of the resulting spectra making them field-strength invariant and thereby allowing comparisons of spectra from different machines (Fig. 65.11). A given metabolite is thus always found at the same ppm chemical shift regardless of field strength, aiding accurate peak identification. Peak areas are usually calculated by fitting a smoothed "ideal spectrum" to the measured one, adjusting the relative heights and areas of the main peaks and then integrating the area under the fitted peaks. Signals are usually plotted as peaks on a normalized frequency scale (ppm on the x-axis) with the intensity of resonances on the y-axis; the area under each peak is proportional to the relative concentration of nuclei that gave rise to it.

Technical Limitations

MRS signals can only be generated from mobile molecules with molecular weights of a few thousand Daltons and even small molecules may not be detectable if there is significant binding to macromolecules. Since many of these "visible" molecules are involved

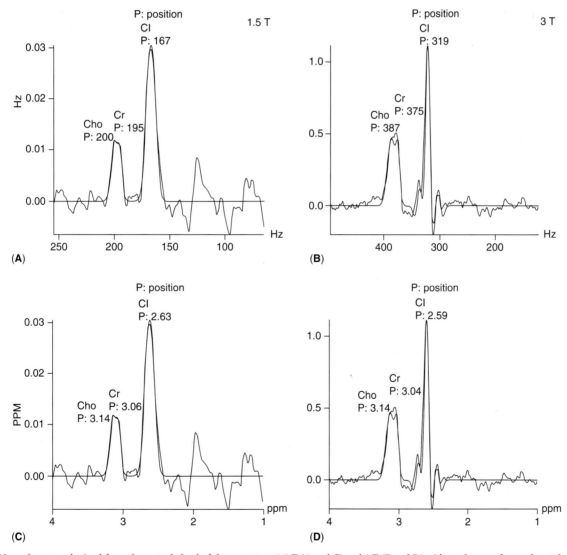

Figure 65.11 Normal spectra obtained from the central gland of the prostate at 1.5 T (A and C) and 3 T (B and D) without the use of an endorectal coil. Spectra are displayed with the x-axis as a frequency scale (Hz) in (A) and (B), or as parts per million (PPM) (C) and (D). Note the superior signal-to-noise ratio of spectra obtained at 3 T. The resonance frequencies of choline (Cho), creatine (Cr), and citrate (Ci) are dependent on field strength which makes comparisons between 1.5 and 3 T spectra difficult. However, after conversion to ppm, comparisons between field strengths are facilitated. Peak areas are usually calculated by fitting a smoothed "ideal spectrum" to the measured one, adjusting the relative heights and areas of the main peaks and then integrating the area under the fitted peaks.

in intermediate metabolism, MRS is said to be able to detect metabolites but importantly not to be able to measure metabolic rates. The greatest weakness of MRS is its low sensitivity, about 10^4 to 10^5 lower than MRI (depending on the nucleus in question). This is mainly because molecules of interest are present at much lower concentrations than tissue water, but also because nuclei other than ^{1}H give rise to inherently weaker signals. Consequently, only a small number of higher concentration metabolites can be detected. As a rule of thumb, metabolite concentration has to be in the millimolar (mM; millimole/liter) to micromolar (μm; micromole/liter) range to be detectable by MRS, thus requiring that voxel size be adjusted to have enough molecules for detection. Fortunately, some metabolites [ATP, (phospho)choline, (phospho)creatine, lactate, N-acetylaspartate] of biological importance are within this concentration range.

The random movement of electrically charged particles (e.g., sodium ions) within tissues is responsible for the random noise detected on the baseline of MR spectra. The signal-to-noise ratio of spectra can be improved by obtaining multiple averages; this method is useful for increasing SNR because the desired signal is identical on each repeat, whereas the noise is random and therefore differs for each repetition and this procedure thus results in destructive noise cancellation.

There is a working requirement that clinical MRS studies are performed on static magnetic fields greater than 1.5 T and that the magnetic field be very homogeneous (less than 100 parts per billion over the intended examination volume). Anatomical features inducing susceptibility can therefore severely interfere with the ability to obtain successful spectra; the latter includes blood from biopsies and even contrast agents (Fig. 65.12). MRS allows the

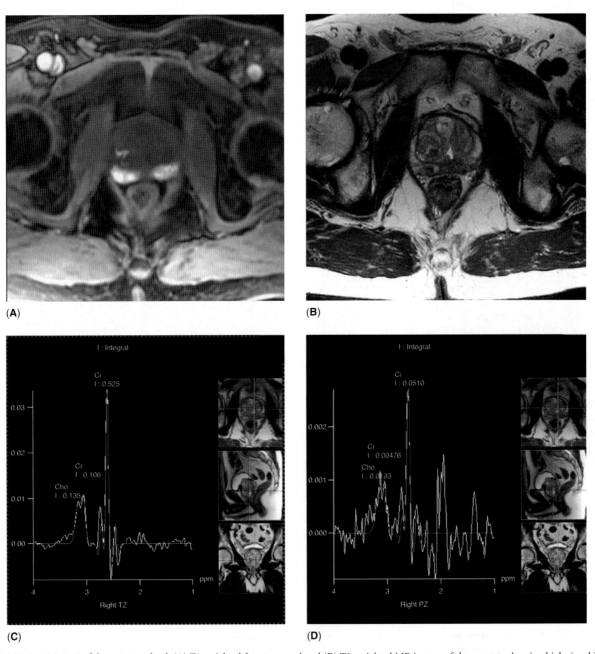

(A) (B)

(C) (D)

Figure 65.12 MR spectroscopy of the prostate gland. (A) T1-weighted fat suppressed and (B) T2-weighted MR images of the prostate showing high signal intensity in the transitional zone and in the peripheral zone due to hemorrhage following recent biopsy. Spectra at 3 T with no endorectal coil obtained from (C) the right transition zone (TZ) and (D) the peripheral zone (PZ). The voxels are indicated on (B). High variability of the baseline signal is due to blood products. Similar effects can be seen shortly following injection of intravenous contrast medium.

detection of signals above the noise level from metabolites and relative concentrations can be estimated but the measurement of absolute metabolite concentration is problematic. It is for this reason that many studies report on the ratio of metabolites.

Cancer Biochemical Processes Depicted by MRS

MRS studies of cancers have revealed that proliferating cells and many tumors display elevated choline signals. This alteration is related to altered phospholipid metabolism which is ultimately related to cell membrane synthesis. Choline abnormalities can be depicted on both ^{1}H- and ^{31}P-MRS. In ^{1}H-MRS, signals produced by choline, phosphocholine (PCho), and glycerolphosphorylcholine (GPC) cannot be resolved (and so are collectively denoted as simply "Cho"), thus it is impossible to be certain of the underlying cause for elevated choline seen in a particular tumor (although cell extracts are helpful and do show that increased intracellular PCho is the dominant molecule via increased anabolism) (55,56). The analogous finding of raised choline in ^{31}P-MRS is elevation of phosphomonoesters in neoplasms and proliferating cells (57–59).

It is well known that tumors have altered glucose metabolism. Initial metabolism of glucose to pyruvate occurs without oxygen (also called anaerobic glycolysis) with further catabolism to carbon dioxide and water requiring oxygen (the aerobic citric acid/Krebs cycle). Tumors frequently have defects which lead to the inefficient operation of the aerobic portion of the pathway. The latter occurs because tumor microenvironmental features lead to cellular hypoxia (as already described in the section "Hypoxia Imaging") and therefore the suboptimal use of the aerobic pathway. Tumors also have altered mitochondrial activity where the aerobic pathway is regulated. As a result of deranged feedback loops between aerobic and anaerobic pathways, high levels of pyruvate and lactate are produced even when adequate levels of intracellular oxygen are present. These derangements lead to elevated lactate levels on ^{1}H-MRS and acidic readings on ^{31}P-MRS (60–63).

MRS studies also make use of the fact that normal metabolites may be absent or reduced when cancer is present. For example, normal prostate tissues contain relatively large amounts of citrate and polyamines which are detectable on ^{1}H-MRS and neoplastic lesions show reduced levels of these metabolites (64–66). Another common example is N-acetylaspartate (NAA) which is readily detectable by ^{1}H-MRS. NAA is produced only within normal neurons (60,67) and brain tumors of glial origin (Fig. 65.13). Metastatic deposits do not contain NAA and this metabolite is therefore much reduced or not detectable by ^{1}H-MRS.

Phosphorus MRS

This is the second most commonly observed nucleus in MRS studies of extra-cranial tumors. ^{31}P-MRS has been evaluated in

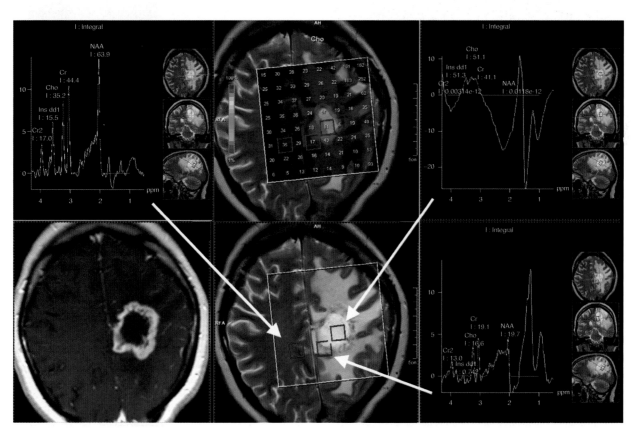

Figure 65.13 ^{1}H-MRS (TE 35 msec) of the brain showing spectra derived from normal brain and from the edge and center of a glioblastoma. The locations of the measured volumes are shown on the T2-weighted images. The spectra from normal brain and enhancing tumor edge are similarly scaled (note that metabolite levels are lowered in the tumor). Free lipids in the area of central necrosis account for the broad peak seen at 1 to 2 ppm. The choline color map if interpreted in the absence of spectral information is misleading particularly in the centre of the lesion. The major resonances are labeled. Cho, choline (peaks 3.24, 3.56, and 3.62 ppm); Cr, creatine (peaks 3.93 and 3.04 ppm); Ins, myoinositol (peaks 3.54, 4.06, 3.63, and 3.28 ppm); and NAA, N-acetylaspartate (peaks 2.02, 2.52, 2.7, and 4.4 ppm).

some clinical MRS studies but examinations are technically more difficult compared to ¹H-MRS, as they require specialist hardware. ³¹P spectra are relatively simple and easy to interpret. Importantly, metabolically-significant phosphorus-containing compounds occur in living systems at high enough concentrations to be detectable by ³¹P MRS, thus providing an ideal method of monitoring tumor energetics (58). Observed energy metabolites typically include the three resonances of γ, α, and β phosphates of NTP (predominantly ATP), inorganic phosphate (Pi), and phosphocreatine (PCr) (Fig. 65.14). Readers are reminded that ATP is the central provider of energy for all energy-demanding processes in cells. PCr functions as an energy reserve and is used to maintain/replenish ATP pools via creatine kinase when demand exceeds mitochondrial ATP production. Other detected metabolites include the pyridine dinucleotides (NAD⁺ and NADH). Phospholipid metabolites observed include phosphomonoesters (PME) (consisting primarily of phosphorylcholine, PC and phosphorylethanolamine, PE) and phosphodiesters (PDE) (glycerolphosphorylcholine, GPC, and glycerolphosphorylethanolamine, GPE).

Tumor intracellular pH can be calculated from the chemical shift of the Pi signal from the PCr and using this observation it is has been established that tumor pH is slightly alkaline (63). The acidic tumor pH, measured by microelectrode techniques appears to arise from lactic acid in the extracellular space (68). Apparently, tumor cells maintain neutrality by pumping acidic ions into the extracellular compartment. Thus, the pH gradient across the tumor cell membrane is the reverse to that seen in normal cells, which are more acidic than their extracellular environment. Tumor acidification is compounded by poor clearance of lactic acid due to poor vascularization.

Human cancers are characterized by elevated PME, elevated PDE, and an alkaline pH (mean 7.2). Animal studies have shown that ³¹P spectra acquired during initial rapid tumor growth phases are quite different from spectra acquired during the nutritionally-deprived phase when there are regional areas of decreased blood flow and the development of hypoxia (69). As PME (PC+PE) and PDE (GPC+GPE) resonances are related to cell membrane turnover in tumors (PC and PE are membrane synthesis substrates and GPC and GPE are membrane breakdown products), alteration of these resonances can be used to probe membrane turnover (58). ³¹P MRS has also been used to study changes in the energy and phospholipid metabolism during therapy (59,70).

Hydrogen MRS

Protons (¹H) produce the most easily detected MRS signals and are convenient for use in routine clinical MRS because the same hardware is used as for conventional MR imaging. ¹H-MRS allows observations of several metabolites that are not detected by MRS of phosphorus. The major obstacle for ¹H-MRS is the high concentrations of tissue water and lipids, which must be suppressed to observe other metabolites. Tissue water signals are very large compared with signals from tissue metabolites which makes metabolite signals hard to identify and measure. The fatty acyl components of lipid triglycerides in fat cells also produce strong overlapping signals whereas other lipids such as the phospholipids do not produce large interfering MRS signals. These considerations mean that effective strategies for suppressing fat and water are needed for ¹H-MRS studies. Most ¹H-MRS studies have therefore focused on the brain and intra-cranial pathologies, because little motion is present and many brain pathologies exhibit no lipid signals. However, technical advances have led to work in other organs particularly the prostate gland where there is now a well-developed literature, and more recently in the breast.

Typical resonances observed in brain at long echo times (e.g., 135–270 msec) include N-acetylaspartate (NAA), total creatine (tCr), total choline (tCho), alanine, and lactate. An echo time of 135 msec is commonly used to observe an inverted lactate peak, while resonances attributed to inositol, glucose, and mobile lipids may appear at short echo times (e.g., 20–50 msec) (Fig. 65.13). A number of studies have shown that ¹H-MR spectra of human brain tumors differ significantly from those of normal brain tissue. NAA is a specific neuronal marker that is not found in tumor tissue and tCho is elevated in tumors. Creatine is used as a marker of normal brain cell density and the creatine content of glioma tissue is considerably reduced. Alanine is often observed in meningiomas suggesting that metabolism involves transamination pathways and partial oxidation of glutamine rather than via glycolysis (71).

Lactate, the end-produce of anaerobic respiration, has been observed in cerebral metastases and astroglial brain tumors distinguishing them from meningiomas, neurinomas, and lymphomas.

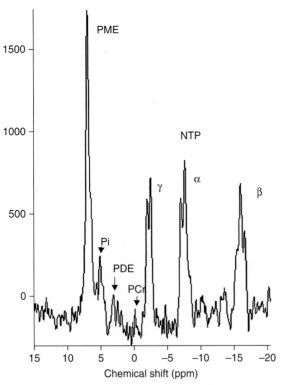

Figure 65.14 ³¹Phosphorus MR spectroscopy of non-Hodgkin's lymphoma. The phoshomonoester peak (PME approximately 7 ppm; primarily phosphocholine and phosphoethanolamine) is the most relevant for cancer because most cancers show elevations of this peak reflecting up-regulated cell proliferation. Phosphodiesters (PDE) (primarily glycerolphosphocholine, and glycerolphosphoethanolamine) are cell membrane breakdown products. The location of the inorganic phosphate signal (Pi) relative to phosphocreatine (PCr) depends on the pH value (with increasing pH value, the chemical shift decreases). Signals from nucleoside triphosphate (NTP) and other metabolites associated with tissue metabolism are shown. *Source*: Courtesy of Dr. G Payne, Institute of Cancer Research, London.

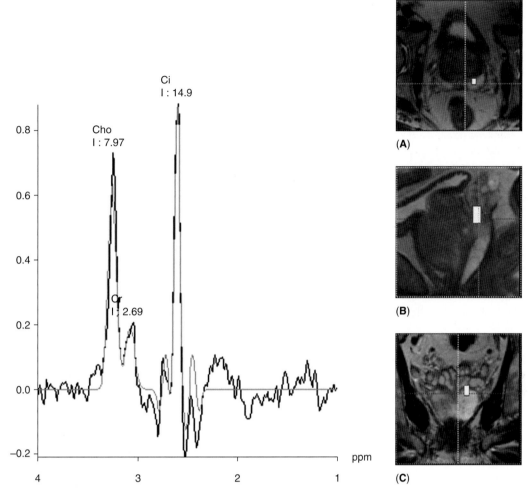

Figure 65.15 Hydrogen MRS of the prostate gland. (A) Axial, (B) sagittal, and (C) coronal T2-weighted MR images. The voxel is apparently placed in the left peripheral zone on the axial image. The raised choline signal (Cho) is due to through-plane contamination arising from the adjacent seminal vesicles superiorly. Note the positions of the MRS voxels in the sagittal and coronal planes. *Abbreviations*: Ci, citrate; Cr, creatine.

Lactate levels appear to correlate with grade and type of tumor, though lactate levels are largely dependent on the balance between production and clearance (72). Lipid resonances are frequently observed in brain tumor with the amount of lipid correlating with the extent of necrosis and grade of malignancy (73). Using a combination of all of these observations, ¹H-MRS can be used to establish non-invasively the diagnosis of tumor and to grade brain gliomas (74).

There is a large body of work showing that ¹H-MRSI of the prostate is a promising method for the metabolic evaluation of prostate cancer extent and aggressiveness (75,76). In particular, the addition of ¹H-MRSI with anatomical information can improve tumor localization, help determine tumor staging, and is useful for tumor volume estimation (77–80). Furthermore, ¹H-MRSI enables assessments of tumor aggressiveness and the detection of metabolically active tumor recurrence after therapy, both of which are observations that cannot frequently be made with morphological MR imaging when used alone (81).

With respect to prostate metabolites, ¹H-MRS yields spectra that depict the relative concentrations of choline (3.2 ppm), polyamines (3.1 ppm), creatine (3.0 ppm), and citrate (2.6 ppm)

(Fig. 65.12) (64). Prostate cancer is characterized by combinations of elevated choline and reduced citrate (citrate is a constituent of normal prostatic tissue). These changes are frequently reported as the metabolic ratios of choline plus creatine to the citrate (Cho+Cr/Ci; elevated in cancer) (65,76,81). This does not imply that interpretation of prostate ¹H-MRSI can be done by observing Cho+Cr/Ci ratios by themselves because calculated ratios do not always take into account the effects of noise and spectral contamination from adjacent voxels. Furthermore individual voxel spectra should never be reviewed in isolation but in the context of the adjacent voxels. A voxel with elevation of choline may be more or less suspicious depending on the choline level in the neighboring voxels (82). Elevated choline in the prostate spectra may be seen from contamination arising from seminal vesicles, ejaculatory ducts, in periurethral areas and cross contaminations may be seen from adjacent muscles of the pelvic floor (Fig. 65.15). Also, there is a need for a dedicated technician to perform post-acquisition processing of ¹H-MRSI data in order to detect and censor all sources of artefacts which represent an additional impediment to the widespread implementation of prostate ¹H-MRSI.

Key Points: MR Spectroscopy

- MRS is a powerful non-invasive method for studying tissue metabolism from chemical compounds that are present at millimolar concentration
- ^{1}H-MRS is the most commonly used technique because it produces the strongest signals and requires no modification of conventional high field MRI systems
- ^{1}H-MRS conveys information on cell membrane synthesis and degradation, thus reflecting cellular proliferation and necrosis. ^{31}P MRS provides information on tissues energetics and pH
- MRS interpretations are done by noting elevations of metabolites such as choline (increased in most tumors) or by the absence of metabolites that should be present such as N-acetylaspartate (reduced in brain tumors) and citrate (reduced in prostate cancer)
- MRS has been slow to develop as a clinical tool because of the need for specialist hardware (for non-hydrogen MRS) and software for data acquisition and analysis; measurement times are also relatively long compared to MR imaging examinations

FUTURE TRENDS

There are extraordinary opportunities for functional MRI/MRS techniques to evolve into biomarkers that could be useful clinically, for pharmaceutical drug development and for predicting therapeutic efficacy. As already noted, functional MRI/MRS could have clinical utility at all stages of a cancer patient's journey: for detection to diagnosis, for staging and assessing therapy response, and finally for assessing relapsed disease. As pharmacodynamic biomarkers, functional MRI/MRS techniques also have the potential to impact on pharmaceutical drug development significantly. It should be recognized that pharmaceutical drug development and clinical therapeutic efficacy assessments are related but are nonetheless different. In pharmaceutical development, questions revolve around whether a drug produces a measurable effect, on the magnitude of effects and the potential biological meanings of observations. For clinical utility, questions revolve around whether changes in individual patients can be measured reliably and reproducibly and whether they predict important clinical outcomes related to therapy.

It is likely that future radiological practice will increasingly incorporate functional and molecular imaging into "routine" patient studies in order to obtain information on physiological and molecular derangements in individual patients. Development frameworks outlining the practical steps that are needed for the qualification of functional imaging in these roles are needed.

It is difficult to predict the pace at which new MR imaging techniques will be deployed into clinical practice. Experience has shown us that some technologies are adopted faster than others (currently it appears as though DW-MRI will come into clinical usage faster than DCE-MRI or MRS), with factors such as clinical demand, ease of use, availability of technology, and cost all driving the pace of change. Trends of what the future may look like are beginning to emerge. Thus we can expect: (*i*) Fusion of imaging techniques (in hardware and in software) with the increased utilization of techniques such as perfusion PET-CT, functional CT/SPECT, functional MRI/MRS/PET, and others, yielding multi-dimensional imaging datasets. (*ii*) Imaging will become increasingly quantitative with imaging measurements being related mechanistically to disease processes. (*iii*) Imaging diagnoses will increasingly require the use of information technology for the analysis of multilayered datasets (multispectral data processing) and computed aided diagnosis (CAD). To truly realize this potential it is imperative for functional techniques to become more robust so as to provide similar information at different institutions using differing equipments. As new imaging technologies make the transition from development to bedside, accepted standards in measurement or analysis methods have to be established. There has to be transparency about how data are acquired and processed on machines from different vendors. Most importantly, the education of imaging physicians will need to incorporate the fundamentals of physiology, biochemistry, and molecular biology as well as the physical and chemical sciences.

Summary

- Well-oxygenated cells are three times more sensitive to radiation than the same cells when they are hypoxic
- The effectiveness of radiotherapy becomes progressively limited as tumor pO_2 levels fall
- Perfusion-related (acute) hypoxia results from inadequate blood flow in tumors which result from structural and functional abnormalities of tumor neovasculature
- Diffusion-related (chronic) hypoxia is caused by increased oxygen diffusion distances due to tumor growth which increases the distance between blood vessels
- Anemic hypoxia is related to the reduced O_2-carrying capacity of the blood
- ^{18}F-MISO, $^{60/64}$Cu-ATSM PET, and BOLD-MRI are non-invasive techniques which have the potential to measure hypoxia status as clinical tools
- Hypoxia imaging may allow better selection of those cancer patients who may benefit from novel anti-hypoxia directed therapies
- Diffusion-weighted MR imaging (DW-MRI) displays information related to the thermally driven, random (Brownian) motion of water molecules in tissues
- Recent technical advances have enabled DW-MRI to be applied for tumor evaluation extracranially and have led to the clinical development of whole body DW-MRI
- Whole body DW-MRI shows promise in identifying malignant disease on the basis of high signal intensity on high b-value images
- In general, tumors have lower ADC values whereas normal/benign/reactive tissues have correspondingly higher values
- DW-MRI may be an effective early biomarker for treatment outcome for therapies that induce tumor cell apoptosis with successful treatment generally causing increases in ADC values
- ^{1}H-MRS is the most commonly used technique because it produces the strongest signals and requires no modification of conventional high field MR imaging systems
- MRS has been slow to develop as a clinical tool because of the need for specialist hardware (for non-hydrogen MRS) and software for data acquisition and analysis; measurement times are also relatively long compared to MR imaging examinations

REFERENCES

1. Gray LH, Conger AD, Ebert M. The concentration of oxygen dissolved in tissues at the time of irradiation as a factor in radiotherapy. Br J Radiol 1953; 26: 638–48.

2. Vaupel P. The role of hypoxia-induced factors in tumor progression. Oncologist 2004 2004; 9(Suppl 5): 10–17.

3. Hall EJ, Giaccia AJ. Oxygen effect and reoxygenation. In: Hall EJ, Giaccia AJ, eds. Radiobiology for the Radiologist. Philadelphia: Lippincott Williams & Wilkins, 2006: 85–105.

4. Ciocca DR, Calderwood SK. Heat shock proteins in cancer: diagnostic, prognostic, predictive, and treatment implications. Cell Stress Chaperones 2005; 10: 86–103.

5. Kallinowski F, Zander R, Hoeckel M, Vaupel P. Tumor tissue oxygenation as evaluated by computerized-pO2-histography. Int J Radiat Oncol Biol Phys 1990; 19: 953–61.

6. Vaupel P, Schlenger K, Knoop C, Hockel M. Oxygenation of human tumors: evaluation of tissue oxygen distribution in breast cancers by computerized O_2 tension measurements. Cancer Res 1991; 51: 3316–22.

7. Brizel DM, Rosner GL, Harrelson J, Prosnitz LR, Dewhirst MW. Pretreatment oxygenation profiles of human soft tissue sarcomas. Int J Radiat Oncol Biol Phys 1994; 30: 635–42.

8. Hockel M, Schlenger K, Aral B, et al. Association between tumor hypoxia and malignant progression in advanced cancer of the uterine cervix. Cancer Res 1996; 56: 4509–15.

9. Nordsmark M, Bentzen SM, Rudat V, et al. Prognostic value of tumor oxygenation in 397 head and neck tumors after primary radiation therapy. An international multi-center study. Radiother Oncol 2005; 77: 18–24.

10. Vaupel P, Harrison L. Tumor hypoxia: causative factors, compensatory mechanisms, and cellular response. Oncologist 2004; 9(Suppl 5): 4–9.

11. Bussink J, Kaanders JH, van der Kogel AJ. Tumor hypoxia at the micro-regional level: clinical relevance and predictive value of exogenous and endogenous hypoxic cell markers. Radiother Oncol 2003; 67: 3–15.

12. Padhani AR, Krohn KA, Lewis JS, Alber M. Imaging oxygenation of human tumours. Eur Radiol 2007; 17: 861–72.

13. Tatum JL, Kelloff GJ, Gillies RJ, et al. Hypoxia: importance in tumor biology, noninvasive measurement by imaging, and value of its measurement in the management of cancer therapy. Int J Radiat Biol 2006; 82: 699–757.

14. Howe FA, Robinson SP, McIntyre DJ, Stubbs M, Griffiths JR. Issues in flow and oxygenation dependent contrast (FLOOD) imaging of tumours. NMR Biomed 2001; 14: 497–506.

15. Hoskin PJ, Carnell DM, Taylor NJ, et al. Hypoxia in prostate cancer: correlation of BOLD-MRI with pimonidazole immunohistochemistry-initial observations. Int J Radiat Oncol Biol Phys 2007; 68: 1065–71.

16. Robinson SP, Rijken PF, Howe FA, et al. Tumor vascular architecture and function evaluated by non-invasive susceptibility MRI methods and immunohistochemistry. J Magn Reson Imaging 2003; 17: 445–54.

17. Kostourou V, Robinson SP, Whitley GS, Griffiths JR. Effects of overexpression of dimethylarginine dimethylaminohydrolase on tumor angiogenesis assessed by susceptibility magnetic resonance imaging. Cancer Res 2003; 63: 4960–6.

18. Taylor NJ, Baddeley H, Goodchild KA, et al. BOLD MRI of human tumor oxygenation during carbogen breathing. J Magn Reson Imaging 2001; 14: 156–63.

19. Rijpkema M, Kaanders JH, Joosten FB, van der Kogel AJ, Heerschap A. Effects of breathing a hyperoxic hypercapnic gas mixture on blood oxygenation and vascularity of head-and-neck tumors as measured by magnetic resonance imaging. Int J Radiat Oncol Biol Phys 2002; 53: 1185–91.

20. Rajendran JG, Krohn KA. Imaging hypoxia and angiogenesis in tumors. Radiol Clin North Am 2005; 43: 169–87.

21. Fujibayashi Y, Taniuchi H, Yonekura Y, et al. Copper-62-ATSM: A new hypoxia imaging agent with high membrane permeability and low redox potential. J Nucl Med 1997; 38: 1155–60.

22. Dearling JLD, Lewis JS, Mullen GED, et al. Design of hypoxia-targeting radiopharmaceuticals: Selective uptake of copper-64 complexes in hypoxic cells in vitro. Eur J Nucl Med 1998; 25: 788–92.

23. Dearling JLJ, Lewis JS, Welch MJ, McCarthy DW, Blower PJ. Redox-active complexes for imaging hypoxic tissues: structure-activity relationships in copper(II)bis(thiosemicarbazone) complexes. Chem Commun 1998; 22: 2531–3.

24. Lewis JS, McCarthy DW, McCarthy TJ, Fujibayashi Y, Welch MJ. The evaluation of ^{64}Cu-diacetyl-bis(N^4-methylthiosemicarbazone)(^{64}Cu-ATSM) in vivo and in vitro in a hypoxic tumor model. J Nucl Med 1999; 40: 177–83.

25. Lewis JS, Sharp TL, Laforest R, Fujibayashi Y, Welch MJ. Tumor uptake of copper-diacetyl-bis(N^4-methylthiosemicarbazone): Effect of changes in tissue oxygenation. J Nucl Med 2001; 42: 655–61.

26. Dearling JL, Lewis JS, Mullen GE, Welch MJ, Blower PJ. Copper bis(thiosemicarbazone) complexes as hypoxia imaging agents: structure-activity relationships. J Biol Inorg Chem 2002; 7: 249–59.

27. Lewis JS, Herrero P, Sharp T, et al. Delineation of hypoxia in canine myocardium using PET and copper(II)-diacetyl-bis(N^4-methylthiosemicarbazone). J Nucl Med 2002; 43: 1557–69.

28. Maurer RI, Blower PJ, Dilworth JR, et al. Studies on the mechanism of hypoxic selectivity in copper bis(thiosemicarbazone) radiopharmaceuticals. J Med Chem 2002; 45: 1420–31.

29. Dehdashti F, Mintun MA, Lewis JS, et al. In vivo assesment of tumor hypoxia in lung cancer with ^{60}Cu-ATSM. Eur J Nucl Med Mol Imaging 2003; 30: 844–50.

30. Dehdashti F, Grigsby PW, Mintun MA, et al. Assessing tumor hypoxia in cervical cancer by positron emission tomography with ^{60}Cu-ATSM: relationship to therapeutic response-a preliminary report. Int J Radiat Oncol Biol Phys 2003; 55: 1233–8.

31. Koh DM, Collins DJ. Diffusion-weighted MRI in the body: applications and challenges in oncology. AJR Am J Roentgenol 2007; 188: 1622–35.

32. Patterson DM, Padhani AR, Collins DJ. Technology insight: water diffusion MRI-a potential new biomarker of response to cancer therapy. Nat Clin Pract Oncol 2008; 5: 220–33.

33. Koh DM, Takahara T, Imai Y, Collins DJ. Practical aspects of assessing tumors using clinical diffusion-weighted imaging in the body. Magn Reson Med Sci 2007; 6: 211–24.

34. Taouli B, Vilgrain V, Dumont E, et al. Evaluation of liver diffusion isotropy and characterization of focal hepatic lesions with

two single-shot echo-planar MR imaging sequences: prospective study in 66 patients. Radiology 2003; 226: 71–8.

35. Parikh T, Drew SJ, Lee VS, et al. Focal liver lesion detection and characterization with diffusion-weighted MR imaging: comparison with standard breath-hold T2-weighted imaging. Radiology 2008; 246: 812–22.

36. Sinha S, Lucas-Quesada FA, Sinha U, DeBruhl N, Bassett LW. In vivo diffusion-weighted MRI of the breast: potential for lesion characterization. J Magn Reson Imaging 2002; 15: 693–704.

37. Guo Y, Cai YQ, Cai ZL, et al. Differentiation of clinically benign and malignant breast lesions using diffusion-weighted imaging. J Magn Reson Imaging 2002; 16: 172–8.

38. Woodhams R, Matsunaga K, Iwabuchi K, et al. Diffusion-weighted imaging of malignant breast tumors: the usefulness of apparent diffusion coefficient (ADC) value and ADC map for the detection of malignant breast tumors and evaluation of cancer extension. J Comput Assist Tomogr 2005; 29: 644–9.

39. Sumi M, Sakihama N, Sumi T, et al. Discrimination of metastatic cervical lymph nodes with diffusion-weighted MR imaging in patients with head and neck cancer. AJNR Am J Neuroradiol 2003; 24: 1627–34.

40. Park SW, Lee JH, Ehara S, et al. Single shot fast spin echo diffusion-weighted MR imaging of the spine; Is it useful in differentiating malignant metastatic tumor infiltration from benign fracture edema? Clin Imaging 2004; 28: 102–8.

41. Nakanishi K, Kobayashi M, Nakaguchi K, et al. Whole-body MRI for detecting metastatic bone tumor: diagnostic value of diffusion-weighted images. Magn Reson Med Sci 2007; 6: 147–55.

42. Hamstra DA, Rehemtulla A, Ross BD. Diffusion magnetic resonance imaging: a biomarker for treatment response in oncology. J Clin Oncol 2007; 25: 4104–9.

43. Pickles MD, Gibbs P, Lowry M, Turnbull LW. Diffusion changes precede size reduction in neoadjuvant treatment of breast cancer. Magn Reson Imaging 2006; 24: 843–7.

44. Yankeelov TE, Lepage M, Chakravarthy A, et al. Integration of quantitative DCE-MRI and ADC mapping to monitor treatment response in human breast cancer: initial results. Magn Reson Imaging 2007; 25: 1–13.

45. Theilmann RJ, Borders R, Trouard TP, et al. Changes in water mobility measured by diffusion MRI predict response of metastatic breast cancer to chemotherapy. Neoplasia 2004; 6: 831–37.

46. Kamel IR, Rayes DK, Liapi E, Bluemke DA, Geschwind JF. Functional MR imaging assessment of tumor response after 90Y microsphere treatment in patients with unresectable hepatocellular carcinoma. J Vasc Intervent Radiol 2007; 18: 49–56.

47. Cui Y, Zhang XP, Sun YS, Tang L, Shen L. Apparent diffusion coefficient: potential imaging biomarker for prediction and early detection of response to chemotherapy in hepatic metastases. Radiology 2008; 248: 894–900.

48. Hayashida Y, Yakushiji T, Awai K, et al. Monitoring therapeutic responses of primary bone tumors by diffusion-weighted image: Initial results. Eur Radiol 2006; 16: 2637–43.

49. Uhl M, Saueressig U, van Buiren M, et al. Osteosarcoma: preliminary results of in vivo assessment of tumor necrosis after chemotherapy with diffusion- and perfusion-weighted magnetic resonance imaging. Invest Radiol 2006; 41: 618–23.

50. Mardor Y, Pfeffer R, Spiegelmann R, et al. Early detection of response to radiation therapy in patients with brain malignancies using conventional and high b-value diffusion-weighted magnetic resonance imaging. J Clin Oncol 2003; 21: 1094–100.

51. Batchelor TT, Sorensen AG, di Tomaso E, et al. AZD2171, a pan-VEGF receptor tyrosine kinase inhibitor, normalizes tumor vasculature and alleviates edema in glioblastoma patients. Cancer Cell 2007; 11: 83–95.

52. Patterson DM, Padhani AR, Collins DJ. Technology Insight: water diffusion MRI—a potential new biomarker of response to cancer therapy. Nat Clin Pract Oncol 2008; 5: 220–33.

53. Alger JR. Magnetic resonance spectroscopy in Cancer. In: Padhani AR, Choyke P, eds. New Techniques in Oncologic Imaging. Boca Raton, FL: Taylor and Francis, 2006: 193–211.

54. Kwock L, Smith JK, Castillo M, et al. Clinical role of proton magnetic resonance spectroscopy in oncology: brain, breast, and prostate cancer. Lancet Oncol 2006; 7: 859–68.

55. Ackerstaff E, Pflug BR, Nelson JB, Bhujwalla ZM. Detection of increased choline compounds with proton nuclear magnetic resonance spectroscopy subsequent to malignant transformation of human prostatic epithelial cells. Cancer Res 2001; 61: 3599–603.

56. Sabatier J, Tremoulet M, Ranjeva JP, et al. Contribution of in vivo 1H spectroscopy to the diagnosis of deep-seated brain abscess. J Neurol Neurosurg Psychiatry 1999; 66: 120–1.

57. Ronen SM, Leach MO. Imaging biochemistry: applications to breast cancer. Breast Cancer Res 2001; 3: 36–40.

58. Podo F. Tumour phospholipid metabolism. NMR Biomed 1999; 12: 413–39.

59. Negendank W. Studies of human tumors by MRS: a review. NMR Biomed 1992; 5: 303–24.

60. Alger JR, Frank JA, Bizzi A, et al. Metabolism of human gliomas: assessment with H-1 MR spectroscopy and F-18 fluorodeoxyglucose PET. Radiology 1990; 177: 633–41.

61. Herholz K, Heindel W, Luyten PR, et al. In vivo imaging of glucose consumption and lactate concentration in human gliomas. Ann Neurol 1992; 31: 319–27.

62. Griffiths JR, McIntyre DJ, Howe FA, Stubbs M. Why are cancers acidic? A carrier-mediated diffusion model for H+ transport in the interstitial fluid. Novartis Found Symp 2001; 240: 46–62; discussion 62–7, 152–3.

63. Gillies RJ, Raghunand N, Garcia-Martin ML, Gatenby RA. pH imaging. A review of pH measurement methods and applications in cancers. IEEE Eng Med Biol Mag 2004; 23: 57–64.

64. Thomas MA, Lange T, Velan SS, et al. Two-dimensional MR spectroscopy of healthy and cancerous prostates in vivo. Magma 2008; 21: 443–58.

65. Shukla-Dave A, Hricak H, Moskowitz C, et al. Detection of prostate cancer with MR spectroscopic imaging: an expanded paradigm incorporating polyamines. Radiology 2007; 245: 499–506.

66. Kurhanewicz J, Vigneron DB, Nelson SJ, et al. Citrate as an in vivo marker to discriminate prostate cancer from benign prostatic hyperplasia and normal prostate peripheral zone: detection via localized proton spectroscopy. Urology 1995; 45: 459–66.

67. Di Costanzo A, Scarabino T, Trojsi F, et al. Multiparametric 3T MR approach to the assessment of cerebral gliomas: tumor extent and malignancy. Neuroradiology 2006; 48: 622–31.

68. Griffiths JR. Are cancer cells acidic? Br J Cancer 1991; 64: 425–7.

69. Hockel M, Vaupel P. Tumor hypoxia: definitions and current clinical, biologic, and molecular aspects. J Natl Cancer Inst 2001; 93: 266–76.

70. Leach MO, Verrill M, Glaholm J, et al. Measurements of human breast cancer using magnetic resonance spectroscopy: a review of clinical measurements and a report of localized 31P measurements of response to treatment. NMR Biomed 1998; 11: 314–40.

71. Yue Q, Isobe T, Shibata Y, et al. New observations concerning the interpretation of magnetic resonance spectroscopy of meningioma. Eur Radiol 2008; 18: 2901–11.

72. Oshiro S, Tsugu H, Komatsu F, et al. Quantitative assessment of gliomas by proton magnetic resonance spectroscopy. Anticancer Res 2007; 27: 3757–63.

73. Astrakas LG, Zurakowski D, Tzika AA, et al. Noninvasive magnetic resonance spectroscopic imaging biomarkers to predict the clinical grade of pediatric brain tumors. Clin Cancer Res 2004; 10: 8220–8.

74. Preul MC, Caramanos Z, Collins DL, et al. Accurate, noninvasive diagnosis of human brain tumors by using proton magnetic resonance spectroscopy. Nat Med 1996; 2: 323–5.

75. Huzjan R, Sala E, Hricak H. Magnetic resonance imaging and magnetic resonance spectroscopic imaging of prostate cancer. Nat Clin Pract Urol 2005; 2: 434–42.

76. Mueller-Lisse UG, Scherr MK. Proton MR spectroscopy of the prostate. Eur J Radiol 2007; 63: 351–60.

77. Coakley FV, Kurhanewicz J, Lu Y, et al. Prostate cancer tumor volume: measurement with endorectal MR and MR spectroscopic imaging. Radiology 2002; 223: 91–7.

78. Scheidler J, Hricak H, Vigneron DB, et al. Prostate cancer: localization with three-dimensional proton MR spectroscopic imaging–clinicopathologic study. Radiology 1999; 213: 473–80.

79. Yu KK, Scheidler J, Hricak H, et al. Prostate cancer: prediction of extracapsular extension with endorectal MR imaging and three-dimensional proton MR spectroscopic imaging. Radiology1999; 213: 481–8.

80. Wang L, Mullerad M, Chen HN, et al. Prostate cancer: incremental value of endorectal MR imaging findings for prediction of extracapsular extension. Radiology 2004; 232: 133–9.

81. Zakian KL, Sircar K, Hricak H, et al. Correlation of proton MR spectroscopic imaging with gleason score based on step-section pathologic analysis after radical prostatectomy. Radiology 2005; 234: 804–14.

82. Westphalen AC, Coakley FV, Qayyum A, et al. Peripheral zone prostate cancer: accuracy of different interpretative approaches with MR and MR spectroscopic imaging. Radiology 2008; 246: 177–84.

Index

Note:
Imaging techniques for individual cancers are located under the specific cancers; entries under the imaging modalities refer to general imaging issues.

Abbreviations
To save space in the index the following abbreviations have been used:
ACTH - adrenocorticotrophic hormone
AJCC - American Joint Committee on Cancer-Union Internationale Contre Le Cancer
CNS - central nervous system
CT - computed tomography
MALT - mucosa-associated lymphoid tissue
MRI - magnetic resonance imaging
NSGCTs - non-seminomatous germ cell tumors
PET - positron emission tomography
PTLD - post-transplant lymphoproliferative disorder/disease
SPECT - single-photon emission computed tomography
STIR - short tau inversion recovery
TRUS - transrectal ultrasound
TVUS - transvaginal ultrasound

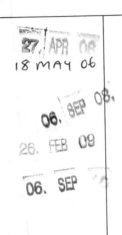